Clinical Pulmonary Medicine

Clinical Pulmonary Medicine

Edited by
Lyle D. Victor, M.D.
Clinical Assistant Professor of Medicine
Wayne State University School of Medicine, Detroit
Director, Transitional Year Residency
Oakwood Hospital, Dearborn, Michigan

Foreword by
Roger C. Bone, M.D.
Dean, Rush Medical College of Rush University
Vice President for Medical Affairs
The Ralph C. Brown, M.D., Professor
Chairman, Department of Internal Medicine
Chief, Section of Pulmonary Diseases
Rush-Presbyterian-St.Luke's Medical Center, Chicago

Little, Brown and Company
Boston/Toronto/London

First Edition

Library of Congress Cataloging-in-Publication Data

Clinical pulmonary medicine/edited by Lyle D. Victor.—1st ed.
p. cm.
Includes bibliographical references and index.
ISBN 0-316-90246-2
1. Respiratory organs—Diseases. 2. Respiratory organs—Physiology.
[DNLM: 1. Lung—physiology. 2. Lung Diseases. WF 600 C6417]
RC731.C62 1992
616.2′4—dc20
DNLM/DLC
for Library of Congress 92-23693
CIP

Printed in the United States of America
EB

To my father, Arthur Van Victor, D.D.S.
Still practicing, he never compromised for quality

Contents

Foreword ix
Preface xi
Contributing Authors xiii

1. Pulmonary Physiology Simplified 1
Bernhard F. Muller
2. Office Pulmonary Function Testing 19
John Haapaniemi, Barry Lesser, and Ernest L. Yoder
3. Clinical Diagnosis of Respiratory Disorders and Physical Examination 43
Charles G. Todoroff
4. Dyspnea 53
James V. Palazzolo and Lyle D. Victor
5. Cough 65
Angela DeSantis
6. Hemoptysis 73
Barry Lesser, John Haapaniemi, and Ernest L. Yoder
7. Chest Discomfort 91
Adil Karamali and Lyle D. Victor
8. Asthma 105
James G. Fordyce
9. Chronic Obstructive Pulmonary Disease 139
Daniel L. Maxwell
10. Pulmonary Embolus and Deep Vein Thrombosis: Prevention, Diagnosis, and Treatment 157
Bradford K. Grassmick and Donald J. Conn
11. Chronic Interstitial Pulmonary Disorders 193
Joseph P. Lynch III and Anthony D. Chavis
12. Restrictive Lung Diseases of Extrapulmonary Origin 265
Barry Lesser, John Haapaniemi, and Ernest L. Yoder
13. Pleural and Diaphragmatic Diseases 283
Robert Sharon, Angela DeSantis, and Lyle D. Victor
14. Occupational Lung Disease 305
Walter J. Talamonti and William H. Heckman
15. Pulmonary Rehabilitation 317
Willane S. Krell
16. Pulmonary Infections: Upper Respiratory Tract Infections 331
Nancy M. McGuire
17. Community-Acquired Pneumonia 347
Nicholas J. Lekas
18. Tuberculosis 379
Dana G. Kissner
19. Blunt Chest Trauma 401
Thomas Siegel
20. Pulmonary and Mediastinal Neoplasms 407
Enrique Signori and Oscar Signori
21. Normal Sleep and Biologic Rhythms 425
Sheldon Kapen
22. Clinical Evaluation of Excessive Daytime Sleepiness 439
Robert Wittig
23. Sleep Disorders: Insomnia 461
Edward J. Stepanski

24. Pulmonary Diseases in Pregnancy 477
Scott B. Ransom, Randall Kelly, and Federico Mariona

25. Preoperative Pulmonary Evaluation 489
Ernest L. Yoder, John Haapaniemi, and Barry Lesser

26. Basic Chest Radiograph Interpretation 497
David S. Yates and Mark Lukens

27. Pulmonary Physiology at Altitude and Depth 519
Michael S. Eichenhorn

Appendix: The Health History Questionnaire 532
Lyle D. Victor

Index 543

Foreword

Clinical Pulmonary Medicine is intended as a complete reference to the clinical aspects of pulmonary medicine. The primary care physician will appreciate the organization and clarity of this effort by the editor, Dr. Lyle D. Victor. Previously Dr. Victor has been the editor of two texts on critical care; his experience and thoroughness will be recognized by readers of this book. Previous journal articles by Dr. Victor concern such important issues as the function of bronchodilating agents, critical care, and pulmonary function tests. His current interest in sleep disorders is reflected here; three chapters in this book cover the subject, from the timely topic of sleep apnea to the essential physiology of the endogenous circadian rhythms.

A novel approach to the essential physiology of the pulmonary system is presented in the first chapter, which utilizes an easy-to-understand pictorial format. Diagnostics are covered in the next two chapters. Pulmonary function testing receives much attention—from equipment purchase to the interpretation of the results. The next chapters cover the breadth and scope of pulmonary diseases, including the increasingly important subjects of occupational lung disease and obstructive airways disease. Finally, a text such as this would not be complete without a section on the special subject of the effects of altitude and depth on the physiology of the pulmonary system, such as is found in the last chapter.

This book is tuned to the problems of today's physician: the effects of rising health care costs and increasing governmental regulation are changing the way health care is performed. Increasing patient self-management and changes in outpatient care are examples of the effects of this new manner of thinking that are frequently encountered in pulmonary medicine. *Clinical Pulmonary Medicine* discusses these issues with the goal of avoiding unnecessary hospital stays and alleviating the suffering of the sick.

Roger C. Bone, M.D.

Preface

Family practitioners, internists, pediatricians and obstetricians frequently encounter a variety of pulmonary problems as part of primary care to their patients. The wheezing patient is encountered from infancy to pregnancy to the geriatric age group. Occupational lung disease can be an important part of worker's compensation and disability litigation, often involving the primary care physician's expertise. Uncommon but disabling lung diseases such as cystic fibrosis, kyphoscoliosis, and interstitial fibrosis cross age and sex barriers and are encountered in many office practices. Accurate screening pulmonary function studies are performed too infrequently in primary care practice.

Clinical Pulmonary Medicine is a practical book written to fill the large void in pulmonary texts directed at the primary care physician. As a board-certified family practitioner and pulmonologist, I have edited this volume to include liberal uses of basic pathophysiologic descriptions, and simple illustrations and photographs to help clarify complex topics. Each chapter covers pulmonary disorders often encountered in primary care practice. The initial chapters, covering the basics of pulmonary physiology and chest examination, will be instructive to the medical student or house officer and will act as a ready reference for the busy practitioner. Four most common respiratory complaints of dyspnea, cough, hemoptysis, and chest discomfort are covered in individual chapters as focal problems. Areas inadequately covered in other texts are emphasized, as with the chapter on pulmonary function testing, which offers important tips on purchasing pulmonary function testing equipment, as well as a simplified approach to interpreting lung function studies. Other topics that may not be encountered in other primary care pulmonary texts include the pregnant pulmonary patient, sleep disorders, chest roentgenograph interpretation, and disorders due to altitude and depth. The very practical appendix offers purchasers of this book a patient health-history questionnaire to copy for use in their own practice.

The recent dramatic increase in the cost of health care has changed the practice patterns of nearly every physician. The arrival of diagnostic-related groups, capitation, and increased governmental intervention has placed a new emphasis on outpatient management for many pulmonary patients who formerly would have been hospitalized for their problems. Respiratory ailments frequently cause much discomfort and anxiety for both the patient and the practitioner. A thoughtful and logical approach to these problems will help the physician to relieve suffering and to avoid unnecessary hospitalization.

I wish to acknowledge the people who gave institutional support for this project: Kenneth Aird, Chairman, Oakwood Health Services Corporation Board of Trustees; Rodney C. Linton, Chairman, Oakwood Hospital Corporation Board of Trustees; Edward H. Bovich and the late Michael Adray, Co-Chairmen, Oakwood Hospital Foundation; Gerald D. Fitzgerald, M.H.A., Chief Executive Officer, and Martin Farber, M.D., Director of Medical Education, Oakwood Hospital Corporation Administration.

I particularly want to thank the following individuals for their invaluable assistance in the preparation of this book: Diane A. Victor, art editing; Martha Berriman, photography; Mike Beebe, computer applications assistance; Lisa Gorman, M.H.S.A., office organization; Pam Zbikowski and Pamela Archibald, secretarial assistance; Sharon Phillips,

A.M.L.S., Director of Library Services; Michael Middleton and Patricia Vick, Oakwood Downriver Sleep Disorders Center; and Kimberly Corsi, R.R.T., Director, and Cathy Jo Ponzi, R.R.T, Assistant Director, Department of Respiratory Care, Oakwood Hospital.

L. D. V.

Contributing Authors

Anthony D. Chavis, M.D.
Attending Physician, Pulmonary Department, G.H.M.A. Medical Centers, Tucson, Arizona

Donald J. Conn, M.D.
Radiology Resident, Department of Radiology, Oakwood Hospital, Dearborn, Michigan

Angela DeSantis, M.D.
Fellow in Critical Care Medicine, Wayne State University School of Medicine; Attending Physician, Department of Critical Care, Detroit Medical Center, Detroit

Michael S. Eichenhorn, M.D.
Clinical Associate Professor of Internal Medicine, University of Michigan Medical School, Ann Arbor; Senior Staff Physician, Pulmonary and Critical Care Medicine, Henry Ford Hospital, Detroit

James G. Fordyce, M.D.
Clinical Instructor of Pediatrics, Wayne State University School of Medicine, Detroit; Attending Physician, and Chief, Section of Allergy, Oakwood Hospital, Dearborn, Michigan

Bradford K. Grassmick, M.D.
Associate Director, Cardiac Surgical Unit, Providence Hospital, Southfield, Michigan

John Haapaniemi, D.O.
Clinical Assistant Professor of Medicine, Wayne State University School of Medicine; Section Chief, Pulmonary Medicine, Grace Hospital, Detroit

William H. Heckman, M.D.
Attending Physician, Department of Medicine, Oakwood Hospital, Dearborn, Michigan

Sheldon Kapen, M.D.
Associate Professor of Neurology, Wayne State University School of Medicine, Detroit; Chief of Neurology, Veterans Affairs Medical Center, Allen Park, Michigan

Adil Karamali, M.D.
Clinical Assistant Professor of Medicine, Wayne State University School of Medicine, Detroit; Intensivist, Oakwood Hospital, Dearborn, Michigan

Randall T. Kelly, M.D.
Assistant Professor of Obstetrics and Gynecology, Wayne State University School of Medicine, Detroit; Associate Perinatologist, and Director, Antenatal Testing Unit, Oakwood Hospital, Dearborn, Michigan

Dana G. Kissner, M.D.
Assistant Professor of Medicine, Wayne State University School of Medicine; Interim Chief, Division of Pulmonary Medicine, Harper Hospital, Detroit

Willane S. Krell, M.D.
Assistant Professor of Medicine, Wayne State University School of Medicine; Director, Pulmonary Diagnostic Services, Harper Hospital, Detroit

Nicholas J. Lekas, M.D.
Clinical Associate Professor of Medicine, Wayne State University School of Medicine, Detroit; Chief of Infectious Diseases and Director of Internal Medicine Residency Program, Oakwood Hospital, Dearborn, Michigan

Barry A. Lesser, M.D.
Clinical Assistant Professor of Medicine, Wayne State University School of Medicine; Director, Medical Intensive Care Unit, and Staff Physician, Section of Pulmonary and Critical Care Medicine, Grace Hospital, Detroit

Mark Lukens, M.D.
Diagnostic Radiology Resident, Department of Radiology, Oakwood Hospital, Dearborn, Michigan

Joseph P. Lynch III, M.D.
Associate Professor of Internal Medicine, University of Michigan Medical School; Attending Physician, Division of Pulmonary and Critical Care Medicine, University of Michigan Hospitals, Ann Arbor, Michigan

Federico G. Mariona, M.D.
Professor of Obstetrics and Gynecology, Wayne State University School of Medicine, Detroit; Director of Maternal-Fetal Medicine, Oakwood Hospital, Dearborn, Michigan

Daniel L. Maxwell, D.O.
Assistant Professor of Medicine, Eastern Virginia Medical School of the Medical College of Hampton Roads, Norfolk; Head, Department of Critical Care, Naval Hospital, Portsmouth, Virginia

Nancy M. McGuire, M.D.
Assistant Professor of Medicine, Wayne State University School of Medicine; Chief of Infectious Disease, Harper Hospital, Detroit

Bernhard F. Muller, M.D.
Assistant Professor of Medicine, Wayne State University School of Medicine, Detroit; Chief, Pulmonary Disease Section, Veterans Affairs Medical Center, Allen Park, Michigan

James V. Palazzolo, M.D.
Fellow, Pulmonary and Critical Care Medicine, George Washington University School of Medicine and Health Sciences, Washington, D.C.

Scott B. Ransom, D.O.
Department of Obstetrics and Gynecology, Bixby Medical Center, Adrion, Michigan

Robert Sharon, M.D.
Attending Emergency Room Physician, Department of Emergency Medicine, Oakwood Hospital, Dearborn, Michigan

Thomas S. Siegel, M.D.
Clinical Assistant Professor of Surgery, Wayne State University School of Medicine, Detroit; Active Staff Surgeon, and Director, Surgical Education, Oakwood Hospital, Dearborn; Active Staff Surgeon, Harper Hospital, Detroit; Consulting Staff Surgeon, Veterans Affairs Medical Center, Allen Park, Michigan

Enrique E. Signori, M.D.
Director, Cancer Center, Oakwood Hospital, Dearborn, Michigan

Oscar R. Signori, M.D.
Clinical Instructor of Medicine, Wayne State University School of Medicine, Detroit; Chief, Section of Hematology/Oncology, Oakwood Hospital, Dearborn, Michigan

Edward J. Stepanski, Ph.D.
Director, Insomnia Clinic, Sleep Disorders and Research Center, Henry Ford Hospital, Detroit

Walter J. Talamonti, M.D., M.P.H.
Physician-in-Charge, Rouge Medical Services, Ford Motor Company; Attending Physician, Department of Internal Medicine, Oakwood Hospital, Dearborn, Michigan

Charles G. Todoroff, M.D.
Attending Physician, Department of Internal Medicine, Oakwood Hospital, Dearborn

Lyle D. Victor, M.D.
Clinical Assistant Professor of Medicine, Wayne State University School of Medicine, Detroit; Director, Transitional Year Residency, Oakwood Hospital, Dearborn, Michigan

Robert M. Wittig, M.D.
Staff Physician, Sleep Disorders and Research Center, Henry Ford Hospital, Detroit

David S. Yates, M.D.
Associate Director of Residency, Department of Radiology, Oakwood Hospital, Dearborn, Michigan

Ernest L. Yoder, M.D.
Assistant Professor of Medicine, Wayne State University School of Medicine; Director of Critical Care, Grace Hospital, Detroit

Clinical Pulmonary Medicine

Notice

1

Pulmonary Physiology Simplified

Bernhard F. Muller

Deranged pulmonary physiology forms the basis of much of the pulmonary pathology encountered by the primary care physician. Understanding the static and dynamic pulmonary physiology discussed in this chapter will improve the reader's comprehension of the chapters that follow. This chapter is designed to present fundamental physiologic information in an intuitively understandable way. An intuitive grasp of the complex and dynamic interrelationships that exist in the normal and diseased lung can often lead to successful diagnostic and therapeutic efforts. For those readers interested in a more in-depth discussion of physiologic concepts, no reference is more detailed or complete than the *Handbook of Physiology* [1].

The characteristics of the lung can be divided into those that are measurable with the lung at rest, and those that are important when air is actively moving in and out of the lung. Those with the lung at rest are called *static characteristics,* and those with the lung in motion are called *dynamic characteristics.*

Static Characteristics

Conceptually, the lung can be divided into volumes that have little to do with anatomic subdivisions, describing the state of the lung under different conditions of inflation.

In Fig. 1-1, each large rectangular block represents the volume of the lung when it is fully inflated at total lung capacity (TLC). The sinusoidal curve represents the volume change during quiet breathing, called the tidal volume. Block (a) in Fig. 1-1 depicts the functional residual capacity (FRC) as the amount of air remaining in the lung at the end of a normal tidal expiration. Block (b) shows that the FRC can be further subdivided into the expiratory reserve volume (ERV) and the residual volume (RV). The RV is that volume remaining in the lungs after a maximum effort to expel as much air as possible from the lungs. Block (c) depicts the vital capacity (VC) as the difference between TLC and RV. Each of these lung volumes measures different aspects of the status of the respiratory system.

The TLC is the volume of gas that the lung contains at the time of maximal voluntary inspiration. Variations in measured TLC reflect lungs that are abnormally sized, stiff, or compliant, as well as neuromuscular disorders that weaken the muscles of inspiration. An abnormally large TLC is often found in emphysema, a disorder in which the lungs are very compliant and easily inflated. Conversely, in diffuse interstitial fibrosis, the lungs are stiff, and the TLC is generally reduced.

The FRC is the volume of gas that the lungs contain at the end of a normal inspiration-expiration cycle, when the respiratory muscles are all at rest in normal persons. The volume of the lungs at FRC is determined by the balance of forces between the lung's propensity to deflate and the chest wall's elastic properties that tend to resist the collapse of the lungs. A very stiff lung or a very compliant chest wall leads to a reduced FRC; a compliant lung or a more elastic and stiff chest wall tends to increase the FRC.

The RV is the volume of gas remaining in the lung at the end of a maximal effort to expel all of the air possible. In young persons, the volume of the RV is determined by the balance of forces between the strength of the expiratory muscles and the force needed to collapse the chest wall. Neuromuscular weakness, for example, leads to an increase

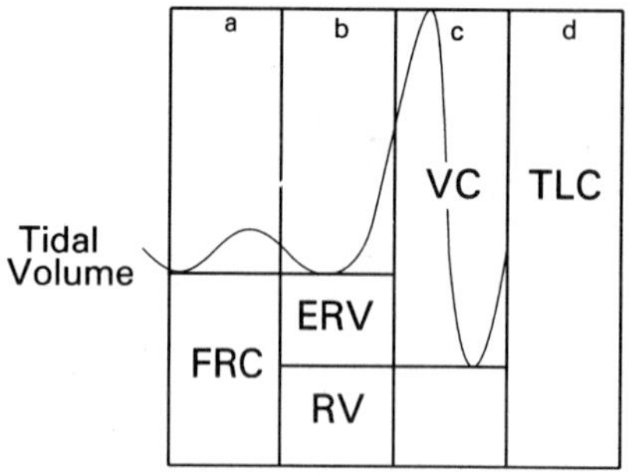
a
b
c
d
VC
TLC
Tidal Volume
ERV
FRC
RV

Fig. 1-1. Schematic depiction of the physiologic lung volumes. VC, vital capacity; FRC, functional residual capacity; ERV, expiratory reserve volume; RV, residual volume; TLC, total lung capacity. See text for details.

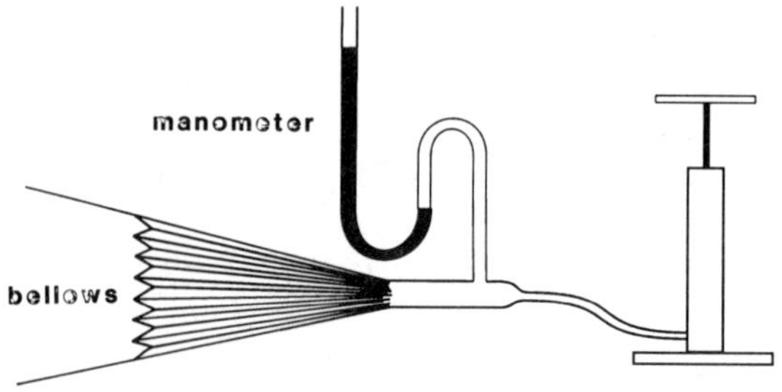
manometer
bellows

Fig. 1-2. The bellows as a lung analogy. See text for details.

in the RV because the chest wall cannot be compressed as much as normal by the weak muscles. RV may be increased in individuals older than 35 because of impaired exhalation of gas due to premature closing of small airways at low lung volumes. A number of factors are responsible for this situation including the age-related loss of lung-supporting structures as well as damage from cigarette smoking.

The VC is the volume of gas contained in the largest breath possible from full inspiration to full expiration: the difference between TLC and RV. Almost any lung disease can reduce the size of the VC, and the amount of reduction can help estimate the amount of disability to be expected from that lung disease.

The ERV is the volume of gas that can be expelled voluntarily from the lungs following a normal breath: The difference between FRC and RV. The expiratory reserve volume is typically reduced in morbid obesity. The RV is determined by the closure of small airways, and the FRC is reduced by the layer of fat on the chest and the layer of fat on the abdominal wall pushing up the diaphragm.

Compliance and Elastance

Imagine a bellows such as is depicted in Fig. 1-2. Blowing air into these bellows increases their volume, stretching the springiness that returns the bellows to the closed state when air is released. Stretching occurs as more air is forced into the bellows and the pressure inside as measured by the manometer increases. As the gas is released from the bellows, the pressure drops until the bellows are fully contracted; a small amount of gas remains inside, the RV.

The graph in Fig. 1-3 depicts the pressure-volume relationship of two different sets of bellows or lungs. The volume is changed by a small amount, while the change in the pressure across the wall of the lung or bellows is measured. This series of volumes and pressures is plotted in Fig. 1-3. The slope of the pressure volume line, the change of volume divided by the change of pressure, is called the *compliance* of the system: compliance = volume change/pressure change. The dashed line in Fig. 1-3 represents a bellows with a lower compliance than that with the solid line.

The dimensions of compliance are volume divided by pressure; in pulmonary physiology, volume is usually measured in liters and pressure in centimeters of water, so the dimensions would be liters per centimeter of water.

The reciprocal of the compliance is called the *elastance* and is given by the equation, elastance = pressure change/volume change. It is important to remember that any structure that exhibits elastic behavior also exhibits compliant behavior, and that a highly elastic structure has a low compliance, and a highly compliant structure has a low elastance. The term *elastic recoil pressure* refers to the specific pressure between the inside and the outside

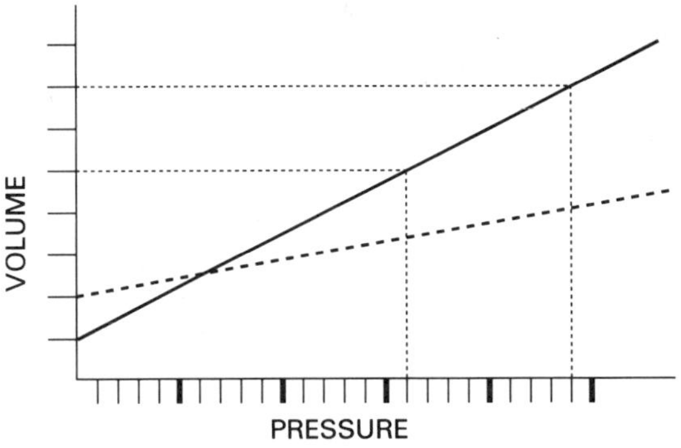
VOLUME
PRESSURE

Fig. 1-3. The volume-pressure curves of two different complaint systems. See text for details.

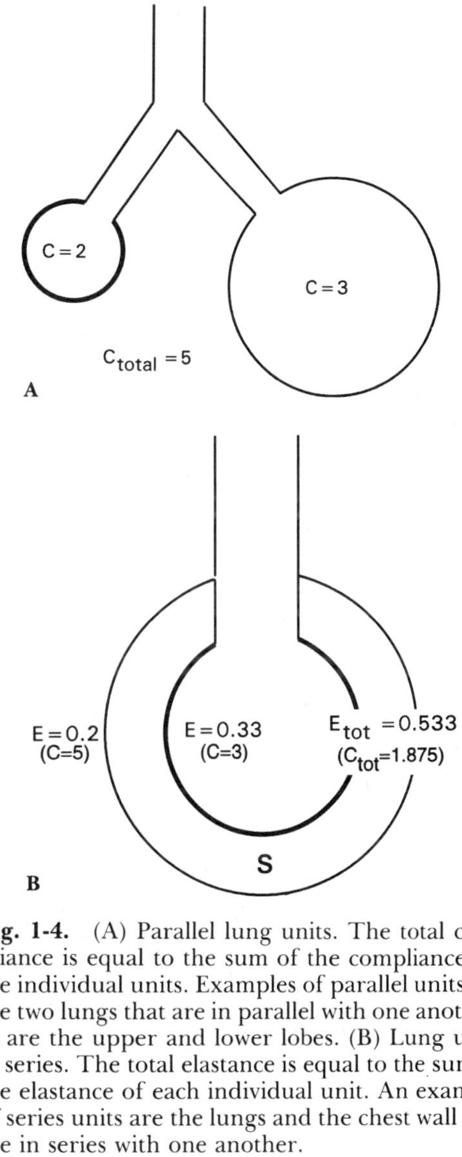
C = 2
C = 3
C total = 5
A
E = 0.2
(C=5)
E = 0.33
(C=3)
E tot = 0.533
(C tot=1.875)
S
B

Fig. 1-4. (A) Parallel lung units. The total compliance is equal to the sum of the compliances of the individual units. Examples of parallel units are the two lungs that are in parallel with one another, as are the upper and lower lobes. (B) Lung units in series. The total elastance is equal to the sum of the elastance of each individual unit. An example of series units are the lungs and the chest wall that are in series with one another.

of the lung at the volume in question, whereas the term *elastance* refers to the reciprocal of the compliance. The elastic recoil pressure of the unit depicted by the solid line in Fig. 1-3 at 7 L volume is 24 pressure units. The elastic recoil pressure of this same unit at 5 L volume is 16 pressure units. The elastance, then, is 24 − 16 = 8 divided by 7 − 5 = 2 or 4 pressure units per liter. The compliance is the reciprocal of this or 0.25 L change per pressure unit change. The term elastic refers to the tendency of an object to restore itself to its initial state after being deformed. So a tennis ball is more elastic than a foam rubber ball, and the foam rubber ball is more compliant than the tennis ball. Diseases in which collagen is laid down in the lung, such as sarcoidosis, lead to an increase in the elastic recoil or elastance of the lung, with a concomitant decrease in the compliance. Emphysema, with its loss of elastic fibers, leads to a loss of elastance and an increase in the compliance of the lung.

Parallel and Series

The terms *parallel* and *series* describe two ways of arranging structures. In a parallel arrangement, the structures can all be filled with the same pressure. For example, the pressure required to fill one lung is the same as the pressure needed to fill the other lung. In a series arrangement, the structures are so arranged that the pressures needed to fill them increase with the addition of more structures. The lung and the chest wall are in series, and require more pressure to expand than either alone. The system in Fig. 1-4A shows compliant structures depicted schematically as balloons arranged in parallel. Compliant structures arranged in parallel may be added for a total system compliance.

The pressure in the two balloons or compliances must be equal because otherwise air would just flow from the higher pressure to the lower pressure device until the pressures were equal. Assume the compliances of the two devices are 2 and 3 as indicated in Fig. 1-4A. If 5 additional liters is added to the system, the gas would distribute itself according to the compliances of the individual devices and the formula

Pressure change = volume change/C

So the compliance 3 device would receive 3 L, and the compliance 2 device would receive 2 L. According to the previous equation, the pressure in each device would increase by 1 pressure unit, and the pressure in the entire system would also increase by 1 unit. The total compliance of the entire system consisting of the two units in parallel can be calculated from the compliance equation as a volume change of 5 divided by the pressure change of 1 for a total compliance of 5. This is the same value we would get from adding the compliances of the component parts of the system. The two lungs are in parallel, and the total pulmonary compliance is equal to the sum of the compliances of each lung alone.

The structures in Fig. 1-4B are in series; a series arrangement is defined as one where the elastances (the reciprocal of the compliances) of each structure must be added together to calculate the total elastance of the system. Assuming the compliance of the outer structure is 5, its elastance is 0.2, and if the compliance of the inner structure is 3, its elastance is 0.33. The total elastance then is 0.33 + 0.2 or 0.53. The overall compliance is then 1/0.53 or 1.875. An analysis of pressures similar to that given for Fig. 1-4A confirms that this is true. The pressure across the inside structure is given by the inside pressure minus the pressure in space *s*. The pressure across the outside structure is given by the pressure in space *s* minus the outside pressure. If we add 15 L of air, both structures stretch by that volume, and the pressure across the outside structure increases by 15/5 pressure units, and the pressure across the inside structure increases by 15/3 pressure units. The total pressure across both structures increases by 15/5 + 15/3 or 8 pressure units. Therefore, the compliance of the entire system is given by 15/8 or 1.875. Note that this is a smaller value than either balloon alone. The lungs and the chest wall are effectively in series, so that the elastances of the lungs and the chest wall add, making the total elastance greater than the elastance of either one alone. Therefore, the compliance of the lung/chest wall system is smaller than the compliance of either the lungs or chest wall alone.

Surface Tension

If an excised lung is filled with air, a volume pressure curve can be constructed, as shown by the dashed line in Fig. 1-5. The slope of this volume pressure curve is the compliance of the lung. Notice, however, that the slope is not constant, so that the compliance of the lung varies with its inflation. Pulmonary physiologists usually measure the compliance of the lung at FRC to avoid variation due to volume change alone. Notice also, that when the lung is filled with saline rather than with air as indicated by the solid line in Fig. 1-5, the slope of the curve (the compliance) increases markedly. This increase of compliance in the saline-filled lung indicates that the compliance (and elastance) in the air-filled lung is determined to a large extent by the presence of an air–water interface. The alve-

Fig. 1-5. Volume-pressure curves for air-filled (dotted line) and water-filled lungs (solid line).

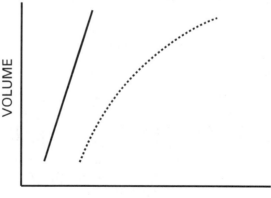

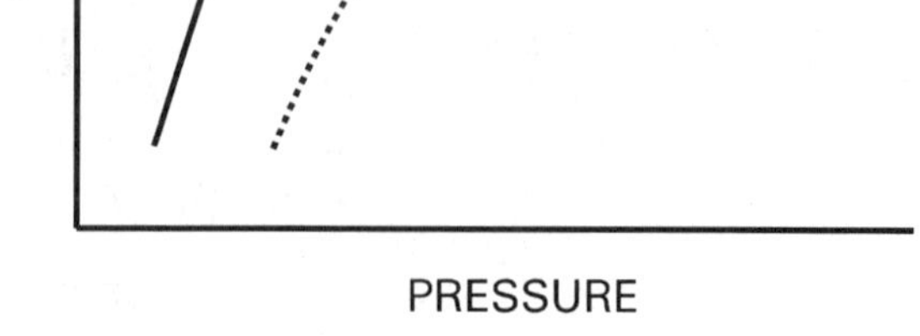
VOLUME
PRESSURE

oli are lined by alveolar fluid, which is mainly water. Filling the alveoli with water eliminates the interface, and decreases the elastance (increasing the compliance) of the lung.

Whenever dissimilar fluids (such as air and water) are in contact with one another, the phenomenon of surface tension appears. Surface tension is caused by the mutual attraction of the water molecules for one another; the interface between the water and the air acts as if there were a membrane under tension stretched between the two substances. The amount of tension in this pseudomembrane is dependent only on the chemical nature of the two substances in contact with each other, and unlike a rubber membrane, is independent of the amount the surface is stretched. A rubber sheet increases its tension as it is stretched, but a surface tension film does not. The water-lined alveolus acts as if its water–air interface were a stretched membrane of constant tension that tries to collapse the alveolus to a smaller volume; similarly, the rubber wall of a child's balloon tries to collapse the balloon to a smaller volume.

The LaPlace relationship describes how the pressure inside a spherical container such as an alveolus may be influenced by surface tension. LaPlace's law states that the pressure inside a sphere is equal to twice the tension in the wall divided by the radius of the sphere.

$$P = 2t/r$$

Where P is pressure in the container, r is the radius, and t is the tension in the wall (Fig. 1-6).

Remember that in a soap bubble, as in a rubber balloon, it is the tension in the wall that generates the pressure inside. In a soap bubble, as in an alveolus at small volume, the tension in the wall (and hence, the pressure inside the alveolus) is caused by the surface tension of the air–water interface. The value of t is independent of bubble or alveolar size because surface tension is dependent only on the chemical nature of the fluids, not on how much they are stretched. Therefore, pressure inside such a sphere is inversely proportional only to its size. Given the two unequal sized air-filled alveoli of Fig. 1-7, it follows that the smaller has a greater pressure inside than the larger one and would empty its contents into the larger alveolus. If all small alveoli tended to empty into larger ones, eventually the lung would consist only of a very few distended alveoli, with the majority of the alveoli collapsed. This highly unstable situation would be incompatible with normal respiration. This unstable situation would not occur in a system consisting of rubber balloons, since in a rubber balloon the tension in the wall in-

Fig. 1-6. Schematic depiction of the LaPlace relationship in a sphere.

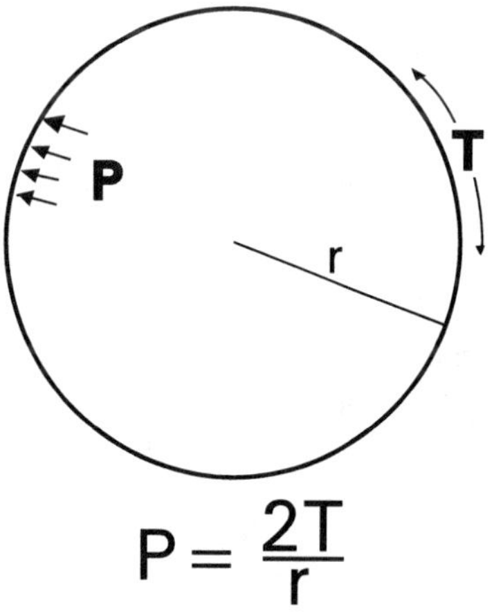
P
T
r
P = 2T/r

Fig. 1-7. Air-filled alveoli of unequal size. In the absence of surfactant, the smaller tends to empty into the larger.

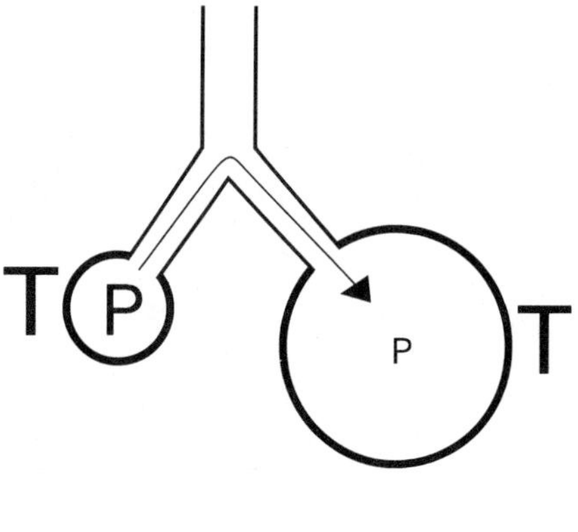
T
P
P
T

creases as the balloon gets larger, thus increasing the pressure inside and counteracting the tendency of the smaller balloon to empty into the larger.

Surfactant is a unique chemical that serves to stabilize alveoli. Not only does surfactant lower the surface tension of the alveolar fluid much as a detergent might, but surfactant has the unique characteristic of changing its surface tension characteristics as the surface is stretched (Fig. 1-8) [2, 3]. The dashed line represents the surface tension of a water–air interface. Adding a detergent to the water decreases the surface tension, as indicated by the dotted line. The solid line represents the surface tension of a water-surfactant solution, which varies with the area of the alveolus. As an alveolus increases in size, the internal pressure tends to decrease according to the LaPlace relationship. However, when the fluid contains surfactant, the surface tension is no longer constant, but increases as the surface area of the alveolus is increased, opposing the effect on pressure of the increasing radius; the internal pressure no longer decreases. The pressure inside small alveoli is no longer greater than that in larger alveoli, so the lung is stable (Fig. 1-9).

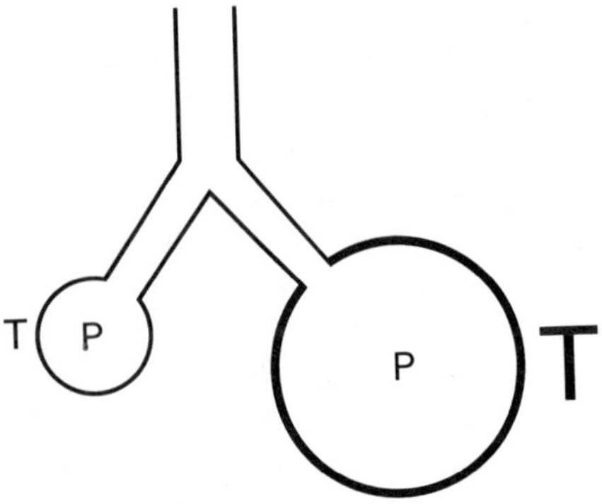
T
P
P
T

Fig. 1-9. The increasing surface tension with size characteristic of surfactant helps to stabilize alveoli of unequal size.

Hysteresis is the phenomenon exhibited by the lung in which the inflation and deflation volume-pressure curves are different (Fig. 1-10) [4]. All the graphs of volume-pressure curves up to this point in the discussion have shown only the deflation branch of the complete curve. In clinical practice, only the deflation branch is considered when measuring compliance. Surfactant also exhibits the characteristic of hysteresis where the area pressure relationship is different during stretching than during shrinking; in fact, surfactant is responsible for almost all the hysteresis the intact lung exhibits since in a saline-filled lung, little hysteresis is seen. It is controversial whether the hysteresis exhibited by surfactant is a significant contributor to lung stability or not.

Fig. 1-8. Surface tension versus area plots for water (dashed line), detergent solution (dotted line), and surfactant solution (solid line).

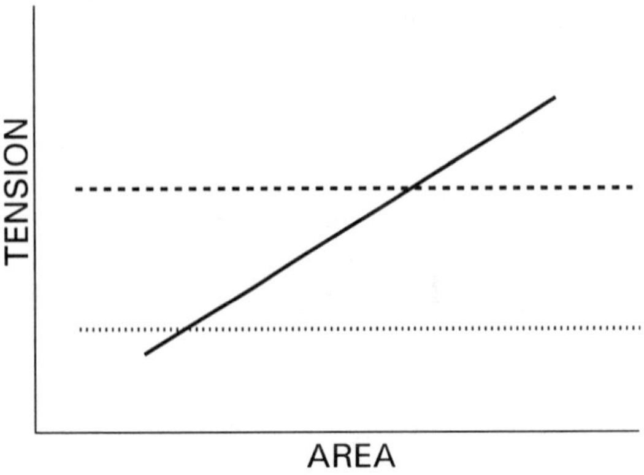
TENSION
AREA

Areas of atelectasis seen in hyaline membrane disease of newborns are caused by the insufficient surfactant in the lungs of these infants with the concomitant instability of alveoli that results. In utero, the lungs are filled with amniotic fluid, so surface tension plays no role in lung inflation. But with the first breaths, surface tension becomes important as the lungs fill with air, and absence of sufficient surfactant leads to widespread microatelectasis. The areas of plate-like atelectasis seen in pulmonary embolism are also thought to be due to localized surfactant deficiency.

The various pressures in the thorax that relate to lung expansion are depicted in Fig. 1-11 [5]. The relationship between various intrathoracic pressures is given by the formula

$$Palv = Pel + PPl$$

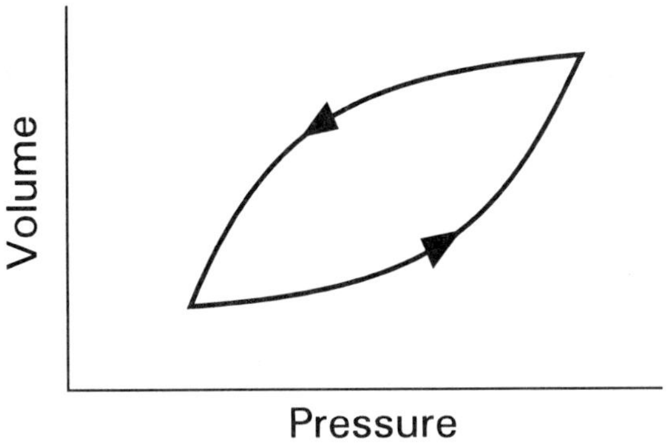
Volume
Pressure

Fig. 1-10. Volume-pressure curve of normal lung. The phenomenon of differing curves on inflation and deflation is called hysteresis.

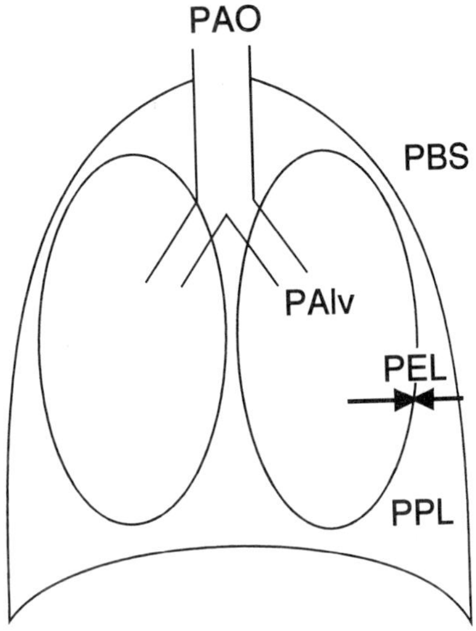
PAO
PBS
PAlv
PEL
PPL

Fig. 1-11. Important thoracic pressures. PBS, barometric pressure at the body surface; PAO, pressure at the airway opening; PAlv, pressure inside the alveolus (usually expressed as a pressure difference from the body surface); PEL, pressure difference between the inside and outside of the lung (in this case, the pressure outside the lung is equal to the pleural pressure); PPL, pleural pressure (usually expressed as a pressure difference from the body surface). See text for explanation.

Where Palv is the pressure difference between the alveolus and the body surface, Pel is the pressure of elastic recoil, and PP1 is the pleural pressure referred to the body surface.

Pel represents the pressure of elastic recoil and is measured as the pressure difference between the inside of the alveolus and the outside. Since the elastic tissue of the lung together with surface tension forces make the intra-alveolar pressure higher than the surrounding pressure, Pel is always a positive number. PPl is usually negative during quiet breathing, but can become positive during forced expiration.

When the respiratory muscles are relaxed and in the absence of the lungs' collapsing force, the chest wall assumes a volume that is somewhat larger than FRC, but slightly smaller than TLC. At FRC, then, the lungs are stretched and elastic forces attempt to collapse them; the chest wall, on the other hand, is being compressed or made smaller by the negative pleural pressure. The pleural space, by virtue of its negative pressure, binds the lung and the chest wall together, despite the lung's attempt to get smaller and the chest wall's tendency to enlarge. The volume of the lung at FRC is determined by the balance between the forces tending to collapse the lung and the forces tending to expand the chest wall (Fig. 1-12). In diseases such as emphysema, the elastic forces of the lung are much diminished, and the FRC increases. In diffuse interstitial fibrosis, the opposite happens.

As the inspiratory muscles inflate the chest, they become shorter, thus reducing the maximum force they can exert. At the same time, the force required to inflate the lung gets greater. Near TLC, the inspiratory muscles also have to work actively against the chest wall, which has a natural volume somewhat smaller than TLC and has been "helping" to inflate the lungs below its natural volume. Eventually, the force required to inflate the lungs and chest wall becomes greater than the force that the inspiratory muscles can generate, and expansion ceases at TLC. So TLC is determined by the balance between inspiratory muscles and the elastic properties of the lungs and chest wall.

During expiration, the lungs and expiratory muscles both act to compress the chest

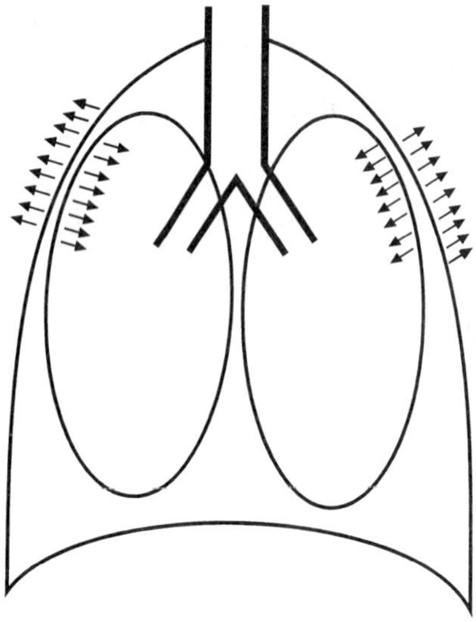

Fig. 1-12. The thorax at FRC. The tendency of the lungs to collapse exactly balances the tendency of the chest wall to expand. The negative intrapleural pressure keeps the pleural surfaces together.

wall. In young individuals (< 20 or 25 years) RV is determined by the balance between the elastic properties of the chest wall on the one hand, and the force of the expiratory muscles and the elastic recoil of the lungs on the other. In older individuals at small lung volumes small airways collapse trapping air behind them. This phenomenon, which occurs at higher lung volumes as we age, determines the volume of the lungs at RV rather than the balance of forces.

Dynamic Characteristics

The flow of air or water through a pipe is determined by a variant of Ohm's law, which states that the flow is proportional to the driving pressure and inversely proportional to the resistance to flow:

$$\dot{V} = (P1 - P2)/R$$

Where $\dot{V}$ is flow, $P1$ is the pressure at the inflow to the pipe, $P2$ is the pressure at the outflow, and R is the resistance (Fig. 1-13).

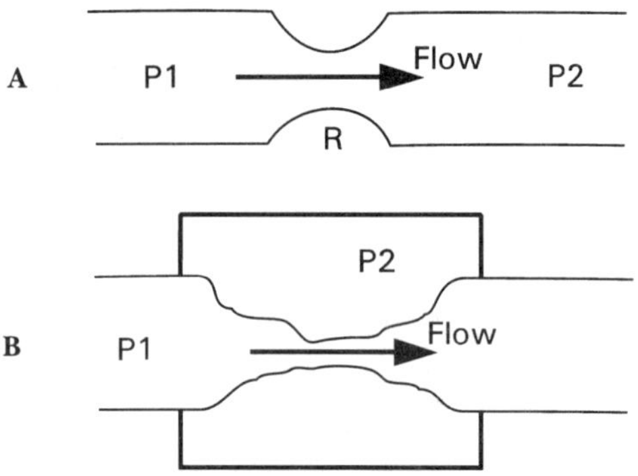
A
P1
Flow
P2
R
B
P2
P1
Flow

Fig. 1-13. (A and B) Schematic representation of the factors determining flow in a pipe. R, resistance; P1 and P2, pressures at the inlet and outlet of the pipe, respectively.

The driving pressure is the pressure difference between the inlet to the resistance and the outlet. In pulmonary physiology driving pressure is usually measured in centimeters of water and the flow rate is measured in liters per second. The units of resistance are centimeters of water per liter per second. Flow always occurs from a region of greater pressure to one of lower pressure and is also proportional to the pressure difference. If both ends of the resistor are at the same pressure, no flow occurs. The converse is also true; in an open airway without flow, there is a pressure drop of zero.

Although Ohm's law is very useful when understanding and describing the function of the airways, it is something of a simplification. The actual cause of the resistance referred to in Ohm's law is based in thermodynamics. During conditions of laminar flow, which is in general slow and smooth as might be found in an airway, the resistance to flow is influenced by the length and size of the pipe and the nature of the fluid (its viscosity) [6].

$$R = \mathrm{K}\, l\mu/r^4$$

Where R is the resistance, K is a proportionality constant, l is the length of the pipe, μ is the viscosity of the fluid, and r is the radius of the pipe.

The fact that the radius of the pipe is raised to the fourth power means that small changes in the diameter of the airways lead to large changes in the resistance to flow; a halving of the diameter leads to a 16-fold increase in the resistance to flow. A similar mechanism occurs in blood vessels; the body uses this characteristic to regulate blood flow and air flow to the appropriate tissues.

Under conditions of turbulent flow, which is the state of affairs in most regions of the lungs, the actual resistance becomes even more dependent on the radius of the pipe and becomes somewhat dependent on the flow rate as well. As shown in Fig. 1-14, when flow is turbulent the pressure required to sustain a certain flow rate increases much faster than under laminar conditions.

Starling Resistors

The Starling resistor consists of a collapsible tube placed inside a pressurizable chamber (Fig. 13B). As the pressure inside the chamber is increased, the tube is compressed, and the resistance to flow through it is increased. It can be shown that in the case of a Starling resistor, the pressure drop of Ohm's law is not the pressure difference between the ends of the tube, but rather the difference between the inlet pressure and the pressure inside the chamber pressing on the tube. If the inlet pressure is much greater than the chamber pressure, a large flow can occur. As the chamber pressure is increased, the total flow is decreased proportionately, until the chamber pressure is made equal to or greater than the inlet pressure, when flow is shut off entirely. Many bodily systems are influenced by the Starling resistor effect: blood flow is modified by tissue pressure, which acts like the chamber pressure, and air flow is modified by pleural pressure, which also acts like the chamber pressure in a Starling resistor (see following).

Fig. 1-14. When flow is laminar, the flow rate is directly proportional to the pressure difference between the inlet and outlet of a pipe (solid line). When flow is turbulent, a greater pressure is required for a similar flow (dashed line).

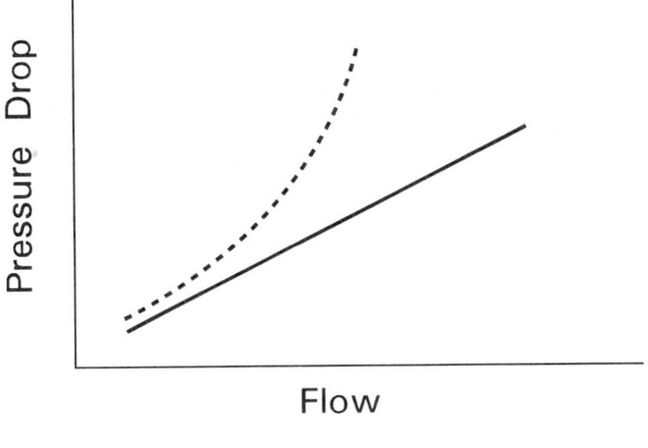
Pressure Drop
Flow

Series Resistors

If two resistors are connected in series so that the outflow from one flows into the inflow of the next one (Fig. 1-15), the total resistance of the system is equal to the sum of the two resistances. If we add a third resistor, the total resistance is equal to the sum of all three. This is the situation where the resistance of the nose, pharynx, and the trachea are in series and add to one another to form part of the total respiratory resistance. It is important to note that the flow through each of the resistors in a series arrangement is exactly the same as all the others, even if the resistances are different. This becomes intuitively obvious when we recognize that the total output of the first resistor in line must pass through the second, and that no air is added or lost en route. Since the flow through all the resistors is the same, we can calculate the pressure drops across them (Fig. 1-16).

Assume P_4 to be zero or ambient
Flow = $P_3 - P_4/R$ from Ohm's law.
Since Flow = 30, and $R = 8$
$30 = (P_3 - 0)/8$
and P_3 is calculated to be 240.

Fig. 1-15. The total resistance to flow is equal to R1 + R2. See text for further explanation.

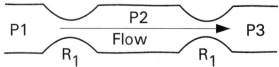

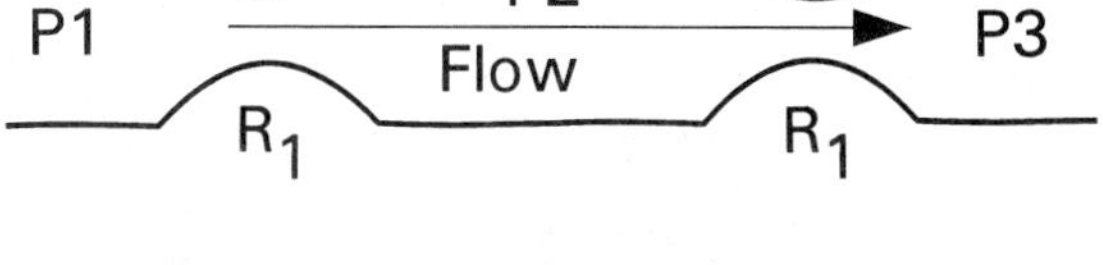
P1
P2
Flow
P3
R1
R1

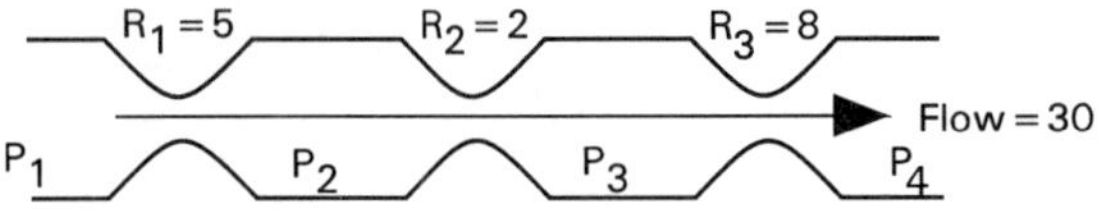
R1 = 5
R2 = 2
R3 = 8
Flow = 30
P1
P2
P3
P4

Fig. 1-16. Three resistors in series. See text for explanation.

If we go through a similar exercise, we find that P_2 is 60 pressure units greater than P_3 or 300 pressure units. P_1 is 150 units greater than P_2 and therefore is 450 pressure units.

The total pressure drop through the pipes in Fig. 1-16 is $P_1 - P_4$ or 450 pressure units. The flow is given as 30, so by Ohm's law, the total resistance is 450/30 or 15 units. This corresponds to 5 + 2 + 8, the sum of the resistors as described previously.

It is notable that the largest pressure drop occurs across the largest resistor, and the smallest across the smallest resistor. That portion of the airway with the largest resistance dissipates the greatest pressure drop. Patients with sleep apnea can have a very high upper airway resistance, requiring a great respiratory effort to generate enough pressure to pass sufficient air through the upper airway for respiration. Notice also, how the airway pressure diminishes downstream. In the airway, during forced expiration, the pressure is greatest in the alveolus and becomes progressively less, until it is 0 or ambient at the mouth.

Parallel Resistors

Imagine you are filling a large swimming pool in the springtime. It will take a very long time to fill it from the garden hose because the resistance of the hose and the pressure available will not generate a large enough flow rate. Is there a way to speed up the process? One that comes to mind is to connect hoses to several outside faucets at a time, or better yet, attach several hoses to faucets on the homes of all your neighbors! Each additional hose you attach will increase the flow rate available to fill your pool. The hoses are now connected in parallel, a connection that increases flow, in contrast to the series connection (all the hoses connected end to end), which serves to decrease flow.

Just as the reciprocal of elastance is compliance, the reciprocal of resistance is conductance, and the symbol is G (since C is already taken up by the symbol for compliance). All resistors are also conductors, and all conductors are also resistors; however, a good resistor is a poor conductor, and a good conductor is a poor resistor. A series connection can be defined as one in which the resistances of the individual units are added together to calculate the total resistance; a parallel connection can likewise be defined as one in which the conductances in the individual units are added together to calculate the total conductance. In Fig. 1-17, the two pipes are connected in parallel. The resistance through the upper branch is R_1, and the conductance through that branch is $G_1 = 1/R_1$. Flow through the upper branch is given by $\text{Flow}_1 = G_1 (P_1 - P_2)$. The total flow through both pipes is simply the sum of the two flows.

$$\text{Flow}_{\text{total}} = \text{Flow}_1 + \text{Flow}_2$$
$$\text{Flow}_{\text{total}} = (P_1 - P_2) * G_1 + (P_1 - P_2) * G_2$$
$$\text{Flow}_{\text{total}} = (P_1 - P_2) * (G_1 + G_2)$$

And since the total conductance is given by

$$G_{\text{total}} = \text{Flow}_{\text{total}} / (P_1 - P_2)$$
$$G_{\text{total}} = G_1 + G_2$$

The total conductance in a parallel system is simply the total of all the conductances, just as the total resistance in a series system is equal to the sum of all the series resistances.

Fig. 1-17. Two conductors in parallel. G_1 and G_2 are equal to $1/R_1$ and $1/R_2$, respectively. See text.

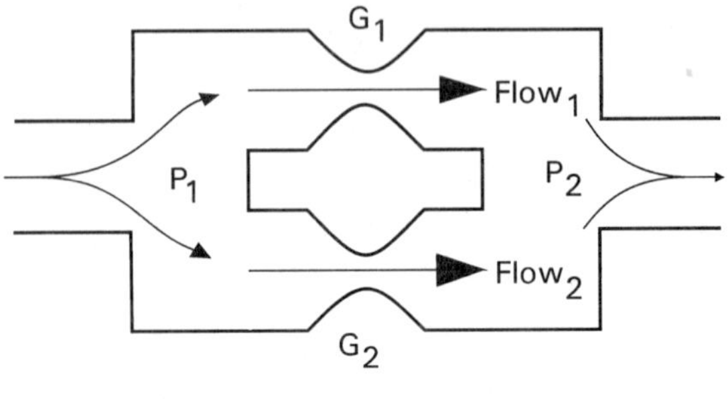
G1
Flow1
P1
P2
Flow2
G2

When conductors are connected in parallel (Fig. 1-17), the conductances add, and the total resistance decreases. Note that in a parallel system, the flow through each branch is proportional to the conductance in that branch.

Time Constant

Imagine a balloon emptying through a resistor (Fig. 1-18). How long will it take for the balloon to empty? At first, the balloon empties with a flow rate given by the pressure difference between the inside of the balloon and the outside, divided by the resistance. As the balloon empties, however, the pressure inside it decreases according to the change in volume divided by the compliance. The smaller pressure causes a smaller flow rate through the resistor, and so, as the balloon gets smaller, the flow decreases as well. Theoretically, at least, the balloon can never completely empty itself. Systems such as this have an exponential filling and emptying curve and can best be described using a number called the time constant (Fig. 1-19).

$$\text{Time constant} = RC$$

Where R is resistance, and C is compliance. The time constant, appropriately enough, has the units of time. In a time interval equal to one time constant, the balloon will empty to 37% of its initial volume. In another such interval it will empty to 37% of the volume at the end of the first interval, or 13.5% of the initial volume, and so forth. Lung units that have a long time constant fill and empty slowly, and units that have a short time constant fill and empty quickly. In diffuse interstitial fibrosis, the lungs and their subunits are stiff, i.e., they have a low compliance. Since the resistance is usually not changed greatly in this condition, the time constant of the lung units is small, indicating rapid emptying and filling. In emphysema, the lungs are very compliant owing to the loss of elastic tissue. Airway resistance is often near normal. But due to the greatly increased compliance of all the individual lung units, their time constants are long. In chronic bronchitis, the elastic tissue is nearly normal, but the resistance of the smaller airways is greatly increased, so, once again, the time constants of these lungs units is increased, leading to slow filling and emptying. If these effects happened uniformly, there would be minimal hypoxemia as a result. However, as we will see, the damaged lung is rarely uniformly damaged, and the nonuniformity leads to problems.

Fig. 1-18. A compliant structure emptying through a resistor.

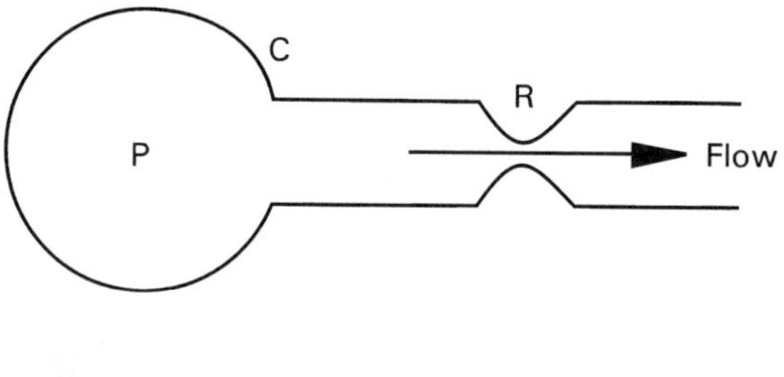
C
R
P
Flow

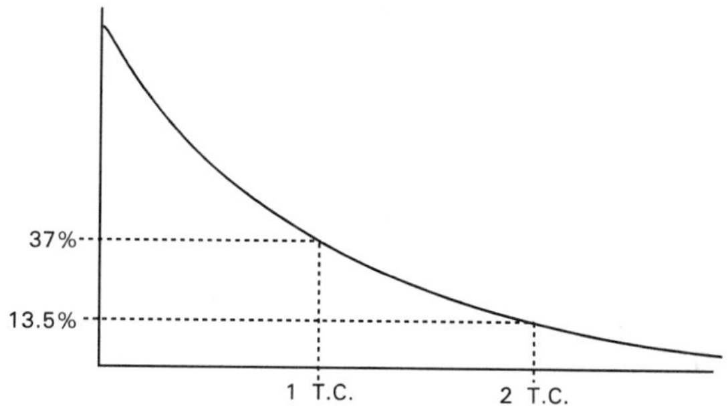
37%
13.5%
1 T.C.
2 T.C.

Fig. 1-19. Exponential volume-time curve of the unit in Fig. 1-18 showing two time constant intervals.

Distribution of Ventilation

Even in normal lungs, ventilation is not uniformly distributed, but favors the bases of the lungs [7]. There are both static as well as dynamic reason for this nonuniformity. During full inspiration (Fig. 1-20A), all the alveoli in the lung are fully distended; however, at maximal expiration (Fig. 1-20B), the alveoli at the bases are fully deflated whereas those at the apex are still partially inflated; the volume change, hence ventilation, of the basal alveoli is thus greater than those at the apex. Why this happens is not fully understood, but

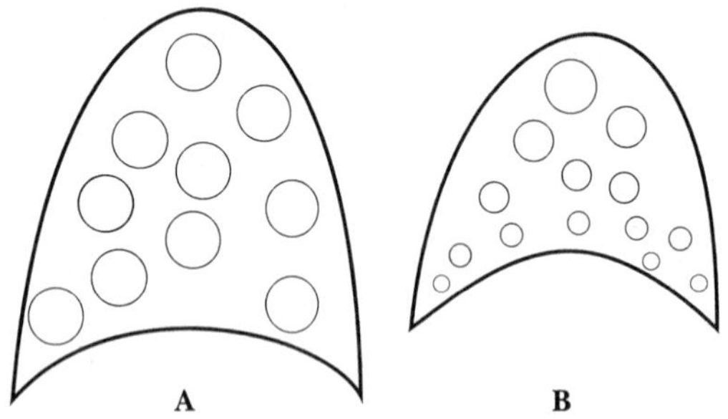
A
B

Fig. 1-20. The lung units at the bases change volume to a greater degree than units at the apices during a respiratory cycle. (A) The lung at TLC. (B) The lung below FRC.

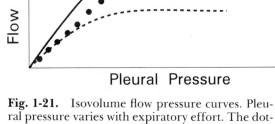

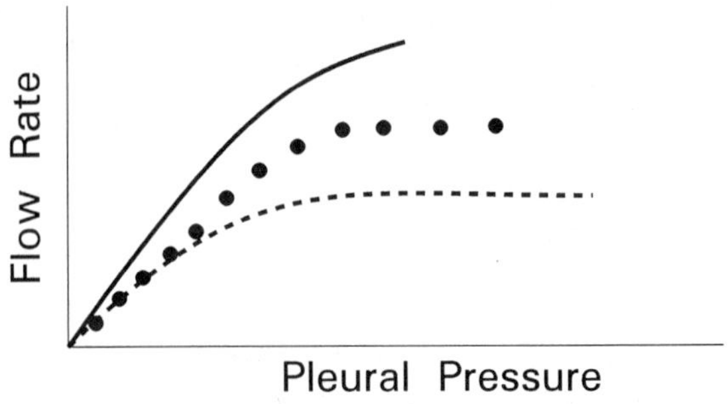
Flow Rate
Pleural Pressure

Fig. 1-21. Isovolume flow pressure curves. Pleural pressure varies with expiratory effort. The dotted curve is measured near FRC, the solid curve near TLC, and the dashed curve near RV.

a pleural pressure gradient caused by gravity effects, the shape of the chest wall, and regional compliance variations all probably contribute to the cause.

Dynamically, variation in time constants can cause scattered regional areas of nonuniform ventilation. In addition, respiratory muscles play a role in the distribution of ventilation. If inspiration is limited to the diaphragm, the bases are preferentially ventilated. If the accessory muscles of the shoulder girdle are used, more of the ventilation goes to the apex of the lung. Nonuniformity of ventilation is a major contributor to the hypoxia often seen in lung disease.

Flow Limitation

A normal individual performing a series of forced expiratory maneuvers with successively greater efforts will have a leveling of flow rates irrespective of increasing effort (Fig. 1-21) [8–10]. It is seen that at low levels of effort, successive breaths result in an increase in flow rate as effort is increased. Above a certain level of effort, however, increases in effort do not result in an increase in flow rate at any but the largest lung volumes. This maximum, effort-independent flow rate is called V_{max} and several models have been proposed to explain its existence. In patients with various kinds of obstructive lung disease, the airflow demonstrates a similar plateau effect, but at lower flow rates than in normal individuals.

In 1967, Mead et al [11] proposed the equal pressure point (EPP) model to explain the plateau phenomenon (Fig. 1-22). The model assumes a collapsible airway and an elastic source of pressure (the alveolus). The model provides a simple and elegant equation:

$$V_{max} = Pel/Rus$$

Where V_{max} is the maximum flow achievable at a given lung volume, Pel is the elastic recoil pressure of a lung segment, and Rus is the resistance of the "upstream" segment of airway between the alveolus and the equal pressure point.

Fig. 1-22. The Equal Pressure Point (EPP) model for airflow limitation. The intra-airway pressures diminish progressively from 30 at the alveolar end of the airway to 0 at the mouth. The EPP is the point where intra-airway pressure equals the pleural pressure. R_{us} is the resistance of the airway segment from the alveolus to the EPP.

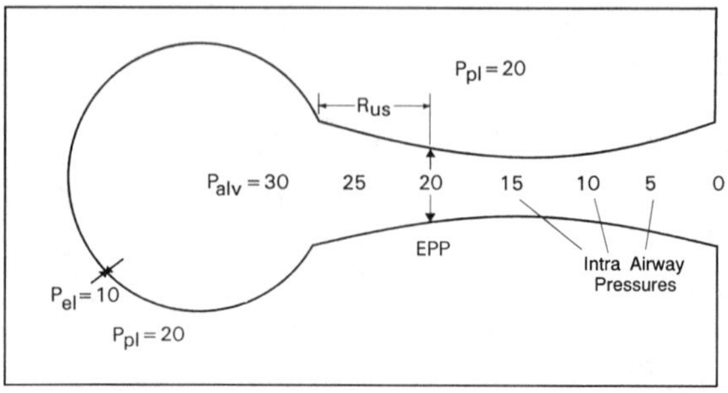
Ppl = 20
Rus
Palv = 30
25
20
15
10
5
0
EPP
Intra Airway Pressures
Pel = 10
Ppl = 20

The equal pressure point is the point in the airway where the pressure inside the airway equals the pleural pressure. Remember that the alveolar pressure equals the pleural pressure plus the elastic recoil pressure. During forced expiration, the pleural pressure is positive, and the alveolar pressure is greater than the pleural pressure. The pressure at the mouth is defined as 0. Inside the airway, there is a gradient from the alveolar pressure to the mouth pressure, and a location exists where the pressure is the same as pleural pressure. This is called the equal pressure point. However, the model suffers from the fact that the equal pressure point does not necessarily correspond to a segment of the airway where the actual flow limitation is occurring and so does not explain physically what is actually happening in the airway. The equation does suggest, however, that both a loss of elastic recoil and an increase in upstream resistance can have deleterious effects on V_{max}, a fact that is easily observable.

The waterfall model of Pride et al (Fig. 1-23) [12] attempts to explain what is actually happening by analyzing the area of collapse, "the flow limiting segment," in terms of how rigid the airway is and the internal and external pressures acting on it. This collapsing segment is a kind of Starling resistor, and equations become complex. Analysis is compounded by the problem of knowing just how rigid the airway is during forced expiration. Furthermore, the static pressures invoked ignore the Bernoulli phenomenon, which tends to reduce intra-airway pressures below those predicted on the basis of airway resistance alone. The Bernoulli phenomenon is the physical property of fluid flow that dictates that as flow rate goes up, pressure within the fluid goes down. This is the basis of action of perfume atomizers and most respiratory therapy nebulizers.

The latest model to be proposed has the benefits of actually explaining what is going on together with equations that are relatively simple [13]. The concept itself, however, is somewhat more complex (Fig. 1-24). The wavespeed model states that the maximal flow rate occurs when the speed of the gas through the airway equals the speed of sound at any point in that airway. The speed of sound is simply the maximum speed at which air molecules can get out of each others' way. In a collapsible tube the speed of sound is considerably slower than in open air. The more easily collapsible the tube, the slower the speed at which a pressure or sound wave propagates through the tube. The slowing of a pressure wave in a collapsible tube may be due to a partial collapse of the tube secondary to the restive pressure drop along with a pressure reduction caused by the Bernoulli phenomenon. The location of this partial collapse is the choke point.

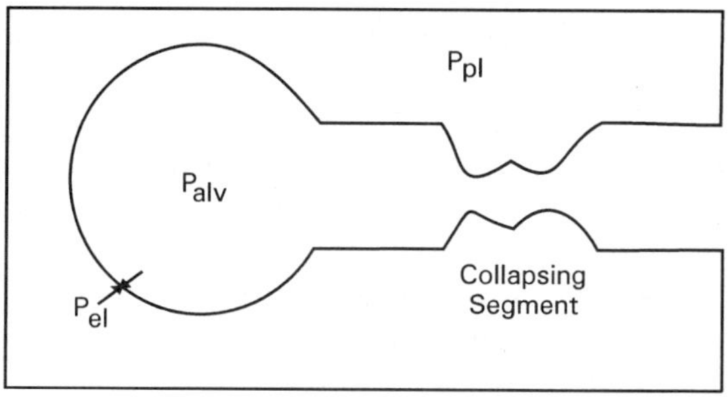
P_{pl}
P_{alv}
P_{el}
Collapsing Segment

Fig. 1-23. The waterfall model of airflow limitation. At some point in the airway, the extramural pressure on the airway is sufficiently greater than the intramural pressure to cause collapse of the airway and consequent airflow limitation.

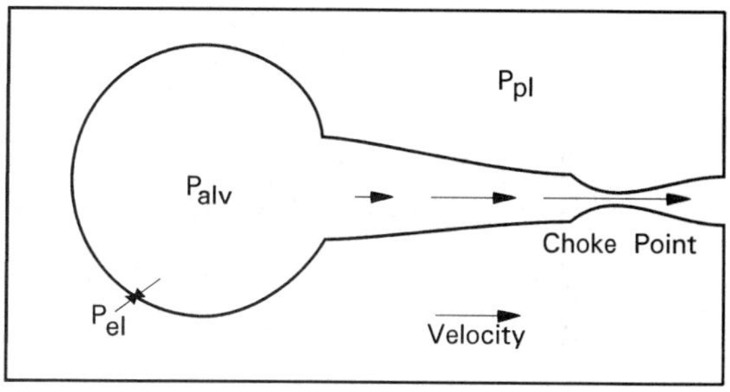
P_{pl}
P_{alv}
P_{el}
Choke Point
Velocity

Fig. 1-24. The wavespeed model. As the cumulative cross-sectional area of the airways decreases toward the mouth, the particle speed of the air increases, until, as some point in the airway, the speed of the air particles equals the speed of sound in the airway. At that point, the speed of airflow can increase no further.

All three models assume that a location in the airways actually collapses partially at the maximal flow rate, but the explanation of why this happens differs among the models.

Blood Flow

The ventilation of air to the lung is non-uniform because of the resistive and elastic properties of the lung and chest wall. Blood flow to the various regions of the lung is non-uniform as well such that there is relative matching of ventilation to perfusion. There is a gradient of blood flow from the top of the lung to the bottom very similar to air flow gradients seen in ventilation [14]. This gradient of blood flow is due to the effects of gravity.

It is useful to consider that the lung can be divided into three perfusion zones as described by West and Dollery (Fig. 1-25) [14]. The capillaries at the apex of the lung are well above the level of the heart in the upright posture, and the systolic pressure of the pulmonary system is not great enough to pump blood that high. This region is called zone 1 and the capillaries are not usually perfused in the upright posture.

At midlung levels, the pulmonary systolic pressure is great enough to fill the capillaries, but the pulmonary venous pressure is not high enough to fill the venous end of the capillaries. The capillaries act as if they were a Starling resistor; the alveolar pressure is the force compressing the venous end of the capillaries. Blood flow is determined by the difference between arterial pressure at that point in the lung and the alveolar pressure, which is nearly constant. Gravity causes an increase in arterial pressure and blood flow rate at lower levels in the lung. This arterial blood has pulsatile characteristics. In zone three, both pulmonary venous and arterial pressures are greater than alveolar pressure, and the capillaries are continuously filled. At less than full lung inflation, a fourth zone appears at the base of the lung [15]. In this zone, perfusion decreases from the top of the zone to the bottom owing to the relative compression of the lung tissue and vessels by gravity with concomitant compression of the extra-alveolar vessels.

The pulmonary arterioles have only a small amount of smooth muscle in their walls and are not very active in regulating blood flow under normal circumstances. However, the stimulus of alveolar hypoxia is a powerful vasoconstrictor [16], and this vasoconstriction serves to deflect blood away from underventilated alveoli in normal persons.

Fig. 1-25. Blood flow through the three zones of the lung. In zone 1, the pressure generated by the right ventricle is less than the hydrostatic pressure needed to counteract gravity. In zone 2, the systolic pressure of the right ventricle is greater than the hydrostatic pressure, but the left atrial pressure is less than the hydrostatic pressure. The flow is pulsatile. In zone 3, both right ventricular and right atrial pressures are greater than the hydrostatic pressure.

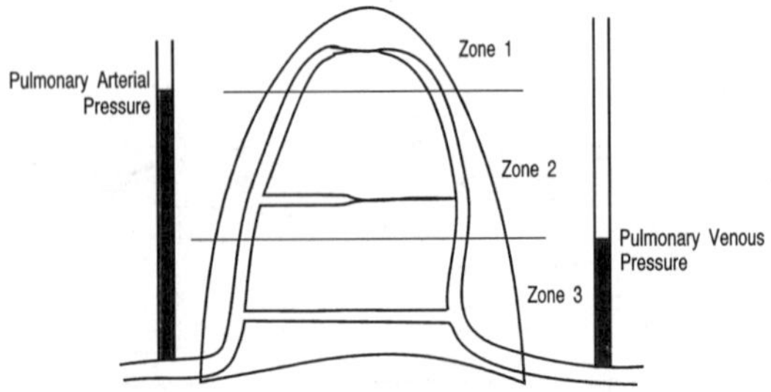
Zone 1
Pulmonary Arterial Pressure
Zone 2
Pulmonary Venous Pressure
Zone 3

Diffusion

Diffusion refers to the process in which respiratory gases pass through the alveolar walls into the red blood cell (Fig. 1-26) [17]. The path through which respiratory gases must pass includes the alveolar lining fluid, alveolar lining cells, alveolar basement membrane, capillary basement membrane, capillary endothelial cell, blood plasma, erythrocyte cell wall, and erythrocyte cytoplasm. The rate at which gases pass through from the alveolus to the capillary is dependent on several factors: the partial pressure difference between the alveolus and the capillary for the gas in question; the chemical nature of the gas and its solubility in the interstitium; the linear distance between the capillary and the alveolus; and finally, the surface area available for diffusion. It is generally thought that only the surface area of the interface between the al-

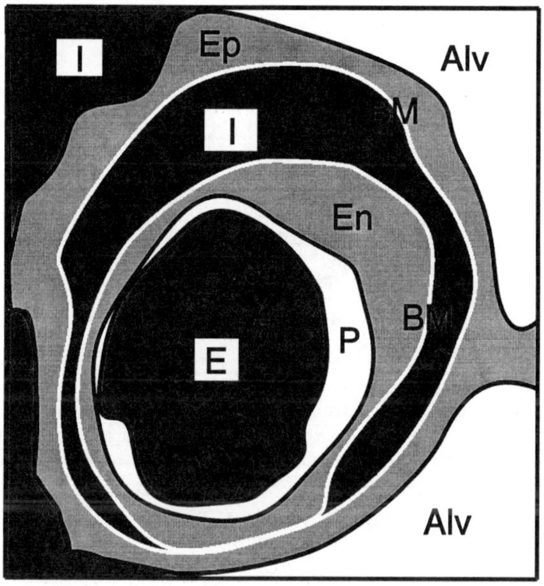
I
Ep
Alv
I
BM
En
BM
P
E
Alv

Fig. 1-26. The diffusion path. The layers gases must traverse between the alveolus and the erythrocyte. E = erythrocyte; Alv = alveolar; P = blood plasma; Ep = the alveolar epithelium; En = the capillary endothelium; BM = basement membranes of the capillary endothelium and the alveolar epithelium; I, interstitium (collagen, ground substance, etc.). (Adapted from an electron micrograph.)

veolus and capillary is an important factor in limiting diffusion of gases in human illness. In such diseases as emphysema, a considerable loss of surface area occurs due to the loss of alveolar walls, and very profound defects in diffusion occur. In fibrosing disorders there is also a loss of surface area because of the replacement of alveolar-capillary tissue with collagen.

Causes of Hypoxemia

The result of deranged pulmonary physiology is hypoxemia or an abnormally low partial pressure of oxygen. There are only five true physiologic causes of hypoxemia: (1) hypoventilation, (2) low inspired PiO_2, (3) ventilation-perfusion ($\dot{V}/\dot{Q}$) mismatch, (4) shunt, and (5) diffusion limitation.

Alveolar-Arterial Gradient

A useful concept to an understanding of arterial oxygen levels is the idea of the alveolar to arterial oxygen gradient (A-a gradient). The A-a gradient is simply the difference between the oxygen tension in an average alveolus and that in the arterial blood. In normal young persons, the gradient can be up to 10 mm Hg pressure difference. With increasing age the gradient increases slightly so that a normal 70-year-old person might have a gradient of 15 or 20. This gradient is calculated from the arterial oxygen tension as measured by arterial blood gases and the simplified alveolar air equation:

$$P_AO_2 = P_IO_2 - (PaCO_2/R)$$

Where P_AO_2 is the alveolar oxygen tension, P_IO_2 is the dry inspired oxygen tension, $PaCO_2$ is the arterial carbon dioxide tension, and R is the respiratory exchange ratio (usually about 0.8 in normal people on a normal diet).

The P_IO_2 can be calculated as

$$P_IO_2 = (P_{atm} - 47) * F_IO_2$$

Where P_{atm} is ambient atmospheric pressure (760 at sea level), 47 is the vapor pressure of water at body temperature, and F_IO_2 is the fraction of inspired oxygen, 0.21 on room air and 1.0 on 100% oxygen.

The P_IO_2 can be taken to be about 150 for most practical purposes. Applying the above formulas, then, gives an alveolar P_AO_2 as follows:

$$P_AO_2 = 150 - (40/0.8)$$
$$P_AO_2 = 100$$

at sea level on room air. The A-a gradient normally is less than 15, so the normal young individual has an arterial oxygen tension of greater than 85. The "normal" A-a gradient is not 0 because of the physiologic shunt. Deoxygenated blood is admitted to the left atrium through the thebesian veins, which drain the myocardium directly into the left atrium, and through the bronchial veins, which likewise drain directly into the left atrium. This deoxygenated blood mixes with fully oxygenated blood from the lungs, and this desaturated hemoglobin contributes to a lower arterial PaO_2.

Hypoventilation and Low P_IO_2

Hypoventilation is defined as ventilation insufficient to maintain a normal $PaCO_2$ in the range of 38 to 42 at sea level. As the concentration of carbon dioxide in the blood increases, the concentration in the alveoli increases also. This elevated alveolar P_ACO_2 effectively displaces oxygen from the alveolar gas, leading to a low alveolar, and hence low arterial, oxygen tension. Hypoventilation can be voluntary, or due to such disease states as severe chronic obstructive pulmonary disease, neuromuscular disease, or drug overdose. Supplemental oxygen administration will correct the hypoxemia due to hypoventilation because the alveolar O_2 tension is increased, but will not correct the hypercarbia.

A low P_IO_2 occurs principally at high altitude or during conditions where the oxygen percentage is reduced below the usual 20.9%. Oxygen administration reverses this hypoxemia also.

Ventilation-Perfusion Mismatch

The most important cause of hypoxemia in human disease is $\dot{V}/\dot{Q}$ mismatch (Fig. 1-27). Normally, the perfusion of blood and the ventilation of alveoli is fairly well matched. In some disease states, however, the lung becomes variably nonuniform, and some areas of the lung become relatively underperfused and others are relatively underventilated. Areas that are underperfused contribute small amounts of well-oxygenated blood to the circulation and are not responsible for hypoxemia. However, for all the areas that are underperfused, there are concomitant areas that are correspondingly poorly ventilated. In these alveoli, there is insufficient oxygen being introduced into the alveolus because of the inadequate ventilation to properly oxygenate the blood circulating there. The result is the contribution of a certain amount of poorly oxygenated blood to the systemic circulation. The overall ventilation to the entire lung can usually be increased sufficiently to avoid hypercarbia in this situation. However,

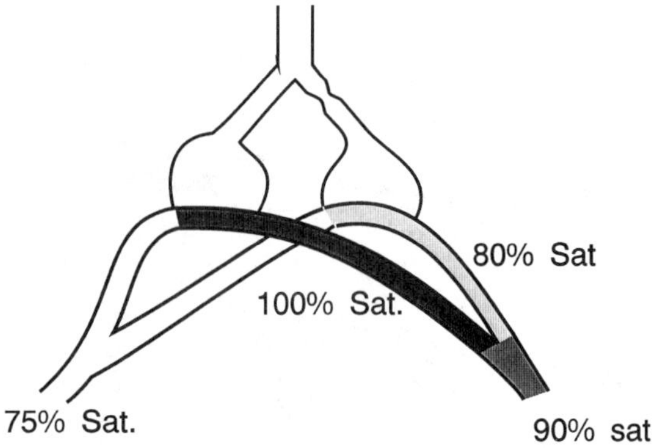
80% Sat
100% Sat.
75% Sat.
90% sat

Fig. 1-27. $\dot{V}/\dot{Q}$ mismatch. The blood from the poorly ventilated alveolus contributes a little additional oxygen to the mixture; additional oxygen administered to the patient finds its way to the poorly ventilated alveolus as well as to the well-ventilated one.

the fact that the hemoglobin in the well-ventilated alveoli cannot be saturated more than 100%, no matter how much that alveolus is hyperventilated, means that there is a limit to how much oxygen the well-ventilated alveoli can contribute. This well-oxygenated blood from well-ventilated alveoli is then diluted in the pulmonary veins by the poorly oxygenated blood from the poorly ventilated alveoli, so that the resulting arterial blood has a lower than normal overall saturation.

Shunt

Shunt describes a situation in which blood completely bypasses any ventilated alveoli and contributes venous blood to the arterial system (Fig. 1-28). Shunt represents the extreme case of low $\dot{V}/\dot{Q}$ ratio. At what level of low ventilation does it cease being a $\dot{V}/\dot{Q}$ defect and become "shunt?" Practically speaking, when ventilation is so low that 100% oxygen administration no longer provides enough oxygen to the affected capillaries to oxygenate the blood in them, it is considered a shunt. By this concept, then, $\dot{V}/\dot{Q}$ mismatch hypoxemia is correctable by oxygen administration, and shunt hypoxemia is not. In normal individuals, up to 5% of the cardiac output is shunted away from alveolar capillaries, predominantly through the cardiac thebesian

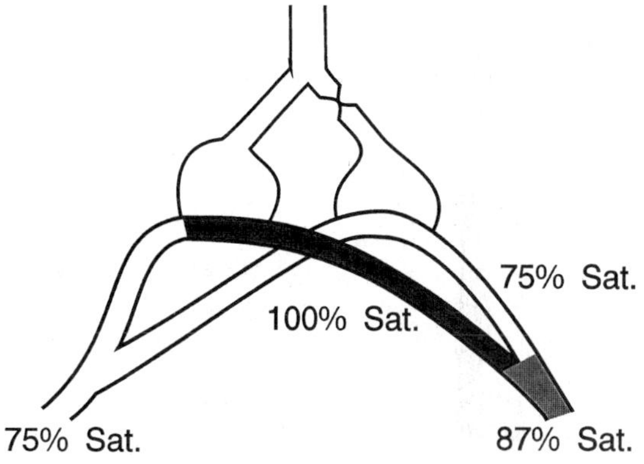
75% Sat.
100% Sat.
75% Sat.
87% Sat.

Fig. 1-28. Schematic depiction of a shunt (note that the right lung unit is totally obstructed). The desaturated blood from the shunt dilutes the fully saturated blood from the ventilated alveolus. Additional oxygen does not get to the unventilated alveolus, and the blood from the well-ventilated one is already fully saturated.

veins and the bronchial veins. A large variety of disease states can significantly increase the amount of shunted blood, including alveolar edema, as in pulmonary edema and adult respiratory distress syndrome, alveolar filling diseases such as lobar pneumonia, and collapse of lung (atelectasis) due to endobronchial obstruction.

Diffusion Defect

Diffusion abnormality represents the last physiologic cause for hypoxemia, in which the diffusion path is so poor (due to small surface area) that the oxygen cannot diffuse into the bloodstream fast enough to meet demand. This never occurs in normal humans at rest, but could be a factor under extreme conditions such as mountain climbing [18]. In disease states, diffusion abnormality rarely contributes materially to hypoxemia at rest, but can become significant during exercise. Exercise induced arterial desaturation is a sensitive test for early diffusion defects. Oxygen administration reverses the hypoxemia of diffusion limitation by increasing the diffusion pressure gradient from alveolus to capillary, and so increasing the amount of gas that can diffuse per unit time.

Conclusion

The static and dynamic characteristics of the lungs are differently deranged by various diseases. Understanding how different diseases affect these characteristics can help make a diagnosis and suggest treatment. The end result of most pathologic processes in the lungs is an increase in the A-a gradient due to a $\dot{V}/\dot{Q}$ mismatch. If the defect proves to be due to a shunt, as demonstrated by a relative resistance to oxygen administration, another set of diagnoses is suggested. An understanding of the physiology of the lung is clinically useful in both the diagnosis as well as the treatment of a wide variety of lung disorders.

References

1. Handbook of Physiology, American Physiological Society, 1986
2. Schuerch S: Surface tension at low lung volumes: Dependence on time and alveolar size. *Respir Physiol* 48:339–355, 1982
3. Brown ES, Johnson RP, Clements JA: Pulmonary surface tension. *J Appl Physiol* 14:717–720, 1959
4. Clements JA, Hustead RF, Johnson RP, et al: Pulmonary surface tension and alveolar stability. *J Appl Physiol* 16:444–450, 1961
5. Rahn H, Otis AB, Chadwick LE, et al: The pressure-volume diagram of the thorax and lung. *Am J Physiol* 146:161–178, 1946
6. Poiseuille JLM: Recherches experimentales sur le mouvement des liquides dans les tubes de tres petits diametres. *C R Acad Sci* 11:961–967, 1041–1048, 1840
7. Rodarte JR, Fung YC: Distribution of stresses within the lung. *In* Macklem PT, Mead J (eds): Handbook of Physiology, Section 3. The Respiratory System, vol 3, part 1. Bethesda, MD, *American Physiological Society,* 1986, pp 233–246
8. Fry DL, Hyatt RE: Pulmonary mechanics. A unified analysis of the relationship between pressure, volume and gas flow in the lungs of normal and diseased human subjects. *Am J Med* 29:672–689, 1960
9. Hyatt RE, Flath RE: Relationship of air flow to pressure during maximal respiratory effort in man. *J Appl Physiol* 21:477–482, 1986
10. Hyatt RE: The interrelationships of pressure, flow and volume during various respiratory maneuvers in normal and emphysematous subjects. *Am Rev Respir Dis* 83:676–683, 1961
11. Mead J, Turner JM, Macklem PT, et al: Sig-

nificance of the relationship between lung recoil and maximum expiratory flow. *J Appl Physiol* 22:95–108, 1967
12. Pride NB, Permutt S, Riley RL, et al: Determinants of maximal expiratory flow from the lungs. *J Appl Physiol* 23:646–662, 1967
13. Dawson SV, Elliot EA: Wave-speed limitation on expiratory flow—A unifying concept. *J Appl Physiol* 43:498–515, 1977
14. West JB, Dollery CT: Distribution of blood flow and the pressure-flow relations of the whole lung. *J Appl Physiol* 20:175–183, 1965
15. West JB, Dollery CT, Heard BE: Increased pulmonary vascular resistance in the dependent zone of the isolated dog lung caused by perivascular edema. *Circ Res* 17:191–206, 1965
16. Lloyd TC Jr: Pulmonary vasoconstriction during histotoxic hypoxia. *J Appl Physiol* 20:488–490, 1965
17. Roughton FJW, Forster RE: Relative importance of diffusion and chemical reaction rates in determining rate of exchange of gases in the human lung, with special reference to true diffusing capacity of pulmonary membrane and volume of blood in lung capillaries. *J Appl Physiol* 11:290–302, 1957
18. West JB, Hackett PH, Maret KH, et al: Pulmonary gas exchange on the summit of Mount Everest. *J Appl Physiol* 55:678–687, 1983

2

Office Pulmonary Function Testing

John Haapaniemi, Barry Lesser, and Ernest L. Yoder

Pulmonary specialists rely on pulmonary function laboratories in their evaluation of patients with mild-to-severe lung disease. However, the greatest value of testing lung function may be in its ability to detect disease before it is otherwise clinically evident. The place for such screening tests is in the setting of the primary practitioner. The spirogram with associated flow volume loop is the single most valuable test in the pulmonary function laboratory and can be performed by office personnel with minimal training and little expense. This test can be performed serially to evaluate progression of disease and response to therapy.

The goal of this chapter is to allow the primary care practitioner to set up an office pulmonary function laboratory, ensure quality testing, and interpret results. A basic understanding of pulmonary physiology and mechanics is required and is covered in the previous chapter. More extensive testing is generally done in a referral laboratory, such as a hospital or specialists' clinic. Even though this more elaborate testing is not recommended for a primary care setting because of cost effectiveness and quality of testing considerations, some discussion of lung volumes, diffusing capacity, and other special tests is covered for better illustration of certain disease processes that affect spirometry.

Indications

The terms *pulmonary function test, complete pulmonary function test,* or *routine pulmonary function test* mean different things to different physicians. Specific terms are listed in Table 2-1. A summary of tests available in the pulmonary function laboratory is shown in Table 2-2. The indications for each test vary depending on the problem, but spirometry is generally the starting point.

About 10 million Americans have chronic obstructive pulmonary disease (COPD), accounting for as many as 165,000 deaths annually in the United States [1]. In COPD, abnormal spirometry often precedes symptoms of dyspnea, abnormal physical findings, chest radiographic changes, or arterial blood gas alterations. The hope with early detection of disease is that identification will lead to earlier treatment and thus reduce morbidity and mortality. COPD alone accounts for billions of dollars of the health care budget, social and economic losses, and disability [2, 3]. Whether COPD or the full spectrum of lung disease, the goal should be to identify disease early, treat or remove the cause, and alter the course of disease [4–6].

Parameters measured with all pulmonary function tests are compared with values obtained from similar "normal" individuals. Performing spirometry early as a screening test supplies a baseline study to which subsequent tests can be compared. This may be analogous to an individual who has an old electrocardiogram for comparison. Arguments have even been made for the performance of spirometry on most patients as part of a complete physical examination [2, 7].

Pulmonary function tests are indicated in the evaluation of lung disease, although they usually do not make a specific diagnosis. Examples include confirmation of airflow limitation in asthma, chronic bronchitis, and emphysema or demonstration of decreased volume in restrictive diseases such as pulmonary fibrosis, sarcoidosis, pleural disease, neuromuscular disease, and kyphoscoliosis. Spirometry has even been employed in serial evaluation of patients with congestive heart

Table 2-1. Terms and abbreviations

PFT	Pulmonary function test
COPD	Chronic obstructive pulmonary disease
OAD	Obstructive airway disease
ATS	American Thoracic Society
VC (SVC)	Vital capacity (slow vital capacity)
FVC	Forced vital capacity
FEV_1	Forced expiratory volume, 1st second
FEV_3	Forced expiratory volume, 1st 3 seconds
FEV_1/FVC	FEV_1 to FVC ratio called the FEV_1 percent or percent FEV_1
$FEF_{25\text{-}75}$	The mean forced expiratory flow during the middle half of the FVC maneuver (also mid-maximal expiratory flow rate [MMFR])
FEF_{max}	The maximal forced expiratory flow achieved during the FVC maneuver (L/s) Maximum expiratory flow (MEF)
PEF	The highest expiratory flow measured with a peak flow meter (L/min)
MVV	Maximum voluntary ventilation. The volume of air exhaled during a 12-second maximum respiratory effort (sum of volumes of each breath $\times$ 5 = L/min) (also called maximum breathing capacity [MBC])
TLC	Total lung capacity
FRC	Functional residual capacity
RV	Residual volume
IC	Inspiratory capacity
ERV	Expiratory reserve volume
TGV	Thoracic gas volume
STPD	Standard temperature (0°C), pressure (760 mm Hg), dry
ATPD	Ambient temperature, pressure, dry
ATPS	Ambient temperature, pressure, saturated
BTPS	Body temperature, pressure, saturated
P_B	Barometric pressure
PD_{20}	Provocative dose. The dose of methacholine required to generate a 20% drop in FEV_1
D_LCO	Diffusing capacity of the lung for carbon monoxide
SE	Standard error
CI	Confidence interval
LLN	Lower limit of normal

failure [8]. In addition to identification of characteristic patterns seen on pulmonary function tests, severity may be graded. Pulmonary function tests may be employed in screening patients at risk for developing lung disease, such as smokers, or in the evaluation of patients with respiratory symptoms such as cough or dyspnea [9–12]. Variant asthma has been described where the sole presenting manifestation is cough [12a]. Preoperative testing allows evaluation of risk in patients prone to pulmonary complications of surgery [13, 14]. Disability is a term that implies a patient has a condition that prevents him or her from performing a certain task. This may or may not correlate with the medical evaluation of impairment. In the case of respiratory disability, the patient must meet a constellation of parameters in the clinical evaluation that includes pulmonary function testing [3].

Objective evaluation of functional impairment can be followed over the course of a disease, and measurement of those parameters can assist in decisions regarding response to therapy and prognosis. Airway responsiveness can be evaluated with prebronchodilator and postbronchodilator studies.

This type of evaluation has become the

Table 2-2. Methods of pulmonary function testing

Procedure	*Method*	*Measurement*
Routine tests		
Spirometry*	Volume or flow-sensing device	FVC, IC, ERV FEV_1, FEV_1/FVC, FEF_{25-75}, FEF_{max}, and others Flow/volume loop MVV
Prebronchodilator and postbronchodilator*	Spirometry before and after bronchodilator	Change in volume and flow as above
Lung volumes	Nitrogen washout Helium dilution Body plethysmography	FRC, TLC, RV
Diffusing capacity	Single breath Carbon monoxide	Transfer of carbon monoxide across alveolar-capillary membranes
Special tests		
Bronchoprovocation†	Spirometry before and after methacholine aerosol (screen or quantified)	Change in flow (FEV_1) (hyperreactive airways)
Cardiopulmonary exercise test	Monitoring of heart rate and exhaled gas analysis during graded exercise	Oxygen consumption, CO_2 production, and other parameters (distinguishes ventilatory from cardiovascular limitation)
Polysomnography	Multiple parameters monitored during sleep	Characterizes and quantifies sleep apnea
Others (various methods)	Lung compliance and elastic recoil, frequency dependence of compliance, volume of isoflow, single breath N_2 washout (closing volume), multiple inert gas studies, dead space, calorimetry, ventilatory drive, etc. (not commonly done or reserved for research laboratories)	

See Table 2-1 for definitions of abbreviations.
*Should be done in primary care setting
†May be done in primary care setting

standard of care in a pulmonary specialist's practice, and elaborate equipment is employed in the assessment of lung volumes, diffusing capacity, and other parameters such as airways resistance, lung elastic recoil, and cardiopulmonary exercise testing. In spite of the well-established use of pulmonary function tests, testing in general and spirometry in particular are underemployed in the practice of medicine. Over the past several years some of the cumbersome aspects of the test, the finicky nature of the equipment, and the time-consuming hand calculations have been improved or simplified with electronic advancements. It is reasonable for a primary practitioner to perform spirometry in the office. The equipment is not prohibitively expensive and will generally pay for itself with only modest testing [2]. Office personnel can be trained either by the manufacturer of the equipment or often by the technicians in a referral laboratory. When viewed from the point of cost-effectiveness, simple spirometry with flow/volume loops yields a wealth of information for very little expenditure relative to more sophisticated tests available in a hospital laboratory. An analogy may be made by comparing routine electrocardiography to real-time B-mode echocardiography with Doppler, stress thallium, and so on. While spirometry may be considered a screening test, it is also a useful diagnostic tool much the same as is an electrocardiogram. Spirometry may be included in the routine complete history and physical examination as is electrocardiography and chest radiography. There is no doubt this test should be used to evaluate anyone at risk for developing lung disease, specifically cigarette smokers [15, 16]. Other groups may also be at risk such as those with occupational exposure to asbestos or silica [17]. In such cases, abnormalities may be found on screening.

Very often the earliest detectable abnormality in the development of lung disease is found on pulmonary function tests. In the natural history of COPD, disease begins in the small airways, but in the earliest stages is evident only histologically. Even though significant lung damage may occur before abnormality is seen on routine spirometry, these abnormalities usually precede symptoms (dyspnea or cough), physical findings (wheezing), radiographic changes, or arterial blood gas alterations [2]. Even so, this is a crude test and significant disease may be present, but not detectable by pulmonary function tests. Several tests, including volume of isoflow, closing volume, and frequency dependence of compliance, have been developed to look specifically for small airways disease, but have not been found to be clinically useful. Mid-maximum flow rate or FEF_{25-75} is a much simpler measurement and has been used to identify small airways disease [18].

In spite of the usefulness of such testing, it is fraught with certain limitations. Pulmonary function tests will not make a specific diagnosis. The purpose is to characterize certain patterns of abnormality and determine their severity. This is largely why the term COPD has become so commonplace rather than referring specifically to chronic bronchitis or emphysema. Typical patterns might suggest a specific disease but are not pathognomonic and interpretation is by no means standardized. Significant disease may be present, yet not be detectable on pulmonary function tests. Comparisons are made to normal, yet there is significant variation from one author's predicted values to another's [19]. In addition, statistical aberrations also occur, making precise cutoff points or thresholds impossible. For example, a patient may have a normal forced vital capacity (FVC) at 110% of normal, and a normal forced expiratory volume in 1 second (FEV_1) of 90% of predicted, yet obstruction exists.

Principles of Testing

Normal and abnormal lung mechanics have been discussed in the previous chapter. Disease states may alter airway resistance or elastic properties of the lung. Chest cage alterations also have superimposed effects. Complex alterations in mechanics result in abnormal spirometry, yet this simple test performed during forced expiration will only show certain patterns of abnormality. The pathophysiology of chronic bronchitis and emphysema are quite different and asthma is another disease all together, yet they all have similar appearances on spirometry. A pneumonectomy may be indistinguishable from a pleural effusion or a pneumonia. A knowledge of lung mechanics and an overview of some of the other tests performed in the pulmonary function laboratory will help in the understanding of spirometry.

Lung volume as shown in Fig. 2-1 can be measured by various techniques. Static lung volume measurements are generally performed in a hospital pulmonary function laboratory. Functional residual capacity is measured, and that value, plus the spirometric tracing shown in Fig. 2-1, allows determination of residual volume (RV), total lung capacity (TLC), and the other lung subdivisions. The spirometric tracing alone can be measured with a simple spirometer, a device that measures exhaled volume and plots it against time. Of the volumes measured on the tracing—vital capacity (VC), tidal volume, inspiratory capacity, and expiratory reserve volume—the most useful is the VC.

This volume (VC), when measured as a forced expiratory maneuver, from TLC to

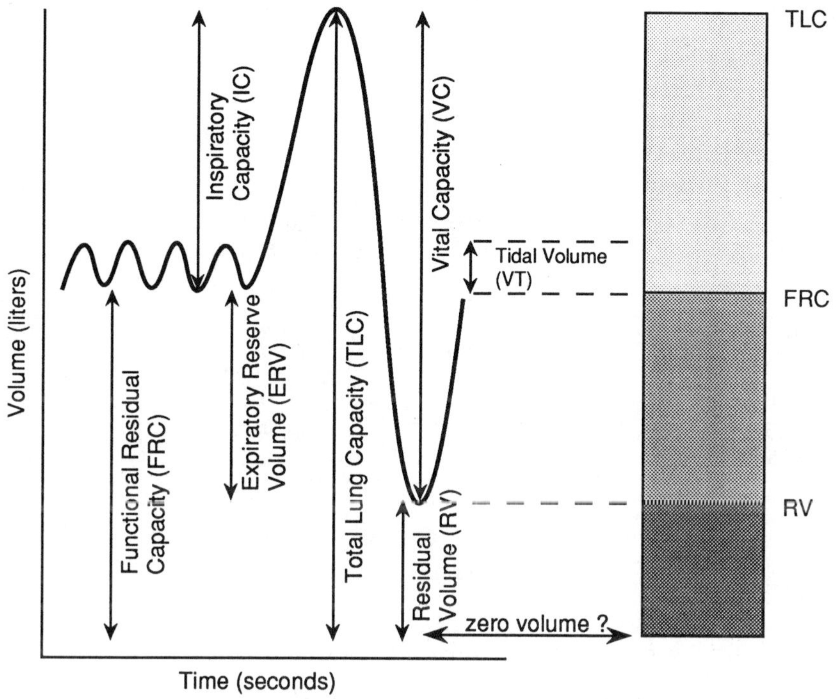
Volume (liters)
Time (seconds)
Inspiratory Capacity (IC)
Vital Capacity (VC)
Tidal Volume (VT)
Functional Residual Capacity (FRC)
Expiratory Reserve Volume (ERV)
Total Lung Capacity (TLC)
Residual Volume (RV)
zero volume ?
TLC
FRC
RV

Fig. 2-1. Lung subdivisions. The tracing shown here illustrates the graph that can be generated with a spirogram. VC, IC, and ERV can be measured, but TLC, FRC, and RV are measured from an unknown zero point. The VC performed as a forced maneuver is the basis for spirometry, the FVC tracing. Measurement of all lung subdivisions requires identification of the zero point, or more extensive static lung volume testing shown in the bar graph.

RV, forms the basis of clinical spirometry, the FVC. The tracing that is derived is often inverted relative to Fig. 2-1 simply by convention so that it looks like Fig. 2-2. Certain brands of spirometers may display the same information with a different orientation. In addition to the standard volume/time tracing, the same test can be displayed as a flow/volume curve. The flow/volume curve is displayed during forced inspiration as well as forced expiration to produce the flow/volume loop (Fig. 2-3). The time/volume tracing is only shown during forced expiration.

Measurements reported with spirometry are generally taken directly from the volume/time tracing. But, remember, the expiratory limb of each curve is just a mathematic derivation of the other. The information can be collected with a volume displacement device or a flow-sensing device and then the other curve derived from the first.

Definitions of Spirometry Testing

Very specific criteria have been set by the American Thoracic Society for acceptable accuracy of instrumentation [20]. Precise criteria have been made for each specific parameter such as FVC, FEV_1, $FEF_{25\text{-}75}$, flow, forced expiratory time, maximum voluntary ventilation (MVV), etc. In general, no more than a 3% margin of error is acceptable when comparing machine measurements to a 3-L calibration syringe. In selecting a spirometer you should insist on equipment that meets American Thoracic Society standards. Specific recommendations have been made for standardization of testing [20, 21].

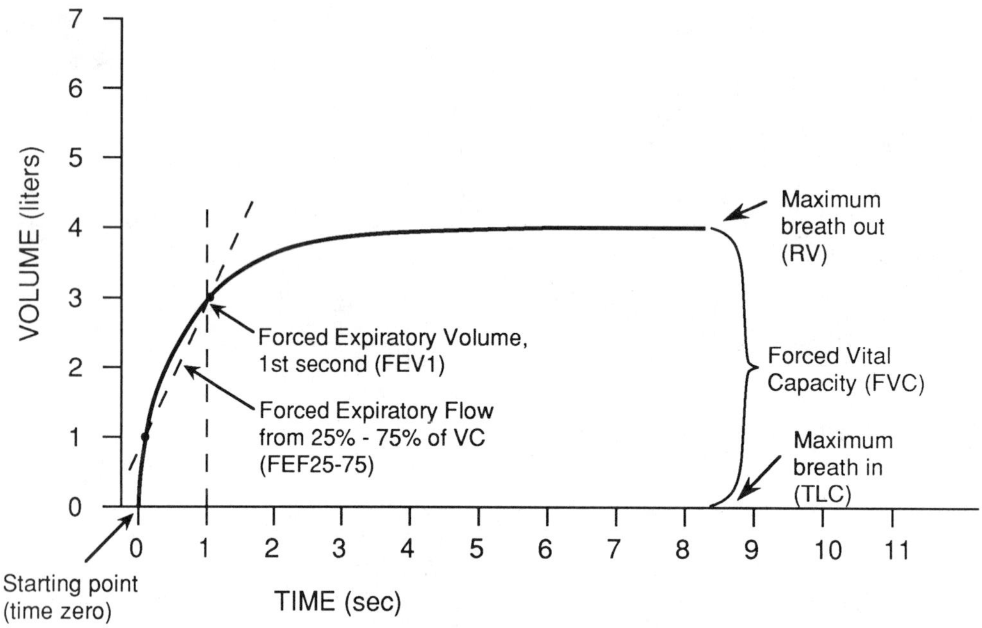
VOLUME (liters)
7
6
5
4
3
2
1
0
Maximum
breath out
(RV)
Forced Expiratory Volume,
1st second (FEV1)
Forced Expiratory Flow
from 25% - 75% of VC
(FEF25-75)
Forced Vital
Capacity (FVC)
Maximum
breath in
(TLC)
0 1 2 3 4 5 6 7 8 9 10 11
Starting point
(time zero)
TIME (sec)

Fig. 2-2. Spirogram. The FVC maneuver is performed by maximum expiratory effort from TLC to RV. Volume is plotted against time. FEV_1 is the volume exhaled during the first second of the test. $FEF_{25\text{-}75}$ is the average flow over the middle half of the test, from 25% to 75% of the FVC. Flow (V/T) can also be derived from the slope of the curve at any point.

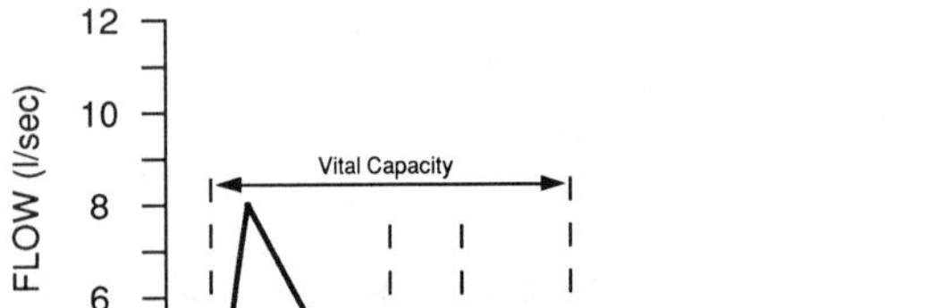
FLOW (l/sec)
12
10
8
6
4
2
0
-2
-4
-6
Expiration
Inspiration
Vital Capacity
Inspiratory
Capacity
Expiratory
Reserve
Volume
first second mark
Tidal
Volume
0 1 2 3 4 5 6 7
VOLUME (liters)
TLC
RV

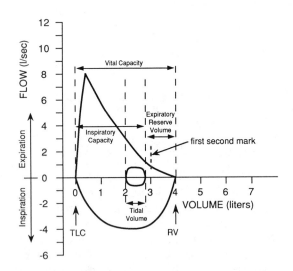

Fig. 2-3. The flow/volume loop is generated from the same patient effort that creates the time/volume tracing. Expiration is shown on the upper half of the loop. The lower half is inspiratory flow, not shown on the V/T tracing. The small inner circle represents flow and volume during quiet tidal breathing. The FVC maneuver is shown as the larger outer loop. Lung subdivisions are also shown for comparison to Fig. 2-1.

Time/Volume Tracing

The volume of a forced expiration, from maximum breath in, to maximum breath out (TLC to RV), is plotted against time as shown in Fig. 2-2. Volume (FVC) and flow (FEV_1, $FEF_{25\text{-}75}$, and others) are measured from the tracing. The FVC is often different than the slow vital capacity (SVC), especially in obstructive lung disease where the FVC is significantly less than the SVC. This occurs because positive intrathoracic pressure during forced expiration causes airways to collapse.

Flow/Volume Loop

In addition to plotting volume against time in the standard spirogram, the same patient effort is plotted flow against volume during both expiration and inspiration as shown in Fig. 2-3. These loops are most useful for typical pattern recognition. The inspiratory portion of the test is not generally shown on the time/volume tracing. Both inspiration and expiration are shown with flow in opposite directions on the flow/volume loop.

Slow Vital Capacity

As in the FVC maneuver the patient exhales from TLC to RV, but this is not a forced maneuver. The patient still needs coaxing to empty as much as possible. This measurement is often made in the pulmonary function test laboratory during measurement of static lung volumes as shown in Fig. 2-1, but may be measured with a simple spirogram.

Peak Flow

Peak or maximum expiratory flow rate may be measured by a specific device called a peak flow meter. This spring-loaded instrument shown in Fig. 2-4 is simple and can approximate the maximal expiratory flow as measured on the flow/volume loop. Its most com-

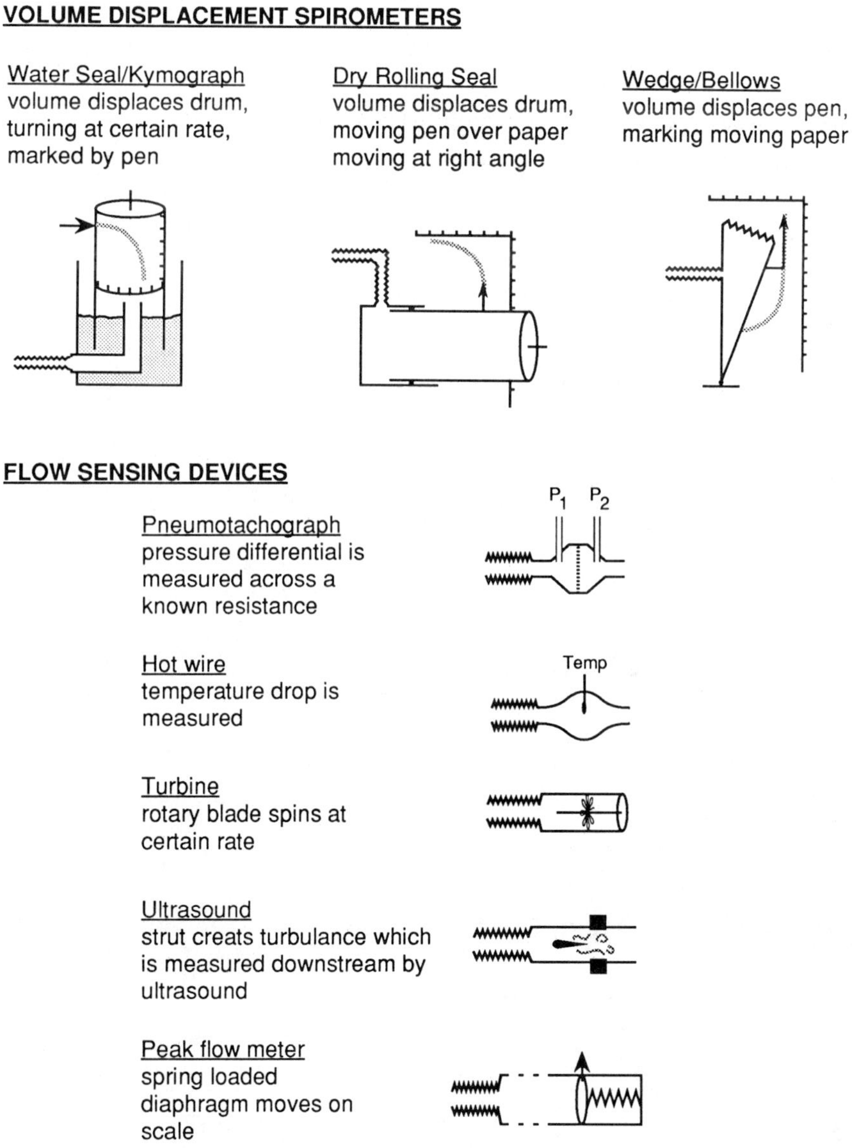
VOLUME DISPLACEMENT SPIROMETERS
Water Seal/Kymograph
volume displaces drum, turning at certain rate, marked by pen
Dry Rolling Seal
volume displaces drum, moving pen over paper moving at right angle
Wedge/Bellows
volume displaces pen, marking moving paper
FLOW SENSING DEVICES
Pneumotachograph
pressure differential is measured across a known resistance
P_1 P_2
Hot wire
temperature drop is measured
Temp
Turbine
rotary blade spins at certain rate
Ultrasound
strut creats turbulance which is measured downstream by ultrasound
Peak flow meter
spring loaded diaphragm moves on scale

Fig. 2-4. Spirometers.

mon use is at the bedside and at home for estimation and monitoring severity of disease and response to therapy.

Maximum Voluntary Ventilation

MVV (Fig. 2-5) or maximum breathing capacity is usually included with spirometry. The patient breathes the largest volume at the fastest rate for 12 seconds. The volume measured is multiplied by 5 to get liters per minute. MVV will be reduced in both obstructive and restrictive disease. An MVV is sometimes reported by multiplying $FEV_1 \times 35$ or 40, but this may not equal the measured MVV. Myasthenia gravis, for example, may show a good FEV_1, but MVV will be reduced because the patient tires as the test is carried out. This parameter is particularly useful in preoperative evaluation of pulmonary patients [14].

Prebronchodilator and Postbronchodilator Testing

Spirometry is performed as a baseline, then an aerosol bronchodilator is administered and spirometry is repeated. If the FEV_1 or the FVC improves by 15% or more, the patient is said to be acutely responsive to bronchodilators.

Bronchoprovocation

Spirometry is performed as a baseline, then an aerosol bronchoconstrictor, such as methacholine, is administered and spirometry is repeated. If the FEV_1 drops by 20%, the patient is said to have hyperreactive airways.

Performing Spirometry

Specific protocols have been defined and outlined for testing in a pulmonary function laboratory [20]. Patients should be instructed ahead of time to wear comfortable loose clothing and refrain from using alcohol, tobacco, or drugs that may affect testing. The test is performed with the patient in the sitting position.

Fig. 2-5. MVV or maximum breathing capacity is usually included with spirometry. The patient breathes the largest volume at the fastest rate for 12 seconds. The volume measured is multiplied by 5 to get liters per minute.

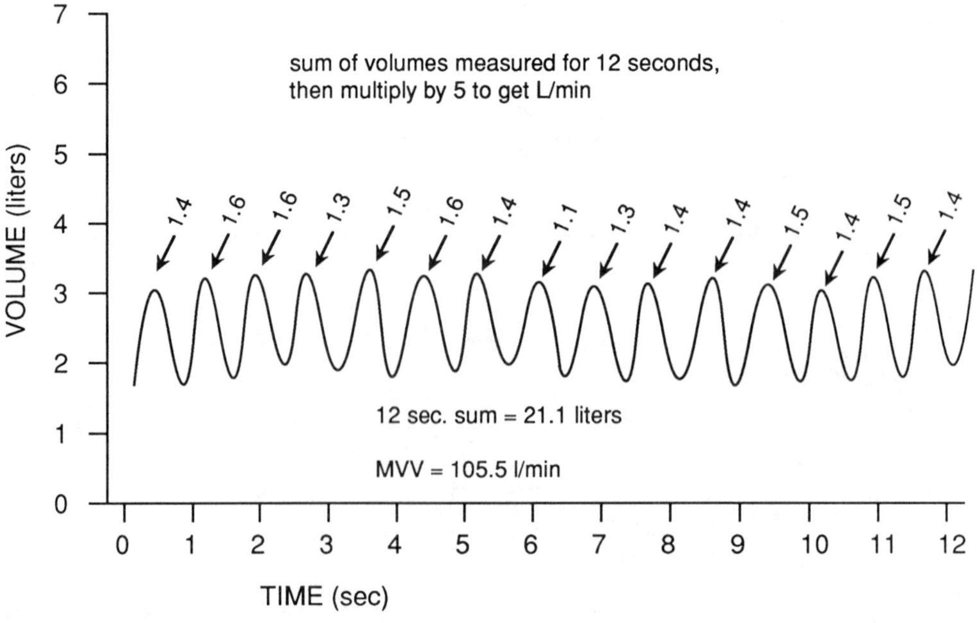
sum of volumes measured for 12 seconds,
then multiply by 5 to get L/min
1.4
1.6
1.6
1.3
1.5
1.6
1.4
1.1
1.3
1.4
1.4
1.5
1.4
1.5
1.4
12 sec. sum = 21.1 liters
MVV = 105.5 l/min
VOLUME (liters)
0
1
2
3
4
5
6
7
TIME (sec)
0
1
2
3
4
5
6
7
8
9
10
11
12

What Makes a Good Test?

A good test is not easy to obtain. It requires great effort on the part of the patient, enthusiastic coaching on the part of the technician, reliable accurate equipment, and an interpreter who can recognize a good from a bad test. Anybody can have the patient blow into the spirometer and generate numbers and a report. However, the old computer maxim applies: GIGO (garbage in, garbage out). Examples of poor quality tests are shown in Fig. 2-6.

Need for Graphics

Once again the machine will spit out a test on almost anybody. The technician performing the test and the interpreter must be able to see the time/volume tracing and/or the flow/volume curve in order to evaluate the quality of the test. Specific requirements have also been outlined for scale of time, volume, and flow graphs. The importance of graphics cannot be overstressed. In selecting a spirometer you should insist on equipment that meets American Thoracic Society standards for graphic display. A device that simply prints out numbers but no graphics is not acceptable. The graphics must be analyzed to determine whether or not the test was good and to evaluate whether or not efforts are reproducible.

Beginning the Test

The patient is instructed to take a maximum breath in (to TLC), then on command exhale as forcefully as possible until no more can be exhaled (to RV). The beginning of the test is seen on time/volume tracing as a sharp increase from the baseline. If there is a slow initial increase followed by the sharp increase, the test may still be useful if the sharp slope can be used to back extrapolate to baseline, identifying the zero point or starting time as shown in Fig. 2-7. The expiratory limb of the flow/volume loop should show a sharp increase and peak flow at high lung volume, and then a progressive decrease in flow as the tracing falls to zero flow.

End of the Test

The patient must continue the expiratory effort until flow ceases. The test must go for at least 6 seconds, and flow must diminish to a slope less than 50 cc over the last 2 seconds. Some patients will exhale for a long period, 15 seconds or more, and still not level out in the case of obstructive lung disease. In this case the patient has given a valiant effort, but by formal criteria this is labeled poor terminal effort. This distinction is meant to say that the FVC may not represent the true VC (see discussion of SVC).

Number of Trials

The test should be repeated at least three times and give two similar, reproducible tracings on both the flow/volume and the time/volume tracings. Inconsistent efforts yield unreliable results and may indicate an uncooperative, fatigued, or malingering patient.

Setting up a Laboratory

Several factors need to be considered when making a decision about setting up a laboratory. Computer technology is rapidly changing and by the time this chapter is written it will be obsolete. Therefore, rather than making specific recommendations about what brand of equipment you should buy, we stress certain basic principles that you should consider when purchasing equipment. Recent literature attempting specific recommendations has been published [2, 22, 23]. Even though such sources are rapidly outdated, they serve as a reference to which more recent claims may be compared. Individual manufacturers are more than willing to bring their product to you for evaluation. Several brands of equipment can be seen in one place during large medical conferences as well as state and national respiratory therapy meetings.

Equipment

Several types and several brands of spirometers are available and sorting through the differences can be confusing. They can be

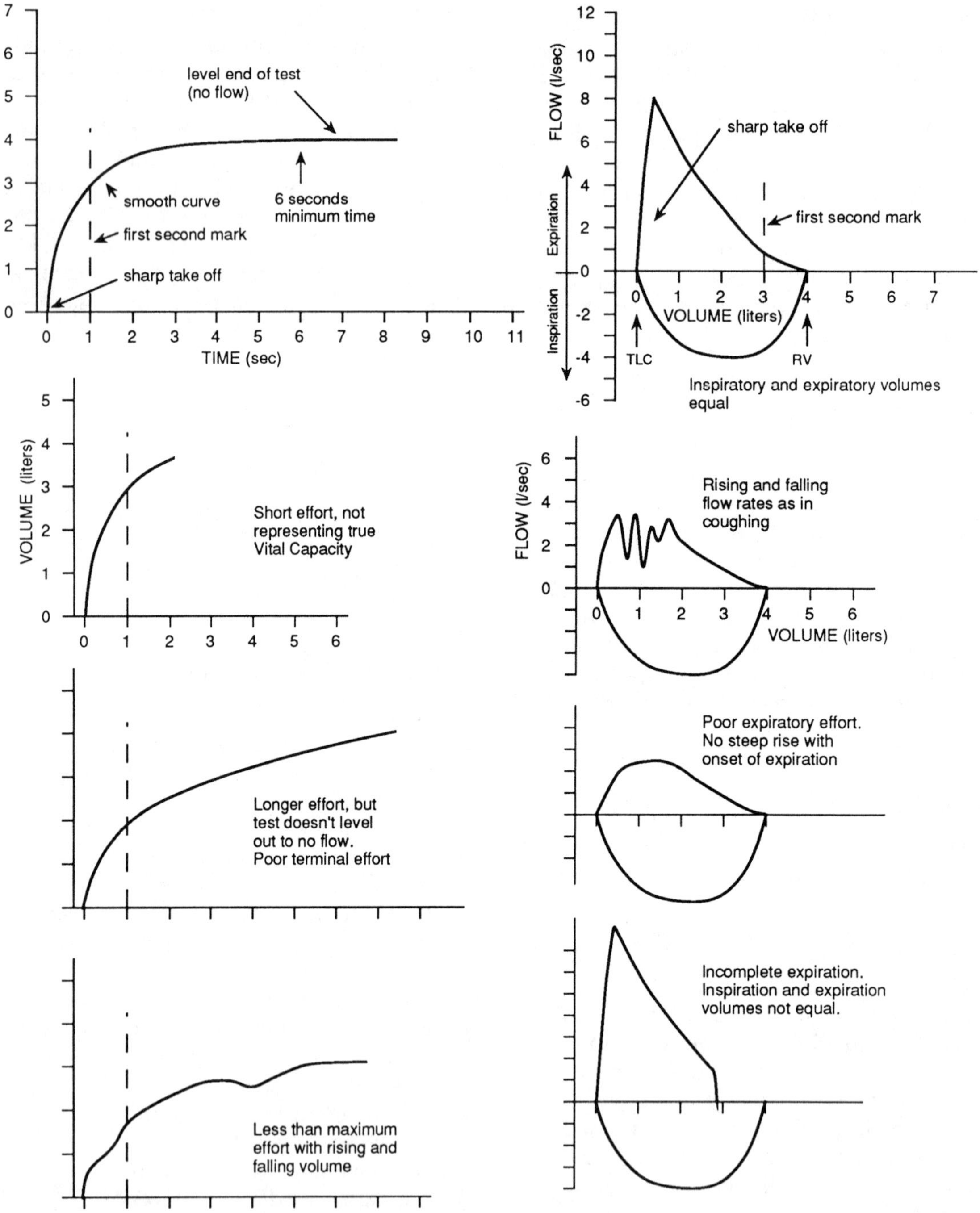
level end of test
(no flow)
smooth curve
6 seconds
minimum time
first second mark
sharp take off
TIME (sec)
VOLUME (liters)
Short effort, not
representing true
Vital Capacity
Longer effort, but
test doesn't level
out to no flow.
Poor terminal effort
Less than maximum
effort with rising and
falling volume
FLOW (l/sec)
Expiration
Inspiration
sharp take off
first second mark
VOLUME (liters)
TLC
RV
Inspiratory and expiratory volumes
equal
FLOW (l/sec)
Rising and falling
flow rates as in
coughing
VOLUME (liters)
Poor expiratory effort.
No steep rise with
onset of expiration
Incomplete expiration.
Inspiration and expiration
volumes not equal.

Fig. 2-6. Good and bad tests. An acceptable test requires vigorous coaching by the tester in order for the patient to generate a curve with a good start and good end. Features of acceptable time/volume and flow/volume graphics are shown on the top tracings. Examples of poor effort are shown below.

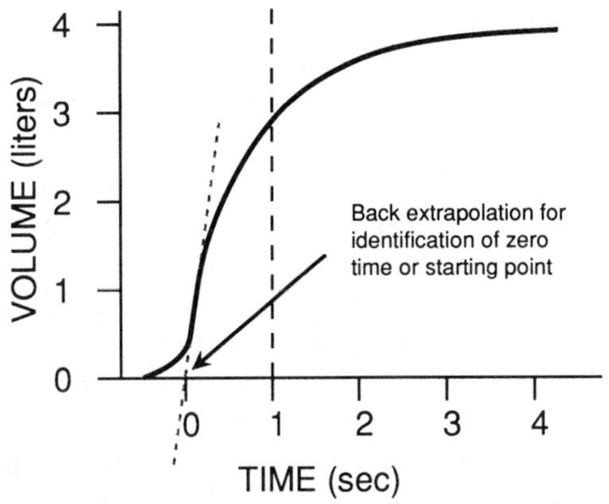
4
3
2
1
0
VOLUME (liters)
Back extrapolation for identification of zero time or starting point
0 1 2 3 4
TIME (sec)

Fig. 2-7. The start of the test should have a sharp take off from the baseline. If there is a gradual start (<10% of the FVC) followed by a steep flow, the starting time can be identified by back-extrapolation.

placed generally in two categories: volume displacement devices and flow-sensing devices. The first spirometers to be used were volume displacement devices such as the water seal spirometer. As the patient exhales into this water seal chamber a certain volume is displaced. The drum turns at a specific speed, generating a graph with volume on the Y-axis and time on the X-axis. From this graph, volume (FVC) and all of the various flow rates may be directly measured. Over time, several modifications have been made and several different volume displacement spirometers have become available. There are also several types of flow-sensing devices. Examples of various spirometers are shown in Fig. 2-4. The development of flow-sensing devices such as the pneumotachograph led to the generation of the flow/volume loop, which has become a standard part of spirometry graphics. Either graph can be generated from the other. Whether volume or flow is the initial parameter being measured, most instruments available today are computerized and easily derive the graph that is not being directly measured. A recent study reviewed 62 different spirometers. In this evaluation 95% of the instruments were computerized [22]. The readout device may be a direct hard copy tracing obtained from the kymograph of the water seal spirometer or the monitor display and computer printout of a computerized system.

Personnel

The American Thoracic Society has also made very specific recommendations regarding personnel qualifications [24]. Their strict criteria for strong mathematics training, more than 1 year of college, and 6 months training in a supervised pulmonary function laboratory seems prohibitive. These strict requirements need not necessarily be applied to simple office spirometry; however, adequate testing depends largely on the individual performing the test. It is important that the person doing the testing spend the time to learn the principles of testing, understand what makes a good test, and be capable of instructing and coaching a patient through difficult maneuvers. Several excellent training manuals have been prepared [20].

Computers

Even if the measuring device being used has been shown to be accurate and acceptable by American Thoracic Society standards, the computer and software used to integrate that measurement add an additional source of error. The computerization of this equipment has made testing much simpler and less time consuming than it had been in the past, but this technologic advance has significant limitations. Specific computer guidelines have been defined [25]. In an older study evaluating several commercially available spirometers [23], more than 60% of the instruments tested had acceptable accuracy. One would think that as technology advances, our instrumentation would become more accurate. However, in a more recent study by Nelson, only 56% of instruments tested were found to be acceptable [22]. A significant component of the unacceptable characteristics in this study was related to computer software problems. This is not to say that the computerized spirometers are not useful. In fact, most devices available today are computerized and such an automated system is recommended. One must be careful, however, in selecting a specific piece of equipment. A basic scheme of microprocessor logic has been described where selections are shown for calibration, FVC, MVV, etc. [15]. Each manufacturer has their own proprietary software and there is no standardization. A practical factor to consider is whether computers are used elsewhere in your office. If so, it may be possible to tie in with the spirometer. Several manufacturers have employed universally accepted computers in their pulmonary function test package.

Some manufacturers also provide interpretation software. A simplified scheme of such logic is shown in Fig. 2-8. A word of caution, even the best frequently give erroneous interpretations. Even when they allow you to customize the summary to your preferences, the proprietary nature of such software may prohibit you from really knowing the interpretation logic. Each test must be reviewed for errors and corrected. This takes away the time that should be saved by such programs. You will stay in practice and do a better job if you simply interpret the tests yourself.

Quality Control

Accuracy of instruments cannot be taken for granted. The review by Nelson et al. [22] found that only 35 of 62 spirometers evaluated (56.5%) performed acceptably. In this study, computer software errors accounted for 25% of the errors identified [22]. The internal "black box" nature of computerized systems often confounds attempts at true quality assurance.

Quality control protocols should be followed for ensuring accuracy and reproducibility of the equipment. A 3-L calibration syringe is often used for this purpose. However, a simple maneuver performed with a calibration syringe may not identify deficiencies in equipment or software accuracy [22]. Periodic checks should also be made against a biological standard. This may be done by having one or more of the individuals in the office tested, using their results as a standard value.

Maintenance includes troubleshooting as problems arise as well as preventive or scheduled checks. Calibration is the process of comparing a known standard measurement with that being measured by the instrument tested. Such calibration checks evaluate accuracy or closeness of measurements as well as precision or reproducibility. Proficiency testing evaluates the overall accuracy of testing in unknown samples and includes evaluation of both equipment and personnel. Strict criteria for maintenance of quality assurance have been described elsewhere [20, 25]. When a calibration syringe is used, measurements are made at saturated ambient temperature and pressure. Appropriate conversions should be made since patients are tested at saturated body temperature and ambient pressure. Such correction factors are generally incorporated in the computer software and should be defined by each specific manufacturer.

Infection control precautions need to be taken. Diseases such as tuberculosis, hepatitis, and possibly others may be transmitted through equipment, and appropriate precautions need to be taken. This includes cleaning of parts outlined by the manufacturer as well as use of disposable mouthpieces and tubing when appropriate.

If contraindications to testing exist, those should be identified. The most common contraindication to testing is an uncooperative patient or a patient who cannot understand the instructions for testing. Recent acute myocardial infarction or chest or abdominal surgery may be relative contraindications. If medications are to be used, such as bronchodilators or bronchoconstrictors, facilities should be available for treating the complications of administration of such substances.

Predicted Normal Values

A particular value that is measured on a spirogram is not very meaningful until it is compared with normal values. The measured value is then divided by the predicted value to get the percent predicted. Such normal or predicted values may be obtained from sev-

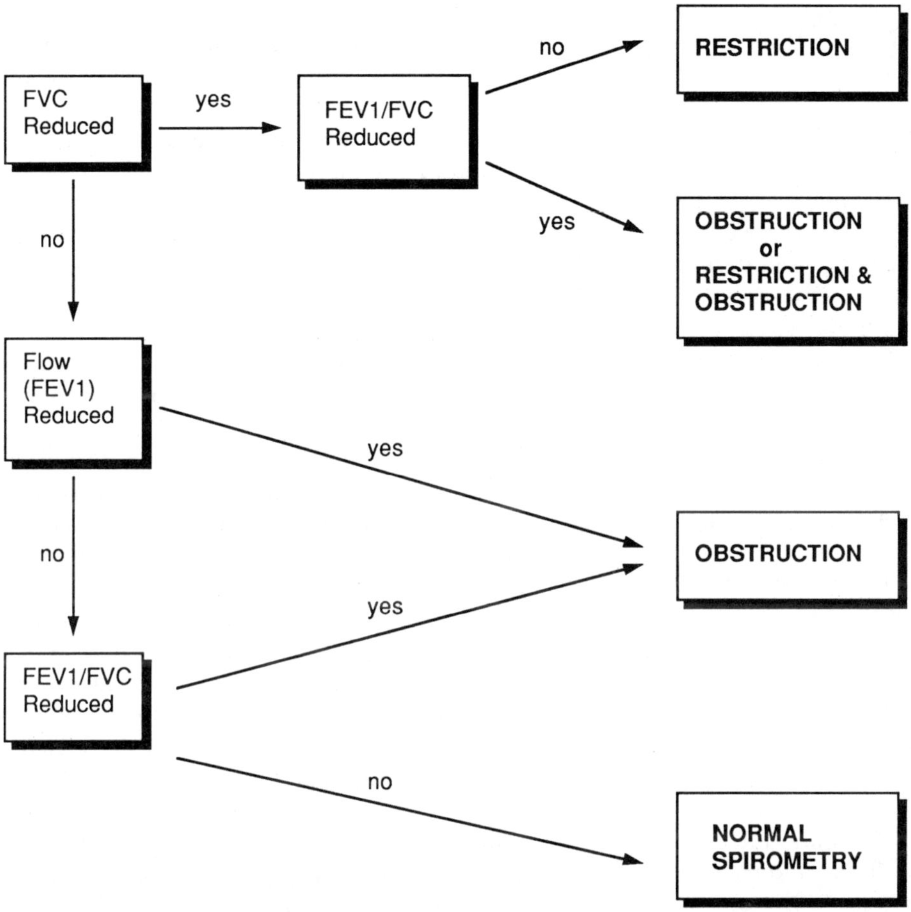
FVC
Reduced
yes
FEV1/FVC
Reduced
no
RESTRICTION
yes
OBSTRUCTION
or
RESTRICTION &
OBSTRUCTION
no
Flow
(FEV1)
Reduced
yes
OBSTRUCTION
no
yes
FEV1/FVC
Reduced
no
NORMAL
SPIROMETRY

Fig. 2-8. This is a simplified example of computer logic that may be used for interpretation of spirometry. Specific normal values must be selected, qualifying statements may be added, and the operator or the program must be able to distinguish a good test from a bad test.

eral different sources [26–29]. Many large studies have been performed on nondiseased individuals who are matched for sex, age, and size (generally height). Arm span can also be used for acquired causes of decreased height [30]. Even though pulmonary function testing has been refined over several years, there is no set standard or universally accepted set of normal values [19, 31]. A handful of authors account for most of the values used in most laboratories, but even among these there is significant variation from one predicted value to another. Several variables account for this discrepancy including race [32–34], weight [35], altitude [26], smokers versus nonsmokers [34], air pollution, and urban versus rural dwellers [36, 37].

When a large population is studied for any given value, the distribution of measurements will fall over a range, and the shape of that distribution is usually a bell-shaped curve. The extreme ends of that curve are still normal individuals, but deviate significantly from the mean or average individual. Generally, a threshold, somewhat arbitrary, is drawn, and individuals who fall below that level are labeled abnormal. Different methods are available for determining that threshold. One of the most widely accepted and commonly used is described in standard pulmonary text books and assumes that normal is between 80% and 120% of the mean predicted value [1, 38]. This method also describes adjectives of severity for abnormal values as shown in Table 2-3. The statistical validity of this method has been questioned. Certain parameters may fall in a rather tight distribution while others are widely distributed. Other methods have been recommended that consider the standard error or the 95% confidence interval [26]. The lower limit of normal is sometimes reported along with or instead of the percent predicted. Extremes of population being tested also broaden the curve, making normal more difficult to evaluate. Examples include very tall or very short individuals and the very young or very old. This is particularly true of pediatric values. A tighter range of predicted normal can be used for the FEV_1/FVC (the $FEV_1\%$) because this is essentially comparing the patient with him- or herself rather than a large population of normal individuals. Even so, it is not valid to say that anyone below 75% is obstructed and anyone over 75% is not obstructed. This ratio changes with age in normal individuals [39].

These statistical and individual limitations of using predicted normal values should be understood, but this is still a useful way to evaluate the measurements taken from a pulmonary function test. Very tight, dogmatic interpretation, however, may be unreasonable. Borderline studies may be interpreted as normal or abnormal, but those evaluations need critical thinking. The final interpretation in such a test should include clinical correlation. For example, a borderline test could be considered abnormal in a patient with the symptom of cough. On the other hand, if the test was done as a screen in an asymptomatic individual, the test could be considered normal. As in so many areas of medicine, it is often more reasonable to follow trends than absolute values when evaluating laboratory results. This emphasizes the importance of serial testing and the value of having a baseline study available.

When you select a given set of predicted values to use in your office there are several factors that need to be taken into account. What are the predicted values used in your hospital or referral laboratory? What is the racial and ethnic makeup of the area where you practice? Are there geographic and environmental factors to consider? What choices are you given by your equipment manufacturer (programmed predicted values in the case of a computerized system)?

Once you choose a set of predicted normal values, you must also select a method of defining abnormal and adjectives of severity. Whatever set of predicted values and method of determining normal you use depend on your evaluation of the advantages and disadvantages of each. The first method described previously offers ease and widespread use. The latter methods are based on sounder scientific rationale. Whatever the method, the raw data do not change. Whenever comparisons are made between tests, the measured values should be used.

Table 2-3. Interpretation of adjectives used to describe degree of pulmonary abnormality

Term	%
Normal*	≥80% of predicted
Mild impairment	65%–79% of predicted
Moderate impairment	50%–64% of predicted
Severe impairment	<50% of predicted

*See text for discussion of percent of predicted, 95% confidence interval, standard error, and lower limit of normal.

Interpretation

Pathophysiology: Diseases that alter pulmonary function tests can be divided into obstructive and restrictive disorders. Obstructive diseases include asthma and COPD (chronic bronchitis and emphysema). Restrictive diseases include all of the interstitial lung diseases, chest wall and pleural derangements, and neuromuscular disease.

Airway obstruction or flow limitation occurs because the lumen of the bronchus is diminished and airway resistance is increased. This may be because of bronchospasm in the case of asthma, secretions and mucosal edema in asthma or bronchitis, or dynamic collapse of airways because of loss of supporting elastic structure in emphysema.

Flow/volume loops are especially useful for evaluation of various forms of obstruction by pattern recognition [40, 41]. Extrathoracic obstruction has a more profound flow limitation during inspiration. Intrathoracic obstruction (including lung disease) has a more profound flow limitation during expiration. Flattening of either portion of the flow/volume loop has characteristic patterns shown in Fig. 2-9. Upper airway obstruction can also be distinguished from lower airway disease [42].

Restrictive defects result in diminished lung volumes. This is most evident when static volumes are measured. Parenchymal lung disease, such as idiopathic pulmonary

Fig. 2-9. Flow/volume loops are useful for typical pattern recognition. See text for discussion.

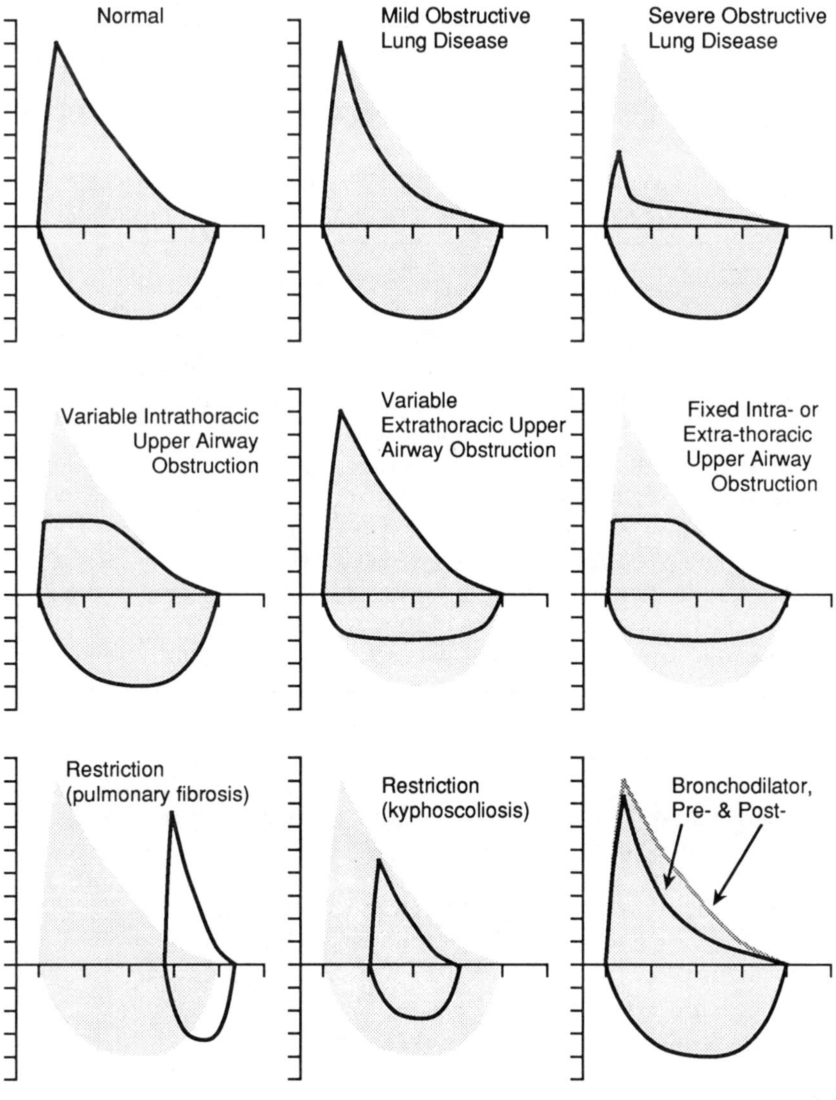
Normal
Mild Obstructive Lung Disease
Severe Obstructive Lung Disease
Variable Intrathoracic Upper Airway Obstruction
Variable Extrathoracic Upper Airway Obstruction
Fixed Intra- or Extra-thoracic Upper Airway Obstruction
Restriction (pulmonary fibrosis)
Restriction (kyphoscoliosis)
Bronchodilator, Pre- & Post-

fibrosis, increases the elastic recoil and reduces the compliance of the lung so that TLC and all of its subdivisions are reduced. In the other causes of restriction listed previously, the mechanical properties of the lung are normal, but the surrounding chest cage causes TLC to be reduced. TLC cannot be measured on a spirogram, but the volume FVC can.

Basic abnormalities on spirometry are divided into obstructive, restrictive, and combination patterns seen in Fig. 2-10. The key feature of obstructive disease is reduced *flow rates.* The key feature of restrictive disease is reduced *volume.* Even though this sounds simple, there is not a uniformly accepted method of interpretation [43–45].

Patient results are compared with predicted normal values taken from a nomogram as described in the previous section. In addition to comparing the patient with a large population of normal people to get percent predicted, we also look at the FEV_1/FVC, which essentially compares the patient with him- or herself. Adjectives defining the degree of abnormality are also commonly used, i.e., mild, moderate, and severe [1, 38].

The FVC and flow rates are measured from a forced expiratory effort. The only volume measured on spirometry is the FVC. This is not the same as the VC (or SVC). All of the other measurements made from a spirometric tracing are flow rates such as the FEV_1, FEV_1/FVC (the FEV_1%), FEV_3, FEV_3/FVC (the FEV_3%), $FEF_{25\text{-}75}$, maximal expiratory flow rate (or peak flow), $FEF_{800\text{-}1200}$, etc. Of these flow rates, the most useful, reliable, and widely accepted measurements are the FEV_1 and the FEV_1% [26, 46–48].

When examining a spirogram, the first step is to determine whether or not it is a good test. The graphics must be analyzed. Was there a sharp takeoff on the time/volume tracing? Can you identify zero time or the starting point? Is there a smooth change in the slope of that curve? Did the patient reach the end of the test (did the effort last for at least 6 seconds and did the tracing level out to the point at which there was no flow)? The next step is also made from the graphics (see Performing Spirometry). In addition to deciding if this was a good test, you can also use the curves for pattern recognition. This is especially true of the flow/volume loop as seen in Fig. 2-9. Characteristic shapes are seen with obstructive lung disease, upper airway obstruction, and restrictive diseases.

The next step is to analyze the numbers derived from the curves, i.e., the specific volume and flow rates, and compare them with the predicted normal values expressed as a percent of predicted. If you see reduced volume and normal flow, this is an obvious restrictive defect. By the same token, if you see normal volume and reduced flow, it is easy to identify that as an obstructive defect. The difficulty comes when the much more common scenario is seen, reduced volume and reduced flow. It is very common for obstructive lung disease to reduce the FVC. Other lung volumes such as RV and FRC are increased in obstructive airway disease, but these cannot be measured on spirography. As airways close early in obstructive airway disease and during forced expiration, the FVC will be decreased. So, the combination of reduced volume and reduced flow is often seen in obstructive airway disease. In the case of restrictive defects, the volume is always reduced, but flow will most often be reduced as well. For example, if there is a pure restrictive disease such as myasthenia gravis reducing the FVC from 4 to 2 L, can the FEV_1 be the normal 3 L? Of course not. So in this case of restriction, flow rates are reduced in proportion to volume.

How then can we distinguish obstruction from restriction when flow and volume are reduced? This is where the FEV_1/FVC (FEV_1%) is so important [49]. In the case of a restrictive defect with a reduced FVC and FEV_1, the FEV_1% will be normal or greater than predicted [39]. That is, flow is reduced, but only in proportion to the reduced volume. In the case of obstruction, flow is reduced to a greater degree than volume, so the FEV_1% is less than predicted. This rationale is summarized in Fig. 2-11 [26].

Several comments are in order here. Poor terminal effort will underestimate the sever-

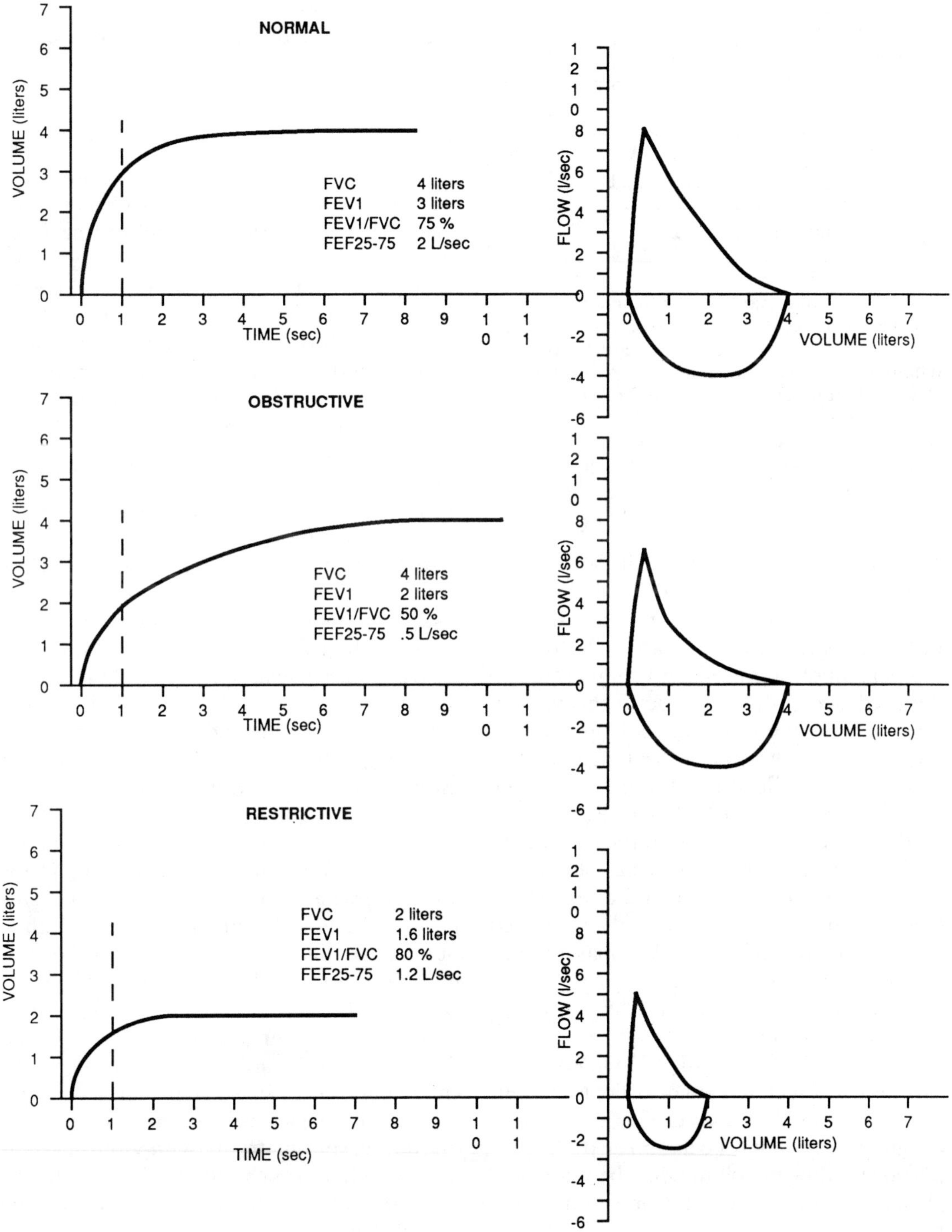
NORMAL
VOLUME (liters)
TIME (sec)
FVC 4 liters
FEV1 3 liters
FEV1/FVC 75 %
FEF25-75 2 L/sec
FLOW (l/sec)
VOLUME (liters)
OBSTRUCTIVE
VOLUME (liters)
TIME (sec)
FVC 4 liters
FEV1 2 liters
FEV1/FVC 50 %
FEF25-75 .5 L/sec
FLOW (l/sec)
VOLUME (liters)
RESTRICTIVE
VOLUME (liters)
TIME (sec)
FVC 2 liters
FEV1 1.6 liters
FEV1/FVC 80 %
FEF25-75 1.2 L/sec
FLOW (l/sec)
VOLUME (liters)

Fig. 2-10. Normal, obstructed, and restricted spirograms and flow/volume loops.

		OBSTRUCTION	RESTRICTION	COMBINED
Spirometry	FVC	NORMAL or ↓	↓	↓
	FEV_1	↓	NORMAL or ↓	↓
	$\frac{FEV_1}{FVC}$	↓	NORMAL or ↑	↓
Lung Volumes	TLC	NORMAL or ↑	↓	↓

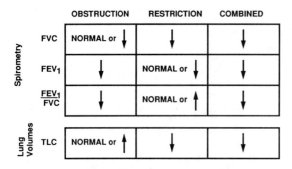

Fig. 2-11. Pulmonary function interpretation. The key feature of obstruction is reduced flow. The key feature in restriction is reduced volume. When volume and flow are reduced the ratio of FEV_1/FVC separates obstruction from restriction. In the case of combined obstruction and restriction it may not be possible to distinguish on spirometry alone. TLC may have to be measured.

ity of obstruction (the FEV_1 will be an accurate measurement, but the FVC will be artificially reduced, increasing the ratio). The $FEV_1\%$ is expressed as a measured value, not as a percent of predicted, and compared with the predicted (to put a value in the percent predicted column would be looking at a percent of a percent which is meaningless). The $FEV_1\%$ is either less than the predicted (obstruction), or it is greater than or equal to the predicted (no obstruction). In the case where obstruction and restriction coexist, it may not be possible to be certain about the restriction. Obstruction is evident by the reduced $FEV_1\%$, but the reduced FVC may or may not represent restriction. In this case it may be necessary to measure static lung volumes and look at the TLC.

In pulmonary fibrosis the term *super-normal flow rates* is sometimes used to depict the effect of increased elastic recoil. Even though the absolute flow may be diminished, the proportionate flow to volume may be increased, giving the appearance of elongation of the flow/volume loop as shown in Fig. 2-9.

Other clues to obstruction are response to bronchodilators (acute or chronic), concavity of the expiratory limb of the flow/volume loop, and significant reduction in the FVC compared with the SVC.

Special Tests

Prebronchodilator and Postbronchodilator Testing

Bronchodilator drugs are useful in treating patients with obstructive airway disease. Predicting how useful might be done with prebronchodilator and postbronchodilator testing. Acute responsiveness to bronchodilators is also useful in distinguishing asthma from other forms of airway obstruction [50]. An important point to be made here relates to those patients who do not respond. All patients with obstruction should be given a trial of bronchodilators whether they show acute reversibility or not. Many patients only respond slowly over a period of days, weeks, or even months [51]. Do not take away the message that "no significant response to bronchodilators" means the patient should not be treated with bronchodilators. Acute response to bronchodilators is an imperfect guide to bronchodilator therapy [52]. This test is generally performed when we want to evaluate the reversible component of airway obstruction. For example, not only is it common to see chronic bronchitis and emphysema in association with one another, but they may also occur in the presence of asthma. A patient with COPD who shows acute improvement with bronchodilator drugs is more likely to respond to treatment and may have a better prognosis. The test is also performed on those individuals suspected of having asthma. Even if the baseline pulmonary function test is normal or borderline, a postbronchodilator study may be done for comparison.

Several different parameters may be followed in the evaluation of response to bronchodilators [53, 54]. We limit the discussion here to those parameters that are available on routine spirometry. Baseline spirometry is performed, a bronchodilator drug is administered, and spirometry is repeated. Any bronchodilator drug can be used, but this test is conventionally performed with sympathomimetic drugs. Aerosolized β-agonist stimulation is given by various methods [55]. These medications are preferred because of their rapid onset of action. Isoproterenol (Isuprel) is the most rapidly acting (peak effect, 5 to 10 minutes), but has β_1 side effects of tachycardia and palpations. β_2-specific drugs such as metaproterenol (Alupent), albuterol (Ventolin and Proventil), isoetharine (Bronchosol), or terbutaline (Brethine) are often used, but have a slower onset of action, necessitating approximately 20 minutes delay before the second spirogram is performed. The medication can be delivered with a metered dose inhaler (with or without a spacer device) or various aerosol devices [56, 57]. A compressor-driven nebulizer is commonly used. In any case, it is critical that the tester ensures adequate aerosol delivery. The dosage of medication used is generally the standard therapeutic dose.

Testing is often performed after bronchodilator drugs have been discontinued for 12 hours or more, but this may not be necessary. If this is a patient with known obstructive disease and we are trying to evaluate the usefulness of additional medications, it may be acceptable to test the patient without stopping any other medications. If, on the other hand, we are trying to evaluate any reversible component, then the test should be performed without other bronchodilator drugs present. The most commonly used and widely accepted parameters to follow with this test are the FVC and the FEV_1 [53, 58]. Other spirometric values such as the $FEF_{25\text{-}75}$, peak flow, and isovolume $FEF_{25\text{-}75}$ have also been used [59, 60].

If the drugs are effective, it is intuitive that flow rates should improve. Improvement in volumes (FVC) is also significant since this may be seen as airways being open. Airway closure does not occur as early, and residual volume decreases. Significant response includes FVC greater than or equal to 15% improvement [26, 61], and FEV_1 greater than or equal to 15% improvement (with at least 200 cc absolute improvement) [62, 63]. Significant controversy exists regarding $FEF_{25\text{-}75}$ and other aspects of this test [64–66].

Bronchoprovocation

Patients with mild asthma typically complain of paroxysms of cough, shortness of breath, and wheezing. Between attacks these patients are normal. When spirometry is performed in such individuals they very often have completely normal studies [67]. The term *occult asthma* has been used for those individuals presenting with cough only. The term *reactive airways dysfunction syndrome* has also been used for patients who have hyperreactive airways believed to be nonimmunologic in nature [68]. In any case, it is not uncommon to see patients with respiratory symptoms suggestive of asthma but no objective evidence can be found on routine testing. These are the patients in whom bronchoprovocation is most useful. Provocative tests have been available for several years and have been employed largely in research settings. They have been used to quantify reversibility in patients with known airway obstruction as well as evaluation of the patients described previously in whom airway obstruction is in question [69].

Various substances have been used as provocative agents. Cold air, exercise, histamine, specific antigens, and methacholine have been employed in bronchial challenge testing [70–72]. The most widely accepted provocative test has been a tedious study done with methacholine [73]. This cholinergic drug is administered in increasing doses until a significant drop in flow rate occurs as determined by serial spirometry. A much simpler screening study has been described and proved to be very useful in the first group of patients described previously [74]. This screening methacholine challenge can be administered in a physician's office if performed carefully [75].

This specific study is not designed for quantification of airway responsiveness in patients with known airway obstruction. It is a screening test to be used in patients with normal or near normal spirometry looking for reactive airways disease or occult asthma.

Bronchodilator drugs, caffeine, and cigarettes are withheld for 1 day before testing. The patient should not have a history of an upper respiratory tract infection within the past 6 weeks since these individuals may have increased responsiveness to methacholine, giving a false-positive result. The office where the test is performed should be fully equipped to treat acute bronchospasm.

Baseline spirometry is performed and should be normal or near normal. The patient is then advised that he or she will receive varying doses of inhaled medication, which may precipitate symptoms of cough and wheezing. In our laboratory we first administer five breaths of aerosolized sterile water and repeat spirometry. Lower doses of methacholine than those described here may also be used for this first step. If there is no significant decrease in flow rates, the next aerosol challenge is given as a single breath of aerosolized methacholine at a concentration of 25 mg/cc. Spirometry is again repeated, looking for a significant decrease in FEV_1. If no significant decrease occurs, the patient is given four additional breaths of aerosolized methacholine at the same concentration and spirometry is again repeated. If there has been no significant decrease in the FEV_1, this is determined to be a negative bronchoprovocation test. If a marginal decrease in FEV_1 occurs after the first breath of aerosolized methacholine, an intermediate step may be added where two breaths are given, but a total of five breaths should not be exceeded during the entire test. A decrease of less than 15% is determined to be a negative test, a decrease between 15% and 20% is termed equivocal, and a decrease of 20% or greater is determined to be a positive test result.

If there has been a significant decrease in flow rates, or if the patient is symptomatic, aerosolized bronchodilator may be administered. Spirometry can also be performed again after this treatment to document responsiveness. This latter step is not necessarily part of the test and may be employed on an individual basis.

Referral Laboratory

Complete testing in many laboratories includes spirometry, flow/volume loops, static lung volumes, diffusing capacity, prebronchodilator and postbronchodilator spirometry, and arterial blood gases. Special tests such as bronchoprovocation, polysomnography, and cardiopulmonary exercise testing may also be available. Other special tests such as lung compliance, elastic recoil, airways resistance, density dependent V_{max} (volume of isoflow), multiple inert gas studies, frequency dependence of dynamic compliance, single breath nitrogen washout (closing volume), and ventilatory drive are not commonly performed or limited to research laboratories. Further elaboration is available elsewhere [31, 57].

Lung Volumes (Static Lung Volumes)

Several methods are available for determination of functional residual capacity. Once functional residual capacity is known and lung subdivisions have been measured on a spirometer, TLC and RV can be calculated. Helium dilution and nitrogen washout are two similar methods for determining lung volumes that depend on distal air spaces communicating with central airways. Therefore, obstructive airways disease may cause erroneous results with these methods. With helium dilution, the patient breathes a known concentration of helium and a steady state is reached where exhaled helium concentration is measured. The degree of dilution indicates lung volume. With nitrogen washout the patient breathes 100% oxygen until all of the nitrogen is washed out. The volume of exhaled nitrogen indicates lung volume. Body plethysmography (body box) employs Boyle's law to determine functional residual capacity or thoracic gas volume. The patient is enclosed in a box of known volume (V_1). Pressure in the box (P_1) and pressure at the mouth (P_2) (airway) are measured as the patient pants, but airflow is stopped by a shutter at the mouth. Boyle's law is then used to calculate the unknown thoracic gas volume (V_2) where [$P_1 \times V_1 = P_2 \times V_2$]. Measurement of these "static lung volumes" is most useful in patients with restrictive disease such as pulmonary fibrosis.

Diffusing Capacity

Diffusing capacity, also called transfer factor, is a test that attempts to measure the efficiency of gas exchange across the alveolar-capillary membrane. A known concentration of carbon monoxide, which has more than 200 times the affinity for hemoglobin as oxygen, is inhaled. The concentration of exhaled carbon monoxide is measured after a single breath hold of 10 seconds. A drop in concentration is due to hemoglobin taking up carbon monoxide (diffusion or transfer). Conditions that reduce the diffusing capacity are diseases that affect the alveolar-capillary membrane such as pulmonary fibrosis, pulmonary emphysema, and pulmonary vascular disease.

Cardiopulmonary Exercise Test

Cardiopulmonary exercise testing is performed by analyzing exhaled gases and heart rate during graded exercise [76, 77]. Oxygen consumption, carbon dioxide production, ventilation, and heart rate are measured to identify the limiting cause in unexplained shortness of breath. Tremendous amounts of information are obtained noninvasively. Patterns of abnormality on this test allow separation into cardiovascular or pulmonary causes of limitation. This type of testing was very cumbersome and difficult in the past, but has become much more practical in clinical practice with the advent of rapid gas analyzers and computers to handle large amounts of information.

In this chapter we have reviewed the indications, methods of testing, and interpretation of office spirometry. This is an inexpensive, noninvasive tool that can be very helpful in diagnosing and treating patients with lung disease. Many patients with pulmonary problems never see a pulmonary specialist. Therefore, it falls on the primary practitioner to employ this modality in his or her armamentarium.

References

1. Murray JF, Nadel JA: Textbook of Respiratory Medicine. Philadelphia, W.B. Saunders, 1988, pp 666–671
2. Enright PL, Hyatt RE: Office Spirometry: A Practical Guide to the Selection and Use of Spirometers. Philadelphia, Lea & Febiger, 1987
3. Kass I, Bell CW, Epler GE, et al: Evaluation of impairment/disability secondary to respiratory disease. *Am Rev Respir Dis* 126:945–951, 1982
4. Black LF: Subject review: Early diagnosis of COPD. *Mayo Clin Proc* 57:765–772, 1982
5. Kanner RE: The relationship between airways responsiveness and chronic airflow limitation. *Chest* 86:54–57, 1984
6. Tashkin DP, Clark VA, Coulson AH, et al: Comparison of lung function in young nonsmokers and smokers before and after initiation of the smoking habit. *Am Rev Respir Dis* 128:12–16, 1983
7. Zamel N, Altose MD, Speir WA: Statement on spirometry. A report of the section on respiratory pathophysiology. *Chest* 83:547–550, 1983
8. Light RW, George RB: Serial pulmonary function in patients with acute heart failure. *Arch Intern Med* 143:429–433, 1983
9. Irwin RS, Rosen MJ, Braman SS: Cough: A comprehensive review. *Arch Intern Med* 137:1186, 1977
10. Kieth W, Morgan C: Clinical significance of pulmonary function tests: Disability or disinclination? *Chest* 75:712–715, 1979
11. Dosman JA, Cotton DJ, Graham BL, et al: Sensitivity and specificity of early diagnostic tests of lung function in smokers. *Chest* 79:6–11, 1981
12. Poe RH, Israel RH, Utell MJ, et al: Chronic cough: Bronchoscopy or pulmonary function testing? *Am Rev Respir Dis* 126:160–165, 1982

12a. Corrao W, Braman SS, Irwin RS: Chronic cough as the sole presenting manifestation of bronchial asthma. *N Engl J Med* 300:633, 1979

13. Tisi GM: Preoperative evaluation of pulmonary function: Validity, indications, and benefits. *Am Rev Respir Dis* 119:293–310, 1979
14. Zibrak JD, O'Donnell CR, Marton K: Indications for pulmonary function testing. *Ann Intern Med* 112:763–771, 1990
15. Black KH, Mitchell EE, Petusevsky ML, et al: A general purpose microprocessor for spirometry. *Chest* 78:605–612, 1980
16. Nemery B, Moarero NE, Brasseur L, et al: Changes in lung function after smoking cessation: An assessment from a cross-sectional study. *Am Rev Respir* Dis 125:122–124, 1982
17. Brooks SM: Task group on screening for respiratory disease in occupational settings. Official ATS statement. *Am Rev Respir Dis* 126:952–956, 1982
18. McFadden ER Jr, Linden DA: A reduction in mid maximal flow rate: A spirometric manifestation of small airways disease. *Am J Med* 52:725–737, 1972
19. Becklake MR: Concepts of normality applied

to the measurement of lung function. *Am J Med* 80:1158–1164, 1986
20. Gardner RM, Hankinson JL, Clausen JL, et al: ATS statement on standardization of spirometry—1987 uptake. *Am Rev Respir Dis* 136:1285–1298, 1987
21. Laszlo G: Standardized lung function testing. *Thorax* 39:881–886, 1984
22. Nelson SB, Gardner RM, Crapo FO, et al: Performance evaluation of contemporary spirometers. *Chest* 97:288–297, 1990
23. Gardner RM, Hankinson JL, West BJ: Evaluating commercially available spirometers. *Am Rev Respir Dis* 121:73–82, 1980
24. Gardner RM, Clausen JL, Epler G, et al: Pulmonary function laboratory personnel qualifications. *Am Rev Respir Dis* 134:623–624, 1986
25. Gardner RM, Clausen JL, Cotton DJ, et al: Computer guidelines for pulmonary laboratories. *Am Rev Respir Dis* 134:628–629, 1986
26. Morris AH, Kanner RE, Crapo RO, et al: Clinical Pulmonary Function Testing: A Manual of Uniform Laboratory Procedures. Salt Lake City, UT, Intermountain Thoracic Society, 1984
27. Morris JF, Koski A, Johnson LC: Spirometric standards for healthy nonsmoking adults. *Am Rev Respir Dis* 103:57–67, 1971
28. Goldman HI, Becklake MR: Respiratory function tests; normal values at median altitudes and the prediction of normal results. *Am Rev Tuberc* 79:457–467, 1959
29. Knudson RJ, Lebowitz MD, Holberg CJ, et al: Changes in the normal maximum expiratory flow-volume curve with growth and aging. *Am Rev Respir Dis* 127:725–734, 1983
30. Hepper NGG, Black LF, Fowler WS: Relationship of lung volume to height and arm span in normal subjects and in patients with spinal deformity. *Am Rev Respir Dis* 91:356–362, 1965
31. Clausen J (ed): Pulmonary Function Testing Guidelines and Controversies. New York, Academic Press, 1982
32. Lapp NL, Amandus HE, Hall R, et al: Lung volumes and flow rates in black and white subjects. *Thorax* 29:185–188, 1974
33. Schoenberg JV, Beck GJ, Bouhuys A: Growth and decay of pulmonary function in healthy blacks and whites. *Respir Physiol* 33:367–393, 1978
34. Seltzer CC, Siegelaub AB, Friedman GD, et al: Differences in pulmonary function related to smoking habits and race. *Am Rev Respir Dis* 110:598–608, 1974
35. Ray CS, Sue DY, Bray G, et al: Effects of obesity on respiratory function. *Am Rev Respir Dis* 128:501–506, 1983
36. Cohen CA, Hudson AR, Clausen JL, et al: Respiratory symptoms, spirometry, and oxidant air pollution in nonsmoking adults. *Am Rev Respir Dis* 105:251–261, 1972
37. Kilburn KH, Warshaw R, Thornton JC: Pulmonary functional impairment and symptoms in women in the Los Angeles Harbor area. *Am J Med* 79:23–28, 1985
38. Snider GL, Kory RC, Lyons HA: Grading of pulmonary function impairment by means of pulmonary function tests. *Dis Chest* 52:270–271, 1967
39. Morris JF, Temple WP, Koski A: Normal values for the ratio of one-second forced expiratory volume to forced vital capacity. *Am Rev Respir Dis* 108:1000–1003, 1973
40. Golish JA, Ahmad M, Yarnal JR: Practical application of the flow-volume loop. Cleveland *Clinic Quarterly* 47:39–45, 1980
41. Jayamanne DS, Epstein H, Goldring RM: Flow-volume curve contour in COPD: Correlation with pulmonary mechanics. *Chest* 77:749–757, 1980
42. Acres JC, Kryger MH: Clinical significance of pulmonary function tests: Upper airway obstruction. *Chest* 80:207–211, 1981
43. Cary J, Hueseby J, Culver B, et al: Variability in interpretation of pulmonary function tests. *Chest* 76:389–390, 1979
44. Colp CR: Interpretation of pulmonary function tests. *Chest* 76:377–378, 1979
45. Thómas HM III, Garrett RC: Clinical significance of pulmonary function tests: Interpretation of spirometry. *Chest* 86:129–131, 1984
46. Kanner RE, Morris AH, et al: Clinical Pulmonary Function Testing: A Manual of Uniform Laboratory Procedures. Salt Lake City, UT, Intermountain Thoracic Society, 1975
47. Detels R, Tashkin DP, Simmons MS, et al: The UCLA population studies of chronic obstructive respiratory disease. 5. Agreement and disagreement of tests in identifying abnormal lung function. *Chest* 82:630–638, 1982
48. Gelb AF, Williams AJ, Zamel N: Clinical significance of pulmonary function tests, spirometry. *Chest* 84:473–474, 1983
49. Crapo RO, Morris AH, Gardner RM: Reference spirometric values using techniques and equipment that meet ATS recommendations. *Am Rev Respir Dis* 123:659–664, 1981
50. Anthonisen NR, Wright EC, and the IPPB Trial Group: Bronchodilator response in chronic obstructive pulmonary disease. *Am Rev Respir Dis* 133:814–819, 1986
51. Gross NJ: COPD: A disease of reversible airflow obstruction. *Am Rev Respir Dis* 133: 725–726, 1986
52. Guyatt GH, Townsend M, Nogradi S, et al: Acute response to bronchodilator: An imper-

fect guide for bronchodilator therapy in chronic airflow limitation. *Arch Intern Med* 184:1949–1952, 1988
53. Berger R, Smith D: Acute postbronchodilator changes in pulmonary function parameters in patients with chronic airways obstruction. *Chest* 93:541–546, 1988
54. Ramsdell JW, Tisi GM: Determination of bronchodilation in the clinical pulmonary function laboratory. *Chest* 76:622–628, 1979
55. Wilson AF (ed): Pulmonary Function Testing Indications and Interpretations. Orlando, Grune & Stratton, 1985
56. Shim C, Williams MH Jr: The adequacy of inhalation of aerosol from canister nebulizers. *Am J Med* 69:891–894, 1980
57. Mahler DA (ed): Pulmonary function testing. Clin Chest Med 10:2, 1989
58. Light RW, Conrad SA, George RB: The one best test for evaluating effects of bronchodilator therapy. *Chest* 72:512–516, 1977
59. Cockcroft DW, Berscheid BA: Volume adjustment of maximal midexpiratory flow. Chest 78:595–600, 1980
60. Sherter CB, Connolly JJ, Schilder DP: The significance of volume adjusting the maximal midexpiratory flow in assessing the response to a bronchodilator drug. *Chest* 73:568–571, 1978
61. Girard WM, Light RW: Should the FVC be considered in evaluating response to bronchodilator? *Chest* 84:87–89, 1983
62. Snider GL, Woolf CR, Kory RC, et al: Criteria for the assessment of reversibility in airways obstruction. Report of the Committee on Emphysema, American College of Chest Physicians. *Chest* 65:552–553, 1974
63. Ries A: Response to bronchodilators. *In* Clausen JL (ed): Pulmonary Function Testing: Guidelines and Controversies. New York, Academic Press, 1982, pp 215–221
64. Sourk RL, Nugent KM: Bronchodilator testing: Confidence intervals derived from placebo inhalations. *Am Rev Respir Dis* 128: 153–157, 1983
65. Dales RE, Spitzer WO, Tousignant P, et al: Clinical interpretation of airway response to a bronchodilator. *Am Rev Respir Dis* 136:317–320, 1988
66. Tweeddale PM, Alexander F, McHardy GJR: Short term variability in FEV_1 and bronchodilator responsiveness in patients with obstructive ventilatory defects. *Thorax* 42:487–490, 1987
67. Pratter MR, Irwin RS: The clinical value of pharmacologic bronchoprovocation challenge. *Chest* 85:260–265, 1984
68. Brooks SM, Weiss MA, Bernstein IL: Reactive airways dysfunction syndrome (RADS). *Chest* 88:376, 1985
69. Fetters LJ, Matthews JI: Methacholine challenge test. *Arch Intern Med* 144:938–940, 1984
70. Assoufi BK, Dally MB, Newman-Taylor AJ, et al: Cold air test: A simplified standard method for airway reactivity. *Bull Eur Physiopathol Respir* 22:349, 1986
71. Stanescu DC, Frans A: Bronchial asthma without increased airway reactivity. *Eur J Respir Dis* 63:5, 1982
72. Heaton RW, Henderson AF, Costello JF: Cold air as a bronchial provocation technique. *Chest* 86:810–814, 1984
73. Myers JR, Corrao WM, Braman SS: Clinical applicability of a methacholine inhalational challenge. *JAMA* 246:225, 1981
74. Chatham M, Bleecker ER, Norman P, et al: A screening test for airways reactivity. *Chest* 82:15, 1982
75. Rebuck AS: Methacholine and airway reactivity. *Chest* 82, 1982
76. Hansen JE: Cardiopulmonary exercise testing. *In* Clausen JL (ed): Pulmonary Function Testing: Guidelines and Controversies. New York, Academic Press, 1982, pp 259–279
77. Neuberg GW, Friedman SH, Weiss MB, et al: Cardiopulmonary exercise testing, the clinical value of gas exchange data. *Arch Intern Med* 148:2221–2226, 1988

Clinical Diagnosis of Respiratory Disorders and Physical Examination

Charles G. Todoroff

Recent decades have produced advancements in the technology used to diagnose and manage respiratory disorders. As our knowledge increases, we have a growing body of opinion that the respiratory system is limited in its variety of physical manifestations. In many illnesses the early diagnosis of respiratory disease rests not on clinical signs and symptoms, but on radiographic and pathophysiologic criteria alone. How then may we justify using a time-consuming and potentially ambiguous sequence of maneuvers in this group of illnesses? The answer lies in the experience of virtually every clinician who has correctly detected pneumonia before the chest radiograph became abnormal, or who recognized effort-induced asthma when spirometry was not diagnostic. Furthermore, careful elicitation of signs and symptoms may provide a dimension of specificity when selecting expensive investigations in the laboratory or radiography suite.

The purpose of this chapter is to systematize the experience of clinical assessment of patients with respiratory disease so as to assist the clinician who must make such assessments rapidly or under adverse circumstances. This is not an introductory text and it is outside the scope of this discussion to reiterate the fundamentals of history taking and the mechanics of physical examination, which are covered in great detail elsewhere [1, 2].

Recently, inquiries into the sensitivity and interobserver reproducibility of physical findings elicited by clinicians and trainees have produced disquieting results [3, 4]. This is true both in the United States, where it is widely believed that medical technology has supplanted expert clinical assessment as a diagnostic tool, and elsewhere in the world. Of particular importance is the need to standardize the nomenclature involved such that observer error is reduced [5].

Enhancing Reliability

Pulmonary diagnosis rests on the ability to distinguish the abnormal from a broad range of normal manifestations. More important, perhaps, is the need to differentiate what is normal for an individual given the wide spectrum in age, size, body habitus, physical fitness, and psychic or emotional factors to which a patient may be predisposed. To these considerations must be added the fact that respiratory disease is widespread in our society, and our patients often present with background conditions such as emphysema or heart disease, which must be placed in some kind of context.

What factors, then, can provide a measure of reliability?

History

Historical factors such as cough, dyspnea, chest discomfort, and expectoration often form the basis for the chief complaint. However, many of these symptoms can be denied, adapted to, and concealed to a surprising degree. The reliability of the history is enhanced when the patient is asked to cite how his or her symptoms have progressed in concrete units (e.g., flights of stairs, blocks) over time. Since the lung has a limited repertoire of symptoms it may produce, it is necessary to proceed to augment the history systematically.

The pulmonary review can be vast if key

bits of information are not elicited heuristically [6], i.e., groups of information are unlocked when key questions are asked based on certain rules of thumb or shortcuts. The occupational history bears particular importance because the work environment often contains the most noxious substances. Some effort should be made to understand how the patient does the job and to explore his or her understanding of the risks involved. A smoking history is standard, but few clinicians seem to inquire whether others in the house also smoke.

Of course the pulmonary system cannot be adequately evaluated if other organ systems are not considered as well. A history suggesting cardiac, gastrointestinal, collagen-vascular, or immune deficiency disease may provide the necessary clue to accurate diagnosis. In children and young adults the birth history may suggest inherited or congenital illness. The childhood history as it relates to atopy, physical fitness, and communicable illness may be useful. The family history may suggest protease deficiency, atopy, and common source exposures such as tuberculosis or asbestos.

Physical Examination

Physical findings are variable, frequently insensitive and often nonspecific. A large man may have considerably more attentuated breath sounds than a smaller individual. Some findings are demonstrable only with higher respiratory rates or deeper breaths. Reliability can be enhanced when physical findings are asymmetric on examination. Pneumonic infiltrates, effusions, localized bronchial stenosis, and other processes may be present bilaterally, but seldom to the same degree. Therefore, deviations from what is considered normal attain a degree of significance when they differ from the contralateral interspace. Figure 3-1 is a diagrammatic view of the chest as seen from the back. Because the upper and lower lobes of the lung are stacked on one another in an oblique fashion, breath sounds from the lower lobes are heard best from the back. Sounds from the upper lobes are heard best by ascultation of the front of the chest.

Inspection usually begins during the earliest portion of the examination. The rate and depth of the respiratory cycle are helpful in assessing the patient with suspected respiratory disease, provided modifying influences are not present. Counting respirations over 30 to 60 seconds is of major importance and yet infrequently noted by physicians. Counting the respirations with one's finger on the radial pulse or engaging the patient in conversation during the counting period en-

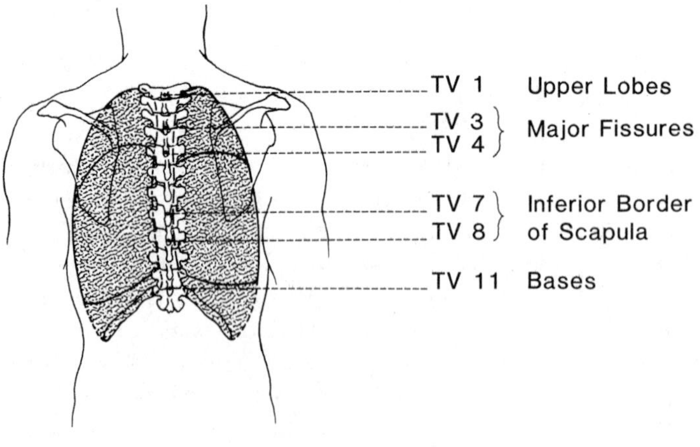
TV 1
Upper Lobes
TV 3
TV 4
Major Fissures
TV 7
TV 8
Inferior Border of Scapula
TV 11
Bases

Fig. 3-1. Diagrammatic view of the chest as seen from the back. The lower lungs lobes have a greater surface area adjacent to the back and therefore breath sounds from the lower lobes are best appreciated posteriorly. TV, thoracic vertebral level of the anatomic part.

hances the reliability of this measurement. A respiratory rate is clearly abnormal if greater than 24 bpm and normal if less than 22 bpm [7].

Traditionally, the expiratory phase of the respiratory cycle is prolonged over the inspiratory phase when airways obstruction is present, although this varies according to the level of activity. Controversy exists as to whether the rate and depth of respirations can be used as a reliable tool to differentiate eucapneic individuals from hypercapneic patients in chronic obstructive lung disease [8].

Cheyne-Stokes respiration is said to occur when the respiratory cycle is interrupted by periods of apnea, usually followed by a period of crescendo-decrescendo respiratory depth [8]. Observation of the patient in a supine position may reveal abnormal diaphragmatic movement. Flattening or dropping of the abdominal wall during inspiration implies diaphragmatic dysfunction due to fatigue, muscular disease, or paralysis [8].

Palpation of the chest may sometimes be useful as the patient phonates, producing so-called "vocal fremitus"; the results, however, are imprecise and I seldom use this clinically. On the other hand, asymmetric and paradoxic motion of the chest wall, tumors and fractures involving the underlying ribs, and the motions of the precordium are best appreciated in this fashion.

Percussive findings can be described as dull, resonant, or tympanitic, and are meaningful as when they demonstrate the drumlike qualities of the normal chest. Figure 3-2 shows that the chest is normally composed of air-filled baffles (alveoli) in close contact with the chest wall. When vibrations in the chest wall produced by percussion reach the airspaces, the frequency decreases and the sound is attenuated. A similar sequence of events occurs when the airspaces themselves are obliterated as might be seen in consolidation from pneumonia. On the other hand, the sound may be enhanced as when air fills the pleural space as in pneumothorax.

Figure 3-2 also depicts the events that occur when the lung is auscultated. The origin of what we call *vesicular* breath sounds is

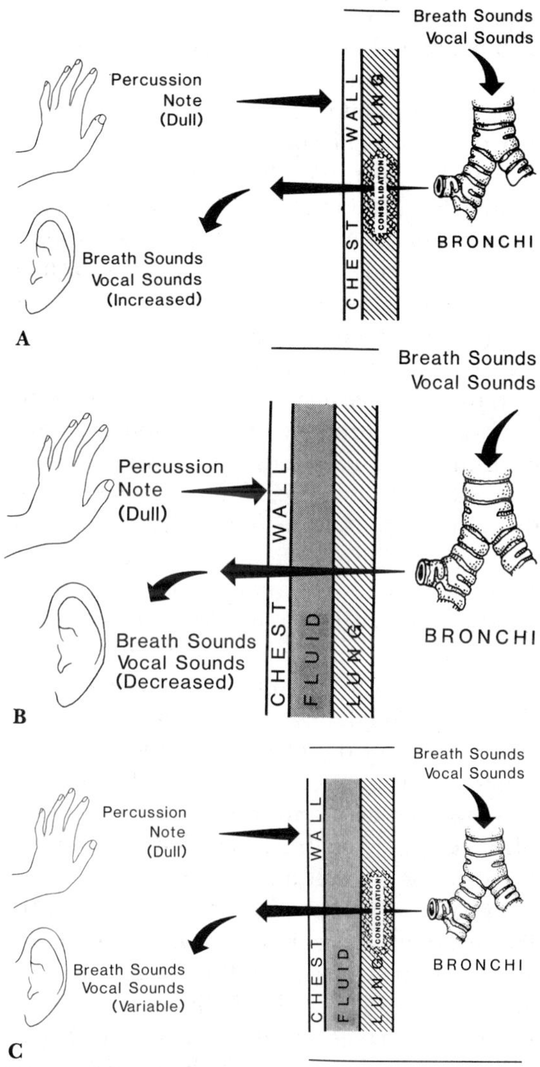
Breath Sounds
Vocal Sounds
Percussion
Note
(Dull)
CHEST WALL
LUNG
CONSOLIDATION
BRONCHI
Breath Sounds
Vocal Sounds
(Increased)
A
Breath Sounds
Vocal Sounds
Percussion
Note
(Dull)
CHEST WALL
FLUID
LUNG
BRONCHI
Breath Sounds
Vocal Sounds
(Decreased)
B
Breath Sounds
Vocal Sounds
Percussion
Note
(Dull)
CHEST WALL
FLUID
LUNG
CONSOLIDATION
BRONCHI
Breath Sounds
Vocal Sounds
(Variable)
C

Fig. 3-2. Stylized frontal (coronal) section through mid-lung showing transmission of percussion notes, fremitus and breath sounds. (A) Consolidation is shown by cross-hatching. Although the percussion note is dull because the pneumonia acts as a barrier to sound transmission, effectively thickening the chest wall at the site, bronchial and vocal sounds are enhanced by their continuity with the fluid density sound transmission in the pneumonic medium. (B) Pleural fluid. The pleural effusion is discontinuous with both the percussion note and auscultatory sounds from within, effectively damping all sound transmission and reducing the loudness of the bronchial and vocal sounds. (C) Pleural fluid and consolidation. Combined effusion and consolidation. The presence of fluid and consolidated lung may result in normalization of bronchial and vocal sounds while the percussion note remains dull.

poorly understood, but probably arises from turbulence within the upper airways, trachea, and central bronchi as airflow beyond that level in the pulmonary tree is insufficient to provide sound energy to transmit to the surface of the chest [9]. That breath sounds are related to turbulence is demonstrated by a drop in intensity when helium is substituted for air [10, 11]. Sound moving through a fluid medium, as in pneumonia, is less attenuated and has more high-frequency content [12]. Consequently, sounds generated from within the upper airways, larynx (vocal resonance), and bronchi (bronchophony) are transmitted to the stethoscope with greater fidelity. However, when fluid or air expands the pleural space, the sound is attenuated once again. The degree to which these effects counterbalance one another is, of course, variable. Of particular importance is the inclusion of the transmitted vocal sound (vocal resonance) in the auscultatory examination of the chest. While the examiner places the stethoscope on the chest the patient speaks. *N* and *M* sounds seem to transmit throughout the chest the best, and the word *ninety-nine* is often used for this purpose. Vocal resonance is enhanced when fluid fills the airspaces and attenuated when the distance from chest surface to airspace is increased as in pleural effusion. Disparity between the breath sounds and vocal resonance is of diagnostic importance; the former are attenuated out of proportion to the latter in focal bronchial stenosis, illustrating that breath sounds tend to vary with regional ventilation, whereas vocal resonance is independent of airflow [13].

The adventitial sounds have been the subject of controversy since the time of Laennec [14]. What has become clear is that the reliability and reproducibility of these sounds is diminished by the use of adjective qualifiers (e.g., fine crackles) and disparate terminology [5, 15, 16]. Therefore, a simplification of our understanding of adventitial sounds is in order.

Crackles are staccato sounds generally associated with the rapid opening of airways proximal to the terminal alveoli [17]. They are apparent in an upright position, usually at the bases, and may disappear in recumbency, but are unmodified by coughing [18]. Although crackles are generally easy to detect and are reproducible under ideal circumstances, other mechanisms may produce a crackling sound, including pleuritis, subcutaneous emphysema, or pericarditis. Crackles may, nevertheless, be considered sensitive but nonspecific signs of regional lung disease. Any mechanism that raises the opening pressure of small airways, such as edema fluid, pus, or surrounding pulmonary inelasticity as in fibrosis, can produce crackles. The uncertain reproducibility of these findings among examiners seems to derive largely from uncertain modifiers such as dry, moist, fine, coarse, etc. Although these descriptive associations may be legitimate components of one's personal repertoire, improving one's recollection of these sounds, they are too subjective to be reliable when describing diagnostic findings [10].

Likewise, wheezes, once called rhonchi and squeaks, are best left as quantal entities—either present or absent—but seldom usefully modified. They are produced by bronchi at or near closure, and their frequency may reflect little more than the native diameter of the airway and the velocity of airflow along its length. Wheezes are also a product of airflow turbulence and can be produced by bronchial smooth muscle constriction, fixed mechanical obstruction, accumulations of viscous secretions, a partially obstructing foreign body, and transmission from other sites in the respiratory tract (i.e., whistling). These sounds are differentiated from crackles by virtue of their continuous nature, predominating in the expiratory phase of respiration.

Stridor is a continuous inspiratory sound that is similar in frequency to wheezing and louder over the neck than the chest—the opposite of wheezing [19]. Its importance rests in the fact that serious upper airway disease is present, potentially compromising the entire respiratory tree. Stridor and wheezing can both be heard at the mouth.

Extrapulmonary Physical Findings

These signs may occasionally provide a diagnosis where one lacks pulmonary findings. Cyanosis is the perceptual equivalent of detectable deoxyhemoglobin concentration. It has been said to occur when the arterial deoxyhemoglobin concentration exceeds 5.0 g [9]. However, more recent data have suggested that deoxyhemoglobin concentrations as low as 1.5 g may be reliably detected [20]. Pallor, on the other hand, is undefined and easily masked by skin pigmentation. Both observations are inexact because either may be influenced by local capillary blood flow, ambient temperature, and the presence of abnormal hemoglobins. When present both signs are useful; when absent, nothing is excluded.

Sarcoidosis is a systemic disorder of unknown etiology whose distribution often includes the lung. Cutaneous features of sarcoidosis may be present in 20% to 35% of patients [21]. The most common nonspecific manifestation is erythema nodosum. Erythematous or violaceous firm papules may be present on the face. Annular plaques may be present anywhere on the body. Lupus pernio, however, is most frequently associated with active pulmonary disease. This appears as violaceous plaques located on the nose, cheeks, and ears. In descending order of frequency peripheral lymphadenopathy, cardiomyopathy, splenomegaly, hepatomegaly, and neuromuscular disease are organ-specific findings in this disorder.

Table 3-1. Some Conditions Known to Be Associated with Digital Clubbing

Bronchogenic carcinoma
Mesothelioma
Metastatic cancer in the thorax
Familial (congenital) clubbing
Lung abscess
Pulmonary alveolar proteinosis
Cystic fibrosis
Pneumoconiosis
Empyema
Arteriovenous malformations
Cyanotic congenital heart disease
Infective endocarditis
Infected vascular prosthesis
Leukemia
Cancer of the nasopharynx, esophagus, thyroid, thymus, liver
Small intestinal tumors
Inflammatory bowel disease, sprue
Amyloidosis
Hodgkin's disease
Hyperparathyroidism
Cirrhosis
Tuberculosis
Familial polyposis

Clubbing and Osteoarthropathy

Digital clubbing and hypertrophic osteoarthropathy are often confused with one another, especially because they may coexist [22, 23]. Although many clinicians associate them with bronchogenic carcinoma, they can be found less frequently in several other conditions (Table 3-1). Clubbing is said to occur when one observes a rounded curving nail, increased thickness and spongy consistency at the base of the nail, a loss of the normal concave curvature where the nail base meets the proximal digit (referred to as Lovibond's angle), and bulbous enlargement of the digital pad (Fig. 3-3) [9]. In early clubbing, one may observe some, but not all, of these findings. Schamroth's sign may be useful in difficult cases [22]: the dorsa of the distal phalanges are apposed and the space normally seen between them may be obliterated (Fig. 3-4).

Hypertrophic osteoarthropathy is seen most frequently in pulmonary malignancy and may be confused with arthritis. One observes thickening of the affected digits, often accompanied by periarticular and synovial swelling, excess warmth, edema, bony tenderness, limited range of motion, and increased sweating. The patient may complain of deep-seated aching or burning along the shafts of long bones and noxious peripheral paresthesiae. Osteoarthropathy may precede

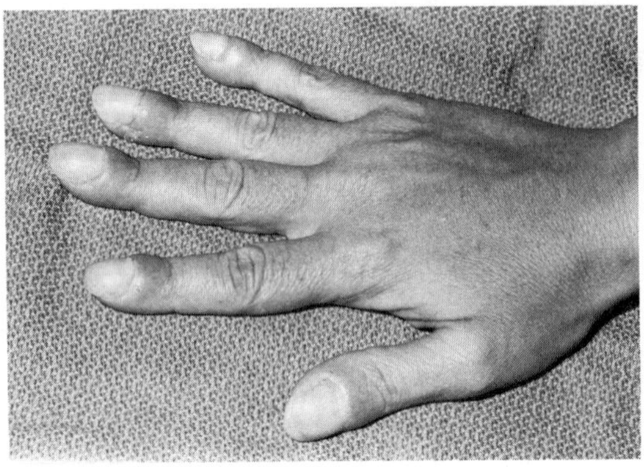

A

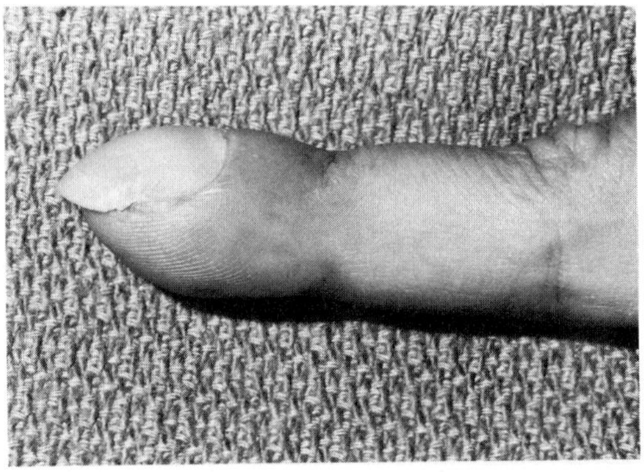

B

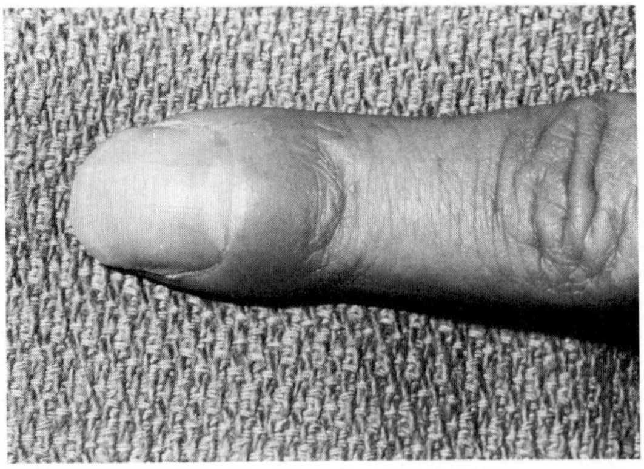

C

Fig. 3-3. (A) Photograph of hand showing digital clubbing in a patient with advanced interstitial pulmonary fibrosis. (B) Digital clubbing. Close lateral view. Note flattening of nail bed. (C) Digital clubbing. Close view from the top. Note widening of the distal phalanx.

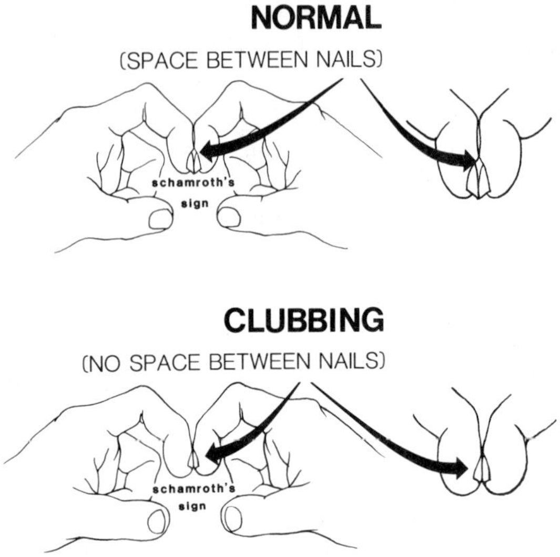
NORMAL
(SPACE BETWEEN NAILS)
schamroth's sign
CLUBBING
(NO SPACE BETWEEN NAILS)
schamroth's sign

Fig. 3-4. Differentiating normal digits from clubbed fingers using Schamroth's sign. Note the loss of space between apposed distal phalanges.

the radiographic appearance of lung malignancy by several months and is insidious in onset, a feature that may be helpful when differentiating from acute arthritis. In addition to long bones and digits, shoulders, clavicles, and temporomandibular joints may be affected as well.

Chest Wall Syndromes

The configuration of the chest wall is an important observation. Pectus excavatum is said to occur when the sternum forms a depression with the anterior rib ends, instead of a gently curving contour [24]. It is usually present at birth and may exacerbate during adolescence. Associations have been shown with rib deformities, dorsal lordosis, scoliosis, and visceral abnormalities. A family history of pectus excavatum may be present in as many as 37% of cases. Some controversy exists as to underlying visceral abnormalities; several clinical series have shown limited ventilatory capacity and impaired ventricular filling that improved following an operation [25]. Other associations are seen with a variety of congenital heart deformities, Marfan's syndrome, and congenital diaphragmatic hernia.

Pectus carinatum, an anterior displacement of the sternum and ribs, appears during childhood and may also be associated with vertebral malformations.

Thoracic outlet syndrome is a generic term applied to any situation in which the brachial plexus, subclavian artery, or subclavian vein is compressed as a result of anatomic anomalies [26]. Nerve compression in the plexus is more common than vascular occlusion. Painful neuropathies may be as widespread as the face, ipsilateral ear, upper chest, upper posterior thorax, and via the radial nerve dermatome to the arm, wrist, and hand. Weakness and temperature change may be more characteristic of lower plexus involvement than upper involvement in which dysesthesiae predominate. Vascular symptoms include venous congestion, swelling, and aching in venous disease. In arterial disease, peripheral embolization and ischemia of the affected digits may occur.

Congenital deformities of the spine and acquired defects may affect the contour or motion of the chest wall and produce restricted lung disease. The visceral implications of this situation are similar to pectus excavatum, with cardiovascular abnormalities predominating. Ankylosing spondylitis may abnormally straighten the spine while osteoporosis with anterior wedging may bow it.

Disorders of chest musculature may be suspected in primary muscle disorders such as polymyositis, in myoneural disorders such as myasthenia gravis, and in neurologic diseases such as multiple sclerosis. Additionally, poor nutrition, a variety of drugs, and disuse atrophy may affect the muscles as well. Abnormal rib-abdominal movements may signal respiratory muscle fatigue in patients with respiratory failure. Hoover's sign, retraction and inward movement of the lower ribs during inspiration, may signal a severely flattened diaphragm [8]. Unilateral diaphragmatic paralysis may be suspected by comparing the percussion note in deep inspiration with full exhalation. Often the dullness moves superiorly on the affected side during inspiration.

The tracheal and mediastinal contents must be considered in patients with dyspnea. The upper airways, trachea, and larynx may produce inspiratory noise or stridor, which is heard better over the neck than the chest. The implication is obstruction due to edema, foreign body, tumor, secretions, etc. Laryngotracheal shift suggests severe atelectasis, hydrothorax, or pneumothorax, causing these structures deviate to the contralateral side. Fixation due to fibrosis or carcinoma causes the trachea to deviate toward the affected side.

Mediastinal sounds include a variety of crackling and rubbing sounds in synchrony with the respiratory cycle, the cardiac cycle, or both. These sounds generally imply inflammation, infection, or infiltration of the serosal surfaces in apposition. Mediastinal crunch implies pneumomediastinum which can result from ruptured viscus, infection with gas-forming organisms, penetrating trauma, or severe vomiting. Cervical subcutaneous emphysema may accompany the crunch due to dissection through the fascial planes by air or gas.

Obstructive Respiratory Syndromes

Obstructive lung disease may be acute or chronic with exacerbations. In the young asthmatic patient, the respiratory rate may be rapid, and wheezing may be audible across the room. There is no correlation between the loudness of the wheezes and the degree of air trapping. Indeed, severe obstruction may reveal an entirely silent chest. Pulses paradoxus may be present and severe (>18 mm) in a particularly severe attack [27]. Pulsus paradoxus reflects left ventricular filling pressure abnormalities in relation to negative intrathoracic pressure during deep inspiration. The product of these pressures, or the transmural pressure, is increased. This in turn increases left ventricular afterload, excessively reducing cardiac output and blood pressure during inspiration [28].

Prolonged hyperinflation as in severe chronic airways disease may produce an expanded chest volume and evidence of diaphragmatic dysfunction. Whether the diaphragm functions poorly as a result of fiber length distortions, metabolic abnormalities, or hypoxemia is a matter of inquiry. Three respiratory patterns may be seen in these circumstances. Asynchronous breathing is defined as a time lag between outward motion of the chest wall and the abdominal wall. Respiratory alternans is alternating motions of the chest wall abdomen with successive breaths. Paradoxical motion occurs when the chest and abdomen move in opposite directions.

Pneumonia

Infective lung disease, especially pneumonia, comprises a mixed group of disorders spanning a spectrum between acute pyogenic infections and more atypical or indolent varieties. The classic pneumonias are the most striking in their presentation [29]. The time of onset is often heralded by strong rigors and high fevers. The patient often experiences changes in sensorium, including agitation, stupor, or coma. Tachypnea and tachycardia are common. Congestive heart failure may be present along with wheezes due to bronchospasm. Herpes labialis may be present. The skin is warm, flushed, and moist until profound shock occurs. Mucosal cyanosis reflects the degree of hypoxemia.

Chest wall expansion may be asymmetric due to large empyema or tension pneumothorax (in which case tracheal deviation may also be present) or splinting caused by pain. The earliest auscultatory findings are focal crackles, following which percussion dullness and enhanced vocal resonance may also be present. When empyema supervenes, the crackles and vocal resonance may diminish in intensity but remain asymmetrically enhanced nevertheless. Because of the enhanced fidelity brought about by alveolar airspace consolidation and the passage of a wider frequency spectrum of sound, "bronchial breathing," whispered pectoriloquy, and egophony are said to occur [30]. Other specific findings of complicating syndromes are discussed elsewhere.

The appearance of the sputum may be useful diagnostically. Lobar disease such as *Streptococcus pneumoniae* pneumonia may produce a rusty sputum while *Staphylococcus* may cause a salmon-colored specimen and *Klebsiella* a red gelatinous sputum.

Carcinoma of the Lung

Tumor growth in the lung is often clinically silent until metastases have occurred [31]. This is especially true of small-cell carcinoma. Pulmonary symptoms are often ignored but consist of cough, hemoptysis, dyspnea, chest wall pain, and wheezing. Auscultatory findings may suggest focal obstruction with wheezing or stridor, pleural effusion, friction rubs, or classic consolidation.

Extrapulmonary findings may include regional lymphadenopathy, hoarseness, dysphagia, or weight loss. Nearly every organ system has been reported to be affected by metastatic spread of the tumor. Paraneoplastic syndromes may be present without direct invasion by tumor, including anorexia, fever, ectopic hormone production, clubbing and osteoarthropathy, myasthenic syndromes, coagulopathies, dermatologic syndromes, and renal disease, in descending order of frequency. Paraneoplastic syndromes may precede the onset of detectable tumor by years.

Pulmonary Arterial Embolic Disease

Pulmonary thromboembolism is a common disease that is underdiagnosed. It is made more difficult in that the presentation is diverse and physical findings are absent or nonspecific in most cases [32]. Recognition of the patient at risk is of major importance. Predisposing conditions include immobilization, congestive heart failure, fractures of the lower extremities, malignancy, pregnancy, oral contraceptive drugs, previous thrombosis or thromboembolism, and the postoperative state. Patients may present with one of three clinical syndromes related to thromboembolism: acute, pleuritic pain, dyspnea, friction rub, and hemoptysis, signaling a pulmonary infarction; acute right-sided heart failure with a loud second pulmonic sound, dyspnea, and cyanosis; and unexplained dyspnea with tachypnea, which is most common. Occasionally the patient may be febrile or present with generalized wheezing.

Pulmonary fat embolism may occur in 0.5% to 2% of patients suffering a long bone fracture and 5% to 10% of those with multiple fractures including the pelvis [33]. Most patients with severe fat emboli present with respiratory distress, tachypnea, altered sensorium, and multiple petechiae covering the upper thorax. In addition, fever, tachycardia, jaundice, and retinal embolization may be observed. Coagulopathy and hemoptysis are reported variably.

The early recognition of respiratory disease depends not only on the presentation of a patient with dyspnea or cough. Many respiratory syndromes present insidiously and their presence must be elicited by careful clinical inquiry. Histories of exposures to airborne particulate matter are often forgotten; low-grade infections may be ignored in their earlier stages; pulmonary emboli may produce few striking changes in hospitalized patients who are already ill; and self-denial plays a role in patients who engage in self-destructive behaviors. In evaluating such patients the clinician is best served who always asks the question "Why?" Why is there weakness or fatigue; why is the respiratory rate increased; why is there fever or tachycardia? Often fundamental knowledge coupled with a spirit of inquiry will provide avenues for diagnosis and management.

References

1. DeGowin EL, DeGowin RL: Bedside Diagnostic Evaluation, ed 2. New York, MacMillan, 1976
2. Burnside JW: Adam's Physical Diagnosis, ed 15. Baltimore, Williams & Wilkins, 1979
3. Mulrow CD, Dolmatch BL, Delong ER, et al: Observer variability in the pulmonary examination. *J Gen Intern Med* 1:364–367, 1986
4. Oboler SK, LaForce M: The periodic physical examination in asymptomatic adults. *Ann Intern Med* 110:214–226, 1989
5. Mikami R, Murao M, Cugell DW, et al: International symposium on lung sounds. Synopsis of proceedings. *Chest* 92:342–345, 1987
6. Kassirer JP: Diagnostic reasoning. *Ann Intern Med* 110:893–900, 1989
7. Gravelyn TR, Weg JG: Respiratory rate as an indicator of respiratory dysfunction. *JAMA* 244:1123–1125, 1980
8. Goldberg P, Roussos C: Assessment of respiratory muscle dysfunction in chronic obstructive lung disease. *Med Clin North Am* 74: 643–660, 1990
9. Fraser RG, Pare JA: Diseases of the Chest. Philadelphia, W.B. Saunders, pp 399, 403–406
10. Loudon R, Murphy RL Jr: Lung sounds. *Am Rev Respir Dis* 130:663–673, 1984
11. Forgacs P, Nathoo AR, Richardson HD: Breath sounds. *Thorax* 26:288–295, 1971
12. Ploysongsang Y, Michel RP, Rossi A, et al: Early detection of pulmonary congestion and edema in dogs by using lung sounds. *J Appl Physiol* 66:2061–2070, 1989
13. Jones FL: Poor breath sounds with good voice sounds: A sign of bronchial stenosis. *Chest* 93:312–313, 1988
14. Laennec RTH: De l'auscultation mediate ou traite du diagnostic des maladies des poumons et du coeur, fonde principalement sur nouveau moyen d'exploration, ed 1. Paris, Brosson et Chaude, 1819
15. Say ninety-nine (editorial). *Lancet* 2:1258–1259, 1986
16. Pasterkamp H, Montgomery M, Wiebicke W: Nomenclature used by health care professionals to describe breath sounds in asthma. *Chest* 92:346–352, 1987
17. Munkata M, Homma Y, Matsuzaki M, et al: Production mechanism of crackles in excised normal canine lungs. *J Appl Physiol* 66: 2061–2070, 1989
18. Forgacs P: Crackles and wheezes. *Lancet* 2:203–205, 1967
19. Baughman RP, Loudon RG: Stridor: Differentiation from asthma or upper airway noise. *Am Rev Respir Dis* 139:1407–1409, 1989
20. Goss GA, Hayes JA, Burdon JG: Deoxyhaemoglobin concentrations in the detection of central cyanosis. *Thorax* 43:212–213, 1988
21. Hanno R, Callen JP: Sarcoidosis. *Med Clin North Am* 64:847–866, 1980
22. Hansen-Flaschen J, Nordberg J: Clubbing and hypertrophic osteoarthropathy. *Clin Chest Med* 8:287–298, 1987
23. Alberts WM: A clinician's guide to clubbing. *J Respir Dis* 10:37–40, 1989
24. Welch KJ, Shamberger RC: Chest wall deformities. *In* Shields TW (ed): General Thoracic Surgery, ed 3. Philadelphia, Lea & Febiger, 1983, pp 515–543
25. Robicsek F: Pectus excavatum and carinatum.

In Grillo HC, et al (eds): Current Therapy in Cardiothoracic Surgery. Toronto, B.C. Decker, 1989, pp 87–90

26. Roos DB: Operative management of the thoracic outlet syndrome. *In* Grillo HC, et al (eds): Current Therapy in Cardiothoracic Surgery. Toronto, BC Decker, 1989, pp 91–94
27. Hall JB, Wood LD: Management of the critically ill asthmatic patient. *Med Clin North Am* 74:779–796, 1990
28. Buda AJ, Pinsky MR, Ingels NB Jr: Effect of intrathoracic pressure on left ventricular performance. *N Engl J Med* 301:453–459, 1979
29. Lerner AM, Jankauskas K: The classic bacterial pneumonias. Dis Mon 1975
30. Farr BM, Mandell GL: Gram positive pneumonias. *In* Pennington JE (ed): Respiratory Infections: Diagnosis and Management, ed 2. New York, Raven Press, 1989, pp 298–313
31. Minna JD, Pass H, Glatstein E, et al: Cancer of the lung. *In* DeVita VT, Hellman S, Rosenberg SA (eds): Cancer: Principles & Practice of Oncology, ed 3. Philadelphia, JB Lippincott, 1989
32. Sharma GV, Sasahara AA: Diagnosis and treatment of pulmonary embolism. *Med Clin North Am* 63:239–250, 1979
33. Heitzman ER: Pulmonary fat embolism. *In* Heitzman ER (ed): The Lung, ed 2. St. Louis, CV Mosby, 1984, pp 131–136

4

Dyspnea

James V. Palazzolo and Lyle D. Victor

Diagnosing dyspnea, or shortness of breath, can prove to be clinically challenging for the primary care physician because of the subjective nature of this symptom. Whereas shortness of breath may result from normal activity such as strenuous exercise, it may just as likely be the symptom of an existing pathology. In the athlete who has just finished a race, dyspnea is an appropriate and predictable occurrence, but shortness of breath in an individual who is sitting at rest reading or watching television would be an abnormal symptom [1]. Many times the circumstances surrounding the diagnosis of dyspnea are not as clear as those just described, and therefore, determining whether an underlying pathology exists becomes more difficult [2].

Although dyspnea may be quantitated with some accuracy [2a], there remains considerable descriptive verbiage associated with the symptom including such terms as breathlessness, air hunger and inability to get a deep breath. A recent study showed that different disease processes may be associated with different descriptions of dyspnea. For example, "shallow" breathing seemed to be associated with neuromuscular disorders, "tight" with asthma and "suffocating" with CHF [2b].

The physiology of dyspnea is complex. In order to understand the origin of the symptom it is useful to begin with a discussion of the control of ventilation. Most investigators believe that the control of ventilation involves three basic components, as described by West (see Table 4-1) [3]. The first component is composed of the sensors, which gather appropriate information regarding respiration. The second component is the control center, which is located in the medulla and pons of the brainstem. This area processes the information it receives from the sensors and coordinates the actions of the respiratory muscles. These respiratory muscles comprise the third component and are responsible for respiration. Checks and balances are provided through the negative feedback that results from the increased activity of the respiratory muscles.

Sensors

Chemoreceptors

There are numerous sensors that relay vital information to the brain concerning the status of respiration (Fig. 4-1). One such sensor is the chemoreceptor, which is of two types: central and peripheral. Central chemoreceptors are located in three distinct areas of the medulla and respond primarily to changes in PCO_2 and pH of the blood and cerebrospinal fluid [4, 5]. Peripheral chemoreceptors are another name for the carotid and aortic bodies that are located at the bifurcation of the common carotid arteries and along the aortic arch, respectively. They are highly vascular and primarily responsible for hypoxic drive. In addition, they respond to changes in blood pH and, to a lesser extent, PCO_2 [4–6].

Mechanoreceptors

The second group of sensors is the mechanoreceptors, which are located in the lung and airways. These receptors respond to changes in airway pressure and volume in their surrounding environment. Until recently it was thought that these receptors only responded to mechanical stimuli. It is now theorized that their response to endogenous chemical stimuli such as histamines, prostaglandins, bradykinins, etc. may constitute the basis of certain pathologic pulmonary states [5]. Included in

Table 4-1. Control of Respiration

I. Sensors
   A. Chemoreceptors
      1. Central
      2. Peripheral
   B. Mechanoreceptors
      1. Stretch
      2. Irritant
      3. J receptors (C fiber)
      4. Muscle spindles and Golgi tendon organ
II. Control center
   A. Medulla oblongata
   B. Pons
   C. Cerebral cortex
III. Effectors (the respiratory muscles)
   A. Intercostals
   B. Diaphragm
   C. Accessory muscles

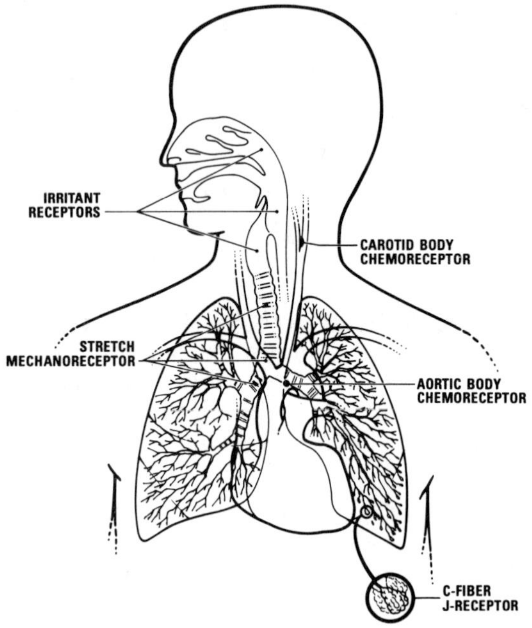
IRRITANT
RECEPTORS
CAROTID BODY
CHEMORECEPTOR
STRETCH
MECHANORECEPTOR
AORTIC BODY
CHEMORECEPTOR
C-FIBER
J-RECEPTOR

Fig. 4-1. Peripheral Sensors. A number of receptors may be responsible for the sensation of dyspnea including irritant, chemo, mechanical and airway (J-receptors).

the mechanoreceptors are the stretch receptors, irritant receptors, C fiber or J receptors, and muscle spindle and Golgi tendon organ.

Stretch receptors are thought to be located among the smooth muscles of the airways [7]. It is believed that they are more prominent in the extrathoracic airways and distributed in a scattered manner [7, 8]. They respond to mechanical changes in lung volumes.

Irritant receptors are distributed predominantly in the upper airway, from the nasal passages to the larynx. Responding to stimuli, they are responsible for many reflexes such as cough and bronchospasm [9].

The C fiber receptors, previously called the J receptors, are located in the lung parenchyma and airways. These fibers have been described as nonmyelinated and closely adherent to the pulmonary capillaries and bronchi [10]. Such a position allows them to respond to various chemical stimuli from the vasculature, as occurs in pulmonary congestion and anaphylaxis, as well as mechanical stimuli from the parenchyma.

The last type of mechanoreceptor is located in the muscles of respiration—the diaphragm, intercostal muscles, and accessory muscles. It is composed of the muscle spindle and the Golgi tendon organ. The exact distribution of each of these in the muscles of respiration is dependent on the additional functions of each muscle. The muscle spindle lies parallel to the normal extrafusal muscle fiber and the Golgi tendon organ lies in a series [1, 2, 4–6].

Control Center

The central nervous system elements involved in the control of respiration and cyclic inspiratory impulses originate in the brain stem. Neurons responsible for inspiratory impulses originate in the dorsal respiratory group, located in the medulla. They are of two types: inhibitory and excitatory, and are stimulated in response to lung inflation [5, 11]. Also located in the medulla are neurons that are associated with both inspiratory and expiratory impulses known as the ventral respiratory group [5, 11]. The ventral respiratory group is responsible for the stimulation of the intercostal and abdominal respiratory motoneurons. The dorsal respiratory group, on the other hand, influences both the phrenic motoneurons and the cells of the ventral respiratory group [5]. It is for these reasons that the dorsal respiratory group has been thought to be the rhythm generator of respiration. Both the dorsal and the ventral respiratory groups are influenced by the impulses arriving from the chemoreceptors and mechanoreceptors and from the cerebral cortex.

The cyclic rhythm of respiration is theorized through the modulation of inspiratory impulses from the dorsal respiratory group. Cells composing the pneumotaxic center in the upper pons have been found to terminate inspiration when stimulated [5, 11]. The exact role of cells in the pneumotaxic center in the modulation of respiratory rhythm is not entirely understood [3, 4, 5, 11].

Theoretical Origins of Dyspnea

Although there is no universally accepted theory to explain the mechanism(s) responsible for the sensation of dyspnea under all circumstances, most authorities believe that dyspnea develops when there is an imbalance between ventilatory demand and ventilatory capacity [12]. This principle of supply and demand is referred to as the oxygen-debt theory. Theoretically, dyspnea occurs when the demand placed on the respiratory muscles exceeds their circulatory supply. This may result in the anaerobic metabolism of glycogen and the production of lactic acid. This anaerobic threshold results in compensatory increases in ventilation and heart rate through neurogenic and humoral stimuli of acidosis and hypercapnia [13, 14]. This threshold is higher than normal in athletes and lower than normal in patients with cardiopulmonary disease. Despite its simplicity, this theory fails to explain the dyspnea experienced by paralyzed patients on total ventilatory support with reduced work of breathing. Further, studies have demonstrated no connection between anaerobic metabolism and the sensation of dyspnea [12].

Increased work of breathing is another theoretical explanation for dyspnea. It is well known that when the work of breathing is changed, the body resets both tidal volume and respiratory rate to minimize this work. Breathlessness is then encountered when an individual senses the change in the amount of work required. This theory suggests that the patient in pulmonary edema who is dyspneic at rest would have a comparable intensity of breathlessness to a normal patient at his or her maximal exercise peak [15–17].

Another theory suggests that the sensation of dyspnea arises from the uninterrupted inspiratory impulses originating in the respiratory center of the medulla. These impulses are normally inhibited via vagal impulses originating from the stretch receptors in the pulmonary parenchyma [18]. Dyspnea, according to this theory, would be due to an overactive medulla or an underactive stretch receptor. This theory is inapplicable to many situations. It does not explain the absence of dyspnea after vagotomy nor why this reflex is almost inoperable at resting tidal volumes [18–20].

The most widely accepted theory which explains the majority of cases of clinical dyspnea is the length-tension inappropriateness relationship developed by Campbell and Howell [1, 2]. This theory suggests that dyspnea occurs when an imbalance exists between the volume of breath achieved (length) and the force of the muscles required to produce it (tension) [1, 2]. A consideration of some basic principles of respiratory physiology is helpful in understanding this theory.

The normal architecture of striated muscle is composed of muscle fibers (referred to as extrafusal muscle fibers) that, through a series of chemical reactions, are responsible for contraction of the muscle. These extrafusal muscle fibers are innervated by large alpha motoneurons that originate in the spinal cord. Strategically enmeshed throughout the muscle are muscle spindles composed of an annulospiral body (the sensory unit), which is attached to its own smaller muscle fibers, called intrafusal muscle fibers (Fig. 4-2). The intrafusal fibers run parallel to the extrafusal fibers and are innervated by gamma motoneurons from the spinal cord. The gamma neurons in turn run parallel to the larger

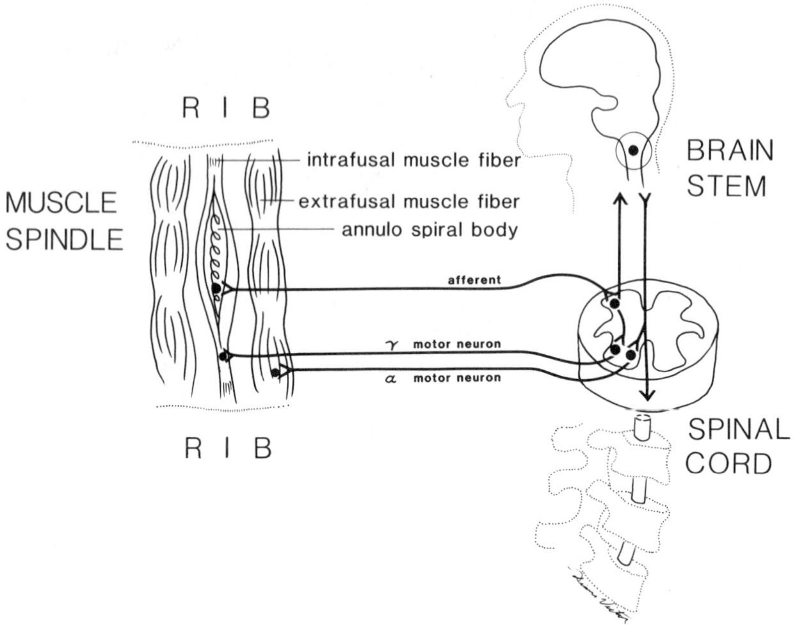
R I B
MUSCLE
SPINDLE
intrafusal muscle fiber
extrafusal muscle fiber
annulo spiral body
afferent
γ motor neuron
α motor neuron
R I B
BRAIN
STEM
SPINAL
CORD

Fig. 4-2. Peripheral Sensor. The muscle spindle. The sensation of dyspnea may occur when the muscle spindle, gamma loop and central nervous system stimulation are dis-synchronous.

alpha motoneurons, both being components of spinal nerves. In addition, each muscle spindle has a sensory afferent communicating with higher centers and the spinal cord.

In normal respiration, contraction of the intrafusal and extrafusal muscle fibers is proportional and synchronous. Intrafusal fiber contraction stretches the muscle spindle, increasing its discharge. Through central communication this increases extrafusal fiber contraction.

It is this function of the gamma loop that Campbell and Howell propose is responsible for the sensation of dyspnea [1, 2]. Accordingly, ventilation is set on the basis of stimuli from various sites throughout the body. Once processed, a tidal volume and frequency are determined to minimize the work of breathing. Impulses are then discharged to the muscles via the alpha and gamma efferent neurons. Normal tidal volume and rate are maintained based on the feedback received. Once there is disproportionate activity between the two muscle fiber groups (extrafusal and intrafusal) the muscle spindle, being contracted more than expected, is activated. This increased activity alerts the respiratory center to alter extrafusal muscle contraction appropriately in an effort to restore equivalence between the two systems. When the discrepancy between the desired and actual muscle length cannot be corrected, the resulting increased spindle discharge is interpreted as dyspnea.

Pathophysiology

There are three main sources of dyspnea. The following is an adaptation of Snider's classification [21].

Classification of Dyspnea

I. Discomfort due to increased ventilatory demand
    A. Proportionate to metabolic stimulation
    B. Disproportionate to metabolic stimulation

1. Organic hyperventilation
2. Psychogenic hyperventilation

II. Discomfort due to decreased ventilatory capacity
   A. Obstructive respiratory disease
      1. Upper airway obstruction
      2. Asthma
      3. Chronic bronchitis, emphysema, and bronchiectasis
   B. Restrictive respiratory disease
      1. Inspiratory muscle impairment
      2. Chest wall impairment
      3. Pulmonary parenchymal disease

III. Discomfort due to insufficient ventilation
   A. Reduction of accustomed ventilation
   B. Breath holding

Cardiac Causes of Dyspnea

Dyspnea develops when there is an imbalance between ventilatory demand and ventilatory capacity [12]. This imbalance involves disruption of either oxygen delivery, carbon dioxide elimination, or both. Oxygen delivery to the tissues is primarily a function of the circulatory system through cardiac output. Cardiac diseases (atherosclerotic, pericardial, and valvular) have as their common disturbance a reduced stroke volume, which is compensated for by an increased heart rate (see Table 4-2) [22]. The increased rate helps to maintain a normal cardiac output. Dyspnea occurs when the increased heart rate can no longer compensate the continued loss in stroke volume.

Dyspnea appears to be the most frequently reported symptom in patients with congestive heart failure (CHF) [23–25]. As the left ventricle fails, there is an increase in the left ventricular diastolic pressure, leading to an increase in left atrial pressure, pulmonary venous pressure, and finally pulmonary capillary pressure. This engorgement of the pulmonary capillary-venous bed is believed to be primarily responsible for the sensation of dyspnea [26]. In this instance the length-tension theory explains shortness of breath because pulmonary congestion increases the resistance to inspiration and alters existing length-tension relationships in the lung [12]. With further leakage of fluid into the interstitial and alveolar areas, additional reductions in the compliance of the lungs result. Ultimately, the Hering-Breuer reflex terminates full inspiration early, which is believed to be responsible for the increased shallow respirations observed.

Another mechanism for breathlessness in congestive heart failure is hypoxemia. The lack of oxygen delivered to the peripheral tissues (brain, kidneys, muscles, etc.) causes a shift to anaerobic metabolism. The accumulation of anaerobic metabolites (lactate and carbon dioxide) are sensed by the chemoreceptors, and an increase in respiratory rate is observed in an attempt to maintain a normal pH.

Patients with high output heart failure experience dyspnea as well, despite low central

Table 4-2. Common Causes of Dyspnea

Cardiac
Acute pulmonary edema
Arrythmias
Congestive heart failure
Myocardial ischemia
Pericarditis
Valvular heart disease
Pulmonary
Acute bronchitis
Asthma
Bronchiectasis
Chronic bronchitis
Emphysema
Interstitial lung disease
Lung cancer
Pleural effusion
Pneumonia
Pneumothorax
Pulmonary embolism
Pulmonary hypertension
Other
Anemia
Cerebral vascular accident
Chest wall/neuromuscular disease
Cirrhosis
Metabolic acidosis
Obesity
Pregnancy
Psychogenic disorder
Thyrotoxicosis

venous pressures. This form of cardiac failure is found in severe anemia, hyperthyroidism, beriberi, arteriovenous malformations, Paget's disease, and sepsis [27, 28]. Initially, these patients do not complain of dyspnea, although they are observed to have rapid, deep respirations similar to Kussmaul's respirations. As the CHF continues, these patients experience dyspnea due to the fatigue of the respiratory muscles.

A second cause of cardiac dyspnea is ischemia and infarction. These events potentially decrease myocardial compliance, leading to increased filling pressures and, as in congestive heart failure, increased elastic resistance of the lung to inspiration. The alteration in the length-tension relationship produces dyspnea.

Valvular heart disease and cardiac arrhythmias are other causes of cardiac dyspnea. Valvular dysfunction may be congenital or acquired, as in rupture of a papillary muscle. In both instances dyspnea follows similar increases in filling pressures, pulmonary congestion, reduced compliance, and dyspoenia. Cardiac arrhythmias, on the other hand, may cause breathlessness by inadequate ventricular filling and/or performance, resulting in decreased cardiac output.

The sensation of breathlessness associated with pericardial disease is less well understood. Patients with as few as 50 to 100 mL of pericardial fluid can experience shortness of breath. The mechanism by which this is sensed remains unclear.

Pulmonary Causes of Dyspnea

Increased ventilation and increased resistance to ventilation are responsible for most of the dyspnea of pulmonary diseases [12]. In pulmonary dyspnea there is an imbalance between external respiration and internal or cellular respiration that results in dyspnea.

For much of pulmonary dyspnea there is a length-tension disparity. As with cardiac dyspnea, several mechanisms may contribute to breathlessness in pulmonary disease. Acute obstructive airways disease such as asthma causes an increased resistance to ventilation through bronchospasm [29]. The resulting increase in the transthoracic pressure gradient requires an increased inspiratory effort to maintain the previously normal tidal volume [12]. Patients experience dyspnea and eventual respiratory failure due to an inability to achieve a new length-tension equilibrium.

Chronic obstructive airways disease such as emphysema, through destruction of lung parenchyma, causes chronic air trapping and increases physiologic dead space (the amount of air left in the lung after a maximal expiration) [30, 31]. Despite a slow accommodation process to the developing length-tension disparity, these patients experience exacerbations with minimal exertion. Respiratory rates are usually increased, with little room for reserve. Their progressive dyspnea is due to an inability to increase mechanical ventilation sufficiently to maintain an adequate alveolar ventilation.

Restrictive lung disease such as interstitial fibrosis and infiltrative disease such as pneumonia affect length-tension relationships in a similar pathophysiologic fashion. Both fibrosis and infiltrative processes increase the elastic recoil of the lung which is normally responsible for passive exhalation [1, 32, 33]. As the elasticity of the lung increases, the compliance reduces and results in increased inspiratory effort to expand a "stiffer" lung. The resulting length-tension alteration causes the sensation of dyspnea.

The acute onset of breathlessness at rest is the dominant feature of pulmonary embolism and is one of the few pulmonary diseases manifested so abruptly. The blockage of a pulmonary segment produces perfusion inequalities such that the contralateral lung may experience pulmonary congestion. Atelectasis can form on the ipsilateral side and on occasion may be seen on chest radiography. These events alter the previous length-tension relationship and require an increased work of breathing, producing dyspnea [1, 34]. Increased airway resistance also has been hypothesized to contribute to the sensation of dyspnea in pulmonary emboli [12].

Primary and secondary pulmonary hypertension may cause right-sided heart failure and pulmonary congestion. This alters previous length-tension relationships and increases the work of breathing and results in breathlessness. Previous theories proposed the existence of pulmonary vasculature receptors that produced dyspnea when stimulated [35].

Other causes of pulmonary dyspnea are pleural effusion and pneumothorax. Pleural effusion has been found to reduce total lung capacity, diffusing capacity, and chest wall and total lung compliance [36]. A pneumothorax may also reduce lung capacity and compliance similarly. Both alter existing length-tension mechanics and produce breathlessness.

Neurologic Causes of Dyspnea

Neurologic disease that produces dyspnea is seldom seen in primary care practice. However, alterations in breathing patterns are common pulmonary manifestations that identify specific neurologic lesions. For example, Cheyne-Stokes respirations usually signify either a lesion in the forebrain or congestive heart failure [37]. Other changes in breathing patterns associated with the forebrain are posthyperventilation apnea [38] and respiratory apraxia, which is the inability to voluntarily change respiratory patterns [39]. Lesions of the midbrain produce hyperventilation and coma [40]. Destruction of the pons usually results in coma, whereas damage to the medulla may destroy all autonomic control [41].

Neurologic diseases of the spinal cord and peripheral nerves produce dyspnea through the paralysis of the respiratory muscles [2]. Diaphragmatic paralysis has been found to produce a more marked dyspnea than intercostal and accessory muscle paralysis alone [21]. In either instance one would then conclude that mechanical ventilation would relieve this sensation of breathlessness. On the contrary, these patients were still found to experience dyspnea despite adequate oxygenation and carbon dioxide elimination [42]. This sensation was relieved with adjustments in tidal volume and the frequency with which the patient hyperventilated. If the rate and depth of this increased ventilation was maintained, the patient was found to tolerate increases in arterial PCO_2. Thus, reducing the tidal volume initiates breathlessness more effectively than changes in the PCO_2 content of the blood. This further supports the case for the role of the length-tension relationship over that of chemical mediation in the sensation of dyspnea.

Other Causes

Another common clinical cause of dyspnea is anemia. It is well known that dyspnea on exertion is experienced in patients with hemoglobin concentrations less than 7 g [43, 44]. The younger age groups are more resilient, and in our experience some patients tolerate decreases in hemoglobin up to 5 g before complaining of breathlessness. Breathlessness in these instances might result from both an increased work of breathing and altered length-tension relationships. The resulting tachycardia and tachypnea observed are compensatory increases in response to the inadequate supply of oxygen due to the anemia.

Various psychological states may manifest themselves through complaints of dyspnea. Frequently a diagnosis of exclusion psychogenic dyspnea occurs predominately at rest and may become worse in crowded areas or be accompanied by the feeling of an inability to fill the lungs [45, 46]. The anxious or hysterical patient may experience shortness of breath during times of emotional unrest [12, 14]. Even after careful questioning about the patient's lifestyle, the etiology may not be uncovered. Such patients may also claim to experience associated chest pains, palpitations, and excessive fatigability. Resolution of the precipitating events usually eliminates all symptoms of dyspnea, although psychotherapeutic treatment may be necessary.

Differential Diagnosis

Much uncertainty is associated with the diagnosis and treatment of dyspnea, according to recent studies. Therefore, patients admitted to hospitals with shortness of breath are often given multiple modes of treatment [47]. The difficulty is in differentiating heart failure from exacerbations of existing lung disease, asthma, or pulmonary embolism. Similar studies, on the other hand, propose that the correct diagnosis can be determined with an accuracy approaching 74% using history alone and 88% by doing a bedside Valsalva's maneuver [48, 49].

In the outpatient setting too, dyspnea presents a major clinical challenge. In most cases, it is caused by cardiac, pulmonary, or emotional disorders, or a combination of these. The initial evaluation should focus on potential organic etiologies for the patient's breathlessness. The possibility of a psychological component is considered after likely organic causes have been ruled out. This of course means that the comprehensive history taken by the primary care physician is of essential importance.

In most instances, dyspnea that is due to cardiac disease can usually be distinguished from other etiologies with a careful history. Shortness of breath that occurs when the patient is lying flat and is relieved when he or she is sitting upright (orthopnea) is characteristically a manifestation of cardiac disease [50, 51]. Awakening at night with shortness of breath (paroxysmal nocturnal dyspnea) may be reported in pulmonary as well as cardiac diseases, but when associated with orthopnea it usually indicates a cardiac event. Other symptoms that suggest a cardiac origin for a patient's dyspnea include substernal chest pain and intermittent swelling in the legs.

There are additional symptoms that help distinguish between dyspnea caused by cardiac disease and that with its origin in a pulmonary disorder. One of these is the character (pressure producing or pleuritic) and nature of the chest pain. The gradual onset of shortness of breath is usually seen in patients with a form of parenchymal lung disease [52–54]. Wheezing is most often associated with asthma (see Chap. 8), although it may be occasionally confused with the wheezing associated with cardiac failure [24, 55]. White, frothy sputum may be seen in heart failure, whereas purulent, yellow and green sputum usually indicates an infectious pulmonary process.

The physical examination may further help differentiate cardiac from pulmonary etiologies of breathlessness. Physical findings such as distention of neck veins, the presence of an S_3 gallop, bilateral rales, and dependent edema are seen in congestive heart failure. Chronic inflammatory lung disease and fibrosis have associated rales, which are often high pitched and of a crackling nature. Isolated S_3 gallops of the right side of the heart may be found in patients with cor pulmonale, the right-sided heart failure associated with pulmonary disease. Audible wheezing may be noted in patients with both heart failure and asthma, but prolonged expiration is usually seen in obstructive lung disease [29, 30, 51].

Hyperresonance to percussion and an increased anteroposterior diameter are found exclusively in obstructive airways disease. Dullness to percussion, on the other hand, may be found in many unrelated problems such as pneumonic consolidation, pleural effusion, or fibrosis. When such dullness is associated with fever and bronchial breath sounds, it is most likely a pneumonic process. Finally, clubbing in the middle-aged or elderly population is usually associated with advanced lung disease, although it may also be seen in cyanotic heart disease.

Ancillary measures may help to differentiate situations where the history and physical examination are less clear. For example, the chest radiograph of an individual with obstructive lung disease will have varying degrees of a small cardiac silhouette, flattened diaphragms, and avascularity of peripheral lung fields, with possible bullae formation. In comparison, the chest radiograph of a patient with cardiac dyspnea may show evidence of an enlarged heart, pulmonary vessel engorgement, Kerley's lines, pleural effusions, or the classic butterfly pattern of interstitial edema (see Chap. 26).

Electrocardiograms also may be helpful. Patients with long-standing lung disease may show evidence of enlarged p waves over the inferior limb leads, suggesting P-pulmonale of advanced lung disease. Arterial blood gases can be of use because carbon dioxide retention may suggest advanced lung disease and elevation of the alveolar-arterial gradient may support a clinical diagnosis of pulmonary embolus. Pulmonary function studies give useful objective and diagnostic information as evidence of obstructive or restrictive disease (see Chap. 2).

The exercise test is useful to differentiate cardiac, pulmonary, and psychogenic dyspnea [56]. Significant hyperventilation at low workloads is highly suspicious of pulmonary disease. On the other hand, a disproportionate increase in heart rate at all workloads is highly suggestive of cardiac disease [14, 15, 22, 45, 57]. In psychogenic dyspnea patients display an inappropriate initial elevation in ventilation and heart rate and, as the workload increases, ventilation and heart rate become entirely normal and appropriate [45, 58–60].

As previously mentioned, the psychological aspects of disease processes are important in all patients. If the history, physical examination, and ancillary tests have proved negative in establishing a diagnosis on an organic basis, then the physician must consider possible psychosocial etiologies and formal exercise testing [45, 58–60].

Dyspnea can be thought of as the conscious sensation of the inability to breathe comfortably in a given setting. In all instances breathlessness appears due to an imbalance between ventilatory capacity and ventilatory demand. Although there appears to be agreement as to the probable neural and sensory pathways involved in the control of respiration, there is no single theory explaining the mechanism responsible for the sensation of breathlessness. Many situations are best explained by more than one theory. It has been the purpose of this chapter to review the common disease processes involved in the generation of dyspnea for the primary care physician.

References

1. Howell JBL, Campbell EJM: Breathlessness in pulmonary disease. *Scand J Respir Dis* 48:321, 1967
2. Campbell EJM, Howell JBL: The sensation of breathlessness. *Br Med Bull* 19:36, 1963
2a. Borg GAV, Psychological basis of perceived exertion. *Med Sci Sports Exerc* 14:377–81, 1982
2b. Simon PM, Schwartzstein RM, Weiss JW, et al; Distinguishable types of dyspnea in patients with shortness of breath. *Am Rev Respir Dis* 142:1009–1014, 1990
3. West JB: Respiratory Physiology—The Essentials, ed 2. Baltimore, Williams & Wilkins, 1979, p 114
4. Seaton A, Seaton D, Leitch AG: Crofton and Douglas's Respiratory Diseases, ed 4. Boston, Blackwell Scientific, 1989, pp 55–56
5. Berger AJ: Control of Breathing. *In* Murray JF, Nadel JA (eds): Textbook of Respiratory Medicine, ed 1. Philadelphia, WB Saunders, 1988, pp 149–164
6. Lahiri S, Delaney RG: Stimulus interaction in the response to carotid body chemoreceptor single afferent fibers. *Respir Physiol* 24:249, 1975
7. Widdingcombe JG: The site of pulmonary stretch receptors in the cat. *J Physiol* 125:336, 1954
8. Bartlett D Jr, Jeffrey P, Sant'Ambrogio G, et al: Location of stretch receptors in the trachea and bronchi of the dog. *J Physiol* 258:409, 1976
9. Widdingcombe JG: Reflex control of airway smooth muscle. *Postgrad Med J* 51(suppl):7, 1975
10. Coleridge JCG, Coleridge HMG: Afferent vagal C-fiber innervation of the lungs and airways and its functional significance. *Rev Physiol Biochem Pharmacol* 99:1, 1984
11. Mitchell RA, Berger AJ: Neural regulation of respiration. *Am Rev Respir Dis* 111:206, 1975
12. Rappaport E: Dyspnea: Pathophysiology and differential diagnosis. *Prog Cardiovasc Dis* 13:532, 1971
13. Wasserman K, Whipp B, Koyal S, et al: Anaerobic threshold and respiratory gas exchange during exercise. *J Appl Physiol* 35:236, 1973
14. Wasserman K, Whipp BJ: Exercise physiology in health and work. *Am Rev Respir Dis* 112:219, 1975
15. Killian KJ, Gandevia SC, Summers E, et al: Effect of increased lung volume on perception of breathlessness, effort, and tension. *J Appl Physiol* 57:686, 1984
16. Killian KJ: The objective measurement of breathlessness. *Chest* 88:85s, 1985
17. Bowie DM, Killian KJ, Summers E, et al:

Breathlessness—The sense of respiratory effort. *Clin Invest Med* 7s:80, 1983
18. Wright GW, Branscomb BV: The origin of the sensation of dyspnea. *Trans Am Clin Climatol Assoc* 66:116, 1954
19. Guz A, Noble M, Widdingcombe JG, et al: The role of vagal and glossapharyngeal afferent nerves in respiratory sensation, control of breathing, and arterial pressure regulation in man. *Clin Sci* 30:161, 1966
20. Guz A, Noble M, Trenchard D, et al: Studies on the vagus nerve in man. Their role in respiratory and circulatory control. *Clin Sci* 27:293, 1964
21. Snider GL: Physiologic causes of dyspnea. Advances in Cardiopulmonary *Disease* 4:145, 1969
22. Wasserman K: Dyspnea on exertion. *JAMA* 248:2039, 1982
23. Braunwald E: Heart failure. *In* Braunwald E (ed): Harrison's Principles of Internal Medicine, ed 11. New York, McGraw-Hill, 1987, p 908
24. Ingram RH, Braunwald E: Dyspnea and pulmonary edema. *In* Braunwald E (ed): Harrison's Principles of Internal Medicine, ed 11. New York, McGraw-Hill, 1987, pp 141–147
25. Cohn J: Approach to the patient with heart failure. *In* Kelley W (ed): Textbook of Internal Medicine, ed 1. Philadelphia, Lippincott, 1989, p 380
26. Hughes R, May AJ, Widdingcombe JG: The effect of pulmonary congestion and edema on lung compliance. *J Physiol* 142:306, 1958
27. Smith TW: Heart failure. *In* Wyngaarden JB, Smith LH (eds): Cecil's Textbook of Internal Medicine, ed 11. Philadelphia, WB Saunders, 1988, p 215
28. Fowler NH: High output cardiac states. *In* Hurst JW (ed): The Heart, ed 6. New York, McGraw-Hill, 1986, p 395
29. Woolcock A: Asthma. *In* Murray JF, Nadel JA (eds): Textbook of Respiratory Medicine, 1988, p 1030
30. Seaton A, Seaton D, Leitch AG: Chronic bronchitis and emphysema. *In* Seaton A, Seaton D, Leitch AG (eds): Crofton and Douglas' Respiratory Diseases, ed 4. Boston, Blackwell, 1989, p 490
31. Snider GL: Chronic bronchitis and emphysema. *In* Murray JF, Nadel JA (eds): Textbook of Respiratory Medicine. Philadelphia, WB Saunders, 1988, p 1069
32. Crystal RG: Idiopathic pulmonary fibrosis. *Ann Intern Med* 85:769, 1976
33. Hay JG, Turner-Warwick M: Interstitial pulmonary fibrosis. *In* Murray JF, Nadel JA (eds): Textbook of Respiratory Medicine. Philadelphia, WB Saunders, 1988, p 1445
34. Goff AM, Geansler EA: Respiratory pathophysiology in chronic progressive pulmonary vascular disease. *Ir J Med Sci* 6:213, 1967
35. Luce J: Vasculitis, primary pulmonary hypertension and arteriovenous fistulas. *In* Murray JF, Nadel JA (eds): Textbook of Respiratory Medicine. Philadelphia, WB Saunders, 1988, p 1328
36. Yoo OH, Ting EY: The effects of pleural effusion on pulmonary function. *Am Rev Respir Dis* 89:55, 1964
37. Brown HW, Plum F: The neurologic basis of Cheyne-Stokes respiration. *Am J Med* 30:849, 1961
38. Plum F, Brown HW, Snoep E: Neurologic significance of post-hyperventilation apnea. *JAMA* 181:1050, 1962
39. Hebertson W, Talbert OR, Cohen ME: Respiratory apraxia and anosognosia. *Tran Am Neurol* A 84:176, 1959
40. Plum F, Swanson AG: Central neurogenic hyperventilation in man. *AMA Archives of Neurol. and Psychiat.* 81:535, 1959
41. Plum F, Swanson AG: Abnormalities in central regulation of respiration in acute and convalescent poliomyelitis. *AMA Archives of Neurol. and Psychiat.* 80:267, 1958
42. Smith SM, Brown HO, Toman JEP, et al: The lack of cerebral effects of d-tubocurarine. *Anesthesiology* 8:144, 1947
43. Porter WB, James GW: The heart in anemia. *Circulation* 8:111, 1953
44. Bunn HF: Anemia. *In* Braunwald E (ed): Harrison's Principles of Internal Medicine. New York, McGraw-Hill 1987, p 262
45. Whipp BJ, Wasserman K: Exercise. *In* Murray JF, Nadel JA (eds): Textbook of Respiratory Medicine. Philadelphia, WB Saunders, 1988, p 191
46. Partridge M: Symptoms that depress the doctor: Difficulty in breathing. *Br J Hosp Med* 84:288, 1984
47. Pearson SB, Pearson EM, Mitchell JRA: The diagnosis and management of patients admitted to the hospital with acute breathlessness. *Postgrad Med J* 57:419, 1981
48. Zema MJ, Masters AP, Margouleff D: Dyspnea: The heart or the lungs? *Chest* 85:59, 1984
49. Schmitt BP, Kushner MS, Weiner SL: The diagnostic usefulness of the history of the patient with dyspnea. *J Gen Intern Med* 1:389, 1986
50. Williams ES: Essential features of the cardiac history and physical examination. *In* Kelley W (ed): Textbook of Internal Medicine. Philadelphia, Lippincott, 1989, p 284
51. Braunwald E: Symptoms of heart failure. *In* Braunwald E (ed): Heart Disease, ed. Philadelphia, WB Saunders, 1988, p 475
52. Logue RB, Robinson PH: Differential diagno-

sis of congestive heart failure. *Prog Cardiovasc Dis* 13:55, 1970
53. ALA/ATS Committee on Disability Criteria: Evaluation of impairment/disability secondary to respiratory disease. *Am Rev Respir Dis* 126:945, 1982
54. Fishman AP, Szidan PJ: Approach to the pulmonary patient with respiratory signs and symptoms. *In* Fishman AP (ed): Pulmonary Diseases and Disorders, ed 2. New York, McGraw-Hill, 1988, p 325
55. Reynolds HY, Bashaer RE: Approach to the patient with respiratory disease. *In* Stein JH (ed): Internal Medicine, ed 3. Boston, Little, Brown, 1990, p 631
56. Becklake MR: Organic or functional impairment. *Am Rev Respir Dis* 129:s96, 1984
57. Jones NL, Jones G, Edwards RHT: Exercise tolerance in chronic airway obstruction. *Am Rev Respir Dis* 103:477, 1971
58. Jones NL: Exercise testing in pulmonary evaluation: Rationale, methods and the normal respiratory response to exercise. *N Engl J Med* 293:541, 1975
59. Jones NL: Exercise testing in pulmonary evaluation: Clinical applications. *N Engl J Med* 293:647, 1975
60. Jones NL: Exercise testing. *Br J Dis Chest* 61:169, 1967

Cough

Angela DeSantis

Cough is an important physiologic reflex that acts to protect the lung from various injuries. However, cough can also be an initiating pathologic event that may be the only manifestation of underlying disease. The two most important aspects in diagnostic evaluation of a patient with cough are the history and physical examination. When a specific cause for a cough is found, treatment should be directed at that cause. This chapter outlines the pathophysiology of the cough reflex, specific causes of cough commonly seen in primary care practice, and basic guidelines as to the evaluation and treatment of cough.

Functions of Cough

Cough begins with stimulation of cough receptors. It is believed that nerve endings are the mechanoreceptors and chemoreceptors responsible for cough and other respiratory defense mechanisms such as bronchoconstriction and increased mucous secretion [1, 2]. Three categories of cough stimuli are often involved: mechanical, inflammatory, and psychogenic. Acute or chronic exposure to environmental irritants, dusts, and gases may directly trigger the cough reflex or induce inflammatory changes in the respiratory mucosa. Mechanical stimuli of cough include those conditions that cause distortion of airways [3]. Finally, a diagnosis of psychogenic cough should be considered only as a diagnosis of exclusion.

Mediators of the Cough Reflex

Coughing can easily be stimulated by mechanical or chemical stimulation of the mucosa of the larynx, trachea, and large bronchi, where most of the receptors are found (Fig. 5-1). These neuroreceptors are thought to mediate their responses through afferent vagal pathways [4]. Almost nothing is known of the central nervous system organization of the cough reflex, although a medullary cough center has been postulated. The musculoskeletal effectors of the cough reflex include the muscles of the larynx, trachea, bronchi, accessory respiratory muscles, abdominal lumbar muscles, and the diaphragm. It has also been suggested that increased amounts of inflammatory mediators such as bradykinin, prostaglandins, and histamine attribute to increased cough reflex [5].

Mechanism

Initiation of reflex coughing begins with irritation of a receptor. There are three phases of the cough mechanism involved in producing high velocity airflow that is important for an effective cough. First, the inspiratory phase involves inhaling a large volume of air to allow maximum expiratory flow rates. Next, the compressive phase begins with closure of the glottis and involves raising intrathoracic pressure enough to produce high flow rates. Finally, in the expiratory phase, the glottis opens and the forced release of air results in removal of undesired material from the respiratory tract [6]. Glottic closure is not essential however for an effective cough because the muscles of expiration can produce enough increase in intrathoracic pressures even with an open glottis. In reviewing these mechanisms, it may be more apparent that patients with various skeletal and neuromuscular disorders may not cough effectively when their efforts are limited due to pain,

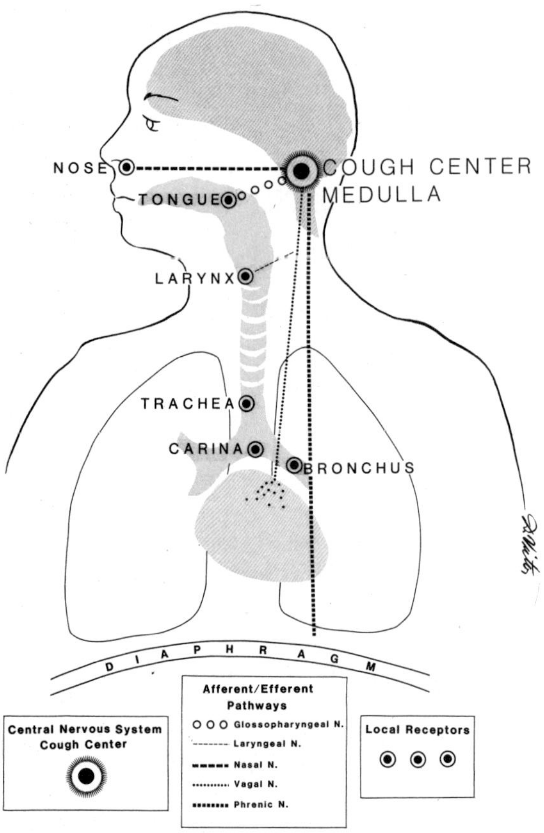
NOSE
TONGUE
COUGH CENTER
MEDULLA
LARYNX
TRACHEA
CARINA
BRONCHUS
DIAPHRAGM
Central Nervous System Cough Center
Afferent/Efferent Pathways
Glossopharyngeal N.
Laryngeal N.
Nasal N.
Vagal N.
Phrenic N.
Local Receptors

Fig. 5-1. Mediators of the cough reflex. Neuroreceptors and pathways generating cough.

weakness, or central nervous system depression [7].

Specific Etiologies of Cough

Acute Infections

The most common cause of an acute self-limiting cough is the common cold (Table 5-1). Viral upper respiratory infections are the most common cause of cough in all age groups [8]. This cough is typically paroxysmal and worse at night and is most commonly caused by postnasal drip of mucus that stimulates receptors in the pharynx [7]. Bacterial infections of the upper respiratory tract causing sinusitis and tracheobronchitis may also cause cough. *Streptococcus pneumoniae* and *Hemophilus influenzae* are most commonly cultured, but *Mycoplasma* and *Legionella* are also found [2]. Cough is a very common symptom of patients who have pneumonia, being present in almost every patient at some time during their illness. This cough usually produces a purulent sputum and is associated with fever, chills, sweats, or other constitutional symptoms such as weakness, fatigue, and generalized malaise.

Chronic Infections

In patients with chronic lower respiratory tract infections, a cough may be the only symptom that brings the patient to the physician. Bronchiectasis is a relatively uncommon condition encountered in clinical practice today. However, before the development of antibiotics, it was second only to tuberculosis in incidence as a cause for cough [2]. Often present since childhood, the cough in bronchiectasis is productive of large amounts of foul, purulent secretions. When the sputum is allowed to settle, it separates into three layers: a foamy top layer, a serous intermediate layer, and bottom layer of pus and debris. Tuberculosis, fungal infections, and lung abscesses may also present with persistent cough for weeks to months, often with blood-tinged sputum [3].

Chronic Obstructive Pulmonary Disease and Chronic Bronchitis

Cough is seen in most patients with chronic obstructive lung disease. Smoking is the most commonly implicated factor in chronic cough [9]. Cigarette smokers have the highest prevalence of cough, followed by pipe and cigar smokers [7]. In patients with chronic bronchitis, cough may be the result of any or all of the following mechanisms. First, cigarette smoke may directly stimulate cough receptors and second, it may cause production of secretions.

It has recently been suggested that chronic cough may be an indicator of worsening lung function in cigarette smokers [36]. The smoker's cough is characteristically increased in the morning, producing a mucoid sputum. When the quality of the cough changes and persists for several weeks, bronchogenic carcinoma should be considered [2, 10].

Table 5-1. Cough: Causes and Diagnostic Clues

Cause	*History*	*Diagnostic Test*
Acute infection	Fever, chills, rhinorrhea	Sputum evaluation, chest radiography
Chronic infection	Night sweats, weight loss; hemoptysis may be present	Sputum evaluation, chest radiography
Chronic bronchitis	Cigarette smoker; loose productive cough increased in the morning	Obstructive airways disease by pulmonary function tests
Tumors	Change in cough or new cough in a smoker; hemoptysis is common	Mass lesion on chest radiograph, sputum cytology, bronchoscopy, laryngoscopy
Parenchymal disease	Nonproductive cough worse on deep inspiration	Abnormal chest radiograph, restrictive pattern by pulmonary function tests, diagnosis by open lung biopsy
Foreign body	Sudden onset of cough after choking	Abnormal chest radiograph, radiopaque object
Cardiovascular	Dyspnea on exertion, orthopnea, P.N.D.	Cardiomegaly, pleural effusion on chest radiograph, two-dimensional echocardiogram
Drug induced	Specific drug by history	Cough improves after stopping drug
Sinusitis	Postnasal drip, throat clearing, headache	Sinus radiography, nasal smear, fiberoptic rhinoscopy
Asthma	Associated with wheezing, dyspnea, nonproductive, paroxysmal	Reversible airways obstruction by spirometry, methacholine challenge helpful, eosinophilia, IgE level
Aspiration syndrome	Choking history; elderly patients with swallowing difficulties	Barium swallow
Psychogenic cough	Pediatric/adolescent population, honking or barking, disruptive, no nocturnal cough	Diagnosis of exclusion

Tumors

Various benign and malignant tumors of the airways may produce cough. Benign tumors of the larynx and laryngeal carcinoma must be considered in a patient with a new cough, especially when associated with hoarseness. Cough is a common symptom in patients with bronchogenic carcinoma, occurring in 70% to 90% of patients. Cough may also be the earliest sign in up to 20% of patients [11]. The character of the cough may be nonproductive to productive and be present for weeks to months. Recurrent small amounts of hemoptysis is common and may be seen in 50% of cases [2]. Patients may have other symptoms, including anorexia, weight loss, malaise, and fever. The chest radiograph is almost always abnormal, with some evidence of a mass lesion, adenopathy, or pleural effusion. The presence of an isolated cough, without other clinical or roentgenographic evidence of lung cancer, is rarely due to tumor [12].

Parenchymal Diseases

Cough is present in most patients with interstitial lung disease [13]. Common disorders in this group include interstitial lung disease associated with the collagen vascular disorders, sarcoidosis, and idiopathic pulmonary fibrosis. Most other causes are relatively uncommon. Idiopathic pulmonary fibrosis is the classic interstitial lung disease of unknown etiology. A current or distant inflammatory process has caused fibroblasts to proliferate, resulting in distortion and distention of the airways from the fibrotic tissue. Cough is usually worsened by deep breathing because of further distention of the airways. Typical chest radiographic findings are usually present and the diagnosis requires an open lung biopsy (see Chapter 11) [13].

Foreign Body

A trapped foreign body may cause an acute and later chronic cough if not expelled. The foreign material causes an immediate cough while still in the upper airway and may result in progressive asphyxiation. Later when the foreign body becomes lodged in the lower airway, it often results in a persistent nonproductive cough associated with localized wheeze [3].

Cardiovascular

More common cardiovascular etiologies for cough include left ventricular failure, with resultant pulmonary edema. The cough in left ventricular failure intensifies when the patient is supine, along with worsening of the dyspnea. In cases of pulmonary infarction, cough is often associated with hemoptysis and pleural effusion. There have also been case reports of cough caused by diseases of the pericardium and even pacemaker wires [7].

Drug Induced

There are rare case reports in the literature of cough being secondary to specific drugs. Drug-induced cough may be a manifestation of bronchial hyperreactivity in the absence of wheezing [14]. Nonproductive cough may also be a prominent symptom in drug-induced pulmonary injury. Bleomycin and amiodarone cause direct lung injury. With bleomycin, this is a dose-limiting toxic effect that may occur in up to 10% of patients. Amiodarone use may cause pulmonary fibrosis and persistent nonproductive cough [15]. Both selective and nonselective β-blockers have been associated with cough. Examples of these include such drugs as Lopressor (metoprolol tartrate), Sectral (acebutolol hydrochloride), Tenormin (atenolol), and Inderal (propranolol hydrochloride). The proposed mechanism is by increasing bronchial tone.

The cough associated with angiotensin-converting enzyme inhibitors, captopril and enalapril has been extensively reported in the literature. This cough is characterized as persistent and nonproductive, with an irritating sensation in the throat. It may become worse on lying down and has been reported to cause sleep disturbances. The cough usually takes several weeks to appear. However, it may show within hours of the first dose or be delayed for months [16–18]. The cough has been reported as a side effect of at least four angiotensin-converting enzyme inhibitors and occurs more frequently in women [19].

The exact mechanism by which angiotensin-converting enzyme inhibitors cause cough is still unknown. It has been suggested that it is related to the accumulation of bradykinins, prostaglandins, or to a sensitizing process [10, 19, 21]. Recent literature concludes that the development of cough secondary to angiotensin-converting enzyme inhibitors is not associated with airflow obstruction or airway hyperresponsiveness [20, 22]. It is important to recognize cough as a possible side effect of the angiotensin-converting enzyme inhibitors and reduce the dose or discontinue treatment with these drugs. In this instance, discontinuing the drug usually eliminates the cough.

Cough Variants

Asthma

The three cardinal symptoms of asthma are wheezing, dyspnea, and cough. Although wheezing is considered the sine qua non of asthma, McFadden [23] reported cases where cough was the predominant or at times the only presenting symptom of asthma. Cough in these patients was described as nonproductive, intractable, and paroxysmal [23]. Despite the absence of wheezing, reversible airways obstruction can be shown by pulmonary function testing. Cough in these patients disappears with bronchodilator therapy. Unlike patients with typical asthma, cough variant asthmatic patients do not show obvious obstruction unless stimulated by bronchoconstricting agents or exercise [24]. The degree of coughing induced by these agents also seems to be more pronounced than that in other asthmatic patients. Cough variant asthma has been identified as a common cause of cough in children and young adults. Often the cough is worse at night and following vigorous exercise. A therapeutic trial of bronchodilator such as theophylline or β-agonist can be given. If this eliminates the cough, a presumptive diagnosis can be made [25, 26].

Aspiration Syndrome

This syndrome may present with chronic cough, with or without sputum production. It is most commonly seen in elderly patients but may also be seen in patients with neuromuscular disorders interfering with normal swallowing or in patients with primary esophageal disease. The patient may give a history of choking on liquids or solids. The modified barium swallow is increasingly being used to diagnose aspiration syndromes, especially in the elderly. A high index of suspicion is necessary to consider this diagnosis in a patient with no other cause of cough [2].

Psychogenic Cough

Psychogenic habit cough is a debilitating condition that is described mostly in pediatric and adolescent populations, but has been reported in adults. This cough is a persistent barking or honking that is disruptive to normal daily activity. Although the condition is not rare, this is a diagnosis of exclusion. There is no objective laboratory evidence of disease. Patients are usually best treated with combination psychotherapy, relaxation, and speech therapy [27].

Chronic Cough

Most of the previously mentioned conditions can result in chronic persistent cough if they go untreated for a period of time. However, it has been shown that more than 90% of cases of chronic cough are due to four common diagnoses: postnasal drip syndrome, asthma, chronic bronchitis, and gastroesophageal reflux. First, chronic postnasal drip is the most common cause of cough in nonsmokers. It is seen in persons with allergic rhinitis, chronic sinusitis, and nasopharyngeal obstruction by enlarged adenoids. These patients often respond well to antihistamines [28, 29].

Next, asthmatic patients and patients with chronic obstructive pulmonary disease are often treated with bronchodilators that may decrease the lower esophageal sphincter tone and encourage reflux. Therefore, in patients with refractory asthma, recurrent pneumonia, or chronic cough, an evaluation for reflux would be necessary, especially in cases that are poorly responsive to therapy.

Finally, cough may be the sole presenting manifestation in gastroesophageal reflux. It has been reported to cause chronic cough with frequencies between 9% and 21% [29, 30]. Lung and airway involvement during reflux may take several forms, including chronic cough, asthma, pneumonia, and interstitial fibrosis. Recurrent lung injury and pneumonia may result from direct contact with gastric acid. Also, aspirated gastric, esophageal, or pharyngeal bacteria may contribute to further lung injury. It has been suggested that vagal mechanisms are responsible for generation of the cough and actual aspiration of gastric contents is not required for stimulating bronchospasm or chronic cough [30].

Complications of Cough

Complications of cough more commonly involve musculoskeletal problems. These may include painful muscle strain, muscle rupture, and even rib fractures along the lateral margins of the rib cage. Pneumomediastinum and pneumothorax are examples of more severe complications. Chronic cough has also been associated with constitutional symptoms such as fatigue, insomnia, headache, and anorexia [7].

Cough syncope is an alarming symptom that sometimes follows a coughing spasm.

This usually occurs within a few seconds after the onset of cough and is usually without major consequence. However, there have been reports of high-grade heart block caused by increase in vagal tone associated with cough [31]. Cough syncope is more common in men, usually of stocky build and who are heavy smokers [32]. Cough is a modified Valsalva maneuver. There is increased intrathoracic pressure, decreased venous return, decreased cardiac output, and then cerebral hypoxia, which results in syncope.

Diagnostic Evaluations

History and Physical Examination

The most common causes of cough can usually be established by a history and physical examination. Specific questions concerning the duration and character of cough, smoking history, environmental and occupational exposures, asthma, and allergies are essential. Special attention to the nose, throat, ears, sinuses, and lower respiratory tract may yield vital information.

Character of the Cough

Timing of the cough may be useful in determining its origin. Most people with chronic cough complain that it is worse at night, especially those with postnasal drip. The patient with chronic bronchitis expectorates on arising in the morning. The character and quality of expectorated sputum may also suggest the diagnosis.

Supplemental Tests

When the history and physical examination do not reveal the cause of a cough, laboratory tests may be appropriate. A complete blood count as well as total eosinophil count may be helpful in diagnosing infections or allergic conditions. Sinus and chest radiography may reveal disease not apparent on physical examination. When chest radiography is normal, it is unlikely that the cause of the cough is anything other than postnasal drip, chronic bronchitis, asthma, or gastroesophageal reflux.

Pulmonary Function Tests and Bronchoscopy

Pulmonary function tests may show obstructive and restrictive disease even when the physical examination is normal. These are most helpful in assessing asthma as a cause for chronic cough. Pulmonary function tests should be performed with methacholine challenge (see Chap. 2) in an attempt to identify hyperreactive airways consistent with asthma [33].

To date, most studies suggest that bronchoscopy is of limited value in determining the cause of chronic cough unless the chest radiograph is abnormal. Sputum cytology examination should be considered early in evaluating a patient with persistent cough and a normal chest radiograph. In smokers and those over 50 years of age, it can be a cost-effective tool in deciding whether or not bronchoscopy should be performed. Bronchoscopy may be reserved for the patient in whom the cause of the cough cannot be identified by history, physical examination, chest radiography, and pulmonary function testing [34].

Therapy

Definitive Treatment

After a careful history, physical examination, and a specific cause of cough has been identified, therapy should be directed at that cause. It may involve antibiotics for pneumonia and sinusitis or cessation of smoking in patients with chronic bronchitis. Antihistamines may be needed in patients with allergic rhinitis and postnasal drip, whereas bronchodilators are the mainstay of therapy for cough variant asthma. Only when the cause of the cough is unknown and persists, causing great discomfort to the patient, should symptomatic treatment be considered (Table 5-2) [2].

Symptomatic Treatment

Antitussive Agents

These agents are designed to suppress cough that serves no useful purpose. They may be classified as either centrally or peripherally

Table 5-2. Symptomatic Treatment of Cough

	Dosage	*Side Effects*	*Commercial Preparations*
Antitussives			
Opioids			
Codeine phosphate Codeine sulfate	10–20 mg every 4–6 h (maximum 120 mg/d)	Nausea, vomiting, constipation, dizziness, rarely respiratory depression	Actifed with Codeine Naldecon-CX Phenergan with Codeine Robitussin AC/DAC Tussi-Organidin
Hydrocodone bitartrate	5–10 mg every 6–8 h	Stronger dependence liability than codeine	Hycodan Tussend Tussinex
Nonopiates			
Benzonatate	100–200 mg every 6–8 h	Rash, constipation, headache	Tessalon
Dextromethorphan hydrobromide	10–20 mg every 4–6 h	Drowsiness, nausea, dizziness	Benylin DM Robitussin DM Rondee-DM Tussi-Organidin
Expectorants			
Guaifenesin (glyceryl guaiacolate)	200–400 mg every 4 h (maximum 2.4 g/d)	Drowsiness, nausea, false-positive 5-HIAA, VMA (vanillylmandelic acid)	Breonesin Glycotuss Robitussin

acting. Central cough suppression acts at the medullary centers, whereas peripheral cough suppression acts at the site of irritation or at the cough receptor. The centrally acting group includes the opioid derivatives and the nonopioid, nonnarcotic agent, dextromethorphan. The peripherally acting group includes agents with local anesthetic and analgesic activity as well as expectorants and mucolytics [35].

Expectorants

This class of drugs increase sputum volume, promoting the expulsion of secretions. Glyceryl guaiacolate (Guaifenesin) is a frequent ingredient in combination cough medicines. Guaifenesin is currently the most widely used, and this agent as well as ammonium salts and iodide salts are common ingredients of many cough mixtures [34].

Mucolytics

The solubilizing action of these agents may make thick, tenacious secretions easier to eliminate. They are usually given by inhalation and therefore generally used in hospital settings. The one most widely used is acetylcysteine (Mucomyst). However, these agents are often irritating and may induce bronchospasm, and for this reason must usually be given simultaneously with a bronchodilator. Most commercial cough preparations are combinations of antitussives, expectorants, sympathomimetics, and antihistamines [5, 35, 36, 37].

Conclusion

Thus, cough is an essential mechanism of respiratory defense. As a general rule, cough represents some organic disease. For this reason, the evaluation and treatment of cough is of great importance.

References

1. Korpas J: Recent advances concerning the cough reflex. *Acta Physiol Hung* 70:161–165, 1987
2. Braman SS, Carrao WM: Cough differential diagnosis and treatment. *Clin Chest Med* 8: 177–188, 1987
3. Fishman AP: Pulmonary Diseases and Disorders, ed 2. New York, McGraw-Hill, 1988, pp 342–346
4. Sant'Ambrogio G: Afferent pathways for the cough reflex. *Bull Eur Physiopathol Respir* 19–23, 1987
5. Choudry NB, Fuller RW, Pride NB: Sensitivity of the human cough reflex: Effect of inflammatory mediators prostaglandin E2, bradykinin, and histamine. *Am Rev Respir Dis* 140:137–141, 1989
6. Leith DE: The development of cough. *Am Rev Respir Dis* 131:39–42, 1985
7. Irwin RS, Rosen MJ, Braman SS: Cough: A comprehensive review. *Arch Intern Med* 137: 1186, 1977
8. Curley FJ, Irwin RS, Pratter MR, et al: Cough and the common cold. *Am Rev Respir Dis* 138:305–311, 1988
9. Loudon RG: Smoking and cough frequency. *Am Rev Respir Dis* 114:1033, 1976
10. Power JT, Stewart IC, Connaughton JJ, et al: Nocturnal cough in patients with chronic bronchitis and emphysema. *Am Rev Respir Dis* 130:999, 1984
11. Hyde L, Hyde CI: Clinical manifestations of lung cancer. *Chest* 65:299, 1974
12. Poe RH, Harder RV, Israel RH, et al: Chronic persistent cough. *Chest* 95:723–728, 1989
13. Crystal RG, Fulmer JD, Roberts WC: Idiopathic pulmonary fibrosis. *Ann Intern Med* 85:759, 1976
14. Kaufman J, Casanova JE, Riendl P, et al: Bronchial hyperactivity and cough due to angiotensin-converting-enzyme inhibitors. *Chest* 95:544–548, 1989
15. Rakita L, Sobol SM, Mostown, et al: Amiodarone pulmonary toxicity. *Am Heart J* 106:1983
16. Caruthers SG: Severe coughing during captopril and enalapril therapy. *Can Med Assoc J* 135:217, 1986
17. Hallwright GP, Maling TBT, Toun GI: Enalapril and cough: Case report. *NZ Med J* 99:66, 1986
18. Sesoko S, Kaneko Y: Cough associated with the use of captopril. *Arch Intern Med* 145: 1524, 1985
19. Berkin KE: Respiratory effects of angiotensin converting enzyme inhibition. *Eur Respir J* 2: 198–201, 1989
20. Lindgren BR: New aspects on inflammatory reactions and cough following inhibition of angiotensin-converting-enzyme. *Acta Physiol Scand* 1–60, 1988
21. Rumore MM: Cough induced by angiotensin-converting-enzyme inhibitors. *Clin Pharm* 8: 11–12, 1989
22. Boulet LP, Milot J, Lampron N, et al: Pulmonary function and airway responsiveness during long-term therapy with captopril. *JAMA* 261:413–416, 1989
23. McFadden ER Jr: Exertional dyspnea and cough as preludes to acute attacks of bronchial asthma. *N Engl J Med* 292:555, 1975
24. Corrao LOM: Chronic cough as the sole presenting manifestation of bronchial asthma. *N Engl J Med* 300:633, 1979
25. Braman S, Pordy W, Corrao WM, et al: Cough variant asthma: A 3–5 year follow-up. *Am Rev Respir Dis* 125:133, 1982
26. Frans A: Cough as the sole manifestation of airway hyperreactivity. *J Laryngol Otol* 103: 680–682, 1989
27. Gay M, et al: Psychogenic habit cough: Review and case reports. *J Clin Psychiat* 48: 483–486, 1987
28. Irwin RS, Curley FJ, French CL: Chronic persistent cough in the Adv H: The spectrum and frequency of causes and successful outcome of specific therapy. *Am Rev Respir Dis* 123:413, 1981
29. Rodney WM: Diagnosis of chronic cough. *JAMA* 242:14–91, 1979
30. Deschner WK, Benjamin SB: Estraesophageal manifestations of gastroesophageal reflex disease. *Am J Gastroenterol* 84:1–5, 1989
31. Baron SB, Huang JK: Cough syncope presenting as mobitz type II atrioventricular block—An electro-physiologic correlation. *PACE* 10:65–69, 1987
32. Fraser RG: Diagnosis of Diseases of the Chest, ed 3. Philadelphia, WB Saunders, 1988, pp 70–71, 389–391
33. Krzyzanowski M, et al: Relationships between pulmonary function and changes in chronic respiratory symptoms. *Chest* 98:62–70, 1990
34. Poe RH, Israel RH, Utell MJ, et al: Chronic cough: Bronchoscopy or pulmonary function testing? *Am Rev Respir Dis* 126:160, 1982
35. Irwin RS, Curley FJ, Pratter MR: The effects of drugs on cough. *Eur J Respir Dis* 153: 173–181, 1987
36. Goodman and Gilman: The Pharmacological Basis of Therapeutics. New York, MacMillan, 1985, pp 174–175, 500–501
37. Irwin RS, Curley FJ: The treatment of cough: A comprehensive review. *Chest* 99: 1477–1484, 1991

6

Hemoptysis

Barry Lesser, John Haapaniemi, and Ernest L. Yoder

The expectoration of blood, or hemoptysis, is a symptom that often evokes significant apprehension by both the patient and the physician and may be seen in 7% to 15% of patients presenting to a busy chest clinic [1–3]. It often causes the patient to seek prompt medical attention because of the fear of an underlying devastating disease. For centuries hemoptysis was most commonly due to pulmonary tuberculosis. However, since the advent of chemotherapy for tuberculosis, bronchitis/bronchiectasis, aspergillomas, and neoplastic disorders are now primarily responsible for most cases of hemoptysis [1] unless the patient is from a region endemic for tuberculosis [4].

Our ability to evaluate the exact cause of hemoptysis has greatly improved over the last 50 years. With the advent of nuclear imaging techniques, pulmonary and bronchial angiography, and most importantly the fiberoptic bronchoscope, we are in most circumstances able to determine the exact diagnosis. In this chapter we review the diagnostic approach to patients with hemoptysis, emphasizing the use of appropriate imaging techniques to make a timely diagnosis. We also review the treatment and discuss specific disease entities commonly associated with hemoptysis (Table 6-1).

Initial Diagnostic Approach and Evaluation

Clinical assessment of the patient with hemoptysis must be directed by the urgency and life-threatening nature of the bleeding. Once the patient who has life-threatening massive hemoptysis is separated from the patient with nonmassive hemoptysis, a logical approach can be taken to obtain the proper diagnosis. This chapter primarily deals with the patient with nonmassive hemoptysis where one generally has ample time to obtain the appropriate diagnostic studies.

If time permits one should proceed in a logical manner when attempting to isolate the cause of hemoptysis. The initial evaluation should include a thorough history and physical examination, chest roentgenogram, hematologic studies, examination of expectorated sputum, and urinalysis. These studies are usually easily performed and results can be known within minutes or hours.

History

The history should be quite detailed in order to determine the source of bleeding and if true hemoptysis exists. One needs to pay attention specifically to the upper airway, including the nasal and oropharynx, the tracheobronchial tree, and the gastrointestinal tract in differentiating hemoptysis from other sources of bleeding (Table 6-2). The age of the patient is quite helpful as an elderly patient is more likely to suffer from lung cancer, and the typical constitutional symptoms of weight loss, weakness, and hemoptysis may be present [5]. In the younger patient disorders such as bronchiectasis, mitral valvular disease [6], rheumatic heart disease [7], would tend to be more likely and questions should be directed in this fashion. The time course also may be very helpful. Someone who has had small amounts of hemoptysis with blood streaking for several years most likely would have a benign condition such as chronic bronchitis with a superimposed acute bronchitis. Bronchiectasis may present with hemoptysis on a background of

Table 6-1. Etiology of hemoptysis

Abnormal Chest X-ray	*Normal Chest X-ray*
Infectious	
TB	Tracheobronchitis
Fungal	Bronchiectasis
Aspergilloma	Endobronchial TB
Actinomycosis	
Histoplasmosis	
Coccidioidomycosis	
Cryptococcosis	
Lung abscess	
Parasitic	
Amebiasis	
Ascariasis	
Paragonimiasis	
Bacterial/viral pneumonia	
Neoplastic	
Bronchogenic carcinoma	Endobronchial tumor
	Tracheal tumor
Metastatic cancer	
Cardiovascular	
CHF	Valvular heart disease
Aneurysm	(Mitral stenosis)
Mitral stenosis	Aegenis of pulmonary artery
Pulmonary A-V malformation	
Pulmonary embolism	
Congenital heart disease	
Collagen vascular	
Wegener's granulomatosis	
Goodpasture's syndrome	
SLE	
Scleroderma	
Miscellaneous	
Cystic fibrosis	Endobronchial endometriosis
IgA nephropathy	
Idiopathic pulmonary hemosiderosis	Coagulopathy
	Thrombocytopenia
Amyloid	Amyloidosis
Broncholithiasis	
Pulmonary endometriosis	
Pulmonary sequestration	
Trauma/Iatrogenic	
Pulmonary contusion	Bronchoscopy
Penetrating lung injury	Pulmonary artery catherization
	Foreign body aspiration

chronic purulent sputum production and a history of recurrent pneumonia. Risk factors for serious disease such as smoking in lung cancer, the use of birth control pills or obesity in pulmonary embolic disease, and occupational exposure with increased risk for bronchogenic carcinoma such as with asbestos and chromium need to be addressed.

If one pays attention to the upper airway, a history of sinusitis, nose bleeds, or foreign bodies within the nasopharynx, may elucidate the true cause of hemoptysis. A careful review of systems is also necessary, looking for systemic disease such as vasculitis and collagen vascular disease, as well as looking into the possibility of bleeding disorders. A drug history is important to ensure the patient is not on any platelet-inhibiting agents, anticoagulants for thromboembolic disease or other agents that may inhibit coagulation. Hemoptysis seen in patients who are using anticoagulants may herald the presence of an underlying endobronchial lesion [8].

Physical Examination

The physical examination should be directed specifically at finding a diagnosis for hemoptysis. If time permits, a thorough examination should be undertaken; however, in the case of massive hemoptysis, the examination must be tailored to ensure the stability of the patient. In most circumstances an adequate physical examination can be undertaken.

A careful inspection of the upper airway including the nasal pharynx and oral cavity may detect foreign bodies, laryngeal masses, or telangiectasias suggestive of hereditary hemorrhagic telangiectasia (Fig. 6-1; see color plate). If there is evidence of sinus disease or perforation of the nasal septum, Wegener's granulomatosis should be considered. If the amount of bleeding is small, examination of the lungs may be normal. However, evidence of obstructive lung disease may be present, with hyper-resonance on percussion and diffuse expiratory wheezing. If a localized wheeze is found, an obstructing lesion should be considered. Classic signs of consolidation may also be found, but caution is suggested in interpreting these findings because this may

Table 6-2. Differentiation of hemoptysis and hematemesis

Hematemesis	*Hemoptysis*
Blood is vomited	Frothy blood expectorated
Blood is dark (coffee grounds)	Blood is usually bright red
Blood is acidic	Blood is alkaline
Vomited blood may contain food particles	Sputum shows WBC, hemosidero-laden macrophages
Anemia is usually present	Anemia may or may not be present
History of nausea and vomiting	History of cough

represent aspirated blood or postobstructive pneumonia. Tracheal shift may be detected, suggesting atelectasis and volume loss from an obstructing lesion. Evidence of valvular heart disease such as mitral stenosis or rheumatic heart disease should be sought. Congestive heart failure and alveolar flooding is perhaps more commonly detected. Hepatomegaly or abdominal masses, if detected, may reveal an underlying malignancy, suggesting metastatic spread to the lungs and subsequent hemoptysis, although hemoptysis from metastatic lung cancer is unusual [9]. Splenomegaly may suggest an underlying hematologic disorder, leading to a blood dyscrasia. Examination of the skin and extremities may reveal ecchymosis and petechiae, again suggestive of a hematologic disorder. Telangiectasia may also be seen peripherally. Evidence of arthritis and joint effusions may suggest an underlying collagen-vascular disease such as systemic lupus erythematosis.

Chest Roentgenogram

The chest roentgenogram is perhaps the most important diagnostic study to obtain in the initial work-up. Frequently, the abnormality leading to the hemoptysis is readily apparent on careful examination of the chest film. However, one must be careful not to ascribe old or chronic findings to the hemoptysis and review of old chest radiographs may be quite useful. Frequently, a normal chest radiograph is obtained, implying pathology in the larger more central bronchi such as bronchitis or an endobronchial tumor.

When abnormal, several possible roentgenographic findings may be found. An infiltrate suggestive of pneumonia or aspirated blood may be detected. If more of an alveolar filling process is found, Goodpasture's syndrome or idiopathic hemosiderosis need to be considered. Coagulopathies may also lead to a similar radiographic pattern. If the infiltrate is more of an interstitial pattern, congestive heart failure and pulmonary edema should be considered. Peripheral wedge-shaped densities are highly suggestive of pulmonary embolic disease, whereas infiltrates confined to specific anatomic distributions suggest a postobstructive pneumonitis from any endobronchial lesion. Masses or hilar adenopathy are quite suggestive of neoplastic disorders. Fleeting infiltrates that may cavitate are suggestive of vasculitides such as Wegener's granulomastosis or septic pulmonary emboli, which may be seen in patients who are intravenous drug abusers with bacterial endocarditis. Cavitary lesions that have free-floating densities suggestive of fungus balls may be seen in diseases such as old tuberculosis and sarcoidosis. Broncholithiasis may or may not be easily detectable on a chest film but might easily be seen at the time of bronchoscopy. The chest roentgenogram commonly shows calcifications, and hemoptysis may be seen in 50% of patients. Broncholithiasis should be considered if the patient has a history of a gritty sensation in expectorated sputum [10, 11]. Regardless of the abnormality on chest roentgenography, most patients need a confirmatory study such as a bronchoscopy to determine if the lesion seen on the chest film is directly responsible for the hemoptysis.

A normal chest radiograph may be seen in approximately 20% to 50% of patients with hemoptysis [12–15] and presents an interesting dilemma [16, 17]. In these patients further diagnostic studies must be considered, depending on the patient's history. Bronchoscopy may elicit the presence of an endobronchial lesion, bronchitis, or bronchiectasis. Other conditions associated with a normal chest radiograph and hemoptysis include endobronchial tuberculosis, endotracheal trauma during intubation or suctioning, hemorrhagic disorders, and anticoagulant usage (Table 6-1). If no other abnormality can be found, closer inspection of the chest radiograph may suggest a Westermark's sign or focal oligemia seen in pulmonary embolic disease.

Laboratory Assessment

Any patient with a history of hemoptysis deserves a complete blood count, routine coagulation profile (prothrombin time, partial thromboplastin time), sputum examination, and urinalysis. Often the only abnormality found, if any, is a slight reduction in the patient's hemoglobin and hematocrit levels. If the bleeding is massive, significant anemia may be detected. If the remainder of the hematologic and coagulation profiles is normal, no further studies are necessary. In patients who have abnormalities of different cell lines, including the white cells and platelets, a primary hematopoetic origin for the patients' hemoptysis such as leukemia or disseminated intravascular coagulation may need to be considered. In patients with coagulation defects, specific coagulopathies should be sought. A careful drug history is also quite useful to ensure that the patient is not taking any antiplatelet agents or anticoagulants. Sputum examination should include a routine Gram stain and culture, acid fast stain and culture, as well as cytologic examination. Urinalysis should be performed to look for evidence of glomerulonephritis (red blood cell, red blood cell casts), which may be associated with Goodpasture's disease or Wegener's granulomatosis.

Specific Diagnostic Studies

In this section we specifically present both invasive and noninvasive imaging studies that may be directed toward specific diagnoses. Once the routine investigation has been completed, further studies may be indicated for accurate diagnosis as well as management. In patients who have recurrent hemoptysis, accurate localization of the site of bleeding, which may be lifesaving, is necessary in order to plan a therapeutic strategy should the patient develop massive hemoptysis. This can be accomplished during bronchoscopy where a thorough examination of the tracheobronchial tree can be undertaken, localization of site of bleeding can be determined, and biopsies can be performed, time permitting, to make a tissue diagnosis. Bronchial arteriography may be necessary to localize the site of bleeding for subsequent therapeutic embolization. Lung scintigraphy and/or pulmonary angiography are indicated in patients with suspected pumonary embolic disease.

Bronchoscopy

With the introduction of the flexible fiberoptic bronchoscope, the evaluation of hemoptysis has changed. It is well recognized that bronchoscopy is a safe procedure and can be highly informative [12, 18–21]. If one can separate the patient with non–life-threatening hemoptysis from the patient with massive hemoptysis, a diagnostic algorithm can be employed. In a patient with non–life-threatening hemoptysis the use of a flexible fiberoptic bronchoscope is usually preferred for adequate localization of the site of bleeding in a distal segment as well as providing a diagnosis. It is controversial whether bronchoscopy should be performed during the period of active bleeding or postponed until the bleeding has subsided. Gong and Salvatierra [22] looked at 129 patients and concluded that although a bleeding site was determined more frequently with early bronchoscopy, clinical outcome was not altered when comparing early versus late bronchoscopy.

In cases of massive hemoptysis, it is controversial whether flexible fiberoptic bronchoscopy is superior to rigid bronchoscopy. Most patients need to be individualized at the time of actual bronchoscopy. The benefit of fiberoptic bronchoscopy is entering more distal segments, isolating the source of bleeding, and potential therapy during bronchoscopy by tamponade with Fogarty balloon occlusion or intrabronchial coagulation. The main advantage of rigid bronchoscopy is a larger diameter scope, thus enabling evacuation of blood and clots more readily. In those patients with massive hemoptysis it is imperative that the site of bleeding be determined in order to direct a thoracic surgeon at the time of surgery. However, with the use of a flexible bronchoscope and Fogarty balloon occlusion, the patients can be stabilized and possibly avoid surgery. If surgery is still necessary the situation is more controlled if the bleeding has been successfully tamponaded. Although bronchoscopy is perhaps the most valuable diagnostic technique in the evaluation of hemoptysis, not all patients with hemoptysis require bronchoscopy. If the diagnosis is readily apparent by other means, patients can be managed more conservatively and followed on a clinical basis. However, if hemoptysis is recurrent, diagnostic bronchoscopy should be performed to rule out the presence of an underlying malignancy.

Lung Scintigraphy

The ventilation-perfusion scan has aided in assessing the patient with suspected pulmonary embolic disease. The ventilatory portion was added to the perfusion scan in the early 1970s in hopes of differentiating primary embolic events, which would cause perfusion defects, with normal ventilation [23]. By using both ventilation and perfusion in performing the study, a high likelihood of pulmonary embolic disease can be determined by the finding of a segmental or greater mismatched defect. Unfortunately, the majority of patients have lung scans that are interpreted in the low or indeterminate probability category. This brings up a diagnostic dilemma since the presence of pulmonary emboli is uncertain and the risk of subsequent anticoagulation is high. Several studies have specifically addressed this question [24–26]. Hull et al [27] have suggested that patients with low or indeterminate probability lung scans and negative impedance plethysmography can be followed clinically without anticoagulation, with the risk of subsequent embolization quite low. The PIOPED study clarified the utility of the high and low probability scan. A high probability scan is 97% specific for the presence of pulmonary embolism, while a low probability scan with a low clinical suspicion makes the likelihood of pulmonary embolism remote [26]. Duplex ultrasound scanning of the lower extremities has been used with ventilation-perfusion scans to determine the presence of thromboembolic disease. The specificity in several studies is 97% to 100% [28]. A negative duplex or impedance plethysmography result in combination with a low probability ventilation-perfusion scan and a low clinical suspicion virtually exclude pulmonary embolic disease. Because of the uncertainty in those patients with low to indeterminate lung scans and a high clinical suspicion, pulmonary angiography may be required for definitive diagnosis.

Angiography

Pulmonary angiography remains the gold standard for the definitive diagnosis of pulmonary embolic disease. In patients who have uncertain results based on lung scintigraphy, the clinical situation may dictate performing pulmonary angiography. Besides determining the presence or absence of embolic disease, angiography provides an assessment of the pulmonary arterial bed and evaluation for the presence of arteriovenous malformations, which may be seen in Osler-Weber-Rendu disease. During angiography pulmonary hemodynamics can be obtained that may detect the presence of pulmonary arterial hypertension or cardiogenic failure.

Selective bronchial arteriography has also been used as a diagnostic and therapeutic modality to identify the source of bleeding

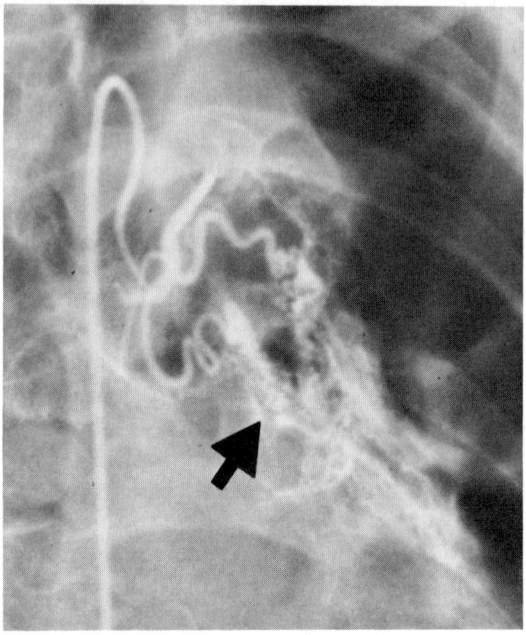

A

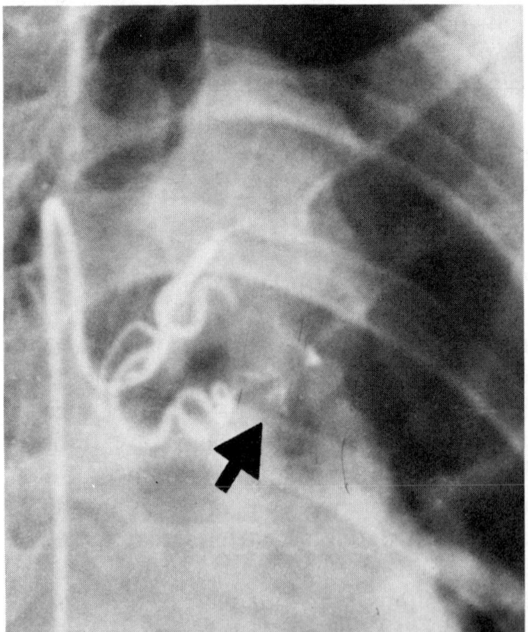

B

Fig. 6-2. (A) Selective bronchial arteriogram before embolization, demonstrating extravasation of contrast (arrow). (B) Selective bronchial arteriogram after embolization, demonstrating no extravasation of contrast (arrow).

(Fig. 6-2A and B). Subsequent embolization with thrombin, wire coils, balloons, or other devices may serve to control further bleeding. This approach is often used in conjunction with bronchoscopy to localize the site of bleeding. The main complication is spinal cord injury if the anterior spinal artery is inadvertently embolized. This can be prevented by ensuring adequate visualization of the anterior spinal artery before embolization. Bronchial artery embolization is usually successful in arresting the bleeding. However, in approximately 20% of patients [29–31] rebleeding may occur during the 6 months following embolization. Mycetoma has been associated with the highest recurrence of bleeding [32]. In patients who rebleed, a combined surgical and medical approach may prove beneficial in long-term outcome.

In those patients with massive hemoptysis, initial embolization may allow the patient to stabilize, thus improving surgical outcome [33]. In those patients who have absolute contraindications for surgery, a combined approach of repeated embolizations with or without endobronchial tamponade may be lifesaving.

Computerized Tomography of the Chest

Computerized tomography (CT) scanning of the chest is not useful as a primary modality in the evaluation and management of hemoptysis. However, it is often used as an adjunct in the work-up of suspected malignancy. Parenchymal abnormalities may be further clarified and the proximal bronchi are easily evaluated via CT imaging. Evaluation of the mediastium is excellent and can readily distinguish vascular structures from abnormally enlarged lymph nodes and lung masses from surrounding tissue. In patients who have an otherwise unremarkable chest radiograph and evidence of severe bronchitis or history of recurrent pneumonia, bronchiectasis may be easily detected, thus negating the need for bronchography [34]. In a study of 32 patients by Haponik [34a] comparing the results of CT versus chest radiography, the CT provided additional information in over 50% of the patients. However, this information did not alter clinical management. For these reasons CT scanning should be used on an individual basis and not in the routine evaluation of hemoptysis.

Specific Diseases Associated with Hemoptysis

Tracheobronchitis and Chronic Bronchitis

It is well known that patients with bronchitis may produce sputum with blood streaking. Chronic bronchitis is perhaps the most common cause of hemoptysis and occurs in 60% to 70% of patients who present with hemoptysis [9]. Although blood streaking is usually seen, occasionally the hemoptysis may be quite significant as reported by Lewis et al [35] in a patient with severe tracheitis secondary to influenza A. Besides the inflammatory component of the bronchitis, small superficial blood vessels may also be ruptured during severe coughing paroxysms. At times direct trauma, such as endotracheal intubation may be the culprit, leading to hemoptysis commonly seen with intubated patients.

Bronchiectasis

Hemoptysis may be seen in approximately 20% to 45% of patients with bronchiectasis [1, 36]. This diagnosis should be suspected in patients who have recurrent pneumonias, usually dating back to childhood or adolescence. These patients typically give a history suggestive of chronic bronchitis. The chest radiograph may be normal; however, tubular shadows or cystic changes may be seen. The classic "gloved-finger" shadow is seen when bronchiectatic segments fill with retained mucus. Although bronchiectasis usually is found in the bases, it has been reported in patients who have had tuberculosis that primarily affects the apices. Although bronchography has been the diagnostic procedure of choice, it is now being recognized that CT may be preferred in documenting the presence of bronchiectasis [34]. Therapy is usually supportive, with broad-spectrum antibiotics; however, occasionally surgical resection may be necessary.

Tuberculosis

It has been reported that approximately 8% to 10% of patients with tuberculosis have evidence of hemoptysis. Usually the amount of hemoptysis is small; however, it can be seen with copious sputum production and occasionally massive hemoptysis with exsanguination has been reported [37]. In almost all cases of pulmonary tuberculosis associated with hemoptysis, there are abnormalities detected on the routine chest radiography. The diagnosis can usually be easily confirmed by positive acid fast smears and positive purified protein derivative (PPD) test; however, bronchoscopy occasionally is necessary to confirm the diagnosis. In patients with more significant degrees of hemoptysis, pulmonary resection may be required. In 1868, Rasmussen [38] originally described patients with massive hemoptysis originating from the erosion of an artery within a residual thick-walled cavity (Rasmussen's aneurysm) from old tuberculosis. Subsequently the arterial supply was found to be of bronchial origin [39]. Other sources of bleeding in old inactive tuberculosis include bronchiectasis, fungal infection usually with mycetoma secondary to *Aspergillus,* broncholithiasis, and scar carcinoma [40].

Pneumonia

Hemoptysis may be associated with severe pneumonias, usually of a necrotizing variety. Classic rusty colored sputum may be seen with lobar pneumococcal pneumonia. Postobstructive pneumonitis may be suspected, with a typical radiographic picture of an infiltrate emanating from the hilum. In patients who develop lung abscess in association with their pneumonia, hemoptysis may be seen but usually to a minor extent. These patients must be investigated not only for anaerobic processes but for tuberculosis, fungal diseases, and the possibility of bronchogenic carcinoma. A good travel history may be helpful in diagnosing patients with hemoptysis. Pneumonia associated with hemoptysis in patients emigrating from South Vietnam, the Philippines, and India may be due to the lung fluke (*Paragonimus westermani*). The diagnosis may be suspected in persons with hemoptysis living in an endemic area. Chest radiography usually shows an infiltrate and 21% of the patients may have an elevated eosinophil count [41].

Pulmonary Mycetoma

Mycetomas have been shown to form in preexisting lung cavities, which are most commonly caused by tuberculosis (Fig. 6-3). The most common organism is usually *Aspergillus* and a diagnosis can easily be established by serologic testing and sputum cultures [42]. Radiographically if one does two projections, including an upright and decubitus view, the mycetoma can be observed to move within the cavity. The pathogenesis of hemoptysis related to a mycetoma is not entirely understood. It has been suggested that friction caused by movement of the mycetoma may be responsible. Varkey and Rose in 1976 [43] suggested that there was release of an anticoagulant and a trypsin-like proteolytic enzyme from the fungus that eventually caused the bleeding. The therapeutic options are few. It has been suggested that all mycetomas should be surgically removed; however, there have been several reports demonstrating that a conservative approach coupled with therapeutic bronchial artery embolization [29, 44] has been quite successful in arresting further bleeding episodes. In one series a third of the cases eventually required surgery because all other methods failed. Those patients had several postoperative complications related to the severity of the underlying lung disease [44].

Fig. 6-3. Chest roentgenogram demonstrating cavitary lesion in left upper lobe with mycetoma (arrow).

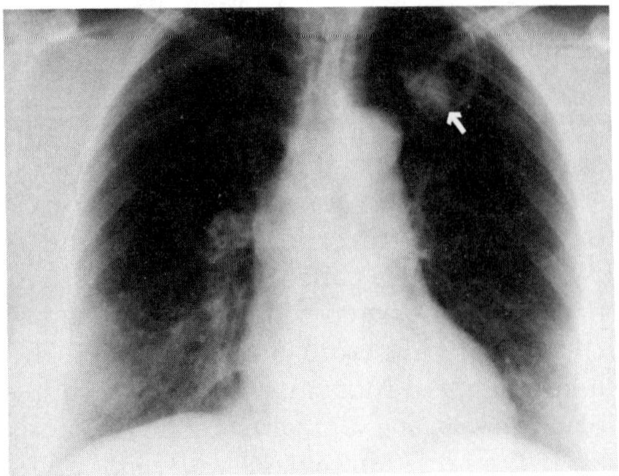

Pulmonary Sequestrations

Pulmonary sequestrations are unusual but when present may occasionally be associated with hemoptysis. The diagnosis should be suspected in lower lobe lesions that are recurrent and present clinically like pneumonia. These lesions are usually adjacent to the hemidiaphragm or mediastinum. Definitive diagnosis requires angiographic visualization of the anomalous vascular supply. Definitive treatment usually involves resection of the sequestration to prevent further pneumonic episodes as well as hemoptysis [45].

Pulmonary Infarction

Pulmonary infarction is commonly associated with pulmonary embolic disease. Pulmonary infarctions typically occur with peripheral emboli and present with pleuritic chest pain, fever, and chest wall tenderness. There may be an associated pleural friction rub. The hemoptysis associated with pulmonary infarction is usually minimal but may last several days. Typically the radiograph demonstrates the presence of a peripheral wedge-shaped lesion that may or may not be associated with a pleural effusion. Ventilation-perfusion scans are usually diagnostic in this situation; however, in a scan that is interpreted as low or indeterminant probability, pulmonary angiography may be warranted to definitively make the diagnosis of pulmonary embolism if clinical suspicion is high. Once confirmed, systemic heparinization followed by therapy with Coumadin (sodium warfarin) is indicated.

Neoplastic Disorders

Bronchogenic carcinoma is often heralded by the presence of hemoptysis. In some series up to 40% of patients had hemoptysis at one point during their course [13]. It is because of this diagnostic possibility that a thorough investigation of hemoptysis is necessary. The chest radiograph may be normal in patients who have endobronchial disease or may be abnormal with a multitude of findings, including collapse, masses, adenopathy, and solitary well-circumscribed nodules. Tumors of the trachea are extremely uncommon, but when present usually are of the squamous cell variety. Bronchial carcinoids tend to be highly vascular and are associated with hemoptysis in 18% of patients [46]. Metastatic involvement of the bronchi is extremely unusual and occurs in approximately 2% of patients. It is heralded by cough and hemoptysis in the majority of patients [47].

The diagnosis of neoplastic disorders is usually relatively simple employing the fiberoptic bronchoscope. At the time of bronchoscopy, samples taken for cytology as well as histopathology are often diagnostic. If bronchoscopy fails to determine a diagnosis, percutaneous needle biopsy may be helpful. Thoracotomy may be necessary for diagnosis and at times provide a cure as in the case of a solitary pulmonary nodule [48, 49].

Alveolar Hemorrhage Syndromes

There are a wide variety of diseases in which alveolar hemorrhage may develop. The symptoms and radiographic features are quite similar in all of these diseases. The findings of hemoptysis, dyspnea, diffuse alveolar infiltrates, anemia, and hypoxemia are common to all forms of alveolar hemorrhage syndromes. Often renal involvement is seen and is manifested by glomerulonephritis [50, 51].

Goodpasture's syndrome is probably the most well-known syndrome causing alveolar hemorrhage. The pathologic process involves antibodies directed to the glomerular basement membrane. Deposits of IgG and complement, specifically C3, have been found within the basement membranes of both the kidney and lung. With immunofluorescent staining there is a linear deposit of both IgG and C3 along the glomerular capillary walls. For this reason a renal biopsy is usually the preferred method of establishing an adequate tissue diagnosis. The prognosis of patients with Goodpasture's syndrome is excellent. Therapy is directed toward removing the circulating antiglomerular basement membrane antibodies via plasmapheresis and preventing further elaboration of antibodies by a combination of cytotoxic therapy, usually with cyclophosphamide and high-dose corticosteroids.

Patients with immune complex diseases that present with alveolar hemorrhage and glomerulonephritis make up an interesting group. The diseases associated with this group of patients include systemic lupus erythematosus [52], Wegener's granulomatosis [53, 54] (Fig. 6-4), and other vasculitides such as Henoch-Schönlein purpura. Wegener's granulomatosis is usually diagnosed by open lung biopsy showing the typical necrotizing vasculitis. Once confirmed, response to therapy is usually excellent, with a combination of steroids and cyclophosphamide.

There is a subgroup of patients with renal disease and alveolar hemorrhage who have no demonstrable immune complex disease. Most of these patients have end-stage uremia and develop a coagulopathy that has been attributed to the uremia. With the advent of dialysis, bleeding is rarely seen as a complica-

Fig. 6-4. Chest roentgenogram demonstrating necrotizing lesion in upper lobe (arrow) in patient with Wegener's granulomatosis.

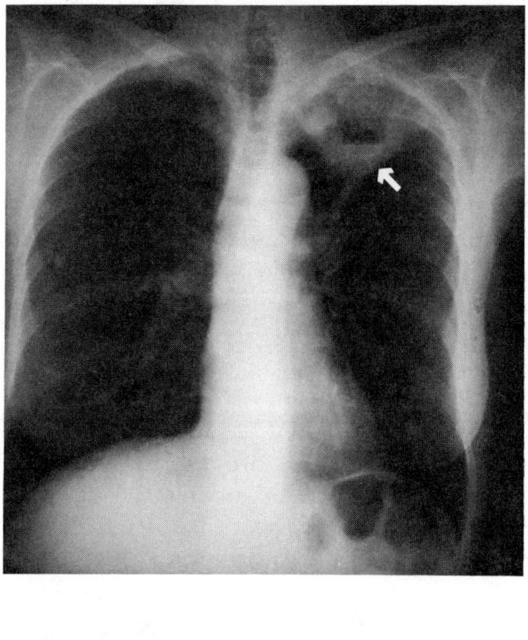

tion of renal disease. In this group of patients as compared with those with Goodpasture's syndrome, the renal disease precedes the pulmonary disease.

The last major group of patients with alveolar hemorrhage have no evidence of either renal disease or immune complex disorders. These include blood dyscrasias such as disseminated intravascular coagulation [55], leukemia [56], thrombocytopenia [57], and anticoagulant usage [58]; patients with acute lung injury including adult respiratory distress syndrome; and miscellaneous causes such as mitral stenosis or blunt trauma. Idiopathic pulmonary hemosiderosis is quite rare, usually presenting in children and young adults. It is associated with fleeting pulmonary infiltrates, hemoptysis, and anemia, with no evidence of renal disease. There is some controversy as to the exact pathologic process, but some groups have found abnormalities of the capillary basement membrane. Some patients have responded to steroids and/or immunosuppressive therapy, but most patients die within 2 to 3 years after diagnosis.

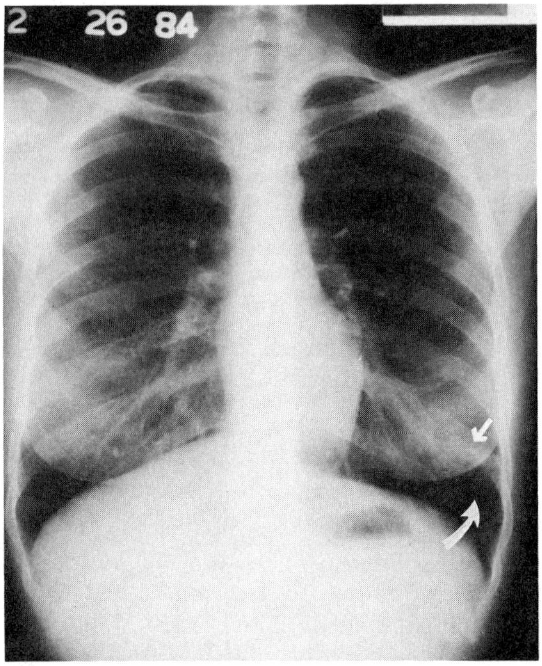
2 26 84

A

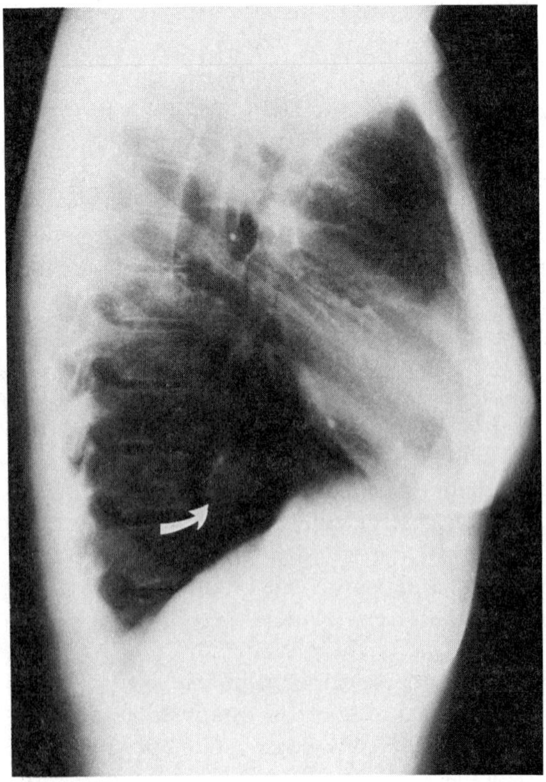

B

Arteriovenous Malformations

Most patients found to have arteriovenous malformations within the lung have subsequently been diagnosed as having Osler-Weber-Rendu disease [59]; however, trauma has been implicated in several of these cases. Commonly these patients have epistaxis and lesions of the skin and mucous membranes showing the typical telangiectasias. Hemoptysis is uncommon, occurring in less than 10% of patients [60]. Patients should be investigated for the presence of a right-to-left shunt if clubbing, cyanosis, and polycythemia are present. The pulmonary arteriovenous malformations usually appear as a lobulated mass (Fig. 6-5A and B), and if one auscultates over the region a bruit can usually be appreciated. The diagnosis is confirmed by angiography (Fig. 6-5C), and therapy either includes resection or more recently embolization via any of a number of techniques including balloon occlusion, wire coil, Gelfoam, or nonresorbable tissue adhesives [61, 62].

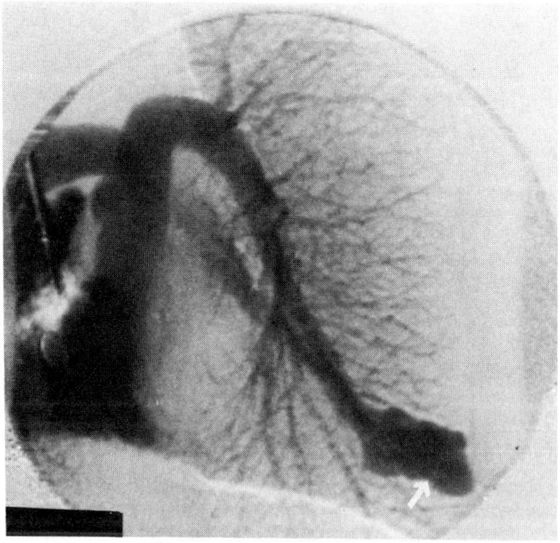

C

Fig. 6-5. (A) Posteroanterior chest roentgenogram demonstrating lobulated mass in left lower lobe in patient with Osler-Weber-Rendu disease. (B) Lateral chest roentgenogram demonstrating lobulated mass in left lower lobe in patient with Osler-Weber-Rendu disease. (C) Digital subtraction angiography demonstrating pulmonary arteriovenous malformation in patient with Osler-Weber-Rendu disease.

Iatrogenic

Several reports of iatrogenically induced hemoptysis have appeared in the literature. In most circumstances this has coincided with the tendency toward more invasive diagnostic and therapeutic interventions. The bleeding may be minor or major. During bronchoscopy [18, 19] hemoptysis may be seen to be associated with friable mucosa typically seen with bronchitis or neoplastic disorders. Frank hemorrhage may occur during endobronchial or transbronchial biopsy. Bleeding is more easily controlled if it is related to a transbronchial biopsy as the distal airway can be tamponaded with the bronchoscope.

Percutaneous fine needle aspiration biopsy, usually with a small gauge Zavala biopsy needle, may result in minimal bleeding. Occasionally massive hemoptysis may occur and at times has been fatal [63, 64]. Rupture of the pulmonary artery with resulting hemoptysis has been observed with flow-directed balloon-tipped pulmonary artery catheters. Two mechanisms that have been proposed include overinflation of the balloon in a small branch artery and a "spear" effect of the catheter tip, causing perforation of the pulmonary artery [65, 66]. The association of pulmonary hypertension, hypothermia, and anticoagulation may increase the risk.

Endotracheal tubes may cause inflammation and pressure necrosis of the trachea, leading to hemoptysis. With the newer low-pressure highly compliant endotracheal tubes this is seen less frequently [67]. Suctioning via endotracheal tube may traumatize the trachea, resulting in minor bleeds.

Unusual Causes

Once the common causes have been effectively excluded, more unusual disorders may need to be considered. In young women, hemoptysis associated with menstruation or catamenial hemoptysis usually occurs in a cyclical fashion associated with menses [68–70]. This is due to the deposition of endometrial tissue in the lung. Therapy at this time is primarily anecdotal, but hormonal manipulation appears to have had some success, especially with progesterone or danazol. Factitious hemoptysis, which may be a form of Munchausen's syndrome, has been reported [71, 72]. Aspiration of foreign bodies in the tracheobronchial tree may result in hemoptysis [73–75], usually due to secondary bronchiectasis. Recently there have been a few reports linking crack cocaine abuse and hemoptysis [76]. The hemoptysis is usually mild blood streaking, but diffuse pulmonary hemorrhage has also been seen. It has been suggested that the intense vasoconstriction induced by cocaine has led to the pulmonary hemorrhage. Hemoptysis in this setting at times has mimicked pulmonary embolic disease and before ascribing the hemoptysis to cocaine, pulmonary embolism and other disorders need to be primarily investigated.

Management

In order to manage patients with hemoptysis it is often helpful to categorize the type and

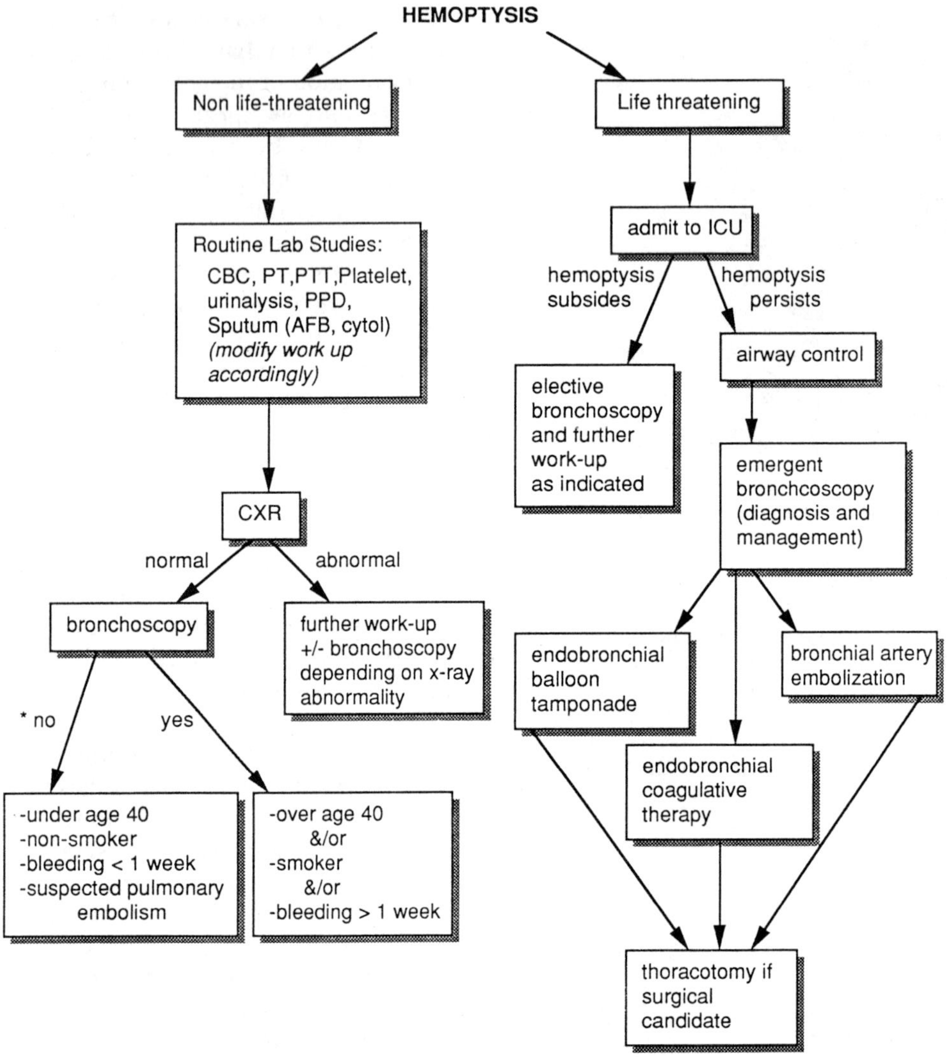
HEMOPTYSIS
Non life-threatening
Life threatening
Routine Lab Studies:
CBC, PT,PTT,Platelet,
urinalysis, PPD,
Sputum (AFB, cytol)
(modify work up
accordingly)
admit to ICU
hemoptysis subsides
hemoptysis persists
airway control
elective
bronchoscopy
and further
work-up
as indicated
emergent
bronchcoscopy
(diagnosis and
management)
CXR
normal
abnormal
bronchoscopy
further work-up
+/- bronchoscopy
depending on x-ray
abnormality
endobronchial
balloon
tamponade
bronchial artery
embolization
* no
yes
endobronchial
coagulative
therapy
-under age 40
-non-smoker
-bleeding < 1 week
-suspected pulmonary
embolism
-over age 40
&/or
-smoker
&/or
-bleeding > 1 week
thoracotomy if
surgical
candidate

* although several studies support this, patients must be individualized.
If bronchoscopy is performed and is normal, the risk of serious disease is minimal.

Fig. 6-6. Management algorithm for patients with mild-to-moderate and massive hemoptysis.

amount of bleeding present. If one separates those patients with massive hemoptysis from those with mild-to-moderate hemoptysis the management strategies can be easily defined (Fig. 6-6). Patients can be classified into three prominent groups. The first being massive hemoptysis, the second being mild-to-moderate hemoptysis with normal chest radiography, and the third group being mild-to-moderate hemoptysis with abnormal chest radiography.

The focus of this chapter is the outpatient management of patients with hemoptysis and with this in mind we make only a few references to the patient who presents with massive hemoptysis. The next section therefore deals with those patients who present with mild-to-moderate hemoptysis. Conventional therapy in all patients with hemoptysis includes supportive measures with bed rest, antitussive agents, and blood transfusions if indicated. Further therapy is individualized once the diagnosis is obtained.

Hemoptysis with a Normal Chest Radiograph

A clinical history is very important in this group of patients as it will usually dictate the investigations necessary. Hemoptysis is generally mild in nature, and emergent bronchoscopy is often unnecessary. Most of these patients are found to have either bronchitis or bronchiectasis; however, endobronchial disease may be present. If the patient is over age 40, has a significant smoking history, and the hemoptysis persists for more than 1 week [13, 14], bronchoscopy is indicated. If the patient does not fulfill these criteria no further interventions may be necessary [13].

Further investigation should be dictated on clinical grounds, but some routine studies may be appropriate in all patients with normal chest radiography. These include complete blood count, prothrombin time, partial thromboplastin time, platelet count, sputum analysis for tuberculosis and cytology, PPD, and urinalysis. If the results of these studies are not diagnostic, more specific investigation is necessary.

In the patient with positive sputum cytology, a negative chest radiograph, and a normal bronchoscopic examination, a thorough evaluation for carcinoma in situ is necessary. This may include laser bronchoscopy in combination with hematoporphyrin derivative to identify the site. Hematoporphyrin is taken up by malignant cells and can be visualized by fluorescence [77]. The tumor can then be ablated by argon dye laser.

Normal radiography may be present in 24% of patients with pulmonary embolic disease [78]. If clinical suspicion is high, noninvasive studies of the lower extremities and venous perfusion studies may be warranted. If cardiovascular disease is suspected, echocardiography and perhaps right or left heart catheterization may be necessary to confirm the presence of valvular heart disease. Medical management often suffices, especially in patients with left ventricular failure and pulmonary edema. However, surgery may be required for valvular heart disease.

Coagulopathies secondary to drug overdose may herald the presence of an underlying lesion. If the patient has any risk factors for the development of an underlying malignancy bronchoscopy should be performed. However, if the coagulopathy is severe, clinical correlation is necessary and these patients may benefit from observation alone.

If no obvious pathology is detected, a clinical decision regarding the need for bronchoscopy is necessary. If there is no predisposing risk factor for neoplastic disease, tuberculosis, etc., bronchoscopy may not be necessary as previously discussed. However, the complication rate from bronchoscopy is quite low [18–20]. If bronchoscopy rules out serious pathology, the prognosis in these patients is quite good [79].

Hemoptysis with an Abnormal Chest Radiograph

When the chest radiograph is abnormal the source of the hemoptysis is usually self-evident. Infectious causes are usually apparent, with consolidation in bronchopneumonia, apical infiltrates in a patient with tuberculosis, and cavitary lesions in patients with lung abscesses, tuberculosis, or mycetomas. These diagnoses usually do not require any further investigation; however, if the source of the bacteriologic diagnosis cannot be made, bronchoscopy may be indicated to obtain adequate specimens for microbiologic assessment.

Bronchoscopy is further required when histopathologic sampling is needed for accurate diagnosis. Percutaneous fine needle aspiration may be preferred, depending on the location of the tumor or if the bronchoscopy is nondiagnostic.

Recurrent or Life-threatening Hemoptysis

Usually hemoptysis is self-limiting; however, there are times when bleeding is persistent. In those circumstances when hemoptysis cannot be controlled by routine means, further investigation and management may be required. Bronchoscopy helps localize the site of bleeding in combination with chest radiography. If specific therapy is ineffective and the patient continues to bleed, both diagnostic and therapeutic intervention may need to be carried out simultaneously. Therapeutic options include endobronchial tamponade, bronchial artery embolization, endobronchial irradiation, intrabronchial coagulative therapy, and/or thoracotomy.

Bronchial artery embolization is used for emergent hemostasis and must be carried out by an experienced angiographer who is familiar with the bronchial artery anatomy. Often bleeding can be controlled and negate the need for future thoracotomy; however, it must be realized that this procedure is palliative, and if there are no contraindications to thoracotomy elective resection may be safely performed at a later date. Katoh et al [32] found a 21.2% recurrence rate after initial successful embolization. No deaths occurred in this group, but four patients eventually required elective surgery.

Intraluminal irradiation using high activity sources with remote afterloading techniques (brachytherapy) [80, 81] have been increasingly used in the last several years. This form of therapy is reserved for patients with symptomatic airway disease from bronchogenic carcinoma. Recurrent hemoptysis often can be arrested with local radiation, which is well tolerated by the patient. Because of rapid dose falloff, surrounding lung tissue is spared. For this reason, even if patients have received maximal external beam radiation they are still candidates for brachytherapy.

Recently intrabronchial selective coagulation with fibrin, thrombin, or other agents have been successfully employed with excellent results [82, 83]. These agents are instilled via a fiberoptic bronchoscope, with special catheters in order to prevent premature coagulation in the bronchoscope. This approach is less invasive and easily performed in the emergency room setting.

In cases of massive life-threatening hemoptysis several of these options may be used in order to stabilize the patient. An additional option includes balloon tamponade with a Fogarty catheter placed into the bleeding subsegment via bronchoscopy [84, 85]. This allows time for intrabronchial coagulative therapy, bronchial artery embolization, or indeed thoracotomy to be performed under more stable conditions. This form of therapy is only palliative and should be performed through a controlled airway either with an endobronchial or tracheostomy tube. Gourin and Garzon [86] have described a method of selective intubation of the main stem bronchi in association with balloon occlusion when bleeding is from the left lung. This is used for emergency stabilization of the airway. Once that stabilization is achieved, surgery versus embolization, either intra-arterial [33] or intrabronchial, should be performed on an individual basis.

Surgical therapy carries significant risks and complications. Most patients have marginal lung reserve with potential postoperative respiratory insufficiency. The most serious postoperative complication is persistent bronchopleural fistula, occurring in 10% to 14% of patients. Other less common problems include postoperative hemorrhage, lung infarction, and wound infections. Although surgical resection remains the only definitive form of therapy, patients must be assessed individually. The majority of patients can be conservatively managed, but when bleeding remains uncontrolled surgery may be lifesaving [87].

In order to ensure optimal management of the patient with hemoptysis, a team approach, involving the primary care physician in conjunction with a pulmonologist or thoracic surgeon, is necessary. We have attempted to offer a practical approach to the timely diagnosis of both life-threatening and non–life-threatening hemoptysis, using the most advanced diagnostic studies. The initial work-up of non–life-threatening hemoptysis can be accomplished on an outpatient basis using noninvasive methods. However, if the diagnosis cannot be established, more invasive studies need to be undertaken, such as bronchoscopy or pulmonary angiography. In those patients with life-threatening massive hemoptysis, time is of the utmost concern in ensuring proper diagnosis and management in order to reduce morbidity and mortality.

References

1. Wolfe JD, Simmons DH: Hemoptysis: Diagnosis and management (medical progress). *West J Med* 127:383–390, 1977
2. Chaves AD: Hemoptysis in chest clinic patients. *American Review of Tuberculosis* 63:194–201, 1951
3. Smiddy JE, Elliott RC: The evaluation of hemoptysis with fiberoptic bronchoscopy. *Chest* 64:158–162, 1973
4. Ofoegbu RO, Anah OO, Jarikre LN, et al: Changing significance of haemoptysis in the tropics: Experience from Benin City, Nigeria. *Tropical Doctor* 14:188–189, 1984
5. Cohen MH: Signs and symptoms of bronchogenic carcinoma. *In* Straus MJ (ed): Lung Cancer: Clinical Diagnosis and Treatment. New York, Grune & Stratton, 1983, pp 97–111
6. Diamond MA, Genovese PD: Life-threatening hemoptysis in mitral stenosis. *JAMA* 215:441, 1971
7. Wolf L, Levine HB: Hemoptysis in rheumatic heart disease. Am Heart J 21:163–171, 1941
8. Williams WJ, Beutler E, Erslev AJ, et al: Antithrombic Therapy. Hematology, ed 4. New York, McGraw-Hill, 1990, pp 1575–1576
9. Petersdorf RG, Adams RD, Brannwald E, et al, (eds): Harrisons Principles of Internal Medicine, ed 10. New York, McGraw-Hill, 1983, pp 157–158
10. Dixon GF, Donnerberg RL, Schonfeld SA, et al: Clinical commentary: Advances in the diagnosis and treatment of broncholithiasis. *Am Rev Respir Dis* 129:1028–1030, 1984
11. Lin C-S, Becker WH: Broncholith as a cause of fatal hemoptysis. *JAMA* 239:2153, 1978
12. Rath GS, Schaff JT, Snider GL: Flexible fiberoptic bronchoscopy: Techniques and review of 100 bronchoscopies. *Chest* 63:689–693, 1973
13. Weaver LJ, Solliday N, Cugell DW: Selection of patients with hemoptysis for fiberoptic bronchoscopy. *Chest* 76:7, 1979
14. Poe RH, Israel RH, Marin MG, et al: Utility of fiberoptic bronchoscopy in patients with hemoptysis and a nonlocalizing chest roentgenogram. *Chest* 92:70–75, 1988
15. Peters J, McClung HC, Teague RB: Clinical medicine: Evaluation of hemoptysis in patients with a normal chest roentgenogram. *West J Med* 141:624–626, 1984
16. Santiago SM, Lehrman S, Williams AJ: Bronchoscopy in patients with haemoptysis and normal chest roentgenograms. *Br J Dis Chest* 81:186–188, 1987
17. Kallenbach J, Song E, Zwi S: Haemoptysis with no radiological evidence of tumour: The value of early bronchoscopy. *S Afr Med J* 59:556, 1981
18. Credle WF, Smiddy JF, Elliott RC: Complications of fiberoptic bronchoscopy. *Am Rev Respir Dis* 109:67–72, 1974
19. Zavala DC: Diagnostic fiberoptic bronchoscopy: Techniques and results of biopsies in 600 patients. *Chest* 68:12–19, 1975
20. Mitchell DM, Emerson CJ, Collyer J, et al: Fiberoptic bronchoscopy: Ten years on. *Br Med J* 281:360–363, 1980
21. Suratt PM, Smiddy JF, Gruber B: Deaths and complications associated with fiberoptic bronchoscopy. *Chest* 69:747, 1976
22. Gong H, Salvatierra C: Clinical efficacy of early and delayed fiberoptic bronchoscopy in patients with hemoptysis. *Am Rev Respir Dis* 124:221, 1981.
23. Denardo G, Goodwin DA, Ravasini R, et al: The ventilatory lung scan in the diagnosis of pulmonary embolism. *N Engl J Med* 282: 1334–1336, 1970
24. Hull RD, Hirsh J, Carter CJ, et al: Diagnostic value of ventilation-perfusion lung scanning in patients with suspected pulmonary embolism. *Chest* 88:819, 1985
25. Hull RD, Hirsh J, Carter C, et al: Pulmonary angiography, ventilation lung scanning, and venography for clinically suspected pulmonary embolism with abnormal perfusion lung scan. *Ann Intern Med* 98:891, 1983
26. PIOPED Investigators: Value of the ventilation/perfusion scan in acute pulmonary embolism. Results of the prospective investigation of pulmonary embolism diagnosis (PIOPED). *JAMA* 263:2753–2759, 1990
27. Hull RD, Raskob GE, Coates G, et al: A new noninvasive management strategy for patients with suspected pulmonary embolism. *Arch Intern Med* 149:2549–2555, 1989
28. White RH, McGahan JP, Daschbach MM, et al: Diagnosis of deep-vein thrombosis using duplex ultrasound. *Ann Intern Med* 111:297–304, 1989
29. Remy A: Treatment of hemoptysis by embolization of bronchial artery. *Radiology* 122: 33–37, 1977
30. Ulflacker R, Kaemmerer A, Neeves C, et al: Management of massive hemoptysis by bronchial artery embolization. *Radiology* 146: 627–634, 1983
31. Ulflacker R, Kaemmerer A, Picon PD, et al: Bronchial artery embolization in the management of hemoptysis: Technical aspects and long term results. *Radiology* 157:637–644, 1985

32. Katoh O, Kishikawa T, Yamada H, et al: Recurrent bleeding after arterial embolization in patients with hemoptysis. *Chest* 97:541–546, 1990
33. Magilligan DJ Jr, Ravipati S, Zayat P, et al: Massive hemoptysis: Control by transcatheter bronchial artery embolization. *Ann Thorac Surg* 32:392, 1981
34. Naidich DP, McCauley DI, Khouri NF, et al: Computed tomography of bronchiectasis. *J Comput Assist Tomogr* 6:437, 1982
34a. Haponik EF, Britt J, Smith PL, et al: Computed chest tomography in the evaluation of hemoptysis: Impact on diagnosis and treatment. *Chest* 91:80–85, 1987
35. Lewis M, Kallenbach J, Kark P, et al: Severe haemoptysis, associated with viral tracheitis. *Thorax* 37:869, 1982
36. Lyons HA: Differential diagnosis of hemoptysis and its treatment. *Basics RD* 5:1–5, 1976
37. Middleton JR, Sen P, Lange M, et al: Death-producing hemoptysis in tuberculosis. *Chest* 72:601, 1977
38. Rasmussen V: On hemoptysis, especially when fatal in its anatomical and clinical aspects (translated from the Hospitalis-Tidende, 11th year, No 9-13, Copenhagen, 1868, by Wilham Daniel Moore). *Edinburgh Med J* 14:385, 1868
39. Cudkowicz L: The blood supply of the lung in pulmonary tuberculosis. *Thorax* 7:270–276, 1952
40. Stinghe RV, Mangiulea VG: Hemoptysis of bronchial origin occurring in patients with arrested tuberculosis. *Am Rev Respir Dis* 101:84, 1970
41. Fischer GW, McGrew GL, Bass JW: Pulmonary paragonimiasis in childhood: A cause of persistent pneumonia and hemoptysis. *JAMA* 243:1360, 1980
42. Freundlich IM, Israel HL: Pulmonary aspergillosis. *Clin Radiol* 24:248, 1973
43. Varkey B, Rose HP: Pulmonary aspergilloma—A rational approach to treatment. *Am J Med* 61:626–631, 1976
44. Johns CJ: Management of hemoptysis with pulmonary fungus balls in sarcoidosis. *Chest* 82:400, 1982
45. Sade RM, Clouse M, Ellis FH Jr: The spectrum of pulmonary sequestration. *Ann Thorac Surg* 18:644, 1974
46. McCaughan BC, Martini N, Bains MS: Bronchial carcinoids: Review of 124 cases. *J Thorac Cardiovasc Surg* 89:8–17, 1985
47. Braman SS, Whitcomb ME: Endobronchial metastasis. *Arch Intern Med* 135:543–547, 1975
48. Stoller JK, Ahmad M, Rice TW: Solitary pulmonary nodule. *Cleve Clinic J Med* 55:68–74, 1988
49. Chaffey MH: The role of percutaneous lung biopsy in the workup of a solitary pulmonary nodule. *West J Med* 148:176–181, 1988
50. Albelda SM, Gefter WB, Epstein DM, et al: Diffuse pulmonary hemorrhage: A review and classification. *Radiology* 154:289, 1984
51. Leatherman JW, Davies SF, Hoidal JR: Alveolar hemorrhage syndromes: Diffuse microvascular lung hemorrhage in immune and idiopathic disorders. *Medicine* 63:343–361, 1984
52. Marino CT, Pertschuk LP: Pulmonary hemorrhage in systemic lupus erythematosis. *Arch Intern Med* 141:201, 1981
53. Fauci AS, Haynes BF, Katz P, et al: Wegener's granulomatosis: Prospective clinical and therapeutic experience with 85 patients for 21 years. *Ann Intern Med* 98:76–85, 1983
54. Cordier JF, Valeyre D, Guillevin L, et al: Pulmonary Wegener's granulomatosis. A clinical and imaging study of 77 cases. *Chest* 97:906–912, 1990
55. Robboy SJ, Minna JD, Colman RW, et al: Pulmonary hemorrhage syndrome as a manifestation of disseminated intravascular coagulation: Analysis of ten cases. *Chest* 63:718–721, 1973
56. Golde DW, Drew WL, Klein HZ, et al: Occult pulmonary haemorrhage in leukaemia. *Br Med J* 2:166–168, 1975
57. Fireman Z, Yust I, Abramov AL: Lethal occult pulmonary hemorrhage in drug-induced thrombocytopenia. *Chest* 79:358, 1981
58. Finley TN, Aronow A, Cosentino AM, et al: Occult pulmonary hemorrhage in anticoagulated patients. *Am Rev Respir Dis* 112:23–29, 1975
59. Dines DE, Seward JB, Bernatz PE: Pulmonary arteriovenous fistulas: *Mayo Clin Proc* 58:176, 1983
60. Peery WH: Clinical spectrum of hereditary hemorrhagic telangiectasia (Osler-Weber-Rendu disease). *Am J Med* 82:989–997, 1987
61. Barth KH, White RI Jr, Kaufman SL, et al: Embolotherapy of pulmonary arteriovenous malformations with detachable balloons. *Radiology* 142:599, 1982
62. Terry PB, Barth KH, Kaufman SL, et al: Balloon embolization for treatment of pulmonary arteriovenous fistulas. *N Engl J Med* 302:1189–1190, 1980
63. Pearce JG, Patt ML: Fatal pulmonary hemorrhage after percutaneous needle aspiration biopsy. *Am Rev Respir Dis* 110:346, 1974
64. Milner LB, Ryan K, Bullo J: Fatal intrathoracic hemorrhage after percutaneous aspiration lung biopsy. *Am J Roentgenol* 132:280–281, 1979
65. Haapaniemi J, Gadowski R, Naini M, et al: Massive hemoptysis secondary to flow-directed thermodilution catheters. *Cathet Cardiovasc Diagn* 5:151–157, 1974

66. Rosenblum SE, Ratliff NB, Shirley EK, et al: Pulmonary artery dissection induced by a swan-ganz catheter. *Cleve Clin Q* 51:671–675, 1984
67. Stauffer JL, Olson DE, Petty TL: Complications and consequences of endotracheal intubation and tracheotomy: A prospective study of 150 critically ill adult patients. *Am J Med* 70:65, 1981
68. Harkaway PS, Eichenhorn MS: Catamenial hemoptysis: A case report. *Henry Ford Hosp Med J* 34:68–69, 1986
69. Elliot DL, Barker AF, Dixon LM: Catamenial hemoptysis: New methods of diagnosis and therapy. *Chest* 87:5, 1985
70. Woellner RC, Wedel MK: Hemoptysis during orgasm (letter). *JAMA* 240:637, 1978
71. Bush A, Collins JV: Pulmonary Munchausen's syndrome. *Postgrad Med J* 58:564, 1982
72. Feinsilver SJ, Raffin TA, Kornei MC, et al: Factitious hemoptysis: The case of the red towel. *Arch Intern Med* 143:567–568, 1983
73. Limper AH, Prakash UB: Tracheobronchial foreign bodies in adults. *Ann Intern Med* 112:604–609, 1990
74. Rees JR: Massive hemoptysis associated with foreign body removal. *Chest* 88:475–476, 1985
75. Hillman BC, Kurzweg FB: Aspiration of grass inflorescene as a case of hemoptysis. *Chest* 78:306–309, 1980
76. Justiniani FR, Cabeza C, Miller BA: Cocaine-associated rhabdomyolysis and hemoptysis mimicking pulmonary embolism. *Am J Med* 88:317–318, 1990
77. Mehta AC, Ahmad M, Nunez C, et al: Newer procedures using the fiberoptic bronchoscope in the diagnosis of lung cancer. *Cleve Clin J Med* 54:195–203, 1987
78. Stein PD, Willis PW, DeMets DI, et al: Plain chest roentgenogram in patients with acute pulmonary embolism and no preexisting cardiac or pulmonary disease. *American Journal of Non-Invasive Cardiology*, 1986
79. Adelman M, Haponik EF, Bleecker ER, et al: Cryptogenic hemoptysis. *Ann Intern Med* 102: 829, 1985
80. Nori D, Hilaris BS, Martini N: Intraluminal irradiation in bronchogenic carcinoma. *Surg Clin North Am* 67:1093–1102, 1987
81. Seagren SL, Harrell JH, Horn RA: High dose rate intraluminal irradiation in recurrent endobronchial carcinoma. *Chest* 88:810–814, 1985
82. Tsukamoto T, Sasaki H, Nakamura H: Treatment of hemoptysis patients by thrombin and fibrinogen-thrombin infusion therapy using a fiberoptic bronchoscope. *Chest* 96:473–476, 1989
83. Bense L: Intrabronchial selective coagulative treatment of hemoptysis. *Chest* 97:990–996, 1990
84. Feloney JP, Balchum OJ: Repeated massive hemoptysis: Successful control using multiple balloon-tipped catheters for endobronchial tamponade. *Chest* 74:683, 1978
85. Thomas R, Siproudhis L, Laurent JF, et al: Massive hemoptysis from iatrogenic balloon catheter rupture of pulmonary artery; successful early management by balloon tamponade. *Crit Care Med* 15:272–273, 1987
86. Gourin A, Garzon AA: Operative treatment of massive hemoptysis. *Ann Thorac Surg* 18:52–69, 1974
87. Bobrowitz ID, Ramakrishna S, Shim YS: Comparison of medical vs. surgical treatment of major hemoptysis. *Arch Intern Med* 143: 1343–1346, 1983

7

Chest Discomfort

Adil Karamali and Lyle D. Victor

Chest pain is a common presenting complaint in the primary care physician's office. This symptom is often confusing and perplexing because of its many causes. Even more frustrating may be the nonspecific description of this symptom; being variously described not as pain but as a disagreeable sensation, feeling, or pressure. As many of the most life-threatening causes of chest discomfort seen in an ambulatory setting are of cardiac origin, the physician naturally focuses on the heart and may subject the patient to an extensive battery of tests without obtaining a clear diagnosis.

Thoracic pain may originate in various structures and organs within the thoracic cavity and below the diaphragm. Pain arising in the superficial tissues is easily localized by the patient. However, pain that arises in deeper structures may be difficult to localize and have uncharacteristic associated symptoms that usually mislead the physician. A careful history that elicits the location, character, radiation, and precipitating and alleviating factors is the most important key to establishing a correct diagnosis.

The purpose of this chapter is to assist physicians in establishing a differential diagnosis of chest pain and to suggest a systematic approach toward the correct diagnosis. A major challenge to the diagnostician is the fact that the causes of thoracic pain are many and varied (Table 7-1).

Pathophysiology of Chest Pain

There is an apparent lack of association between the location of chest pain and the organ involved [1]. This is explained by the fact that all major thoracic structures are supplied by the same sensory fibers. The dermatomal distribution for the thoracic cavity involves T1–T6, with extension down the anteromedial aspect of the arm and forearm. Sensory pathways from viscera in this region are interconnected and as such produce a similar pattern of chest pain. Dermatomes T1–T4 serve practically all thoracic viscera: myocardium, pericardium, aorta, pulmonary artery, esophagus, and mediastinum. Pain originating in these organs presents with the same quality: deep, visceral, and poorly localized. The point of maximal intensity is usually the retrosternal area, with radiation to the neck and arms. Dermatomes T5–T6 constitute the lower thoracic wall, diaphragm, pancreas, duodenum, and stomach. Pain originating in these structures is similar to that of areas supplied by dermatomes T1–T4; however, it is localized mainly in the subxiphoid region, with radiation to the back.

In order to determine the cause of deep chest pain the physician must use the location of the pain as a clue to the dermatomal distribution and shorten the list of causes by asking the appropriate historical questions followed by precise testing. The following discusses the causes of chest pain by systems.

Cardiovascular Causes of Chest Pain

Angina pectoris is the most common serious cause of chest pain seen by the primary care physician. The pain is commonly described as a heaviness, a sense of pressure, tightness, or squeezing located in the substernal area. Often radiation to the neck, left shoulder, and down the ulnar aspect of the arm is described. Some patients may describe the sensation along with the associated gesture of a

Table 7-1. Causes of Chest Discomfort

- Cardiovascular
  - Myocardial infarction
  - Coronary spasm and ischemia
  - Valvular diseases
  - Pericardial diseases
- Vascular
  - Aortic dissection and aneurysm
- Pulmonary
  - Pleuritis
  - Pulmonary embolus
  - Pulmonary hypertension
  - Tracheobronchitis
  - Pneumonia/abscess
  - Pneumothorax/pneumomediastinum
  - Neoplasm
- Gastrointestinal
  - Cholecystitis
  - Hepatic disease
  - Abdominal infection (abscess, perforation)
  - Peptic ulcer disease
  - Esophageal diseases
  - Hiatal hernia
- Musculoskeletal
  - Chest wall syndrome
  - Rib cage diseases
  - Intercostal myositis
  - Muscular strain
  - Cervical disk disease
  - Bone tumor
- Neurologic
  - Intercostal neuralgia
  - Herpes zoster
  - Cervical radiculopathy
- Psychological
  - Anxiety/depression
  - Hypochondriasis
  - Somatization syndrome
- Miscellaneous
  - Breast disease
  - Obesity
  - Mondor's disease

clenched fist (Levine's sign) [2]. A distinguishing factor may be provocation of the discomfort by exercise and resolution by rest. Sublingual nitroglycerin may differentiate a coronary artery etiology by abating pain within a few minutes of using nitrates. Another characteristic of angina is that the intensity of effort required to incite pain seems to vary from day to day and time of the day in the same patient. The anginal threshold is lower in the morning than at any other time of the day. Meals consumed, weather, and stress may be responsible for inconsistent pain reporting patterns. Coronary artery spasm (Prinzmetal's angina) may also be responsible for inconsistent reports of pain. Dyspnea may be the first sign of angina. The patient usually describes the midchest as the site of the shortness of breath. True dyspnea is not as well localized. Other associated symptoms of chest pain associated with myocardial disease (infarction) include nausea, vomiting, diaphoresis, and, by definition, pain that is present for 20 minutes or more [3].

In clinical practice the difficulty arises in those without the classical symptoms of angina pectoris. Patients may use different words to describe their discomfort and may perceive their pain in an atypical location. For example, atypical chest pain may be described as sharp while unusual locations of discomfort may be found in the neck, jaw, or teeth. Surprisingly benign precipitating events may include nothing more than rising in the morning or eating a large meal. Some patients may perceive pain early in the course of their physical activity that improves as the physical activity continues. Confusing the issue is the fact that other cardiac disorders may show ischemic symptoms that produce pain identical to angina pectoris. Aortic valvular stenosis and idiopathic hypertrophic subaortic stenosis may cause pain identical to angina pectoris.

A practical question to ask all patients complaining of chest discomfort is whether a doctor has previously evaluated their pain. Often, another physician has ordered an exercise stress test or upper gastrointestinal series. Knowledge of negative prior examinations will help the primary care physician to direct diagnostic studies into more productive areas. Physical examination may help sort out the cause of chest pain when used in conjunction with appropriate testing [4]. For example, the acute onset of an S_4 gallop or the systolic murmur of acute papillary muscle dysfunction suggests acute myocardial dysfunction, whereas palpable chest pain suggests a more musculoskeletal origin. [5]

Valvular and Septal Disease

Coronary ischemia is not the only cardiac cause of chest discomfort. The often encountered valvular heart disease, aortic stenosis, may present as chest pain. There are three etiologies of aortic stenosis: congenital, rheumatic, and degenerative [5]. Congenital aortic stenosis secondary to a biscuspid valve is most common in patients under 50 years of age. Many patients with this lesion have an audible ejection click along with a short systolic murmur. Rheumatic fever should be considered a cause when coexisting mitral valve disease is evident. Physical examination reveals a normal blood pressure unless coexistent hypertension or aortic regurgitation is evident. Inspection of the thorax may reveal a localized systolic pulsation in the second right intercostal space due to poststenotic dilatation of the aorta. Examination of the carotid arterial pulse may show a slow rising, small volume arterial pulse sometimes called pulsus parvus et tardus. The detection of an aortic click, at the apex and to the right of the sternum, confirms the diagnosis. Additionally, in approximately two thirds of elderly patients, the second heart sound is single. The second heart sound (S_2) is paradoxic in about 25% of patients and may be quite normal in others. Aortic stenosis produces a classic systolic ejection murmur: a crescendo-decrescendo sound that begins after the first heart sound (S_1) and ends before S_2. The murmur sounds harsh and is typically heard best at the second left interspace.

Another cause of chest pain is idiopathic hypertrophic subaortic stenosis, sometimes known as hypertrophic cardiomyopathy, which usually presents secondary to a massively enlarged intraventricular septum associated with displacement of the anterior leaflet of the mitral valve during ventricular systole. Idiopathic hypertrophic subaortic stenosis has two variants: obstructive and nonobstructive. Presenting symptoms of idiopathic hypertrophic subaortic stenosis vary, including dyspnea on exertion, dizziness, syncope, angina, and palpitations. Chest pain is similar to classic angina pectoris and is related to an imbalance between oxygen supply and demand as a consequence of the increased myocardial mass [6]. Malignant arrhythmias may cause sudden death, often in young adults. Physical examination of patients with idiopathic hypertrophic subaortic stenosis must include observation of the jugular venous pulses. A prominent a wave as a result of a noncompliant right ventricle and powerful atrial contraction is characteristic. The systolic murmur of idiopathic hypertrophic subaortic stenosis is a long ejection murmur heard best at the apex and frequently variable in intensity. The Valsalva maneuver usually increases the intensity of the murmur, whereas squatting or leg raising usually decreases its intensity because the associated increase in right-sided heart return increases left ventricular volume. The apparent obstruction to the left ventricular outflow is thereby reduced and the systolic murmur is softened.

Mitral valve prolapse (MVP) and mitral stenosis are other valvular disorders that may be associated with symptoms indistinguishable from classic angina. MVP is the most common anomaly of the mitral valve, affecting as much as 5% to 10% of the population [7]. Affected individuals may have a variety of symptoms such as palpitations, chest pain, and dyspnea. Chest discomfort may be similar to angina pectoris, but most often is atypical in that it is prolonged, not clearly related to exertion, and usually described as short episodes of sharp stabbing pain at the apex. The discomfort is secondary to the tension on the papillary muscles. Physical examination of the patient may suggest the diagnosis as individuals with familial MVP are often red-haired women with fair skin [8]. They may have an increased incidence of associated musculoskeletal abnormalities such as kyphoscoliosis, Marfan's syndrome, Ehlers-Danlos syndrome, osteogenesis imperfecta, and Duchenne's muscular dystrophy [8]. The presence of a single click or multiple clicks in mid to late systole is specific for MVP. This should be differentiated from a systolic ejection: the MVP click occurs distinctly after the beginning of the upstroke of the carotid pulse. There may be an associated holosystolic murmur following the click that continues to A2. The murmur is similar to that produced by papillary muscle dysfunction. The duration of the murmur is related to the severity of the regurgitation, and when confined to the latter portion of systole, regurgitation is usually not severe. Clicks are best heard at the apex with the patient in the left lateral decubitus position. Electrocardiographic evaluation of patients with MVP is most commonly within normal limits. In a small minority of asymptomatic patients and in a majority of symptomatic patients, the electrocardiogram (ECG) characteristically shows inverted T waves and nonspecific ST-segment changes in leads II, III, and aV_F [8]. A wide variety of arrhythmias, including atrial and ventricular premature contractions and supraventricular and ventricular tachyarrythmias and various forms of bradyarrhythmias, have been observed in association with MVP. The most common sustained tachyarrhythmia is paroxysmal supraventricular tachycardia [9].

Diagnostic criteria for MVP are divided into major and minor criteria and nonspecific findings [10]. The presence of one or more major criteria establishes the diagnosis of MVP. Minor criteria only raise the suspicion of MVP but in themselves are not sufficient to establish a diagnosis.

Mitral stenosis uncommonly presents with the symptom of chest pain as thoracic discomfort is seen in only 15% of cases. The pain is indistinguishable from angina pectoris. It is most likely the result of right ventricular hypertension and may be further complicated by coronary atherosclerosis [11, 12]. The principal symptom of mitral stenosis is dyspnea secondary to a reduction in compliance of the lungs. Hemoptysis is another frequent symptom caused by mitral stenosis. Physical examination may reveal a small volume arterial pulse and a prominent a wave on examination of the jugular venous pulse. Auscultation of the heart may reveal an opening snap that is heard best at the cardiac apex with the diaphragm of the stethoscope. There may be an accompanying accentuated first heart sound. The diastolic murmur of mitral stenosis is a low-pitched, rumbling murmur, heard best at the apex with the bell of the stethoscope. The murmur usually starts immediately after the opening snap. ECG may reveal left atrial enlargement in those patients in sinus rhythm.

Pericardial Disease

The pericardium has few pain fibers, yet cardiac discomfort may be felt because of pain generated from the adjacent parietal pleura. There may be a distinct pleuritic component to the chest discomfort that changes with respiration. Exacerbations of pericardial pain are also related to coughing and inspiration. Pericarditis may cause pain that is sharp and stabbing, which varies in intensity and may last for hours. Pericardial pain is commonly localized to the left shoulder, arm, and retrosternal areas, frequently radiating to the trapezius ridge and neck. The pain is often aggravated by lying supine, coughing, deep inspiration, and swallowing. It is relieved by sitting up and leaning forward. Sometimes the pain is noted with each heartbeat [13].

There may be a history of a recent viral syndrome or inflammatory disorders such as systemic lupus erythematosus and rheumatoid arthritis. Pericarditis is also associated with uremia. Auscultation of the heart reveals the pathognomonic pericardial friction rub. The rub is classically described as having three components: atrial systolic, ventricular systolic, and early diastolic. The atrial systolic component is present in approximately 70% of affected individuals and the ventricular component is present in almost all cases [14]. An important feature of the rub is that it is transitory and may change in quality from one examination to the next. A pericardial rub may be confused with a murmur, air in the mediastinum, or the artifact of skin scratching against the stethoscope. Rubs may be differentiated from murmurs by physical maneuvers, timing of the rub, and ECG changes. Serial ECGs are extremely helpful in diagnosing pericarditis. ECG changes associated with pericarditis are divided into four stages [15]. Stage I accompanies the onset of chest pain and is virtually diagnostic of acute pericarditis. These changes include ST-segment elevation that is concave upward and is present in all leads except aV_R and V_1. The T waves are usually upright. Stage II changes manifest several days later and are accompanied by the return of the ST segments to baseline and T-wave flattening followed by T-wave inversions. This is in contrast to changes in acute myocardial infarction where the T waves often become inverted before the return of the ST segments to baseline. Stage III involves inversion of the T waves without loss of R-wave voltage or the appearance of Q waves. Stage IV represents the normalization of T-wave changes, which may take up to weeks or months. Occasionally T-wave inversions persist indefinitely, usually in patients with chronic pericardial inflammation due to tuberculosis, uremia, or neoplastic disease. A word of caution: stage I changes may be confused with early repolarization changes usually seen in young men in whom the characteristic symptoms of pericardial inflammation are absent. The ECG in early repolarization does not evolve through the four stages described for pericardial disease [16]. The most common arrythmia associated with pericardial disease is sinus tachycardia. Other atrial arrhythmias suggest underlying myocardial disease [17].

The management of acute pericarditis is based on its cause and usually includes bed rest and observation in the hospital to exclude underlying myocardial infarction and the possibility of cardiac tamponade. The pain of pericarditis usually responds to nonsteroidal anti-inflammatory agents, although corticosteroid therapy may be warranted for failure of treatment after 48 hours. Antibiotics should only be used to treat a confirmed purulent cause of pericarditis. Oral anticoagulants should never be administered in the acute phase of pericarditis because of the risk of pericardial bleeding and tamponade. If anticoagulation is necessary (such as in the presence of prosthetic valves), then intravenous heparin should be employed. Pericarditis secondary to viral, idiopathic, postmyocardial infarction, or postpericardiotomy syndromes are usually self-limited and abate in 2 to 6 weeks. Disabling chest pain and fever may recur over a period of years and require steroid administration for pain relief [18].

Other Cardiovascular Diseases

Aortic vascular disease such as dissecting aneurysm may present with tearing chest pain and radiation to the back. As most of these patients are hemodynamically unstable, presentation to an outpatient facility is rare.

Taking an adequate history is most important in differentiating the various etiologies of chest pain. For example, chest discomfort similar to previous episodes of ischemic pain suggests angina. Atypical chest pain is frequently nonanginal in origin as up to 80% of these patients may have normal coronary angiograms [19]. The ECG may also be useful in diagnosing the cause of chest pain. The suspicion of angina may be aroused if nonspecific S- and T-wave changes are found. Sometimes ECG findings of left ventricular hypertrophy or ST-T wave changes indicate underlying coronary ischemia and epicardial disease. Valvular heart disease and pericardial effusions are readily detected with the aid of echocardiography. An exercise test combined with coronary angiography may give further definitive answers depending on the clinical assessment and validity of the initial testing.

Pulmonary Etiologies of Chest Pain

Although the visceral pleura of the lung contains no pain fibers, the parietal pleural reflection is richly innervated. Stimulation of these fibers by adjacent pulmonary pathology is seen in many disorders of the thorax. Chest pain secondary to pulmonary diseases is characterized by relatively acute onset and a pleuritic quality. Pleuritic chest pain is restricted in its location and is usually one sided, following a distribution of the intercostal nerves. Pulmonary chest pain is frequently described as sharp or a catch and is worsened by taking a deep breath or coughing. The pain is often superficial in nature. Associated symptoms include dyspnea, especially with exertion [20]. Specific entities causing pleuritic chest pain are listed in Table 7-1.

Dyspnea is the most common symptom seen in pulmonary embolus, occurring in approximately 84% of patients in one series [21]. Pulmonary embolism presents with pleuritic chest pain about 75% of the time. Dyspnea frequently accompanies the onset of chest pain. The findings of acute cor pulmonale, accentuated pulmonic closure sound, jugular venous distention, and systemic hypotension are characteristic of massive pulmonary embolus and may subsequently be fatal [22]. Hypoxia on arterial blood gases and ECG findings may aid in the diagnosis. The correct use of an isotope lung scan followed, if necessary, by pulmonary angiography can confirm the diagnosis (see Chap. 10). Pulmonary artery embolism and infarction present with pain in the dermatomal distribution T1 to T4 as discussed in the introduction to this chapter. Inability to confirm an embolus by diagnostic testing should prompt an investigation for other conditions, such as asthma, bronchopneumonia, pleurisy, pericarditis, pneumothorax, myocardial infarction, or perforated peptic ulcer. Recurrent pulmonary embolus can increase pulmonary artery pressure and may be mistaken for pulmonary hypertension [23]. Similar symptoms between these two disease entities include fatigue, dyspnea on exertion, chest pain, syncope, hemoptysis, and cyanosis. Their clinical course is one of progressive dyspnea, leading to right-sided heart failure. Some major differences help separate these two clinical entities. Recurrent pulmonary embolus usually manifests in persons older than 50 years with a female to male ratio of 1:1. Pulmonary hypertension on the other hand is most commonly manifested in persons between the ages of 20 to 40 years, with women being affected four times as often. Lung scanning shows classic perfusion defects in the setting of pulmonary embolus whereas no defects are seen in pulmonary hypertension [24].

The pulmonary circulation is a low resistance system and is not prone to elevated pressures. Most cases of pulmonary hypertension are caused by another illness. As a rule the signs and symptoms of this secondary pulmonary hypertension are those manifested by the underlying disease process. However, primary pulmonary hypertension is encountered occasionally and represents a clinical challenge of exclusion. Its diagnosis is based on the clinical, radiographic, and hemodynamic findings in addition to the inability to find a probable cause clinically. Primary pulmonary hypertension is responsible for about 1% of all causes of cor pulmonale. The only clue to the disorder in its early stages is roentgenographic evidence of prominent pulmonary arteries. However, pulmonary hypertension is clearly developed by this time and the most common evoked symptoms are easy fatigability and nondescript chest discomfort. In a study done by Fuster et al [25], consisting of the long-term follow-up of 120 patients with pulmonary hypertension, it was shown that the mean age at diagnosis was 34 years, with 73% of the patients being women. The four most frequent clinical symptoms at the time of diagnosis were exertional dyspnea, a loud second heart sound, roentgenographic abnormalities including cardiomegaly and prominent pulmonary arteries, and ECG changes such as right ventricular hypertrophy, right axis deviation, and large P waves. Chest pain was usually associated with exertion and was noted in only 8% of the patients studied. As the disease progresses, dyspnea with exertion is common, with most patients presenting with tachypnea. Other symptoms include weakness and syncope on effort. Right-sided heart failure eventually develops as the disease progresses. The physical examination of patients with pulmonary hypertension may show a jugular venous pulse with a prominent a wave, a palpable impulse over the main pulmonary artery, and an accentuated second heart sound. An audible S_4 gallup may be appreciated secondary to right atrial contraction into a hypertrophied right side of the heart. The murmur of pulmonic valvular insufficiency may be present as the right side of the heart dilates in advanced disease.

Pulmonary infection including bronchopneumonia, abscess, and tracheobronchitis are discussed at great length in other chapters.

Gastrointestinal Causes of Chest Pain

Evaluation of chest pain should begin with the exclusion of the most life-threatening etiologies, including coronary artery disease, aortic dissection, cardiac tamponade, and esophageal rupture. Each one of these problems has distinguishing clinical features. Esophageal syndromes are common causes of chest pain in many patients who do not have cardiac disease. Colgan et al [26] demonstrated esophageal disorders in 51% of patients with evidence of coronary artery disease. Unfortunately, cardiac and esophageal causes of chest pain may be quite similar in presentation and may coexist. Esophageal causes of chest pain include those listed in Table 7-2. Most often symptoms other than chest pain accompany the various disorders (Table 7-3).

Sympathetic nerve fibers richly innervate the esophagus. Regulation of smooth muscle is probably due to α- and β-sympathetic fibers. β-Adrenergic agonists relax and α-agonists contract the smooth muscle of the lower esophageal sphincter. As early as 1940 Morrison and Swaim [27] demonstrated chest pain and ischemia on balloon dilatation of the esophagus. The complexity of esophageal motility disorders is related to smooth muscle dysfunction.

Table 7-2. Chest Pain of Esophageal Origin

GERD
Esophageal motility disorders
Nutcracker esophagus
Diffuse esophageal spasm
Achalasia
Malignancy

Table 7-3. Symptoms Suggestive of Esophageal Origin of Chest Pain

Heartburn
Dysphagia
Pain relief with antacids
Postprandial pain
Sleep-interrupting pain
Symptoms in the absence of exertion
Symptoms lasting >20 minutes
Retrosternal pain without lateral radiation

Gastroesophageal reflux disease (GERD) is the most common cause of noncardiac chest pain [28]. Symptomatic GERD is manifested by heartburn; however, chest pain indistinguishable from angina may be of esophageal origin [29]. Reflux may further result in chronic cough, aspiration pneumonia, and most notably, reflex bradycardia [30]. Furthermore, pathologic reflux disease may occur without pain or other sensation of heartburn [30]. Garcia-Pulido et al [31] studied patients with documented coronary artery disease and concluded that up to 70% of episodes of chest pain were secondary to esophageal disorders. Mild, transient reflux occurs in many normal individuals after a meal. Clearance of the acid material occurs quickly. The episodes of reflux that are prolonged with slow clearance times are more serious and may be associated with significant pain. Most serious are the episodes occurring at night because of very prolonged acid clearing times that result in the significant complication of aspiration.

Achalasia is a term that refers to a failure to relax the lower esophageal sphincter. The disorder occurs as a result of a lack of smooth muscle innervation of the esophageal body and lower esophageal sphincter. Symptoms are caused by failure of the lower esophageal sphincter to relax during swallowing. Most often achalasia is associated with progressive dilatation of the esophageal body and may be associated with chest pain in its early stages [32]. Although dysphagia is the most common symptom, achalasia may be associated

Table 7-4. Esophageal Chest Pain: Tests and Findings

Disorder	*Test*	*Finding*
GERD	Barium swallow	Reflux of barium
	Endoscopy	Stricture, ulcer, Barrett's
	Bernstein's test	Symptoms reproduced with acid
	24-hour pH	Detect, quantitate reflux
Achalasia	Barium swallow	Esophageal dilatation
	Endoscopy	Secondary causes (gastric cancer)
	Manometry	Incomplete lower esophageal sphincter relaxation
Esophageal spasm	Barium swallow	Uncoordinated simultaneous contractions
	Manometry	Increased amplitude and duration
Nutcracker	Manometry	Peristaltic amplitude > 180 mm Hg

with chest pain. In a series of 910 patients, Katz et al [33] showed that 255 were secondary to esophageal motility disorders, with 2% of patients having achalasia.

Esophageal spasm disorders are accompanied by intermittent dysphagia. The most common form of spasm is the nutcracker esophagus. The prolonged contraction associated with this disorder produces chest pain and dysphagia [34]. Table 7-4 lists the various types of spasm and motility disorders and their associated findings.

Diagnostic Tests

Many authors recommend ruling out a cardiac cause of chest pain before performing tests to diagnose esophageal disease as an etiology to unexplained chest pain [35, 36]. A barium swallow may document GERD and show evidence of stricture, ulcer, and Barrett's (a precancerous) epithelium. Bernstein's test, using a nasogastric tube to perfuse the esophagus with alternating solutions of isotonic saline and 0.1 N-hydrochloric acid, may be especially helpful in distinguishing esophageal pain because pain is provoked by infusion of the acid. Bernstein's test has a sensitivity of 50% and a predictive value of 38%. However, the 24-hour ambulatory esophageal pH monitoring may have rendered Bernstein's test obsolete [37]. Achalasia and scleroderma are often evident on esophageal fiberoptic endoscopy, which may be especially useful in excluding other causes of chest pain such as carcinoma, candida, and herpetic esophagitis. Endoscopy may further aid in identifying complications of GERD such as erosive esophagitis, Barrett's esophagus, and esophageal ulceration.

Since GERD is the most common cause of esophageal chest pain, empiric therapy is warranted for symptoms suggestive of this disorder [38]. Relief of symptoms with antacids alone or in combination with H_2-receptor antagonists leads one to suspect a diagnosis of GERD. In addition to medications, conservative therapy may be of great help, including elimination of late night snacks, elevation of the head of the bed, and avoidance of alcohol, chocolate, fat, and tobacco, agents that are known to reduce lower esophageal sphincter pressure.

The treatment of achalasia is more complex. The calcium channel blockers have been shown to decrease contractions of smooth muscles, resulting in relaxation of the distal two thirds of the esophagus [39]. Other studies have shown that the amplitude and duration of contraction is inhibited by nitrates and hydralazine, which subsequently reduce lower esophageal sphincter pressure [40]. However, this effect was shown to be transient and may not be reproducible with oral or topical nitrates [41]. Of the calcium channel blockers, only nifedipine has been shown to be efficacious in the treatment of achalasia [42]. Other treatment options for achalasia include pneumatic dilation and surgical myotomy.

Management of any esophageal disorder should be instituted in a step-wise fashion. It is important to recognize coexistent disorders that may require additional therapy. Esophagitis and carcinoma classically produce chest pain and dysphagia, may coexist, and are diagnosed with the aid of a barium swallow and endoscopy.

Nonesophageal Gastrointestinal Causes of Chest Pain

Diaphragmatic hernia (hiatal hernia) presents as a dull, steady or burning pain located in the retrosternal or xiphoid region. This pain may be confused with angina except that it is not relieved with the administration of nitroglycerin and has no associated ECG findings. The pain is usually worse in the recumbent position. Physical findings are limited, however, as one of the only findings may be the auscultation of peristaltic sounds over the left hemithorax. Diagnosis with the aid of plain radiography and barium studies is readily available. The defect is twice as common in women and affects approximately 70% to 80% of the population older than 60. If a hiatal hernia is associated with reflux then therapy should be directed as for GERD. However, those defects not associated with reflux disease probably do not warrant any specific therapeutic measures [43].

Zenker's diverticulum is an outpouching in the posterior hypopharynx that produces dysphagia and regurgitation of food. Occasionally it may produce retrosternal chest pain. It is easily visualized with the aid of esophagraphy. Other important symptomatology includes gurgling sounds in the neck, halitosis, and a sour metallic taste in the mouth. Complications of Zenker's diverticulum may be potentially serious. These vary and include regurgitation and aspiration, leading to tracheobronchial irritation and aspiration pneumonitis. Occasionally, food may become trapped in the diverticulum and lead to perforation. Treatment is usually surgical [44].

At times cholecystitis may present as substernal chest pain. Classically it is described as an acute onset of pain following a large meal. This relationship of pain after meals rather than after exertion may be used as a clue in the differentiation of chest discomfort from anginal causes versus cholestatic causes. Most commonly the pain from acute cholecystitis is localized to the right upper quadrant. An ultrasound of the abdomen that shows stones is useful in differentiating cholecystitis from other abdominal sources of discomfort. Differential diagnosis includes abdominal angina, peptic ulcer disease, acute pancreatitis, and, on occasion, the Fitz-Hugh-Curtis syndrome associated with acute gonococcal infection. Peptic ulcer disease is suggested by a history of epigastric pain relieved with food. It is aggravated by aspirin and alcohol and usually flares in the early morning.

Neuromuscular Causes of Chest Pain

Chest wall muscular pain is one of the most common causes of chest discomfort [45]. Unfortunately, the diagnosis is often one of exclusion and requires a meticulous history and physical examination. Too often patients undergo extensive work-ups for what proves to be chest pain of musculoskeletal origin [46]. Chest wall pain may originate in muscles, bones, joints, ligaments, and nerves. There are very few specific laboratory tests to aid in the diagnosis. Levine and Mascette [47] demonstrated that musculoskeletal tenderness that reproduces chest pain combined with testing suggestive of low probability of coronary artery disease may be useful in ruling out ischemic coronary disease. Furthermore, they suggest that local injection of tendon sheaths, bursae, and trigger points with anesthetics and corticosteroids is both beneficial diagnostically and therapeutically.

Tietze's syndrome, or costochondritis, is characterized by swelling, redness, and warmth of the anterior chest. Most often the diagnosis is suggested by a history of minor trauma or new or unusual physical activity. The ache associated with Tietze's syndrome may last for hours and is commonly relieved by heat, anti-inflammatory medications, and analgesics.

The chest wall twinge syndrome is one of the more frequent complaints bringing patients to seek medical attention. The patient experiences brief episodes of sharp pain or "catches" in the left anterior chest. This symptom last from 1 to 3 minutes and may be aggravated in the bent over posture. It is worsened with deep breathing and is relieved by shallow respirations [48]. A rarer cause of palpable chest pain is a bone tumor.

Sharp, stabbing pain along an intercostal nerve produces the nonspecific syndrome of intercostal neuralgia. The pain worsens on deep inspiration and motion of the trunk. Tenderness along the nerve is diagnostic. Intercostal neuralgia may be associated with tabes dorsalis, mediastinal neoplasms, neurofibroma, and vertebral caries. Rib disease includes fracture and periostitis. Fractures cause well-localized sharp pain, especially with breathing and coughing. Many cases of rib fractures have a prior history of blunt trauma. Point tenderness and crepitations are suggestive of the diagnosis. Periostitis can also produce sharp, localized tenderness affected by motion that persists for hours and is worse at night. Severe coughing and sneezing may lead to rib fractures, especially when a destructive local process is present such as metastatic cancer. Mondor's disease or thrombophlebitis of the thoracoepigastric vein presents with chest pain along with palpable tenderness. The pain is felt along the anterolateral chest wall, with radiation to the axilla or inguinal region. A tender cord is usually palpable. The disease is self-limited and lasts 2 to 4 weeks [49].

Cervical spine disease may cause upper infraclavicular, anterior chest wall pain. The mechanism of this referred pain is not clearly defined. Pain referred from cervical spine disease may be felt at the base of the neck, across the top of the shoulder, the medial aspect of the upper arm and forearm, and across the deltoid muscle.

Herpes zoster is a common, often self-limited disease characterized by pain and dermatomal vesicular rash caused by reactivation of the varicella zoster virus. Its clinical onset is usually documented by pain, with the rash generally appearing a few days later [50]. In most patients the rash and pain completely disappear [51]. Pain that persists or recurs beyond the period of active skin disease is referred to as postherpetic neuralgia. Postherpetic neuralgia is a constant deep pain that is recurrent and accompanied by allodynia. The mechanism of this recurrence is unknown [52]. Three different components of postherpetic neuralgia are described: (1) constant deep burning or aching discomfort called continuous, (2) brief, spontaneous, recurrent, shooting, or shocking pain called neuralgic, and (3) sharp radiating dysesthetic pain elicited by light mechanical stimulation called allodynia [52]. Pain relief using local infiltration of anesthetics is of rapid onset and long duration even in chronic pain situations. Rowbotham and Fields [52] found skin infiltration easy to perform and sufficient to eliminate pain in a majority of cases.

Psychological Causes of Chest Discomfort

Chest pain is a common somatic symptom of emotional illness and is quite often associated with anxiety disorders. It is estimated that psychiatric illness is present in up to 50% of patients presenting for a cardiac evaluation [53]. Atypical chest discomfort secondary to psychiatric causes is also a frequent cause of admission to the coronary care unit [54]. Lavey and Winkle [55] demonstrated a lack of patient reassurance and consolability associated with a high cost of disability secondary to chest discomfort of noncardiac origin. Overall, however, psychiatric disorders are considerably more common than in the general population and occur with a higher incidence in those patients with other chronic diseases [56].

Clinical features of atypical chest pain

include a noncardiac description of chest pain, breathlessness, hyperventilation, previous history of psychiatric disorder, and a conviction of heart disease. Atypical chest pain may be associated with a history of chronic stress, coincide with life events, and a recognition of a family history of chest discomfort [57]. Other symptoms include palpitations, fatigue, sweats, sighs, parasthesias, and syncope. Physical signs accompanying atypical chest pain include more than one site of localization or diffuse areas of tenderness. Other features that point toward a psychiatric cause include association with dizziness, anxiety, depression, and an extreme concern with somatic complaints. The etiology for such a syndrome is multifactorial, frequently complicated by the patient's misinterpretation of their significance [58]. This frequently leads to an exacerbation of the underlying disease process, thus creating a vicious cycle. Treatment on initial presentation should include a negative work-up for organic causes followed by reassurance that none was found. In cases where patients are not satisfied, repeated reassurances may actually worsen the symptoms [59]. In these cases it is important to elicit the patient's fears and concerns about the pain. Hyperventilation should be explored thoroughly by performing a hyperventilation provocation test [53]. The test is performed by asking the patient to breathe at a rate of 30 to 40 breaths per minute for 3 minutes and then asking the patient to stop. If the symptoms were reproduced during this period of hyperventilation then the test is considered positive. Additionally, in a positive test, dizziness and parasthesias of the digits may precede chest pain. Treatment ranges from psychological therapy to medical intervention. Medications include tricyclic antidepressants, β-blocking agents in those with palpitations, and benzodiazepine anxiolytic drugs in those who have significant anxiety.

Other Causes of Chest Discomfort

Chest wall pain is a common occurrence after thoracotomy. This pain is generally attributed to (1) postthoracotomy pain syndrome or (2) pain of musculoskeletal origin, including infection, sternal nonunion, sternal dehiscence, fractured ribs, or painful sternal wires [60]. The postthoracotomy pain syndrome is described as an aching sensation in the distribution of the incision. The discomfort is usually present beyond 2 months after the surgical procedure and may recur as parasthesias. It is usually accompanied by tenderness, sensory loss, and absence of sweating along the scar [61]. Mailis et al [62] further described 11 patients seen 4 months to 5 years after internal mammary artery bypass grafting with a specific cluster of signs and symptoms confined to the site of internal mammary artery harvesting and postulated that internal mammary artery bypass surgery was associated with a specific pain syndrome. The syndrome develops after injury to the anterior branches of the intercostal nerves at the site of harvesting the graft. They also noted severe tenderness on palpation of the sternum and costosternal junction. The majority of these patients were also noted to have delayed healing of their sternal wounds. Treatment is similar to other causes of chest wall pain, i.e., sympathetic blockade, and analgesics.

A recent entry to the list of causes of chest pain is the use of "crack" cocaine. Most users present with chest pain and dyspnea. In a study by Eurman et al [63], 72% of cases complained of chest pain alone, 11% complained of dyspnea, and 17% complained of both symptoms. A large number of complications associated with the use of cocaine are described, including arrhythmias, myocardial infarction, myocarditis, and sudden death [64]. Pneumomediastinum and pneumothorax are further pulmonary complications of cocaine use that present with chest discomfort.

One of the most difficult diagnostic tasks for the primary care physician is to distinguish anginal and nonanginal chest pain. As many as 30% of patients diagnosed as having anginal chest pain were found to have normal coronary angiograms [65]. Furthermore, up to 50% of patients with angina also have concurrent musculoskeletal pain [66]. Attributing chest pain to a coronary cause is common. For example, Goldman et al [36] have stated that only 30% of patients admitted to the coronary care unit are eventually diagnosed as having a myocardial infarction. They developed a protocol that "performed as well as the physicians." Using this protocol, computer-assisted programs for the evaluation of chest pain in the emergency department have been derived [67].

Generally speaking, cardiac causes of chest pain should be investigated initially. To determine if the pain is of anginal origin it must meet certain criteria: it lasts longer than 20 to 30 minutes, is relieved with sitting up, which reduces the venous return to the heart, and is of a crescendo-decrescendo nature and not short stabbing pain [68]. Once cardiac causes of chest discomfort have been eliminated, pulmonary causes for chest discomfort should be sought. A chest pain that increases with inspiration is usually nonanginal. An exception is the fact that hyperventilation can worsen chest pain by increasing venous return to the heart by causing coronary vasoconstriction [69]. One of the most common nonanginal symptoms missed is pain brought on by arm movement. This type of pain is frequently nonanginal and usually related to musculoskeletal disorders. The occasional patient, however, may have anginal pain exacerbated by performing work with the arms stretched over the head. Furthermore, these patients have chest tenderness on palpation. Gastrointestinal disorders such as from esophageal causes should be investigated next. Pain that is reproduced by stooping forward is classically esophageal in origin [70]. Once these causes have been satisfactorily ruled out a psychosomatic cause of chest discomfort must be sought. With the rising cost of medical care it is increasingly important for physicians to recognize the various causes of chest discomfort and be able to diagnose it with reasonable accuracy. With continued experience, it is possible to label a patient's symptoms as nonanginal even in the face of significant coronary artery disease by angiography.

References

1. Wall P: Heart pain. *In* Textbook of Pain, ed 2. New York, Churchill Livingstone, 1989, p 410
2. Levine HJ: Difficult problems in the diagnosis of chest pain. *Am Heart J* 100:108, 1980
3. Sampson JJ, Cheitlin MD: Pathophysiology and differential diagnosis of cardiac pain. *Prog Cardiovasc Dis* 13:507, 1971
4. Stein PD, Sabbah HN: Intensity of heart sounds in the evaluation of patients following myocardial infarction. *Chest* 75:679, 1979
5. Abrams J: Synopsis of Cardiac Physical Diagnosis. Philadelphia Lea & Febiger, 1989
6. Sutton MG, Tajik AJ, Smith HC, et al: Angina in idiopathic hypertrophic subaortic stenosis. A clinical correlation of regional left ventricular dysfunction. A videometric and echocardiographic study. *Circulation* 61:561, 1980
7. Savage DD, Garrison RJ, Devereux RB, et al: Mitral valve prolapse in the general population. I. Epidemiologic features: The Framingham study. *Am Heart J* 106:571, 1983
8. Barlow JB: Perspectives on the Mitral Valve. Philadelphia, F.A. Davis, 1987, pp 45–112
9. Josephson ME, Horowitz LN, Kastor JA: Proximal supraventricular tachycardia in patients with mitral valve prolapse. *Circulation* 57:111, 1978
10. Perloff JK, Child JS, Edwards JE: New guidelines for the clinical diagnosis of mitral valve prolapse. *Am J Cardiol* 57:1124, 1986
11. Wood P: An appreciation of mitral stenosis. Br Med J 1:1051, 1954
12. Ross RS: Right ventricular hypertension as a cause of precordial pain. *Am Heart J* 61:134, 1961
13. Fowler NO: Acute pericarditis. *In* Fowler NO (ed): The Pericardium in Health and Disease. Mt. Kisco, NY, Futura Publishing Co., 1985
14. Spodnick DH: Pericardial rub: Prospective, multiple observer investigation of pericardial friction rub in 100 patients. *Am J Cardiol* 35:357, 1975
15. Spodick DH: Diagnostic electrocardiographic sequences in acute pericarditis: Significance of PR segment and the PR vector changes. *Circulation* 48:575, 1973
16. Wanner WR, Schaal SF, Bashore TM, et al: Repolarization variant vs. acute pericarditis. A prospective electrocardiographic evaluation. *Chest* 83:180, 1983
17. Spodick DH: Frequency of arrhythmias in acute pericarditis determined by Holter monitoring. *Am J Cardiol* 53:842, 1984
18. Fowler NO, Harbian AD: Recurrent pericarditis: Follow-up of 31 patients. *J Am Coll Cardiol* 7:300, 1986

19. Lim HF, Dreifus SL, et al: Chest pain, coronary artery disease and coronary cinearteriography. *Chest* 57:41–46, 1970
20. Christie LG Jr, Conti CR: Systemic approach to evaluation of angina-like chest pain. *Am Heart J* 102:897, 1981
21. Bell WR, Simon TL, DeMets DL: The clinical features of submassive and massive pulmonary emboli. *Am J Med* 62:355, 1977
22. Stein PD, Willis PW III, DeMets DL: History and physical examination in acute pulmonary embolism in patients without pre-existing cardiac or pulmonary disease. *Am J Cardiol* 47: 218, 1981
23. Rich S, Pietra GG, Kieras K, et al: Primary pulmonary hypertension: Radiographic and scintigraphic patterns of histologic subtypes. *Ann Intern Med* 105:499, 1986
24. Goldharber SZ: Strategies for diagnosis. *In* Goldharber SZ (ed): Pulmonary Embolism and Deep Venous Thrombosis. Philadelphia, W.B. Saunders, 1985, p 89
25. Fuster V, Steele PM, Edwards WD, et al: Primary pulmonary hypertension: Natural history and the importance of thrombosis. *Circulation* 70:580, 1984
26. Colgan SM, Schofield PM, Whorell PJ, et al: Angina-like chest pain: A joint medical and psychiatric investigation. *Postgrad Med J* 64: 743, 1988
27. Morrison LM, Swaim WA: Role of the gastrointestinal tract in production of cardiac symptoms: Experimental and clinical observations. JAMA 114:217, 1940
28. Janssens J, Vantrappen G, Ghillebert G: Twenty-four hour recording of esophageal pressures and pH in patients with non-cardiac chest pain. *Gastroenterology* 90:1978–1984, 1986
29. Mellow WH, Simpson AS, Watt L: Esophageal acid perfusion and coronary artery disease: Induction of myocardial ischemia. *Gastroenterology* 85:306, 1983
30. Deschner KW, Benjamin SB: Extraesophageal manifestation of gastroesophageal reflux disease. *Am J Gastroenterol* 84:1–5, 1989
31. Garcia-Pulido J, Patel PH, Hunter WC, et al: Esophageal contribution to chest pain in patients with coronary artery disease. *Chest* 98: 806, 1990
32. Fulp SR, Richter JE: Esophageal chest pain. *Am Fam Physician* 40:101, 1989
33. Katz PO, Dalton CB, Richter JE, et al: Esophageal testing of patients with non-cardiac chest pain or dysphagia. Results of three years experience with 1161 patients. *Ann Intern Med* 106:593–597, 1987
34. Orr WC, Robinson MG: Hypertensive peristalsis in the pathogenesis of chest pain: Further exploration of the "nutcracker" esophagus. *Am J Gastroenterol* 77:604–607, 1982
35. Rustgi AK, Chopra S: Chest pain of esophageal origin. *J Gen Intern Med* 4:151–159, 1989
36. Goldman L, Weinberg M, Weisberg M, et al: A computer-derived protocol to aid in the diagnosis of emergency room patients with acute chest pain. *N Engl J Med* 30:588–596, 1982
37. Hewson EG, Sinclair JW, Dalton CB, et al: Acid perfusion test: Does it have a role in the assessment of non-cardiac chest pain? *Gut* 30:305–510, 1989
38. Lieberman D: Noncardiac chest pain. *Postgrad Med* 86:207, 1989
39. Richter JE, Dalton CB, Bradley LA, et al: Oral nifedipine in the treatment of non-cardiac chest pain in patients with the nutcracker esophagus. *Gastroenterology* 93:21–28, 1987
40. Swamy N: Esophageal spasm: Clinical and manometric response to nitroglycerin and long acting nitrates. *Gastroenterology* 72:23–27, 1977
41. Kikendall JW, Mellow MH: Effect of sublingual nitroglycerin and long acting nitrate preparations on esophageal motility. *Gastroenterology* 79:703, 1980
42. Berger K, McCallum RW: Nifedipine in the treatment of achalasia. *Ann Intern Med* 96: 61, 1982
43. Tucker HJ: Disorders of the esophagus: Dysphagia and gastroesophageal reflux. *In* Barker LR (ed): Principles of Ambulatory Medicine, ed 2. Baltimore, Williams & Wilkins, 1986, p 427
44. Palmer ED: Disorders of the cricopharyngeus muscle: A review. *Gastroenterology* 71:510, 1976
45. Mayou R: Invited review: Atypical chest pain. *J Psychosom Res* 33:393–406, 1989
46. Epstein SE, Gerber LH, Borer JS: Chest wall syndrome: A common cause of unexplained cardiac pain. *Am J Cardiol* 29:154, 1972
47. Levine PR, Mascette AM: Musculoskeletal chest pain in patients with "angina": A prospective study. *South Med J* 82:580, 1989
48. Miller AJ, Taxidor TA: The "precordial catch," a neglected syndrome of precordial pain. JAMA 159:1364, 1955
49. Thomford NR, Holaday WJ: Mondor's disease (phlebitis of the thoracoepigastric vein). *Ann Surg* 170:1035, 1969
50. Peto T: Shingles in the general practice. Practitioner 233:398, 1989
51. Demoragas JM, Kierland RR: The outcome of patients with herpes zoster. *Arch Dermatol* 75:193, 1957
52. Rowbotham MC, Fields HL: Post-herpetic neuralgia: The relation of pain complaint,

sensory disturbance and skin temperature. *Pain* 39:129, 1989
53. Bass C: Non-cardiac chest pain. *Practitioner* 233:352, 1989
54. Herlitz J, Hjalmarson A, Karlson BW, et al: Long-term morbidity in patients where the initial suspicion of myocardial infarction was not confirmed. *Clin Cardiol* 11:209, 1988
55. Lavey EB, Winkle RA: Continuing disability of patients with chest pain and normal coronary arteriograms. *J Chronic Dis* 32:191, 1979
56. Bass C, Wade C: Chest pain with normal coronary arteries: A comparative study of psychiatric and social morbidity. *Psychol Med* 14:51, 1984
57. Katon W, Hall ML, Russo J, et al: Chest pain: Relationship of psychiatric illness to coronary arteriographic results. *Am J Med* 84:1–8, 1988
58. Kellner R: Hypochondriasis and somatization. JAMA 258:2718, 1987
59. Warwick HMC, Salkovskis PM: Reassurance. *Br Med J* 290:1028, 1985
60. Weber LD, Peters RW: Delayed chest wall complications of median sternotomy. *South Med J* 79:723, 1986
61. International Association for the Study of Pain Subcommittee on Taxonomy: Classification of chronic pain. *Pain 3* (suppl):S138, 1986
62. Mailis A, Chan J, Basinski A, et al: Chest wall pain after aortocoronary bypass surgery using internal mammary artery graft: A new pain syndrome: *Heart Lung* 18:553, 1989
63. Eurman DW, Potash HI, Eyler WR, et al: Chest pain and dyspnea related to "crack" cocaine smoking: Value of chest radiography. *Radiology* 172:459, 1989
64. Cregler LL, Mark H: Medical complications of cocaine abuse. *N Engl J Med* 315:1495–1500, 1986
65. Pasternak RC, Thiibault GE, Savoia M, et al: Chest pain with angiographically insignificant coronary arterial obstruction: Clinical presentation and long term follow-up. *Am J Med* 68:813, 1980
66. McElroy JB: Angina pectoris with coexisting skeletal chest pain. *Am Heart J* 66:296, 1973
67. Doyle DJ: Diagnosis of acute chest pain. *MD Computing* 62:97–99, 1989
68. Merrill AJ Jr: Chest pain—The diagnostic dilemma. *J Med Assoc Ga* 65:395–399, 1976
69. Neill WA, Hattenhaver M: Impairment of myocardial oxygen supply due to hyperventilation. *Circulation* 52:854, 1975
70. Roberts R, Henderson RD, Wigle ED: Esophageal disease as a cause of severe retrosternal chest pain. *Chest* 67:523, 1975

Asthma

James G. Fordyce

Practitioners of the art of medicine have been treating bronchial asthma for thousands of years. Initially, the term *asthma* was used to describe simple shortness of breath. Laennec [1] emphasized in his works that asthma was a symptom and doubted the existence of a specific disease process. Over the years, the term asthma has evolved to describe a separate disease process. Basically, asthma is a physical condition in which airways respond to a number of factors, resulting in a reversible increase in airway resistance. A number of factors affect this disease, including genetic, environmental, immunologic, and neuropsychiatric [2]. In this chapter recent concepts and treatment regimens for the patient with bronchial asthma are discussed.

Prevalence, Morbidity, and Mortality

Because the definition of asthma varies among physicians, the true prevalence of asthma is difficult to determine. A study of data by Evans et al [3] of the National Center for Health Statistics for the period 1965 to 1984 showed that from 7 to 20 million individuals in the United States had asthma. The number of children with asthma in the United States was estimated at 2 to 5 million [3]. The prevalence rate for children aged 6 to 11 increased by 58% from 1976 to 1980, with a prevalence rate of 6.7% [4]. It is estimated that the total cost of illness related to asthma in 1990 was $6.2 billion [4a].

Studies indicate an increase in prevalence and morbidity of asthma. For the period 1965 to 1983 the hospitalization rate for adults increased by 50%. The rate for children increased by 200% during this period [3]. A study of admissions to Children's Hospital of Pittsburgh showed a 40% increase in the rate of admissions for bronchial asthma from 1960 to 1980 [5].

Mortality due to asthma has also been increasing. Review of data of the National Center for Health Statistics showed an increase in death rates due to asthma from 1.2 per 100,000 to 1.5 per 100,000 from 1979 to 1984. The rate of death for black individuals showed a greater proportionate increase [6]. In Massachusetts, the death rate rose from 0.66 per 100,000 to 1.8 per 100,000 from 1979 to 1986. The rate for the previous 10 years was stable [7]. A study of data from other nations also indicates that mortality due to asthma has gradually increased since the 1970s [8].

In 1979, the World Health Organization International Classification of Diseases, Ninth Revision, was put into use, raising the question that changes in diagnostic classification have artificially increased asthma mortality figures. A review of this question supports the view that the increase is real [9]. Possible causes of the increase include increased frequency of diagnosis of asthma, increased severity of the disease, and undertreatment of asthma by physicians fearing side effects of medications [10]. This increase in mortality is a far cry from Osler's opinion that in asthma "death during the attack is unknown [11]."

Pathophysiology: Pathways to Bronchoconstriction

Hyperresponsiveness, or hyperreactivity, of asthma leads to airway obstruction. This obstruction is a result of edema of the walls of airways, increased mucus production, and contraction of smooth muscle found in the airways. These changes are a result of an inflammatory process as well as altered neurologic function in the airway. The asthmatic response can be divided into an immediate, or early response, and a delayed, or late response.

Early and Late Asthmatic Responses

The early response in bronchial asthma begins within minutes after exposure to a stimulus. The decrease in volume of air expired in the first second of a forced maneuver (FEV_1) is usually 20% of baseline or greater. Treatment with bronchodilators usually improves FEV_1. Improvement may occur without any specific treatment, however, and flow rates usually improve to preattack levels within 1 to 2 hours.

The classic example of the early phase of bronchial asthma occurs during an acute allergic response following antigen challenge. This phase is the result of release of mediators from cells found in the airways and surrounding tissue. Reflex bronchospasm by neural mechanisms may also play a role in the early phase of asthma.

The late or delayed phase of bronchial asthma usually begins 3 to 4 hours after exposure to a stimulus and progresses to a peak decrease in FEV_1 at 5 to 8 hours after exposure. The flow rates may stay depressed for 12 hours or longer. This phase is related to continued mediator release, neural mechanisms, and inflammatory products from cells recruited to the area by early response mechanisms. Persistence of inflammation and hyperresponsiveness related to this phase may represent the ongoing process in those individuals with chronic asthma.

Occasionally a patient may present with a dual type asthmatic response after challenge with a stimulus (Fig. 8-1). Following the early response, flow rates may improve transiently only to again decrease to low, often more severe levels. This delayed phase may persist for prolonged periods and respond poorly to bronchodilators. A recurrent, nocturnal pattern of asthma may also occur.

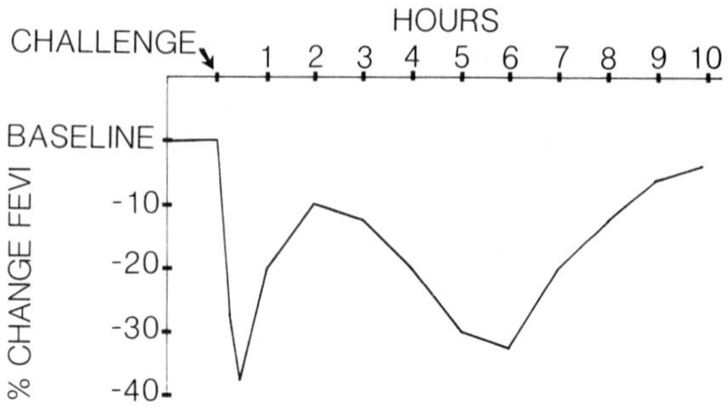
HOURS
CHALLENGE
1 2 3 4 5 6 7 8 9 10
BASELINE
-10
-20
-30
-40
% CHANGE FEVI

Fig. 8-1. Example of early and late phase asthma response following antigen challenge at hour 0.

Anatomic Elements

Airway smooth muscle is spirally arranged within the lamina propria, extending from the trachea and continuing throughout the bronchi, bronchioles, terminal bronchioles, and terminal alveolar ducts. These muscles are innervated by both sympathetic and parasympathetic nerve fibers, the latter originating in the vagus nerve [12]. Specific staining techniques have shown that there are very few noradrenergic nerve fibers in the smooth muscles of the airways [13]. This indicates that sympathetic stimulation of the airways, leading to muscle relaxation, is not significant compared with the cholinergic input promoting smooth muscle contraction.

Nonadrenergic noncholinergic innervation also has been demonstrated. The nonadrenergic effector nerves relax smooth muscle, possibly by way of the neurotransmitter vasoactive intestinal peptide. Smooth muscle receptors for vasoactive intestinal peptide are found primarily in the larger bronchi, suggesting a lack of bronchodilation of small airways in response to vasoactive intestinal peptide [14]. Noncholinergic bronchoconstriction is caused by the neuropeptide substance P as well as nerve-stimulated release of mast cell mediators. Afferent nerves, including irritant and stretch receptors and nonmyelinated C-fiber nerve endings, are found in the walls of the airways, and irritation of these nerve endings can lead to reflex bronchospasm or mediator release [15].

Cellular Elements

The mast cell is the primary cell associated with the acute hypersensitivity response. On activation, this cell releases preformed as well as newly generated substances called mediators that are responsible for the early asthmatic response. Mast cells are found throughout the respiratory tract. They are a heterogeneous group of cells, with subsets differing morphologically as well as functionally [16]. For example, bronchial mast cells are sensitive to the action of cromolyn sodium, but parenchymal mast cells are relatively insensitive [17]. After antigen challenge, bronchoalveolar lavage fluid from asthmatic patients shows elevated levels of histamine and tryptase in atopic but not nonatopic asthmatic patients [18]. Mast cells of the same subset from different individuals therefore can respond differently, having a direct effect on individual response to a stimulus.

Activation of mast cells classically occurs when IgE combines with antigen and attaches to receptors on the cell membrane. When two of these receptors are bridged by antibodies and attached antigen, the cell releases mediators. Other stimulants of activation include products of the immune response, inflammation, neural activation, and some drugs.

In the lumen of the airways and alveoli, more than 90% of all cells are alveolar macrophages, 6% mononuclear cells, 2% neutrophils, and only 0.4% mast cells [19]. This suggests that, within the airways, cells other than mast cells play a role in asthma. Macrophages, mononuclear cells, and neutrophils are part of the lung's defense system. Alveolar macrophages can be activated to release inflammatory mediators and chemotactic factors. Their activity has direct correlation with the degree of airway responsiveness. After IgE-dependent stimulation, alveolar macrophages appear to have an inhibitory role on the immune response [20]. Decreased functional activity of alveolar macrophages in asthmatic subjects correlates with numbers of eosinophils in the sample [21]. Elevated neutrophil counts are associated with airway hyperresponsiveness [22]. These cells participate in and have a regulatory role in airway hyperreactivity.

Increased numbers of eosinophils are found in bronchoalveolar lavage samples of patients with asthma, either atopic or nonatopic [22]. Eosinophils are recruited to the airways as a result of the early asthmatic response and have a role in the ongoing hyperreactive state. The proteins found in the eosinophil granule, particularly major basic protein, have a direct effect on bronchial smooth muscle reactivity and respiratory epithelium function [23].

These are the major cells found in the airways associated with asthma (Table 8-1). Their usual function is important in the genesis of the asthmatic response. In addition, their activity and response pattern is different in asthmatic individuals. Asthma, therefore, presents with pulmonary symptoms,

Table 8-1. Major cellular elements involved in asthma

Cell Type	*Role in Asthma Response*
Mast cell	Primary cell, early asthma response Involved in both allergic and nonallergic response Release of mediators and chemotactic factors
Alveolar macrophage	Phagocytosis and antigen processing Release of mediators of inflammation
Eosinophil	Appear in late asthma response Damage to respiratory epithelium
Neutrophil, monocyte	Appear in late asthma response Release of mediators of inflammation
Epithelial cell	Possible source of a relaxing factor
Nerve cell	Reflex and direct muscle contraction or relaxation Mediator release from mast cell

but the differences between an asthmatic and nonasthmatic individual involves systems other than the lung.

Mediators Involved in Asthma

The interaction of the cells involved in asthma and their effect on airway reactivity are dependent on a number of mediators (Table 8-2). Histamine, a preformed mediator released primarily from the granules of activated mast cells, plays a significant role in the early asthmatic response. Stimulation of histamine receptors in lung tissue results in smooth muscle contraction, arterial vasoconstriction, and increased epithelial permeability [24]. Histamine causes bronchoconstriction by irritation of vagal afferents, which can be inhibited by anticholinergic agents such as atropine. Histamine also has a role in the regulation of the immune response [25].

In addition to histamine, the enzyme kininogenase is released, which generates bradykinin. Bradykinin causes bronchoconstriction in asthmatic but not nonasthmatic persons [26]. Preformed eosinophil and neutrophil chemotactic factors are released, causing the influx of these cells seen in the late asthma response. These recruited cells contribute to the hyperresponsiveness and pathologic changes of bronchial asthma [27]. Serum levels of high molecular weight neutrophil chemotactic activity have been noted to vary inversely with improvement in lung function in hospitalized asthmatic patients [28].

When inflammatory cells are activated, arachidonic acid is released from their plasma membrane phospholipid. The arachidonic acid is then acted on by two enzyme systems, either cyclo-oxygenase or lipoxygenase, to produce newly formed mediators that are released from the cell.

The products of the cyclooxygenase system include both prostaglandins and thromboxanes. These mediators affect smooth muscle, mucus secretion, vasoconstriction or dilation, and chemotaxis. The lipoxygenase enzyme system gives rise to the leukotrienes or hydroxyeicosatetraenoic acids. These products were initially known as slow reacting substances of anaphylaxis. These mediators are powerful bronchoconstrictors, affect vascular tone and permeability, increase mucus production, and have chemotactic properties.

Table 8-2. Primary Mediators Involved in Asthma

Mediator	*Function*
Histamine	Bronchoconstriction, partially mediated by vagus nerve Arterial vasoconstriction Edema
Proteases	Tissue damage Formation of bradykinin
Bradykinin	Bronchoconstriction
Chemotactic factors	Recruitment of eosinophils and granulocytes
Arachidonic acid–derived products Prostaglandins Thromboxanes Leukotrienes	Bronchoconstriction Mucus secretion Chemotaxis Increased hyperreactivity Some may lead to bronchial relaxation
Platelet-activating factor, acether	Bronchoconstriction Increased hyperreactivity
Adenosine	Bronchoconstriction in asthmatic patient
Epithelial-derived relaxing factor	Decreased hyperreactivity
Neuropeptides	
Vasoactive intestinal peptide	Smooth muscle relaxation
Substance P	Smooth muscle constriction

Platelet-activating factor, also called PAF-acether, is derived from membrane phospholipid. It can cause bronchoconstriction and has also been shown to sensitize normal, but not asthmatic, airways to methacholine challenge [29]. Adenosine, a nucleoside released from adenosine monophosphate during inflammation, can cause bronchoconstriction in asthmatic, but not normal, patients [30]. Superoxide and hydrogen peroxide cause bronchoconstriction and increased vascular permeability [26].

The epithelial damage seen in bronchial asthma contributes to airway obstruction. Decreased mucus clearance and loss of protection of underlying tissues, including nerves, can lead to increased bronchoconstriction as well as inflammation. Intact bronchial epithelium plays a role in the effect of both bronchodilators and bronchoconstrictors [31]. Studies suggest that epithelial damage or dysfunction leads to decreased amounts of an epithelial-derived relaxing factor, contributing to increased bronchial hyperreactivity [32].

Therefore, a general overview of bronchial asthma consists of an initial stimulus, leading to release of mediators from cells found in the airways and lung parenchyma. Neural mechanisms come into play, with a direct effect on airways as well as amplification of the initial, or early, response. These mechanisms and mediators contribute to early inflammation, bronchospasm, and mucus production. In addition, chemotactic factors recruit inflammatory cells. As these cells arrive and become activated, release of more mediators amplify the inflammatory process. Ongoing inflammation contributes to the recurrent obstruction and hyperreactivity of chronic asthma. Indeed, asthma is often described as chronic eosinophilic inflammation of the airways.

Inflammation is only part of the complex process of this disease. Not all early asthmatic responses lead to the late response and chronic asthma. Hyperresponsiveness is the platform for asthma. Inflammation builds on this base, resulting in the signs and symptoms of clinical asthma.

Changes at the Cellular Level

Changes in the microscopic appearance of the airways in bronchial asthma reflects the effects of the mediators discussed earlier. Eosinophils, macrophages, and increased numbers of epithelial cells are seen in the lavage fluid of asthmatic subjects. Activated eosinophils as well as collagen deposition due to fibroblast stimulation are seen in the mucosa [33, 34]. Epithelial destruction in the airways at all levels is seen, with resultant exposure of intraepithelial nerves. Ciliated cells appeared to suffer the most damage [35]. Microscopic examination of asthmatic airways demonstrates greater wall area due to increased epithelial, mucosal, and submucosal areas, making the amount of smooth muscle shortening needed to occlude the lumen less in these airways [36]. This supports the theory that ongoing inflammation is important in the genesis of the chronic asthmatic state. These changes, in combination with increased mucus production and decreased clearance of mucus due to loss of ciliary function [37], are the basis for the airway obstruction of asthma (Table 8-3).

Gross Pathology

Classically, postmortem findings in bronchial asthma reveal hyperinflated lungs that stay inflated due to the widespread obstruction of airways secondary to mucus plugging as well as bronchial wall thickening. On cut section the mucus plugs may protrude from the bronchi and are thick and tenacious [38]. In chronic asthma the walls of the airways are

Table 8-3. Pathways to Bronchoconstriction

Airway hyperreactivity
Mediator release
Neural stimulation
Inflammation, acute and chronic
Increased mucus production
Decreased mucus clearance
Edema
Smooth muscle contraction
Epithelial damage

grossly thickened due to both long-term and acute inflammatory changes [38a]. The obstruction of the airways can lead to impaired ventilation and atelectasis of the distal lung tissue. These changes result in ventilation perfusion inequalities, the major physiologic abnormality present in asthma.

Manifestation of Bronchial Asthma

Natural History of Asthma

Two questions are frequently heard by physicians caring for patients with bronchial asthma: "Will my child grow out of asthma?" and "How and why did I get asthma?"

The concept that asthma in early childhood will probably resolve as the child grows older is false. In one prospective study, children who initially had only infrequent wheezing had but a 50% chance of being free of wheezing by early adult life. More than 50% of young adults with wheezing had onset of wheezing before 2 years of age [39]. Physicians should not trivialize early-onset asthma by giving the false hope that the child will grow out of it.

Asthma in childhood has long been associated with a genetic tendency to develop hypersensitivity reactions (atopy). However, in young children, acute episodes of bronchial asthma are often precipitated by viral episodes. There is an association with croup and the development of bronchial hyperreactivity as well as IgE antibodies against various respiratory viruses [40]. This further emphasizes the relationship of asthma and atopy in childhood, although not all children with asthma are atopic.

A study of over 600 asthmatic adults with a mean age of 51 demonstrated that the longer the duration of asthma, the more persistent the obstruction, with poorer response to treatment. In this study the severity of asthma did not correlate with the presence of atopy [41]. A prospective study of asthmatic children into adulthood showed increased numbers of positive skin tests correlating with age and persistence of symptoms. However, they were not predictive for the outcome of childhood asthma [42]. As with children, atopy is not a prerequisite for asthma in adults.

The answer to the "how and why" a patient develops bronchial asthma is elusive. Bronchial hyperreactivity appears to be an inherited characteristic, but why it expresses itself in different individuals at different times is unknown. Obviously, the concurrent inheritance of atopic characteristics plays a role in childhood, as well as the development of viral infections. Environmental factors, such as exposures to various irritants or chemicals, may play a role in the development of asthma. Maternal smoking of as little as one half of a pack of cigarettes per day leads to higher rates of asthma as well as earlier onset of asthma in children [43]. "Internal" factors, such as stress and autonomic imbalance, can also influence the onset of asthma.

Intrinsic and extrinsic asthma are commonly used terms. Classically, extrinsic asthma is used to describe asthma that is related to atopy, while intrinsic asthma is associated with the nonatopic state. However, there is a good deal of crossover. Atopic asthmatic individuals are affected by non-atopic factors, and atopy may be present but not clinically relevant in those with intrinsic asthma.

To summarize, asthma can appear at any age. The earlier the onset, the more pronounced and the more likely it is to persist into adult life and be associated with atopy. Adult onset asthma has less association with atopy, and acute episodes are more likely to be associated with factors other than atopy.

Patient History and Chief Complaint

The range of symptoms and complaints can vary greatly in asthma. Cough, especially at nighttime, may be present without any shortness of breath. Exertional dyspnea of varying degrees may be present, and individuals who routinely exercise may complain of a gradual decrease in endurance. Parents may notice that the child does not keep up with other children at play or has coughing episodes with exertion. Persistent coughing or wheezing following viral infections in children and adults may in reality be asthma. These episodes may be mild and intermittent, and the patient may not initially seek medical attention. As the degree of asthma increases, the frequency, duration, and severity of symptoms increase. Coughing, wheezing, and shortness of breath become more pronounced, and at this point the patient may seek some type of medical intervention, either with proprietary medication or presentation to a physician.

The hallmark of the acute episode of asthma is shortness of breath. The patient complains of tightness of the chest. Occasionally a symptom of chest pain is given. This may be related to coughing or the use of accessory muscles during the acute attack of asthma. Children often complain of abdominal pain. A report of wheezing with or without exertion is given, and inability to "catch one's breath" may also be present. With the severe attack, a sense of impending doom and panic may set in, with the patient being very restless and unable to voice complaints easily.

Physical Findings

The physical findings in asthma are the result of airway obstruction. The more severe and longer the duration of obstruction, the more severe and persistent the physical findings. The sequela of airway obstruction and the patient's efforts to overcome the obstruction and meet the body's oxygen demand results in the increased work of breathing observed during the acute attack of asthma.

Physical findings in bronchial asthma may vary greatly. With very mild episodes, good air exchange may be present, with no wheeze or rhonchi at rest, but the patient complains of tightness of the chest. With forced expiration to residual volume, a high pitched, expiratory wheeze characteristic of asthma is heard. This may lead to an episode of coughing. The patient may present with recurrent coughing, harsh and wet in nature, and auscultation reveals both inspiratory and expiratory rhonchi, with diffuse expiratory wheeze that may progress to inspiratory and expiratory wheezes. Biphasic wheezing with increased pitch and volume as well as increased respiratory rate is associated with greater airways obstruction. These signs, however, should not be substituted for objective measurements of respiratory flow rates [44, 45]. With increasing obstruction, the expiratory phase of ventilation becomes prolonged. Sputum is usually present, thick and tenacious, and may be difficult to clear. The wheeze is often audible without the use of a stethoscope. The heart rate becomes elevated, increasing as dyspnea increases.

With increasing severity of asthma, the patient uses accessory muscles as wheezing becomes more pronounced. The patient prefers to sit up with arms braced on the legs or chair, using the straight arms as support during the prolonged expiration of an acute attack. Retractions, both intercostal and supraclavicular, are seen as severity of obstruction increases, and an audible expiratory grunt may be heard at the end of expiration. The chest becomes hyperinflated and hyperresonant due to air trapping and increased residual volume. Airway resistance is lower at higher lung volumes, and this hyperinflation may be a functional attempt to decrease airway resistance. Diaphragm excursion may decrease. Pulsus paradoxus (see Chapter 3) may develop as hyperinflation increases. The patient appears more apprehensive and may become diaphoretic. Hypoxia may lead to confusion and restlessness as well as circumoral cyanosis. With increasing severity, airflow may decrease to the point where no wheeze is audible by auscultation. This is a grave sign and calls for immediate and intensive treatment. Acute pain in the midchest area, with crepitus over the thoracic inlet and medial ends of the clavicles, is compatible with pneumomediastinum. These same findings in a patient who suddenly worsens or shows poor response to treatment may represent a pneumothorax. A patient who becomes lethargic or unconscious with signs of respiratory failure requires ventilatory support.

Infants and very young children with asthma may be very irritable, with wet, harsh coughing and audible wheeze. Nasal congestion may be profuse. The clinician may diagnose croup, which is often difficult to differentiate from asthma. High-pitched, diffuse expiratory wheeze by auscultation accompanied by an end-expiratory grunt and increased respiratory rate is more indicative of asthma than uncomplicated croup. As the attack progresses, nasal flaring and retraction occur, and the irritability of the infant gives way to fatigue and lethargy. The progress from a mild attack of asthma to the symptoms of respiratory failure may be quite rapid, requiring aggressive therapy. The infant with acute asthma must not be approached simply as an asthmatic in a small body.

Laboratory Findings

The most consistently useful diagnostic laboratory study is the pulmonary function test. These studies are useful not only to monitor the progress of asthma, but also to assess the acute episode and as a diagnostic tool.

The routine use of a home peak flow monitor, used properly, can give the patient and physician information regarding progress of the disease and guide medication changes. Since a peak flow measurement is an effort-dependent maneuver, the patient's technique should be observed frequently. Predicted values are available, although the asthmatic patient may not attain these values. Each patient should chart his or her normal values and monitor the changes in flow rates relative to these values. Since peak flow values are not as sensitive as FEV_1 or $FEF_{25\text{-}75}$ values (see Chap. 2), peak flow rates may be normal even in the presence of obstruction [46]. Peak flow readings should not take the place of regular spirometry.

Spirometry is the most common office laboratory study performed in asthma. As with peak flow rates, predictive values are available but often not attainable in the asthmatic patient. An asymptomatic patient may show decreased pulmonary function findings and be clinically stable. The findings of airway obstruction-decreased FEV_1/forced vital capacity, peak flow rate, and $FEF_{25\text{-}75}$, as well as decreased forced vital capacity, are present during episodes of bronchial asthma and are covered in Chapter 2.

Spirometry performed in the emergency room during an acute episode of bronchial asthma has been used as a guideline for admission. However, pulmonary function studies do not have good predictive values as to relapse after discharge from the emergency room [47]. Indeed, ventilation-perfusion abnormalities can persist even in the face of normal spirometry for weeks after an acute attack, supporting the concept that spirometry reflects large airflow rates rather than terminal airway obstruction. This terminal airway obstruction is the major factor in gas-exchange abnormalities [48].

Spirometry is useful in establishing the diagnosis of asthma. Airway response to bronchodilator is a simple procedure to document reversible airway obstruction. If possible, the patient should not use bronchodilators for at least 12 hours prior to pulmonary function testing. After baseline studies, aerosolized bronchodilator is given, and repeat studies are done 15 to 30 minutes later. An improvement in FEV_1 by 15% or $FEF_{25\text{-}75}$ by 25% is compatible with reversible obstruction. These studies are most useful in patients already demonstrating diminished flow rates.

In patients with a history suggesting asthma but with normal flow rates, nonallergic bronchoprovocation studies may be performed, providing evidence of bronchial hyperresponsiveness. Exercise, cold air, or medications may be used to provoke bronchospasm. In these studies, the provocative dose of medication needed to decrease the FEV_1 by 20% from baseline is measured. Methacholine or histamine may be used, and guidelines for these studies are available for both adults and children [49–51]. Bronchoprovocation studies are valuable as research tools and are also useful in cases of occupational asthma. It has been recommended that individuals entering employment with a high risk of occupational asthma undergo methacholine or histamine challenge. Those demonstrating nonspecific bronchial hyperreactivity are at higher risk to develop occupational asthma.

Bronchoprovocation studies using allergens and industrial materials are also valuable. These studies not only document hyperreactivity but establish a specific inciting agent of asthma. Both early and late asthma responses may be demonstrated with these types of challenge studies. Guidelines and methods are available for these types of studies [52, 53].

Preexposure and postexposure determination of pulmonary function values is useful in other circumstances. Measurements of workers on the job with suspected occupational asthma can be performed with portable spirometry, and exercise challenges can be done in the laboratory or in the field. Determination of response to medication taken before exposure can guide medication selection in these situations.

Challenge testing, whether with bronchoprovocating drugs, allergens, exercise, or other agents, is not without risk. Severe, life-threatening bronchial asthma may occur with bronchoprovocation. These studies should be performed by personnel familiar with the risks and able to respond quickly. They are not routine procedures and the patient should be warned of the potential risks.

Chest radiographs in asymptomatic asthmatic patients are usually normal. Children with acute asthma may demonstrate increased perihilar markings, often confused with an infiltrate or bronchopneumonia. During severe attacks, increased thoracic volume and hyperinflation with flattening of the diaphragm is seen (see Figure 9-1). Atelectatic areas representing complete obstruction of terminal airways may also be noted. Complications including pneumomediastinum or pneumothorax may also be observed.

Sputum from an asthmatic patient is usually thick and tenacious. Grossly, mucus casts may be seen, and if numerous fine, brown casts are seen, allergic bronchopulmonary aspergillosis must be considered. Microscopically, bronchial ciliated epithelial cells may be seen, often in clumps. Eosinophils are noted in stained samples. Curschmann's spirals, which are mucus casts of terminal bronchioles, are found in asthmatic sputum (Fig. 8-2). Charcot-Leyden crystals, octahedral and elongated in shape, represent protein from the eosinophil. Neutrophils and bacteria may be present, usually in cases with concurrent infection.

Arterial blood gas determinations are very valuable in the acute asthmatic patient, and many advocate blood gas measurements in all episodes of acute asthma. Those with severe or poorly responsive asthma should have determinations done. Supplemental oxygen may be given to patients with acute asthma, without predetermination of arterial blood gases providing there is not a history of chronic obstructive pulmonary disease and CO_2 retention.

The changes in arterial blood gas measurements in acute bronchial asthma reflect the ventilation-perfusion abnormalities and respiratory rate. Initially, PaO_2 is reduced. The $PaCO_2$ may be decreased due to an increased respiratory rate. As the attack worsens, CO_2 retention occurs, and $PaCO_2$ may return to normal levels, with PaO_2 staying low or decreasing further. With progression of the attack, $PaCO_2$ levels increase above predicted normal levels. Decreasing PaO_2 and increasing $PaCO_2$ levels are ominous signs and assisted ventilation must be considered, especially when PaO_2 has the same value as $PaCO_2$. $PaCO_2$ levels greater than PaO_2 levels absolutely require assisted ventilation. Arterial pH findings reflect the blood gas changes in the progress of the attack as well as the level of alveolar ventilation.

Complete blood counts during acute bronchial asthma are usually unremarkable, except for the presence of elevated eosinophil counts in those with atopy. White blood cell counts may be elevated in patients who have been on corticosteroids or who have concurrent infection. Electrolytes and renal function studies may be needed in acute asthmatic patients who are dehydrated.

Serum IgE levels may be elevated in atopic individuals [54]. The higher the serum IgE, the closer the relationship with asthma [55]. Atopy by IgE or skin or in vitro tests was found in 58% of asthmatic adults [56]. These

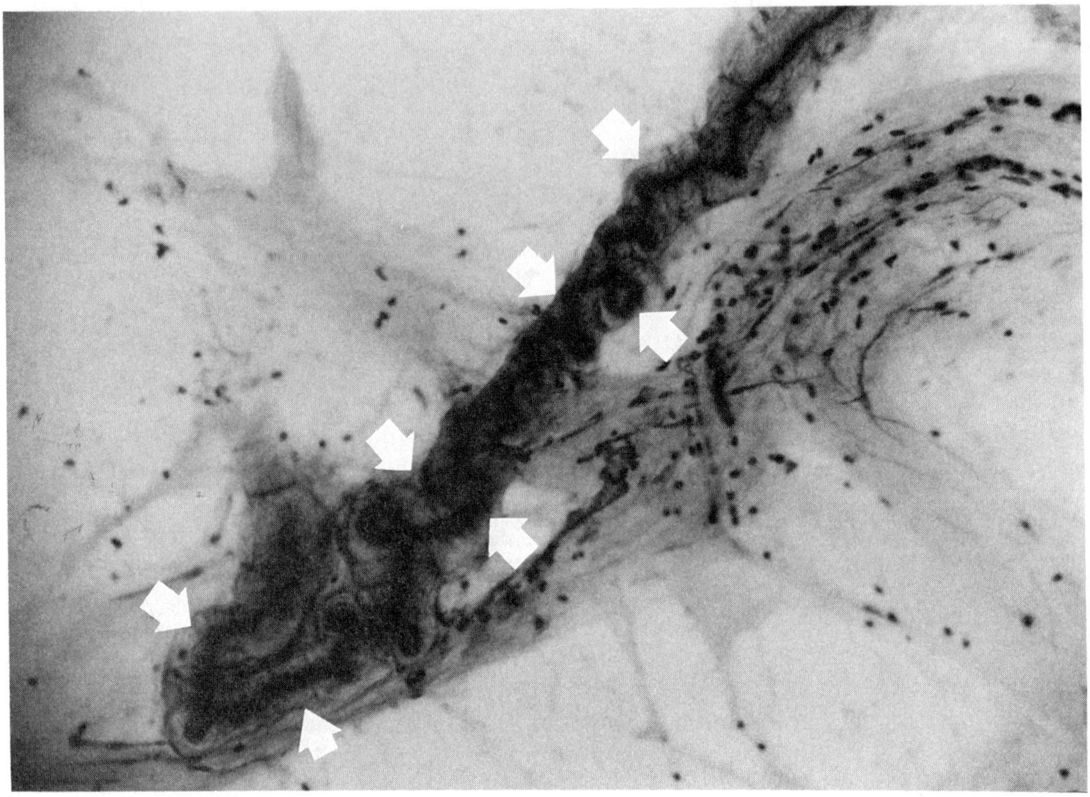

Fig. 8-2. Curschmann's spirals found in sputum (arrows outline structure). These are coiled bronchiole casts. (Courtesy of Joseph T. Powaser, MD, Oakwood Hospital.)

studies suggest that the majority of asthmatic patients have some type of IgE disease.

Do all asthmatic patients need an allergy evaluation? A good history can give important clues to the role of allergy in the patient's asthma. If asthma is infrequent or mild and easily controlled with medication taken as necessary, complete allergy evaluation is probably not warranted. If asthma is more frequent, a serum IgE can give evidence of an atopic process. Caution must be used in the interpretation of in vitro allergen studies, as they are not as sensitive as skin tests. If chronic medications are necessary and asthma is not well controlled, allergy evaluation is a logical step in the evaluation and care of the patient. This is especially true in the pediatric population, where allergy plays a greater role in more severe asthma [57].

Differential Considerations

Children

Conditions in children that must be differentiated from asthma include any potential cause of airway obstruction. In infants this includes anatomic anomalies, including laryngeal or tracheal stenosis, vascular rings, tracheoesophageal fistula, and tumors. Croup is probably the most common problem to differentiate in infants and is often associated with the onset of asthma in infancy. Recurrent episodes of croup are rare and are more compatible with asthma.

Acute dyspnea not responding to a bronchodilator in children without a history of asthma requires aggressive investigation. Epiglottitis may present with airway obstruction and wheezing, but usually these children have signs of systemic illness, including fever, malaise, and irritability. Direct visualization may be dangerous, and facilities for prompt intubation should be available. Foreign body aspiration in children must always be considered. In children with recurrent coughing, mucus production, and radiographic changes, sweat chloride determinations should be performed to rule out cystic fibrosis. Immotile cilia syndrome may be considered in those patients having recurrent sinus and ear infections as well as situs inversus.

Obviously, there are a multitude of differential diagnoses in children. The presence of expiratory wheezing, often associated with a viral respiratory illness, as well as a family history of atopy or asthma, usually is associated with asthma. If respiratory distress is noted on inspiration or the onset is sudden in an otherwise healthy child, other causes of obstruction must be ruled out. Long-term respiratory problems that are poorly responsive to aggressive medication therapy, including steroids, should be evaluated for diagnoses other than asthma.

Adults

In adults, chronic obstructive pulmonary disease, infection, and congestive heart failure (cardiac asthma) are the primary differential diagnoses of asthma. History, other physical findings, and radiography can usually clarify the diagnosis. Tumors, aneurysm, and foreign body may present with obstruction and wheezing, and pulmonary function studies may be necessary to evaluate the nature and source of obstruction.

Diffuse pulmonary disease, including hypersensitivity pneumonitis and other types of interstitial fibrosis, may present with wheezing and shortness of breath. The hyperventilating patient may also have wheezing. Anaphylactic reactions to food, medication, or insect stings can cause respiratory distress, and in this situation injected epinephrine rather than inhaled bronchodilator is required. Less common causes of wheezing include pulmonary parasites, carcinoid syndrome, collagen vascular disease, and shellfish poisoning [58]. Factitious asthma must be considered in patients with symptoms not responsive to therapy [59]. Refractory wheezing may actually be vocal cord dysfunction arising from anatomic or functional problems. Direct visualization may demonstrate adduction of the vocal cords on inspiration. These patients often require speech therapy or psychotherapy [60]. A thorough history and physical findings can usually establish the cause of airway obstruction.

Factors Associated with Asthma

In the majority of cases, acute episodes of asthma can be related to specific exposures or situations. It is important that the patient is aware of his or her triggers so that they can be avoided or altered. Patients with chronic asthma, daily wheezing, and diminished flow rates can have chronic exposures that are stimulating asthma on a constant basis. In all patients with asthma a thorough evaluation of the environment, including occupational history, lifestyle, and stress, must be performed. One factor, or a combination of factors, can be involved in the acute episode of asthma (Table 8-4).

Table 8-4. Common Triggers of Acute Asthma

Allergens
Inhaled: house dust, animal danders, pollens, mold spores, some industrial dusts
Ingested: foods, medications
Irritants
Particulates, smoke
Fumes: perfumes, formaldehyde
Pollutants: ozone, sulfur and nitrogen dioxide
Dry air, cold air, abrupt weather changes
Infection
Viral: respiratory syncytial virus, parainfluenza, adenovirus, rhinovirus
Bacteria: *Mycoplasma*
Psychological
Stress
Laughter, crying
Exercise
Medications
Nonsteroidal anti-inflammatory drugs, aspirin
Radiocontrast media
Tartrazine, sulfites
β-Blocker drugs

Allergic Factors

Allergic factors must always be evaluated in persons with asthma, especially in atopic patients. The most important allergens are the inhalants. Outdoor inhalants include pollens, which give rise to seasonal variations in the patient's asthma. Depending on geographic location, trees pollinate in early spring, grasses in late spring, and weeds in late summer and fall. Mold spores are prevalent during times of higher humidity and heat. Indoor inhaled allergens include house dust, animal danders, and mold spores. The major allergen in house dust is fecal matter of the house dust mite, *Dermatophagoides*. Increased exposure to house dust is associated with increased activity of asthma, and aggressive control of house dust leads to clinical improvement of asthma [61]. Inhaled allergens from occupational exposures may also contribute to asthma.

Other allergens, including foods or drugs, are also capable of triggering asthma. Allergy elimination diets may be helpful in evaluating foods, but double-blind food challenges may be necessary to determine specific food allergy [62]. Following ingestion of a specific food, airway response to histamine may be enhanced, even if the initial histamine challenge was negative [63]. Challenges should never be done if the food in question has triggered an anaphylactic, life-threatening response.

Physical Factors

Inhaled irritants can cause worsening of asthma. These include physical irritants, such as particulates or fumes, cold air, or dry air. With the push for energy efficient buildings, less fresh outside air may be allowed to enter, leading to an increase in indoor pollutants. Building-related illness is related to inadequate ventilation. Pollutants include tobacco and wood smoke, nitrogen dioxide, formaldehyde, and other volatile agents [64]. Although smoking may not be a strong risk factor for asthma in adults [65], studies indicate that passive smoke exposure in children increases the risk of respiratory tract infection [66]. This has led the American Academy of Pediatrics to declare this exposure a definite health hazard [67]. Nitrogen dioxide may come from gas stoves or malfunctioning propane engines [68]. Formaldehyde may be liberated from urea-formaldehyde foam insulation or as an occupational exposure.

Outdoor air pollutants include ozone, sulfur dioxide, and nitrogen dioxide from the burning of fossil fuels and other pollutants. These may be difficult to measure and determine as factors in the patient's asthma. Sulfur dioxide is a known trigger of bronchoconstriction [69].

Cold air and dry air have been shown to trigger asthma and are used experimentally in the laboratory. Cold air during winter months and dry air in nonhumidified buildings can pose a hazard to susceptible patients.

Infection

Infections are important triggers of acute asthma in children. Respiratory syncytial virus, parainfluenza virus, and adenovirus are the most common viruses, with *Mycoplasma pneumonia* the most common bacteria [70]. Viral infections have also been shown to cause exacerbations of asthma in adults. Those exacerbations related to viral episodes are often more severe than those caused by other factors [71]. Rhinovirus infections induced in volunteers can produce increased airway reactivity and persistence of the late asthmatic response [72]. The exact mechanism by which infection produces asthma has not yet been determined. Possibilities include reflex bronchoconstriction due to irritation of receptors in airways, viral IgE production, decreased adrenergic response, interferon, and direct tissue damage [73].

Stress

Stress may be associated with exacerbations of bronchial asthma in both adults and children, possibly through increased vagal tone. Relaxation techniques may be beneficial in these episodes [74]. Persons with asthma may have a higher incidence of anxiety disorders, and trials of antidepressant medications have been advocated [74a]. Vigorous medication treatment, including steroids, may be needed by asthmatic individuals experiencing emotional stress.

Exercise

Exertion, even for short periods of time, may lead to acute exacerbations of asthma. The exact mechanism of this trigger is not known. Airway cooling and drying have been postulated as causes. Exercise-induced bronchospasm is a specific type of bronchial asthma and is covered later in this chapter.

Medications

Various medications have been associated with bronchial asthma. Patients with a history of bronchial asthma should not receive β-blocking agents, such as propranolol (Inderal) or atenolol (Tenormin) because of possible blocking of adrenergic-induced bronchodilation. Eye drops such as Timolol (Timoptic) and Levobunolol (Betagan) used to treat glaucoma may induce bronchospasm. Patients with cardiac problems or hypertension as well as a history of asthma should be placed on medications other than β-blockers.

Tartrazine, also known as FD&C Yellow No. 5, has been implicated as a cause of asthma. It is found in numerous foods, including pickles, candies, and soft drinks. This sensitivity has been related to aspirin sensitivity in some patients, but a European study of 156 aspirin-sensitive patients challenged with oral tartrazine showed only four patients reacting to tartrazine [75]. Asthma may not occur until 1 or 2 hours after ingestion. Controlled challenges may confirm the diagnosis.

Sulfites are used as food and drug preservatives because of their antioxidant properties. They may be sprayed on vegetables at salad bars, on shellfish, in wine, and in sausage and dried fruits. In susceptible persons, sulfites are broken down into sulfur dioxide, leading to asthma due to a vagal irritant mechanism. These patients appear to have a deficiency of sulfite oxidase [76]. Monosodium glutamate, a food enhancer often used in Chinese restaurants, has often been associated with exacerbations of asthma, but a double-blind study has not confirmed this association [77]. Oral provocation studies have been advocated to document sensitivity to additives [77a].

Sinusitis

Sinusitis has been associated with bronchial asthma. Patients with poor response to medications should be evaluated for sinus disease, especially if they exhibit rhinorrhea or mucopurulent discharge. Radiographs may show thickening of the lining of the sinus, opacification, or an air–fluid level. Children at risk may exhibit these findings as well as atopy and middle ear problems [78]. Possible mechanisms relating sinusitis and asthma include intermittent seeding of the airways with bacteria from the sinusitis, β-blockade enhancement, and reflex bronchospasm from nerve endings in the sinus through vagal efferents to the lung [78a]. Aggressive therapy, either with antibiotics or surgical drainage or ablation of the sinus, must be done if asthma is to improve in these patients [79].

Aspirin and the Aspirin Triad

Aspirin and aspirin-related nonsteroidal anti-inflammatory drugs may produce acute asthma in both adults and children [80, 81]. Patients with recurring asthma should be questioned regarding use of these medications. The incidence of aspirin sensitivity is unknown. It is not IgE mediated but may be a result of increased arachidonic acid metabolites available for leukotriene production, since aspirin blocks cyclooxygenase activity and subsequent prostaglandin production. Mediator release and platelet activation have been postulated as a mechanism, as well as acetylation of proteins. None of these theories have been proved [82]. Polyps, a complication of chronic sinusitis, may also be found. This finding should raise the possibility of the so-called aspirin triad of asthma, polyps, and aspirin sensitivity. One study showed that 90% of asthmatic patients with sinus disease had nasal polyps, and 50% of these patients were aspirin sensitive [78a]. These patients may exhibit nasal eosinophilia without atopy as well as urticaria [83]. Polypectomy does not cure this condition, and strict avoidance of aspirin and related drugs is necessary. In aspirin-sensitive patients requiring aspirin, the use of nonacetylated salicylates has been suggested, although these patients may react to these drugs [84]. Acetaminophen may be used for febrile episodes. If aspirin is needed, aspirin desensitization protocols are available, with gradual increasing doses of aspirin being given until a maintenance dose is tolerated. If aspirin is discontinued, sensitivity returns [85].

Gastroesophageal Reflux

Gastroesophageal reflux can also contribute to bronchial asthma in adults and children. Esophageal dysfunction has been demonstrated to be higher in children with asthma than in healthy children [86]. The effect of reflux may be due to aspiration or irritation of the esophagus by gastric acid. Barium swallow studies can confirm this diagnosis.

Hormonal Effects

Hormonal changes can have modulating effects on asthma. Asthma symptoms may be more pronounced during the 7- to 10-day period before menses, and it is estimated that one third of women with asthma experience this worsening of their asthma. One study showed that this increase in wheezing and shortness of breath was not related to hormonal levels or spirometric values [87]. Asthma during pregnancy is reviewed in Chapter 24.

Treatment of Bronchial Asthma

Avoidance of Precipitators

The logical means of treating any disease is to prevent it. Triggers of asthma should be avoided. Avoidance of tobacco smoke is mandatory. Passive smoking increases the incidence of respiratory illness in infants [88] and increases the severity of asthma in older children [89]. Avoidance of fumes, irritants, particulates, and temperature extremes should be attempted. Psychological factors in the patient's asthma should be approached and counseling provided when warranted. In atopic individuals any food, medication, or inhalant triggering allergic asthma must be strictly avoided.

Mite allergy has been found to be an important factor in asthma. Antigens from the house dust mite, *Dermatophagoides* species, are the major allergens of house dust. These mites live in carpeting, bedding, stuffed furniture and toys, and mattresses. Their numbers are increased by high humidity. The antigen of these mites are found in fecal pellets and are found in the home air in higher concentrations when windows are closed.

Control of house dust is an important part of the treatment of asthma, especially in atopic individuals. It is usually carried out in the bedroom and includes washable pillows or plastic covers over pillows, washable bedding, airtight covers over mattress and box springs, and bare floors, if possible. Books, plants, and stuffed toys should be kept out of the patient's bedroom, and furniture and other fixtures in the room should be easy to clean. Frequent dusting with oiled dust cloths is helpful. Filtration of air from furnace ducts should be carried out as well as frequent cleaning of the furnace and ducts. Dehumidifiers help keep mite growth as well as mold growth to a minimum. Humidification of the air is necessary during the heating months, but should be kept below 35% to 40% relative humidity.

Pets in the home can complicate asthma in atopic patients. Removing pets from the home is advised but usually not heeded in families attached to their pet. Pets should not be allowed in bedrooms, and, if possible, kept out of the house. Removal of cat dander from the home may take 5 or more months of vacuuming after the pet is gone [90]. Patients often insist that certain pets do not bother them, even if allergy is documented. This may be due to variability of shedding of antigen [91] but the patient must be informed that there is no such thing as a "hypoallergenic pet."

Medications

With the explosion of knowledge regarding the immunology of asthma and the inflam-

Table 8-5. Medications Used to Control Asthma

Adrenergic drugs: direct relaxation of airways, possible interference with mediator release
Epinephrine, isoproterenol, isoetharine, ephedrine, metaproterenol, albuterol, terbutaline, pirbuterol, bitolterol
Theophylline: direct relaxation of airways, possible anti-inflammatory effect, mucus clearance, other effects
Anhydrous theophylline, theophylline salts, aminophylline
Cromolyn sodium: inhibition of mediator release, other effects possible
Atropine: inhibition of cholinergic-induced bronchospasm
Atropine sulfate, ipratropium bromide
Corticosteroids: anti-inflammatory, inhibition of immune response, increased sensitivity to bronchodilators, other effects
Hydrocortisone, prednisone, prednisolone, methylprednisolone, triamcinolone, betamethasone, dexamethasone, beclomethsasone, flunisolide
Other drugs possibly used
Antihistamines, troleandomycin, antimetabolites, expectorants

matory response, there has also been a rapid increase in medications available for the control of asthma. Theories have changed, but the main goal of medication is to allow the patient to lead as normal a lifestyle as possible, prevent the attacks of acute asthma, and reverse the attacks when they do occur. In the last 20 years, new and more effective adrenergic agents, corticosteroid products, and theophylline preparations have been made available in the United States. Cromolyn sodium has been introduced as well as atropine derivatives. New concepts in anti-inflammatory pharmacology are being studied. The following is an overview of currently available drugs (Table 8-5).

Adrenergic Drugs

Adrenergic drugs cause bronchodilation. The archetypical drug, epinephrine, was first used in the early 1900s and is the basic drug on which the adrenergic type drugs are based. Adrenergic receptors are divided into β_1- and β_2-receptors. β_1-Receptors are associated primarily with cardiovascular responses, while β_2-receptors are primarily respiratory responses.

Because epinephrine has both β_1 and β_2 activity, sympathetic responses, including tachycardia, irregular heartbeats, and blood pressure changes, are common side effects. Epinephrine is rapidly broken down by catecholomethyltransferase and therefore is short acting and not effective orally. To circumvent these problems, various changes to the structure of epinephrine result in drugs with higher β_2 specificity as well as longer duration of action. These changes also enable the drugs to be used orally.

β_2-Agonist drugs stimulate β_2-receptors on cell membranes. These receptors appear to be closely related to the enzyme adenylcyclase. This enzyme acts on adenosine triphosphate to produce cyclic adenosine monophosphate (cAMP). Increased intracellular cAMP is responsible for the cellular effects and bronchodilation. These effects are seen in the lung, heart and blood vessels, uterus, and on blood levels of insulin, potassium, and lipids [92]. In the lung, effects include decreased mediator release, increased mucociliary clearance, decreased microvascular permeability, and decreased cholinergic activity [93]. β_2-Agonist drugs are effective in inhibiting the early phase but not the late phase of asthma. The most important clinical effect is bronchodilation by smooth muscle relaxation in the airways.

Epinephrine is available for subcutaneous injection in a 1 mg per mL solution. The dose is 0.01 mL/kg body weight up to a maximum of 0.25 mL in children or 0.50 mL in adults. Lower doses may be repeated every 20 to 30 minutes if needed, and adjustment to lower doses should be made in the patient with a history of cardiovascular disease. A long-acting suspension of epinephrine (Susphrine) is also available with a dose one half that of aqueous epinephrine. Inhaled epinephrine is available as an over-the-counter drug, but because of short action and side effects and possibility of overuse, is not usually recommended for the routine treatment of asthma. Epinephrine in a diluted form of 1 to 10,000 has been recommended for slow intravenous use in intractable asthma, but this can be quite dangerous because of cardiovascular effects.

Ephedrine is available orally for asthma, but is not routinely used for asthma because of availability of other, more potent medications. It is thought to be safe during pregnancy, used at a dose of 25 mg three times daily [94].

β_2-Specific agonist drugs available in the United States include albuterol (Proventil, Ventolin), terbutaline (Brethine, Bricanyl), metaproterenol (Alupent, Metaprel), pirbuterol (Maxair), and bitolterol (Tornalate). Isoproterenol (Isuprel) and isoetharine (Bronkometer, Bronkosol) are also available, but are less β_2-specific and have a shorter duration of action.

Albuterol and terbutaline are available in oral and aerosolized metered dose inhaler forms. Albuterol solution can be used in nebulizers, and terbutaline is available for injection. In equipotent doses both are equally effective in producing bronchodilation by mouth, with fewer side effects noted with albuterol [95]. Both are effective by inhalation, with fewer side effects than by the oral route. The use of albuterol by metered dose inhaler has fewer side effects than by the nebulized route [92]. Inhaled albuterol is effective in protecting against bronchoconstriction induced by hyperventilation of cold, dry air, but a higher than recommended dose for terbutaline is necessary for equal effectiveness.

The dose of oral albuterol is 2 to 4 mg three to four times daily, and for terbutaline is 2.5 to 5 mg three times daily. The use of oral terbutaline has not been established in children under 12. Albuterol syrup is available for children at doses of 0.1 mg/kg three times daily up to 2 mg three times a day. Metered dose inhalers for both drugs are available in the dose of two puffs every 6 hours. Albuterol solution 0.5% may be given, 0.25 to 0.5 mL diluted in saline four times daily. Its use has not been established in children under 12. Injectable terbutaline, 1 mg/mL, may be given in a dose of 0.01 ml/kg, up to a limit of 0.25 mL subcutaneously.

Metaproterenol is available in oral, metered dose inhaler and nebulizer solution forms. Children over 6 years of age may be given 10 mg three or four times daily. Adults and children over 60 pounds may receive 20 mg three or four times daily. Metered dose inhaler use in patients over age 12 is limited to 12 inhalations per day. A 5% solution for nebulization is dosed at 0.2 to 0.3 mL in 2 to 3 mL of saline four times daily.

Pirbuterol is available in a metered dose inhaler and appears to be as effective as albuterol [96]. One to two puffs every 4 to 6 hours is used in patients over 12 years of age. Bitolterol is a prodrug, used in a metered dose inhaler. Esterases necessary for its transformation to active form are present in the lung [97]. Two puffs every 8 hours is the dose in those over age 12.

The side effects noted with β_2-agonist drugs reflect their sympathetic-like activity. These include tachycardia, arrhythmias, tremor, and blood sugar changes. Decreased serum potassium has been noted with inhaled β_2-agonists, including albuterol and terbutaline [98]. The addition of theophylline does not seem to have an effect on serum potassium. Because of the potential additive effect of theophylline and β_2-agonists on the heart, use of this combination of drugs in the patient with a history of cardiovascular disease should be done with caution. It has been shown in children that low-dose therapy with a combination of oral theophylline and terbutaline is effective in the control of asthma [99]. Central nervous system effects may occur, although these agents do not easily enter into the central nervous system.

The choice of product and route of administration will depend on the clinical assessment of the patient. Since inhaled forms of these medications have fewer systemic side effects, it may be argued that this is the preferred method. Metered dose inhalers have been shown to have an effect for up to 6 hours and have faster onset of action than oral forms. In some patients, compliance with oral forms may be better, with resultant improved clinical response. The correct technique for use of metered dose inhalers is discussed elsewhere in this book.

β_2-Agonist agents are the first-line drugs in

acute asthma, usually in inhaled form, and play a significant role in the long-term treatment of asthma.

Methylxanthines

Xanthines have been advocated for the treatment of asthma since the middle of the nineteenth century. The naturally occurring xanthines include caffeine, theobromine, and theophylline. They are found in coffee, tea, and cocoa. Caffeine has been shown to be an effective bronchodilator and may be used temporarily if other bronchodilators are not readily available. It is not recommended for regular use [99a].Theophylline, the xanthine most effective for asthma, has been in use for over half a century. Since theophylline is poorly soluble, intravenous theophylline is given in the form of aminophylline, which is approximately 85% theophylline. Theophylline has been used in the United States as a primary drug for the treatment of asthma and chronic obstructive pulmonary disease. With increasing knowledge of the inflammatory changes of asthma, other drugs, including cromolyn and steroids, have started to replace theophylline as the first-line drug for chronic asthma. Theophylline is not as potent or rapid a bronchodilator as β_2-agonists, and its routine use intraveneously during an acute attack has been questioned [100].

The bronchodilating effect of theophylline has been attributed to its ability to inhibit the enzyme phosphodiesterase, which catalyzes the breakdown of cAMP. Increased cAMP within the smooth muscle is related to relaxation. Thus, with higher intracellular levels of cAMP, smooth muscle relaxation and bronchodilation should occur. However, bronchodilation occurs at concentrations that do not inhibit phosphodiesterase, and this mechanism is no longer accepted as the reason for bronchodilation in asthmatic patients. Phosphodiesterase inhibition has been proposed as a mechanism by which theophylline inhibits release of arachidonic acid–derived mediators of inflammation [101]. Theophylline may compete with adenosine on cell membrane adenosine receptors [102]. Adenosine has been shown to cause bronchoconstriction by inhalation in asthmatic patients [30]. The exact cellular mechanism of action of theophylline bronchodilation has not been determined.

Theophylline has a number of effects on the lung and other organs. It directly relaxes the smooth muscle of both large and small airways [103] and appears to inhibit airway inflammation [104]. It inhibits the early and late asthmatic responses, perhaps through its ability to inhibit mediator release by allergen challenge [105]. However, it has not been shown to be effective in protecting against hyperreactivity to cold, dry air challenge [106]. Theophylline facilitates mucus clearance by increasing fluid content of mucus and stimulation of ciliary activity [107]. At one time it was thought that theophylline improved respiratory muscle function in patients with chronic obstructive pulmonary disease [108]. This effect has not been demonstrated in subsequent studies [109, 110].

Theophylline has a number of effects outside the lung. In the central nervous system it causes vasoconstriction, stimulates respiration, and may cause headache and nausea. It increases gastric secretion and relaxes the lower esophageal sphincter. This effect may not be significant when sustained-release theophylline products are used [111]. Theophylline can cause a mild diuresis. Theophylline has positive chronotropic and inotropic effects on cardiac muscle and can cause peripheral vasodilation [112].

The bronchodilating effect of theophylline is proportional to its serum concentration. However, theophylline has a narrow therapeutic index. The accepted therapeutic blood level of theophylline is 5 to 15 μg/mL. Above this level, side effects include nausea, vomiting, headache, and tachycardia or tachyarrhythmias. Agitation, hyperreflexia, and seizures may occur. The more severe side effects are seen in patients with blood levels of 40 μg/mL or higher. Cardiac arrest and permanent brain damage may occur. Prompt emergency treatment, including repeated doses of activated charcoal, correction of metabolic disturbances, and hemoperfusion or hemodialysis may be required [113].

The blood level present in a patient at any time is determined by the amount and rate of theophylline absorbed versus the rate of clearance of drug from the bloodstream. These rates are affected by a number of factors. The timing of blood sampling relative to medication administration must be taken into consideration for blood values to be valid.

Rapid-release theophylline products are available in tablet and liquid form. They can raise blood levels rapidly, which may or may not be desirable, and, depending on rate of clearance, may result in wide fluctuations in blood levels. Aminophylline is used for intravenous purposes and can give the same fluctuations, unless given as a constant intravenous infusion.

Sustained- (controlled) release products were introduced in the early 1970s. They have the advantages of requiring less frequent dosing and exhibiting fewer variations in blood levels. Capsules with beads may be opened and sprinkled on food such as applesauce and given to children. However, not all products release the same amount of theophylline (bioavailability), and each has its own variability in rate of release. Factors influencing rate of release include age of the patient, dosing interval, presence of food, and type of food (fat, protein, carbohydrate) [114, 115]. Rates of absorption may vary according to morning versus evening dosing [116]. All these effects vary between products and patients.

Studies have been performed on the effect of food on the absorption of specific sustained-release products. Increased absorption was noted when Theo-24 and Uniphyl, two once-a-day products, were taken with food, especially if taken with a fatty meal [117, 118]. This increase in absorption may be significant in children in whom rapid absorption can lead to elevated blood theophylline levels. Theodur Sprinkle, a capsule meant to be opened and spread on food for children unable to swallow whole capsules, showed a significant decrease in bioavailability when given with food [119]. Theodur tablets and Theolair SR have slightly decreased bioavailability with food, but Slobid, Theobid, and Somophyllin SR do not appear to be affected by food [120].

It is best that clinicians use two or three preparations with which they are thoroughly familiar regarding these variables, and use only those products. Generic products are available, but may cause problems because of bioavailability variations. Stipulating "dispense as written" may be necessary.

Patient factors have an effect on the metabolism of theophylline. Conditions affecting liver metabolism, including liver disease and congestive heart failure, slow clearance of theophylline. Viral illnesses can also have this effect [121]. Patients with chronic renal failure may develop toxic levels [122]. Younger individuals and young smokers have increased rates of clearance. This effect may not be seen in older smokers [123]. A number of drug interactions have been described with theophylline (Table 8-6). There is a great deal of patient to patient variability in the clearance of this drug, making monitoring of blood theophylline levels necessary as larger doses are used [124].

In starting a patient on theophylline, the variations in products, patient absorption and clearance, and food and drug interactions must be considered [125]. Side effects may occur at lower blood levels of theophylline, as not all patients tolerate the therapeutic range. Accurate blood measurements are necessary. Once the patient is stable, repeat blood levels may be clinically necessary. The primary goal should be patient stability, not laboratory value stability. A good number of patients are clinically stable on blood theophylline levels

Table 8-6. Effects of Drugs on Theophylline Clearance

Increased Clearance	*Decreased Clearance*
Rifampin	Birth control pills
Phenobarbital	Erythromycin
Carbamazepine	Cimetidine
Phenytoin	Troleandomycin (TAO)
	Isoniazid
	Ciprofloxacin

Ref: Jonkman J Allergy Clin Immunol 1986; Tenenbein J Emerg Med 1989; Torrent DICP 1989; Cremer J Clin Pharmacol 1989; Adebayo Clin Exp Pharmacol Physio 1988 below the usual therapeutic range, and a few require and tolerate levels above 20 μg/mL.

A number of regimens have been suggested in dosing theophylline. These are guidelines, and individualization of dosing is necessary, with monitoring of blood levels for best results. A frequently suggested starting dose of 16 mg/kg/d, or 400 mg/d, whichever is lower, is used, with increases up to 18 to 24 mg/kg/d [126]. This regimen may be used when using sustained-release products and should be given in two or three divided doses. Children less than 1 year of age should be given a lower dose and blood levels followed closely. Intravenous doses of theophylline in patients already taking theophylline are best determined by using existing blood theophylline as a guide. Mitenko and Ogilvie [127] determined that a loading dose of 5.6 mg/kg followed by a maintenance dose of 0.9 mg/kg/h resulted in a blood theophylline level of 10 μg/mL. Blood theophylline levels should be followed closely in patients on a constant infusion of aminophylline.

Salts of theophylline have no advantage over anhydrous theophylline. The amount of theophylline available in these products must be considered when dosing is determined. For example, aminophylline is about 85% theophylline, and oxtriphylline (Choledyl) is about 63% theophylline. The relative amount of theophylline in theophylline salts should be determined before their use over anhydrous theophylline products.

Rectal suppositories of theophylline are available, but because of toxicity [128], are not recommended. Rectal solutions of aminophylline have very few indications because of variable absorption.

Theophylline is effective and safe in the treatment of chronic bronchial asthma. Because compliance with inhalers can be a problem and many patients prefer oral medications, these patients are good candidates for long-term theophylline use [129]. Once-a-day and twice-a-day medications are available. Blood levels are more consistent with twice daily dosing, but compliance is better with once-a-day dosing, making this mode more advantageous [130]. Some patients may require three times daily dosing.

Theophylline has been used in the treatment of chronic obstructive pulmonary disease. Beneficial effects have been ascribed to the bronchodilating effect, increased cardiac ejection fraction, decreased pulmonary artery resistance, increased central respiratory drive, and improved mucociliary function [131, 132]. These effects are controversial, but since many patients show improvement, the gradual introduction of long-acting theophylline may be used in these patients, with cessation of theophylline if no objective or subjective improvement is seen [132a]. Combining oral theophylline with inhaled β_2-agonists in patients with chronic obstructive pulmonary disease appears to give more bronchodilation than either drug alone [133], but this is controversial [134].

Cromolyn Sodium

Disodium cromoglycate (Intal), also called cromolyn, is a poorly absorbed and rapidly cleared drug that is used only in the inhaled form for asthma. Cromolyn is effective in blocking both the early and late asthmatic response. It is described as a mast cell stabilizer, thus, its effect on the early response. It has also been shown to inhibit activation in vitro of human neutrophils, eosinophils, and monocytes [135]. This may explain the inhibition of the late asthmatic response. No other drug, in suggested doses, has been shown to be effective in blocking both early and late asthmatic responses. Cromolyn is effective in blocking the effect of inhaled allergen and preventing exercise-induced asthma when used 15 to 30 minutes before exercise. Treatments may have to be repeated with prolonged exertion or exposure to allergen. The mechanism of action of cromolyn is unknown.

The primary use of cromolyn is the long-term management of bronchial asthma. It is effective in the control of chronic asthma and may decrease bronchial hyperreactivity [136]. When used properly, it has few adverse effects. Side effects may include dermatitis, myositis, and gastroenteritis. These are easily reversed by discontinuing the drug [137]. Cromolyn can decrease or eliminate the need for other bronchodilators and is thought by many to be the first choice in the treatment of asthma [138].

Patient education and compliance is very important if cromolyn is to be successful. The patient must understand that cromolyn is not a bronchodilator and will not be effective if taken during an acute episode of asthma.

Cromolyn is available as a metered dose inhaler and may be used in a dose of 2 puffs three to four times daily.

Proper technique for inhalation of cromolyn must be taught and reviewed with the patient. When using the spinhaler, the sleeve should be pulled down and returned only once, the neck extended and head held back while inhaling. Deep inhalations should be taken until the capsule is emptied. If patients are experiencing some mild asthma, the use of an inhaled β_2-agonist may be beneficial when used just before using cromolyn. When starting a patient on cromolyn, it may be necessary to use aggressive bronchodilator or steroid therapy. The patient has to understand that regular use of cromolyn, even when feeling well, is necessary for continued control of asthma.

Atropine and Related Drugs

Cholinergic innervation to the airways can be responsible for bronchoconstriction. This effect is seen primarily in the larger, central airways. Stramonium, from the *Datura stramonium* plant, and belladonna, from the *Atropa belladonna* plant, were used in the form of cigarettes for the relief of asthma [11]. The active agent released from these plants is atropine.

Atropine and related drugs antagonize cholinergic (muscarinic) nerve impulses through competitive inhibition of acetylcholine, the neurotransmitter of postganglionic fibers. With decreased cholinergic tone, bronchial relaxation occurs, primarily in larger airways.

Atropine, unfortunately, is easily absorbed, short acting, and has side effects including tachycardia, dry mouth, and blurring of vision. Ipratropium bromide (Atrovent), a derivative of atropine, is available in inhaled form. It is poorly absorbed and longer acting and thus can be used when anticholinergic bronchodilation is desired [139]. The usual dose of ipratropium bromide by metered dose inhaler is two puffs, equivalent to 36 μg, four times daily. Some patients may need twice this dose of ipratropium to realize bronchodilation [140].

Ipratropium bromide is effective in blocking the effect of methacholine challenge and may be useful in the face of β-blockade, as when patients are taking β-blocking agents. Psychogenic causes of asthma, with bronchospasm due to increased cholinergic tone, may also respond to this agent. Ipratropium is effective in the prevention of exercise-induced asthma, but has less effect in protecting against bronchospasm due to antigen exposure. It has been advocated in the treatment of emphysema and chronic obstructive pulmonary disease [141].

Corticosteroids

Because asthma is a chronic inflammatory airway disease, corticosteroids, with their anti-inflammatory properties, are primary drugs in the treatment of chronic asthma. The introduction of inhaled corticosteroids, with fewer side effects, has stimulated interest in this group of drugs as a first-line medication in the treatment of asthma.

The mechanism of action of corticosteroids is still being clarified. They are potent anti-inflammatory drugs. Given systemically, they cause a redistribution of leukocytes, with an increase in blood neutrophils and a decrease in eosinophils, monocytes, and lymphocytes. There is a decrease in movement of neutrophils into inflammatory sites, and the activity of granulocytes is decreased. Lymphocyte activity is also decreased [142]. Vasoconstriction is also noted, as is decreased vascular permeability. Corticosteroid administration does not usually inhibit the early asthma response, but does suppress the late asthma response and subsequent long-term bronchial hyperresponsiveness. In high doses, corticosteroids may suppress the early asthmatic response [143]. Corticosteroids also reverse the decreased sensitivity of cell receptor sites for β-adrenergic agents [144].

Corticosteroids are used in both emergency treatment of acute asthma as well as the long-term treatment of chronic asthma. In acute asthma, systemic corticosteroids are indicated, especially in those patients who initially are not responsive to therapy. Systemic hydrocortisone in high doses has been shown to speed the recovery of patients with severe asthma, although the effect may not be seen until 6 to 12 hours after administration [145].

Prednisone, an oral, short-acting corticosteroid, may be used in adults and children at a dose of 1 to 3 mg/kg/24 hours in two divided doses for 3 to 5 days. The afternoon dose may then be discontinued and the morning dose continued as clinically appropriate. In preschool children, early introduction of prednisone, 1 mg/kg/d, at the first sign of a viral infection has been shown to decrease morbidity, emergency room visits, and hospitalizations [146]. In both children and adults only the most severe cases of asthma require more than 60 mg of prednisone per day as a starting dose outside of the hospital. This dose may be tapered off or abruptly stopped. Abrupt cessation of steroids used less than 14 days is not associated with adrenal problems, and it is rarely necessary to use steroids more than 10 to 14 days in patients who have not been on regular systemic steroid therapy. If the patient is not stable off corticosteroids, consideration must be given to the use of chronic corticosteroid therapy [147].

Chronic corticosteroid therapy can usually be established using regular inhaled corticosteroid preparations. If inhaled preparations, even in high doses, do not give good control, chronic oral steroids may be indicated. Corticosteroid side effects are usually associated with doses greater than the equivalent of prednisone, 10 mg daily. The lowest dose of oral, short-acting corticosteroid, usually in the form of prednisone, should be used. Side effects are minimized using alternate day prednisone, giving the equivalent of 2 days' doses every other morning [148]. This dosage varies between 10 to 60 mg of prednisone given every other morning, depending on patient response. Because of diurnal endogenous cortisol secretion controlled by the hypothalamic-pituitary-adrenal axis, evening doses of prednisone may give rise to decreased adrenal function if used on a long-term basis. The short half-life of prednisone given in the morning minimizes this effect. Other medications, including cromolyn, should be continued to keep the asthma as stable as possible so that the lowest effective dose of predisone is used. Frequent assessment of clinical condition, progress, and pulmonary function studies should be performed and the prednisone dose adjusted accordingly. Patient education and compliance are extremely important with this regimen.

Many different corticosteroid preparations are available. These forms can be either short- or long-acting, depending on their rate of clearance and duration of effect on the hypothalamic-pituitary-adrenal axis. Inhaled preparations, when used at recommended doses, do not affect this axis, but may have an effect at higher doses [149].

The common short-acting corticosteroids include hydrocortisone, prednisolone, prednisone, and methylprednisolone. Hydrocortisone and methylprednisolone are available for intravenous administration. Hydrocortisone may be used as a bolus of 100 to 250 mg and methylprednisolone as a bolus of 40 to 125 mg. These may be repeated every 6 hours. No good evidence exists that higher doses are more effective, although higher doses probably will not cause adverse effects. Prednisone is the most commonly used oral corticosteroid. Prednisolone and methylprednisolone have no real advantage over prednisone, except that methylprednisolone has fewer sodium retention properties. Prednisone and prednisolone are available in tablet and syrup form, and methylprednisolone is available in tablets.

Long-acting systemic corticosteroids are not usually used for chronic asthma. Betamethasone and dexamethasone are available in tablet and syrup forms and may be used for short, 3- to 5-day bursts of corticosteroid. These drugs are about six to eight times more potent than prednisone. They have no role in the long-term oral management of asthma. Long-acting injections of triamcinolone, 40 mg, or betamethasone, 6 mg, may be considered in patients who are not compliant or unable to take oral corticosteroids [150]. This route of administration is rarely needed, although it may have a role in the patient with seasonal asthma due to high pollen counts.

Inhaled corticosteroids are available in various forms. Beclomethasone metered dose inhaler (Vanceril, Beclovent) delivers 42 μg per actuation. The usual dose is two puffs four times daily. Flunisolide metered dose inhaler (Aerobid) delivers 250 μg per actuation, with a usual dose of two puffs twice daily. Triamcinolone metered dose inhaler (Azmacort) delivers 100 μg from the unit per actuation and is dosed at two puffs three to four times a day.

When patients are being changed from oral or systemic corticosteroids to inhaled corticosteroids, the systemic corticosteroids are tapered slowly and the patient observed for any sign of adrenal insufficiency. Withdrawal from systemic corticosteroids may take months or longer, depending on the dose and length of time the patient has taken these drugs.

The side effects of corticosteroids include cushingoid features, increased blood sugar, fluid retention, osteoporosis, and ocular changes [142, 151]. Muscle wasting and weakness may occur. Growth suppression has been a concern in children, although not at the usual doses. Triamcinolone aerosol for 1 year in children was not related to decreased growth rate [152]. These side effects are time and dose dependent. Inhaled corticosteroids may lead to dysphonia or oral candidiasis, the latter usually prevented by rinsing the mouth and gargling after use. Patients must be thoroughly educated in the use of corticosteroids. Documentation of discussion of use and possible side effects should be made in the patient's chart.

Inhaled corticosteroids are important drugs in the long-term care of asthma. They are effective in the control of chronic bronchial hyperreactivity. The beneficial effects on flow rates over a period of time are equal to or greater than cromolyn sodium [153]. Higher than recommended doses (1500 μg/d) of beclomethasone have been shown to maintain flow rates that have been stabilized by a short course of oral prednisone [154]. Metered dose inhalers delivering higher doses of corticosteroid are available outside the United States. In view of our knowledge of the inflammatory process and long-term bronchial hyperreactivity in asthma, inhaled corticosteroids are first-line drugs for asthma.

Other Drugs

Since histamine is a major mediator involved in bronchial asthma, investigations into the potential use of antihistamines have been made. With the introduction of newer antihistamines, some benefits have been noted [24]. Terfenadine (Seldane), in doses of 60 to 180 mg/d, has a bronchodilating as well as protective effect against exercise-induced asthma [155]. Antihistamines may also have a beneficial effect on the late asthma response [156]. Ketotifen, a drug used outside the United States, has antihistamine and antiasthma properties [157]. Based on these findings, the classic admonition of not allowing patients with asthma to use antihistamines is unwarranted [158]. Antihistamines are not presently viewed as a regular drug in the treatment of asthma, but ongoing research may lead to a more important role in asthma treatment.

Expectorants and mucolytic drugs and their effect on clearance of secretions would seem to be beneficial for the asthmatic patient with thick, tenacious mucus. Guaifenesin has been combined with theophylline for this purpose, and potassium iodide and terpin hydrate also are used. Iodinated glycerol may help in the clearance of mucus in asthmatic patients and was found to be effective in patients with chronic obstructive pulmonary disease [159]. In general, expectorants do not occupy an important role in the treatment of asthma. To be effective, adequate hydration is necessary, and hydration by itself leads to easier mucous clearance. The inhaled mucolytic, acetylcysteine (Mucomyst), should be used with caution in asthmatic patients because of the possibility of bronchospasm.

Troleandomycin, an antibiotic, decreases the rate of methylprednisolone clearance, resulting in decreased methylprednisolone requirements. It has no effect on other oral corticosteroids. Troleandomycin also decreases the rate of theophylline clearance. It should be reserved for use in patients requiring high-dose corticosteroids. Liver enzymes must be regularly monitored because of possible hepatic toxicity. The use of troleandomycin, 250 mg every other morning, with decreased dosage of theophylline has been shown to be effective in decreasing methylprednisolone to an alternate day dosing schedule [160].

Methotrexate in severe cases of corticosteroid-dependent asthma has been shown to be effective in decreasing corticosteroid requirements [161]. However, because of the toxicity of this drug, it should be used only in specially selected cases by physicians familiar with its actions and side effects [162].

General Considerations in the Medical Approach to Asthma

Medical treatment of asthma should be aggressive enough to control the disease but logical enough to not interfere greatly with the patient's lifestyle. In the adult, chronic smoking, fume exposure, and other chronic cardiac or pulmonary diseases must be considered.

Mild, intermittent asthma can be treated with inhaled β_2-agonists by inhalation [163]. This can be administered by metered dose inhaler or nebulizer. Some patients do well with daily theophylline for short periods of time. More severe exacerbations usually require corticosteroids. Short-term use of inhaled corticosteroids at presently available doses is rarely effective.

Patients with chronic asthma or recurrent exacerbations require regular medications, either cromolyn sodium or theophylline. Chronic use of inhaled corticosteroids should also be considered a first-line type of treatment, especially if theophylline or cromolyn sodium is ineffective or not tolerated. Regular inhaled corticosteroids alone may be effective in the control of asthma. β_2-Agonists are added as needed or on a chronic basis, but these patients should be observed for any side effects with this combination, including tachycardia or hypokalemia with chronic β_2-agonist use. Increased risk of death or near death has been associated with regular use of β_2-agonist metered dose inhalers [163a]. Ipratropium bromide can be used on an as needed basis as well as a daily basis, especially in patients with chronic lung disease.

Regular use of inhaled corticosteroids is indicated in patients who are on regular bronchodilators but still are experiencing symptoms of asthma. Considering the inflammatory nature of asthma, their use should be considered early in the formulation of the medical regimen for the asthmatic individual. Alternate day prednisone is used if the inhaled route is ineffective, with daily use in the most severe asthmatic patients. If there is an inability to change corticosteroid use to alternate day therapy, one may consider troleandomycin and methylprednisolone.

Education and regular follow-up of the patient is necessary for successful treatment. Patients should never be given a short course of medication for asthma without a subsequent visit being scheduled. Treatment regimens should allow the patient to be as active as desired without hindrance from asthma. Recommendations of an expert panel on bronchial asthma were published by the National Institutes of Health in 1991 to improve the diagnosis and management of bronchial asthma [163b].

Allergic Considerations

Controversy exists regarding the necessity of allergy evaluation and therapy for allergy-induced asthma. Optimal dose immunotherapy should be considered in those patients in whom pharmacologic treatment has been maximal and corticosteroids are required, allergens have been identified and are playing a role in the asthma, or the course of asthma has become more unstable [164]. Immunotherapy has been shown to be effective in children in the treatment of allergic disease [165]. Immunotherapy with cat extract results in decreased bronchial response to cat extract [166]. Immunotherapy with birch pollen resulted in blunted bronchial hyperresponsiveness during the birch pollen season as well as increased flow rates and less use of medication [167]. The selection of patients for immunotherapy rests on the history of atopy and pattern of asthma. This therapy should be carried out by physicians experienced in immunotherapy. Unproven or controversial techniques have no role in the treatment of allergic asthma.

Acute Asthma or Status Asthmaticus

Acute bronchial asthma is a common medical emergency (Fig. 8-3). It is estimated that 1 million emergency room visits are for acute asthma, with over 10% of these visits resulting in admission to the hospital [168]. The treatment of acute bronchial asthma has as its goals lessening of airway obstruction and improvement in ventilation-perfusion inequalities. The usual approach to this condition is β_2-agonist administration by inhalation or injection [169]. The concurrent administration of intravenous aminophylline is no more effective than a β_2 drug by itself at maximum dose, although the combination may be indicated when submaximal doses of a β_2-agonist is used [170]. The use of ipratropium bromide or inhaled atropine in patients with poor response to inhaled bronchodilators may be of benefit. Hydration to facilitate mucus clearance is often necessary, and supplemental oxygen is indicated for hypoxia. If the patient does not improve with these initial medications, he or she is said to be in status asthmaticus.

Patients in status asthmaticus have already shown little or no response to β_2-agonists. These patients need aggressive therapy and monitoring in the hospital as the patient can deteriorate rapidly. Risk factors for death from asthma include previous history of respiratory failure, poor initial monitoring, poor or no response to initial treatment, history of poor compliance, and failure to appreciate the seriousness of the attack by both the patient and physician [171]. If possible, spirometric studies should be obtained as well as blood gases when indicated. Signs of deterioration include decreasing PaO_2 and increasing $PaCO_2$ levels and greatly reduced flow rates and vital capacity. Intravenous corticosteroids, such as methylprednisolone, 40 to 125 mg every 6 hours, should be administered as early as possible, and intravenous aminophylline started. Inhaled bronchodilators are continued, and fluid and electrolyte abnormalities are corrected. Respiratory failure, including PaO_2 decreasing and $PaCO_2$ increasing to equal levels, altered consciousness, pulsus paradoxus, and electrocardiographic changes require intubation and ventilation. Corticosteroids, aminophylline, and bronchodilators are continued. The general approach to respiratory failure from asthma includes standard treatment and precautions as well as ongoing efforts to decrease inflammation, resolve obstruction, and correct ventilation-perfusion inequalities.

Special Types of Bronchial Asthma

Exercise-Induced Asthma

Asthma following exercise may occur in any asthmatic individual, but in some individuals exercise is the primary trigger for asthma. Exercise initially leads to bronchodilation. In exercise-induced asthma, bronchoconstriction occurs after the initial bronchodilation, usually 3 to 15 minutes after exercise has begun. Occasionally the patient is able to "run through their asthma," and, if able to continue or resume exercise, there appears to be a refractory period during which the patient can exercise without asthma. This may also occur if the patient warms up slowly before exercise [172]. The asthma may be severe, but often resolves after 1 to 2 hours. Relapses similar to a late asthma response may be seen.

The specific cause of exercise-induced

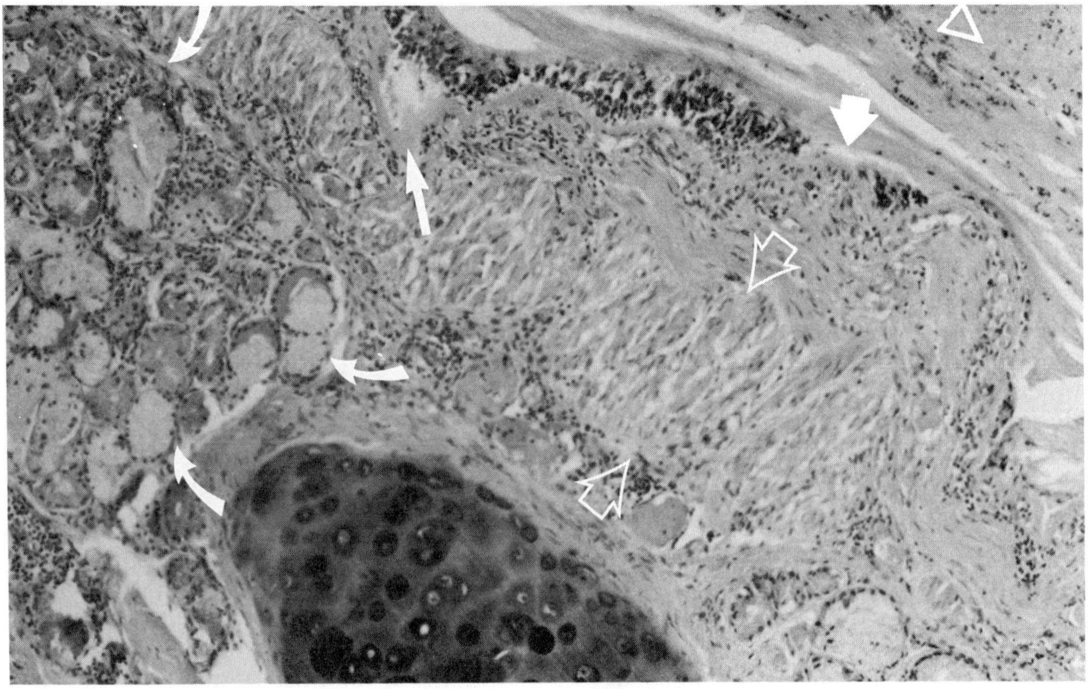

Fig. 8-3. Microscopic section of airway of patient who expired in status asthmaticus. Curved arrows outline glandular hypertrophy. The straight solid arrow points to thickened basement membrane. The blunt, solid arrow points to loss of epithelium. The area between open arrows demonstrates hypertrophy of the muscularis mucosa. The open triangle is placed in the lumen of the airway, which is filled with mucus. Note the inflammatory cells in submucosa and in luminal mucus. (Courtesy of Joseph T. Powaser, MD, Oakwood Hospital.)

asthma is not known. It is probably not due to heat loss, but may be due to water loss from the epithelial environment, leading to a hypertonic microenvironment, which can cause mediator release [172a]. Gradual warming up gives more time for fluid losses to be corrected, thus the blunted effect if the patient warms up slowly. Using a foam rubber type of cold weather mask while running, especially during cold weather, helps prevent heat and fluid loss. Medical treatment is directed toward prevention of the attack. β_2-Agonists, specifically albuterol, before exercise are effective, as well as cromolyn sodium. A combination of both may be used, and ipratropium bromide may be added to these medications [173]. The diagnosis of this condition is based on history, but pre-exercise and post-exercise spirometry can verify questionable cases.

Nocturnal Asthma

Asthmatic patients and their physicians agree that asthma often occurs at night. This may be in the form of an overt attack or recurrent coughing and sleep disturbance. Numerous theories have been proposed to explain the phenomenon of nocturnal asthma. Diurnal variations, with resultant decreased epinephrine, decreased cortisol, and increased blood histamine at night, have been noted, all of which may contribute to bronchospasm [174]. Increased vagal tone is present at night, and airway cooling, sleep, increased nighttime airway hyperreactivity, and decreased mucociliary activity can also contribute to nocturnal asthma [175].

Patients with nocturnal asthma may experience more problems than simple nighttime cough and sleep disturbances. Patients experiencing nocturnal asthma show greater daytime airflow restriction as well as increased airway hyperresponsiveness [175a]. Hospitalized patients with wide diurnal variations in flow rates are at higher risk for fatal asthma, which appears to be more common in the early morning hours [176]. Good overall control of asthma with regular medications can help control nocturnal asthma, but often other measures and medication changes must be made.

Since nocturnal asthma may occur later than 6 hours after onset of sleep, and other asthma medications given orally or by inhalation do not have a duration of action longer than 6 hours, sustained-release theophylline products have been evaluated for the control of nocturnal asthma. Theophylline has been found to be effective in controlling nocturnal asthma and oxygen saturation without adversely affecting sleep quality [177]. In one study, the use of a once-a-day sustained-release theophylline preparation (Uniphyl) after the evening meal resulted in better morning peak flow rates as well as less nighttime awakening when compared with a twice-a-day theophylline regimen [178]. Given in this manner, theophylline levels are adequately elevated during the early morning hours to control the bronchospasm without interfering with sleep. This method of controlling nocturnal asthma will also benefit daytime asthma as long as theophylline levels remain adequate during the day. The use of other medications may be needed through the day in addition to the evening theophylline.

Allergic Bronchopulmonary Aspergillosis

Allergic bronchopulmonary aspergillosis is a hypersensitivity response to *Aspergillus* molds. These patients are asthmatic and have *Aspergillus* organisms growing in the airways without tissue invasion. An immune response, involving both IgE and IgG antibody, is mounted by the patient, resulting in inflammation of the airways with cellular infiltrates, thick exudate, and mucus production as well as interstitial and alveolar fibrosis [179]. Features of this disease include asthma, positive immediate skin test and precipitating antibodies to *Aspergillus*, elevated IgE and peripheral blood eosinophil counts, infiltrates on chest radiography, proximal bronchiectasis, and elevated IgE and IgG titers against *Aspergillus* [180]. Examination of sputum may reveal brown casts of small airways, which, when viewed microscopically, reveal the hyphae of *Aspergillus*.

Early diagnosis and treatment is necessary to prevent the bronchiectasis and fibrosis that can occur in this disease. Patterson et al [181] have proposed that patients with allergic bronchopulmonary aspergillosis be divided into two groups, those with and those without bronchiectasis. Total serum IgE is measured every 1 to 2 months. If this level doubles, prednisone is given at a dose of 0.5 mg/kg/d for 2 weeks, then every other day for 3 months, then discontinued as tolerated [181]. This is the same regimen for patients who have exacerbations with radiographic infiltrates. This aggressive treatment is used to prevent the progression of allergic bronchopulmonary aspergillosis without bronchiectasis to allergic bronchopulmonary aspergillosis with lung damage and bronchiectasis.

Since these patients have asthma, regular treatment of their bronchial asthma should be continued. Bronchodilators and inhaled or alternate day steroids may be used. However, with exacerbations of allergic bronchopulmonary aspergillosis, aggressive prednisone therapy is the treatment of choice. Since the *Aspergillus* in the airway is not invasive, antifungal treatment is not indicated.

Occupational Asthma

Over 200 agents have been implicated in causing bronchial asthma [182]. Those who develop occupational asthma may have nonspecific bronchial hyperreactivity that can be documented by methacholine challenge [183]. Occupational asthma is reviewed in the chapter on occupational lung diseases (Chap. 14).

Long-Term Considerations of Bronchial Asthma

Bronchial asthma, by itself, rarely results in permanent morphologic damage to the lung. As with any chronic disease, the major long-term problem is the impact on that person's lifestyle and growth. This is especially important in the pediatric population.

Children with chronic bronchial asthma view health and asthma in different ways. Where a physician's and parent's concept of health may mean absence of symptoms, almost 75% of responses of a group of 9- to 11-year-old children with asthma viewed health as the ability to be active or happy. Less than 10% of the responses defined health as a lack of asthma symptoms [184]. The physician must explore the child's concept of asthma and encourage the child to take an active part in the control of his or her disease [185].

Adolescents with chronic illness may be very difficult to care for because of the stresses of growth and development and their search for identity [186]. Asthma has been associated with delayed puberty [187]. Chronic illness is a risk factor for behavioral problems in children and adolescents [188]. The adolescent may be angry because of his or her illness, and compliance with medication programs may be poor. Long-term hospitalization in specialized centers caring for both physical and psychological problems associated with asthma may be of benefit to selected children [189]. The physician may have to take on the role of patient advocate when dealing with overprotective or harsh parents.

The stresses of chronic illness on the asthmatic adult, both physical and emotional, must be dealt with vigorously. Fears regarding loss of job, inability to care for or support the family, and even death must be discussed openly. The role of stress in asthma in adults and the need for relaxation techniques should be discussed. Unless the total impact of asthma is approached, medical treatment will be ineffective.

The need for education of the patient has been stressed in this chapter. A National Heart, Lung, and Blood Institute workshop has been held to formulate a national program to educate not only patients but physicians and the general public [190]. Numerous educational programs have been formulated, but a review of programs for children indicated that their effectiveness may be small [191]. The responsibility for education of the patient and parents lies with the physician.

Bronchial asthma is a reversible obstructive airway condition of the lungs, involving both inflammatory processes and hyperreactivity of the airways. There is no permanent cure. Asthma can present differently in the same patient and between patients. Physicians caring for patients with asthma must tailor a specific treatment regimen for each person. The goal should be a lifestyle unencumbered by respiratory difficulties, with a minimum of interference caused by the treatment regimen. As the mysteries of this condition unfold, the physician must stay abreast of new findings and treatments so that he or she may better care for the asthmatic patient. An informed and caring physician is the best medicine for the patient with asthma.

References

1. Laennec RTH: A Treatise on the Diseases of the Chest (translated by Forbes J.). London, T. and G. Underwood, 1821, pp 75–76
2. Freour P: Definition of asthma. *Chest* 91: 191S–192S, 1987
3. Evans R, Mullally DI, Wilson RW, et al: National trends in the morbidity and mortality of asthma in the U.S. *Chest* 91:65S–74S, 1987
4. Gergen PJ, Mullally DI, Evans R: National survey of prevalence of asthma among children in the United States, 1976 to 1980. *Pediatrics* 81:1–7, 1988

4a. Weiss KB, Gergen PJ, Hodgson TA: An Economic Evaluation of Asthma in the United States. *N Engl J Med* 326:862–6, 1992

5. Friday GA, Fireman P: A review of asthma admissions and deaths at Children's Hospital of Pittsburgh from 1968 to 1985: A sequel

to a previous review from 1935 to 1968. *Pediatric Asthma Allergy Immunology* 3:13–19, 1989
6. Sly RM: Mortality from asthma, 1979–1984. *J Allergy Clin Immunol* 82:705–717, 1988
7. Hannaway PJ: Asthma deaths in Massachusetts 1971–1987. *Pediatric Asthma Allergy Immunology* 2:99–104, 1988
8. Jackson R, Sears MR, Beaglehold R, et al: International trends in asthma mortality: 1970–1985. *Chest* 94:914–919, 1988
9. Sears MR: Increasing asthma mortality—Fact or artifact? *J Allergy Clin Immunol* 82: 957–960, 1988
10. Buist AS: Asthma mortality: What have we learned? *J Allergy Clin Immunol* 84:275–283, 1989
11. Osler W: The Principles and Practices of Medicine. New York, Appleton and Company, 1892, pp 500–501
12. Junqueira LC, Carneiro J, Kelley RO: Basic Histology, ed 6. Norwalk, CT, Appleton & Lange, 1989, pp 340–344
13. Sheppard MN, Kurian SS, Henzen-Logmans SC, et al: Neuron-specific enolase and S-100. New markers for delineating the innervation of the respiratory tract in man and other animals. *Thorax* 38:333–340, 1983
14. Barnes PJ: Neuropeptides in the lung: Localization, function, and pathophysiologic implications. *J Allergy Clin Immunol* 79:285–295, 1987
15. Barnes PJ: Neural control of human airways in health and disease. *Am Rev Respir Dis* 134: 1289–1314, 1986
16. Barrett KE, Metcalfe DD: Heterogeneity of mast cells in the tissues of the respiratory tract and other organ systems. *Am Rev Respir Dis* 135:1190–1195, 1987
17. Peters SP, Schleimer RP, Naclerio RM, et al: The pathophysiology of human mast cells. *Am Rev Respir Dis* 135:1196–1200, 1987
18. Wenzel SE, Fowler AA, Schwartz LB: Activation of pulmonary mast cells by bronchoalveolar allergen challenge. *Am Rev Respir Dis* 137:1002–1008, 1988
19. Lee TH: Interactions between alveolar macrophages, monocytes, and granulocytes. *Am Rev Respir Dis* 135:S14–S17, 1987
20. Gosset P, Lassalle P, Tonnel AB, et al: Production of an interleukin-1 inhibitory factor by human alveolar macrophages from normals and allergic asthmatic patients. *Am Rev Respir Dis* 138:40–46, 1988
21. Godard P, Chaintreuil J, Damon M, et al: Functional assessment of alveolar macrophages: Comparison of cells from asthmatics and normal subjects. *J Allergy Clin Immunol* 70:88–93, 1982
22. Kelly C, Ward C, Stenton CS, et al: Number and activity of inflammatory cells in bronchoalveolar lavage fluid in asthma and their relation to airway responsiveness. *Thorax* 43: 684–692, 1988
23. Gleich GJ: The eosinophil and bronchial asthma: Current understanding. *J Allergy Clin Immunol* 85:422–436, 1990
24. Rafferty P, Holgate ST: Histamine and its antagonists in asthma. *J Allergy Clin Immunol* 84:144–151, 1989
25. Beer DJ, Rocklin RE: Histamine-induced suppressor-cell activity. *J Allergy Clin Immunol* 73:439–452, 1984
26. Barnes PJ, Chung KF, Page CP: Inflammatory mediators and asthma. *Pharmacol Rev* 40:49–84, 1988
27. Church MM, Lai C, Beasley R, et al: The mediator and cellular basis of the allergic response. *Allergy* 43(suppl 8):26–29, 1988
28. Buchanan DR, Cromwell O, Kay AB: Neutrophil chemotactic activity in acute severe asthma (status asthmaticus). *Am Rev Respir Dis* 136:1397–1402, 1987
29. Rubin AE, Smith LJ, Patterson R: The bronchoconstrictor properties of platelet-activating factor in humans. *Am Rev Respir Dis* 136: 1145–1151, 1987
30. Cushley MJ, Tattersfield AE, Holgate ST: Inhaled adenosine and guanosine on airway resistance in normal and asthmatic subjects. *Br J Clin Pharmacol* 15:161–165, 1983
31. Cuss FM, Barnes PJ: Epithelial mediators. *Am Rev Respir Dis* 136:S32–S35, 1987
32. Vanhoutte PM: Epithelium-derived relaxing factor(s) and bronchial reactivity. *Am Rev Respir Dis* 138:S24–S30, 1988
33. Beasley R, Roche WR, Roberts JA, et al: Cellular events in the bronchi in mild asthma and after bronchial provocation. *Am Rev Respir Dis* 139:806–817, 1989
34. Roche WR, Williams JH, Beasley R, et al: Subepithelial fibrosis in the bronchi of asthmatics. *Lancet* 1:520–524, 1989
35. Laitinen LA, Heino M, Laitinen A, et al: Damage of the airway epithelium and bronchial reactivity in patients with asthma. *Am Rev Respir Dis* 131:599–606, 1985
36. James AL, Pare PD, Hogg JC: The mechanics of airway narrowing in asthma. *Am Rev Respir Dis* 139:242–246, 1989
37. Lundgren JD, Shelhamer JH: Pathogenesis of airway mucus hypersecretion. *J Allergy Clin Immunol* 85:399–412, 1990
38. Bhaskar KR, De Feudis O'Sullivan D, Coles SJ, et al: Characterization of airway mucus from a fatal case of status asthmaticus. *Pediatr Pulmonol* 5:176–182, 1988
38a. Spencer H. Pathology of the Lung, New York, Pergamon Press, 1985, pp 758–764.
39. Phelan PS: The natural history of childhood

asthma into adult life. *Immunology Allergy Practice* 10:334–341, 1988
40. Pearlman DS: The relationship between allergy and croup. *Allergy Proc* 10:227–231, 1989
41. Connolly CK, Chan NS, Prescott RJ: The relationship between age and duration of asthma and the presence of persistent obstruction in asthma. *Postgrad Med J* 64:422–425, 1988
42. Gerritsen J, Koeter GH, deMonchy JGR, et al: Allergy in subjects with asthma from childhood to adulthood. *J Allergy Clin Immunol* 85:116–125, 1990
43. Weitzman NM, Gortmaker S, Walker DK, et al: Maternal smoking and childhood asthma. *Pediatrics* 85:505–511, 1990
44. Shim CS, Williams MH: Relationship of wheezing to the severity of obstruction in asthma. *Arch Intern Med* 143:890–892, 1983
45. Kesten S, Maleki-Yazdi MR, Sanders BR, et al: Respiratory rate during acute asthma. *Chest* 97:58–62, 1990
46. Ferguson AC: Persisting airway obstruction in asymptomatic children with asthma with normal peak expiratory flow rates. *J Allergy Clin Immunol* 82:19–22, 1988
47. Worthington JR, Ahuja J: The value of pulmonary function tests in the management of acute asthma. *Can Med Assoc J* 140:153–156, 1989
48. Roca J, Ramis L, Rodriguez-Roisin R, et al: Serial relationships between ventilation-perfusion inequality and spirometry in acute severe asthma requiring hospitalization. *Am Rev Respir Dis* 137:1055–1061, 1988
49. Cockcroft DW: Bronchial inhalation tests. I. Management of nonallergic bronchial responsiveness. *Ann Allergy* 55:527–533, 1985
50. Rosenthal RR: Approved methodology for methacholine challenge. *Allergy Proc* 10:301–312, 1989
51. Shapiro GG: Methacholine bronchoprovocation challenge in children. *Allergy Proc* 10:332, 1989
52. Chai H, Farr RS, Froehlich LA, et al: Standardization of bronchial inhalation challenge procedures. *J Allergy Clin Immunol* 56:323–327, 1975
53. Cockcroft DW: Bronchial inhalation tests. II. Measurement of allergic (and occupational) bronchial responsiveness. *Ann Allergy* 59:89–98, 1987
54. Abdullah AK, El-Hazmi MAF, Uz-Zaman AU, et al: Serum IgE levels in adults with asthma. *J Asthma* 24:207–213, 1987
55. Burrows B, Martinez FD, Halonen M, et al: Association of asthma with serum IgE levels and skin-test reactivity to allergens. *N Engl J Med* 320:271–277, 1989
56. Kalliel JN, Goldstein BM, Braman SS, et al: High frequency of atopic asthma in a pulmonary clinic population. *Chest* 96:1336–1340, 1989
57. Zimmerman B, Feanny S, Reisman J, et al: The dose relationship of allergy to severity of childhood asthma. *J Allergy Clin Immunol* 81:63–70, 1988
58. Amin NM: Unusual causes of wheezing in adults. *Immunol Allergy Prac* 8:17–25, 1986
59. Downing ET, Braman SS, Fox MJ, et al: Fictitious asthma—physiological approach to diagnosis. *JAMA* 248:2878–2881, 1982
60. Christopher KL, Wood RP, Eckert RC, et al: Vocal-cord dysfunction presenting as asthma. *N Engl J Med* 308:1566–1570, 1983
61. Platts-Mills TAE, Chapman MD: Dust mites: Immunology, allergic disease, and environmental control. *J Allergy Clin Immunol* 80:755–775, 1987
62. Bousquet J, Michel FB: Food allergy and asthma. *Ann Allergy* 61:70–74, 1988
63. Silverman M, Wilson N: Clinical physiology of food intolerance in asthma. Proceedings of the XII International Congress of Allergology and Clinical Immunology. *J Allergy Clin Immunol* 457–462, 1986
64. Samet JM, Marburn MC, Spengler JD: Respiratory effects of indoor air pollution. *J Allergy Clin Immunol* 79:685–700, 1987
65. Vesterinen E, Kaprio J, Koskenvuo M: Prospective study of asthma in relation to smoking habits among 14729 adults. *Thorax* 43:534–539, 1988
66. Chesebro MJ: Passive smoking. *Am Fam Physician* 37:212–218, 1988
67. Committee on Environmental Hazards—American Academy of Pediatrics: Involuntary smoking—A hazard to children. *Pediatrics* 77:755–757, 1986
68. Hedberg K, Edberg CW, Iber C, et al: An outbreak of nitrogen dioxide-induced respiratory illness among ice hockey players. *JAMA* 262:3014–3017, 1989
69. Koenig JQ: Pulmonary reaction to environmental pollutants. *J Allergy Clin Immunol* 79:833–843, 1987
70. Busse WW: Respiratory infections: Their role in airway responsiveness and the pathogenesis of asthma. *J Allergy Clin Immunol* 85:671–683, 1990
71. Beasley R, Coleman ED, Hermon Y, et al: Viral respiratory tract infection and exacerbations of asthma in adult patients. *Thorax* 43:679–683, 1988
72. Lemanske RF, Dick EC, Swenson CA, et al: Rhinovirus upper respiratory infection increases airway hyperreactivity and late asthmatic reactions. *J Clin Invest* 83:1–10, 1989

73. Li JTC, O'Connell EJ: Viral infections and asthma. *Ann Allergy* 59:321–331, 1987
74. Weiner HM: Stress, relaxation and asthma. *Int J Psychosom* 34:21–24, 1987
74a. Yellowlees PM, Kalucy RS: Psychological aspects of asthma and the consequent research implications. *Chest* 97:628–34, 1990
75. Virchow C, Szczeklik A, Bianco S, et al: Intolerance to tartrazine in aspirin-induced asthma: Results of a multicenter study. *Respiration* 53:20–23, 1988
76. Settipane GA: The restaurant syndromes. *NER Allergy Proc* 8:39–46, 1987
77. Schwartzstein RM, Kelleher M, Weinberger SE, et al: Airway effects of monosodium glutamate in subjects with chronic stable asthma. *J Asthma* 24:167–172, 1987
77a. Genton C, Frei PC, Pecoud A: Value of oral provocation tests to aspirin and food additives in the routine investigation of asthma and chronic urticaria. *J Allergy Clin Immunol* 76:40–45, 1985
78. Shapiro GG: Role of allergy in sinusitis. *Pediatr Infect Dis J* 4:S55–S58, 1985
78a. Slavin RG: Relationship of nasal disease and sinusitis to bronchial asthma. *Ann Allergy* 49:76–80, 1982
79. Minor MW, Lockey RF: Sinusitis and asthma. *South Med J* 80:1141–1147, 1987
80. Slepian IK, Mathews KP, McLean JA: Aspirin-sensitive asthma. *Chest* 87:386–391, 1985
81. Tan Y, Collins-Williams C: Aspirin-induced asthma in children. *Ann Allergy* 48:1–5, 1982
82. Morassut P, Yang W, Karsh J: Aspirin intolerance. *Semin Arthritis Rheum* 19:22–30, 1989
83. Zeitz HJ, Jarmoszuk I: Nasal polyps, bronchial asthma, and aspirin sensitivity: The Samter syndrome. *Comp Ther* 11:21–26, 1985
84. Chudwin DS, Strub M, Golden HE, et al: Sensitivity to non-acetylated salicylates in a patient with asthma, nasal polyps, and rheumatoid arthritis. *Ann Allergy* 57:133–134, 1986
85. Mathison DA, Stevenson DD, Simon RA: Precipitating factors in asthma—aspirin, sulfites, and other drugs and chemicals. *Chest* 87(suppl):50S–54S, 1985
86. Gustafsson PM, Kjellman NIM, Tibbling L: Oesophageal function and symptoms in moderate and severe asthma. *Acta Paediatr Scand* 75:729–736, 1986
87. Pauli BD, Reid RL, Munt PW, et al: Influence of the menstrual cycle on airway function in asthmatic and normal subjects. *Am Rev Respir Dis* 140:358–362, 1989
88. Pedreira FA, Guandolo VL, Feroli EJ, et al: Involuntary smoking and incidence of respiratory illness during the first year of life. *Pediatrics* 75:594–597, 1985
89. Murray AB, Morrison BJ: Passive smoking by asthmatics: Its greater effect on boys than on girls and on older than on younger children. *Pediatrics* 84:451–459, 1989
90. Wood RA, Chapman MD, Atkinson NF, et al: The effect of cat removal on allergen content in household-dust samples. *J Allergy Clin Immunol* 83:730–734, 1989
91. Wentz PE, Swanson MC, Reed CE: Variability of cat-allergen shedding. *J Allergy Clin Immunol* 85:94–98, 1990
92. Price AH, Clissold SP: Salbutamol in the 1980's. *Drugs* 78:77–122, 1989
93. Marsac JH, Vlastos FD, Lacronique JG: Inhaled beta adrenergic agonists and inhaled steroids in the treatment of asthma. *Ann Allergy* 63:220–224, 1989
94. Fitzsimons R, Greenberger PA, Patterson R: When asthmatic patients become pregnant. *J Respir Dis* 7:40–46, 1986
95. Wolfe JD, Yamate M, Biedermann AA, et al: Comparison of the acute cardiopulmonary effects of oral albuterol, metaproterenol, and terbutaline in asthmatics. *JAMA* 253: 2068–2072, 1985
96. Richards DM, Brogden RN: Pirbuterol: A preliminary review of its pharmacological properties and therapeutic efficacy in reversible bronchospastic disease. *Drugs* 30:6–21, 1985
97. Walker SB, Kradjan WA, Bierman CW: Bitolterol mesylate: A beta-adrenergic agent. *Pharmacotherapy* 5:127–137, 1985
98. Deenstra M, Haalboom JRE, Struyvenberg A: Decrease of plasma potassium due to inhalation of beta-2-agonists: Absence of an additional effect of intravenous theophylline. *Eur J Clin Invest* 18:162–165, 1988
99. Chow OKW, Fung KP: Slow release terbutaline and theophylline for the long term therapy of children with asthma: A latin square and factorial study of drug effects and interactions. *Pediatrics* 84:119–125, 1989
99a. Becker AB, Simons KJ, Gillespie CA, et al: The bronchodilator effects and pharmacokinetics of caffeine in asthma. *N Engl J Med* 310:743–6, 1984
100. Self TH, Ellis RF, Abou-Shala N, et al: Is theophylline use justified in acute exacerbations of asthma? *Pharmacotherapy* 9:260–266, 1989
101. Kuehl FA, Zanetti ME, Soderman DD, et al: Cyclic AMP-dependent regulation of lipid mediators in white cells. *Am Rev Respir Dis* 136:210–213, 1987
102. Church MK, Featherstone RL, Cushley MJ, et al: Relationships between adenosine, cyclic nucleotides, and xanthines in asthma. *J Allergy Clin Immunol* 78:670–675, 1986
103. Svedmyr N: Theophylline. *Am Rev Respir Dis* 136:568–571, 1987

104. Pauwels R: The effects of theophylline on airway inflammation. *Chest* 92(suppl):32S–37S, 1987
105. Pauwels R: New aspects of the therapeutic potential of theophylline in asthma. *J Allergy Clin Immunol* 83:548–553, 1989
106. Merland N, Cartier A, L'Archeveque JL, et al: Theophylline minimally inhibits bronchoconstriction induced by dry cold air inhalation in asthmatic subjects. *Am Rev Respir Dis* 137:1304–1308, 1988
107. Ziment I: Theophylline and mucociliary clearance. *Chest* 92(suppl):38S–43S, 1987
108. Aubier M: Effect of theophylline on diaphragmatic and other skeletal muscle function. *J Allergy Clin Immunol* 78:787–792, 1986
109. Kongragunta VR, Druz WS, Sharp JT: Dyspnea and diaphragmatic fatigue in patients with chronic obstructive pulmonary disease. *Am Rev Respir Dis* 137:662–667, 1988
110. Foxworth JW, Reisz GR, Knudson SM, et al: Theophylline and diaphragmatic contractility. *Am Rev Respir Dis* 138:1532–1534, 1988
111. Hubert D, Gaudric M, Guerre J, et al: Effect of theophylline on gastroesophageal reflux in patients with asthma. *J Allergy Clin Immunol* 81:1168–1174, 1988
112. McEvoy GK (ed): American Hospital Formulary Service Drug Information 90. Bethesda, American Society of Hospital Pharmacists, 1990, p 2098
113. Stavric B: Methylxanthines: Toxicity to humans. 1. Theophylline. *Food Chem Toxicol* 26: 544–565, 1988
114. Szefler SJ: Erratic absorption of theophylline from slow-release products in children. *J Allergy Clin Immunol* 78:710–715, 1986
115. Hendeles L, Weinberger M: Selection of a slow-release theophylline product. *J Allergy Clin Immunol* 78:743–751, 1986
116. Smolensky MH, Scott PH, Kramer WG: Clinical significance of day-night differences in serum theophylline concentration with special reference to theodur. *J Allergy Clin Immunol* 78:716–722, 1986
117. Pedersen S: Effects of food on the absorption of theophylline in children. *J Allergy Clin Immunol* 78:704–709, 1986
118. Karim A: Effects of food on the bioavailability of theophylline from controlled-release products in adults. *J Allergy Clin Immunol* 78:695–703, 1986
119. Vaughan LM, Milavetz G, Weinberger MM, et al: Oral bioavailability of slow-release theophylline from unencapsulated beads in preschool children with chronic asthma. *Ther Drug Monit* 10:395–400, 1988
120. Jonkman JHG: Food interactions with sustained-release theophylline preparations. *Clinic Pharmacokinet* 16:162–179, 1989
121. Jenne JW: Effect of disease states on theophylline elimination. *J Allergy Clin Immunol* 78: 727–735, 1986
122. Nicot G, Charmes JP, Lachatre G, et al: Theophylline toxicity risks and chronic renal failure. *Int J Clin Pharmacol Ther Toxicol* 27: 398–401, 1989
123. Samaans S, Fox R: The effect of smoking on theophylline kinetics in healthy and asthmatic elderly males. *J Clin Pharmacol* 29: 448–450, 1989
124. Lesko LJ: Dose-dependent kinetics of theophylline. *J Allergy Clin Immunol* 78:723–727, 1986
125. Bernocchi D, Castiglioni CL: Guide to therapy with theophylline for the treatment of obstructive lung disease. *J Int Med Res* 16: 1–18, 1988
126. Weinberger M, Hendeles L: Therapeutic effect and dosing strategies for theophylline in the treatment of chronic asthma. *J Allergy Clin Immunol* 78:762–768, 1986
127. Mitenko PA, Ogilvie RI: Rational intravenous doses of theophylline. *N Engl J Med* 289:600–603, 1973
128. Nolke AC: Severe toxic effects from aminophylline and theophylline suppositories in children. *JAMA* 161:693–697, 1956
129. Rossing TH: Methylxanthines in 1989. *Ann Intern Med* 110:502–504, 1989
130. Jordan TJ, Reichman LB: Once-daily versus twice-daily dosing of theophylline. *Am Rev Respir Dis* 140:1573–1577, 1989
131. Sharp JT: Theophylline in chronic obstructive pulmonary disease. *J Allergy Clin Immunol* 78:800–805, 1986
132. Matthay RA, Mahler DA: Theophylline improves global cardiac function and reduces dyspnea in chronic obstructive lung disease. *J Allergy Clin Immunol* 78:793–799, 1986
132a. Hill NS: The use of theophylline in 'irreversible' chronic obstructive pulmonary disease. *Arch Intern Med* 148:2579–2584, 1988
133. Jenne JW: Theophylline as a bronchodilator in COPD and its combination with inhaled β-adrenergic drugs. *Chest* 92:7S–14S, 1987
134. Flenley DC: Should bronchodilators be combined in chronic bronchitis and emphysema? *Br Med J* 295:1160–1161, 1987
135. Kay AB, Walsh GM, Moqbel R, et al: Disodium cromoglycate inhibits activation of human inflammatory cells in vitro. *J Allergy Clin Immunol* 80:1–8, 1987
136. Petty TL, Rollins DR, Christopher K, et al: Cromolyn sodium is effective in adult chronic asthmatics. *Am Rev Respir Dis* 139: 694–701, 1989
137. Settipane GA, Klein DE, Boyd GK, et al: Adverse reactions to cromolyn. *JAMA* 241: 811–813, 1979
138. Bernstein IL: Cromolyn sodium in the treatment of asthma: Coming of age in the

United States. *J Allergy Clin Immunol* 76: 381–388, 1985
139. Gross NJ, Skorodin MS: Anticholingeric, antimuscarinic bronchodilators. *Am Rev Respir Dis* 129:856–870, 1984
140. Larsson K: Ipratropium bromide: Bronchodilator action and effect of methacholine-induced bronchoconstriction. *J Asthma* 24:29–35, 1987
141. Gross NJ: Ipratropium bromide. *N Engl J Med* 319:486–494, 1988
142. Fauci AS, Dale DC, Balow JE: Glucocorticoid therapy: Mechanisms of action and clinical considerations. *Ann Intern Med* 84:304–315, 1976
143. Martin GL, Atkins PC, Dunsky EH, et al: Effects of theophylline, terbutaline, and prednisone on antigen-induced bronchospasm and mediator release. *J Allergy Clin Immunol* 66:204–212, 1980
144. Mano K, Akbarzadeh A, Townley RG: Effect of hydrocortisone on beta-adrenergic receptors in lung membranes. *Life Sci* 25:1925–1930, 1979
145. Fanta CH, Rossing TH, McFadden ER: Glucocorticoids in acute asthma. *Am J Med* 74: 845–851, 1983
146. Brunette MG, Lands L, Thibodeau LP: Chlidhood asthma: Prevention of attacks with short-term corticosteroid treatment of upper respiratory tract infection. *Pediatrics* 81:624–629, 1988
147. Woolcock AJ: Use of corticosteroids in treatment of patients with asthma. *J Allergy Clin Immunol* 84:975–978, 1989
148. Harter JG, Reddy WJ, Thorn GW: Studies on an intermittent corticosteroid dosage regimen. *N Engl J Med* 269:591–596, 1963
149. Burge PS, Turner-Warwick M, Nelmes PTJ: Double-blind trials of inhaled beclomethasone diproprionate and fluocortin butyl ester in allergen-induced immediate and late asthmatic reactions. *Clin Allergy* 12:523–531, 1982
150. McLeod DT, Capewell SJ, Law J, et al: Intramuscular triamcinolone acetonide in chronic severe asthma. *Thorax* 40:840–845, 1985
151. Rimsza ME: Complications of corticosteroid therapy. *Am J Dis Child* 132:806–810, 1978
152. Brown DCP, Savacool AM, Letizia CM: A retrospective review of the effects of one year of triamcinolone acetonide aerosol treatment on the growth patterns of asthmatic children. *Ann Allergy* 63:47–51, 1989
153. Svendsen UG, Frolund L, Madsen F, et al: A comparison of the effects of sodium cromoglycate and betamethasone dipropionate on pulmonary function and bronchial hyperreactivity in subjects with asthma. *J Allergy Clin Immunol* 80:68–74, 1987
154. Salmeron S, Guerin J, Godard P, et al: High doses of inhaled corticosteroids in unstable chronic asthma. *Am Rev Respir Dis* 140:167–171, 1989
155. Pierson WE, Furukawa CT, Shapiro GG, et al: Terfenadine blockade of exercise-induced bronchospasm. *Ann Allergy* 63:461–464, 1989
156. Holgate ST, Finnerty JP: Antihistamines in asthma. *J Allergy Clin Immunol* 83:537–547, 1989
157. Medici TC, Radielovic P, Morley J: Ketotifen in the prophylaxis of extrinsic bronchial asthma. *Chest* 96:1252–1257, 1989
158. Collins-Williams C: Antihistamines in asthma. *J Asthma* 24:55–58, 1987
159. Petty TL: The national mucolytic study. *Chest* 97:75–83, 1990
160. Wald JA, Friedman BF, Farr RS: An improved protocol for the use of troleandomycin (TAO) in the treatment of steroid-requiring asthma. *J Allergy Clin Immunol* 78:36–43, 1986
161. Mullarkey MF, Blumenstein BA, Andrade WP, et al: Methotrexate in the treatment of corticosteroid-dependent asthma. *N Engl J Med* 318:603–607, 1988
162. Kaslow JE, Novey HS: Methotrexate use for asthma: A critical appraisal. *Ann Allergy* 62: 541–545, 1989
163. Clark TJH: Efficacy and safety of anti-asthma treatment. *Allergy* 43(suppl 8):32–35, 1988
163a. Spitzer WO, Suissa S, Ernst P, et al: The use of β-agonists and the risk of death and near death from asthma. *N Engl J Med* 326:501–6, 1992
163b. Guidelines for the Diagnosis and Management of Asthma, National Asthma Education Program—Expert Panel Report, National Institutes of Health Publication No. 91-3042, Bethesda, 1991
164. Ohman JL: Allergen immunotherapy in asthma: Evidence for efficacy. *J Allergy Clin Immunol* 84:133–140, 1989
165. Johnstone DE: Immunotherapy in the prevention of allergic disease. *Pediatric Asthma Allergy Immunology* 1:15–30, 1987
166. Van Metre TE, Marsh DG, Adkinson NF, et al: Immunotherapy for cat asthma. *J Allergy Clin Immunol* 82:1055–1068, 1988
167. Rak S, Lowhagen O, Venge P: The effect of immunotherapy on bronchial hyperresponsiveness and eosinophil cationic protein in pollen-allergic patients. *J Allergy Clin Immunol* 82:470–480, 1988
168. Summer WR: Status asthmaticus. *Chest* 87 (suppl):87S–94S, 1985
169. McFadden ER: Therapy of acute asthma. *J Allergy Clin Immunol* 84:151–158, 1989

170. Fanta CH, Rossing TH, McFadden ER: Treatment of acute asthma. *Am J Med* 80: 5–10, 1986
171. Dolen WK, Weber RW: Assessment and management of acute asthma. *Ann Allergy* 63:86–95, 1989
172. Scoggin C: Exercise-induced asthma. *Chest* 87(suppl):48S–49S, 1985
172a. Anderson HR: Is the prevalance of asthma changing? *Arch Dis Child* 64:172–175, 1989
173. Bierman CW: Exercise-induced asthma. *Allergy Proc* 9:193–197, 1988
174. Barnes PJ: Inflammatory mechanisms and nocturnal asthma. *Am J Med* 85(suppl 1B): 64–70, 1988
175. Busse WW: Pathogenesis and pathophysiology of nocturnal asthma. *Am J Med* 85(suppl 1B):24–29, 1988
175a. Martin RJ, Cicutto LC, Ballard RD: Factors related to the nocturnal worsening of asthma. *Am Rev Respir Dis* 141:33–38, 1990
176. Hetzel MR, Clark TJH, Branthwaite MA: Asthma: Analysis of sudden deaths and ventilatory arrests in hospital. *Br Med J* 1:808–811, 1977
177. Zwillich CW, Neagley SR, Cicutto L, et al: Nocturnal asthma therapy. *Am Rev Respir Dis* 139:470–474, 1989
178. Grossman J: Multicenter comparison of once-daily uniphyl tablets administered in the morning or evening with baseline twice-daily theophylline therapy in patients with nocturnal asthma. *Am J Med* 85(suppl 1B): 11–13, 1988
179. Fink JN: Allergic bronchopulmonary aspergillosis. *Chest* 87:81S–84S, 1985
180. Greenberger PA: Allergic bronchopulmonary aspergillosis. *J Allergy Clin Immunol* 74: 645–653, 1984
181. Patterson R, Greenberger PA, Halwig JM, et al: Allergic bronchopulmonary aspergillosis. *Arch Intern Med* 146:916–918, 1986
182. Chan-Yeung M, Lam S: Occupational asthma. *Am Rev Respir Dis* 133:686–703, 1986
183. Butcher BT, Salvaggio JE: Occupational asthma. *J Allergy Clin Immunol* 78:547–556, 1986
184. Kieckhefer GM: The meaning of health to 9-, 10-, and 11-year-old children with chronic asthma. *J Asthma* 25:325–333, 1988
185. Quinn CM: Children's asthma: New approaches, new understandings. *Ann Allergy* 60:283–292, 1988
186. Siegel DM: Adolescents and chronic illness. *JAMA* 257:3396–3399, 1987
187. Balfour-Lynn L: Effect of asthma on growth and puberty. *Pediatrician* 14:237–241, 1987
188. Gortmaker SL, Walker DK, Weitzman M, et al: Chronic conditions, socioeconomic risks, and behavioral problems in children and adolescents. *Pediatrics* 85:267–276, 1990
189. Strunk RC, Fukuhara JT, LaBrecque JF, et al: Outcome of long-term hospitalization for asthma in children. *J Allergy Clin Immunol* 83:17–25, 1989
190. Parker SR, Mellins RB, Sogn DD: Asthma education: A national strategy. *Am Rev Respir Dis* 140:848–853, 1989
191. Howland J, Bauchner H, Adair R: The impact of pediatric asthma education on morbidity. *Chest* 94:964–969, 1988

9

Chronic Obstructive Pulmonary Disease

Daniel L. Maxwell

Chronic obstructive pulmonary disease (COPD) (chronic obstructive lung disease, chronic airflow obstruction), is a nonspecific term denoting a disease process, not associated with bronchiolitis, bronchiectasis, or cystic fibrosis, which is characterized by chronic, predominantly irreversible reduction in maximal airflow velocity, increased respiratory morbidity, and early mortality [1, 2]. The spectrum of disease includes pulmonary emphysema, as well as chronic bronchitis. Some degree of reversible airway obstruction is typically found in addition to the fixed limitation. With very few exceptions, patients with COPD suffer from a mixed form of disease, despite the predominance of one clinical pattern [1]. The following obstructive airway diseases participate in the definition of COPD.

Emphysema is defined anatomically as the abnormal dilation of airspaces distal to the terminal bronchioles due to destruction of alveolar walls, without obvious fibrosis (Fig. 9-1). Emphysema may be further categorized by the location of alveolar destruction, although this is of little clinical significance.

Chronic bronchitis is defined clinically as the presence of a productive cough, on most days of the month, for 3 months in 2 consecutive years, in the absence of other causes for chronic cough (i.e., tuberculosis, lung cancer). This hypersecretory disorder exists with or without airflow limitation, and in the absence of such obstruction is not associated with an increased respiratory morbidity or early mortality, leading Petty and associates [3] to describe chronic obstructive bronchitis as chronic bronchitis associated with demonstrable airflow obstruction and its complications. In this chapter, chronic bronchitis refers to chronic bronchitis with airflow obstruction.

Asthma is characterized by intermittent and variable reductions in airway caliber and airflow velocity, occurring spontaneously or as a result of treatment [4]. Long-standing asthma may progress to the irreversible airflow obstruction of COPD. Nonspecific airway hyperreactivity is common, but may also be seen in chronic bronchitis [2]. Atopy, peripheral eosinophilia, aspirin hypersensitivity, and elevated serum IgE levels may be seen, but are not required for diagnosis. Asthma is considered in detail in Chap. 8. Asthma may coexist with chronic bronchitis or emphysema of unrelated cause.

Bronchiectasis is an abnormal, permanent dilation of subsegmental airways that are typically tortuous and partially filled with mucoid or purulent secretions [5]. Secondary infection is typical and recurrent pneumonias distal to the involved segments are common and frequently lead to scarring. Diffuse bronchiectasis may result from inhalation or aspiration of corrosives, including repeated microaspiration of gastrointestinal contents, intravenous drug abuse, or following diffuse bronchopulmonary infection such as mycoplasma or viral pneumonia. Airflow limitation is not generally seen unless diffuse disease is encountered. Bronchiectasis is not usually considered as part of the definition of COPD.

Therefore, from a clinician's standpoint, COPD is a disorder of chronic airway ob-

Opinions expressed herein are those of the author and do not necessarily represent the official position of the Department of the Navy, Department of Defense, or any other governmental department or agency.

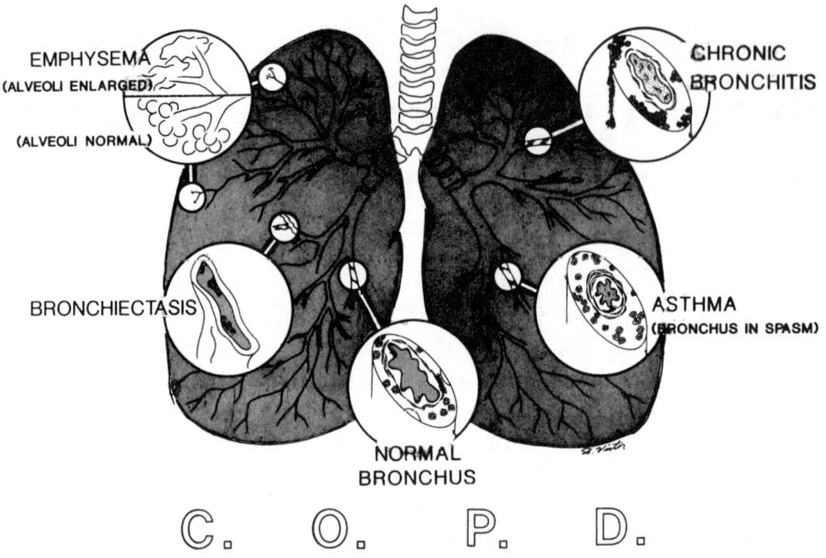
EMPHYSEMA
(ALVEOLI ENLARGED)
(ALVEOLI NORMAL)
CHRONIC
BRONCHITIS
BRONCHIECTASIS
ASTHMA
(BRONCHUS IN SPASM)
NORMAL
BRONCHUS
C. O. P. D.

Fig. 9-1. Figure shows defects found in various types of COPD. Loss of alveolar structure in emphysema; mucus gland hyperplasia, hypersecretion, and inflammation in chronic bronchitis. Bronchial damage and mucus hypersecretion in bronchiectasis and bronchial spasm and inflammation in asthma.

struction that may have components of emphysema, chronic bronchitis, and bronchospasm.

Epidemiology and Pathogenesis

COPD is the most prevalent form of lung disease in the western world, the fifth leading cause of death in the United States, increasing in frequency, and almost totally preventable [6–8]. Cigarette smoking is clearly the most important cause of COPD, although many other factors have been implicated, including urban air pollution, heredity, socioeconomic status, airway hyperreactivity, and occupational exposure.

Clinically significant COPD is extremely rare in the nonsmoking population. Between 10% and 15% of those smoking more than 20 pack-years (packs per day × years smoking) develop airflow limitation. Cigarette smokers have a significantly greater incidence of emphysema, chronic bronchitis/chronic obstructive bronchitis, and respiratory symptomatology, including excessive mucus production, cough, and exertional or resting dyspnea. Pipe and cigar smokers who do not inhale tobacco smoke appear to have an intermediate risk for the development of COPD [8–10]. Recent evidence suggests that marijuana smoking produces similar changes, with a lower exposure threshold [11]. The use of low tar and nicotine cigarettes does not appear to slow the progression of established COPD, although the prevalence of cough and sputum production may be reduced [12–14]. Most smokers tend to compensate for the reduction in nicotine by taking larger puffs from low nicotine cigarettes. Whether the incidence of COPD will be reduced in smokers of low tar and nicotine cigarettes remains to be seen. A single, cross-sectional study, however, has found no differences in pulmonary function between smokers of filtered and unfiltered cigarettes [15].

The contribution of environmental irritants to the development of COPD remains controversial. Many studies have demonstrated an increased incidence of chronic cough and sputum production and minimally reduced pulmonary function in regions with higher levels of air pollution. There are, however, no longitudinal studies showing progressive deterioration in pulmonary function with continued exposure. In our highly mobile society, it is unlikely that one could be done. What is clear, however, is that respiratory morbidity and mortality increase in patients with preexisting lung disease during periods of increased air pollution.

Several studies have demonstrated greater annual declines in forced expiratory volume in 1 second (FEV_1) and other indices of pulmonary function with occupational exposure to various gases, fumes, and organic and inorganic dusts [16–20]. Exposure to dusts that cause pneumoconioses has been shown to cause airflow obstruction and an increased incidence of chronic cough and sputum production in addition to fibrosis [21–23]. Korn et al [24] have also shown an increase in respiratory symptoms and airflow obstruction associated with workplace exposure. What is not clear, however, is whether such exposure, in the absence of other risk factors such as cigarette smoking, leads to clinically significant COPD.

More recently, epidemiologic data have become available documenting the hazards of passive exposure to tobacco smoke [25]. In adults, a negative correlation between degree of environmental tobacco smoke exposure and maximal mid-expiratory flow rates has been described [26, 27]. Although statistically significant, the differences are small in absolute terms, have not been shown to predict similar decreases in FEV_1, and are of uncertain clinical significance. Other authors have failed to demonstrate an association between secondary smoke exposure and lung function [28]. Currently there is insufficient evidence to support a causative role for secondary smoke exposure in the pathogenesis of COPD in adults not otherwise predisposed. Further prospective longitudinal studies will be required to determine the contribution of passive smoke exposure to the development of clinical lung disease in ex-smokers without COPD and the rate of disease progression in those with COPD. In children the evidence is more compelling. Children exposed to sidestream smoke over a period of years suffer from an increased incidence of primary respiratory infections, chronic respiratory symptoms, and reduced pulmonary function. Several cross-sectional studies have demonstrated a greater frequency of respiratory infections and symptoms in children whose parents smoke [29, 30]. Children with a history of lower respiratory tract infection have been shown to have worse lung function during adult life than those without such a history [31]. Maternal smoking has been associated with reduced lung function in children, measured by serial FEV_1 and expiratory flow rates compared with children of nonsmoking parents [32]. Whether these children will develop clinically significant COPD in later life is yet to be determined. What is most clear, however, is that children whose parents smoke are more likely to smoke themselves, and this may be the most important risk factor of all.

Interest has also recently been focused on chronic bronchial irritation due to gastroesophageal reflux (GER) and recurrent microaspiration of gastric and oropharyngeal contents. It has long been established that GER can be an important trigger or exacerbating factor of asthma [14, 33]. Changes in airway tone can be mediated by GER in patients with chronic bronchitis [34, 35]. Installation of small quantities of 0.1 N HCl into the esophagus of known asthmatic patients has provoked both clinically significant bronchospasm and increased airway reactivity to nonspecific bronchoprovocation testing [34, 36]. In animals a similar response is noted and can be ablated by the administration of atropine or pretreatment of the esophagus with topical anesthetics [37]. Recent studies using continuous esophageal pH monitoring, esophageal manometry, and ^{99m}Tc labeled meals have demonstrated both GER and microaspiration of gastric contents in asthma and chronic bronchitis [34, 38–40]. An incidence of GER has been reported as high as 40%–60% in these same patients [34, 41]. Theophylline in therapeutic serum concentrations and, to a lesser extent adrenergic agonists, given systemically, reduce lower esophageal sphincter tone and may predispose to additional reflux [42, 43]. Inhaled sympathomimetics appear to have no effect on lower esophageal sphincter tone [42]. Treatment of symptomatic GER by physical means, H_2-blockers, and antacids is effective in relieving pulmonary symptomatology in many cases. Addition of agents that promote gastric motility and decrease lower esophageal sphincter pressure (i.e., metoclopramide, Reglan) appears to improve the success rate [38]. Gastric reflux surgery may also be effective in selected cases that are refractory to medical management [44].

Other risk factors for the development of COPD have been defined but are far less important than cigarette smoking. There is an association between recurrent respiratory infections in childhood and chronic respiratory symptomatology with airflow obstruction in adult life. Infection with respiratory syncytial virus during infancy has been most clearly implicated [45, 46]. The magnitude of long-term disability and the implications of such infection during adult life have not been adequately studied. Socioeconomic class has been reported as an independent risk factor for the development of COPD. It would seem more likely that this effect can be better described by differences in living conditions, access to health care, and exposure to environmental and occupational irritants [47]. The frequency of cigarette smoking may also be higher in certain socioeconomic groups, further confounding the data. Age and sex do not appear to have an independent effect on the development of COPD except as they relate to duration of exposure to respiratory irritants. Certainly, the continuing increase in smoking among women is contributing to a greater incidence of COPD, as it has to lung cancer. Unfortunately, women indeed appear to have "come a long way" at least in terms of respiratory disease. Familial clustering of abnormal lung function, respiratory disease, and clinically evident COPD is well described, but the effects of environment and genetics are difficult to differentiate [48–50]. Although there appears to be some familial predisposition to the development of COPD, the tendency for children of smokers to smoke themselves is of prime importance [51].

Epidemiologic and experimental evidence has identified several risk factors for the development of COPD. Of these, cigarette smoking has been shown to be the most important by far. No one factor, or combination of risk factors, however, is conclusively predictive of the development of lung disease. Definitive answers await a better understanding of the pathophysiology and defense mechanisms at the organ and cellular levels.

Pathology of Chronic Obstructive Pulmonary Disease

The histopathologic changes associated with COPD involve the airways, lung parenchyma, and pulmonary vasculature. A mixed anatomic appearance is typical, with elements of airway inflammation, mucus plugging, and alveolar destruction. Pathologic studies are hampered by the lack of a good animal model for COPD and the difficulties inherent in postmortem studies.

Chronic irritation of the large airways is manifested by patchy squamous metaplasia of the normal ciliated respiratory epithelium [52] and hypertrophy and hyperplasia of the bronchial submucosal glands with dilation of the ducts and occasional mucus plugging [53, 54]. The Reid index, the ratio of bronchial gland height to the height of the total bronchial wall in cross section, is an insensitive indicator of chronic bronchitis due to the normal variability in the general population. Further, there is no correlation between mucus hypersecretion, bronchial gland enlargement, and airflow obstruction [55]. Reduction of bronchial cartilage, predominantly at the level of the segmental and subsegmental bronchi, has been reported and may also play a role in airflow obstruction [56, 57].

The small airways (< 2 mm internal diameter) have been shown to be the primary site of increased resistance to airflow in COPD [58]. Chronic inflammatory changes of the small airways are manifested by neutrophilic and lymphocytic infiltration of the bronchial wall with hyperplasia of the smooth muscle cells, varying degrees of fibrosis, and squamous metaplasia of the epithelial cells reducing and occasionally obliterating the lumen. Mucus plugging is common. In the terminal and respiratory bronchioles, excessive numbers of intraluminal macrophages may be seen. Destruction of surrounding alveolar walls with loss of radial traction also contributes to reduction of the intraluminal diameter and increases in airway resistance [59].

Emphysematous changes, abnormal dilation of the airspaces distal to the terminal bronchioles due to destruction of alveolar walls with the formation of large, saccular airspaces, are seen to some degree in all cases of COPD. Fibrosis at the alveolar level is essentially absent. In the advanced state it is usually not possible to define in what portion of the acinus the destruction began. In milder cases, several patterns of destruction have been described. These are summarized in Table 9-1, but have little clinical usefulness. Emphysema associated with COPD is seen predominantly in the upper lobes and superior segments of the lower lobes. Hereditary emphysema, due to alpha-1 protease inhibitor (α_1-PI) deficiency, is usually worse in the bases of the lung.

Adjacent emphysematous airspaces may coalesce to form bullae. The distribution of bullae is variable, but tends to follow the emphysematous changes. Bullae can enlarge to dramatic sizes, compressing adjacent lung tissue, or rupture, producing a pneumothorax. Differentiation of a giant bullae from a pneumothorax may be difficult; a paucity of vascular markings is common to both.

Protease-Antiprotease Theory of Emphysema

It is believed that the destruction of alveolar walls characteristic of emphysema is due to enzymatic degradation of the supportive tissue network. Normal cellular inhabitants of the alveolar space, including alveolar macrophages and polymorphonuclear leukocytes, contain proteolytic enzymes. Of these, human neutrophil elastase (HNE), a small glycoprotein, appears to be of primary importance [60]. HNE is released from the granules of the neutrophil during phagocytosis and following stimulation, chemotaxis, or cell death. Cigarette smoke stimulates the release of neutrophil chemotactic factor from alveolar macrophages and HNE from neutrophil granules. The implications are clear: cigarette smoke increases the amount of HNE presented to the lung parenchyma by stimulating both migration of neutrophils to the alveolar space and degranulation with release of HNE [61, 62].

The action of HNE is regulated by a 52-kd serum protein α1-antitrypsin (α_1-PI), which is synthesized in the liver, released into the circulation, and migrates freely into the alveolar spaces [63]. α_1-PI inhibits the action of many proteolytic enzymes, including trypsin, chymotrypsin, pepsin, collagenase, and HNE by the formation of an irreversible covalent bond [60]. The serum level of α_1-PI in smokers is approximately 20% greater than in nonsmokers [64]. Oxidation of a methionine

Table 9-1. Anatomic patterns of emphysema

Pattern	*Location of Injury*	*Clinical Correlation*
Centrilobular	Respiratory bronchioles	Cigarette smoking most common variant seen
Panacinar	Diffuse involvement of entire respiratory unit	α_1-Antiprotease deficiency
Paraseptal	Alveolar ducts and sacs	Linear, focal, may be initial lesion of bullae
Scar	Irregular acinar involvement	Always associated with fibrotic changes

residue at position 358 in the α_1-PI molecule results in inactivation of the enzyme and may be accelerated by oxidants in cigarette smoke or released by polymorphonuclear neutrophils [65].

At least 75 codominant alleles for the α_1-PI gene locus have been described. By far, the most common are those of the M class, which account for over 90% of the gene pool [63]. MM homozygotes produce normal levels of normally functioning α_1-PI, at least 130 mg/dL. S and Z class alleles are seen much less frequently and code for production of an abnormal protein. SS homozygotes, MS and MZ heterozygotes, have intermediate levels of α_1-PI, more than 50 mg/dL [66]. There does not appear to be an excessive incidence of lung disease in these populations [67, 68]. Other alleles are rarely encountered. Clinical α_1-PI deficiency is characterized by early onset of severe emphysema involving primarily the lower lobes and occasionally a cholestatic liver disease that may progress to cirrhosis. Levels of α_1-PI less than 15 mg/dL are typically found. The PIZZ phenotype is identified in the vast majority (>90%) of those cases having severe emphysema [63].

α_1-PI deficiency was first described by Lowell and Erickson in 1963 [69]. The disorder is seen almost exclusively in the Caucasian population, most frequently in persons of Northern European descent [70]. A 2.0 to 2.5:1 male to female ratio is described, but may only reflect smoking patterns [63, 71, 72]. Clinically, α_1-PI deficiency may come to medical attention during infancy or early childhood for evaluation of cholestasis or hepatomegaly. Liver disease in the adult is uncommon, although cirrhosis and hepatic failure have been described [71]. The mechanism of hepatic disease is unclear. Incomplete glycosylation of the protein with intracellular accumulation, interfering with release from the hepatocyte and hepatocellular function, has been demonstrated. The majority of patients are first evaluated for respiratory symptoms, which occasionally present in the teenage years. Onset of symptomatology is typically between 25 and 40 years of age [63, 72]. Dyspnea is by far the most frequent complaint. Bronchospasm is encountered in less than one quarter of the patients. A productive cough is distinctly uncommon [63, 71, 72]. Clinically significant emphysema does not invariably occur in all patients with profoundly low serum levels of α_1-PI. In most studies, clinical lung disease is still associated with a history of cigarette smoking or exposure to other respiratory irritants.

α_1-PI deficiency should be suspected when there is a family history of emphysema occurring at a young age, severe otherwise unexplained pulmonary function abnormalities are found in a young patient, especially a nonsmoker, or there is roentgenographic evidence of bullous emphysema predominating in the bases. α_1-PI accounts for approximately 30% of the proteins that migrate in the α_1-macroglobulin band on serum protein electrophoresis. Although flattening and widening of the band may be seen [70], the diagnosis of α_1-PI deficiency should be made by demonstrating serum levels of α_1-PI less than 50 mg/dL [73]. Pulmonary function studies are consistent with emphysema. Some response to bronchodilators may be seen.

Treatment of patients with symptomatic α_1-PI deficiency should follow the same general guidelines for any patient with emphysema, as detailed below. Discontinuation of cigarette smoking is of even greater importance and must be emphasized.

Replacement therapy with α_1-PI (Prolastin, Miles, Inc., West Haven, CT) has recently become available and holds great promise for reducing the rate of decline in pulmonary function and future morbidity and mortality. Recommendations for use of exogenous α_1-PI are based on demonstration of the safety of the product and improvement in serum α_1-PI levels in affected patients. Studies of clinical efficacy have not been performed. The long-term effect of augmentation therapy will not be known for years. In the absence of exogenous α_1-PI supplementation, however, it is clear that the prognosis for patients with symptomatic α_1-PI deficiency is poor: The FEV_1 decreases more rapidly than in the general population [9, 63, 74] as does the diffusing capacity of the lungs for carbon monoxide [63]. Actuarial survival curves predict a much earlier mortality. In one study the cumulative probability of survival to age 50 was approximately 30% and to age 60 was 10% [74]. Recommendations for augmentation therapy were published by the American Thoracic Society in 1989 and include all patients 18 years and older with abnormal pulmonary function tests and α_1-PI levels less than 11 mg/dL [75]. Augmentation therapy is not indicated in patients with heterozygous α_1-PI phenotypes or emphysema not associated with α_1-PI deficiency. To evaluate the efficacy of treatment with exogenous α_1-PI, a national registry of patients with severe α_1-PI deficiency has been established by the National Heart, Lung and Blood Institute. Enrollment of all eligible patients is strongly suggested whether or not replacement therapy is instituted. The American Thoracic Society position paper contains eligibility criteria and a list of participating centers [75]. Further information on replacement therapy may also be obtained from the manufacturer, Miles, Inc., Biological Products, 400 Morgan Lane, West Haven, CT, 06516, 1-800-288-8378.

Clinical Presentation of Chronic Obstructive Pulmonary Disease

Patients with COPD may come to medical attention for evaluation of nonrelated medical problems. A carefully obtained history and detailed physical examination reveal findings typical of COPD. The majority of patients, however, seek evaluation for chronic symptoms of dyspnea, cough, sputum production, or wheezing [76].

Cough, frequently productive of mucoid nonpurulent sputum, is the most common symptom of COPD. Sputum production usually begins subtly, initially present only on arising due to pooling of secretions in the airways during sleep. With progression of disease, cough and sputum production become more prominent, but are rarely disabling in the absence of a superimposed bacterial infection. The sputum of patients with COPD is typically mucoid and off-white or brownish, nonpurulent, and relatively easy to expectorate. The duration and degree of tobacco exposure does not correlate well with the severity of cough and sputum production, but cessation of smoking is usually associated with a reduction in the volume produced. Yellow, green, or grossly purulent sputum is indicative of a bacterial superinfection. Hemoptysis is distinctly uncommon in uncomplicated COPD, but may be seen with superimposed bacterial infection. Hemoptysis in patients with COPD, however, must prompt a complete evaluation to exclude an underlying carcinoma. Hemoptysis due to acute or chronic bronchitis must be considered a diagnosis of exclusion.

Dyspnea may be a prominent feature. In patients with relatively mild disease, exertional dyspnea may be the initial symptom. As pulmonary function continues to worsen, progressively lesser degrees of exertion are required to produce dyspnea, which in some patients with advanced, severe disease may become disabling and is evoked with minimal activity, or in the most severe cases, is present at rest. Although the severity of dyspnea in a given patient appears to parallel the decline in pulmonary function, variation in individual response precludes prediction of functional limitation based on the FEV_1 or other indicators of airflow obstruction, except in the most severe cases. Similarly, arterial blood gases do not accurately predict severity of dyspnea.

The natural history of COPD is a progressive decline in respiratory status, more rapid than that seen in normal individuals and punctuated by episodes of acute decompensation. These are characterized by worsened dyspnea, increased production of often purulent sputum, and wheezing. Initially exacerbations occur infrequently, once or twice a year, but as the disease progresses, become more common. The period between exacerbations shortens, and baseline symptomatology becomes more apparent. Many patients relate an exacerbation after which they never noted complete recovery and often incorrectly date the onset of their disease from this episode. A careful history, however, reveals multiple similar illnesses over several years. The intermittent nature of exacerbations, and a history of audible wheezing may suggest an erroneous diagnosis of asthma. A history of progressive disease and recurrent similar episodes without complete intercurrent resolution of symptoms, suggests the correct diagnosis. Audible wheezing or rapid decompensation with exposure to cold air or deterioration during times of high pollen counts also suggests asthma or a significant asthmatic component to COPD.

Physical Examination

In most patients with mild COPD, physical examination during relaxed tidal breathing is essentially normal. Rapid, forced expiration or maximal ventilatory trials may evoke wheezing (forced expiratory wheezing) [77]. With more severe disease and increased airway resistance, spontaneous wheezing at rest may be noted. Reduction in distal airspace emptying occurs and pulmonary hyperinflation results, which is manifested in the pulmonary function laboratory as an increase in the closing capacity and functional residual capacity. Clinically, this overinflation presents as a reduction in intensity of breath and heart sounds. The percussion note is hyperresonant. Progressive lung overdistention and incomplete emptying leads to fixation of the rib cage in an inspiratory position. There is an increase in the anteroposterior diameter of the thorax, and the thoracic kyphosis is accentuated, producing the characteristic barrel-shaped chest. The diaphragm is depressed, and contraction is limited. Use of the accessory muscles of respiration is common. The liver border is depressed below the right costal margin without hepatomegaly. Reduction in airflow velocity can be demonstrated at the bedside by prolongation of the forced expiratory time beyond 4 seconds, best measured by auscultating over the larynx while the patient forcibly exhales from total lung capacity to residual volume [78]. Clubbing of the fingers does not occur as a result of COPD and if seen should prompt an evaluation for an undiagnosed pulmonary malignancy, bronchiectasis, or interstitial fibrosis.

The physical findings of pulmonary hypertension and cor pulmonale, which may complicate COPD with chronic hypoxemia, are subtle and usually obscured by the severe lung disease. Occasionally, however, a narrowly split second heart sound with a prominent pulmonic (P2) component, and a right ventricular heave may be found. A right ventricular S_3 may be heard in patients with frank right ventricular failure. Emaciation is not uncommon in the later stages of disease [79].

Laboratory Diagnosis

Laboratory evaluation of patients with COPD serves two important functions. First, quantification of the degree of airflow obstruction and gas-exchange abnormalities and their progression over time may help in prognostication and guide therapy. Of greater importance is the ability to identify airflow obstruction before the development of clinical disease. Diagnosis and intervention at an early stage is the best hope for preventing disability and progressive lung disease. Cessation of smoking does not lead to recovery of lost function, but does reduce the rate of decline compared with continuing smoking. As the incidence of postoperative complications is higher in patients with COPD, appropriate risk assessment and counseling can be offered to these patients.

Pulmonary Function Testing

Pulmonary function tests measure intrathoracic gas volume and expiratory airflow. The increased resistance to airflow characteristic of COPD is manifested primarily at the level of the small airways, bronchioles 2 to 3 mm in internal diameter, which lack direct cartilaginous support [58]. Patency of these airways is maintained by the elastic properties of the surrounding lung tissue. Emphysematous destruction of alveolar septa and the resulting loss of elastic recoil leads to progressive reduction in luminal diameter. Luminal patency is also compromised by the smooth muscle hypertrophy, bronchial mucosal gland hyperplasia, and mucus hypersecretion characteristic of chronic bronchitis [80]. The net effect is collapse or obstruction of the distal airways at higher than normal lung volumes and increased resistance to airflow at all lung volumes, resulting in an increased work of breathing.

Spirometry

Abnormal reductions in expiratory flow may not be apparent during quiet tidal breathing, but can be unmasked by forced expiration. Spirometry assesses airflow and airway dynamics during a forced exhalation from full inspiration (total lung capacity) to full expiration (residual volume). The FEV_1 is the most reproducible and predictable value obtained from spirometry. Normal values are based on the patient's age, sex, height, and race. The FEV_1 is often expressed as the ratio of FEV_1 to forced vital capacity to normalize for variations in measured lung volumes. The peak expiratory flow rate, maximal and average mid and terminal flow rates parallel the FEV_1, but are more variable in a given individual [81]. In patients with COPD progressive airflow obstruction is manifested by progressive declines in FEV_1 and the FEV_1/forced vital capacity ratio. Flow rates are reduced throughout exhalation and the flow/volume loop becomes progressively more convex toward the volume axis. Several sets of regression equations for predicting normal spirometric values have been published. However, all are based on populations of healthy, nonsmoking, Caucasians and ethnocentrically referred to as normal. Lung volumes of almost every other ethnic group average 10% to 15% less than Caucasians [82]. Many, but by no means all, pulmonary function laboratories reduce the normal values by 15% when evaluating non-Caucasians.

Although reversibility of airflow obstruction is considered to be the hallmark of asthma, up to 30% of patients with COPD manifest significant improvement in FEV_1 immediately after administration of an inhaled adrenergic bronchodilator [83]. Even in the absence of an immediate response, some patients improve with extended therapy and/or corticosteroids. An empiric therapeutic trial with serial spirometric evaluation while on therapy is warranted to identify these patients.

Lung Volumes

In patients with COPD, obstruction and early collapse of the distal small airways prevents complete emptying of the alveoli, which is manifested as an increase in the residual volume [84]. Increases in residual volume may be seen before measurable reductions in FEV_1 and be the first indicator of airways disease. In patients with more severe disease, increases in total lung capacity and functional residual capacity may also be seen.

Performance and interpretation of pulmonary function tests is considered in greater detail in Chapter 2.

Roentgenographic Findings

The radiographic changes of COPD are nonspecific, can be extremely variable, and are dependent on the severity of disease, pathophysiologic manifestations, and sequelae. In mild cases, especially those with a predominantly bronchitic presentation, the chest radiograph may be entirely normal [85]. In other cases, and with more severe disease, several roentgenographic changes may be identified.

Pulmonary hyperinflation is most commonly associated with emphysema. Radiographic findings that suggest hyperinflation include the following:

1. Flattening of the diaphragm, which is the most reliable indicator, manifested by an overall height of less than 2.6 cm in the lateral projection [86, 87] or concavity of the diaphragm superiorly [85].
2. An increase in the retrosternal airspace between the posterior aspect of the sternum and the ascending aorta, defined by Nicklaus and coworkers [86] as more than 4.5 cm.
3. An increased angle, usually more than 90 degrees, between the sternum and the

anterior portion of the diaphragmatic leaflets.
4. In the absence of cardiac disease, a long and narrow cardiac silhouette.
5. Rapid proximal tapering of the vascular markings (vascular deficiency pattern) [88], which, if present, may also help to differentiate emphysema from other diseases that also cause hyperinflation, especially asthma, and are not associated with changes in the pulmonary vasculature [85].

Other typical radiologic findings, including widely spaced ribs, accentuation of the thoracic kyphosis, and an increase in the relative anteroposterior thoracic diameter, are less useful.

The increased markings pattern of COPD is characterized by increased prominence of bronchial and vascular markings throughout the lung fields. This produces a "dirty" appearance of the chest radiograph and is associated with varying degrees of emphysema and bronchial gland hypertrophy. Pulmonary hyperinflation and findings associated with pulmonary hypertension may occasionally be seen; bullae are encountered infrequently [88].

Bullae represent locally severe emphysematous changes and may be single or multiple. In the usual case several bullae are represented by areas of increased radiolucency that measure more than 1.0 cm in diameter and are surrounded by a thin hairline shadow or adjacent compressed lung tissue. The number and distribution of bullae throughout the lung fields are variable. The presence of predominantly lower lobe disease should suggest the possibility of α_1-PI deficiency, especially in younger patients. Bullae can enlarge massively and mimic a pneumothorax or rupture, producing a pneumothorax. The presence of bullous changes is pathognomonic of at least localized emphysema. Although often visualized on conventional roentgenograms, bullae are best demonstrated on computed tomographic scans.

Pulmonary hypertension is manifested radiologically by enlargement of the hilar pulmonary arteries. The right ventricular hypertrophy and dilation associated with sustained pulmonary hypertension and ventricular failure, however, may produce either minimal enlargement of the cardiac silhouette on the posteroanterior chest film or a nonspecific cardiomegaly. Frequently the cardiac shadow appears normal on a given chest radiograph and only when compared with previous films can the progressive cardiac enlargement be identified.

Computed tomographic scans of the chest often demonstrate changes of COPD more clearly than the routine chest roentgenogram. Regions of relative oligemia are better defined, bullae are more easily seen, especially in the apices, and adjacent compressed lung tissue is easily demonstrated. With the increased markings pattern of COPD, prominent and frequently tortuous pulmonary vessels and bronchi may be identified [89, 90]. Despite the relative ease with which pulmonary parenchymal lesions can be visualized with computed tomography, the potential risk from additional radiation exposure, intravenous contrast administration, and high cost outweigh the minimal additional diagnostic information that may be obtained. The role of magnetic resonance imaging in the diagnosis of chest disease has yet to be determined.

Therapeutics

There is no specific treatment for COPD. Once established, lung damage is essentially permanent and irreversible. The goal of therapy is to maximize the quality and duration of life by reducing or eliminating further injury, reducing the incidence, length, and severity of intermittent exacerbations, and relief of symptoms, particularly dyspnea. In general, treatment plans should be individualized, interdisciplinary, and structured to meet the particular needs of the patient. An outline of a basic treatment plan is presented in Table 9-2.

Of primary importance is the avoidance of additional injury. Proper use of masks, filters, and respirators in the workplace should

Table 9-2. Components of a treatment plan

Smoking cessation
Pulmonary rehabilitation
Pneumococcal vaccine (one time only)
Annual influenza vaccine
Pharmacotherapy as required. See text
Bronchodilators
Mucolytic agents
Corticosteroids
Oxygen
Treatment of esophageal reflux
Physical means
Medical: antacids, H_2-blockers, metoclopramide, etc.
Surgical

be emphasized, and patients should be instructed to avoid contact with irritating fumes and dusts. Cessation of smoking, however, is the key to treatment. Continued exposure to primary or secondary (side-stream) cigarette smoke leads to progression of COPD. To minimize relapses and maximize the distribution of the considerable health benefits of smoking cessation family members should be encouraged to quit with the index patient [91]. The role of the primary physician cannot be overemphasized. Less than 25% of smokers are advised by their doctor to quit [92], yet in two separate studies significant numbers of patients stopped smoking in response to less than 5 minutes of specific counseling from their primary care physician [93, 94]. Along with advice to quit, referral to smoking cessation programs is often beneficial. The local branches of the American Heart Association, American Lung Association, and American Cancer Society, among others, often have smoking cessation groups or classes, usually free or at a minimal charge. The American Lung Association also publishes self-help books on achieving and maintaining a smoke-free lifestyle. Nicotine replacement therapy with nicotine-polystyrex (Nicorette) gum or slow-release nicotine patches can be an effective adjunct therapy when nicotine dependence is prominent. Close monitoring and frequent support are required. It is important to ensure that the patient does not continue to smoke while receiving nicotine replacement. Once the cigarette habit is broken gradual tapering of the nicotine replacement therapy is required and may also prove difficult, especially gum use, which is regulated by the patient. Other pharmacologic interventions, including the use of benzodiazepines and clonidine patches, have been useful in some patients and hypnosis may be helpful in others. Despite all efforts many ex-smokers relapse. Nonjudgmental support and continued encouragement to quit by physician, friends, and family are required. Most ultimately successful quitters have relapsed at least once on the way to sustained abstinence [95].

In conjunction with attempts at smoking cessation many patients benefit from the mutual support, education, and exercise training of a pulmonary rehabilitation program (see Chap. 15). Although pulmonary rehabilitation has not been shown to prolong life, improvements in patient self-image, quality of life, and reductions in hospital admission rate and length of stay have been demonstrated.

Extremes of temperature and humidity are often associated with increased respiratory discomfort. During winter the provision of adequate humidity through room or furnace humidifiers helps to maintain the normal viscosity of nasal and lower respiratory tract secretions, reducing mucus plugging, inspissation, and resultant airway inflammation and edema. Patients with asthmatic components of their COPD may experience dyspnea when suddenly exposed to cold air. For these patients, protection of the respiratory tract with two or three layers of scarves or a mask covering the mouth and nose is frequently of benefit. Prophylactic use of inhaled cromolyn sodium may also be helpful in a few cases. During hot and humid periods maintenance of indoor temperature between 72°F and 78°F and humidity between 50% and 70% may reduce the sensation of dyspnea and respiratory fatigue. The use of electrostatic or activated charcoal air cleaners is unlikely to be helpful unless they are of a size capable of rapidly exchanging large volumes of air.

Infections are the most frequent cause of

exacerbation of COPD. Ciliary dysfunction and abnormalities in alveolar macrophage phagocytosis due to cigarette smoke predispose to bacterial colonization of the tracheobronchial tree. Clinical decompensation of the previously stable patient may result from simple viral upper respiratory tract infections, viral or bacterial tracheobronchitis, pneumonia, or remote infections. Polyvalent influenza vaccine decreases the incidence of clinical influenza in vaccinated persons. The current recommendations for annual administration include all patients with respiratory disease, including COPD. Although the evidence supporting the use of polyvalent pneumococcal vaccine is less convincing, most pulmonary physicians suggest one-time vaccination of all patients with COPD. Vaccination against *Hemophilus influenzae* serotype b is unlikely to be of benefit in this population. Although *H. influenzae* is a frequent colonizing organism, the majority of isolates are either untypeable or of a different serotype. In patients with a clinical exacerbation suggestive of bacterial infection, low-grade fever, increased dyspnea, and cough productive of purulent sputum, a 10-day course of empiric antibiotics has been shown to be effective in shortening the duration and severity of the exacerbation [96]. The choice of antibiotic was not shown to affect the outcome, but it would seem prudent to cover *Streptococcus pneumoniae* and *H. influenzae*, which are frequently encountered in this patient population, as well as organisms with which the patient is known to be colonized. Indiscriminate use of very broad-spectrum oral antibiotics is discouraged.

Symptomatic therapy is directed at improving airflow throughout the respiratory tract and reducing dyspnea. Three classes of agents are used in the treatment of COPD. These are summarized in Table 9-3. The pharmacology and clinical use of these medications are considered elsewhere in this text. The use of these agents in the treatment of COPD varies from that in asthma. While airway obstruction and symptomatology are, by definition, intermittent in asthma they are essentially continuous in COPD. Airway obstruction in COPD is multifactorial, encompassing chronic mucosal inflammation, excessive bronchial secretions with mucus plugging, bronchial smooth muscle contraction, and loss of elastic recoil. Reduction in bronchial inflammation and secretions is accomplished through removal of irritating factors, especially cigarette smoke. The loss of elastic recoil is due to emphysematous changes and is irreversible. Pharmacologic treatment is directed at reducing bronchomotor tone and lessening the viscosity of bronchial secretions.

Resting bronchomotor tone is maintained, at least in part, by parasympathetic fibers, branches of the vagus nerve. The degree of basal cholinergic stimulation does not appear to be increased in either COPD or asthma. Bronchodilation produced by anticholingeric agents is effected by elimination of this basal tone [97]. In asthmatic individuals, bronchial inflammation appears to be related to excessive stimulation and production of locally acting mediators. The resulting bronchospasm is highly responsive to adrenergic stimulation. In contrast, the airway inflammation of COPD is due to continued mucosal irritation by foreign material, without the formation of inflammatory mediators. The response of patients with COPD to adrenergic bronchodila-

Table 9-3. Classes of pharmacotherapeutic agents

Bronchodilators	
Adrenergic	Albuterol Isoetharine Isoproterenol Metaproterenol
Anticholingeric	Atropine Ipratropium
Methylxanthine derivatives	Aminophylline Theophylline Oxtriphylline
Corticosteroids	
Mucolytic	Acetylcysteine Guaifenesin Iodinated glycerol

tors is less dramatic and similar in magnitude to anticholinergic agents [97]. Either an anticholingeric or adrenergic agent may be chosen as the initial bronchodilator, the other being added if insufficient clinical response is achieved. Theophylline and derivatives are also effective despite the low therapeutic ratio and should be used as a second-line agent when maximal doses of inhaled bronchodilators fail to produce the desired improvement.

The use of corticosteroids in the treatment of COPD is controversial. Despite widespread clinical use there is, at best, scanty evidence supporting this practice. A recent meta-analysis demonstrated significant improvement in FEV_1 in only 10% of cases of stable COPD without an asthmatic component [98]. In view of the significant complications of corticosteroid therapy, indiscriminate use in the COPD population cannot be justified. Following baseline spirometry a 2- to 4-week trial of prednisone, 0.5 mg/kg daily, or the equivalent, may be given to patients with severe COPD who fail to respond to maximal bronchodilator therapy. Spirometry should then be repeated. If no objective improvement can be documented, steroids should be tapered and discontinued. When significant improvement is seen, corticosteroids should be tapered to the minimal effective dosage, given every other day, if possible.

The use of mucolytic agents as adjunctive therapy to enhance clearance of bronchial secretions is gaining greater acceptance in the United States. Iodide, in the form of iodinated glycerol, has recently been shown to enhance mucus clearance in patients with COPD [3]. Use of a saturated solution of potassium iodide has been advocated in the past, but is associated with significant side effects. A therapeutic trial of iodinated glycerol (Organidin), 60 to 120 mg four times daily, is warranted in patients with prominent symptoms related to tenacious bronchopulmonary secretions. The use of inhaled acetylcysteine is associated with significant bronchospasm and has not been shown to be efficacious in the treatment of COPD. Oral forms are currently marketed outside the United States and have been clinically useful [99]. These agents, and derivatives, may soon be marketed within the United States. Adequate hydration is necessary to maintain normal sputum characteristics. No benefit has been shown from additional water intake [100]. Guaifenesin has not been shown to be efficacious in the adjunctive treatment of COPD.

The use of cyclosporin A in advanced immunosuppressive regimens has led to the consideration of lung transplantation in the treatment of patients with end-stage lung disease. Over the last 3 to 4 years patients with severe COPD have undergone single-lung, double-lung, and heart–lung transplantation with gratifying results. Overall 1-year survival exceeds 60% at experienced centers. Acceptance criteria differ between programs, but commonly include prolonged abstinence from tobacco use, oxygen dependency, life expectancy of less than 18 months, and an absence of systemic or other end-organ disease. Patients considered for transplantation are usually required to have been weaned from corticosteroids for at least 1 month. Transplantation candidates are evaluated for psychosocial stability in addition to medical criteria. The choice of operative procedure is dependent on the experience of the transplant surgeon. In most centers single-lung transplantation appears to be the technique of choice. This procedure can often be performed without cardiopulmonary bypass, with lower perioperative morbidity and mortality, and allows a single donor to provide lungs to two recipients. Postoperative exercise performance is identical in groups of single- and double-lung transplant recipients. Lifelong immunosuppressive therapy is required and transplant rejection remains a significant problem [101].

Patients with COPD are best managed by close, frequent contact with their primary care physician. Subspecialty consultation is indicated for very severe disease—an FEV_1 of less than 1.0 L on maximal therapy—refractory symptoms, corticosteroid dependency, frequent hospital admissions for exacerbation, the development of acute or chronic ventilatory failure, or when a review of therapy is desired. Younger patients whose severity of disease appears out of proportion to their age may also benefit from subspecialty evaluation. Patients who have undergone lung transplantation for COPD require close follow-up with the transplant facility and pulmonary physicians familiar with the transplant procedure and immunosuppressive therapy.

References

1. Fletcher CM, Pride NB: Definitions of emphysema, chronic bronchitis and airflow obstruction: 25 years on from the Ciba Symposium. *Thorax* 39:81, 1984
2. Burrows B: Airways obstructive diseases: Pathogenetic mechanisms and natural histories of the disorders. *Med Clin North Am* 74:547–559, 1990
3. Petty TL: The national mucolytic study: Results of a randomized double-blind placebo controlled study of iodinated glycerol in chronic obstructive bronchitis. *Chest* 97:75, 1990
4. Harris HW, Mcneely GR, Renzetti A, et al: Chronic bronchitis, asthma and pulmonary emphysema. *Am Rev Repir Dis* 85:762, 1962
5. Barker AF, Burdana EJ: Bronchiectasis: Update of an orphan disease. *Am Rev Respir Dis* 137:969, 1988
6. Friedman D, Dales LG, Ury HK, et al: Mortality in middle aged smokers and nonsmokers. *N Engl J Med* 300:2134, 1979
7. Ferris B Jr: Chronic bronchitis and emphysema: Classification and epidemiology. *Med Clin North Am* 57:637, 1973
8. Higgins M: Epidemiology of COPD: State of the art. *Chest* 85(suppl):35, 1986
9. Burrows B, Kanelson RJ, Cline MG, et al: Quantitative relationships between cigarette smoking and ventilatory function. *Am Rev Respir Dis* 115:195–205, 1977
10. Higgins MW, Keller JB, Becker M, et al: An index of risk for chronic obstructive pulmonary disease. *Am Rev Respir Dis* 116:195, 1977
11. Tashkin DP, Coulson AH, Clark VA, et al: Respiratory symptoms and lung function in habitual heavy smokers of marijuana alone, smokers of marijuana and tobacco, smokers of tobacco alone and nonsmokers. *Am Rev Respir Dis* 135:209, 1987
12. Freidman S, Fletcher CM: Changes in smoking habits and cough in men smoking cigarettes with 30% NSM tobacco substitute. *Br Med J* 1:1427, 1976
13. Scheaker MB, Samet JM, Speizer FE: Effect of cigarette tar content and smoking habits on respiratory symptoms in women. *Am Rev Respir Dis* 125:684, 1982
14. Sontag S, O'Connell S, Grunlee H, et al: Is gastroesophageal reflux a factor in some asthmatics? *Am J Gastroenterol* 102:119, 1987
15. Higgenbottam T, Shipley MJ, Clark TJH, et al: Lung function and symptoms of cigarette smokers related to the yield and number of cigarettes smoked. *Lancet* 1:409, 1980
16. Attfield MD: Longitudinal decline in FEV, in United States coal-miners. *Thorax* 40:132, 1985
17. Kauffmann F, Drovet D, Lelorich J, et al: Occupational exposure and 12-year spirometric changes among Paris area workers. *Br J Ind Med* 39:221, 1982
18. Medical Research Council (MRC): Chronic bronchitis and occupation. M.R.C. report. *Br Med J* 1:101, 1966
19. Ruckley VA, Gould SJ, Chapman JS, et al: Emphysema and dust exposure in a group of coal workers. *Am Rev Respir Dis* 129:528, 1984
20. Tobona M, Chan-Yeung M, Enarson D, et al: Host factor affecting decline in lung spirometry among grain elevator workers. *Chest* 85:782, 1984
21. Enterline PE, Lainhart WS: The relationship between coal-mining and chronic nonspecific respiratory disease. *Am J Public Health* 57: 484, 1967
22. Morgan WKC: Industrial bronchitis. *Br J Ind Med* 35:285, 1978
23. Stein-Cremer GR, Walters LG, Sichel HS: Chronic bronchitis in miners and nonminers: An epidemiological survey of a community on the gold mining area in the Transvaal. *Br J Ind Med* 24:1, 1967
24. Korn RJ, Dockery DW, Speizer FE, et al: Occupational exposures and chronic respiratory symptoms. A population based study. *Am Rev Respir Dis* 136:298, 1987
25. Jarvis MJ, Russell MAH, Feyeraband C, et al: Absorption of nicotine and carbon monoxide from passive smoking under natural conditions of exposure. *Thorax* 31:829, 1983
26. Kauffman F, Tessier JF, Oriol P: Adult passive smoking in the home environment: A risk factor for chronic airflow limitation. *Am J Epidemiol* 117:269, 1983
27. White JR, Froeb MF: Small airways dysfunction in nonsmokers chronically exposed to tobacco smoke. *N Engl J Med* 302:720, 1980
28. Weiss ST, Tager IB, Schenker M, et al: The health effects of involuntary smoking. *Am Rev Respir Dis* 128:933, 1983

29. Burchfeil CM, Higgins MN, Keller JB, et al: Passive smoking in childhood. Respiratory conditions and pulmonary function in Tecumseh, Michigan. *Am Rev Respir Dis* 133:966, 1986
30. Schilling RSF, Letai AD, Hui SL, et al: Lung function, respiratory disease and smoking in families. *Am J Epidemiol* 106:274, 1977
31. Martinez FD, Morgan WJ, Wright AL, et al: Diminished lung function as a predisposing factor for wheezing respiratory illness in infants. *N Engl J Med* 318:1112, 1988
32. Hankins D, Drage C, Zemel N, et al: Pulmonary function in identical twins raised apart. *Am Rev Respir Dis* 125:119, 1982
33. Deschner WK, Benjamin SB: Extraesophageal manifestations of gastroesophageal reflux disease. *Am J Gastroenterol* 84:1, 1989
34. Ducolone A, VanDevenne A, Jovin H, et al: Gastroesophageal reflux in patients with asthma and chronic bronchitis. *Am Rev Respir Dis* 135:327, 1987
35. Kennedy JH: "Silent" gastro-esophageal reflux: An important but little known cause of pulmonary complications. *Dis Chest* 42:42, 1962
36. Goldman J, Bennett JR: Gastro-oesophageal reflux and respiratory disorders in adults. *Lancet* 2:493, 1988
37. Mansfield LE: Gastroesophageal reflux and respiratory disorders: A review. *Ann Allergy* 62:158, 1983
38. Barish CF, Wu WC, Castell DO: Respiratory complications of gastroesophageal reflux. *Arch Intern Med* 145:1882, 1985
39. Chernow B, Johason LF, Janowitz WR, et al: Pulmonary aspiration as a consequence of gastroesophageal reflux: A diagnostic approach. *Dig Dis Sci* 24:839, 1979
40. Crausaz FM, Favez G: Aspiration of solid food particles into lungs of patients with gastroesophageal reflux and chronic bronchial disease. *Chest* 93:376, 1988
41. May EE: Intrinsic asthma in adults. *JAMA* 236:2626, 1976
42. Schindlbeck NE, Heinrich C, Huber RM, et al: Effects of albuterol (Salbutamol) on esophageal motility and gastroesophageal reflux in healthy volunteers. *JAMA* 260:3156, 1988
43. Stein MR, Towner TG, Weber R, et al: The effect of theophylline on the lower esophageal sphincter pressure. *Ann Allergy* 45:238, 19xx
44. Pevin-Fayolle M, Gormand F, Braillon G, et al: Long-term results of surgical treatment for gastroesophageal reflux in asthmatic patients. *Chest* 96:40, 1989
45. Colley JRT, Douglas JWB, Reid DD: Respiratory disease in young adults: Influence of early childhood lower respiratory tract illness, social class, air pollution and smoking. *Br Med J* 3:195, 1973
46. Pullan CR, Hey EN: Wheezing, asthma, and pulmonary dysfunction 10 years after infection with respiratory syncytial virus in infancy. *Br Med J* 284:1665, 1982
47. Burr ML, Holliday RM: Why is chest disease so common in South Wales? Smoking, social class and lung function: A survey of elderly men in the area. *J Epidemiol Community Health* 41:140, 1987
48. Kauffmann F, Kleishbauer JP, Cambon-de-Mouzon A, et al: Genetic markers in chronic air flow limitation. A genetic epidemiologic study. *Am Rev Respir Dis* 127:263, 1983
49. Lebowitz MD, Knudson RJ, Burrows B: Family aggregation of pulmonary function measurements. *Am Rev Respir Dis* 129:8, 1984
50. Redline S, Tishler PV, Leoritter FI, et al: Genetic and nongenetic influences on pulmonary function. *Am Rev Respir Dis* 135:217, 1987
51. Hubert HB, Fabsitz RR, Feinleib M, et al: Genetic and environmental influences in pulmonary function in adult twins. *Am Rev Respir Dis* 125:409, 1982
52. Auerback O, Stout AP, Hammond EC, et al: Changes in bronchial epithelium in relation to cigarette smoking and in relation to lung cancer. *N Engl J Med* 261:253, 1961
53. Mitchell RS, Silvers GW, Dart GA, et al: Morphologic correlations in chronic airway obstruction. *Am Rev Respir Dis* 97:54, 1968
54. Reid L: Measurement of the bronchial mucous gland layer: A diagnostic yardstick in chronic bronchitis. *Thorax* 15:132, 1960.
55. Peto R, Speizer FE, Cochran AL, et al: The relevance in adults of airflow obstruction, but not of mucus hypersecretion to mortality from chronic lung disease. *Am Rev Respir Dis* 128:491, 1983
56. Nagai A, West W, Paul J, et al: The National Institutes of Health intermittent positive pressure breathing Thai-pathology studies. 1. Interrelationship between morphologic lesions. *Am Rev Respir Dis* 132:937, 1985
57. Thurlbeck WM, Pun R, Toth J, et al: Bronchial cartilage in chronic obstructive lung disease. *Am Rev Respir Dis* 109:73, 1974
58. Hogg JC, Macklem PT, Thurlbeck WM: Site and nature of airway obstruction in chronic obstructive lung disease. *N Engl J Med* 278: 1355, 1968
59. Petty TL, Silvers GW, Stanford RE, et al: Radial fraction and small airway disease in excised human lungs. *Am Rev Respir Dis* 133:132, 1986
60. Janoff A: Elastases and emphysema—cur-

rent assessment of the protease-antiprotease hypothesis. *Am Rev Respir Dis* 132:417, 1985
61. Hunninghake GW, Crystal RG: Cigarette smoking and lung destruction: Accumulation of neutrophils in the lungs of cigarette smokers. *Am Rev Respir Dis* 127:540, 1983
62. Weitz JI, Crowley KA, Landman SL, et al: Increased neutrophil elastase activity in cigarette smokers. *Ann Intern Med* 107:680, 1987
63. Brantly ML, Paul LD, Miller BH, et al: Clinical features and history of the destructive lung disease associated with alpha-1-antitrypsin deficiency of adults with pulmonary symptoms. *Am Rev Respir Dis* 138:324, 1988
64. Idell S, Cohen HB: Alpha-1-antitrypsin deficiency. *Clin Chest Med* 4:359, 1983
65. Hubbard RC, Ogushi F, Fells GA, et al: Oxidants spontaneously released by alveolar mucrophages of cigarette smokers can inactivate the active site of alpha-1-antitrypsin, rendering it ineffective as an inhibitor of neutrophil elastase. *J Clin Invest* 80:1289, 1987
66. Carrell RW, Owen MC: Alpha-1-antitrypsin structure, variation and disease. *Essays Med Biochem* 4:83, 1979
67. Bruce RM, Cohen BH, Diamond EL, et al: Collaborative study to assess risk of lung disease in PIMZ phenotype studies. *Am Rev Respir Dis* 130:386, 1984
68. Morse LO, Lebowitz MD, Knudson RJ, et al: Relations of protease inhibitor phenotypes to obstructive lung disease in a community. *N Engl J Med* 296:190, 1977
69. Lowell CB, Erickson S: The electrophoretic α-globulin pattern of serum in antitrypsin deficiency. *Scand J Clin Lab Invest* 15:132, 1963
70. Erickson S: Alpha-1-antitrypsin deficiency: Lessons learned from the bedside to the gene and back again. *Chest* 95:181, 1989
71. Black LF, Kueppers F: Alpha-1-antitrypsin deficiency in nonsmokers. *Am Rev Respir Dis* 117:421, 1978
72. Tobin MJ, Cook PJL, Hutchinson DCS: Alpha-1-antitrypsin deficiency: The clinical and physiological features of pulmonary emphysema in subjects homozygous for Pi type Z. *Br J Dis Chest* 77:14, 1983
73. Wewers H: Pathogenesis of emphysema: Assessment of basic science concepts through clinical investigation. *Chest* 95:190, 1989
74. Larsson C: Natural history and life expectancy in severe alpha-1-antitrypsin deficiency, PiZ. *Acta Med Scand* 204:345, 1978
75. Buist AS, Burrows B, Cohen A, et al: Guidelines for the approach to the patient with severe hereditary alpha-1-antitrypsin deficiency. *Am Rev Respir Dis* 140:1494–1497, 1989
76. Burrows B, Niden AH, Barclay WR, et al: Chronic obstructive lung disease II. Relationship of clinical and physiologic findings to the severity of airway obstruction. *Am Rev Respir Dis* 92:665, 1965
77. Marks A: Chronic bronchitis and emphysema: Clinical diagnosis and evaluation. *Med Clin North Am* 57:707, 1973
78. Campbell EJM: Physical signs of diffuse airways obstruction and lung distention. *Thorax* 24:1, 1969
79. Boushy SF, Adhikary PK, Sakamoto A, et al: Factors affecting prognosis in emphysema. *Dis Chest* 45:402, 1964
80. Cosco MG, Ghezzo H, Hogg JC, et al: The relations between structural changes in small airways and pulmonary function tests. *N Engl J Med* 298:1277, 1977
81. Beck GJ, Doyle CA, Schacter EN, et al: Smoking and lung function. *Am Rev Respir Dis* 123:149, 1981
82. Rossiter CE, Weill H: Ethnic differences in lung function: Evidence for proportional differences. *Int J Epidemiol* 3:55–61, 1974
83. Anthonisen NR, Wright EC: Bronchodilator response in chronic obstructive pulmonary disease. *Am Rev Respir Dis* 133:814, 1986
84. Hogg JC, Wright JL, Pare PD, et al: Airway disease: Evolution, pathology and recognition. *Med J Aust* 142:605, 1984
85. Fraser RG, Pare JAP, Pare PD, et al: Diagnosis of Diseases of the Chest, ed 3. Philadelphia, W.B. Saunders, 1990
86. Nicklaus TM, Stirrell DW, Christiansen WR, et al: The accuracy of the roentgenologic diagnosis of chronic pulmonary emphysema. *Am Rev Respir Dis* 93:889, 1966
87. Reich SB, Weinshelbaum A, Yee J: Correlation of radiographic measurements and pulmonary function tests in chronic obstructive pulmonary disease. *Am J Radiol* 144:695, 1985
88. Thurlbeck WM, Henderson JA, Fraser RG, et al: Chronic obstructive lung disease: A comparison between clinical, roentgenologic, functional, and morphologic criteria in chronic bronchitis, emphysema, asthma, and bronchiectasis. *Medicine* 49:81, 1970
89. Goddard PR, Nicholson EM, Lazlo G, et al: Computed tomography in pulmonary emphysema. *Clin Radiol* 33:379, 1982
90. Meziane MA, Hruban RH, Zerhouni EA, et al: High resolution computed tomography of the lung parenchyma with pathologic correlation. *Radiographics* 8:27, 1988
91. Coppotelli HC, Orleans CT: Partner support and other determinants of smoking cessation maintenance among women. *J Consult Clin Psychol* 53:455, 1985

92. Bigelow GE, Haines CS, Stitzer ML: Tobacco use and dependence. *In* Barker LR, Burton JR, Zieve PD (eds): Principles of Ambulatory Medicine. Baltimore, Williams & Wilkins, 1986
93. Rose G, Hamilton PJS: A randomized controlled trial of the effect on middle aged men of advice to stop smoking. *J Epidemiol Community Health* 32:275, 1978
94. Russell MAH, Wilson C, Taylor C, et al: Effect of general practitioners' advice against smoking. *Br Med J* 28:231, 1979
95. Fischer EB, Rost K: Smoking cessation: A practical guide for the physician. *Clin Chest Med* 7:551, 1986
96. Anthonisen NR, Manfreda J, Warren CPW: Antibiotic therapy in exacerbations of chronic obstructive pulmonary disease. *Ann Intern Med* 106:196, 1987
97. Gross NJ: Ipratropium bromide. *N Engl J Med* 319:486, 1988
98. Callahan CM, Dittus RS, Katz BP: Oral corticosteroid therapy for patients with stable chronic obstructive pulmonary disease. A meta-analysis. *Ann Intern Med* 114:216, 1991
99. Ziment I: Pharmacologic therapy of obstructive airway disease. *Clin Chest Med* 11:461, 1990
100. Shim C, King M, Williams MH: Lack of effect of hydration on sputum production in chronic bronchitis. *Chest* 92:679, 1987
101. Patterson GA: Lung transplantation for chronic obstructive pulmonary disease. *Clin Chest Med* 11:547, 1990

Pulmonary Embolus and Deep Vein Thrombosis: Prevention, Diagnosis, and Treatment

Bradford K. Grassmick and Donald J. Conn

The "sudden breathless sleep," known today as pulmonary embolism, was described as long ago as the eleventh century when the discovery of thrombi in the lung was recognized to be the cause of symptoms and death in this disorder. The physiologic impact of thrombi in the pulmonary circulation was described by Virchow in the last century, but only in this century has therapy been available for this common and deadly event [1, 2]. It has been estimated that there are as many as 500,000 to 700,000 episodes of pulmonary embolism per year, resulting in approximately 200,000 deaths [1–5]. About one third of these deaths occur in the first hour. Postmortem studies have shown the presence of thrombi in the pulmonary vessels in as many as 64% of autopsies. It has been estimated that pulmonary embolism is the third most common cause of death [6] in the United States and yet is among the most underdiagnosed [7]. Approximately two thirds of the patients who survive their pulmonary embolism acutely, fail to have the diagnosis made, which suggests the difficulty that this entity presents to the clinician. The mortality, if the diagnosis is missed, is four times higher (32% versus 8%) than if therapy is instituted in a timely manner [2]. This chapter concentrates on the diagnosis, treatment, and prevention of this life-threatening, often fatal, yet treatable and preventable disease.

Pathogenesis of Deep Venous Thrombosis and Pulmonary Emboli

The majority of pulmonary emboli arise from thrombus in the deep veins of the lower extremity (deep venous thrombosis [DVT]). Other sites of origin include the pelvic and prostatic veins, the right atrium and ventricle, and the subclavian veins [2]. Although the majority of emboli are composed of platelets and fibrin from thrombus formation, pulmonary embolization may also occur from septic emboli arising from endocarditis involving the tricuspid valve, septic pelvic thrombophlebitis and suppurative phlebitis from intravenous catheters, or intravenous drug abuse [2]. Fat embolization can occur with long bone fractures [8]. Amniotic fluid embolization may occur with labor or delivery [9], and air embolization can occur with intravenous line insertions or during diving accidents [10, 11].

Pulmonary artery thrombosis occasionally may arise de novo as a result of trauma, pulmonary artery stenosis, or sickle cell anemia [10].

The usual scenario is the development of a thrombus in the veins of the lower extremity [12]. Three factors are involved in thrombus formation. Damage to the endothelial lining of the vein, stasis of blood flow, and alteration in the coagulation system comprise the triad described about 150 years ago by Virchow [1].

Damage to the endothelial lining exposes collagen to which platelets adhere via factor VIII and von Willebrand's factor complex. As a result of platelet adherence, adenosine diphosphate and thromboxane A_2 are released, which cause further platelet aggregation and activation of the extrinsic clotting system with the production and cross-linking of fibrin [13]. Continued coagulation is limited by fibrin degradation products such as plasmin, antithrombin III, and protein C, which prevents disseminated coagulation from occurring. Endothelial injury can occur at sites far removed from the initial area of thrombin formation [14]. Release of vasoactive mediators from traumatized tissue causes excessive vasodilation, which results in intimal lacerations and exposure of collagen, which initiates thrombus formation [15, 16]. Mediators may include histamine, serotonin, and bradykinin as well as anesthetic agents [17]. While vascular injury may play a role in some types of DVT (i.e., related to hip fracture or replacement) direct endothelial injury is not necessary in the presence of venostasis for thrombosis to develop. Thrombi usually develop in the deep venous system without preexisting endothelial injury [2].

Reduction in the velocity of blood flow has long been recognized to be a significant factor in venous thrombus formation. Normally small amounts of activated clotting factors are present in the blood, but are cleared by the liver. In areas of diminished blood flow the activated factors such as adenosine diphosphate, factor X, thrombin, and fibrin may remain in contact with the platelets for prolonged periods, causing platelet aggregation and initiating thrombus formation [18]. Bed rest as a predisposing factor for DVT has been well described [1, 4, 7, 19, 20]. Immobility in a supine position results in decreased drainage of the soleal sinuses of the calf and stasis of blood [21]. Clearance times of activated clotting factors from the blood increase from 1 minute in normal patients to over 9 minutes in patients at bed rest. As a result, studies indicate that thrombus formation probably begins in the soleal sinuses and within the valve cusps of the veins of the lower extremity [7, 17, 22]. Anesthesia results in venous smooth muscle dilation and contributes to the stasis of blood in the extremities [17]. The third part of Virchow's triad, hypercoagulability, may be mediated by the release of thromboplastin from injured tissues and activation of procoagulant factors in trauma, shock, childbirth, or surgery [2, 14]. Hypercoagulable states may also be the result of the liver's inability to clear activated clotting factors from the circulation in these states or as a result of decreased fibrinolytic activity [14]. Exogenous drugs such as estrogens and oral contraceptives have been found to be associated with an increased risk of DVT and pulmonary embolism [5]. Primary hypercoagulable states include patients with an antithrombin III deficiency, protein C deficiency, protein S deficiency, or impairment of the fibrolytic system such as hypoplasminogenemia [13, 23]. Deficiency of these naturally occurring anticoagulants and lytic agents results in unopposed thrombosis from the small amounts of activated clotting factors that are normally present in the circulation. Other hypercoagulable states include factor XII deficiency, patients with lupus anticoagulatent, and patients with dysfibrinogenemia, which produces a type of fibrin that resists lysis [13]. Primary hypercoagulable states are relatively rare, with the incidence of antithrombin III deficiency being about 1 in 2000 people. Other conditions known as the secondary hypercoagulable states include malignancy, pregnancy, and nephrotic syndrome, which alter coagulation and fibrinolysis. Abnormalities of platelets such as myeloproliferative disorders, diabetes, hyperlipidemia, as well as abnormalities of blood vessels and blood cells may contribute to a hypercoagulable state. These would include hyperviscosity syndromes such as polycythemia vera, sickle cell disease, multiple myeloma, thrombotic thrombocytopenia purpura, and diseases of the vessels, such as vasculitis or prosthetic vascular grafts [13].

Risk Factors in Medical Patients

Patients who appear to be particularly at risk can be divided into surgical and medical categories (Table 10-1). High-risk medical patients include those patients with prolonged immobility such as paraplegia, severe congestive heart failure, Guillain-Barré syndrome, and other debilitating diseases that limit mobility. Venous flow diminishes with increasing periods of bed rest, reaching a minimum after 7 days of immobility. Venous thrombo-

Table 10-1. Risk Factors for Deep Venous Thrombosis and Pulmonary Embolism

Medical patients
Prolonged immobility
Hip fractures
Paraplegia/paralysis
Stage IV congestive heart failure
Obesity
Advancing age
Malignancies
Breast, stomach, prostate
Colonic, lung, genitourinary
Pancreatic
Pregnancy
Critical illness
Shock
Cardiac failure
Respiratory failure
Surgical patients
Low risk
Age <40 with uncomplicated surgery
Age >40 with surgery <30 minutes
Moderate risk
Obesity
Large bowel surgery
Varicose veins
Extensive dissection
Advanced age
Malignancy
High risk
Patient >40 with history of DVT/pulmonary embolism
Extensive pelvic or abdominal surgery for malignancy
Lower extremity orthopedic procedures

embolism increases in frequency as the duration of bed rest increases [24]. As a result, patients with paralysis have been reported to have as high as a 30% incidence of pulmonary emboli [13, 25–27]. Obesity is a contributing factor as well. Patients who were more than 20% overweight had a 20% incidence of pulmonary emboli when examined at autopsy. Age and sex did not appear to alter the effect of obesity.

Heart failure is one of the major risk factors of the development of pulmonary emboli, particularly with increasing age. If patients with heart disease were less than 30 years old, there was approximately a 5% incidence of pulmonary embolism at autopsy, the same rate as patients under 30 without heart disease. For patients over 30 years of age with heart disease, the incidence of pulmonary embolism jumped to 18.6%, whereas those without heart disease had no change in incidence. Of particular note were older patients with congestive heart failure who had a 25.5% incidence of pulmonary emboli and those with atrial fibrillation of whom 35.9% had evidence of pulmonary emboli at autopsy [13].

Advancing age appears to be correlated with an increased incidence of pulmonary emboli. It is difficult to separate the effect of age from the effect of various disease processes. It does appear that fatal pulmonary emboli are more common in patients over the age of 50. There does not appear to be an effect of gender on pulmonary emboli except as mediated by pregnancy or estrogen use [2].

Malignancies have long been known to be associated with a hypercoagulable state and an increase in the incidence of pulmonary emboli. The magnitude of the risk depends on the type of malignancy. Patients with tumors of the head and neck were found to have pulmonary emboli in only 5.8% of the cases. Patients with breast, stomach, and prostate malignancies had about a 16% incidence of pulmonary embolism. Patients with lung and other genitourinary malignancies had greater than a 20% incidence of emboli. The highest association was in patients with pancreatic malignancies in whom 35% had evidence of pulmonary emboli at autopsy [13]. There was no additive effect of heart disease and malignancy.

Diabetes appears to be a risk factor for pulmonary embolism, although the exact risk is difficult to determine. Twenty percent of the patients with diabetes have evidence of pulmonary emboli at autopsy, but many of those patients also have other risk factors including heart disease, vascular disease, or malignancies.

Pregnancy appears to predispose patients to the development of thromboembolic disorders for a number of reasons. Levels of all coagulation factors except XI or XIII are increased during pregnancy, producing a hypercoagulable state possibly due to thrombin generation and fibrin formation in the placenta. Pregnancy itself may not result in blood vessel damage, but local damage to the pelvic veins may occur during delivery. Pregnancy reduces venous flow in the lower extremities by compression of the inferior vena cava by the gravid uterus. Elevated levels of estrogen during pregnancy also result in venous smooth muscle relaxation and dilatation, which results in further venous stasis. The result is an increase in DVT and pulmonary embolus during pregnancy. Pulmonary embolism was the second leading cause of death in pregnancy over a 27-year period in England ending in 1975 [28].

Critical illness is also a predisposing factor for the development of DVT. Without prophylaxis 29% of patients admitted to a general intensive care unit developed DVT compared with 10.5% of general medical patients [20]. Fifty percent of the intensive care unit patients had shock, cardiac failure, or had suffered a cardiac arrest. Another third of the patients had undergone recent major surgery and 25% had respiratory failure. DVT appeared to be both more common and more severe in the critically ill patients.

Risk Factors in Surgical Patients

Surgical patients can be separated into patients who undergo emergency surgery because of trauma and patients who undergo elective surgery. Patients who undergo elective surgery can be stratified according to their risk, depending on several variables including age, duration of the surgery, type of surgery, and underlying medical problems. Patients at low risk include those under 40 years of age with uncomplicated surgery or patients over 40 with surgery of less than 30 minutes and no identifiable risk factors. In those patients there is less than a 10% risk of calf vein thrombosis and less than a 1% incidence of proximal vein (iliofemoral) thrombosis in the absence of prophylaxis. Less than 1 patient in 10,000 (0.01%) in the low-risk group suffered a fatal pulmonary embolism. Patients over 40 years of age who had surgery that lasted for more than 30 minutes were thought to have a moderate risk of postoperative pulmonary embolism. Risk is further increased if there is obesity, large bowel surgery, varicose veins, extensive dissection, malignancy, advanced age, or prolonged bed rest. As a group those patients had a 10% to 40% incidence of calf vein thrombosis and a 2% to 10% incidence of proximal vein thrombosis. Less than 1% of these patients (0.1% to 0.7%) suffered fatal pulmonary emboli in the absence of prophylaxis. The high-risk group was composed of patients over 40 years of age who had a previous history of DVT or pulmonary embolism. Patients who underwent either extensive pelvic or abdominal surgery for malignancy or major lower extremity orthopedic procedures were also considered to be at high risk. In those patients in the absence of prophylaxis, 40% to 80% have thrombosis develop in the calf and 10% to 20% develop more proximal venous occlusion. Fatal pulmonary emboli occur in from 1% to 5% of those patients [17].

Evaluation of patients for the development of DVT revealed that in general surgical patients the incidence of DVT was between 16% to 42% in various trials and increased with age. Patients who were older than 60 years of age or who had a malignancy had a 40% to 60% incidence of DVT. The majority of thrombi were in the calf. Orthopedic surgery, particularly for hip fracture or total hip replacement, was associated with a 40% to 78% incidence of DVT, which were predominantly proximal as a result of vein injury. Knee operations had a 57% incidence and femur operations a 45% incidence of DVT formation. Gynecologic operations were associated with 6% to 15% incidence of DVT if unrelated to malignancy. If malignancies were involved, however, the incidence doubled to 12% to 35%. Urologic procedures such as transurethral resections of the prostate were associated with a 7% to 10% incidence of DVT while patients who underwent open prosthetectomies had a 21% to 51% incidence of DVT. The rate of DVT formation after craniotomies was between 18% to 40% while laminectomies had 4% to 25% incidence of DVT [5, 17, 29].

Determining the true incidence of pulmonary embolism is difficult, but it has been estimated that 50% or more patients with thrombi in the iliofemoral system will embolize [7]. In patients with documented DVT, but without clinical symptoms of pulmonary embolism, ventilation-perfusion scans revealed 51% of the patients had a high probability of having had a pulmonary embolism. Only 27% of the patients with proximal DVT had a normal lung scan [30].

Patients with accidental trauma appeared to have varying risks for pulmonary embolism depending on their injury, their age, and the duration of survival. Of trauma patients who died, 14% had evidence of emboli in the lungs except if the hip was involved and then the incidence was much higher [19].

Postmortem examinations revealed that patients who underwent emergency surgery of the back or lower extremities had a 40% incidence of pulmonary emboli. Of these the majority had either hip operations or amputations of the lower extremity. By comparison patients with operations of the head and neck had a 20% incidence, operations of the thorax a 9.4% incidence, and abdominal operations a 15.8% incidence [19]. The risk of embolism was increased with age.

In patients with fractures of the hip, 60% had evidence of pulmonary emboli and tended to be more elderly. Patients with burns had an 8% incidence of pulmonary emboli, which did not increase with age. Increasing duration of survival increased the incidence of emboli, however. Patients who died within 24 hours had only a 3% incidence while survival from 1 to 7 days increased the incidence of pulmonary emboli found at autopsy to 22.7% [19].

In view of the high incidence of asymptomatic pulmonary emboli, premorbid determination of pulmonary emboli incited by symptoms probably underestimates the true number of emboli, while postmortem examinations select a subgroup who were more critically ill than the survivors. In addition, thrombus formation is known to occur as a preterminal event. The true incidence of clinically significant pulmonary emboli lies between these two extremes.

The most common risk factors of patients who developed pulmonary embolism were the presence of DVT, prolonged immobilization, postoperative state, and obesity [4].

Sites of Venous Thrombosis

The relative risk related to the site of DVT has produced a great deal of controversy. The predominant opinion has been that proximal popliteal, ileal, or femoral vein thrombosis was associated with a much greater risk of fatal pulmonary emboli than calf vein thrombi [2, 7, 31].

It has been suggested that although many, if not most, thrombi develop in the veins of the calf, it is not until they propagate and enlarge into the more proximal veins of the thigh that they are large enough to become life threatening. Some studies have indicated that embolism occurs only when the clot extends into the popliteal and femoral veins and very rarely if the clot remains in the calf alone [32–34]. Other studies, however, have shown that a significant number of calf vein thromboses may embolize either silently, symptomatically, or fatally [30, 35]. The greater risk for calf vein thrombosis is the propagation of thrombus into the more proximal iliofemoral vessels. It is estimated that approximately 15% to 20% of calf vein thrombi progress and that as many as 50% of iliofemoral thrombi may embolize [7, 30].

Diagnosis of Deep Vein Thrombosis

Detection of the presence of DVT by clinical means is notoriously unreliable, but, when present, may alert the physician to underlying DVT especially when clinical findings develop acutely (Fig. 10-1). Various studies looking at the clinical findings of DVT (leg pain, edema, erythema, venous dilatation, and Homans' sign) reveal that the clinical examination is not terribly diagnostic, with specificities ranging between 36% and 76%

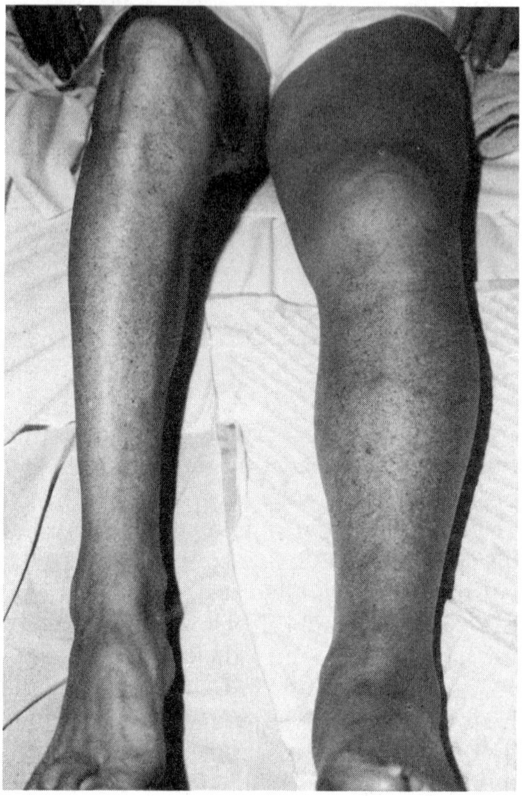

Fig. 10-1. Deep venous thrombosis. Patient had acute onset of left leg pain, erythema, and swelling, which alerted the physician to perform a Doppler flow study of the left leg, verifying clot and sluggish blood flow.

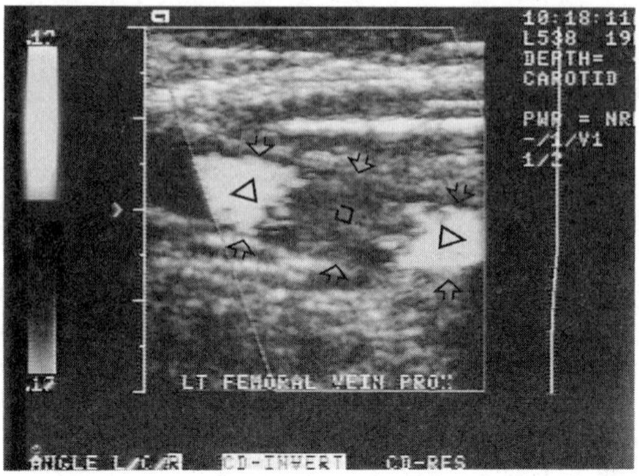
LT FEMORAL VEIN PROX
CAROTID
CD-INVERT
CD-RES

A

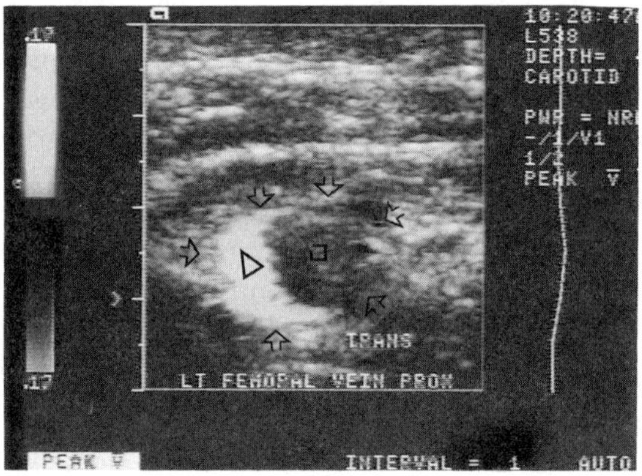
LT FEMORAL VEIN PROX
CAROTID
TRANS
PEAK
INTERVAL = 1
AUTO

B

Fig. 10-2. Doppler flow study of the left femoral vein. Open arrows point to the vessel wall, closed square is in center of blood clot, and open triangles delineate attenuated blood flow. (A) Longitudinal view and (B) transverse view. (Courtesy of Larry Campbell, MD, Denise Sawyer, and Mary Cooke, Oakwood Hospital, Dearborn, MI.)

[33]. Many of the signs of DVT (pain, swelling, etc.) may be present in conditions other than DVT, and many patients with DVT may not have either signs or symptoms [32, 33, 36]. Several imaging modalities have been developed to evaluate the presence of DVT. These include venography, impedance plethysmography, Doppler ultrasonography, I^{123} labeled fibrinogen uptake tests, and real-time B-mode ultrasound (duplex) studies.

Venography

The best diagnostic imaging tool for the diagnosis of a deep venous thrombosis is the contrast venogram (Fig. 10-2) against which all other modalities are compared. Venograms are reliable in that a negative finding has not been associated with any incidence of subsequent pulmonary embolism [33]. A contrast venogram is performed by first cannulating a small vein, usually on the dorsal aspect of the foot. This initial step can be challenging in that there is often a paucity of veins and/or the foot may be very edematous. Once venous access is obtained, tourniquets are placed at the ankle and above the knee to direct the contrast into the deep venous system. During injection and with the patient elevated approximately 30° to 45° when possible, radiographs are obtained of contrast-filled deep venous structures in the anterior-posterior and lateral projections.

The difficulty with venography is that it is invasive and has been associated with post-venographic leg pain and the subsequent development of thrombophlebitis [37]. Other problems include contrast-induced anaphylactic reactions as well as contrast-induced renal failure. While venography is the standard against which other diagnostic imaging techniques are compared, it is labor intensive and can have significant sequelae, which do not make it suitable as a screening technique. Technically, acceptable studies may be impossible to obtain in as many as 7% of attempted venograms [38].

By evaluating several factors, such as the presence of swelling above the knee, swelling below the knee, fever, recent immobility, and the presence of malignancy, the decision to proceed with diagnostic tests may be more productive. A recent study found the presence of one of the previously mentioned factors correlated with only a 5% incidence of DVT documented by venography while two or more factors were associated with a positive venogram in 42% of patients. By limiting venography to those patients with one or more of these factors, 77% of patients with DVT would have been diagnosed and 26% of patients who had normal results could have avoided venography [39].

I^{125} Fibrinogen Scans

I^{125} labeled fibrinogen uptake incorporates a labeled tracer into a developing thrombus. The labeled fibrinogen is injected intravenously and can be found in the major blood vessels of the pelvis and in the bladder as well as in the forming thrombus. This produces a high background activity, which makes evaluation of ileofemoral thrombosis difficult. The utility of the test appears to be in the diagnosis of calf thrombophlebitis, distal thigh, and popliteal vein thrombus where it is both highly sensitive (94%) and specific (90%). False-positive results have been reported with muscle injury, hematomas, arthritis, and infections in the lower extremity [40]. The advantages are that the test is relatively noninvasive, readily repeatable and can be done at bedside if necessary [33, 40]. A disadvantage, however, is the relative lack of availability at many institutions.

Impedance Plethysmography and Doppler Studies

Impedance plethysmography (IPG) uses the electrical impedance properties of the leg to measure the rate of venous drainage of the leg. Obstruction of the ileofemoral veins by thrombi causes a delay in the venous outflow, and many studies have shown high (>90%) sensitivity and specificity [41–43] in the diagnosis of proximal femoral vein thrombosis.

A negative IPG test has a good prognostic value. In a large study of over 300 patients there were no deaths from pulmonary embolism in patients with a negative IPG examination [41]. The test is easily repeated and noninvasive and has been used serially to detect DVTs [42]. The test is not especially sensitive to calf vein thrombosis, however [41].

An improvement in the sensitivity of the IPG is to combine the test with Doppler ultrasound evaluation of venous outflow. The frequency of sound wave directed at a flowing column of blood is altered with changes in blood flow. Venous flow changes with inspiration, leg compression, and Valsalva maneuvers. Characteristic changes in frequency are noted that do not occur when thrombosis is present. The test is noninvasive, but requires that a significant venous obstruction be present. The test cannot distinguish thrombus from extravascular obstruction, and if collateral circulation has developed around the thrombus there may be a false-negative result. The Doppler ultrasound examination is useful in proximal vein thrombosis where sensitivities of 40% to 100% have been found. The overall sensitivity is about 90%. When combined with IPG studies, as is currently the normal procedure in some institutions, the combined sensitivity rate increases to about 97% [33].

Duplex Ultrasound Examinations

A new development is the use of real-time B-mode ultrasound (duplex) to image the proximal femoral veins of the lower extremity. B-mode ultrasound provides two-dimensional images of the blood vessel, both longitudinal and cross sectional (Fig. 10-2). It can detect the presence of thrombosis in the femoral veins and distinguish between new and old (organized) thrombus as well as between sessile clot and those with free floating tails. Thrombi that have a free-floating tail may have a greater tendency to embolize. Using this technique the common femoral, superficial femoral, and greater saphenous veins as well as popliteal and ileal veins may be evaluated with a reliability equal to that of venography for proximal DVT [44, 45, 169, 170, 173].

The advantage of the ultrasound procedure is the repeatability and noninvasive nature of the examination. Four factors should be evaluated by the sonographer when scanning for a DVT. These include the presence of a visible thrombus, inability to compress the vein with the probe, absence of blood flow, and an alteration of the normal cyclic flow pattern with respirations. The combination of the above variables has demonstrated duplex scanning to give a sensitivity of 95% with a 95% confidence level in finding DVTs [187].

There are two disadvantages to duplex studies for DVT. First, isolated thrombi in the iliac vein are difficult to detect because the anatomic location prohibits compression of the vein with the probe. Second is the low sensitivity of the procedure in discovering calf vein thrombosis. However, improved scanners are allowing improved image quality and sensitivity in the calf.

Newer diagnostic modalities include thermography, pedal vein pressures, and radioisotope-labeled urokinase scans, but as of yet none have gained widespread acceptance [33].

Other Sources of Pulmonary Emboli

Although DVTs were the source of pulmonary emboli in 95% or more of reported cases, pulmonary emboli may also arise from thrombi developing in the subclavian veins, the right side of the heart, or from fat or amniotic fluid emboli.

Catheter-Related Emboli

Subclavian vein thrombosis is an uncommon source of emboli and is almost always related to central vein catheterization. Emboli have been reported after short periods of catheterization with pulmonary artery catheters (mean, 40 hours) as well as with chronic indwelling Hickman or Broviac catheters [171, 172]. An autopsy study of patients who had died with a pulmonary artery catheter in place revealed a high incidence of catheter-related thrombosis (53%) and 4 of 32 patients had thrombosis involving the pulmonary artery. The incidence of thrombosis increased significantly after 36 hours of catheterization [45]. Hickman or Broviac catheters have been reported to have a 3.7% incidence of thrombus formation, which may lead to pulmonary embolism [46, 47]. Patients with indwelling catheters for chemotherapy may be particularly at risk, especially if the malignancy is a solid tumor where thrombosis rates were as high as 45% [48].

Other complications of central venous catheters include air embolism and catheter tip embolism. Air embolism occurs most often in the spontaneously breathing patient either during insertion of the catheter or if the catheter becomes disconnected from the intravenous tubing. Air embolism may also occur during removal of a central vein catheter if it has been in place for 2 weeks or longer. During that time a fibrous tunnel may form that may remain patent temporarily after catheter removal. Generation of negative intrathoracic pressure during inspiration draws air into the tunnel and into the venous circulation. Bubbles may lodge in the pulmonary circulation, causing obstruction to blood flow, and death is a possible complication. Care during insertion to occlude the catheter lumen and the use of locking intravenous tubes and occlusive dressings at the time of removal reduce the risk of an embolism [49, 50]. Therapy includes hyperbaric oxygen, left lateral Trendelenburg's positioning, and hemodynamic support.

Catheter embolization can occur with the catheter through the needle technique. If the catheter is withdrawn against the sharp bevel of the needle, the catheter may be severed and lost into the central circulation. Catheter embolization requires immediate intervention under fluoroscopy to retrieve the catheter fragment [49, 50].

Amniotic Fluid Emboli

Pulmonary emboli can occur with the introduction of amniotic fluid into the venous circulation. Most commonly this occurs during labor, but has been reported from 20 weeks of gestation to 90 minutes postpartum [51]. Risk factors include increased age, parity, premature placental separation, intrauterine fetal death, meconium contamination, and hypertonic labor [52]. Uterine contractions may tear amniotic and placental membranes and force amniotic fluid into the venous passages [53]. The onset is noted by the rapid onset of hypotension, pulmonary edema, and coagulopathy due to disseminated intravascular coagulation. Mortality is about 85% and accounts for between 6% and 20% of all maternal deaths or 2.7 to 29.8 deaths per 100,000 live births [53]. Treatment is largely supportive, with particular attention to oxygenation, maintenance of blood pressure, and correcting pulmonary artery hypertension [52].

Fat Embolism

Fat emboli from single long bone fractures have a 9% mortality while emboli from combined tibial and femoral fractures are associated with a 20% mortality. Fat emboli reaching the lung cause platelet activation and release of vasoactive mediators that may cause shock, bronchial constriction, and a consumptive coagulopathy [8]. Symptoms of fat embolism usually develop within 48 hours after the injury. Signs and symptoms include tachypnea, dyspnea, tachycardia, and fever. Delirium is common and petechia may develop. Steroids are used, and patients show predictable improvement within 12 to 72 hours [54]. Heparin may actually be contraindicated since it activates lipoprotein lipase and may increase the level of free fatty acids in the lung.

Prophylaxis of Deep Venous Thrombosis

Prevention or prophylaxis of DVT begins with the recognition of the patient at risk, i.e., bed ridden, hip fracture, hypercoagulable, followed by consideration of relative risks and benefits of the prophylaxis. Studies indicate that prophylaxis for deep vein thrombosis is underused in patients who are at risk [186]. The means by which clot formation and subsequent DVT is prevented include anticoagulation and prevention of venous stasis. Anticoagulation usually involves heparin or warfarin administration, but drugs that inhibit platelet function such as aspirin, dipyridamole, low molecular weight dextran, and hydroxychloroquine sulfate may also be used. Methods to prevent venous stasis include patient positioning, external compression stockings of various lengths, bilateral intermittent pneumatic compression devices, and dihydroergotamine administration [55, 56]. The utility of each of these methods depends in part on patient selection and the relative risks and benefits for the individual patient.

Heparin

Heparin is a heterogeneous group of sulfated mucopolysaccharide molecules usually obtained from beef or pork lung or intestine, which inhibits the action of thrombin. Heparin binds to a plasma protein, antithrombin III, which in turn binds to and inhibits thrombin activity. Thrombin is prevented from catalyzing the conversion of fibrinogen to fibrin and thrombus formation is prevented [174].

Heparin also binds to and forms inactive complexes with factors IX, X, and plasmin. Various fractions of heparin vary in the relative activity binding to antithrombin III. Low molecular weight heparin (fragmin) has been shown to be particularly effective as an anticoagulant. Heparin inhibits phospholipid-mediated platelet activation and increases inactivation of thrombus by another plasma protein heparin cofactor II. Heparin cofactor II may also play a role in inhibiting coagulation factors within the vascular tissues. Other actions of heparin, particularly the low molecular weight variety, include direct binding to platelets and inhibition of aggregation when platelets are exposed to collagen. Heparin also increases fibrinolytic activity, and after transformation within the vascular endothelium, alters the endothelial surface to prevent platelet adherence [57]. Monitoring of therapy involves measuring an activated partial thromboplastin time (APTT), which measures the final activity of a cascade of coagulation proteins in vitro. The prolongation of APTT is proportional to the log of the heparin concentration, but heparin also exerts a number of anticoagulant effects that are not measured by the APTT [57].

In DVT prophylaxis in medical patients heparin is usually administered subcutaneously in a dose of 5000 units every 12 hours. The APTT is not usually altered by this dose of heparin. Increasing the frequency of administration to every 8 hours does not provide additional protection from fatal pulmonary emboli and may increase the risk of bleeding complications [5, 56]. Heparin therapy may be initiated 2 hours preoperatively in surgical patients, but does not provide adequate prophylaxis in patients undergoing major orthopedic procedures such as knee or pelvic operations [56, 57].

Intermittent low-dose subcutaneously administered heparin has been shown to reduce the risk of DVT in critically ill patients and general medical patients. This form of anticoagulation has been shown to decrease the development of DVT from 29% without treatment to 13% with heparin in critically ill medical patients. In less ill general medical patients heparin reduced the incidence of DVT from 10% without treatment to 2% with heparin [20]. Mortality is reduced as has been shown in studies of both medical and general surgery patients [57–59]. While heparin is effective prophylactic therapy in most patients, it does not appear to be adequate in patients undergoing hip replacement, knee surgery, or transurethral urologic procedures [17, 56, 60, 61]. Low-dose heparin may also be relatively contraindicated in patients undergoing procedures where any bleeding could be catastrophic as with patients with a neurosurgical, spinal cord, or ophthalmologic procedure or in patients with an active central nervous system or gastrointestinal bleed.

Recently, studies using adjusted dose heparin or larger fixed dose heparin have been shown to be more effective in reducing the incidence and severity of DVT after hip replacement [62, 63]. In adjusted dose heparin, heparin is given subcutaneously every 8 hours in a dose adequate to prolong the APTT to more than 30 seconds. The average dose was 6000 units every 8 hours (range, 4000 to 10,000 units) and bleeding did not appear to be increased. Using a larger fixed dose of heparin (7500 units twice a day) decreases the incidence and severity of DVT after major thoracic surgery, without an increase in bleeding. Low molecular weight heparin has been evaluated as a prophylactic therapy in patients undergoing elective hip surgery and appears to be promising. Low molecular weight heparin appears to have a greater potentiating effect on the activity of antithrombin III, a longer half-life, and fewer antiplatelet effects than standard heparin [64, 191].

Complications of Heparin

Intermittent low-dose heparin does not alter the APTT and is rarely associated with bleeding or other complications, including thrombocytopenia, osteoporosis and spinal fractures, and paradoxically, thrombotic complications.

Thrombocytopenia Thrombocytopenia is a relatively frequent occurrence in about 5% of patients receiving heparin and may result from several causes. The initial infusion of heparin may produce platelet aggregation and transient thrombocytopenia, but the usual problem is an immune-mediated platelet destruction that occurs after 6 to 12 days of heparin therapy [65, 66, 174]. The incidence of thrombocytopenia appears to range from between 5.8% to 15.6% and may occur earlier in patients with previous exposure to heparin. The immune reaction appears to be related to the binding of heparin to the platelets, which then acts as a hapten, inducing an immune response against the bound heparin and platelets. The diagnosis of heparin-induced thrombocytopenia is usually made by excluding other causes of thrombocytopenia such as disseminated intravascular coagulation. Some researchers have found a heparin-dependent platelet aggregation factor in the serum of patients, but this test is not widely used. Measurement of IgG may show elevation but is nonspecific [66, 67]. Normally the heparin-induced thrombocytopenia is mild, but it has been our policy to discontinue heparin prophylaxis when platelet counts fall below 100,000 per cubic millimeter. There is no evidence, however, that thrombocytopenia is in itself adequate protection against DVT. Platelet counts usually do not fall below 80,000 and usually recover over a few days to 1 to 2 weeks after withholding heparin [12]. Severe thrombocytopenia below 50,000 occurs less frequently, but if associated with bleeding may warrant intervention with intravenous immunoglobulin, which binds to antibody receptors, blocking the reticulothelial destruction of platelets [68]. The use of plasmapheresis to remove IgG has also been reported as treatment for severe heparin-induced thrombocytopenia [69]. Heparin must be discontinued from all sources, including arterial lines and pulmonary artery catheters, to prevent further immune-mediated platelet destruction.

Thrombotic Complications Other complications of subcutaneous heparin therapy include thrombotic injury at the site of injection of the skin as well as more rare systemic thrombotic events. The phenomenon occurs very infrequently, approximately 0.2%, and is usually associated with thrombocytopenia [70]. It appears likely that platelet aggregation is responsible for the thrombus formation and subsequent skin necrosis or systemic arterial or venous occlusion [71, 72]. Complications include stroke, myocardial infarction, extremity necrosis, and pulmonary embolism. Overall mortality of this rare complication appears to be as high as 40% [72]. The diagnosis is made by observing platelet aggregation in vitro with the addition of heparin. It is recommended that platelet counts be obtained regularly during heparin therapy and that if the count drops below 120,000/uL that the test be performed for heparin-induced platelet aggregation [72]. The test is usually done at a reference laboratory and requires both a sample of the patient's serum and a sample of the type of heparin the patient received. If the diagnosis is strongly suspected, then heparin should be discontinued and alternative therapy instituted.

Osteoporosis Heparin has also been associated with the development of osteoporosis and subsequent spinal fractures. The development of the problems appears to be related both to the daily dose of heparin as well as the duration of therapy has not been reported with daily doses of less than 10,000 units. Osteoporosis occurs with increasing frequency after 120 days of therapy. The pathogenesis appears not to be related to alterations in parathyroid hormone, but rather to an increase in collagenolytic activity in the bone. Rats exposed to heparin have lysosomal bodies that contain collagenase which are less stable and may contribute to increased bone reabsorption [69, 73, 74].

Bleeding Complications Bleeding complications are the greatest concern with intermittent low-dose subcutaneous heparin. While most studies indicate a low incidence of bleeding other than small hematomas at the injection site, at least one study found a significant incidence of bleeding with preoperative heparin administration [75, 76]. When the patients received 5000 units of heparin 2 hours preoperatively and every 12 hours postoperatively there was a 27% incidence of bleeding complications, particularly wound hematomas, compared with a 7.5% incidence if heparin was administered only postoperatively and 1.4% if no heparin was administered [76]. Concern with bleeding in the surgical population has prompted some surgeons to avoid heparin or use alternate methods of prophylaxis.

Other Complications Transient increases of hepatic transaminases have been reported in up to 95% of patients receiving heparin, but there is little evidence as to the etiology or clinical significance of this finding [77].

Warfarin

Another form of prophylactic anticoagulation is the use of low-dose warfarin, a vitamin K antagonist, to increase the prothrombin time (PT) to approximately 1.3 to 1.5 times the control value or about 16 to 18 seconds [5]. Warfarin is not a direct anticoagulant, but rather prevents carboxylation of glutamic acid residues of vitamin K dependent factors II, VII, IX, and X [175]. The altered proteins fail to bind calcium and prevent proper interaction of activated clotting factors, resulting in decreased activity of the coagulation system [78]. The vitamin K dependent factors vary in their half-life, with factor VII being the shortest at 4 to 6 hours and factor II the longest at 24 hours. The PT will show alteration 24 hours after a single large dose of warfarin because of inhibition of factor VII, but measured levels of other clotting factors will be maintained for several days until inhibition of synthesis occurs. Several studies have shown the efficacy of warfarin in preventing DVT and fatal pulmonary emboli in patients with hip fractures where heparin has been shown to be ineffective [2, 57, 78, 79]. Warfarin is given preoperatively for 3 to 5 days in doses of 2.5 or 5 mg/d in order to raise the PT by 1 to 2 seconds, but not more, to prevent intraoperative bleeding complications. After surgery the dose is increased to raise the PT to 16 to 18 seconds for 3 weeks or until discharge. An alternative is to begin warfarin as soon as possible after surgery with a dose of 10 mg and strive to obtain a PT of 16 to 18 seconds by the fifth postoperative day. Another variation is the use of fixed minidose warfarin at a dose of 1 mg/d started before major gynecologic surgery. The therapy has been shown to be as effective as full anticoagulation and significantly more effective than placebo in preventing DVT and had fewer bleeding complications than full anticoagulation [80].

Dextran

Low molecular weight dextran (40,000 MW average) has been used as an anticoagulant. Dextran is a branched chain starch polymer that has been shown to inhibit platelet aggregation. The use of low molecular weight dextran has also been shown to decrease levels of factor III [55]. Dextran may also alter the nature of the fibrin clot, making it more easily lysed. The usual regimen is to infuse 500 to 1000 mL of a 10% dextran solution intraoperatively and daily thereafter for 4 more days. The infusion is then repeated every third day until the patient is ambulatory. The incidence of DVT after hip fracture after prophylaxis with dextran was one third of the control group, as was the incidence of pulmonary embolism [55]. Dextran is a plasma volume expander and since about 20% of the molecules are above 50,000 daltons and may not be excreted renally, volume overload and pulmonary edema may occur in the susceptible individual. Anaphylactic reactions and allergic reactions are uncommon, but bleeding complications are not [55]. Dextran is best reserved for the high-risk individual in whom heparin is not effective.

Antiplatelet Agents

Antiplatelet agents such as aspirin, hydroxychloroquine sulfate (Plaquenil), and dipyridamole, which inhibit adenosine diphosphate induced platelet aggregation, have also been used for DVT prophylaxis [55, 78, 79, 81]. Various studies have produced conflicting results regarding the utility of aspirin and dipyridamole in preventing DVTs. While there appears to be some protective effect produced by these agents, the degree of protection provided is controversial, particularly with aspirin. Some studies have found an eightfold decrease in fatal pulmonary emboli, while others have shown no protective effects at all [55, 56, 74, 75, 81]. Dihydroxychloroquine sulfate has shown significant protective effects in postoperative prophylaxis in general, gynecologic, and urologic surgery patients in preventing both DVT and pulmonary emboli, but more studies are needed to confirm its efficacy [56]. Current recommendations for prophylaxis of DVT do not include the use of antiplatelet agents [60].

A number of studies have evaluated the efficacy of dihydroergotamine (DHEA) and heparin in combination [38, 82, 83]. DHEA increases venous smooth muscle tone and as a result the velocity of blood flow in the femoral vein is increased. It is postulated that by avoiding venodilation that endothelial injury is prevented. DHEA also decreases platelet aggregation. The usual dose is 0.5 mg injected subcutaneously every 8 to 12 hours in combination with heparin, 5000 units every 8 to 12 hours. Studies suggest that the combination of DHEA and heparin is more effective in preventing DVT than either agent alone [38, 83]. In particular DHEA and heparin appear to provide protection for patients undergoing hip replacement [82]. The major complication of DHEA is arterial vasospasm, which occurs in about 3 of every 100,000 patients and is reversible in about 50% of patients. The contraindications to DHEA include conditions such as trauma, hypotension, sepsis, or end-stage vascular ischemia where the incidence of side effects may be greater [82].

Mechanical Prophylaxis

Mechanical means of DVT prophylaxis include elastic compression stockings, pneumatic compression devices, and early ambulation. While elastic stockings were used for years to provide external compression of the femoral veins and decrease venous stasis, studies have shown no benefit to their use in a general surgical population [84].

Pneumatic compression devices have gained some acceptance for use intraoperatively and postoperatively in patients at high risk for bleeding with anticoagulation. By applying intermittent external compression approximately once per minute to the calf or calf and thigh, these devices prevent venostasis by providing essentially an external muscle pump. Pressures generated by the device are generally 35 to 55 mm Hg. Numerous studies have demonstrated the efficacy of pneumatic compression devices in preventing DVT and subsequent pulmonary emboli in high-risk patients [81, 82, 85, 86, 87]. The major drawback to this prophylaxis is the cumbersome equipment involved, but in high-risk patients or patients in whom other means of prophylaxis are contraindicated, pneumatic compression devices are both safe and effective.

Early ambulation is the most cost-effective means of preventing DVT and should be encouraged as soon as the patient is medically able to tolerate activity. Ambulation is not only effective in restoring normal venous flow, but also in preventing pulmonary atelectasis that is often a problem for the bedridden patient.

Recommendations for Deep Venous Thrombosis Prophylaxis

The current recommendation for prophylaxis of DVT in medical patients is subcutaneous heparin, 5000 units every 12 hours, unless the patient is actively bleeding or has an intracranial bleed or severe thrombocytopenia, in which case pneumatic compression devices may be used.

Heparin may also be used for prophylaxis in low-risk general surgical patients as long as there are no contraindications. High-risk patients such as those undergoing hip or knee surgery or extensive gynecologic or urologic surgery or patients with extensive risk factors may require more aggressive prophylactic treatment with adjusted dose heparin, full-dose heparin, warfarin, dextran, or pneumatic compression devices [27, 29, 55, 60]. Neurosurgical patients should receive pneumatic compression devices to prevent venous stasis and DVT [81].

Catheter Thrombosis

Venous thrombosis may develop as a result of central venous catheters. Prophylaxis to prevent the development of clot formation includes the use of heparin-bonded catheters, infusion of heparin through the catheter in low doses, and the use of very low-dose warfarin [88]. Patients with femoral intravenous catheters are at particular risk for the development of DVT, and catheters should be removed within 4 days of placement to avoid this development [89, 176]. Patients with permanent indwelling catheters and malignancies are at particular risk, especially if the malignancy is a solid tumor [48, 90]. Low-dose warfarin, 1 mg/d, may be very effective in preventing this complication [88].

Treatment of Established Deep Venous Thrombosis

Once the diagnosis of DVT has been established, therapy should be initiated with three goals in mind: (1) interruption of the hypercoagulable state to prevent further propagation of the thrombus, (2) initiation of clot lysis either by endogenous mediators or by exogenous lytic agents, and (3) prevention of the development of a pulmonary embolis.

Full Dose Heparin Therapy

Interruption of the hypercoagulable state is usually achieved with full anticoagulation with heparin. Heparin is usually given intravenously as a continuous infusion of 1000 units per hour after a 5000- to 10,000-unit bolus. Alternate methods of dosing heparin include an initial bolus of 50 to 100 (average 70) units/kg/h. The goal of heparinization is to maintain a partial thromboplastin time (PTT) 1.5 to 2.5 times the control level or if the patient's control is not available, a PTT of between 50 to 60 seconds. While heparin does not lyse the thrombus, it does prevent clot propagation, while endogenous mediators such as plasmin act on the thrombus and initiate lysis. Several studies indicate the necessity for maintaining the PTT at 1.5 times normal to provide adequate protection from recurrent thromboembolism [23, 91, 92]. The PTT should be measured initially no sooner than 6 to 8 hours after the heparin bolus to avoid the effect of the heparin bolus. If measured too soon after the bolus, the PTT will not reflect the steady state and may be significantly elevated, prompting the clinician to decrease the rate of the heparin infusion, resulting in subtherapeutic PTTs. If the PTT is excessively elevated, i.e., greater than 100 seconds, the infusion should be discontinued for 1 to 2 hours, then restarted at a lower rate. If the PTT is subtherapeutic, then the rate should be increased, and if severely subtherapeutic, the patient may need another intravenous bolus of 1000 to 5000 units of heparin. Usually changes in the heparin infusion rate are made in increments of 100 units/h. The heparin should be infused with a rate controlled pump to prevent inadvertent overadministration. The infusion may be mixed as 25,000 units in 250 mL of D_5W, producing a concentration of 100 units/mL. Initial infusion rates would be 10 mL/h for a total of 1000 units/h. More dilute infusions, i.e., 25,000 units in 500 or 1000 mL, allow for finer adjustments in infusion rates. There is significant interpatient variation in the half-life of heparin, and it appears that the patient with more extensive disease, i.e., pulmonary embolism versus DVT, has a shorter heparin half-life [90, 93, 116]. Because there is a narrow therapeutic range for heparin, PTT should be monitored at least twice a day until the patient is on a stable heparin dose. The duration of heparin therapy is usually 7 to 10 days during which endothelialization of the clot and more secure attachment to the blood vessel will occur [23].

The major complication of heparin therapy is bleeding, which is correlated with the prolongation of coagulation as measured by activated clotting time or PTT [91]. Other risk factors for bleeding include liver dysfunction, cardiac illness, renal insufficiency, malignancy, and advanced age [71, 177]. Bleeding occurs in about 10% of patients receiving heparin and has required either blood transfusions or discontinuing heparin in about half of those patients [94]. Bleeding related to heparin in the urokinase study was found in 27% of patients and occurred at sites of catheterization, the gastrointestinal tract, or the retroperitoneal space and was not necessarily clinically apparent [95]. Daily measurements of hemoglobin or hematocrit as well as platelet count are necessary while patients are receiving full-dose heparin. If significant bleeding occurs while receiving heparin, it may be necessary to reverse the anticoagulation with protamine sulfate, which binds heparin to form an inactive salt. The inactivation is rapid, occurring within 5 minutes after intravenous injection. Each milligram of protamine inactivates from 90 to 115 units of heparin. The dose of protamine depends on the amount of heparin administered, but if unknown, initial doses of 25 to 50 mg infused intravenously over 10 minutes may be used [96]. Care must be taken because the heparin-protamine complex may cause histamine release from the lungs, resulting in hypotension or an anaphylactic reaction in the sensitive or fish-allergic individual. This effect is particularly pronounced when given by a central venous catheter [97]. Coagulation studies should be repeated after administration to guide further doses. Protamine has a weak anticoagulant effect and doses of greater than 100 mg over a short period are not recommended unless clearly indicated by coagulation studies [96].

Other complications of heparin therapy include thrombocytopenia, vascular occlusion, osteoporosis, and liver function abnormalities, already mentioned under low-dose therapy.

Warfarin (Coumadin)

During the period of full-dose heparinization, warfarin is begun to provide long-term anticoagulation for when the patient leaves the hospital. Warfarin is usually started on the fourth or fifth days of heparinization, but may be started on the first day as well and may shorten hospital stays [23]. Initially, warfarin is given as 10 mg/d orally in the afternoon, with daily measurements of the PT the following morning. After 3 days, there is usually a change in the PT and the dose is decreased to 5 or 2.5 mg/d depending on the magnitude of the response. Warfarin inhibits all the vitamin K derived coagulation factors, including the endogenously occurring anticoagulants and protein C. Without heparin, warfarin may actually result in a mildly hypercoagulable state for the first few days of administration [23]. The usual goal for anticoagulation with warfarin is PT 1.5 to 2 times the control or between 18 and 24 seconds. Compared with prolonged therapy with standard low-dose subcutaneous heparin, oral anticoagulation results in a significantly lower recurrence rate of thromboembolic problems [57]. Adjusted dose subcutaneous heparin may be as effective as oral anticoagulation, however [98]. The standard duration of therapy currently is 3 months, but several studies have shown that anticoagulation for periods of 4 to 6 weeks provided the same protection as therapy for 6 months in terms of recurrences and was associated with significantly fewer bleeding complications [61, 99, 100]. The recurrence rate in these shorter studies was somewhat higher, however, than that found in the 3-month studies [98, 101].

Control of Warfarin

The incidence of bleeding while on oral anticoagulation is dependent on the duration of anticoagulation as well as the intensity of anticoagulation [61, 102, 103]. The incidence of major hemorrhage increases with the duration of therapy, with a 10% incidence at 3 months, 18% at 1 year, and 41% by 5 years [61]. Patients who are more aggressively anticoagulated with a PT of 41 seconds have nearly five times the risk of bleeding than patients with a PT of 27 seconds, without any significant difference in the rate of recurrence of thromboembolic problems [102]. The current recommendations are that anticoagulation be continued for 3 months at a dose adequate to raise the PT to 1.2 to 1.5 times the control [23, 104].

Drug Interactions

Warfarin interacts with many other medications as a result of changes in hepatic metabolism and protein binding (Tables 10-2 and 10-3) [175]. In particular drugs that may potentiate the effect of warfarin include salicylates, quinidine, clofibrate, anabolic steroids, thyroxine, acetaminophen overdose, allopurinal, diazoxide, and disulfiram. Drugs that may inhibit warfarin's activity include oral contraceptives, adrenocortical steroids, cholestyramine, and meprobamate. Warfarin

Table 10-2. Interactions with Warfarin: Drugs and Conditions That Increase the Effect of Warfarin

Cancer	Cefoperazone (Cefobid)	Metronidazole (Flagyl)
Collagen disease	Monolactam antibiotics	Miconazole (Monistat)
Congestive heart disease	Chloral hydrate	MAOIs
Diarrhea	Chlorpropamide (Diabinese)	Nalidixic acid
Fever	Cimetidine (Tagamet)	Pentoxifylline (Trental)
Hepatic dysfunction	Clofibrate	Phenytoin (Dilantin)
Hyperthyroidism	Dextran	Pyrazolines
Malnutrition	Thyroxine	Quinidine
Vitamin K deficiency	Diazoxide	Quinine
Alcohol	Diflunisal (Dolobid)	Ranitidine (Zantac)
Allopurinol	Diuretics	Sulfinpyrazone
ASA/nonsteroidal drugs	Disulfiram (Antabuse)	Sulfa drugs
Amiodarone	Glucagon	Sulindac (Clinoril)
Anabolic steroids	Mefenamic acid (Ponstel)	Thyroxine
Inhalation anesthetics	Methyldopa	Tamoxifen (Nolvadex)
Cefamandole (Mandol)	Methylphenidate (Ritalin)	

may also alter the metabolism of other drugs, in particular raising the half-life of drugs such as chlorpropamide, tolbutamide, diphenylhydantoin, and phenobarbital [105]. Outpatient monitoring of PT is mandatory and should be done weekly initially then every other week followed by monthly monitoring if the PT remains stable until the end of therapy.

Table 10-3. Interactions with Warfarin: Drugs and Conditions That Inhibit Warfarin

Edema	Cholestyramine Questran)
Hereditary resistance	Diuretics
Hyperlipidemia	Ethchorvynol
Hypothyroidism	Glutethimide (Doriden)
Adrenocortical steroids	Haloperidol (Haldol)
Aminoglutethimide (Cytadren)	Meprobamate
Antacids	Oral contraceptives
Antihistamines	Paraldehyde
Barbiturates	Primidone (Mysoline)
Carbamazepine (Tegretol)	Ranitidine
Alcohol	Rifampin
Chloral hydrate	Trazadone (Desyrel)
Chlordiazepoxide (Librium)	Vitamin C

Treatment of DVT in the pregnant patient presents a special problem. Warfarin will cross the placenta and can produce bleeding problems and malformation in the fetus [96]. Given the contraindication to warfarin with pregnancy, outpatient management of DVT consists of intermittent subcutaneous heparin, which does not cross the placenta. The usual dose is to inject 10,000 to 15,000 units every 12 hours and measure a PTT 6 hours after injection. The goal is to achieve a PTT that is between 1.5 and 2 times the patient's own control. Pregnancy results in elevated factor VIII levels and the baseline PTT is usually shortened. Failure to appreciate this physiologic change may lead the clinician to suspect resistance to heparin and increase the dose, leading to an increased risk of bleeding [106]. Heparin is usually administered in a concentration of 25,000 μ/mL to minimize the volume of the injection. The site of injection is rotated on the lower abdomen and inner and outer thighs and should be compressed for 5 minutes after injection to minimize bruising [106]. Therapy should be stopped at the time of delivery and a PTT checked and protamine administered if necessary.

Controversy continues whether intermittent adjusted subcutaneous heparin provides the same protection as continuous intravenous administration of heparin, but in the pregnant outpatient there is currently no alternative [28].

Lytic therapy using streptokinase, urokinase, or tissue plasminogen activator (TPA) may have some advantages in more prompt resolution of a DVT and in avoiding postphlebitic syndromes [106, 178, 184] (Table 10-4). The postphlebitic syndrome, venous incompetence, and/or recurrent DVT may affect 30% to 50% of patients with a DVT and be incapacitating in 10% [106]. Lytic agents act by increasing the conversion of plasminogen to plasmin that then actively lyses the fibrin in the clot. The effectiveness of lytic therapy has been well established for DVT [92, 107–109]. Compared with heparin therapy alone, thrombolysis is achieved about four times as often, with a decreased incidence of postphlebitic problems [91, 109]. Clot lysis with streptokinase occurs in 55% to 90% of the patients treated compared with 10% to 70% of patients treated with heparin. Complete clot lysis is far more frequent and valve function is more often preserved with lytic therapy [109]. Concern over bleeding problems is justifiable, but while some studies indicate a greater tendency for bleeding with lytic therapy, the difference between heparin and streptokinase is not statistically significant. The risk of lethal hemorrhage or intracranial bleeding with lytic therapy is under 1% [109, 110]. Bleeding more often occurs at operative sites, intravascular catheter sites, the gastrointestinal tract, the genitourinary tract, or in the retroperitoneal space and is usually minor. Identification of DVTs with free-floating tails may militate against the use of lytic therapy, which could cause release of an embolus as the base of the clot lyses. Clot greater than a week old may be sufficiently organized that lytic therapy may not be effective.

Table 10-4. Potential Advantages of Lytic Therapy

Prevent subsequent embolization by removing thrombus
Normalize hemodynamic disturbances
Prevent venous vascular damage and postphlebitic syndrome
Prevent pulmonary hypertension from recurrent embolization

From Thrombolytic therapy in thrombosis: A National Institute of Health Consensus Development Conference. *Ann Intern Med* 93:141–144, 1980; with permission.

A well-documented proximal femoral vein thrombosis of less than 7 to 10 days duration is the ideal setting for lytic therapy. While clot lysis can be demonstrated experimentally for up to 3 months, the sooner after thrombus formation lytic therapy can be initiated, the higher the success rate [110]. The patient should not have known sensitivity to the agent, or in the case of streptokinase, previous therapy or streptococcal infection in the previous 6 months. Most importantly, the patient should not have an absolute or major contraindication to the use of a lytic agent such as active bleeding, recent stroke, surgery, or hypertension (Table 10-5). Streptokinase has the greatest potential for allergic reactions, but given the potential for bleeding all lytic agents should be administered under close supervision, preferably in an intensive care unit. Streptokinase forms a complex with plasminogen, which then acts as an activator converting plasminogen to plasmin, the active lytic agent. If the initial dose of streptokinase is not adequate to produce a lytic state, the patient may have antistreptococcal antibodies and require an additional loading dose. However, if an excessively large dose of streptokinase is given, then all the plasminogen may be bound to streptokinase, not leaving any to be converted to plasmin to lyse thrombus [111]. Urokinase directly activates plasminogen to plasmin as does TPA, so lower doses are required (Table 10-6). Results of thrombolytic therapy are usually very good, with restriction of normal blood flow in 90% to 95% of cases if therapy is initiated within 5 to 7 days of clot formation [111]. Delay of therapy to more than 10 days after the onset of symptoms will result in only 10%

Table 10-5. Contraindications for Lytic Therapy

Absolute contraindications
Active internal bleeding
Cerebrovascular accident, disease, procedure or process (within 2 months)
Major relative contraindications
Recent (<10 days)
Major surgery
Obstetric delivery
Organ biopsy
Puncture of noncompressible vessels (i.e., subclavian vein)
Serious gastrointestinal bleeding
Serious trauma
Severe arterial hypertension (>220 mm Hg systolic or 110 mm Hg diastolic)
Minor relative contraindications
Recent minor trauma including cardiopulmonary resuscitation
High likelihood of a left heart thrombus (mitral disease with atrial fibrillation)
Bacterial endocarditis
Coagulopathy
Age >75 years
Diabetic hemorrhagic retinopathy

to 15% of patients having a good response [111].

Pulmonary Embolism: Clinical Diagnosis

The diagnosis of pulmonary embolism is difficult since many of the classic signs and symptoms do not occur in the majority of patients. The classic findings are the acute onset of pleuritic chest pain, hemoptysis, and shortness of breath. In a large series of patients with pulmonary emboli, chest pain was present in 88%, but was pleuritic in only 75%. Eighty-four percent of patients experienced dyspnea, but only 30% had hemoptysis. The specificity of these complaints, which often have multiple etiologies, was 76% or less [112]. Even combining 12 multiple clinical variables including risk factors still resulted in a 12% to 18% error rate [56, 112–114].

Table 10-6. Administration of Lytic Agents

All patients
Obtain secure intravenous access for administration and blood sampling
Draw coagulation studies: PT, PTT, TCT, platelets, fibrinogen for baseline
Avoid vascular puncture during infusions
Streptokinase
Infuse 250,000 units intravenously over 30 minutes as a loading dose
Infuse 100,000 units per hour for 24 to 72 hours unless bleeding occurs
Follow coagulation studies after 4 hours to confirm lytic state and hemoglobin to detect bleeding
If values have not changed after 4 hours, reload with 250,000 units and continue infusion
Urokinase
Infuse 2000 units per pound over 10 minutes as a loading dose
Infuse 2000 units per pound per hour for 12 to 24 hours
Follow coagulation studies after 4 hours and hemoglobin periodically to detect bleeding during therapy
Tissue plasminogen activator (not yet approved for DVT)
Infuse 100 mg or 1.25 mg/kg over 2 to 3 hours as a one-time infusion. The dose should not exceed 150 mg
Indication of subsequent anticoagulation
When coagulation studies return to approximately two times the control values, initiate heparin infusion without a loading dose
Repeat ventilation-perfusion scans after 24 hours

The most common symptoms in patients with a pulmonary embolism were, in order of decreasing frequency, chest pain, dyspnea, apprehension, and cough.

Physical examination is generally nonspecific. The patient may be tachypneic, tachycardiac, apprehensive, and either hypertensive or hypotensive. A pleural friction rub occurs in fewer than 20% of patients and wheezing occurs in only about 15%. Approximately 50% of patients have an increase in the intensity of the pulmonic component of the second heart sound, but this is a very subjective finding. A right ventricular S_3 gallop may be heard. Patients are often febrile, exceeding 38°C [2, 7]. Overall, the clinical examination in patients with pulmonary embolism is nonspecific. The most frequent physical findings are a respiratory rate greater than 16 breaths per minute, rales, an increased pulmonic component of the second heart sound, and a heart rate greater than 100 [114].

Laboratory Findings

Laboratory studies usually reveal an altered alveolar-arterial oxygen gradient in the majority of patients, but a normal gradient does not exclude the diagnosis of pulmonary embolism [115].

The chest radiograph may show pleural based wedge-shaped infiltrates, elevation of a hemidiaphragm, or paucity of vascular markings in a portion of the lung, but the most common finding is a normal or nondiagnostic chest radiograph [2, 5]. A normal chest radiograph in the face of severe arterial hypoxemia may be suggestive of pulmonary embolism, however. Pleural effusions may be seen roentgenographically in as many as 96% of pulmonary infarctions, but the most common positive finding was atelectasis [2, 113]. Overall, the sensitivity of chest radiography is about 20% [113].

Electrocardiography frequently is abnormal in both massive (94%) and submassive (77%) pulmonary embolism. The most frequent finding is tachycardia, and the most frequent electrical abnormality is T-wave inversion (42%), followed by ST-segment abnormalities [116]. The classic $S_1Q_3T_3$ pattern associated with pulmonary emboli was only seen in 18% of patients with massive embolus. Right axis deviation and left axis deviation occurs with equal frequency. Overall electrocardiographic changes are transient and tend to resolve within 2 weeks after the event [116].

Laboratory studies are generally nonspecific, but may show an increase in lactate dehydrogenase, and bilirubin with a normal serum glutamic-oxaloacetic transaminase. This pattern was only seen in 4% of patients. Thus, enzymes are of little diagnostic value [2]. Coagulation studies are frequently abnormal, but normal parameters do not exclude a pulmonary embolus. In some patients pulmonary embolism may present as a disseminated intravascular coagulation state, with thrombocytopenia, hypofibrinogenemia, altered coagulation studies, and the presence of fibrin degradation products [117, 118]. The presentation may range from a minor alteration of coagulation studies to a life-threatening bleeding disorder requiring large amounts of blood products.

Physiologic Changes

The acute consequences of pulmonary embolism range from minor asymptomatic alterations in oxygenation to profound cardiovascular collapse and death. The physiologic sequelae of a pulmonary embolus may be separated into the respiratory changes and the hemodynamic consequences.

The respiratory changes involve three important alterations within the lung: (1) alterations in perfusion, causing changes in ventilation-perfusion ratios, (2) release of mediators from the embolus, leading to altered vascular and bronchial reactivity, and (3) decreased surfactant production [31] from alveolar injury that may result in atelectasis.

The obstruction to pulmonary blood flow results in an area of alveolar dead space, a portion of lung that remains ventilated, but does not receive blood flow and so cannot contribute to gas exchange. In addition, the alterations in blood flow result in overperfusion of other areas of the lung, changing the ventilation-perfusion ratio in those areas. The resulting increase in dead space would be expected to cause hypercapnia, but this is an unusual finding even with massive pulmonary emboli [119]. Pneumoconstriction occurs in the affected areas of the lung, which may actually reduce the alveolar dead space [31]. While an increase in the ratio of physiologic dead space to tidal volume has been documented in patients with angiographically proven pulmonary embolism, increased minute ventilation usually results in a respiratory alkalosis and an increased alveolar-arterial oxygen ratio [120].

The most significant major abnormality in the lungs is an increase in intrapulmonary shunt. Intrapulmonary shunt has been demonstrated experimentally and clinically, but does not correlate with either the size of the embolus or the change in pulmonary artery pressure. Shunting may occur from the release of vasoactive mediators such as prostaglandins, serotonin, and histamine [121, 122]. Release of the vasoactive amines also produces bronchoconstriction and the clinical finding of diffuse wheezing on auscultation. In addition, the bronchoconstriction alters the distribution of ventilation and further alters ventilation-perfusion ratios within the lung. Other possibilities include the opening of preexisting pulmonary arteriovenous anastomosis or the development of pulmonary edema from lung injury and the loss of hypoxic vasoconstriction. Intracardiac shunts may develop in the 15% of patients with a patent foramen ovale when right pressure exceeds that of the left atrium [122].

Ventilation-perfusion abnormalities have been demonstrated with pulmonary emboli in experimental animals, but the role in humans is less clear. In several patients who underwent studies involving multiple inert gas washout techniques both large shunts and increased dead space were found, but no areas of diminished ventilation-perfusion ratios were found [123].

The loss of surfactant and subsequent atelectasis occurs after injury to the alveolar type II cells from the pulmonary artery occlusion. The deficit of surfactant results in atelectasis within 24 hours because of the low alveolar stability and subsequent collapse [31]. Atelectasis may produce increases in intrapulmonary shunt, further contributing to hypoxia in the patient as well as producing the elevated hemidiaphragms seen on chest radiography in some patients.

Hemodynamic Alterations

The acute hemodynamic consequences of a pulmonary embolism include acute increase in pulmonary artery pressure as a result of the increased pulmonary vascular resistance. There is extensive reserve capacity in the pulmonary vascular bed, however, and a pulmonary embolism must result in a 50% or greater reduction in the pulmonary vasculature before pulmonary artery pressure increases [31]. In patients without previous cardiac or pulmonary disease, mean pulmonary artery pressures are generally less than 40 mm Hg [124].

In a patient without preexisting cardiopulmonary disease, pulmonary artery pressures appear to be proportional to the magnitude of the obstruction [180]. In patients with preexisting cardiac or pulmonary disease, pulmonary hypertension may be of greater magnitude and occur with less severe occlusion than in a normal patient [124]. The more severe the obstruction, the more likely the development of acute right ventricular failure, which may occur with mean pulmonary artery pressures between 30 and 40 mm Hg. As pulmonary artery pressure increases, the velocity of blood flow from the ventricle decreases. With increasing right ventricular failure, the magnitude of the pulmonary artery hypertension decreases as the ventricle is less able to generate high pressures. Right atrial and ventricular pressures increase with a massive (>40% occlusion) pulmonary embolus, and the right ventricle dilates in response to the increased pressure [125]. There does not appear to be a good correlation between the right atrial and right ventricular end-diastolic pressures, however. Confined within the pericardial sac the enlarged right ventricle shifts the intraventricular septum to the left, compromising the left ventricle end-diastolic volume [126, 127]. The septal shift results in a decrease in the left-sided cardiac output and a decrease in systolic blood pressure [125, 128].

With inspiration in a spontaneously breathing patient, intrathoracic pressure decreases, resulting in an increase in venous return and further distention of the right ventricle. The septal shift in normal patients results in a drop in systolic blood pressure of 10 to 12 mm Hg, the normal pulsus paradoxus. The increased septal shift in patients with a massive pulmonary embolus results in an accentuated drop in systolic blood pressure. The drop in systolic pressure occurs with inspiration in spontaneously breathing patients and during exhalation in patients on mechanical ventilation when venous return is augmented. Contributing further to the diminished cardiac output is a decrease in left ventricular filling because of the obstruction of venous return by the pulmonary embolism. If a pulmonary artery catheter is placed, pulmonary capillary wedge pressures (PCWP) are found to be low. Particularly striking is the gradient between the pulmonary artery diastolic pressure and the PCWP, which may be 20 mm Hg or more (Fig. 10-3) [128]. The hemodynamic profile reveals a low cardiac output and index, decreased systemic arterial pressure, and increased heart rate (Tables 10-7). Sytemic vascular resistance is increased as are pulmonary artery pressures and pulmonary vascular resistance. The PCWP is diminished and the left ventricular stroke work index may be diminished, not because of any inherent defect in the myocardium, but rather as a result of diminished left ventricular filling and inadequate stretch of myofibrils. As a result of the diminished cardiac output oxygen delivery to the tissues is decreased. In order to compensate for the decreased oxygen delivery more oxygen is extracted from the blood and the mixed venous oxygen content and oxygen saturation are diminished [125].

The immediate therapy of a pulmonary embolism is aimed at maintaining adequate arterial oxygenation (>90% saturation) and adequate systemic blood pressure. The magnitude of the hemodynamic compromise and lethality associated with a pulmonary embolism do not appear to be associated with the size of the embolus [129, 131]. The initial therapeutic response to hypotension is usually fluid administration, particularly in situations where the left ventricular filling pressure is suspected to be low. The acute increase in pulmonary artery pressure with pulmonary embolism results in acute right ventricular failure. Fluid administration may further dilate an already overdistended right ventricle and result in worsening of left ventricular function [126]. Experimental evidence shows a marked decrease in left ventricular stroke work with volume loading after pulmonary embolization [132]. The results suggest a worsening of the septal shift caused by right ventricular dilatation and decreased left ventricular filling. Hemodynamic support with inotropic agents and vasode-

Fig. 10-3. Pulmonary artery catheter tracing showing pulmonary hypertension and marked difference between the pulmonary artery diastolic pressure and the pulmonary capillary wedge pressure.

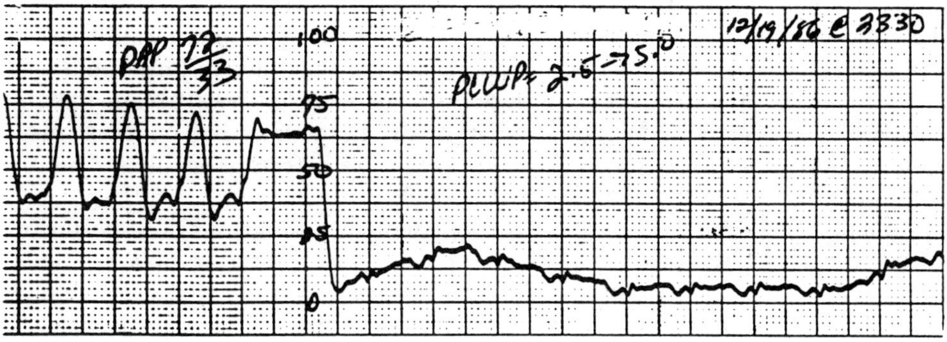
100
75
50
25
0

Table 10-7. Improvement in Hemodynamics in Patients with Pulmonary Embolism with Streptokinase Infusion

	Pretreatment	*2 Hours*	*9 Hours*	*14 Hours*
Blood pressure (mm Hg)	90/40	140/76	168/93	106/58
CO/CI (L/m)	1.84/1.1	5.3/3.1	—	7.8/4.6
Positive airway pressure (mm Hg)	77/30	47/19	42/24	35/19
PCWP (mm Hg)	0–2.5	12.5	10	10
SVO_2 (%)	25–30	50–60	77	73
Fractional inspired oxygen (%)	100	100	30	30
pH	7.12	7.23	7.34	7.40
Partial pressure of oxygen (mm Hg)	102	178	82	77
Partial pressure of carbon dioxide (mm Hg)	33	36	41	34
HCO_3 (mEq/L)	11	15	—	
Lactate (mmol/L)	11.1	12.0	7.2	2.3

pressors such as dopamine and dobutamine have been shown to improve cardiac output and decrease right ventricular overload [31, 126, 128–130, 185]. The use of pulmonary vasodilators in the acute setting of pulmonary embolus has not been advocated since drugs like isoproterenol, hydralazine, or calcium channel blockers also may have deleterious effects on systemic blood pressure. Paradoxically, improving cardiac output with inotropic support initially may have an adverse effect on arterial oxygenation by increasing intrapulmonary shunt. Worsening of ventilation-perfusion matching with improved cardiac output may be the result of recruitment of vessels in poorly ventilated areas that had not been perfused previously [129].

Oxygenation may be maintained by the use of supplemental oxygen either by cannula or mask, depending on the severity of the deficit. Since a significant cause of the hypoxemia may be a function of increased physiologic shunting, arterial oxygenation may not be responsive to supplemental oxygen and endotracheal intubation may be required. Mechanical ventilation may have beneficial effects on ventilation-perfusion matching and improve oxygenation. Detrimental effects on right ventricular function may occur with mechanical ventilation and positive end-expiratory pressure because the increased intrathoracic pressure causes an increase in right ventricular afterload and further septal shifts.

Pulmonary Embolus: Diagnostic Techniques

Nuclear Ventilation-Perfusion Lung Scanning

Ventilation-perfusion lung scans use the injection of ^{99}Te labeled macroaggregated albumin intravenously to determine the distribution of vascular perfusion of the lung. The isotope lodges in the pulmonary capillaries in proportion to the blood flow generally blocking 1 in 1000 capillaries. Meanwhile the radiation of the radioactive tracer is measured. Perfusion defects as small as 2 mm in diameter may be detected. Usually six views are obtained, including anterior, posterior, both anterior and posterior oblique views, and both lateral views (Fig. 10-4). Used alone, radioisotope perfusion lung scans lack speci-

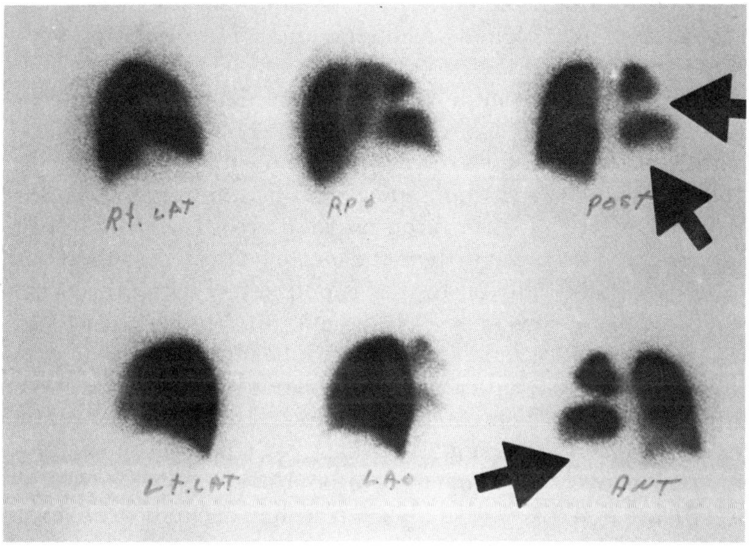
Rt. LAT
RPO
POST
Lt. LAT
LAO
ANT

Fig. 10-4. Perfusion scan showing multiple segmental and subsegmental perfusion deficits consistent with a high probability of pulmonary embolism.

ficity when compared with pulmonary angiography (Fig. 10-5) [7, 31]. In several series of patients with suspected pulmonary embolism and an abnormal perfusion scan, pulmonary embolism was confirmed in between 34% and 71% of patients [133, 135, 168]. Without a ventilation scan a pulmonary embolism can be confirmed only if there is a clear perfusion defect in the patient in whom there is a high clinical suspicion of embolus and a clear chest X-ray [133]. Several factors cause an abnormal perfusion scan in the absence of a pulmonary embolism. These include regional hypoxic vasoconstriction, emphysema, pneumonia, asthma, atelectasis, tumor, pleural effusion, and chronic obstructive pulmonary disease [133, 135]. Chest radiography may increase the utility of a perfusion scan because a matching defect on lung scan and chest radiograph had only a 21% incidence of a pulmonary embolism [135]. Discrimination of perfusion defects into segmental or subsegmental defects also increases specificity. 86% of patients with pulmonary embolism have lobar defects, 70% of patients have segmental defects, while only 37% of patients with subsegmental defects [134, 136]. Pulmonary emboli are multiple 90% of the time and bilateral in 85% of the cases.

Fig. 10-5. Pulmonary angiogram showing a large saddle embolus on the right (straight arrows) that extends into the branches of the right pulmonary artery. There is also a sizeable embolism on the left pulmonary arterial trunk (curved arrows).

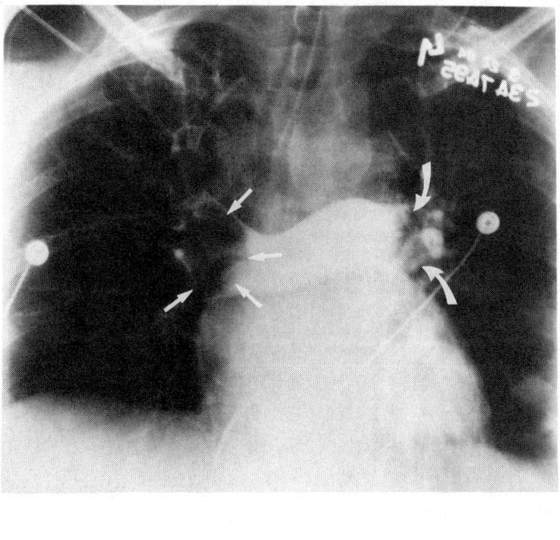

The clinical utility of perfusion lung scanning is markedly improved by obtaining a ventilation scan to improve the specificity of the examination. The ventilation scan involves inhalation of a radioactive gas such as xenon (^{127}Xe or ^{133}Xe) while the gamma camera measures the distribution of the gas from a single posterior view. The ventilation scan requires the patient to rebreathe the gas from a closed circuit and can only be used with spontaneously breathing patients who can cooperate. Patients with severe distress are not usually able to cooperate with the examination. The resolution of ventilation defects outlined by radioactive gases in a single view is less than optimal, and small areas of underventilation may be missed on lung scan [31]. A washout view is usually obtained as well to determine areas of gas trapping suggestive of chronic obstructive pulmonary disease that might correlate with decreased perfusion. A new technique is the use of radiolabeled aerosols, which deposit in the same pattern as the ventilation but remain in the lung for an hour or more, allowing several views to be obtained [117, 188]. It has been demonstrated that aerosol-perfusion scans utilizing Tc-99m-DTPA aerosol are diagnostically comparable with gas-perfusion studies that utilize ^{133}Xe as the ventilation agent [188]. There was over 80% agreement on diagnoses. However, certain very ill or uncooperative patients were left out of this study who may have rendered unsatisfactory images using the aerosol technique. Advantages of Tc-99m is its ready availability, ideal imaging energy, and ability to image in multiple projections. Disadvantages in using aerosol are the small amount of activity delivered to the patient and the inability to obtain washout images.

Ventilation-perfusion lung scans should be obtained within 24 to 48 hours of embolization since spontaneous resolution of the embolus can occur, which will reduce the sensitivity of the test [7, 134]. In patients treated with heparin the urokinase-pulmonary embolism trial found absolute resolution in less than 48 hours was unusual, but progressive resolution occurred with time [95].

Using both ventilation and perfusion lung scans results in of reasonable sensitivity, specificity, and prognostic utility. Perfusion lung scans are graded as to the degree of perfusion impairment anatomically, i.e., lobar, segmental or subsegmental. The perfusion scans are compared with the ventilation scan to determine if an area of decreased perfusion matches an area of decreased ventilation. If it does then it may be due to hypoxic vasoconstriction rather than a pulmonary embolus. If there are ventilated areas that are not perfused, then the probability of a pulmonary embolism that is detectable angiographically increases. Ventilation-perfusion scans are graded as to the probability of a pulmonary embolism: high, intermediate, or low. Ventilation-perfusion scans with multiple segmental or lobar perfusion deficits, but without a corresponding ventilation defect, have been shown to have a high probability (>85%) of having a pulmonary embolus on subsequent pulmonary angiography [31, 134, 135]. Therapy with anticoagulants or lytic therapy may be initiated in those patients without a pulmonary angiogram based on the ventilation-perfusion scan alone. Patients with a low probability have either matching ventilation and perfusion abnormalities or small segmental perfusion defects. The estimated frequency of pulmonary embolism in these patients is less than 10% [7]. Other studies have suggested a higher frequency of between 25% and 40% angiographically detectable emboli in these patients with low probability scans [137]. Even with the possibility of this high incidence of detectable pulmonary embolism, studies have indicated that in follow-up, patients with a normal or low probability ventilation-perfusion scan are at very low risk for fatal thromboembolic disease [134, 136–138]. In patients with a low probability of pulmonary embolism on ventilation-perfusion scan, therapy may be withheld unless another indication for anticoagulation exists [138].

The difficulty arises in patients who have a single segmental defect on perfusion scan without a corresponding ventilation defect or who have multiple segmental defects with matching or mismatching ventilation. Those patients are classified as having an intermediate possibility of pulmonary embolism. Intermediate scans may also be found in patients with severe chronic obstructive pulmonary disease (COPD) where there may be delayed washout of inhaled isotopes, giving the appearance of a ventilation defect, and the parenchyma may be destroyed giving the perfusion deficits. The estimated frequency of pulmonary embolism in this group of patients is approximately 50% [7]. A rational approach to patients who have an intermediate probability of pulmonary embolism on ventilation-perfusion scan would be to evaluate the patient for the potential presence of embolic sources by IPG, duplex ultrasound, or venography. If an embolic source is identified, therapy should be initiated without further studies. Patients without an obvious source of emboli but an intermediate probability ventilation-perfusion scan present the greatest clinical challenge. It is in these patients that a pulmonary angiogram is of the greatest use in determining the need for therapy.

Indeterminate scans are those that are of inadequate sensitivity to be reliably predictive of the presence or absence of pulmonary emboli [133]. This occurs on scans where lobar or segmental perfusion deficits and matching ventilation defects exist. Patients with malignancies involving the lung or lymphangitic spread within the lung, or young patients with small segmental perfusion defects and normal ventilation scans may all have scans that are indeterminate. As with patients with intermediate probability scans, those with indeterminate scans may warrant pulmonary angiography if the clinical diagnosis of pulmonary embolism is highly suspected. The incidence of a positive pulmonary angiogram in patients with an indeterminate scan ranges between 13% and 50% [133].

The definitive diagnosis can be obtained by pulmonary angiography. Using a procedure of this magnitude for every suspected pulmonary embolism is unrealistic because of significant cost, availability, morbidity, and mortality associated with the study. For this reason, Bayes' Theorem as described by McNeil in 1980 [133] was developed, which incorporates clinical suspicion and likelihood ratios to estimate the probability of a patient with a particular ventilation-perfusion scan to have a pulmonary embolism.

Bayes' Theorem uses clinical suspicion and likelihood ratios to establish the degree of probability prior to a patient obtaining a ventilation-perfusion scan. Likelihood ratio is determined by the relative frequency of a certain ventilation-perfusion scan pattern in patients with pulmonary embolism divided by the frequency of the scan pattern in patients without a pulmonary embolism. Ratios greater than 1.0 increase the possibility that the patient has a pulmonary embolism, whereas ratios less than 1.0 lessen the chance. Clinical suspicion for the probability of a pulmonary embolism is determined by the physician and arbitrarily preset values are assigned. If the suspicion is "high," a value of greater than 85% is assigned. If suspicion is "possible," a value between 10% and 85% is assigned, while if "low," a value of less than 10% is given [133, 189].

By a somewhat complex equation, the calculated probability of pulmonary embolism is determined before the ventilation-perfusion scan by using available clinical and laboratory data. This prior probability estimate may help determine and maximize the level of certainty a physician has before establishing a treatment plan or further investigation if necessary.

As a result of the complexity of the equation, clinicians are not using the theory to help diagnose pulmonary embolism. For this reason, a simplified version of Bayes' Theorem was introduced [190]. This form allows calculation of post-test probability by adding "weights." Weights contain information on sensitivity and specificity of a given test. This allows the clinician to consider one value to interpret a certain test. A positive test will have a positive weight. A larger weight will produce a larger increase in the post-test probability of disease process.

Pulmonary Angiography

Pulmonary angiography is the definitive study to determine the presence or absence of pulmonary emboli. The test is invasive, however, and is associated with an approximate 0.2% to 0.7% mortality and 4% morbidity, including arrhythmias, myocardial injury, and hypersensitivity to the contrast medium [7, 31, 139]. Indications for arteriography include patients with an intermediate probability ventilation-perfusion scan, patients in whom an adequate ventilation-perfusion study cannot be performed, such as patients on mechanical ventilation or patients in whom the presence of pulmonary or cardiac disease interferes with a ventilation-perfusion scan. Pulmonary angiography may be technically inadequate for the diagnosis of pulmonary embolism in as many as 11% to 25% of patients studied [139, 140].

The diagnosis of pulmonary embolism is made if an intraluminal filling defect can be seen on several views or if there is an abrupt cutoff of a vessel more than 2.5 mm in diameter. Other nonspecific findings that interfere with vessel filling can be seen with pneumonia, dilatation, pulmonary hypertension, and emphysema. Injection of dye results in some vasodilation and may result in hypertension or arrhythmias. Selective angiography in which small volumes of dye are repeatedly injected decrease the risk of the test. The predictive value of a negative pulmonary angiogram is excellent. In one study of 167 patients during a follow-up period of 6 months, no patient with a negative angiogram result had evidence of pulmonary emboli or death from pulmonary emboli [141].

The standard pulmonary arteriogram is invasive, costly, time consuming, and requires special training. An alternative is digital subtraction angiography. A bolus of dye is injected intravenously and the presence of vessel cutoffs or intraterminal filling defects are evaluated after computer enhancement. Studies have shown a good correlation compared both with radionuclide ventilation-perfusion scans and standard pulmonary angiography [139, 141, 143]. The limits of resolution appear to be emboli approximately 2 to 2.5 mm in diameter, which is comparable to standard angiography [142, 143]. It has been suggested that digital subtraction angiography may make conventional angiography unnecessary in 85% to 90% of patients with suspected pulmonary emboli [139].

For patients who are too unstable to move from the intensive care unit, a technique of bedside pulmonary angiography using a pulmonary artery catheter has been described [144]. A single injection of contrast material was made with the patients positioned on a standard x-ray plate. Immediately after injection the plate was exposed. No complications were reported in a series of nine patients, and the results were confirmed in 80% of the patients [144].

Treatment of Pulmonary Embolism

Beyond simple support of oxygenation and blood pressure, therapy for a pulmonary embolism is aimed at inhibiting the thrombotic process, promoting lysis, and prevention or recurrence of embolism of the clot. A pulmonary embolism that does not cause significant hypoxia or hemodynamic compromise may be treated with heparin alone, whereas more severe thromboembolism may require lytic therapy. Patients who have a contraindication to heparin or lytic agents may require vena caval interruption to prevent a recurrence of pulmonary emboli. Overall treatment of acute pulmonary embolism may reduce mortality to 8% regardless of whether or not shock is present [131]. Full anticoagulation with heparin is the standard treatment at present. Treatment is initiated with an intravenous bolus of 5000 to 10,000 units followed by a continuous infusion adequate to raise the PTT to 1.5 to 2.5 times normal. The indication for treatment is a reasonable suspicion that a thromboembolic event has occurred. Heparin therapy should be initiated while diagnostic tests are being obtained since a delay in treatment may result in a recurrence. There are few absolute contraindications to heparin in the setting of pulmonary embolism, but uncontrolled bleeding, patient sensitivity, intracranial bleeding, severe thrombocytopenia, or heparin-related vascular thrombosis would preclude the use of heparin [78, 94]. Mild gastrointestinal or genitourinary bleeding may be tolerated if low levels of anticoagulation are used [78]. The means of administration of heparin and the degree of anticoagulation have an effect on the incidence of bleeding. Continuous intravenous administration of heparin is associated with a lower incidence of bleeding problems. In some studies the incidence of bleeding has been 0% to 1% whereas in others it has been as high as 48% [94, 145]. If the PTT is elevated between two and three times the control value, the risk of bleeding is increased threefold. Prolongation of the PTT to three times or greater increases the risk of bleeding by eight times [78]. Other conditions that may increase the risk of bleeding include acute cardiac dysfunction and systolic pressure below 90 mm Hg, renal insufficiency, hepatic insufficiency, or cancer, anemia, or other evidence of a debilitated condition.

The use of low molecular weight heparin, which has a greater activity to inhibit factor X activity, has been associated with a decreased incidence of bleeding complications compared with standard heparin [145]. Heparin therapy should be initiated as for the treatment of DVT. As with treatment for DVT the goal is to maintain a PTT between 1.5 and 2 times the patient's pretreatment value. Inadequate anticoagulation results in a high rate of emboli recurrence [92].

While heparin interrupts the hypercoagulable state and prevents the propagation of thrombus and recurrence of emboli, heparin does not cause clot lysis, prevent valvular damage, alter the hemodynamic manifestations of the pulmonary embolus, or prevent the development of chronic pulmonary hypertension [146]. The potential advantages of lytic therapy in the setting of pulmonary embolism are many, but the potential for severe bleeding complications is great as well.

The indications for initiating lytic therapy include patients with pulmonary emboli who have hemodynamic instability, lobar obstruction, or multiple segmental perfusion defects. Patient selection includes patients with documented pulmonary embolism and patients in whom the benefits of lytic therapy outweigh the risks. The more recent the embolic event, the greater the possibility of successful clot lysis. The contraindications to lytic therapy are listed in Table 10-5. In one study, 47% of the patients evaluated were excluded because of contraindications for lytic therapy. The most frequent reason for exclusion was recent surgery or organ biopsy followed by low hematocrit and internal bleeding, either active or significant within 6 months [147]. Other considerations in the use of lytic therapy include the necessity to avoid vascular procedures during therapy and the need for careful monitoring of the patient during therapy. Lytic therapy may be initiated as described in Table 10-6 either by systemic intravenous infusion or by direct infusion of the lytic agent through a pulmonary artery catheter at a lower dose [147, 148].

Lytic therapy has been shown to be effective in reducing pulmonary hypertension, vascular occlusion, and providing more complete clot resolution than heparin. After initiation of lytic therapy, pulmonary hemodynamics usually show improvement within a few hours and maximal improvement occurs within 6 to 12 hours [146, 149] (Table 10-7). Therapy is initiated as for lytic therapy in DVT (Table 10-6). The three agents, streptokinase, urokinase, and tissue plasminogen activator, vary in the duration of infusions and in their effectiveness. Streptokinase is infused for 24 to 72 hours or until bleeding requires cessation of therapy. Urokinase is infused for 12 hours as studies have indicated that 24-hour infusions are not more effective than 12-hour infusions [24, 95]. Studies have also indicated that urokinase may have advantages over streptokinase, particularly in the treatment of massive pulmonary emboli [24, 95]. Recent studies with tissue plasminogen activators have suggested that tissue plasminogen activators may provide more rapid clot resolution with increased safety compared with urokinase [150, 182]. The majority of studies confirm the superiority of all of the thrombolytic agents compared with heparin in clot lysis, but vary in the estimate of the relative risk of bleeding that lytic agents may present [107–109, 111, 150, 151]. In an attempt to reduce the bleeding complications of streptokinase, some investigators have infused boluses of the drug intermittently with some success, but controlled studies have yet to be done [151, 179, 183]. Newer agents are also being evaluated such as acylated plasminogen streptokinase activator complex and single chain urokinase plasminogen activator, but these agents are experimental at present. The overall incidence of severe bleeding complications appears to be approximately 1% for streptokinase compared with about 0.5% with heparin [146, 153]. With any lytic agent invasive vascular procedures need to be kept to an absolute minimum.

With all lytic agents coagulation profiles are monitored after infusion. When coagulation tests decline to two times normal, heparin is started without an initial bolus and continued for 7 to 10 days. During that period, warfarin therapy is initiated and maintained as described for the treatment of DVT.

Pulmonary Embolectomy

Patients who are not candidates for lytic therapy and who are hemodynamically unstable and unresponsive to heparin may require embolectomy.

Unfortunately, mortality for this procedure has been reported to be as high as 30% to 75% [153]. The number of patients who might be expected to benefit from pulmonary embolectomy given this mortality is very low, especially given the high mortality of massive pulmonary emboli in the first hour before a cardiac bypass team can be mobilized [153a]. The criteria for embolectomy include systolic blood pressure less than 90 mm Hg, urine output of less than 22 mL/h, and an arterial PO_2 less than 60 mm Hg after an hour of maximal medical therapy. The exact criteria are impossible to define and depend on many factors, but the embolectomy should be performed on those patients who will die without the procedure [154].

Vena Cava Interruption

Patients who have a recurrence of thromboembolic disease while on anticoagulants or have contraindications to anticoagulants may require mechanical interruption of the vena cava. A variety of devices and procedures have been used with varying degrees of success [155, 156]. The major difficulty with most operative techniques was a relatively high recurrence rate (4.6% to 6.4%) and high intraoperative mortality (7.3% to 15.5%) [155]. Ligation, plication, or external clips on the inferior vena cava also have had a high rate of leg sequelae and problems with maintaining patency [156]. Impairment of venous patency has also been a problem, and development of collateral circulation has developed after vena caval interruption [157]. Exercise intolerance from inadequate venous return has been found in patients who have undergone vena caval interruption [158]. The development of the Greenfield filter, which can be placed percutaneously, has been a major advance in mechanical prophylaxis for thromboembolic disease [159, 160]. The filter has a lower complication rate than previous filters, with a low incidence of impaired patency, filter migration, and caval perforation [159, 161]. The use of the filter requires obtaining a venogram to determine the proximal extent of the thrombus in the location of the renal veins. Concern over perirenal placement of the filter has not been borne out by subsequent experience, and the filter is a reasonable therapeutic device when anticoagulation fails or is contraindicated.

Sequelae of Thromboembolic Disease

The three major sequelae of venous thromboembolic disease are the postphlebitic syndrome, recurrent pulmonary embolism, and chronic pulmonary hypertension.

The postphlebitic syndrome consists of incomplete thrombus resolution, resulting in decreased venous outflow and venous incompetence. The clinical manifestations include peripheral edema, hyperpigmentation, ulceration, and pain. Before anticoagulation this complication occurred in 80% of patients with DVTs. The use of heparin still results in residual disease in 89% of patients and the postphlebitic syndrome in 78% [162]. The use of lytic therapy may result in a lower incidence of postphlebitic syndrome [109].

Recurrent pulmonary emboli occur in more than 18% who were originally admitted for pulmonary embolism and treated with heparin. Pulmonary emboli also occurred in 6% of patients who had been treated with heparin for 8 days. Recurrences were more likely if the venogram revealed a free-floating thrombus. Thirteen percent of patients with DVTs and a free-floating thrombus had a subsequent pulmonary embolus compared with 3% of patients without a free-floating thrombus. Patients with a pulmonary embolism and a free-floating thrombus had a recurrence rate of 38%, while those who did not had an 11% recurrence rate in spite of therapeutic heparin therapy. Venography may be useful in determining those patients at high risk for subsequent complications of thromboembolic disease [163].

Pulmonary hypertension from recurrent pulmonary emboli occurs with an unknown incidence. While 70% to 80% of patients with an acute pulmonary emboli exhibit pulmonary hypertension (mean pulmonary pressure >20 mm Hg), few patients undergo subsequent right-sided heart catheterization. Most patients have resolution of their ventilation-perfusion scans over the course of a year. It is estimated that less than 2% of patients with chronic pulmonary emboli develop chronic pulmonary hypertension. The development of chronic pulmonary artery pressures greater than 30 mm Hg has been associated with a 30% 5-year survival. The diagnosis is usually made on the basis of an abnormal chest radiograph, electrocardiogram, pulmonary function tests to exclude chronic obstructive pulmonary disease, and a ventilation-perfusion scan that may differentiate other primary pulmonary hypertension from thromboembolic disease. The chest radiograph may be normal, but may reveal large pulmonary vessels in the hilar regions, with abrupt cutoff of the vessels of the areas of the periphery. A lateral film usually reveals right ventricular and arterial enlargement. Electrocardiography reveals evidence of right atrial enlargement (P-pulmonale) and right axis deviation suggestive of right ventricular enlargement. A right bundle branch block may also be present. Pulmonary function tests with chronic pulmonary embolus will not reveal obstructive airflow limitations as compared with chronic obstructive pulmonary disease, but diffusing capacity may be diminished and the lung volumes appear to be mildly restrictive. Clinically, patients are usually symptomatic. Arterial blood gases reveal some degree of dyspnea on exertion or at rest and hypoxia [164].

Treatment with lytic agents is generally not successful, and thromboendarterectomy has been advocated for disease that has been present for 6 months or more. Elective operative mortality has been reduced to less than 6%. Complications include right ventricular failure, pulmonary reperfusion injuries, and microemboli. Vasodilators have been tried but with limited success, whereas calcium channel blockers have been somewhat more successful [164].

Pulmonary embolism is an exceedingly common entity that causes a high mortality if untreated. Failure to treat is largely the result of the difficulty in diagnosing the disease. Appreciation of the risk factors and appropriate prophylactic treatment can lower the incidence of pulmonary emboli, and prompt diagnostic procedures and therapy can reduce the mortality from pulmonary emboli. In spite of advances in diagnosis, prevention, and therapy, however, pulmonary embolism remains a major clinical dilemma for physicians and a major cause of death for patients.

Pulmonary Hypertension: Other Etiologies

Other causes of pulmonary hypertension include primary pulmonary hypertension, vasculitides, collagen vascular disease, hypoxic vasoconstriction, and interstitial lung disease.

Primary pulmonary hypertension may be divided into three subsets of pathology. The subgroups are medial hypertrophy, laminar internal proliferation, and microthrombotic lesions. The disease affects women between the ages of 20 and 50 in a 2 : 1 ratio with men. The diagnosis is usually made by exclusion of other causes, and treatment is directed at reducing pulmonary pressure with vasodilators and reducing inflammation with steroids. Heart–lung transplantation holds hope for the future [165].

The vasculitides comprise a diffuse group of diseases involving small to large arteries, including polyarteritis nodosa, hypersensitivity vasculitis, Wegener's granulomatosis, Takayasu's arteritis, temporal arteritis, and Henoch-Schönlein's disease. Therapy involves decreasing the inflammatory response with steroids and other anti-inflammatory drugs.

Secondary pulmonary hypertension may be the result of lung diseases such as cystic fibrosis, hypoventilation, congenital heart disease, and chronic obstructive pulmonary disease.

Clinically, the patient with pulmonary hypertension complains of fatigue and dyspnea on exertion. As the disease progresses, there may be syncope or near syncope on exertion as well as anginal pain from right ventricular ischemia. Hemoptysis is uncommon, occurring in 10% to 15% of patients and is usually scant. Physical findings may reveal an accentuated P_2 and a parasternal heave, indicating right ventricular enlargement. As the process worsens, tricuspid valve insufficiency produces a systolic murmur and pulmonary valve incompetence results in the diastolic murmur known as Graham Steell's murmur [166]. Chest radiography often shows large central pulmonary arteries, with marked attenuation or "pruning" of the vessels in the periphery (see Chap. 26, Fig. 26-31). Therapy is directed at maintaining adequate oxygenation to prevent hypoxic vasoconstriction [166, 167].

References

1. Virchow R: Gesammelte Adhandlungen zur Wissen-schaftlichen. Vol IV, Thrombose und Emboli. Berlin, G-Hamm-Grotesche Buchhandlung, 1862, p 219
2. Bell WR, Simon TL: Current status of pulmonary thromboembolic disease: Pathophysiology, diagnosis, prevention, and treatment. *Am Heart J* 103:239–262, 1982
3. Hayes SP, Bone RC: Pulmonary emboli with respiratory failure. *Med Clin North Am* 67: 1179–1191, 1983
4. Dunmire SM: Pulmonary embolism. *Emerg Med Clin North Am* 7:339–354, 1989
5. West JW: Pulmonary embolism. *Med Clin North Am* 70:877–893, 1986.
6. Freiman DG, Suyemoto J, Wessler S: Frequency of pulmonary thromboembolism in man. *N Engl J Med* 272:1278–1280, 1965
7. Rosenow EC, Osmundson PJ, Brown ML: Pulmonary embolism. *Mayo Clinic Proc* 56: 161–178, 1981
8. Grossling HR, Donohue TA: The fat embolism syndrome. *JAMA* 241:2740–2742, 1979
9. Clark SL: Amniotic fluid embolism. *Clin Perinatol* 13:801–811, 1986
10. Cales RH, Humphreys N, Pilmanis AA, et al: Cardiac arrest from gas embolism in scuba diving. *Ann Emerg Med* 10:585, 1981
11. McGoon MD, Benedetto PW, Greene BM: Complications of percutaneous central venous catheterization. *The Johns Hopkins Medical Journal* 145:1–6, 1979
12. Moser KM: Venous thromboembolism. *Am Rev Respir Dis* 141:235–249, 1990
13. Schafer AI: The hypercoagulable states. *Ann Intern Med* 102:814–828, 1985
14. Shackford SR, Moser KM: Deep venous thrombosis and pulmonary embolism in trauma patients. *J Intensive Care Med* 3: 87–98, 1988
15. Comerota AJ, White JV: The use of dihydroergotamine and heparin in the prophylaxis of deep venous thrombosis. *Chest* 89 (suppl 5):389S–395S, 1986
16. Stewart GJ, Schaub RG, Niewiarkowski S: Products of tissue injury. *Arch Pathol Lab Med* 104:409–413, 1980
17. Merli GJ, Martinez J: Prophylaxis for deep vein thrombosis and pulmonary embolism in surgical patient. *Med Clin North Am* 71:377–397, 1987
18. Williams JW: Venous thrombosis and pulmonary embolism. *Surg Gynecol Obstet* 143: 385–390, 1976
19. Coon WW: Risk factors in pulmonary embolism. *Surg Obstet* 143:385–390, 1976
20. Cade JF: High risk of the critically ill for venous thromboembolism. *Crit Care Med* 10: 448–450, 1982
21. Nicolaicies AN, Kakkar VV, Renney JTG: Soleal sinuses and stasis. *Br J Surg* 58:307, 1971
22. Nicolaicies AN, Kakkar VV, Renney JTG: The soleal sinuses: Origin of deep vein thrombosis. *Br J Surg* 57:860, 1976
23. Mohr DN, Ryn JH, Litin SC, et al: Recent advances in the management of venous thromboembolism. *Mayo Clin Proc* 63:281–290, 1988
24. Havig G: Deep venous thrombosis and pulmonary embolism. *Acta Chir Scand* [Suppl] 478:1, 1977
25. Gracey DR, McMicham JC, Divertie MB, et al: Respiratory failure in Guillain-Barré syndrome. *Mayo Clin Proc* 57:742–746, 1982

26. Raman TK, Blake JA, Harris TM: Pulmonary embolism in Landre-Guillain-Barré-Stokes syndrome. *Chest* 60:555–557, 1971
27. Ropper AH, Kehne SM: Guillain-Barré syndrome: Management of respiratory failure. *Neurology* 35:1665–1667, 1985
28. Lealerc JR, Hirsh J: Venous thromboembolic disorders. *In* Burrow GN, Ferris FF (eds): Medical Complications During Pregnancy. Philadelphia, W.B. Saunders, 1988
29. Rose SD: Prophylaxis of thromboembolic disease. *Med Clin North Am* 63:1205–1224, 1979
30. Huisman MV, Buller HR, tenCate JW, et al: Unexpected high prevalence of silent pulmonary embolism in patients with deep venous thrombosis. *Chest* 95:498–502, 1989
31. Moser KM: Pulmonary embolism. *Ann Rev Respir Dis* 115:829–852, 1977
32. Kakkar VV, Howe CT, Flanc C, et al: Natural history of postoperative deep vein thrombosis. *Lancet* 2:230, 1969
33. Painter TD: Thrombophlebitis: Diagnostic techniques. *Prog Cardiovasc Dis* 17:386–397, 1974–75
34. Moser KM, LeMoine JR: Is embolic risk conditional by location of deep venous thrombosis. *Ann Intern Med* 94:439–444, 1981
35. Menzoran JD, Sequeira JC, Doyle JE, et al: Therapeutic and clinical course of deep vein thrombosis. *Am J Surg* 146:581–585, 1983
36. Mathewson M: A Homans' sign is an effective method of diagnosing thrombophlebitis in bedridden patients. *Crit Care Nurse,* July/Aug, 1983 p. 64
37. Albrechtson V, Olson CG: Thrombotic side effects of lower limb phlebography. *Lancet* 1:723–724, 1976
38. Gent M, Roberts RS: A meta-analysis of the studies of dehydroergotamine plus heparin in the prophylaxis of deep vein thrombosis. *Chest* 89(suppl 5):398S–406S, 1986
39. Landefeld CS, McGuire E, Cohen AM: Clinical findings associated with acute proximal deep vein thrombosis: A basis for quantifying clinical judgement. *Am J Med* 88:382–388, 1990
40. Secker-Walker RH: The use of radioisotopes in the management of venous thromboembolism. *Chest* 89(suppl 5):413S–415S, 1986
41. Hill RD, Hirsh J, Carter CJ, et al: Diagnostic efficacy of impedance plethysmography for clinically suspected deep-vein thrombosis. *Ann Intern Med* 102:21–28, 1985
42. Huisman MV, Buller HR, tenCate, JW, et al: Serial impedance plethysmography for suspected deep venous thrombosis in outpatients. *N Engl J Med* 314:823–828, 1984
43. Wheeler HB, O'Donnell JA, Anderson TA, et al: Occlusive impedance phlebography: A diagnostic procedure for venous thrombosis and pulmonary embolism. *Prog Cardiovasc Dis* 17:199–205, 1974
44. Lensing AWA, Prandoni P, Brandjes D, et al: Detection of deep vein thrombosis by real-time B mode ultrasonography. *N Engl J Med* 320:342–345, 1989
45. Connors AE, Castele RJ, Farhat NZ, et al: Complications of right heart catheterization. *Chest* 88:567–572, 1985
46. Luby JM, Purcell H, Kraut EH, et al: Pulmonary embolism as a result of Hickman catheter related thrombosis. *Am J Med* 86:228–231, 1989
47. Moss JF, Wagman LD, Rirschimaki DV, et al: Central venous thrombosis related to the silastic Hickman-Broviac catheter in an oncologic population. *JPEN* 15:397–400, 1989
48. Wheeler HB, Anderson FA: Diagnostic approach for deep vein thrombosis. *Chest* 89 (suppl 5):407S–412S, 1986
49. Mitchell SE, Clark RA: Complications of central venous catheterization. *AJR* 133:467–476, 1979
50. Parsa MH, Tobira F: Establishment of intravenous lines for long term intravenous therapy and monitoring. *Surg Clin North Am* 65:835–865, 1985
51. Clark SL: Amniotic fluid embolism. *Clin Perinatol* 13:801–811, 1986
52. Peterson EP, Taylor HB: Amniotic fluid embolism. *Obstet Gynecol* 35:787–793, 1970
53. Mulder JI: Amniotic fluid embolism: An overview and case report. *Am J Obstet Gynecol* 152:430–435, 1985
54. Herndon JH: The syndrome of fat embolism. *South Med J* 68:12:1577–1584, 1975
55. Borow M, Goldson H: Postoperative venous thrombosis: evaluation of five methods of treatment. *Am J Surg* 141:245–251, 1981
56. Celi A, Palla A, Petruzzelli S, et al: A prospective study of a standardized questionnaire and improved clinical estimate of pulmonary embolism. *Chest* 95:332–337, 1989
57. Rose SD: Prophylaxis of thromembolic disease. *Med Clin North Am* 63:1205–1224, 1979
58. Hathin H, Goldberg J, Modan M, et al: Reduction of mortality of general medical inpatient by low-dose heparin prophylaxis. *Ann Intern Med* 96:561–565, 1982
59. Collins R, Sarimgevin A, Yusuf S, et al: Reduction in fatal pulmonary embolism and venous thrombosis by perioperative administration of subcutaneous heparin. *N Engl J Med* 318:1162–1172, 1988
60. Hull RD, Raskob GE, Hursh J: Prophylaxis of venous thromboembolism. *Chest* 89(suppl 5):374S–383S, 1986

61. Petitt DB, Shom BL, Melmon KL: Duration of warfarin anticoagulant therapy and the probabilities of recurrent thromboembolism and hemorrhage. *Am J Med* 81:255–259, 1986
62. Leyviaz PE, Richard J, Bachman F, et al: Adjusted versus fixed dose subcutaneous heparin in the prevention of deep vein thrombosis after total hip replacement. *N Engl J Med* 309:954–958, 1983
63. Cade JF, Clegg EA, Westlake GW: Prophylaxis of venous thrombosis after major thoracic surgery. *Aust NZ J Surg* 53:301–305, 1983
64. Turpil AGG, Levine MN, Hirsch J, et al: A randomized controlled trial of low molecular weight heparin to prevent deep vein thrombosis in patients undergoing elective hip surgery. *N Engl J Med* 315:925–929, 1986
65. Bubcock RB, Dumper CW, Scharfman WB: Heparin-induced immune thrombocytopenia. *N Engl J Med* 295:237–241, 1976
66. King DJ, Kellon JG: Heparin-associated thrombocytopenia. *Ann Intern Med* 100: 535–540, 1984
67. Bell WR: Diagnosing and managing heparin-associated thrombocytopenia. *Journal of Critical Illness* 2:11–14, 1987
68. Frame JN, Mulvey KP, Phares JC, et al: Connection of severe heparin-associated thrombocytopenia with intravenous immunoglobin. *Ann Intern Med* 111:946–947, 1989
69. Griffith GC, Nichols G, Asher JD, et al: Heparin osteoporosis. *JAMA* 193:85–88, 1965
70. Atkinson JLD, Sundt TM, Kazmier FJ, et al: Heparin-induced thrombocytopenia and thrombosis in ischemic stroke. *Mayo Clinic Proc* 63:353–361, 1988
71. White PW, Sudd JR, Neusel RE: Thrombotic complications of heparin therapy. *Ann Surg* 190:595–608, 1979
72. Chang JC: White clot syndrome associated with heparin-induced thrombocytopenia: A review of 23 cases. *Heart Lung* 16:403–407, 1987
73. Squires JW, Pinch LW: Heparin induced spinal fractures. *JAMA* 241:2417–2418, 1979
74. Jaffe MD, Willis PW: Multiple fractures associated with long-term sodium heparin therapy. *JAMA* 193:152–154, 1965
75. Rocko JM, Mikhart F, Trilles F, et al: The safety of low-dose heparin prophylaxis. *Am J Surg* 135:798–800, 1978
76. Pachter HL, Riles TS: Low dose heparin: Bleeding and wound complications in the surgical patient. *Ann Surg* 186:669–674, 1977
77. Dukes GE, Sanders SW, Ursso J, et al: Transaminase elevation in patients receiving bovine or porcine heparin. *Ann Intern Med* 100:646–650, 1984
78. Myers TM, Hull RD, Weg JC: Antithrombotic therapy for venous thromboembolic disease. *Chest* 89(suppl 2):26S–35S, 1986
79. Powers PJ, Gent M, Jay RM, et al: A randomized trial of less intensive postoperative warfarin or aspirin therapy in the prevention of venous thromboembolism after surgery for fractured hip. *Arch Intern Med* 149:771–774, 1989
80. Poller L, McKernan A, Thompson JM, et al: Fixed minidose warfarin: A new approach to prophylaxis against venous thrombosis after major surgery. *Br Med J* 298:1309–1312, 1987
81. Chagett GP, Salzman EW: Prevention of venous thromboembolism. *Prog Cardiovasc Dis* 17:345–366, 1975
82. Comerota AJ, White JV: The use of dihydroergotamine and heparin in the prophylaxis of deep venous thrombosis. *Chest* 89 (suppl 5):389S–395S, 1986
83. Kakker VV, Stamatakes JD, Bentley PG, et al: Prophylaxis for postoperative deep vein thrombosis. *JAMA* 241:39–42, 1979
84. Rosengarten DS, Land J, Jeyasingh K, et al: The failure of compressive stockings (Tubigrip) to prevent deep venous thrombus after operation. *Br J Surg* 57:296–299, 1970
85. Coe NP, Collins REC, Klein LA, et al: Prevention of deep vein thrombosis in urological patients: A controlled randomized trial of low-dose heparin and external compression pneumatic compression boots. *Surgery* 83: 230–234, 1978
86. Salzman EW, Ploetz J, Bettman M, et al: Intraoperative external pneumatic calf compression to afford long-term prophylaxis against deep vein thrombosis in urological patients. *Surgery* 87:239–242, 1980
87. Cuprini JA, Chucker SL, Zuckerman L, et al: Thrombosis prophylaxis using external compression. *Surg Gynecol Obstet* 156:599–604, 1983
88. Bern MD, Lockik JJ, Wallack SR, et al: Very low dose of warfarin can prevent thrombis in central venous catheters. *Ann Intern Med* 112:423–428, 1990
89. Panian NG, Kosowsky BD, Gurewich V: Transfemoral temporary pacing and deep vein thrombosis. *Am Heart J* 100:847–851, 1980
90. Anderson AJ, Krasnow SH, Boyer MW, et al: Thrombosis: The major Hickman catheter complication in patients with solid tumor. *Chest* 95:71–75, 1989
91. Hull RD, Raskob GE, Hirsh J, et al: Continuous intravenous heparin compared with in-

termittent subcutaneous heparin. The initial treatment of proximal vein thrombosis. *N Engl J Med* 315:1109–1114, 1986
92. Holm HA, Finnanger B, Harmann A, et al: Heparin treatment of deep venous thrombosis in 280 patients: Symptoms related to dosage. *Acta Med Scand* 215:47–53, 1984
93. Hirsh J, Van Aken WG, Gallus AS, et al: Heparin kinetics in venous thrombosis and pulmonary embolism. *Circulation* 53:691–695, 1976
94. Genton E, Hirsch J: Observations in anticoagulation and thrombolytic therapy in pulmonary embolism. *Prog Cardiovasc Dis* 17: 335–343, 1975
95. Urokinase Pulmonary Embolism Trial Study Group: Urokinase streptokinase pulmonary embolism trial phase II results. *JAMA* 229: 1606–1613, 1974
96. Physician's Desk Reference. Montvale, NJ, Medical Economics Co., 1990, pp 1238–1239
97. Casthety PA, Goodman K, Fryman PN, et al: Hemodynamic changes after the administration of protamine. *Anesth Analg* 65:78–80, 1986
98. Hull R, Delmore T, Carter C, et al: Adjusted subcutaneous heparin versus warfarin sodium in the long-term treatment of venous thrombosis. *N Engl J Med* 306:189–194, 1982
99. Holmgreen K, Anderson G, Fagrell B, et al: One-month versus six-month therapy with oral anticoagulant after symptomatic deep vein thrombosis. *Acta Med Scand* 218:279–284, 1985
100. O'Sullivan EF: Duration of anticoagulant therapy in venous thrombo-embolism. *Med J Aust* 2:1104–1107, 1972
101. Hull R, Delmore T, Genlin E, et al: Warfarin sodium versus low-dose heparin in the long-term treatment of venous thrombosis. *N Engl J Med* 301:L855–858, 1979
102. Hull R, Hirsh J, Jay R, et al: Different intensities of oral anticoagulant therapy in the treatment of proximal-vein thrombosis. *N Engl J Med* 307:1676–1681, 1982
103. Petty GW, Lennihan L, Mohr JP, et al: Complications of long-term anticoagulation. *Am Neurol* 23:570–574, 1988
104. Hirsh J, Deykin D, Polleo L: Therapeutic range for oral anticoagulation therapy. *Chest* 89(suppl):115–159, 1986
105. Koch-Weser J, Sellus EM: Drug interaction with coumadin anticoagulants (parts 1 and 2). *N Engl J Med* 285:#9 pp 407–497 #10 pp 547–557, 1971
106. Hulstuk K, Mahler D, Baker WH: Late sequelae of deep venous thrombosis. *Am J Surg* 147:216–220, 1984
107. Turpie AGG, Levine MN, Hirsh J, et al: Tissue plasminogen activator versus heparin in deep vein thrombosis. *Chest* 97(suppl 4): 1725–1755, 1990
108. Goldhaber SZ: Thrombolysis in venous thromboembolism. *Chest* 97(suppl 4):1765–1815, 1990
109. Rogers LQ, Lutcher CL: Streptokinase therapy for deep vein thrombosis: A comprehensive review of the English literature. *Am J Med* 88:389–395, 1990
110. Schulman S: Studies on the medical treatment of deep vein thrombosis. *Acta Med Scand* [Suppl] 704:1–68, 1985
111. Person AV, Ekdahl KM: Treatment of acute deep venous thrombosis with fibrinolytic agents. *Med Clin North Am* 70:1325–1332, 1986
112. Hoellerick VL, Wigton RS: Diagnosing pulmonary embolism using clinical findings. *Arch Intern Med* 146:1699–1704, 1986
113. Rissanen V, Suomalainen O, Karjalainen P, et al: Screening for postoperative pulmonary embolism on the basis of clinical symptomatology, routine electrocardiography and plain chest radiography. *Acta Med Scand* 215:13–19, 1984
114. Bell WR, Simon TL, DeMets DL: The clinical features of submassive and massive pulmonary emboli. *Am J Med* 62:355–360, 1977
115. Overton DT, Bocka J: The alveolar-arterial gradient in patients with documented pulmonary embolism. *Ann Emerg Med* 16:501, 1987
116. Stein PD, Dalen JE, McIntyre KM, et al: The electrocardiogram in acute pulmonary embolism. *Prog Cardiovasc Dis* 17:247–257, 1975
117. Stahl RL, Javid JP, Lackner H: Unrecognized pulmonary embolism presenting as disseminated intravascular coagulation. *Am J Med* 76:772–778, 1984
118. Perola GR, Carlon GC: Pulmonary embolus-induced disseminated intravascular coagulation. *Crit Care Med* 15:983–984, 1987
119. Bouchania A, Curley W, Al-Dossay S, et al: Refractory hypercapnea complicating massive pulmonary embolism. *Am Rev Respir Dis* 138:466–468, 1988
120. Burki NK: The dead space to tidal volume ratio in the diagnosis of pulmonary embolism. *Am Rev Respir Dis* 133:679–685, 1986
121. Hechtman HB, Huval WV, Lelick S: Use of serotonin antagonists in the treatment of pulmonary embolus. *Resident and Staff Physician* 29:64–78, 1983
122. Dantzker DR, Bower JS: Clinician significances of pulmonary function tests: Alterations in the gas exchange following pulmonary thromboembolism. *Chest* 81:496–501, 1982

123. D'Almzo GE, Bower JS, DeHart P, et al: The mechanisms of abnormal gas exchange in acute massive pulmonary embolism. *Am Rev Respir Dis* 128:170–172, 1983
124. McIntyre KM, Sarhara AA: Hemodynamic and ventricular responses to pulmonary embolism. *Prog Cardiovasc Dis* 17:175–190, 1974
125. Miller GAH, Sutton GC: Acute massive pulmonary embolism. *Br Heart J* 32:518–523, 1970
126. Prewitt RM, Ghignone M: Treatment of right ventricular dysfunction in acute respiratory failure. *Crit Care Med* 11:346–352, 1983
127. Jardin F, Duborg O, Gueret P, et al: Quantitative two-dimensional echocardiography in massive pulmonary embolism: Emphasis in ventricular interdependencies and leftward septal displacement. *J Am Coll Cardiol* 10: 1201–1206, 1987
128. Ozier Y, Duborg O, Farcot JC, et al: Circulatory failure in acute pulmonary embolism. *Intensive Care Med* 10:91–97, 1984
129. Jardin F, Gurdjian F, Derfonds P, et al: Hemodynamic factors influencing arterial hypoxemia in massive pulmonary embolism with circulatory failure. *Circulation* 59:909–912, 1979
130. Calvin JE: Right ventricular afterload mismatch during acute pulmonary hypertension and its treatment with dobutamine: A pressure segment length analysis in a canine model. *J Crit Care* 4:239–250, 1989
131. Alpat JS, Smith R, Carlson J, et al: Mortality in patients treated for pulmonary embolism. *JAMA* 236:1477–1488, 1976
132. Belenkie I, Dani R, Smith ER, et al: Effects of volume loading during experimental pulmonary embolism. *Circulation* 80:178–188, 1989
133. McNeil BJ: Ventilation-perfusion studies and the diagnosis of pulmonary embolism: Concise communication. *J Nucl Med* 21: 319–323, 1980
134. Hull RD, Raskob GE, Coates G, et al: Clinical validity of a normal perfusion lung scan in patients with suspected pulmonary embolism. *Chest* 97:23–26, 1990
135. Hull RD, Hirsh J, Carter CJ, et al: Diagnostic value of ventilation-perfusion scanning in patients with suspected pulmonary embolism. *Chest* 97:23–26, 1985.
136. Dalen JE, Alpert JS: Natural history of pulmonary embolism. *Prog Cardiovasc Dis* 17: 259–270, 1975
137. Kahn D, Bushnell DL, Dean R, et al: Clinical outcome of patients with a "low probability" of pulmonary embolism on ventilation-perfusion lung scan. *Arch Intern Med* 194: 377–379, 1989
138. Kipper MS, Moser KM, Hortman KE, et al: Long-term follow-up of patients with suspected pulmonary embolism and a normal lung scan. *Chest* 82:411–415, 1987
139. Piers DB, Verziglberger F, Westerman CJJ, et al: A comparative study of intravenous digital subtraction angiography and ventilation-perfusion scans in suspected pulmonary embolism. *Chest* 91:837–843, 1987
140. Hull R, Hirsh J, Carter CJ, et al: Pulmonary angiography, ventilation lung scanning and venography for clinically suspected pulmonary embolism with abnormal perfusion lung scan. *Ann Intern Med* 98:891–899, 1983
141. Novellini RA, Baltarowich OH, Athanasoulis CA, et al: The clinical course of patients with suspected pulmonary embolism and a negative arteriogram. *Radiology* 126:561–567, 1978
142. Pond GD, Ovitt TW, Capp MP: Comparison of conventional pulmonary angiography with intravenous digital subtraction angiography for pulmonary embolic diseases. *Radiology* 147:345–350, 1983
143. Ludwig LW, Verhoeven LAJ, Kersbergen JJ, et al: Digital subtraction angiography of the pulmonary arteries for the diagnosis of pulmonary embolism. *Radiology* 174:639–645, 1983
144. Doughtery JE, LaSala AF, Fieldman A: Bedside pulmonary angiography utilizing an existing Swan-Ganz catheter. *Chest* 77:43–46, 1980
145. Albador J, Niewenhaus HK, Sixma JJ: Treatment of acute venous thromboembolism with low molecular weight heparin (fragmin). *Circulation* 80:935–940, 1989
146. Sherry S, Bell WR, Duckert FH, et al: Thrombolytic therapy in thrombosis. *Ann Intern Med* 93:141–144, 1980
147. Terrin M, Goldhaber SZ: Selection of patients with acute pulmonary embolism for thrombolytic therapy. *Chest* 95(suppl 5): 279S–281S, 1989
148. Risius B, Zelch MG, Giaor RA, et al: Catheter-directed low dose streptokinase: A preliminary experience. *Radiology* 150:349–355, 1984
149. PIOPED Investigators: Tissue plasminogen activator for the treatment of acute pulmonary embolism. *Chest* 97:528–533, 1990
150. Goldhaber SZ: Tissue plasminogen activator in acute pulmonary embolism. *Chest* 95(suppl 5):282S–289S, 1989
151. Sharma GVRK, Cella G, Parisi AR, et al: Thrombolytic therapy. *N Engl J Med* 306: 1268–1276, 1982
152. Persson AV, Robichaux WT, Jaxheimer EC, et al: Burst therapy. *Am J Surg* 147:531–536, 1984

153. Marder VJ, Sherry S: Thrombolytic therapy: Current status (Parts 1 & 2). *N Engl J Med* 318:23–24, 1988
153a. Alpert JS, Smith RE, Ochine IS, et al: Treatment of massive pulmonary embolism: The role of pulmonary embolectomy. *Am Heart J* 89:414–418, 1975
154. Saulter RD, Meyers WO, Ray JF, et al: Pulmonary embolectomy: Review and current status. *Prog Cardiovasc Dis* 17:371, March/April 1975
155. Bomalaski JS, Martin GJ, Hughes RL, et al: Inferior vena cava interruption in the management of pulmonary embolism. *Chest* 82:335–339, 1982
156. Kempczinski RF: Surgical prophylaxis of pulmonary embolism. *Chest* 89(suppl 5):384S–388S, 1986
157. Crane C: Venous interruption for pulmonary embolism: Present states. *Prog Cardiovasc Dis* 17:329–333, 1975
158. Miller TD, Staats BA: Impaired exercise tolerance after inferior vena cava interruption. *Chest* 93:776–780, 1988
159. Kanter B, Moser KM: The Greenfield vena cava filter. *Chest* 93:170–175, 1988
160. Welch TJ, Stanson AW, Sheedy PF, et al: Percutaneous placement of the Greenfield vena cava filter. *Mayo Clin Proc* 63:343–347, 1988
161. Mobin-Uddin K, Utley JR, Bryant LR: The inferior vena cava umbrella filter. *Prog Cardiovasc Dis* 17:391–399, 1975
162. Halstuk K, Mahler D, Baker WH: Late sequelae of deep venous thrombosis. *Am J Surg* 147:216–220, 1989
163. Monreal M, Ruiz J, Salvador R, et al: Recurrent pulmonary embolism. *Chest* 976–979, 1989
164. Rich S, Sevitsky S, Brundage BH: Pulmonary hypertension from chronic pulmonary thromboembolism. *Ann Intern Med* 108:425–434, 1988
165. Palevsky HI, Schloo BL, Pretra GG, et al: Primary pulmonary hypertension. *Circulation* 80:1207–1221, 1989
166. Moser KM: Primary pulmonary hypertension. *In* Manual of Clinical Problems in Pulmonary Medicine. Boston, Little, Brown, 1985
167. Ashutosh K, Dunsky M: Noninvasive tests for responsiveness of pulmonary hypertension to oxygen. *Chest* 92:393–399, 1987
168. Prins MH, Hirsh J: A critical review of the evidence supporting a relationship between impaired fibrinolytic activity and venous thromboembolism. *Arch Intern Med* 151:1721–1731, 1991
169. Council on Scientific Affairs: Doppler sonographic imaging of the vascular system. *JAMA* 265:2382–2387, 1991
170. Chance JF, Abbit PL, Tegtmeyer CS, Powers RD: Real-time ultrasound for the detection of deep venous thrombosis. *Ann Emerg Med* 20:494–499, 1991
171. Monreal M, Lafoz E, Ruiz J, et al: Upper-extremity deep venous thrombosis and pulmonary embolism. *Chest* 99:280–283, 1991
172. Becker DM, Philbrick JT, Walker FB: Axillary and subclavian venous thrombosis. *Arch Intern Med* 151:1934–1943, 1991
173. Lensing AW, Leir MM, Buller HR, et al: Diagnosis of deep-vein thrombosis using objective Doppler method. *Ann Intern Med* 113:9–12, 1990
174. Hirsh J: Heparin. *N Engl J Med* 324(22):1565–1574, 1991.
175. Hirsh J: Oral anticoagulant drugs. *N Engl J Med* 324(26):1865–1875, 1991
176. Williams JF, Seneff MG, Friedman BC, et al: Use of femoral venous catheters in critically ill adults: Prospective study. *Crit Care Med* 19:550–553, 1991
177. Landefeld CS, McGuire E, Rosenblatt MW: A bleeding risk index for estimating the probability of major bleeding in hospitalized patients.
178. Francis CW, Marder VJ: Fibrinolytic therapy for venous thrombosis. *Prog Cardiovasc Dis* 34:193–204, 1991.
179. Agnelli G, Parise: Bolus thrombolysis in venous thromboembolism. *Chest* 101(4S):172S–182S, 1992
180. Elliot CG: Pulmonary physiology during pulmonary embolism. *Chest* 101:163S–171S, 1992
181. Prewitt RM: Hemodynamic management in pulmonary embolism and acute hypoxemic respiratory failure. *Crit Care Med* 18(1S):S61–S69, 1990
182. Mitchell JP, Trulock EP: Tissue-plasminogen activator for pulmonary embolism resulting in shock. Two case reports and discussion of the literature. *Am J Med* 90:255–260, 1991
183. Goldhaber SZ: Evolving concepts in thrombolytic therapy for pulmonary embolism. *Chest* 101(4S):183S–185S, 1992
184. Sherry S: Thrombolytic therapy for noncoronary diseases. *Ann Emerg Med* 20(4):396–404, 1991
185. Calvin JE: Acute right heart failure: Pathophysiology, recognition and pharmacological management. *J Cardiothorac Vasc Anesth* 5:507–513, 1991
186. Anderson FA, Wheeler HB, Goldberg RS, et al: Physician practices in the prevention of venous thromboembolism. *Ann Intern Med* 115:591–595, 1991

187. Shandness C Jr: Duplex scanning in vascular disorders. Raven Press, 1990, 167–183.
188. Alderson, PO, et al: Tc-99m-DTPA aerosol and radioactive gases compared as adjuncts to perfusion scintigraphy in patients with suspected pulmonary embolism. *Radiology* 153:515–521, 1984
189. Hull, R, et al: Diagnostic value of ventilation-perfusion lung scanning in patients with suspected pulmonary embolism. *Chest* 88:819–828, 1985
190. Rembold CM: Posttest probability calculation by weights. *Ann Intern Med* 108, 1988
191. Levine MN, Hirsh J, Gent M, et al: Prevention of deep vein thrombosis after elective hip surgery. *Ann Intern Med* 114:545–551, 1990

Chronic Interstitial Pulmonary Disorders

Joseph P. Lynch III and Anthony D. Chavis

The interstitial lung disorders are a heterogeneous group of diseases characterized by a spectrum of inflammatory and fibrotic changes affecting alveolar walls and airspaces [1–5]. Clinical manifestations are protean, but progressive cough, dyspnea, interstitial infiltrates on chest radiographs, and loss of pulmonary function are characteristic. More than 100 causes of interstitial lung disease (ILD) have been identified and include disorders in which specific agents or antigens have been identified (e.g., pneumoconioses, asbestosis, silicosis, berylliosis, granulomatous infections, hypersensitivity pneumonitis, neoplasm) as well as a host of disorders in which the etiology (or inciting stimulus) is not known [1–3]. The wide spectrum of ILD has been well reviewed in previous publications [1–3]. In this chapter, we discuss in detail several specific ILDs, with an emphasis on features common to these disorders, as well as features that distinguish these disease entities. Lung biopsy (transbronchial or open) is usually required as part of the initial evaluation of ILD, as multiple diverse etiologies may display similar clinical and radiographic features (Fig. 11-1A and B). Increased numbers of activated inflammatory cells within alveolar structures may be observed in many ILDs and may be critical to the development of lung injury, pulmonary fibrosis, and late sequelae. Open lung biopsy has traditionally been used as the gold standard to assess the extent of inflammatory and fibrotic components in idiopathic pulmonary fibrosis (IPF) and other ILD [4–6]. More recently, ancillary techniques including bronchoalveolar lavage (BAL) [1–3, 6], gallium scanning [1–3, 6], and thin-section chest computed tomographic (CT) scanning [7–9] have provided significant insights into the pathogenic mechanisms that operate in ILD and a common framework for devising rational therapeutic strategies. In the following section, we discuss in detail data gleaned from BAL, not to imply that strategies should be based on BAL (which they should not), but to provide insight into the evolution of our understanding of these complex and rare disorders. Since many of the distinguishing features of ILD rely on subtle differences in histopathologic features, we also define in detail specific histopathologic features characteristic of each of the various diseases, in order to stress the importance of a close working relationship with a competent pulmonary pathologist. The initial section describes IPF, a disease whose clinical and histopathologic features overlap with several other ILDs. This provides a framework on which the remaining sections of the chapter rest.

Idiopathic Pulmonary Fibrosis

IPF is an inflammatory interstitial lung disease of uncertain etiology in which clinical and radiographic features overlap with many other ILDs [6, 10]. The estimated prevalence is 3 to 5 cases per 100,000, with a slight male predominance [6, 10]. Most cases occur in the fifth through seventh decades of life, although young adults and children may also be affected [1–3, 6]. The literature may be confusing, as a variety of synonymous terms have been applied to this disorder, including diffuse interstitial pulmonary fibrosis, cryptogenic fibrosing alveolitis, interstitial pneumonitis, usual interstitial pneumonitis (UIP),

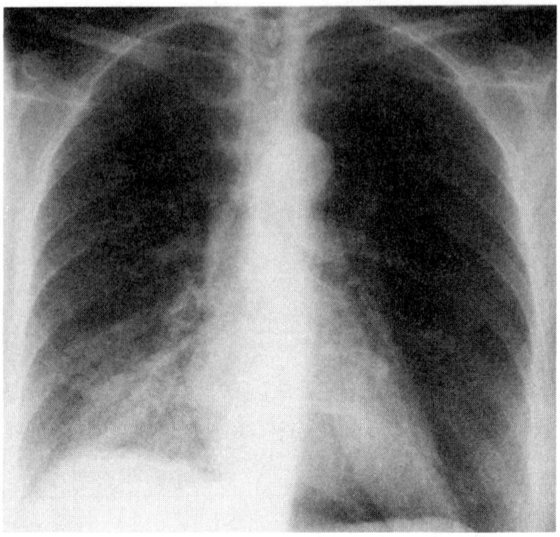

A

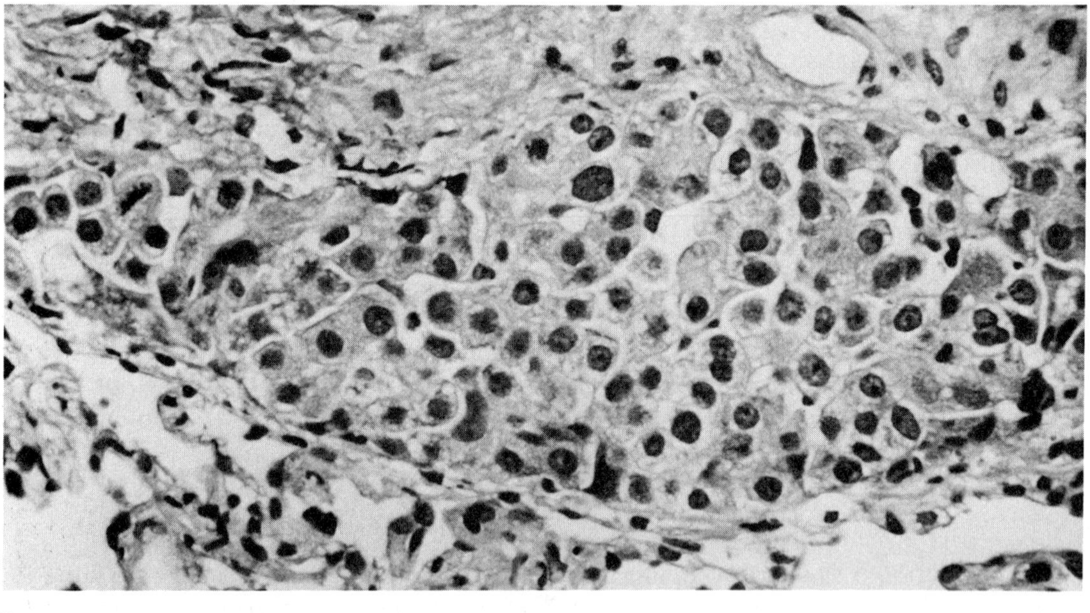

B

Fig. 11-1. (A) Lymphangitic carcinomatosis. Chest radiograph demonstrating an alveolar infiltrate involving the right lower lung field superimposed on a diffuse miliary pattern scattered throughout all lung fields in a 64-year-old woman. One year earlier, an interstitial process involving the right lower lobe had been noted, but no biopsy was obtained. Because of progression of the process to involve both lung fields, she was referred for evaluation. Fiberoptic bronchoscopy with TBB and BAL demonstrated malignant cells consistent with adenocarcinoma. (B) Photomicrograph from transbronchial lung biopsy demonstrating adenocarcinoma cells filling a pulmonary lymphatic (hematoxylin-eosin, high power).

and desquamative interstitial pneumonitis (DIP) [6, 10–18]. As is discussed later, UIP and DIP reflect different histologic stages of the disorder and should not be construed as distinct disease entities.

Clinical Signs and Symptoms

Initial symptoms are dyspnea and a nonproductive cough. Malaise, fatigue, and weight loss may occur, but specific extrapulmonary features are lacking. Fever has been reported in fewer than 5% of cases and usually reflects an alternative diagnosis. A chronic course is characteristic, with progressive cough and dyspnea over several months or years. In many instances, the cough, which can be protracted, paroxysmal, and debilitating, may be the presenting complaint. The development of dyspnea may be insidious. Initially, dyspnea may be noted only with vigorous activity and may result in the patients' curtailing or restricting their activities. With progression of the disease, dyspnea is evident even at rest and may be disabling. Ultimately, patients may be bedridden or wheelchair-bound by the extreme dyspnea and exercise limitation. It is critical for the physician to be diligent and aggressive in recognizing the disease before development of severe and irreversible damage and initiating aggressive therapy. Certain findings on physical examination are helpful clues to the diagnosis. Bibasilar end-inspiratory ("Velcro") rales can be demonstrated in over 90% of cases [6, 10]. Unfortunately, basilar rales are often dismissed by the examining physician as one of the accompaniments of aging, and the diagnosis is missed. The presence of unexplained rales that fail to clear on coughing should prompt a chest radiograph (at a minimum) to exclude ILD. With progression of the disease, the rales may progress to involve all lobes of the lung, extending even into the apices. Digital clubbing (see Chap. 3), a feature rarely found in other ILDs, occurs in 10% to 25% of cases of IPF [6, 10, 16]. Cyanosis, an accentuated pulmonary second sound (P_2), right ventricular heave S_3 gallop, and peripheral edema may be late findings when pulmonary hypertension and cor pulmonale have developed [6, 10, 16].

Natural History

The course of IPF is characterized by gradual, but relentless, progression to respiratory failure and even death, within 2 to 8 years. Mortality at 5 years has been 30% to 50% in most series [6, 10, 14–18], with most deaths occurring as a result of respiratory failure or cor pulmonale. The clinical course is variable, however, and a wide spectrum of disease exists. A fulminant course, with fatal respiratory failure developing within several weeks or months, has also been described and has been termed the Hamman-Rich syndrome. Occasionally the course is benign and the disease stabilizes or "burns out," leading to minimal or no symptoms or pulmonary dysfunction. While such patients likely would not require therapy, it is not possible to identify them at the outset, and we do not advocate withholding therapy because this occurs in a small subset of patients. However, a conservative approach is sometimes justified in patients in whom disease has been present for several years (by retrospective analysis of old radiographs or pulmonary function tests [PFTs]) and stable, with minimal or no symptoms for prolonged periods of time (> 2 years). In such cases, we have sometimes deferred open lung biopsy or therapy and reevaluated symptoms, chest radiographs, and PFTs serially at 6-month intervals. This practice is not recommended for newly diagnosed cases or patients with significant symptoms, pulmonary dysfunction, or disease progression, as the chance for substantial recovery may be lost by excessive delays in therapy. It should be emphasized that spontaneous remissions do not occur in IPF. Thus, in contrast to sarcoidosis, where a period of observation may be warranted before initiation of specific therapy, early diagnosis and treatment are necessary in IPF to avert late fibrosis and mortality.

Chest Radiography

Abnormalities on chest radiographs are present in over 95% of cases [4, 6, 15]. Reduced lung volumes and diffuse interstitial infiltrates on chest radiographs are characteristic, with a bibasilar predominance (Fig. 11-2). The process is usually diffuse and relatively symmetric, and strictly unilateral disease is exceptionally rare. Intrathoracic lymphadenopathy, cavities, and pleural effusions are not found in IPF and suggest an alternative diagnosis. The value of chest radiography as an indicator of extent or activity of disease is limited, as the degree of radiographic changes does not correlate with the degree of fibrosis (as assessed by open lung biopsy), pulmonary dysfunction, or responsiveness to therapy [6, 19]. Distinct patterns of radiographic parenchymal abnormalities (alveolar, reticular, reticulonodular, or honeycombing) have been described, however, and may have prognostic significance. The most com-

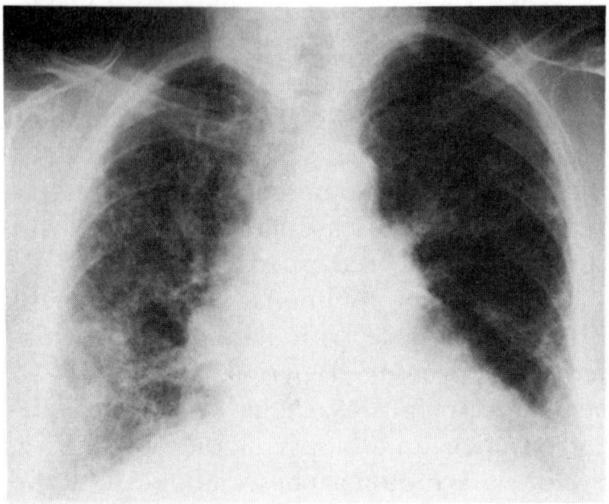

Fig. 11-2. Idiopathic pulmonary fibrosis. Chest radiograph from a 72-year-old woman with IPF demonstrating diffuse reticulonodular and alveolar infiltrates with a slight right-sided predominance.

mon radiographic pattern in IPF is termed *reticular* or *interstitial,* which is characterized by fine, lacy, horizontal lines distributed throughout the lung fields. When small (1 to 3 mm) nodules are superimposed on these horizontal lines, this has been termed *reticulonodular.* These reticular or reticulonodular shadows may reflect either inflammatory cells or fibrosis within the alveolar interstitium and are of uncertain prognostic significance. A more diffuse opacification of the alveolar structures, termed *alveolar, acinar,* or *ground glass,* typifies alveolar filling with inflammatory cells and has been associated with an earlier phase of the disease (alveolitis) and a more favorable response to corticosteroids [6, 20]. Diffuse, cystic radiolucencies, ranging from 3 to 15 mm in diameter, termed *honeycombing,* reflect destruction of the lung architecture and end-stage fibrosis and predict a poor response to therapy. To the extent that a dominant radiographic pattern can be recognized, invaluable prognostic information may be gleaned from chest radiography. However, in many cases, overlapping radiographic patterns coexist. Thus, the ability to predict prognosis or therapeutic responsiveness by chest radiography is poor, as one cannot reliably distinguish alveolitis (which may respond to therapy) from fibrosis (which is unlikely to respond to aggressive therapy). Nevertheless, serial chest radiographs are important, to better assess disease progression, or regression, over time. Thus, when a patient with IPF initially presents to the physician, prior chest radiographs (even dating back for years) should be obtained and scrutinized to determine the course of the disease. The role of chest CT scanning in the staging and management of IPF continues to evolve and remains controversial. Chest CT provides much greater detail than conventional chest radiography and appears to be more accurate in discriminating alveolitis from fibrosis, particularly when thin-section (1 to 3 mm) CT scans are used [7–9]. Because of the limited availability, expense, and radiation exposure with sequential CT scans, the precise application of thin-section CT needs to be defined in prospective studies.

Pulmonary Function

PFTs typically demonstrate reductions in lung volumes (e.g., vital capacity [VC] and total lung capacity [TLC]) and diffusing capacity for carbon monoxide (DLCO) [6, 10, 14, 21, 22]. The DLCO is the most sensitive marker of the disease, and reductions in DLCO may be evident early in the course of the disease when lung volumes are still normal [22]. Expiratory flow rates (FEV_1, $FEF_{25\text{-}75}$) are preserved and often supranormal, which may distinguish IPF from sarcoidosis and other ILDs in which a concomitant obstructive component may coexist. Arterial hypoxemia is present in most patients at rest and can be demonstrated in over 90% of cases following exercise [6, 10, 22]. This nearly invariable hypoxemia observed with IPF also distinguishes this disorder from other ILDs (e.g., sarcoidosis) in which hypoxemia is absent except in far advanced, severe cases. PFTs (e.g., spirometry, lung volumes, DLCO) are important to assess the degree of functional impairment, but cannot differentiate alveolitis from fibrosis [1–3, 6]. More sophisticated measurements of pulmonary function, such as compliance, which requires the use of an esophageal balloon, or exercise testing, may provide a more accurate determination of active inflammation according to some investigators [6, 10, 22], but are cumbersome, moderately difficult for some patients to perform, and their routine applicability in the staging of ILD remains controversial. Watters and coworkers [21] demonstrated that resting alveolar-arterial oxygen gradient, forced vital capacity, and gas exchange at exercise correlated with pathologic changes on open lung biopsy, but combining clinical, radiographic, and pathologic data into a composite scoring index (CRP score) correlated best with pathological findings. CRP score may offer a more quantitative and reproducible method of longitudinally evaluating patients, but additional long-term studies assessing greater numbers of patients are required to determine its role in the management of IPF.

Histopathology

IPF is characterized by thickening, distortion, and eventual destruction of the alveolar septae by a chronic inflammatory alveolitis [3, 6, 15]. A chronic interstitial inflammatory cellular infiltrate, comprised largely of mononuclear cells (lymphocytes, plasma cells, mononuclear phagocytes), but with an admixture of neutrophils and eosinophils, is characteristic [3, 6, 15]. In the early phases of the disease, the alveolar septae may be thickened and edematous by the chronic interstitial inflammatory infiltrate, with overall preservation of the alveolar architecture. However, in late phases, the lung architecture is disrupted, and an exuberant fibrotic scar remains. The process typically is heterogeneous, with areas of intense inflammation as well as dense fibrosis interspersed even within the same biopsy (Fig. 11-3A to 3D). Fibroblasts and excessive deposition of collagen are usually prominent. The deposition of collagen can be best appreciated when special stains with an affinity for collagen (such as Masson's trichrome) are used [6, 10]. With progression of the fibrosis, only remnants of normal alveolar architecture remain. Destruction of the alveolar walls may lead to extensive cysts and microbullae, which are most evident in the periphery of the lung. This final phase of alveolar destruction, referred to as *honeycomb lung,* is not specific for IPF, as this may be observed in any severe destructive ILD leading to extensive fibrosis. While involvement of the pulmonary vasculature is indirect, smooth muscle hyperplasia and changes consistent with pulmonary hypertension may be noted when cor pulmonale is present [6, 10, 15].

The extreme heterogeneity of the disease process, with areas of fibrosis and inflammation present concomitantly in individual patients, has made assessment of disease activity and prognosis difficult, particularly when small biopsy specimens are analyzed. Because of these limitations, transbronchial lung biopsy is not adequate on which to base decisions regarding intensity of alveolar inflammation or fibrosis. For this reason, a surgical (open) lung biopsy is usually appropriate as part of the initial staging of IPF, not only to confirm the diagnosis, but also to better define the inflammatory and fibrotic components [3–6, 20]. Open lung biopsy provides the most information regarding prognosis and potential responsiveness to therapy, but even its value is controversial. The degree of fibrosis on open lung biopsy has been shown to correlate inversely with prognosis by most investigators [1–3, 6, 15, 20], but occasional favorable responses to therapy have been achieved even in the presence of severe interstitial fibrosis. Some studies have demonstrated that biopsies demonstrating an intensely cellular infiltrate suggest an earlier phase of the disease and greater responsiveness to therapy [3, 6], but conflicting data exist [17, 20]. The mix of cellular and fibrotic reactions may be great, with areas of striking cellular infiltration interspersed with areas of severe fibrosis [20]. From a practical standpoint, this makes clinical decisions based solely on open lung biopsy difficult and potentially erroneous. Owing to the limitations in predicting prognosis by conventional histologic criteria, Liebow and associates developed a classification schema that incorporated UIP and DIP as separate entities [11, 13]. UIP referred to the usual or classical his-

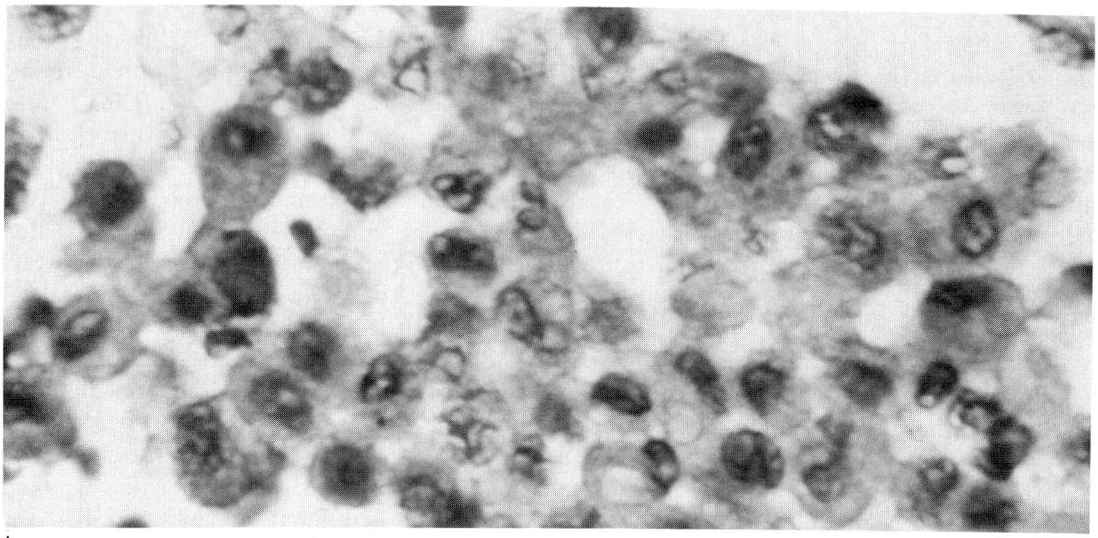
A

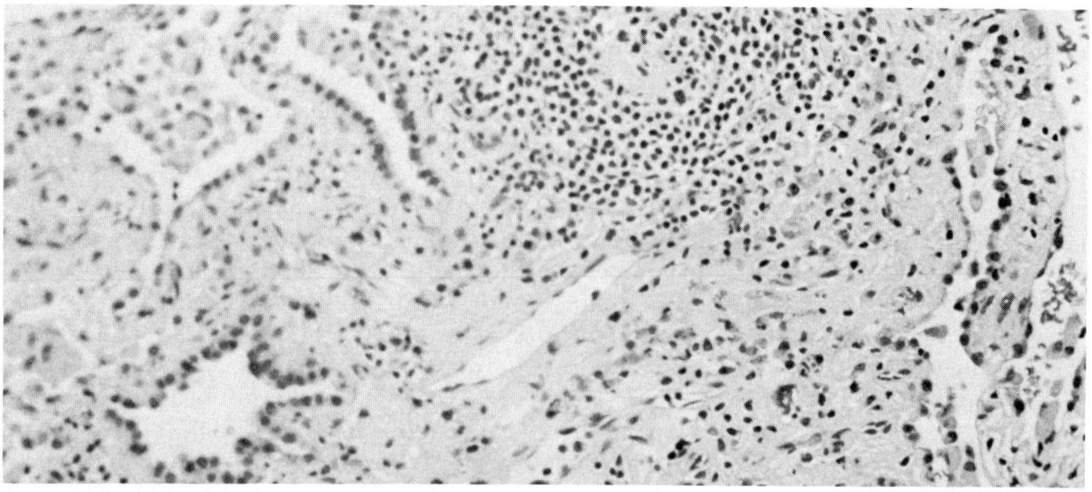
B

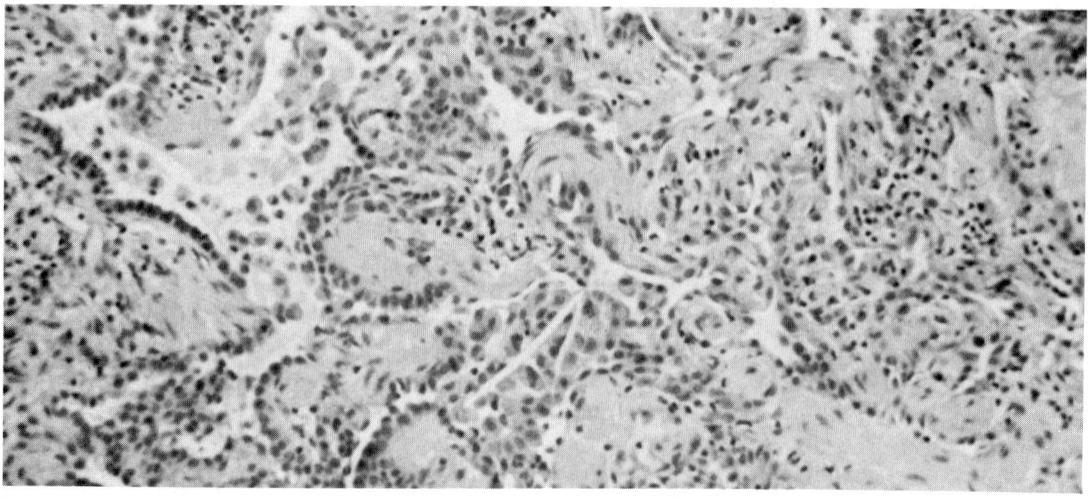
C

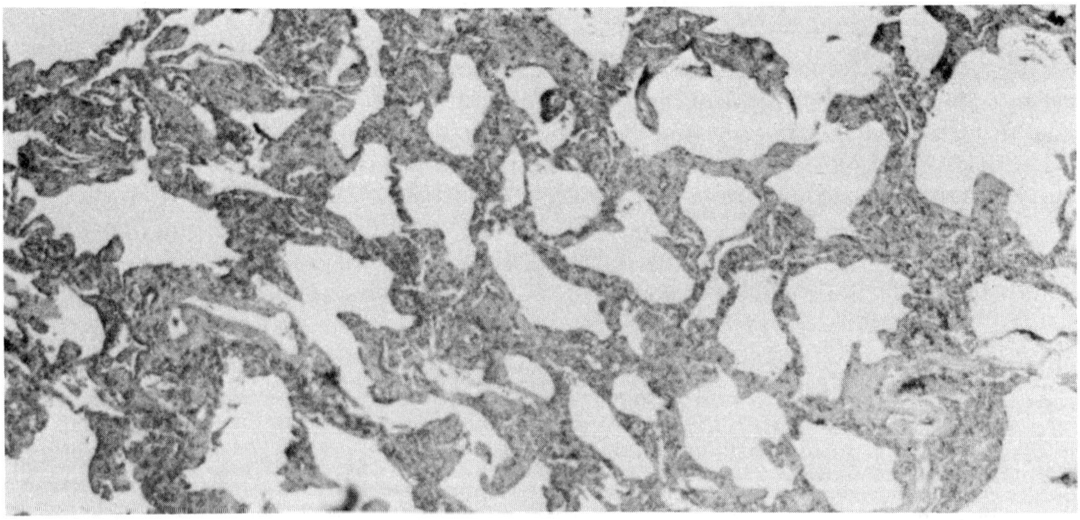

D

Fig. 11-3. (A) Desquamative interstitial pneumonitis. Photomicrograph from open lung biopsy demonstrates filling of alveolar spaces with alveolar macrophages, consistent with an alveolitis phase of IPF (hematoxylin-eosin, oil immersion). (B) IPF. Photomicrograph from open lung biopsy demonstrating thickening and distortion of the alveolar structures, and prominent lymphoid cellular infiltrates. Foci of DIP are also present, with intra-alveolar macrophages (hematoxylin-eosin, high power). (C) IPF. Photomicrograph from open lung biopsy demonstrating distortion of the alveolar architecture, scattered inflammatory cells, and smooth muscle hyperplasia within the alveolar interstitium. These changes are characteristic of IPF in the advanced stages (hematoxylin-eosin, high power). (D) IPF. Photomicrograph from open lung biopsy demonstrating extensive cystic structures from damaged alveolar walls, consistent with honeycomb lung. There is a paucity of inflammatory cells at this late stage (hematoxylin-eosin, low power).

tological variety of IPF, with striking heterogeneity, prominent interstitial mononuclear cell infiltrates, few intra-alveolar cells, and extensive destruction and disruption of the alveolar architecture [11, 13]. By contrast, DIP was a more homogeneous process in which a pronounced intra-alveolar component existed, with collections of free alveolar macrophages within airspaces, associated with minimal or no necrosis and relative preservation of the alveolar architecture [11, 13] (Fig. 11-3A). In a classic study that subdivided cases into those confidently classified as either UIP or DIP, it was shown that DIP had a distinctly more favorable prognosis and responsiveness to corticosteroid therapy compared with UIP [11]. However, as was evident from that and later studies, the differentiation of UIP and DIP is frequently not possible, as foci of both UIP and DIP frequently coexist in individual patients [6, 20]. It has now become apparent that DIP and UIP simply represent different histologic expressions of the same disease. DIP represents an earlier phase of the process, before advanced fibrosis or alveolar destruction, whereas UIP represents a later phase. While we agree that patients exhibiting predominantly DIP are likely to have a better prognosis than those with predominantly UIP, this classification scheme has limited value as an independent prognostic indicator.

Role of Lung Biopsy

Open lung biopsy represents the gold standard for assessing the extent of alveolar inflammatory and fibrotic components and should usually be performed as part of the initial dignostic evaluation. A standard thoracotomy incision, however, is not required because the lung parenchyma can be adequately assessed and sampled via a small (8 to 12 cm) axillary incision (a minithoracotomy) in most instances. In order to provide optimal prognostic information from the surgical biopsy, two or more sites (preferably from separate lobes) should be biopsied. The surgeon should sample representative areas, rather than the most seriously involved or most normal areas. Controversies exist, however, as to the true merits of open lung biopsy in this disorder, given the tremendous heterogeneity of the histopathology of IPF and the possibility of sampling error even when 2 to 3 cm sections of lung are obtained. How much fibrosis on open lung biopsy contraindicates a trial of therapy is far from clear, and most clinicians are unwilling to withhold therapy in patients exhibiting a progressively downhill course, irrespective of findings on open lung biopsy. In addition, open lung biopsy has potential morbidity (including the need for general anesthesia, prolonged discomfort at the thoracotomy site, potential for prolonged air leak, etc.). Following open lung biopsy, corticosteroid therapy usually needs to be deferred for 10 to 14 days to permit wound healing and prevent complications such as wound dehiscence, local infections, and disruption of the suture lines. Percutaneous trephine needle biopsies have been performed in lieu of open biopsy by some investigators, but experience with this procedure is limited and has been associated with a high complication rate, including some fatalities. Before proceeding with open lung biopsy, we usually perform fiberoptic bronchoscopy with transbronchial lung biopsy (TBB), primarily to exclude other causes of ILD. Owing to the small sample size obtained by TBB (2 to 4 mm), TBB is not adequate to determine the extent of alveolitis or fibrosis nor can TBB definitively establish the diagnosis of IPF, as foci of interstitial fibrosis or inflammation may be observed in a wide spectrum of other pulmonary disorders. Despite these important limitations, TBB is a reasonable first step in the invasive evaluation of ILD, as TBB may establish a specific etiologic diagnosis in other ILDs mimicking IPF such as sarcoidosis, eosinophilic granuloma, eosinophilic pneumonia, pulmonary alveolar proteinosis, carcinomatosis, and other disorders to be discussed elsewhere in this chapter. In addition, chronic pulmonary infections due to *Pneumocystis carinii* (in patients with acquired immunodeficiency syndrome), *mycobacteria* (both typical and atypical mycobacteria), and fungi may present with clinical and radiographic features indistinguishable from IPF. All of these diseases may bc diagnosed by TBB. In such cases, substantiation of a specific histologic diagnosis by TBB may eliminate the need for open lung biopsy. However, when a specific etiology is not demonstrated by TBB, an open lung biopsy should be done unless specific contraindications exist. In some cases, however, the morbidity associated with open lung biopsy appears excessive for the anticipated yield; in that context, TBB may be a reasonable alternative. For example, we have often deferred open lung biopsy in very elderly or severely debilitated patients with classical and longstanding clinical and radiographic changes consistent with IPF, in whom alternative diagnoses are highly unlikely. In this context, when patients exhibit progressive disease and therapy is being considered, we proceed with TBB and BAL to include smears and cultures for acid fast bacilli and fungi, and (if no alternative etiology is identified) initiate empirical treatment with corticosteroids and/or immunosuppressive/cytotoxic agents for a 3- to 6-month trial.

Pathogenesis

While the precise mechanisms initiating the fibrotic process in IPF have not been clarified, IPF is characterized by an alveolitis in which activated alveolar macrophages (AMs) and neutrophils appear to have pivotal roles in the pathogenesis of the lung lesion [1–3, 6]. Nonimmune cells, such as fibroblasts, interstitial cells, and endothelial cells, may also play critical (albeit poorly defined) roles in the fibrotic and inflammatory process. BAL has provided invaluable insights into the nature of the inflammatory alveolitis. Increases in the numbers and percent of BAL neutrophils, and occasionally eosinophils, with normal lymphocytes, are characteristic [6, 12, 23, 24]. The neutrophil has a armamentarium of potentially toxic products, including of proteolytic enzymes and oxygen radicals and likely plays some role in the induction of lung injury. Increases in eosinophils have been associated with more extensive fibrosis [23, 25–27]; it is possible that the eosinophil may represent a bystander cell or epiphenomenon, but the eosinophil also is capable of inducing lung injury. Increases in immunoglobulin G (IgG), IgG-secreting cells, immune complexes, neutrophil collagenase, activated AMs, and AM products fibronectin, AM-derived growth factors have also been demonstrated by BAL [1–3]. These latter AM-derived products may amplify the fibrotic process by their ability to recruit fibroblasts and enhance their proliferation [1–3]. Immune complexes have been demonstrated in serum, BAL, and in lung tissue in patients with IPF, particularly when a cellular inflammatory component is present, suggesting that intrapulmonary deposition of immune complexes may be an early event in the pathogenesis of the lung lesion [3, 28, 29]. While the stimulus (or stimuli) that initiates inflammatory cell influx into the lower respiratory tract is not known, inhaled antigen(s) may elicit the formation of immune complexes, which then activate local immune effector cells (e.g., AMs, polymorphonuclear neutrophils [PMNs]) and propagate the inflammatory process. The end result depends on the persistence of the injurious agents (inflammatory cells, mediators, immune complexes, antigens) and the ability of the host to initiate repair.

Role of New Techniques (Gallium Scanning and Bronchoalveolar Lavage)

Gallium Scanning

Since traditional parameters such as clinical scores, chest radiographs, and PFTs do not reliably discriminate between alveolitis and fibrosis, additional staging techniques such as gallium scanning and BAL have been used. Increased intrapulmonary uptake of Ga 67 has been demonstrated in a variety of pulmonary inflammatory disorders (including IPF) and appears to better reflect the degree of alveolitis as compared with clinical scores or chest radiographs [1–3, 6, 19]. The clinical value of gallium scanning, however, has not been demonstrated. Several investigators have confirmed that intrapulmonary uptake of Ga 67 correlates with a more cellular (alveolitis) phase of the disorder [3, 6, 19, 29], but recent studies have failed to demonstrate that gallium scans are useful in predicting prognosis or responsiveness to therapy [29, 30]. Although increased intrapulmonary uptake of gallium may suggest an active inflammatory component, a negative scan result does not exclude alveolitis. We have observed favorable responses to therapy in individual patients despite negative gallium scan results. Thus, a negative gallium scan result is not sufficient to justify withholding therapy in patients with a deteriorating course. Unfortunately, gallium scanning is expensive, inconvenient (scanning is done 48 hours after injection of the radioisotope), and involves exposure to a radionuclide. Moreover, it is difficult to extrapolate data derived from research centers to community hospitals, because of differences in techniques, quantitation, and reproducibility and interobserver variability. For these reasons, we do not believe that routine gallium scanning is warranted in the diagnosis or staging of IPF.

Bronchoalveolar Lavage

Despite initial enthusiasm for the role of BAL as a guide to disease activity and prognosis [6], its clinical value remains highly controversial. An initial study from the National Institutes of Health described the BAL characteristics among 19 patients with IPF; increases in percent PMNs (mean of 33%), eosinophils, and IgG, with normal lymphocytes, were demonstrated on BAL [6]. A subsequent study from that institution of 27 patients with IPF noted similar findings but more importantly, decreases in BAL neutrophils and IgG were observed in six of seven patients after initiation of corticosteroid therapy [24]. This raised the possibility that BAL findings may have prognostic significance. British investigators also reported increases in BAL neutrophil and eosinophil counts in 51 patients with IPF, but noted that BAL cell counts did not reliably predict prognosis or therapeutic responsiveness [14]. BAL neutrophil counts did not discriminate between responders or nonresponders, and BAL eosinophilia suggested a worse prognosis. In addition, occasional patients exhibited BAL lymphocytosis, which was associated with an improved prognosis and greater responsiveness to corticosteroids [14, 23]. The role of BAL in the staging and management of IPF remains a hotly contested area. However, several investigators have corroborated that BAL lymphocytosis has been associated with an improved prognosis, whereas the degree of neutrophilic elevation on BAL does not influence prognosis [14, 23, 27, 29, 31]. Two prospective studies have found that increases in BAL lymphocytes have been associated with improved prognosis and responsiveness to corticosteroids [27, 31]. Watters et al [31] demonstrated that increased BAL lymphocytes correlated with less honeycombing on chest radiography and a more favorable response to corticosteroids. Turner-Warwick and Haslam [27] noted that the absence of BAL lymphocytosis predicted a poor response to corticosteroids (only 3 of 23 responded) whereas more than half of these patients responded to cytotoxic agents. While additional data involving larger numbers of patients would be welcome, it appears that BAL lymphocytosis identifies a more responsive subset of patients. As a corollary, the low rate of steroid responsiveness among subsets of patients failing to exhibit BAL lymphocytosis suggests that cytotoxic agents may be appropriate as first-line therapy in this context.

Therapy

Because chronic inflammatory alveolitis leads to injury and derangement of the alveolar structures, agents that ablate the inflammatory component are the mainstays of therapy. Agents that may inhibit collagen synthesis or cross-linking, such as D-penicillamine, have also been tried, but fewer data are available. Glucocorticoids, which exert potent and relatively global inhibitory effects on immune responses, have been used most often. However, favorable responses have been achieved in only 20% to 30% of cases in most series [8, 10, 14–17, 27, 31], although higher responses have been achieved when treatment is initiated within 12 to 18 months of the onset of symptoms [14, 20]. Results have been variable, however, owing to heterogeneity in patient populations, differences in the timing, dose, and duration of corticosteroid therapy, and criteria for response. The optimal dose and duration of therapy has not been delineated and multiple treatment regimens have been advocated. Most investigators have initiated therapy with prednisone (or the equivalent), 1 mg/kg/d for the first 4 to 12 weeks, with a subsequent taper. Unfortunately, no studies directly comparing doses of steroids have been done, so the optimal dose has not been defined. We believe that doses of corticosteroids in the range of 50 to 80 mg of prednisone (or the equivalent) for the first 4 to 12 weeks are appropriate, as lower doses in the initial phase of therapy may not be adequate to determine a therapeutic effect. However, these high doses of corticosteroids, while reasonably well tolerated in young patients, may be associated with disabling side effects in elderly patients, due to osteoporosis, vertebral compression fractures, glucose intolerance, emotional lability (confusion, depression, disorientation), etc. Owing to the high failure rate with corticosteroids alone and the high rate of steroid complications, other immunosuppressive agents (e.g., azathioprine, cyclophosphamide, D-penicillamine) have also been used, with anecdotal successes [14, 18, 20, 32, 33]. In one early study, Winterbauer and colleagues [20] combined azathioprine with high-dose corticosteroids, and demonstrated a 60% response rate among 20 patients with progressive IPF, all of whom had disease for less than 2 years. By contrast, investigators at the National Institutes of Health [3, 6] failed to find any additional benefit of azathioprine plus corticosteroids over corticosteroids alone, although only the short-term outcome was analyzed. A more recent randomized prospective study by Raghu and colleagues [33] demonstrated a lower mortality at a mean follow-up of 8 years among patients treated with azathioprine plus prednisone as compared with prednisone alone. Cyclophosphamide (Cytoxan) has been used extensively in England for IPF, but experience with this agent in the United States has largely been limited to patients who failed to respond to corticosteroids. In uncontrolled studies, favorable responses to cyclophosphamide (1 to 2 mg/kg/d) were achieved in 50% to 60% of cases, including some who failed to respond to corticosteroids [12, 14, 23, 27]. The high success rate achieved with cyclophosphamide (and its superiority over corticosteroids in other inflammatory disorders such as systemic vasculitis and Wegener's granulomatosis) led to more aggressive use of cyclophosphamide as the initial treatment of IPF. In a recently completed prospective trial in England, patients with IPF were randomized to either oral cyclophosphamide plus low-dose prednisolone (20 mg every other day) or conventional high-dose corticosteroids (prednisolone, 60 mg daily for 1 month, with a gradual taper) [18]. While there appeared to be an improved survival in the cyclophosphamide-treated group, the patient groups were not well matched in terms of extent of disease or pulmonary dysfunction and when these differences were taken into account, the survival advantage with cyclophosphamide was limited to patients with forced vital capacity between 60% and 80% of predicted at entry. Several additional findings were noted in that study: (1) the response to cyclophosphamide may be delayed, as no cyclophosphamide-treated patients improved within the first month of therapy, while some patients treated with corticosteroids did; (2) responses to either agent (prednisolone or cyclophosphamide) were not usually maintained; and (3) neither agent was particularly efficacious (response rates of 10% to 15%) among patients who had previously failed to respond to the other agent. While these data suggested that cyclophosphamide may be superior to corticosteroids in the treatment of IPF, the differences in outcome between these agents are not striking, and additional studies are required to place these agents in perspective. It has been our practice to initiate treatment with high-dose corticosteroids (our usual starting dose is 60 mg daily for the first month, with 10-mg decrements monthly for the next 3 months) and carefully assess clinical status, perform PFTs at 4- to 6-week intervals, and reevaluate at 3 to 4 months. When patients fail to respond to corticosteroids (by objective PFT and/or radiographic criteria), we then taper the steroid to 20 to 40 mg every other day and begin cyclophosphamide, 1 to 2 mg/kg/d, to a maximal dose of 200 mg daily. As the response to cyclophosphamide is usually delayed, we are relatively conservative about the dose and start at 100 mg daily in most patients. At 10 to 14 days, blood counts (complete blood count, differential, and platelet count) are performed and if the counts are adequate (leukocyte count > $4500/mm^3$), platelet count > $100{,}000/mm^3$, Hgb > 11.0 g/dL), the dose is increased to 150 mg and blood counts are checked 10 to 14 days later. As long as the counts are acceptable, an additional increase to 200 mg daily is made at that time, but blood counts are rechecked at 2-week intervals until stability has been ensured. For chronic therapy, leukocyte counts should be maintained greater than $3000/mm^3$ in order to avoid infectious complications. Once the dose has been stabilized for 6 weeks, monthly or bimonthly blood counts may be acceptable for monitoring toxicity. Bone marrow toxicity with cyclophosphamide may be cumulative, so dose reductions may be necessary with prolonged use. Cyclophosphamide is maintained at the maximal dose (according to blood counts, clinical drug toxicity, etc.) for a minimum of 6 months, because a shorter period may be inadequate to judge a therapeutic response. We see little reason to continue cyclophosphamide beyond this point in those who fail to respond, but continue the drug for a minimum of 12 to 18 months in those who do respond. These guidelines are admittedly somewhat arbitrary, as data comparing these various agents and dosage regimens are limited. Alternative regimens combining two or more immunosuppressive/cytotoxic agents (e.g., prednisone/azathioprine, azathioprine/cyclophosphamide, prednisone/cyclophosphamide) have been advocated by some. However, we have not combined high-dose corticosteroids with second immunosuppressive/cytotoxic agents, as an unacceptably high rate of infectious complications has been observed in other conditions treated with aggressive multiagent therapy. Pulse methylprednisolone (Solu-Medrol) therapy has also been tried, but has not been demonstrated to be superior to conventional dose corticosteroids. In one study, patients with IPF in "mid-course of the disease" were randomized to a low-dose corticosteroid (prednisone, 0.25 mg/kg/d) or pulse methylprednisolone (2 g intravenously weekly plus 0.25 prednisone mg/kg/d) group for a 6-month period, and clinical status, PFTs, chest radiography, BAL, and gallium 67 scans were repeated after 6 months of therapy [34]. At 6-month follow-up, there were no differences in PFTs, chest radiography, or symptom scores between groups, although intrapulmonary uptake of gallium and BAL neutrophil counts were less in the pulse methylprednisolone group. While this study has been interpreted as suggesting that pulse methylprednisolone may diminish the alveolitis component and thus have long-term salutary effects, the lack of impact on clinical scores or PFTs raises serious questions as to the role of this mode of therapy in IPF. The role of pulse methylprednisolone has not been clarified and awaits additional long-term studies involving greater numbers of patients.

Ancillary Therapy (Home Oxygen, Vasodilators)

Cardiovascular disease (cor pulmonale, ischemic heart disease, congestive heart failure) accounts for nearly one third of deaths in IPF [6, 10, 15]. Right-sided heart failure may result from progression of the pulmonary inflammatory process, with obliteration of the pulmonary microvasculature, pulmonary vasoconstriction due to chronic hypoxemia, and pulmonary hypertension [6, 10, 15]. In this context, home oxygen therapy may be instrumental in improving quality of life, reducing the need for hospitalization, and improving survival. Vasodilator agents (nitrates, hydralazine, angiotensin-converting enzyme inhibitors, smooth muscle relaxants) have not been proved to have any favorable effect on patients with pulmonary hypertension secondary to IPF but have potential toxicity and therefore are not recommended. Nonetheless, clinical trials are necessary to define the role (if any) of vasodilator agents in the treatment of patients with cor pulmonale or pulmonary hypertension complicating IPF.

Lung Transplantation

Single lung transplantation may be considered a viable option for patients with severe IPF refractory to medical therapy with a limited life expectancy. This procedure was developed in 1986 by the Toronto Lung Transplant Group for patients with end-stage parenchymal pulmonary disease and well-preserved cardiac function, which allowed retention of the native (recipient) heart [35]. By August 1989, 20 single lung transplants had been performed at Toronto for end-stage pulmonary fibrosis, with 11 survivors, including nine who had survived longer than 1 year [36]. Among patients surviving the initial perioperative period, exercise capacity, quality of life, and pulmonary function improved substantially. This procedure has now been adopted in several other transplant centers, with 1-year survivals of 50% to 85%, although the long-term survival is not known [36]. As lung transplantation is currently available in only a few medical centers and donor availability is limited, many patients with severe IPF may be expected to succumb before transplantation. Nevertheless, lung transplantation represents a novel and promising therapeutic advance for relatively young patients with end-stage ILD and without associated debilitating or serious underlying disorders.

Interstitial Pulmonary Fibrosis Complicating Collagen Vascular Disease

The myriad pulmonary complications that occur in the context of rheumatologic disorders has been elegantly reviewed in previous publications [37–45] and is beyond the scope of this text. In this section, we discuss ILD that may complicate collagen vascular disease (CVD) and review some recent data supporting the concept that pathogenic mechanisms and therapeutic strategies of CVD and IPF are similar. IPF associated with CVD resembles IPF clinically, physiologically, and radiographically [1–3, 37]. Pulmonary fibrosis is most common in rheumatoid arthritis (RA), polymyositis/dermatomyositis (PM/DM), progressive systemic sclerosis (PSS), and mixed connective tissue disease (MCTD); by contrast, chronic interstitial disease complicates systemic lupus erythematosus (SLE) or Sjögren's syndrome in fewer than 3% of cases [3, 37]. Pulmonary fibrosis complicating CVD is frequently not recognized due to the predominance of extrapulmonary (articular, systemic) symptoms and the limitation of activity as a result of underlying arthritis or CVD. Chest radiographs may be normal early in the course of the disease, and pulmonary manifestations may be subtle. However, in some cases, pulmonary manifestations are the presenting or predominant feature of the disease. The clinical course is heterogeneous. Typically, the course of interstitial pneumonitis/fibrosis is indolent, with gradual progression of cough and dyspnea over several months or even years [1–3, 37]. However, an acute, fulminant course, progressing to respiratory failure and death within weeks or months, may rarely occur. The activity of the pulmonary process does not necessarily correlate with the extent of articular, systemic, or extrapulmonary involvement. While we see little role for open lung biopsy in the evaluation of ILD in the context of a known CVD, the spectrum of histopathologic changes of CVD-associated IPF mirrors those seen in the idiopathic variety and includes UIP, DIP, bronchiolitis obliterans and organizing pneumonia (BOOP), and varying degrees of cellular infiltrates and fibrosis within the alveolar structures [40, 46]. BAL findings are similar in both idiopathic and CVD-associated pulmonary fibrosis; increases in neutrophils (and occasionally eosinophils or lymphocytes), IgG, immune complexes, activated AMs, and AM products in BAL fluid have been described [1–3]. Increases in BAL neutrophils and/or lymphocytes have been demonstrated even in asymptomatic patients with CVD, suggesting that subclinical alveolitis may exist [47, 48]. The presence of alveolitis may identify patients at risk for subsequent clinical deterioration. Wallaert et al [47] noted abnormal BAL cell differentials, increases in PMNs or lymphocytes or both in 29 of 61 (48%) patients with a variety of CVD, none of whom had pulmonary symptoms. PFTs were normal in all but eight cases. More importantly, BAL cell profiles appeared to correlate with type of CVD and had prognostic significance. A lymphocytic alveolitis (lymphocytes > 18%) was found in 11 of 25 patients with primary Sjögren's syndrome and in four of eight with Sjögren's associated with other CVD. By contrast, a neutrophilic alveolitis (>4% PMNs) with or without increased percentage of lymphocytes occurred in those types of CVD classically associated with pulmonary fibrosis: PSS (6 of 10), RA (1 of 4), DM (2 of 3), and MCTD (3 of 8). On follow-up PFT 12 months later, 11 patients with normal BAL and 10 patients with lymphocyte alveolitis had not deteriorated. By contrast, six of seven with untreated neutrophilic alveolitis deteriorated while all four such patients treated with corticosteroids stabilized [47]. Greene et al [48] performed BAL and gallium scans in 36 patients with CVD and noted that patients with progressive dyspnea and a deteriorating course displayed abnormal gallium scans and BAL neutrophilia. By contrast, patients with BAL lymphocytosis improved or stabilized with corticosteroid therapy. These data suggest that influx of inflammatory cells in the lower respiratory tract precedes the development of pulmonary fibrosis and may be predictive of subsequent deterioration. The role of gallium scans and BAL in the staging and management of CVD, however, remains controversial and of unproven efficacy. Nevertheless, these data are intriguing and suggest that the pathogenesis of pulmonary fibrosis complicating CVD is similar to IPF, and more aggressive therapeutic strategies employing corticosteroids, immunosuppressive/cytotoxic agents, or D-penicillamine may be warranted.

Specific Collagen Vascular Disorders

Rheumatoid Arthritis

Pulmonary complications have long been recognized as a prominent feature of RA. Walker and Wright [43], in a classic article, delineated the major pulmonary complications of RA, which included pleural effusion(s), necrobiotic (rheumatoid) nodules, Caplan's syndrome, pulmonary vasculitis, and chronic ILD. In 1977, Geddes et al [49] described six patients five of whom had classical RA with rapidly progressive dyspnea, a severe obstructive defect on PFTs, and chest radiography demonstrating hyperinflation without infiltrates. Five of the six died of respiratory failure despite corticosteroid/immunosuppressive therapy, and obliterative (constrictive) bronchiolitis was noted at necropsy. Subsequent investigators found that a subset of nonsmoking patients with RA exhibited progressive airways obstruction, associated with bronchiolar inflammatory and fibrotic changes, with a more gradual course [50]. These investigations widened the spectrum of pulmonary complications associated with RA. The later recognition that specific agents used in the therapy of this disorder, such as methotrexate [38, 51, 52] and gold salts [38, 53], were capable of inducing toxic or hypersensitivity pneumonitis emphasized the diversity of immunologic pulmonary disorders associated with RA. In addition, opportunistic pulmonary infections may complicate immunosuppressive therapy in some patients. In this section, we focus on chronic interstitial pneumonitis/fibrosis complicating RA. Interstitial lung disease is more frequent in patients with late-onset rheumatoid arthritis, with a peak incidence in the fifth to sixth decade. In 10% to 20% of cases, ILD antedates the onset of classic joint symptoms [37, 42]. Dyspnea on exertion is a cardinal symptom in rheumatoid ILD, although dyspnea may be masked for prolonged periods due to decreased mobility induced by articular disease. Chest radiographic findings are similar to IPF, with reticulonodular or alveolar infiltrates predominantly affecting the basilar portions of the lungs. Pleural thickening or effusion can be demonstrated in 15% to 20% of patients and may aid in distinguishing rheumatoid lung from IPF. Histopathologic features are usually indistinguishable from IPF. However, on occasion, rheumatoid nodules with characteristic central necrosis and palisading epithelioid cells surrounded by a mixed lymphocyte, plasma cell, and fibroblast infiltrate may be observed [37, 42, 46]. The natural history of rheumatoid ILD has a highly variable course, but classically results in a slowly progressive, unrelenting loss of lung function. The mean survival after onset of symptoms in most series is 3 years, with 5-year mortality of 50% to 60% [37, 42, 54]. Unfortunately, we do not as yet have any gold standard for determining activity of ILD in RA. Open lung biopsy may provide prognostic information, but we have rarely resorted to open lung biopsy in the setting of known underlying CVD.

Pathogenesis and Bronchoalveolar Lavage Findings As with IPF, BAL has permitted significant new insights into the critical cellular and humoral elements involved in the chronic interstitial inflammatory process. BAL fluid from RA patients with clinical and radiographic ILD exhibits increased numbers and percent PMNs (typically in the range of 10% to 25% PMNs) [55–59] and enhanced neutrophil chemotactic, elastase, and myeloperoxidase activity [55–57], supporting a central role for the neutrophil in the pathogenesis of the lung lesion. Increased levels of neutrophil elastase on BAL has been shown to correlate inversely with DLCO in two separate investigations [56, 57]. A subset of patients exhibit BAL lymphocytosis but have no clinical evidence for ILD; the significance of BAL lymphocytosis is not known [55, 58]. AMs from RA patients release increased amounts of oxygen radicals, neutrophil chemotactic activity, and fibronectin, even when no clinical evidence for ILD is present [37]. Thus, increased numbers of inflammatory and immune effector cells are present in the lower respiratory tract of patients with RA and may be responsible for late fibrosis. While these data are intriguing, a firm role for BAL as a tool for establishing prognosis and staging in the clinical setting has not been established.

Therapy The treatment of rheumatoid ILD is controversial. No controlled studies have been done, but we believe that aggressive therapy with corticosteroids, immunosuppressive, or cytotoxic agents is warranted in patients with severe or rapidly progressive rheumatoid ILD. In this context, we have usually initiated high-dose corticosteroids (prednisone, 60 mg/d or equivalent for 1 to 3 months, with a subsequent taper); cyclophosphamide has been reserved for those who fail to respond to corticosteroids.

Progressive Systemic Sclerosis

PSS (scleroderma) is a multisystemic disorder characterized by extensive tissue fibrosis and accompanying vascular abnormalities. The cutaneous abnormalities are the most prominent clinical features of PSS. However, renal, gastrointestinal, and pulmonary involvement contribute significantly to morbidity and mortality from this disease. Pulmonary complications of PSS include recurrent episodes of pneumonia (from patients with severe esophageal dysmotility), chronic ILD, pulmonary hypertension, and rarely, bronchioloalveolar cell carcinoma [39]. ILD, with or without pulmonary hypertension and isolated pulmonary hypertension have emerged as leading causes of death in PSS as a more aggressive approach to controlling systemic hypertension has reduced late renal insufficiency [37, 39]. Pulmonary involvement is rarely the presenting manifestation of PSS [60]. The incidence of ILD in PSS varies depending on the mechanism used to detect it. Autopsy studies have documented ILD in 60% to 100% of patients with PSS [37, 39]. Pulmonary symptoms of dyspnea on exertion or nonproductive cough have been reported in 29% to 60% of scleroderma patients [39, 61–64]. Pleuritic chest pain, a common feature of SLE and RA, rarely occurs in PSS. Rales are appreciated in approximately 50% of patients with ILD; an accentuated P_2 on auscultation of the heart may provide a clue to pulmonary hypertension. Physiologic alterations in lung function are frequent in PSS. A restrictive ventilatory defect (characterized by a reduction in VC, TLC, and DLCO) occurs in 20% to 30% of patients [61–65]. A concomitant obstructive defect (possibly reflecting peribronchiolar fibrosis) is present in 20% to 30% of cases [62, 63]. In addition, one quarter of patients have an isolated reduction in DLCO without alterations in static lung volumes [62, 63]. An abnormal pulmonary vascular response to external cold stimulation has also been reported as evidenced by a reduction in DLCO and an abnormal ventilation-perfusion relationship by nucleotide scanning on cold exposure [65]. The radiographic features of ILD complicating PSS are indistinguishable from IPF. However, mediastinal air–fluid levels suggestive of esophageal achalasia or recurrent alveolar infiltrates as a consequence of aspiration may provide valuable clues to the possibility of PSS. Histopathology of the lung is characterized by a scant mononuclear interstitial infiltrate, an increase in fibroblasts, and collagen deposition. Extensive fibrotic bands replace the normal lung architecture in later stages of lung involvement. Fibromuscular hypertrophy of the media, concentric intimal proliferation, and fibrosis of small muscular arteries and arterioles are also seen [39]. The vascular changes are more commonly noted in the CREST variant of systemic sclerosis (the syndrome of calcinosis, Raynaud's phenomenon, esophageal hypomotility, sclerodactyly, and telangiectasia) [39, 66].

Pathogenesis and Bronchoalveolar Lavage Data Despite the historical dogma that lung involvement in PSS is characterized by progressive fibrosis without an active cellular component, several recent investigations have challenged this hypothesis. Changes consistent with an inflammatory alveolitis (positive gallium scan results, increased inflammatory cells or cellular products on BAL) have been found, even in asymptomatic individuals with PSS [65–69]. In one early study, Silver et al [68] demonstrated increased BAL PMNs or eosinophils in 11 of 19 (58%) patients with PSS; BAL neutrophilia correlated with decreased DLCO. Konig et al [69] noted that 9 of 20 PSS patients exhibited abnormal BAL cell differentials; patients with greater than 20% lymphocytes or greater than 10% PMNs on BAL had more severe impairment in pulmonary function. At long-term follow-up, clinical symptoms and DLCO remained stable in all four patients with normal BAL but deteriorated in all three with abnormal BAL differentials. Edelson et al [70] studied 25 patients with PSS (only eight of whom had chest radiographs consistent with ILD) and noted increased intrapulmonary uptake of gallium in 19 (76%) patients with PSS; BAL cellular differentials were consistent with alveolitis in 11, which was predominantly lymphocytic in seven. Higher mean BAL lymphocyte counts were noted among the eight patients with radiographic evidence for ILD and correlated with positive gallium scan results and a greater degree of restriction on PFTs [70]. Investigators at the National Institutes of Health prospectively assessed 13 patients with PSS and biopsy-proven ILD (average duration of symptoms, 9 years) [67]. Increased intrapulmonary uptake of gallium was noted in 77% and BAL demonstrated mild increases in neutrophils and eosinophils (mean of 6.8% and 2.0% compared with 0.5% and 0.4% in normal subjects); only one had increased percent BAL lymphocytes [67]. Corticosteroids did not influence BAL or gallium scans at 6 to 24 months in four patients. Silver et al [65] observed that 21 of 43 (49%) nonsmoking PSS patients exhibited increased BAL cell count or differentials. Mean percent BAL neutrophils (4.0%) and eosinophils (1.1%) were increased compared with normal control subjects (0.7% and 0.4%, respectively), but differences were slight. The patients with abnormal BAL did not differ in duration of symptoms, skin score, or extrapulmonary involvement except for a slightly higher degree of esophageal involvement, yet displayed worse PFTs, more pulmonary symptoms, and a more rapid decline in forced vital capacity and DLCO [65]. The administration of cyclophosphamide in four patients and prednisone (60 mg/d) in one patient was associated with improvement in dyspnea and less deterioration in PFTs. Increases in BAL neutrophils, eosinophils, lymphocytes, activated AMs, AM products (fibronectin, AM-derived growth factors), neutrophil chemotactic factors, immune complexes, collagenase, IgG, and antibodies to type 1 and 4 collagen have been demonstrated in subsets of patients with PSS on BAL [39, 65–67]. Although preliminary, these data suggest that BAL may identify subsets of patients with alveolitis, although additional prospective studies are required to more fully delineate the utility of BAL as a prognostic tool.

Prognosis and Therapy The natural history of pulmonary involvement in PSS is heterogeneous. The classic course is progressive decline in lung function over many years. Five-year mortality from ILD may be as high as 30% to 50%, once pulmonary symptoms or significant radiographic findings have become apparent [39, 62, 63]. In one study, a DLCO of less than 40% of predicted was associated with a 91% mortality at 5 years compared with a 25% mortality when DLCO exceeded this level [63]. Initial pulmonary symptoms and extent of abnormalities on chest radiographs or PFTs do not predict the course of pulmonary scleroderma, which may be quite variable [62, 63]. Severe Raynaud's phenomenon, peripheral vascular involvement, digital pitting or ulceration, and a history of smoking have been associated with a more rapid decline in DLCO and greater likelihood of developing pulmonary hypertension [62, 63, 71]. Traditionally, an approach to PSS has been one of therapeutic nihilism. No agent has been shown to ameliorate or slow the course of the disease. There have been a few anecdotal cases that have improved with corticosteroids, cyclophosphamide, plasmapheresis, and a variety of immunosuppressive/cytotoxic agents, but controlled studies are lacking. In one 3-year, randomized prospective study, chlorambucil was of no benefit [72]. Corticosteroids, colchicine, and vasodilators have not been shown to be of benefit in retrospective studies [39, 62, 63, 67, 73]. D-penicillamine, an agent that blocks cross-linking of mature collagen, accelerates collagen turnover, and inhibits synthesis and maturation of collagen, has promise [64, 73–75], but its efficacy needs to be more fully evaluated. In one retrospective, uncontrolled study, deClerk et al [73] treated 17 patients with D-penicillamine and compared their course with 10 patients treated with prednisone [73]. Although neither pulmonary symptoms nor PFTs changed following D-penicillamine therapy, greater than 10% deterioration of DLCO at long-term follow-up occurred in only 3 of 17 patients treated with D-penicillamine compared with 5 of 10 treated with prednisone. Steen et al [74] compared 44 PSS patients treated with D-penicillamine compared with 48 untreated patients and noted less progression of dyspnea, rales, and fibrosis in the D-penicillamine group although FVC and FEV_1 did not change. However, DLCO improved in the D-penicillamine group (from 76% to 87% predicted) but not in the control group (73% to 76% prednisone); improvement in DLCO was associated with reduced skin thickening among patients treated with D-penicillamine. Treatment with D-penicillamine was also associated with lower BAL lymphocyte counts in one study [70]. None of these trials are convincing, however, and additional long-term, prospective, double-blinded studies are required to determine the role of corticosteroids, immunosuppressive/cytotoxic agents, and D-penicillamine in the therapy of ILD complicating PSS. In view of the indolent nature of ILD complicating PSS, and the uniform toxicity of therapeutic agents available, we do not advise therapy for the vast majority of patients with PSS. However, we believe that these agents (particularly D-penicillamine) may be appropriate for patients with rapidly progressive or severe ILD complicating PSS, and may be beneficial in subsets of patients with active alveolitis.

Mixed Connective Tissue Disease

MCTD was originally described in 1972 as a distinct overlap syndrome characterized by clinical features of two or more CVD (PSS, RA, PM, SLE) and serologic findings of high titers of serum antibodies to extractable nuclear antigen, ribonucleoprotein, a speckled pattern antinuclear antibody, and absent antibodies to Sm antigen [76]. The original report suggested that the prognosis was generally favorable, and the disease was highly responsive to corticosteroids [76]. Significant pulmonary involvement was not appreciated in the initial report [76], but subsequent studies have demonstrated that 50% to 80% of patients develop pulmonary involvement [45, 77, 78]. Even in patients without pulmonary symptoms, abnormal PFTs or chest radiographs have been detected in over two thirds of patients [45]. Common clinical features of MCTD include Raynaud's phenomenon (80% to 90%), swollen hands/sclerodactyly (85% to 95%), polyarthritis (85% to 90%), myositis (70% to 80%), esophageal dysmotility (30% to 74%), alopecia (30% to 41%), pleuritis (35%), malar rash (29%), and a gamut of clinical manifestations corresponding to the underlying CVD(s) present [45, 77]. The most severe pulmonary manifestation of MCTD is pulmonary hypertension, which occurs in 15% to 30% of cases (typically in patients with features of PSS) and may account for up to 10% of deaths due to MCTD [45, 77]. A scleroderma-like pattern on nail-fold capillary microscopy has been predictive of the subsequent development of pulmonary hypertension [45]. Chronic ILD complicates MCTD in 30% to 85% of cases [45, 77, 78]; clinical features include progressive dyspnea on exertion, pleuritic chest pain, and a nonproductive cough. Bibasilar inspiratory rales are present in 30% to 40% of cases [45, 77]. PFTs reveal abnormalities in at least one parameter in 50% to 85% of patients with MCTD (both symptomatic and asymptomatic patients) [45, 77]. A low DLCO occurs in nearly two thirds of patients, and approximately 40% exhibit reductions in TLC [45]. Chest radiographs demonstrate bibasilar interstitial markings in one third of patients; small pleural effusions have been noted in less than 10% of patients [45, 77, 78]. Histologic specimens obtained by open lung biopsy have shown primarily a proliferative and medial hypertrophy of pulmonary arteries and arterioles; in contrast with PSS, interstitial inflammation or fibrosis has been minimal [45].

Prognosis and Therapy The overall mortality of MCTD as assessed by five series totalling 194 patients is 13%, with a mean duration of disease varying from 6 to 12 years [45]. Most pulmonary deaths have been due to pulmonary hypertension, rather than parenchymal fibrosis [45]. Corticosteroids have often been associated with improvement in the inflammatory manifestations of MCTD (e.g., skin rashes, arthritis, serositis, lymphadenopathy, nephritis, myositis); by contrast, sclerodactyly, PSS skin changes, esophageal hypomotility, pulmonary interstitial disease, and pulmonary hypertension have been less responsive to corticosteroids [45]. Corticosteroids were associated with improvement in dyspnea in 7 of 20 (35%) and PFTs in five of nine (55%) cases in one prospective study [45]. Cyclophosphamide plus steroids resulted in further improvement or stabilization in the PFTs in 7 of 12 patients with severe disease refractory to corticosteroids alone [45]. When serial chest radiographs were analyzed, improvement was noted in only 1 of 11 patients and remained stable in 10 [45]. While optimal therapy has not been defined, we believe that corticosteroids are preferred as initial treatment of pulmonary complications of MCTD; cyclophosphamide (or alternative immunosuppressive/cytotoxic agents) are appropriate for patients failing to respond to corticosteroids or sustaining severe side effects.

Systemic Lupus Erythematosus
Pleuropulmonary manifestations of SLE are protean and include pleuritis with or without effusion, acute interstitial pneumonitis (lupus pneumonitis), pulmonary vasculitis, alveolar hemorrhage reflecting diffuse endothelial cell injury, infections (primarily as a complication of drug therapy), and chronic interstitial pneumonitis [37, 44]. Chronic interstitial pneumonitis complicates SLE in only 3% to 13% of patients with SLE [37, 79]; clinical, radiographic and histologic features are similar to ILD complicating other CVD. While treatment of chronic ILD is rarely necessary in SLE, corticosteroids or immunosuppressive/cytotoxic agents are appropriate for severe or progressive disease.

Polymyositis/Dermatomyositis
A variety of pulmonary complications have been described in PM/DM, including aspiration pneumonitis from weakness of the pharyngeal or esophageal musculature, respiratory failure from global weakness of respiratory muscles, infection secondary to corticosteroid or immunosuppressive therapy, and chronic interstitial pneumonitis/fibrosis. This latter complication occurs in 3% to 10% of cases [40, 41, 80] and exhibits clinical and histopathologic features similar to ILD complicating other CVD. Chronic interstitial pneumonitis may occur (Fig. 11-4A and B) simultaneously with muscle involvement, but may also precede or follow the clinical myopathy. The severity and extent of pulmonary parenchymal involvement may not correlate with the course of the muscle disease, muscle enzymes, or systemic features [40, 41, 80]. Serologic abnormalities are sometimes helpful in identifying patients at risk for IPF complicating PM/DM, as this complication is much more frequent among patients exhibiting circulating serum anti-Jo-1 antibody [81, 82]. Management and therapy of IPF associated with PM/DM is similar to other CVD [40, 41, 83].

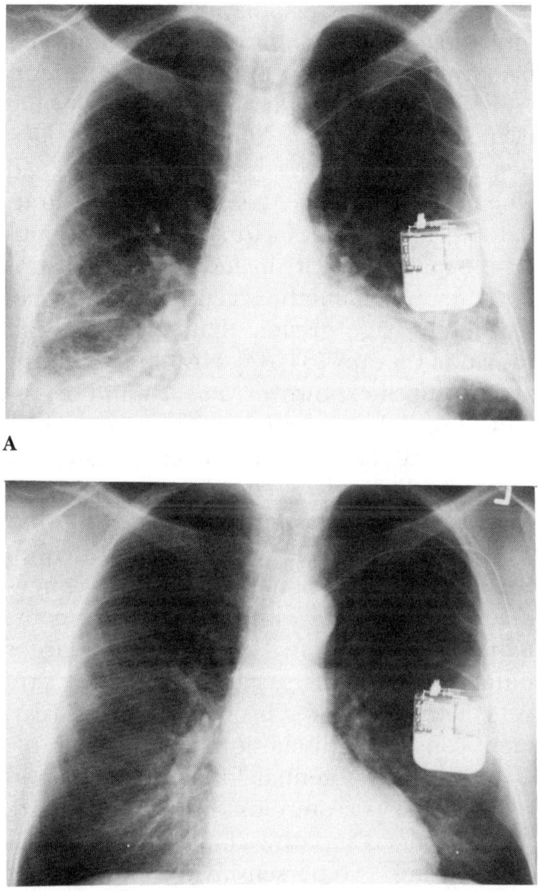

A

B

Fig. 11-4. (A) Polymyositis. Chest radiograph from a 70-year-old man presenting with cough and dyspnea but no muscle symptoms. Bilateral, predominantly basilar, interstitial and alveolar infiltrates are present. Serum CPK was elevated at 1200 IU/L. (B) Polymyositis. Clearing of chest radiograph following 3 months of corticosteroid therapy. The patient was asymptomatic and serum CPK had normalized.

Drug-Induced Interstitial Pneumonitis

Physicians are faced with a growing number of drugs that result directly or indirectly in lung injury. Clinical, radiographic, and physiologic manifestations of drug-induced chronic interstitial pneumonitis/fibrosis may be indistinguishable from IPF. The diagnosis may be extremely difficult in patients with an underlying disease process in which lung involvement is common such as CVD or when patients are receiving several agents concomitantly. The diagnosis of drug-induced pneumonitis requires a high clinical suspicion and the exclusion of alternative etiologies. A careful drug history is always required before labeling a patient as having IPF. This is critical, since discontinuation of the responsible agent may be curative. Interstitial pneumonitis most commonly results from cytotoxic chemotherapeutic agents, but a variety of drugs are capable of causing lung injury. The best recognized agents include nitrofurantoin, hydralazine, procainamide, methotrexate, gold salts, and amiodarone, but a host of others have been implicated [84–90]. Multiple mechanisms of drug-induced chronic interstitial pneumonitis/fibrosis have been demonstrated, including direct cytopathic effects as well as indirect injury related to the influx of inflammatory cells into the alveolar spaces and interstitium [84–87]. The activation of resident inflammatory cells of the lung and the release of inflammatory mediators may be critical for the propagation of pulmonary injury and fibrosis in response to a variety of pulmonary toxic agents [84–87]. The clinical and radiographic features of drug-induced pneumonitis may be similar, irrespective of the agent used. However, certain features may be characteristic of specific drugs such as mediastinal/hilar adenopathy (methotrexate), T-suppressor cell alveolitis on BAL (methotrexate and gold salts), pleural effusions (procainamide, hydralazine), or foamy macrophages (amiodarone) and may be helpful diagnostic clues. Drug-induced chronic interstitial pneumonitis/fibrosis is typically indolent, with worsening dyspnea over several weeks to months. Nonproductive cough, fatigue, and generalized malaise are frequent associated symptoms. A more fulminant course, leading to acute respiratory insufficiency and even death, may also occur. Bibasilar end-inspiratory crackles can usually be appreciated on physical examination. Chest radiographs typically demonstrate diffuse, reticular, or reticulonodular infiltrates. An alveolar filling pattern, with prominent air bronchograms, may also occur. Pleural effusions are rarely seen in drug-induced pneumonitis, but have been described in association with procainamide, hydralazine, mitomycin, busulfan, and bleomycin [84–87]. A restrictive defect on PFTs, with reduced lung volumes and DLCO is characteristic; hypoxemia may be prominent in advanced cases. Clinical features, histopathology, and responsiveness to therapy of pneumonitis secondary to cytotoxic agents and noncytotoxic agents overlap but display salient differences and are discussed separately.

Cytotoxic Drug-Induced Interstitial Pneumonitis/Fibrosis

Several classes of chemotherapeutic agents including bleomycin, alkylating agents, and nitrosoureas may induce acute or chronic interstitial pneumonitis [84, 87, 91, 92]. The prevalence of pulmonary injury varies widely according to the agent used and the presence or absence of cofactors. The histopathologic features of pneumonitis secondary to cytotoxic agents include three cardinal features: (1) type II pneumocyte proliferation with cellular atypia; (2) cellular interstitial and/or alveolar inflammatory cell infiltrates; and (3) varying degrees of fibrosis [87, 91]. Type II epithelial proliferation is a result of destruction of the type I epithelial lining and is characterized by cuboidal cells replacing the previously flat alveolar epithelial surface. As previously quiescent type II epithelial cells begin to proliferate, cytopathic changes (large nuclei, prominent nucleoli, and bizarre chromatin patterns) occur due to interference with normal nucleic acid synthesis. A concomitant interstitial and/or alveolar inflammatory component, consisting predominantly of mononuclear cells, but with occasional PMNs, eosinophils, and fibroblasts, is characteristic. Varying degrees of collagen deposition and fibrosis occur and are important determinants of prognosis [87].

Specific Cytotoxic Agents

Bleomycin

Bleomycin, a cytotoxic chemotherapeutic agent, has been one of the best studied of the pulmonary toxic drugs [84, 87–90]. Chronic interstitial pneumonitis/fibrosis complicates bleomycin therapy in 2% to 10% of patients [84, 87, 89]. Lung injury may occur following even low doses of bleomycin, but the incidence of pneumonitis is markedly increased when the cumulative dose exceeds 450 units [84, 89]. Additional factors that may potentiate bleomycin toxicity include the administration of supplemental oxygen, multidrug chemotherapy, age greater than 70 years, and radiation therapy [84, 89]. Histologic features are nonspecific; however, an early and persistent fibrotic lesion with an exuberant mononuclear cellular infiltrate involving alveolar septae and spaces is characteristic [87, 89]. Increased numbers and percentage of PMNs and eosinophils have been demonstrated on BAL [90]. The prognosis for chronic pneumonitis associated with bleomycin is poor; mortality varies from 1% to 7%, but a larger number of patients sustain serious and irreversible pulmonary fibrosis [84, 87]. Treatment consists of discontinuing drug therapy. Owing to the potential for late fibrosis and sequelae, corticosteroids have been tried, with anecdotal successes, but controlled trials are lacking. Hypersensitivity pneumonitis (HP) may also complicate bleomycin therapy, but is rare. In contrast to the chronic pneumonitis syndrome, the prognosis for patients with HP appears to be favorable, with resolution of disease on cessation of the drug.

Alkylating Agents

Busulfan, cyclophosphamide, melphalan, and chlorambucil all belong to a group of drugs known as alkylating agents [84]. The incidence of lung disease due to alkylating agents varies from 4% of patients treated with busulfan, to less than 1% treated with cyclophosphamide, and only rare case reports associated with melphalan or chlorambucil [84, 87]. Busulfan rarely causes lung disease unless the total dose exceeds 500 mg, except in cases where concomitant or prior pulmonary toxic therapy has been administered [84, 87]. Clinical disease as a result of busulfan therapy is seen on average 3 years after institution of therapy, with a range from 6 weeks to 10 years [84]. A similar course has been noted for cyclophosphamide, with a range from 2 weeks to 13 years [84]. Risk factors for cyclophosphamide-induced lung disease include multidrug chemotherapy and prior or concomitant radiation therapy. The prognosis of alkylating agent-induced lung disease has been poor, with mortality approaching 50% for all agents [84]. The mean survival after diagnosis of busulfan-induced lung disease averages only 5 months and long-term sequelae are common among survivors [84]. The role of corticosteroid therapy has not been clarified, but is recommended for patients with severe or progressive disease once infection has been reliably excluded.

Nitrosoureas

The nitrosoureas include a group of drugs that include the agents carmustine (BCNU), lomustine, and semustine [84, 87]. The incidence of interstitial pneumonitis/fibrosis associated with lomustine and semustine appears to be rare; by contrast, 20% to 30% of patients receiving BCNU develop toxicity [84]. Risk factors contributing to toxicity include the cumulative dose of BCNU and concomitant therapy with cyclophosphamide [84]. The effect of cumulative dose is linear until 1500 mg/m^2 is administered, at which time the incidence of pulmonary fibrosis rapidly increases to approximately 50% [84, 87]. BCNU toxicity typically induces a chronic interstitial pneumonitis, but rare cases of a more fulminant alveolitis resulting in adult respiratory distress syndrome have been described. Unusual features of BCNU-induced chronic pneumonitis include a higher than expected incidence of normal chest radiographs despite histologically documented pulmonary fibrosis [84, 87]. Fibrosis is often patchy and associated with minimal inflammatory cell infiltrates [84, 87]. The mortality among symptomatic patients has varied from 16% to 50% [84, 87]. Pulmonary functional deficits usually persist even after discontinuing therapy. Corticosteroids appear to be of little or no benefit, which may reflect the paucity of inflammatory cells in the histopathology of the lung lesion [84, 87].

Drug-Induced Hypersensitivity Pneumonitis

Several agents, notably methotrexate, nitrofurantoin, and gold salts may induce an HP-like picture by clinical, histologic, and BAL criteria [38, 52, 53, 85, 86, 88]. Histopathologic features include an exuberant inflammatory cellular exudate involving airspaces and interstitium. Although eosinophils and PMNs may be observed, a mixed mononuclear cell infiltrate, with loosely formed granulomas and giant cells, has been more chracteristic of HP due to methotrexate or nitrofurantoin [53, 86–88]. The prognosis for HP is usually favorable, as complete resolution of pneumonitis occurs in most cases following discontinuation of the drug. Corticosteroids may facilitate more rapid clearing and are recommended for severe cases, although controlled trials are lacking.

Methotrexate

Methotrexate, an agent that is being increasingly used in a variety of benign immune-mediated disorders including asthma, RA, and psoriasis as well as for a number of neoplastic and inflammatory disorders, induces pulmonary toxicity in 3% to 7% of cases [51, 84–87]. Pulmonary toxicity has been reported in association with oral, intramuscular, and intrathecal routes of administration [38, 85]. Factors that may enhance or potentiate pulmonary toxicity include combination chemotherapy (especially cyclophosphamide), daily administration of methotrexate, recent corticosteroid taper, or adrenalectomy [84–87]. Methotrexate pneumonitis usually presents as an acute or subacute pneumonia associated with prominent constitutional symptoms, skin rash, and peripheral eosinophilia [38, 51, 87]. Chest radiography demonstrates predominantly alveolar infiltrates, although mixed alveolar and interstitial patterns may occur. Although rare, nodular infiltrates have also been described. Pleural effusions and paratracheal or hilar adenopathy, which are unusual features in most drug-induced pneumonias, can be demonstrated in 10% to 15% of cases [38, 51, 87]. Histologic features typically exhibit a dense mononuclear cell (primarily lymphocytic) infiltrate, although eosinophils may sometimes predominate. Noncaseating granulomata with multinucleated giant cells have been noted in 10% of patients, a feature not seen in other forms of chemotherapy-induced lung disease [38, 51, 87]. The presence of granulomas may provide a clue to methotrexate-induced pneumonitis, but (granulomatous) infectious etiologies should be excluded. Severe pulmonary fibrosis has been uncommon with methotrexate HP. The prognosis associated with methotrexate HP is usually favorable, if the drug is discontinued early. Corticosteroids may facilitate more rapid resolution and should be given in patients with severe or life-threatening disease. Although we believe methotrexate should be discontinued in cases of suspected methotrexate pneumonitis, resolution of the disease has been reported even when the drug has been continued [38, 51]. In addition, rechallenge with methotrexate in patients with resolved methotrexate pneumonitis does not consistently reinduce the syndrome [38, 51]. While the mechanism of pulmonary toxicity induced by methotrexate is controversial, several features support a hypersensitivity reaction [87]; the prominent constitutional symptoms, myalgias, fever, skin rash, peripheral eosinophilia, a lymphocytic/granulomatous reaction on lung biopsy, increased T-suppressor cells on BAL [52], and the low doses of methotrexate necessary to induce disease. However, the fact that some cases spontaneously improve despite continuing methotrexate or do not relapse on rechallenge argue against a simple hypersensitivity reaction.

Amiodarone

Amiodarone is an amphophilic, iodinated antiarrhythmic agent that may be lifesaving in the treatment of refractory ventricular dysrhythmias. The most significant limitation to its clinical utility is pulmonary toxicity, which occurs in approximately 5% to 10% of patients receiving the drug (range, 0% to 27% in various studies) [91–95]. The risk factors for pulmonary toxicity are controversial. Maintenance doses exceeding 400 mg/d have been associated with a higher incidence of toxicity, whereas the total cumulative dose appears to be unrelated to toxicity [91–93]. The presence of preexisting pulmonary disease or an abnormal chest radiograph before initiation of therapy has also been associated with a higher rate of clinical toxicity [91–93]. The most frequent clinical manifestation of amiodarone lung toxicity is chronic interstitial pneumonitis, characterized by slowly progressive dyspnea, nonproductive cough, and weight loss. Chest radiography typically demonstrates diffuse, bilateral reticular infiltrates, with a predilection for the peripheral segments of the upper lobes [91–93]. Uncommon radiographic manifestations include focal consolidation, nodular infiltrates, and pleural effusions. A reduced DLCO is the most sensitive indicator of pulmonary toxicity; with more advanced disease, restricted lung volumes and hypoxemia may be noted. Histologic features are relatively specific and are consistent with an acquired lysosomal storage disorder. Dense lamellar bodies are spread throughout the cytoplasm of AMs (as determined by electron microscopy) and give the AMs a distinct appearance, with abundant pale foamy cytoplasm [91, 92]. Other cells, including type II pneumocytes and bronchial epithelial cells, fibroblasts, and endothelial cells, may be affected. A mixed mononuclear cell interstitial infiltrate and hyperplasia of type II pneumocytes are common associated features. Rarely, amiodarone may give rise to more fulminant injury, characterized by the acute onset of dyspnea and diffuse alveolar infiltrates (Fig. 11-5A and B). In this setting, lung biopsy may demonstrate combinations of diffuse alveolar damage, interstitial inflammation, and the characteristic foamy AMs [86, 91, 94]. Increased numbers of PMNs and/or lymphocytes have been observed on BAL in one third to one half of patients; increased numbers of BAL T-suppressor cells consistent with HP, have also been described [91, 94]. The most effective

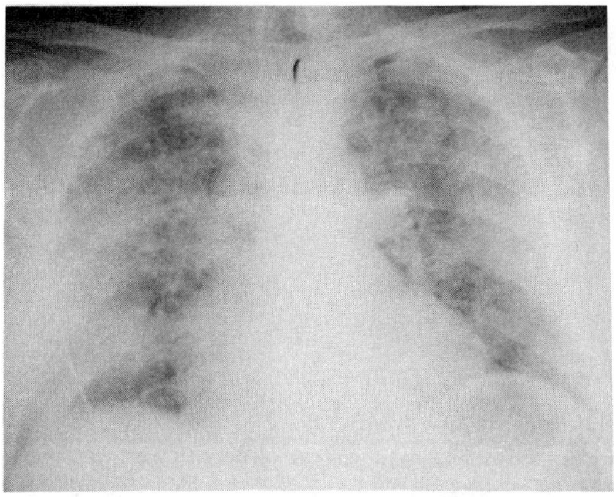

A

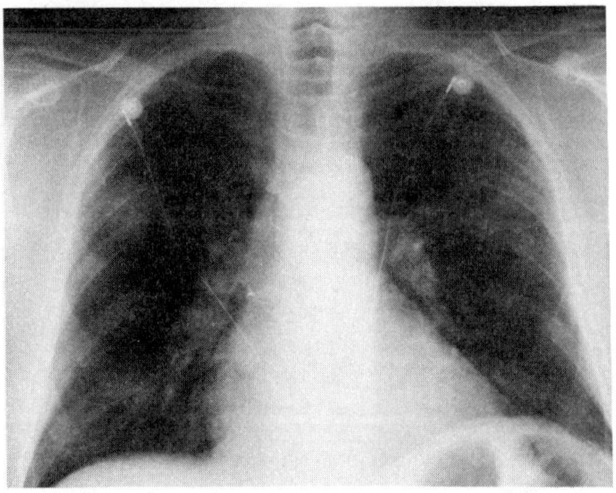

B

Fig. 11-5. (A) Amiodarone acute pneumonitis. Chest radiograph demonstrating extensive alveolar infiltrates in a 66-year-old man who had been taking amiodarone for ventricular arrhythmias. Cardiac function (as assessed by MUGA and clinical examination) was normal; transbronchial lung biopsy demonstrated foamy AMs and extensive interstitial inflammation consistent with amiodarone pneumonitis. Amiodarone was discontinued and prednisone, 80 mg daily, was initiated. (B) Amiodarone pneumonitis (resolving). Chest radiograph 5 days after initiation of prednisone demonstrating marked improvement. Residual infiltrates in the upper lung fields persist, but later disappeared within 4 weeks.

therapy for amiodarone toxicity is discontinuation of therapy. Recovery from amiodarone pneumonitis may be slow, even after the drug has been discontinued. This slow resolution is the result of a prolonged elimination half-life and the fact that concentrations of amiodarone in the lung are 1000 times higher than levels achieved in serum [91]. Unfortunately in many patients alternative effective therapy for their ventricular dysrhythmias may not be available. If amiodarone cannot be discontinued, chronic corticosteroid therapy at the lowest effective doses may limit toxicity [96].

Nitrofurantoin

Nitrofurantoin (Macrodantin), an oral antibiotic used primarily as chronic suppressive therapy for patients with chronic urosepsis, may cause acute or chronic pneumonitis, although pulmonary complications occur in fewer than 1% of patients receiving this medication [85, 88]. The acute form of the disease accounts for 90% of cases [85, 88]. Symptoms begin within 1 month of initiation of nitrofurantoin therapy; fever and dyspnea occur in 80% to 90% of patients [85, 88]. Nonproductive cough is present in two thirds of patients; pleuritic chest pain, rash, myalgias, or arthralgias occur in 15% to 30% [85, 88]. Peripheral eosinophilia and elevated erythrocyte sedimentation rate occur in 70% to 90% of cases. Chest radiography characteristically reveals bibasilar interstitial or alveolar infiltrates; small pleural effusions have been reported in one third of patients [85, 88] (Fig. 11-6A and B). Lung biopsy demonstrates a mixed mononuclear interstitial process predominated by lymphocytes and plasma cells; eosinophils are rarely seen [85, 87, 88] (Fig. 11-6C). For mild cases, simply discontinuing nitrofurantoin may be adequate therapy, as infiltrates usually begin to clear within 24 to 96 hours and resolve without significant functional impairment. Mortality from the acute form of the disease is approximately 1% [85, 88]. For severe or fulminant cases, however, corticosteroids are recommended. Chronic interstitial pneumonitis/fibrosis may also complicate nitrofurantoin. The features of this disorder are indistinguishable from IPF. The onset of symptoms usually occurs within 6 to 12 months of starting nitrofurantoin, but cases of chronic nitrofurantoin pneumonitis have been described in individuals after several years of therapy in the absence of prior

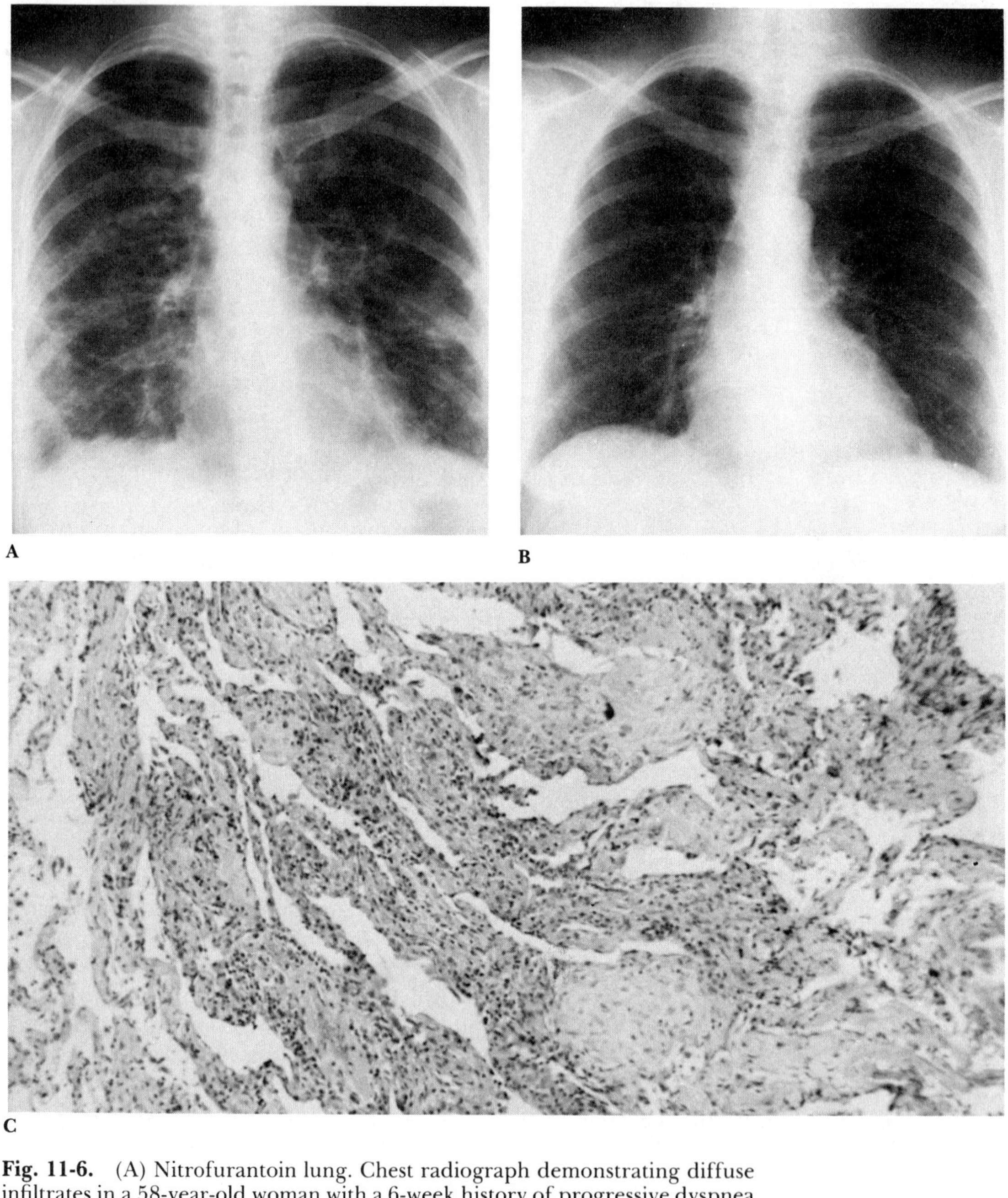
A
B
C

Fig. 11-6. (A) Nitrofurantoin lung. Chest radiograph demonstrating diffuse infiltrates in a 58-year-old woman with a 6-week history of progressive dyspnea and cough, severe restriction on PFTs, and hypoxemia (paO_2 of 48 mm Hg). She had been taking nitrofurantoin intermittently for 8 years before the development of pulmonary symptoms. Nitrofurantoin was discontinued and prednisone, 60 mg daily, was initiated. (B) Nitrofurantoin lung following treatment. Chest radiograph 4 weeks after starting prednisone is essentially normal. The patient was asymptomatic and had normal PFTs. (C) Nitrofurantoin lung. Photomicrograph of transbronchial lung biopsy from same patient demonstrating areas of fibrosis, interstitial inflammation, and occasional foci of granulomatous change. While nonspecific, these findings are compatible with nitrofurantoin-induced interstitial pneumonitis (hematoxylin-eosin, low power).

pulmonary toxicity. Recovery from this chronic form of nitrofurantoin pneumonitis has been poor; mortality approaches 10% and chest radiographic and PFT abnormalities frequently persist after discontinuing the drug [85, 87, 88].

Bronchiolitis Obliterans

Bronchiolitis obliterans (BO) refers to a rare condition in which exuberant granulation tissue and fibrosis may lead to partial or complete obliteration of small bronchioles (terminal and respiratory), with occasional extension into alveolar ducts, resulting in airway obstruction [97–113]. Although BO has been recognized for over a century, the nomenclature has rapidly evolved and changed within the past two decades and may be confusing. A variety of terms of this disorder have been applied, including cryptogenic organizing pneumonitis, organizing-pneumonia–like process, obliterative bronchiolitis, BO fibrosis, and BO organizing pneumonia. When this exuberant inflammatory and fibrotic process extends into the adjacent alveolar airspaces, the term BOOP is applied [97–113]. Several series have included both BO without organizing pneumonia and BOOP in the analysis, which makes interpretation of data difficult. BO should be considered in the differential diagnosis of unexplained obstructive lung disease as well as interstitial lung disease of unknown etiology. In either instance, however, BO is rare. For example, in 1985, Epler and coworkers [97] reported 67 patients with BOOP gleaned from more than 2500 open lung biopsy specimens obtained from 1950 to 1980. In a study from England, Turton and coworkers [105] identified 10 cases of BO (five of which were associated with RA) among 2094 patients referred for obstructive lung disease over a 3-year period. The incidence may be higher than has been appreciated, however, as 16 cases of BO were detected in the pulmonary clinic at Ohio State University over a 4-year period, which represented 4% of all cases of obstructive lung disease seen during that period [106]. BO may also occur in association with specific underlying diseases such as RA [49, 50, 107], bone marrow transplantation [108], heart-lung transplantation [109], toxic fume inhalation [101], and following specific infections [101] but this discussion is limited to the idiopathic variety.

Clinical Findings and Physical Examination

BOOP can affect individuals of any age, although the average age of onset is in the fifth or sixth decade [97–113]. Men and women are affected equally. Nonproductive cough, dyspnea, and constitutional symptoms of fever, malaise, and weight loss are characteristic [97–113]. Sputum production is not a feature of BO, which differentiates this condition from other obstructive lung disorders such as chronic bronchitis, cystic fibrosis, and bronchiectasis. Symptoms are typically of short duration, ranging from 2 weeks to 6 months in most cases [97, 99, 101, 103, 104, 111]. An antecedent flu-like illness within 4 to 12 weeks of the onset of symptoms has been described in one third of cases [97, 101, 105]. The subacute onset, presence of constitutional symptoms, and antecedent flu-like illness may distinguish BO from IPF, in which the onset of symptoms may be protracted over months or even years. Crackles are present on physical examination in more than 60% of cases [97, 103, 104]. Consolidation findings, although uncommon, have been described [97, 103, 104]. Despite the presence of airways obstruction, wheezing is present in only 10% to 30% of cases [97, 101, 103]. A midinspiratory squeak has been described [105] in up to 40% of cases. The physical examination may be normal in up to one third of cases [97, 103, 104, 112]. Clubbing does not occur.

Chest Radiography

Chest radiographic changes in BO are variable [97–113]. Solitary or multiple alveolar opacities occur in 60% to 80% of cases and diffuse reticulonodular infiltrates in 20% to 40%. In 4% to 10% of cases, the chest radiograph may be normal or exhibit only hyperinflation [97–99]. Pleural involvement is not a feature and cavitation does not occur. Lung volumes, as assessed by chest radiography, are preserved. When a prominent component of organizing pneumonia is present, bilateral, patchy alveolar opacities, exhibiting a "ground-glass pattern," often with air bronchograms, are characteristic [97–104] (Fig. 11-7). This ground glass pattern was described in 29 of 42 (62%) and 39 of 52 (79%) patients in two separate studies [97, 98]. The infiltrates may be segmental or lobar in distribution, without predilection for any particular site, and may wax and wane even before initiation of therapy [97–100]. When these radiographic features are present, the distinction from IPF is obvious, as bibasilar reticular or reticulonodular infiltrates and reduced lung volumes are characteristic of the latter entity. The pattern on chest radiography has prognostic significance and depends to a large extent on whether organizing pneumonia is present. The presence of multiple, alveolar infiltrates on chest radiography has been associated with a more acute course and an excellent response to corticosteroid therapy [97, 104]. Since patients with patchy pneumonic infiltrates are often treated empirically for community-acquired pneumonia, the migratory or transient nature of these infiltrates may be mistaken for pneumonia. Other causes of focal airspace disease with air bronchograms include infections (viral, bacterial, mycoplasma) as well as less common disorders such as neoplasm, chronic eosinophilic pneumonia, alveolar hemorrhage, and pulmonary vasculitis. BOOP may also present as solitary, localized pneumonic infiltrates [97, 101]. In this context, surgical resection has often been carried out because of the suspicion of neoplasm, and relapses have been infrequent [97, 98, 101]. A diffuse reticulonodular pattern, indistinguishable from other chronic ILD (including IPF), occurs in 20% to 40% of cases [97, 98, 104] (Fig. 11-8). In this context, the course has been more chronic (ranging from 6 weeks to several

Fig. 11-7. BOOP. Chest radiograph demonstrating dense airspace disease in the periphery of the left upper lobe and mild infiltrate in the right lower lobe. Transbronchial lung biopsy confirmed the diagnosis of BOOP. The patient responded promptly to prednisone, 60 mg daily.

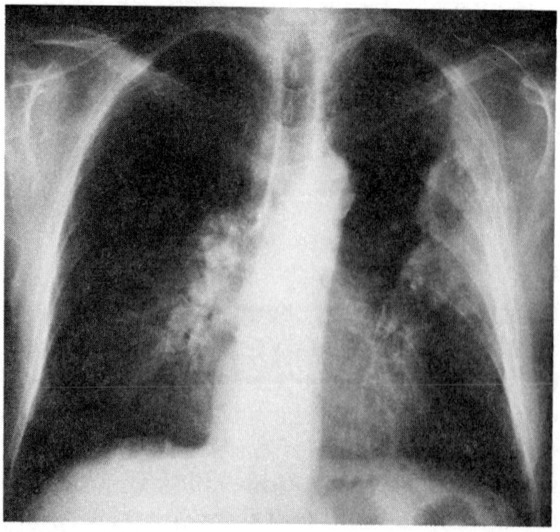

Fig. 11-8. BO. Chest radiograph demonstrating diffuse reticulonodular and nodular infiltrates. No focal airspace disease or consolidation is evident. This 27-year-old woman had noted progressive cough and dyspnea for 2 months and had a moderate combined obstructive-restrictive defect on PFTs. Transbronchial lung biopsy demonstrated changes compatible with BO (no organizing pneumonia was apparent). After 3 months of prednisone therapy, chest radiographs and PFTs had normalized.

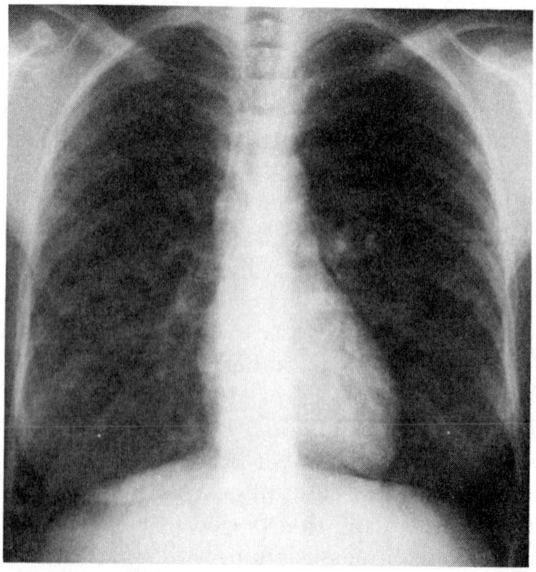

years), is associated with progressively worsening dyspnea, and exhibits less consistent responsiveness to corticosteroids [104]. This clinical and radiographic profile has many more features consistent with IPF as compared with patients exhibiting the more classical alveolar (ground glass) pattern on chest radiography. It is possible that this subset of BOOP reflects a more chronic process in which persistent alveolar inflammation over months or years has led to fibrosis and disruption of the alveolar architecture. In fact, it is likely that many cases previously encompassed under the spectrum of IPF (particularly those exhibiting excellent responses to corticosteroids) may have reflected BOOP. Chest CT scans are more sensitive in detecting abnormalities, compared with conventional chest radiographs, and may dramatically illustrate the alveolar nature of the process [113], but we do not believe that CT scans are required for the diagnosis or staging of this disorder.

Pulmonary Function Tests

Aberrations in PFTs are almost uniformly present, although the type of defect(s) may depend on whether coexisting organizing pneumonia is present. With BOOP, reductions in lung volumes (VC, TLC) and DLCO are characteristic [97–104]. Despite the presence of small airways disease, an obstructive component is usually not evident except in smokers [97, 101]. By contrast, with pure BO, a combined obstructive-restrictive deficit is typical [101, 102]. Bronchodilators have not been shown to improve pulmonary function [101, 112]. Hypoxemia is usually present in both variants of the disorder [97, 101, 106, 112]. PFTs may markedly improve or normalize following corticosteroid therapy [97–112].

Histopathology

The histologic features of BOOP are variable and overlap with several other entities. In fact, a variety of other histopathologic diagnoses are often suggested by the pathologist, including organizing pneumonia, lipoid pneumonia, cholesterol pneumonia, and resolving pneumonia. Often the diagnosis of BOOP is not substantiated until a careful review of the pathologic material has been made, in conjunction with clinical, radiographic, and physiologic data. The histologic hallmark of BO is plugging of the lumens of bronchioles and alveolar ducts by loose connective tissue or polypoid masses of granulation tissue [97–104] (Fig. 11-9A and B). An admixture of inflammatory cells (primarily plasma cells, lymphocytes, and histiocytes, with scattered neutrophils and eosinophils), fibrous connective tissue (fibroblasts, myofibroblasts, collagen), fibrin, edema, and a proteinaceous exudate may be found within the small airway lumens and alveoli [97–104]. Multinucleated giant cells have been detected in a minority of cases. In some cases, the intraluminal process may completely obliterate bronchioles and alveolar ducts, leaving only fibrotic remnants of the airway lumens. A distinctive feature of BO is its patchy nature, which can best be appreciated on low power magnification [97, 100, 104]. In the early phases, the inflammatory and fibrotic process may be confined to the airways, but may extend into the alveolar spaces and interstitium, resulting in an organizing or obstructive pneumonitis. However, even when extensive consolidation is present, the alveolar architecture is usually preserved [97, 100]. Large numbers of foamy macrophages within alveolar spaces may be observed in some cases and may erroneously suggest the diagnosis of DIP [97, 100, 104]. Severe interstitial fibrosis or honeycombing rarely complicates BOOP. Nevertheless, it is easy to understand how BOOP may be mistaken for IPF, particularly when small biopsy specimens are reviewed, and the peribronchiolar nature of the process is not appreciated.

Bronchoalveolar Lavage

Fiberoptic bronchoscopy with BAL may be helpful in suggesting the diagnosis and excluding other obstructive disorders. In an initial study, Dorinsky et al [112] noted striking increases in BAL neutrophils (mean of 53%), with slight increases in eosinophils and normal lymphocytes among four adults with BO.

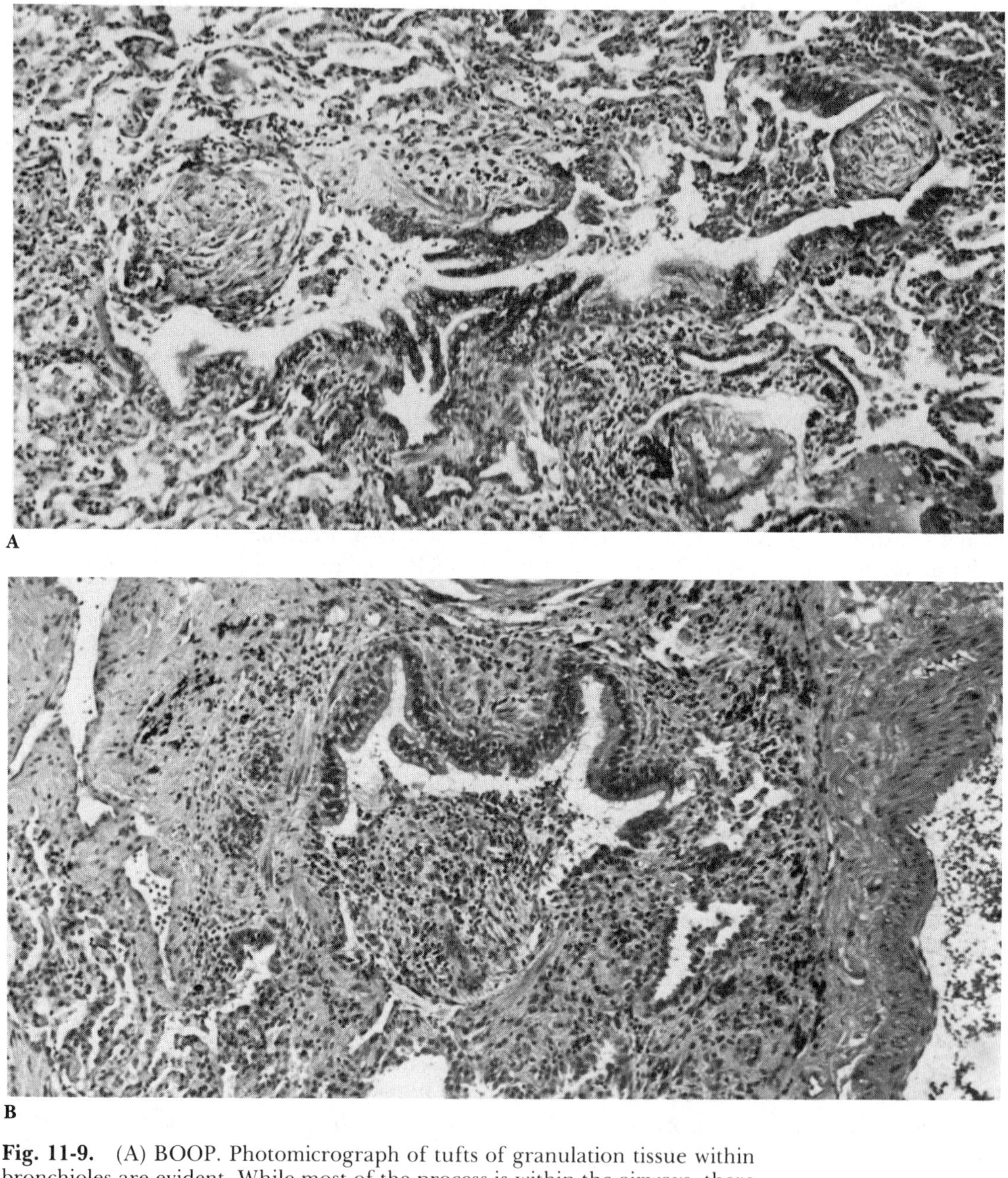

A

B

Fig. 11-9. (A) BOOP. Photomicrograph of tufts of granulation tissue within bronchioles are evident. While most of the process is within the airways, there is extension of the inflammatory process into the pulmonary interstitium as well (hematoxylin-eosin, low power). (B) BOOP. Photomicrograph of a plug of granulation tissue containing neutrophils, mononuclear cells, collagen, and stroma is clearly evident within a bronchiole. This change is classical for BO (hematoxylin-eosin, high power).

These investigators subsequently performed BAL in 16 adults with a prominent component of bronchiolitis on open lung biopsy and noted marked increases in BAL neutrophils (mean of 54%), collagenase activity, and myeloperoxidase activity, with normal lymphocyte counts [106]. Following 3 months of prednisone therapy (1 mg/kg/d), BAL neutrophils decreased from a mean of 46% to 6% among five who responded, whereas slight increases (76% to 59%) were observed among the three who did not respond to steroids [106]. Cordier et al [104] performed BAL in 12 patients with BOOP and noted a more mixed picture on BAL, with increases in BAL lymphocytes, neutrophils, and eosinophils. Striking elevations in BAL lymphocytes (mean of 37.5%) were demonstrated in patients with a more acute course and patchy alveolar infiltrates all of whom were responsive to steroids, whereas BAL lymphocytes were normal (mean, 6.2%) among five patients with a more chronic course and interstitial changes on chest radiography. Increases in BAL neutrophils and eosinophils were seen in both groups. While these data are intriguing, the role of BAL in the management of BO remains controversial. However, bronchoscopic findings (including gross macroscopic changes and BAL cell counts) may be diagnostically helpful, as the absence of bronchitic changes within large airways or purulent secretions may distinguish BO from other pulmonary disorders such as infection, bronchiectasis, or bronchitis due to cigarette smoking. Slight increases in BAL neutrophils (typically < 5%) have been observed among cigarette smokers with chronic bronchitis, but intense BAL neutrophilia is lacking. However, whether sequential BALs offer any advantage over conventional parameters (PFTs, chest radiography) in the follow-up of BOOP has not been clarified.

Pathogenesis

The etiology of idiopathic BOOP is not clear. Several lines of evidence suggest that BOOP represents a distinctive host response to a variety of inflammatory or injurious stimuli or agents [101, 110]. BOOP can occur as a result of drugs or medications, inhalation of toxic fumes, in association with connective tissue disease, organ transplantation, or as a response to infection [101, 110]. The prominence of neutrophils in the histopathology of the lesion, the striking increase in PMNs and neutrophil products (collagenase and myeloperoxidase) on BAL fluid, and the declines in BAL with corticosteroid therapy support a central role for the neutrophil in the pathogenesis of the lung lesion. Neutrophils contain an array of mediators including oxygen radicals, proteolytic enzymes that have the capacity to damage bronchiolar and pulmonary epithelium. The inciting signal(s) responsible for neutrophil recruitment and activation is not clear. However, the uniformity of the histologic stages of the disease, including the fibrotic component, suggests that an initial stimulus, possibly an inhaled antigen or noxious agent, may have initiated an inflammatory process, which is then followed by an attempt to repair [101, 110]. Several stimuli (e.g., viral or bacterial infection, connective tissue disease, graft-versus-host reaction, organ transplant rejection, toxic fume inhalation) may initiate an inflammatory process within the bronchioles. Once damage has occurred, inflammation (neutrophil influx) and reparative mechanisms (fibrosis, remodelling) dictate the evolution of the pathologic lesion.

Therapy

Corticosteroids are the mainstay of therapy. The optimal dose and duration of corticosteroid therapy has not been defined, as prospective, controlled studies have not been done. Prednisone, 1 mg/kg/d for 1 to 3 months, with a subsequent taper, has been advocated by most investigators [97, 101, 106, 112]. Using this regimen, complete remissions have been achieved in 60% to 80% of cases, and progression to severe pulmonary fibrosis has occurred in less than 20% of cases [97, 101, 106, 112]. The response to corticosteroids may be dramatic, with complete resolution of symptoms within hours or days and normalization of chest radiographs within 1 to 4 weeks. The exact rate of taper and duration of therapy needs to be adjusted according to clinical and radiographic parameters, but a 9- to 18-month course of therapy is usually adequate. More prolonged courses may be warranted in patients exhibiting recrudescence or persistence of disease. Immunosuppressive or cytotoxic agents have been used in patients refractory to or experiencing side effects from corticosteroids, with anecdotal successes, but their efficacy has not been evaluated in clinical, prospective trials.

Sarcoidosis

Sarcoidosis, a chronic granulomatosis disease of uncertain etiology, involves the lung in over 95% of cases and may give rise to a wide gamut of manifestations [114–122]. Sarcoidosis is the most common of the immune-mediated interstitial lung disorders, with a prevalence rate of 10 to 20 cases per 100,000 population [114–116]. Over 80% of cases occur in individuals between 20 and 45 years [114–116]. The predominance of sarcoidosis in young adults is a distinguishing feature from IPF, which typically affects older adults. Sarcoidosis is eight times more common in blacks, with a slight female predominance [114–116]. Occasional clustering of cases within families has also been described. These data suggest that a genetic predisposition exists, but no specific gene defect has been identified.

The clinical expression and natural history of sarcoidosis is extraordinarily variable. Pulmonary manifestations usually dominate, but multisystemic involvement is virtually always present, even if no organ-specific symptoms are present. Asymptomatic involvement of liver or spleen has been demonstrated in 40% to 70% of cases, but gives rise to symptoms in less than 5% of cases [114–117]. Virtually any organ can be affected. The most common sites of symptomatic extrapulmonary involvement include skin, lymph nodes (both intrathoracic and extrathoracic), and eye; symptoms due to involvement of the central nervous system, heart, kidneys, skeletal muscle, or bone occur in 2% to 6% of cases [114–117]. The disease is typically indolent and chronic, lasting for several months or even years, and may pursue a relapsing and remitting course. Subacute or acute presentations, although uncommon, may also occur. The prognosis is usually favorable, as spontaneous complete remissions occur in two thirds of patients; however, chronic, progressive sarcoidosis may lead to irreversible end-organ injury, and fatalities due to respiratory failure, cor pulmonale, or extrapulmonary organ failure occur in 1% to 2% of cases [114–121]. Rare, but potentially lethal manifestations of extrapulmonary sarcoidosis include ventricular arrythmias, heart block, congestive heart failure or sudden death due to myocardial involvement, quadriparesis or paresis from involvement of the nervous system, abdominal pain, pancytopenia from massive splenomegaly, fulminant hepatic failure, and chronic nephrocalcinosis secondary to chronic hypercalcemia and hypercalciuria [114–117]. The extrapulmonary features of sarcoidosis have been reviewed in previous publications [114, 116, 117] and are not further addressed in this chapter.

Forty percent to 60% of patients with sarcoidosis are asymptomatic, with incidental changes noted on chest radiography [114–121]. Abnormalities on chest radiography including intrathoracic lymphadenopathy, and parenchymal infiltrates are present in 90% to 95% of cases; cough and dyspnea are the most common symptoms [114–121]. Fatigue and malaise may be prominent nonspecific findings. Early in the course of the disease, a distinct symptom complex of erythema nodosum (EN), polyarthritis, fever, and bilateral hilar lymphadenopathy (BHL), termed Loefgren's syndrome, occurs in 10% to 20% of cases [114–121]. BHL may persist for prolonged periods, but fever, EN, and arthritis typically regress completely within 4 to 12 weeks. Loefgren's syndrome is a favorable prognostic indicator, as sarcoidosis spontaneously remits in more than 85% of cases in this context [114–121]. A similar constellation of symptoms may occur in tuberculosis and mycotic infections, but these features are virtually never seen in other ILD.

The pulmonary lesion in sarcoidosis is characterized by an alveolitis (composed of mononuclear cells (lymphocytes, macrophages, plasma cells) in the early phase of this disorder, which leads to granuloma formation and varying degrees of injury and fibrosis within the alveolar structures [115]. The alveolitis and granulomatous lesions often spontaneously regress without producing any clinically overt damage, but permanent damage and severe fibrosis may be important sequelae in some cases.

Laboratory Features

Laboratory features in sarcoidosis are nonspecific. Hypergammaglobulinemia, reflecting generalized B-cell activation, occurs in 25% to 75% of cases [114–117]. Elevations in the erythrocyte sedimentation rate may occur, but do not consistently correlate with disease activity. Chronic hypercalcemia occurs in 2% to 6% of cases and hypercalciuria in 20% to 50% [114–117]. These derangements in calcium metabolism reflect a heightened sensitivity to vitamin D, associated with increased serum levels of 1,2-dihydrocholecalciferol, and may reverse with corticosteroid therapy [116]. Increases in hepatic enzymes, particularly alkaline phosphatase, occur in 5% to 15% of cases [114–117]. Five percent to 10% of patients display mild leukopenia, but anemia attributable to sarcoidosis has been demonstrated in fewer than 3% of cases [114–117, 122]. Increases in serum angiotensin converting enzyme (SACE) have been described in 30% to 80% of cases and may correlate with disease activity [123–128]. This laboratory parameter is discussed in greater detail later in the section on newer techniques.

Chest Radiography

Abnormalities on chest radiography are present in 90% to 95% of cases [114–121]. BHL is the most characteristic finding and is present in 50% to 75% of cases (Fig. 11-10A) [114–122]. Unilateral hilar adenopathy occurs in fewer than 5% of cases of sarcoidosis and suggests an alternative diagnosis such as bronchogenic carcinoma. Right paratracheal lymphadenopathy accompanies BHL in more

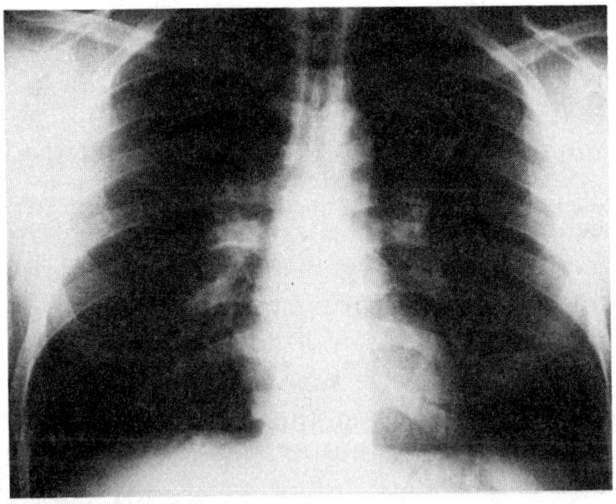

A

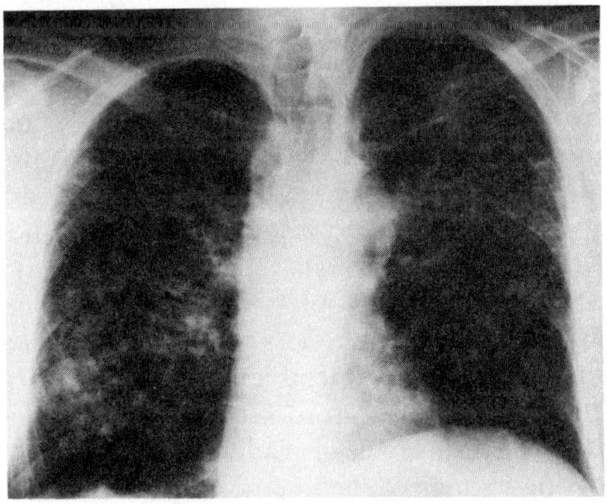

B

Fig. 11-10. (A) Sarcoidosis (stage 1). Chest radiograph demonstrating bilateral hilar lymphadenopathy in a 28-year-old black man with arthritis and erythema nodosum. No pulmonary parenchymal infiltrates are present. Transbronchial lung biopsy demonstrated multiple noncaseating granulomata, consistent with sarcoidosis. Symptoms spontaneously resolved within 4 weeks and he has remained asymptomatic at long-term follow-up. (B) Sarcoidosis (stage 2). Chest radiograph demonstrating bilteral patchy, reticular, and reticulonodular infiltrates with areas of nodularity and coalescence. The hilar structures are elevated, and slight adenopathy is present.

than one third of cases on plain chest radiography, but substantial enlargement of other mediastinal lymph node groups (anterior mediastinum, left para-aortic) is uncommon and suggests an alternative diagnosis, such as lymphoma. However, when more sensitive techniques such as chest CT scanning have been applied, enlargement of left para-aortic, paratracheal, subcarinal, and other mediastinal lymph nodes can often be demonstrated. We do not believe that CT scanning is required, however, in the routine diagnostic evaluation or staging of sarcoidosis. Pulmonary parenchymal infiltrates are present on chest radiography in 30% to 70% of cases [114–122] and may assume a variety of forms. Reticular or reticulonodular infiltrates are characteristic and may be diffuse or patchy (focal) in distribution. A miliary pattern, characterized by diffuse 2- to 4-mm nodular densities and a ground glass appearance, occurs in fewer than 10% of cases, but when present is usually characterized by an active inflammatory phase (alveolitis) and an excellent responsiveness to corticosteroid therapy. When concomitant BHL is present, the demonstration of parenchymal infiltrates irrespective of radiographic pattern strongly suggests the diagnosis of sarcoidosis. However, in the absence of BHL, the radiographic appearance may be indistinguishable from IPF or other ILD. The distribution of infiltrates in sarcoidosis may sometimes be a helpful clue to the diagnosis. In contrast to IPF, which preferentially involves the basilar regions of the lungs, sarcoidosis has a predilection for upper and mid lung zones (Fig. 11-10B). In addition, focal infiltrates, sometimes with an acinar pattern and airbronchograms, may be superimposed on a more diffuse interstitial pattern. These radiographic features (upper lobe predominance, dense focal infiltrates) are rarely present in IPF. Loss of lung substance by the chronic, destructive granulomatous process may lead to "shrinking lungs," with low lung volumes and linear, coarse stranding (reflecting fibrous bands), upward retraction of the hilae (due to contraction of the upper lobes), and honeycombing. Upper lobe cavitation and mycetomas (fungus balls) or severe bullous emphysema have also been described as rare complications of extensive parenchymal destruction. Enlargement of the cardiac silhouette and pulmonary arteries due to cor pulmonale from long-standing pulmonary insufficiency occurs in 1% to 4% of cases. Other unusual radiographic features occurring in 1% to 3% of cases include lobar atelectasis (due to granulomatous stenosis of bronchi), large nodular infiltrates simulating malignant neoplasm, and pleural effusions. In view of the rarity of these radiographic findings, their presence should stimulate a search for an alternative cause before accepting the diagnosis of sarcoidosis.

While chest radiography cannot reliably distinguish between fibrosis and inflammation (alveolitis), the pattern of the chest radiograph at the time of presentation has prognostic importance. The radiographic staging pattern espoused by Siltzbach [117] is useful as a prognostic guide (stage 1, BHL without parenchymal infiltrates; stage 2, BHL plus parenchymal infiltrates; and stage 3, parenchymal infiltrates without BHL). Fifty percent to 90% of patients with radiographic stage 1 disease spontaneously remit, but remissions occur in only 30% to 50% with stage 2 disease, and less than 30% with stage 3 disease [115–121]. In a recent study in Sweden that longitudinally assessed 505 sarcoid patients, both treated and untreated, over a 2-year period, chest radiographs normalized in over 80% of patients with stage 1 disease and only 10.6% progressed to radiographic stage 2 or 3 [121]. By contrast, radiographs normalized in 68% and 37% of stage 2 and 3 patients, respectively. Danish investigators noted similar trends among 210 patients with sarcoidosis followed for 1 to 10 years; among stage 1 patients, complete radiographic resolution occurred in 57% of patients and only 10% progressed to stage 2 (none developed stage 3 disease) [119]. Among patients with stage 2 disease, chest radiographs normalized in 48% and an additional 38% improved or stabilized. By contrast, chest radiographs normalized in only 1 of 10 with stage 3 disease, and 80% remained in radiographic stage 3.

These investigators also found that, with few exceptions, the course of the disease was dictated within the first 2 years. Eighty-five percent of remission occurred within this time, and late relapses were rare in patients exhibiting stable disease for the first 2 years. Only 1 of 63 patients with initial stage 1 disease developed disease progression after the second year. Stability at 2 years also implied a low rate of subsequent resolution. Chest radiographs eventually normalized in only 12% of patients who remained in stage 2 after 2 years of observation [119]. These data suggest that the critical management decisions should be made within the first 12 to 24 months. Treatment should be considered in patients with stage 2 or 3 disease who are symptomatic or exhibit significant pulmonary dysfunction when parenchymal infiltrates fail to clear within 12 to 24 months, since late spontaneous regression is unlikely. Persistence of stage 1 disease does not require therapy in the absence of significant or progressive pulmonary dysfunction or symptoms. In order not to lose this therapeutic window, we believe that follow-up visits (to include chest radiography and PFTs) should be most frequent within the first 2 years of diagnosis. The practice of reassuring patients that sarcoidosis is benign and should "go away in time" should be avoided. It is only through meticulous and consistent follow-up that progressive or persistent disease can be promptly identified and treated before development of irreversible fibrosis. Even in asymptomatic individuals, we schedule follow-up visits at 3- to 4-month intervals during the first year to identify patients who may require therapy, either because of disease progression or persistent infiltrates associated with pulmonary dysfunction. When patients have been stable for 1 year, subsequent visits at 6-month intervals for the next year is reasonable. Since the rate of relapse is low among patients who have been stable for 2 years, follow-up at 1- to 2-year intervals is reasonable in this subset of patients. We have extended follow-up beyond 2 years because we have observed several patients who have demonstrated disease progression (especially those with stage 2 or 3 disease) even after several years of previous stability. The decision to treat should be individualized and should not rest on radiographic findings alone. Factors that should be taken into account include the extent and duration of disease, presence or absence of symptoms, the degree of pulmonary dysfunction, and the potential toxicity of corticosteroids.

Pulmonary Function Tests

Pulmonary function studies are of critical importance in following the course of the pulmonary lesion and identifying patients who may benefit from therapy. Aberrations in pulmonary function may be demonstrated even when no parenchymal infiltrates are apparent on chest radiography, but are more common in radiographic stage 2 or 3 disease. A restrictive ventilatory defect, with reductions in lung volumes (VC, TLC), occurs in 40% to 70% of cases [22, 115, 120]. The DLCO is reduced in a similar percentage of patients, but is usually less severe than the change in lung volumes, and much less severe than the marked reductions observed in IPF [22]. Other differences in patterns of pulmonary functional changes between sarcoidosis and IPF exist. Measurements of resting and exercise gas exchange (DLCO and alveolar-arterial O_2 gradient) are relatively well preserved in sarcoidosis compared with IPF at a comparable degree of reduction in VC and TLC [22]. Hypoxemia, a cardinal feature of IPF, is usually not found in sarcoidosis except in far advanced cases. Thus, we have not found exercise testing to be helpful in the evaluation of sarcoidosis. Reductions in FEV_1 and expiratory flow rates, which are usually well preserved and often supranormal in IPF, are found in 20% to 30% of patients with sarcoidosis, which reflects the predilection of sarcoidosis to involve the airways and bronchial submucosa [115, 129]. A concomitant restrictive defect is usually evident in patients exhibiting airways obstruction, but isolated obstructive defects may also occur. A subset of patients exhibit bronchial hyperreactivity to methacholine or exogenous stimuli and may complain of wheezing, paroxysmal cough, or dyspnea [129]. In such cases, a trial of bronchodilators should be administered, but corticosteroids are often required for symptomatic control in this context.

As with IPF, abnormalities on PFTs cannot discriminate between active alveolitis and fibrosis. Nevertheless, serial measurements may be useful to better delineate the course and prognosis of the disease. Changes in VC appear to be most sensitive as an indicator of disease progression or regression [22]. Thus, sequential spirometry may be adequate among patients with minimally symptomatic or asymptomatic disease. Progressive loss of pulmonary function on longitudinal testing or persistent substantial deficits on repeat examinations, may warrant a trial of corticosteroid therapy even in asymptomatic patients with stable chest radiographs.

Histology

The histologic hallmark of sarcoidosis is the noncaseating or nonnecrotizing granuloma. Characteristically, epithelioid and multinucleated giant cells, derived from monocyte/macrophage precursors, make up the central core of the granuloma, interspersed with collagen (Fig. 11-11A and B) [115]. In the periphery, lymphocytes, occasional plasma cells, mononuclear phagocytes, and fibroblasts may be found. In some cases, the granuloma may be relatively devoid of inflammatory cells, with broad bands of collagen and a dense hyalinized or fibrotic background. In others, dense inflammatory cells, composed largely of lymphocytes and mononuclear phagocytes, may be present [115].

When to Biopsy?

The issue of which patients require biopsy confirmation when sarcoidosis is suspected remains controversial. We agree with other investigators that biopsy is usually not necessary in asymptomatic patients with BHL, for reasons that are discussed shortly. However, we usually attempt to establish a specific tissue diagnosis in patients exhibiting symptoms, pulmonary parenchymal infiltrates, significant organ dysfunction, persistent fever, profound weight loss, or atypical features. Histologic confirmation of the diagnosis is required whenever corticosteroid therapy is contemplated. A variety of sites may be amenable to biopsy. For example, when cutaneous involvement is evident, punch biopsy of an accessible skin lesion may be the preferred procedure to substantiate a diagnosis as it can, be readily performed in the physician's office. Biopsy of clinically involved extrapulmonary sites such as the liver, peripheral lymph nodes, and bone marrow may be appropriate in cases where intrathoracic involvement is not evident (e.g., radiographic stage 0). However, when intrathoracic lymphadenopathy or pulmonary parenchymal infiltrates are present, flexible fiberoptic bronchoscopy with TBB is the initial invasive procedure of choice. TBB can be performed as an outpatient procedure with minimal morbidity (complication rate of $< 2\%$) and diagnostic yields of 70% to 95% [115]. In the appropriate clinical setting, the demonstration of noncaseating granulomata in bronchial submucosa or alveoli is sufficient to establish the diagnosis. Given the predilection of sarcoid granulomas to involve the bronchial submucosa, the diagnosis can sometimes be suspected by the gross endoscopic appearance. While the bronchial mucosa is normal in most cases of sarcoidosis, in occasional patients the bronchial mucosa may be studded, with a distinct cobblestone appearance; in this context, even endobronchial biopsies may be diagnostic (Fig. 11-11B). Scalene node or mediastinal lymph node biopsy are diagnostic in 70% to 100% of cases [114–117]. However, these procedures have greater morbidity than fiberoptic bronchoscopy and are reserved for patients in whom TBB is nondiagnostic. Open lung biopsy is virtually never required to make the diagnosis of pulmonary sarcoidosis. Biopsy of extrathoracic sites may occasionally be rewarding. Noncaseating granulomata may be demonstrated by percutaneous liver biopsy in 40% to 70% of cases, even in the absence of clinical hepatic involvement [114–117]. Some investigators have reported diagnostic yields of 10% to 30% with biopsy of conjunctivae or skeletal

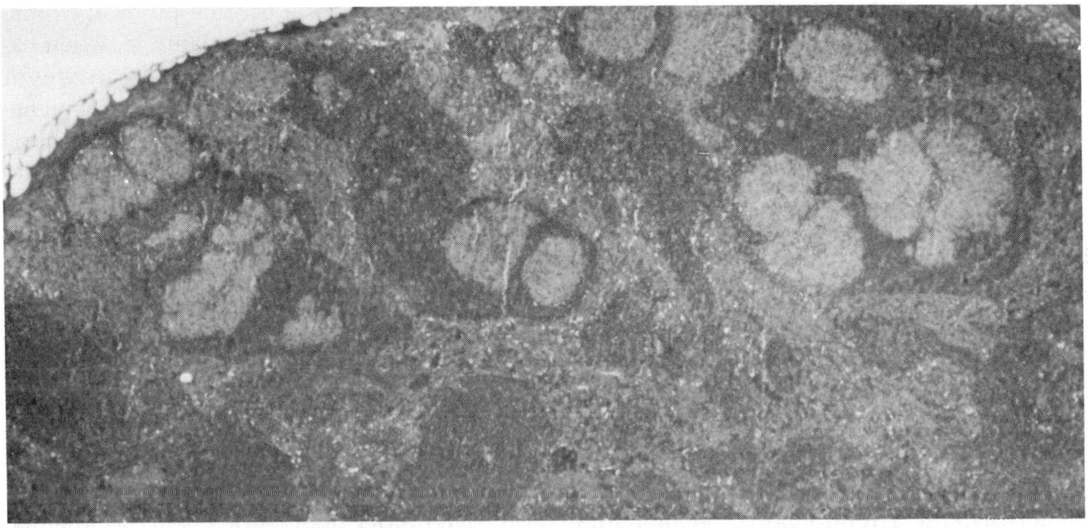

A

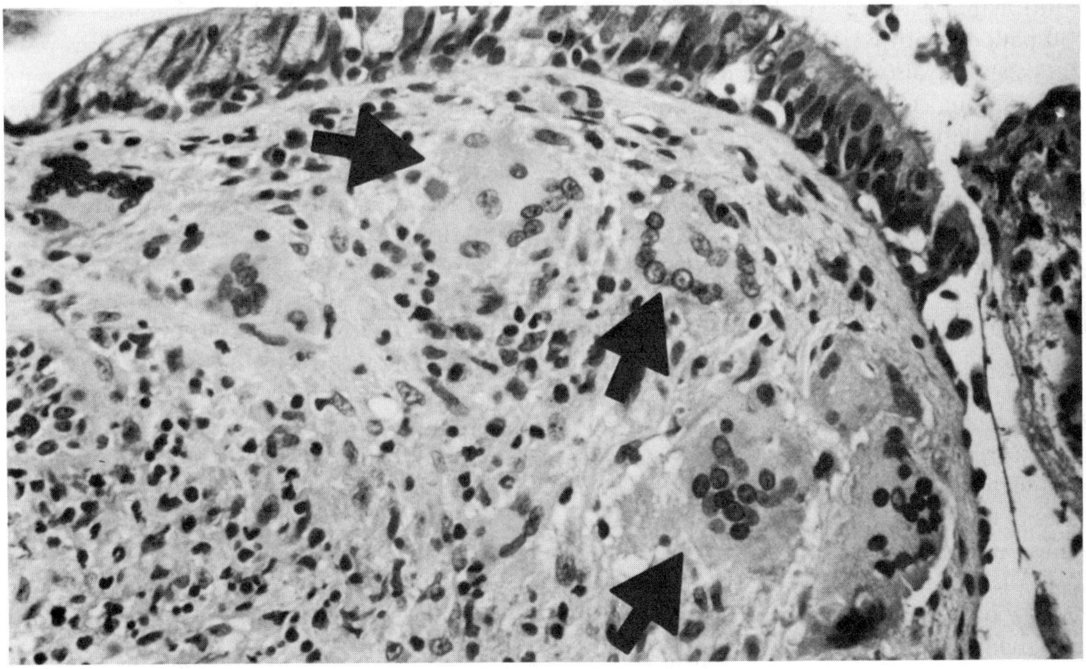

B

Fig. 11-11. (A) Sarcoidosis. Photomicrograph of lymph node biopsy demonstrating multiple, discrete noncaseating granulomata in a patient with extensive sarcoidosis involving mediastinum, liver, spleen, skin, and lung (hematoxylin-eosin, low power). (B) Sarcoidosis. Photomicrograph of endobronchial biopsy from a patient with sarcoidosis demonstrating granulomatous inflammatory changes. Note the multinucleated giant cells in the submucosa beneath the layer of bronchiolar lining cells (*arrows*) (hematoxylin-eosin, high power).

muscle, even in patients without clinically evident involvement of these sites. While our experience with these procedures is limited, we do not believe they offer any advantage over higher yield procedures such as bronchoscopy.

Significance of Bilateral Hilar Lymphadenopathy

Symmetrical BHL in individuals who are asymptomatic or have only EN or uveitis is so commonly due to sarcoidosis that tissue confirmation of the diagnosis is rarely required in this context. Unfortunately, many such patients are needlessly subjected to a variety of invasive procedures and anxiety because of concern about lymphoma or malignancy. This issue was addressed in a classic article by Winterbauer et al [122] in 1973 that reviewed 100 patients with BHL (74 of whom had sarcoidosis) and also analyzed the incidence of BHL among patients with lymphoma and other malignancies. Although 20 of 212 (9.4%) patients with lymphoma displayed BHL at some point in the course of the disease, only eight (3.8%) had BHL at the initial presentation. Of these eight patients, all were symptomatic, seven had easily identifiable extrathoracic tumor on physical examination, and five had anemia. BHL as a manifestation of solid carcinomas was also exceedingly rare. Four of 500 (0.8%) patients with bronchogenic carcinoma had BHL, which was associated with an anterior mediastinal mass in two cases. The remaining two patients were symptomatic and had extrathoracic tumor easily accessible to biopsy. Only 2 of 1201 (0.2%) patients with primary extrathoracic malignancies exhibited BHL; both were severely symptomatic. In summary, all patients in whom BHL was a manifestation of malignancy were symptomatic, and all but two had extrathoracic mass lesions deleted on physical examination. An analysis of the 100 patients with BHL disclosed only 34 who were asymptomatic; all 34 had sarcoidosis. In addition, all 13 patients with EN or uveitis had sarcoidosis. Laboratory studies and physical examination were also useful in distinguishing sarcoidosis from neoplastic causes of BHL. Fifty of 52 patients with a normal physical examination had sarcoidosis. In contrast, when extrathoracic findings other than EN, uveitis, or arthritis were present, nearly 50% had malignancy. Nine of 20 patients with peripheral lymphadenopathy, splenomegaly, or hepatomegaly had neoplasm; the remaining cases had sarcoidosis. Anemia was also a useful differentiating feature. Anemia attributable to sarcoidosis was found in only 1 of 74 cases, but was common in malignancy [122]. Thus, in patients with asymptomatic BHL (or only uveitis or EN), biopsy may not be necessary to determine the etiology of BHL, as long as the physical examination is normal, there is no prior history of malignancy, and significant laboratory aberrations (such as anemia) are absent. This practice has been followed widely in Europe, and misdiagnoses in this context have been rare [119, 121]. This practice of withholding biopsy in asymptomatic patients should not be extrapolated to other groups of patients, such as those exhibiting hectic fevers, a prolonged course, weight loss, or significant constitutional or systemic symptoms. In such cases, biopsy is essential not only to substantiate the diagnosis of sarcoidosis, but to convincingly exclude other causes of BHL. BHL may be a presenting feature of granulomatous infections such as tuberculosis or mycoses. Thus, we routinely perform tuberculin skin testing and serologic studies for fungi (complement fixation or immunodiffusion test) to more definitely exclude these etiologies in all patients with newly diagnosed BHL, irrespective of whether symptoms are present. Certain clinical features (fever, night sweats, weight loss), particularly when persistent, should heighten the suspicion for granulomatous infection. In that context, our practice has been to proceed with TBB including BAL and appropriate smears and cultures for acid fast bacilli and fungi to more convincingly rule out infection (Fig. 11-12). When bronchoscopic findings are nondiagnostic, biopsy of other sites (bone marrow, liver) may be necessary to establish a diagnosis. Smears and cultures of buffy coat blood and bone marrow to look for *Histoplasma capsulatum* should be done in patients

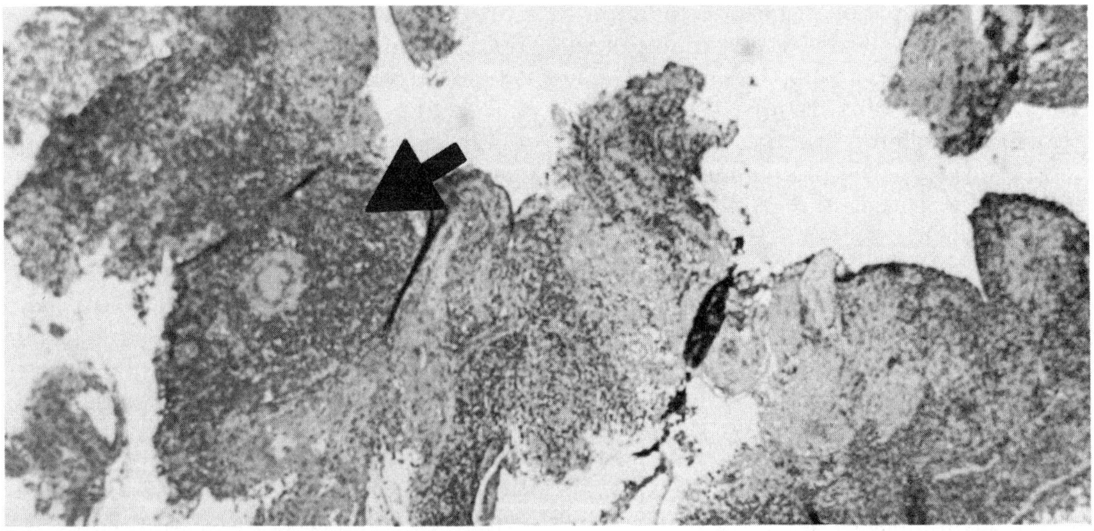

Fig. 11-12. Mycobacteriosis. Photomicrograph of transbronchial lung biopsy from a 75-year-old man with patchy airspace disease involving the left lingula. Note the exuberant lymphocytic infiltrate surrounding a prominent multinucleated giant cell (*arrow*) (hematoxylin-eosin, lower power).

with BHL and chronic fevers who live in endemic areas. It should be emphasized that noncaseating granulomas the histologic hallmark of sarcoidosis are not pathognomonic or specific for this condition. Although infectious granulomas typically exhibit foci of necrosis or caseation, noncaseating granulomas may also be found, even in tuberculous or fungal infections. Thus, special stains for acid fast bacilli and fungi should be done to exclude these organisms.

Newer Staging Techniques

Within the past two decades, newer techniques (gallium scans, BAL, and SACE) have been applied to better assess the activity of sarcoidosis compared with conventional techniques (chest radiography, PFTs, clinical scores). Increased intrapulmonary uptake of gallium or incresed BAL T-lymphocytes are more sensitive indicators of the degree of alveolar inflammation while SACE has been used as a marker of total body granuloma burden [115]. Despite widespread enthusiasm for gallium scanning and BAL shortly after their introduction, we agree with most investigators that neither technique has an established role in the clinical management of sarcoidosis.

Gallium 67 Scanning

Initial studies at the National Institutes of Health demonstrated that increased intrapulmonary uptake of gallium 67 citrate (Ga 67) was observed in a high percentage of patients with sarcoidosis, correlated with proportion of T-lymphocytes on BAL, and provided a more accurate assessment of alveolitis than did chest radiography or PFTs [115, 130]. While multiple investigators have corroborated these findings [124, 125, 127, 131, 132], the value of gallium scanning in predicting prognosis remains controversial. Some studies have shown excellent correlations between degree of intrapulmonary uptake of Ga 67 and responsiveness to corticosteroids [131, 132], but others have not [127, 133]. Interpretation is confounded by varying methodology, interobserver variability, and the lack of a gold standard. In addition, gallium scans are inconvenient as scanning is done 48 hours after injection of the radioisotope, expensive, and result in modest radiation exposure. Thus, while gallium scans may provide adjunctive information regarding the intensity of alveolitis, repeated scans are impractical. Therefore, we do not recommend gallium scans in the routine staging of sarcoidosis. Gallium scanning may have a role, however, in selected patients in whom the clinical activity is uncertain and therapy is being debated.

Bronchoalveolar Lavage

Since its introduction in the mid-1970s, BAL has permitted significant new insights into the pathogenesis of sarcoidosis. However, enthusiasm for its application as a clinical tool has waned. Initial studies at the National Institutes of Health demonstrated striking increases in lymphocytes and T-lymphocytes in BAL fluid among patients with active pulmonary sarcoidosis, with higher numbers seen with more clinically active disease [24, 115]. Further, these cells were activated, spontaneously released lymphokines, and expressed the T-helper/inducer cell phenotype [115]. Subsequent studies from multiple centers confirmed that increased T cells and T-helper cells were characteristic of pulmonary sarcoidosis, but overlap between patients with active and inactive disease existed [115, 128, 133–138]. French investigators reported that high levels of T-lymphocytes were commonly seen with active disease, but that occasional patients responded to corticosteroid therapy even though BAL cell profiles were normal [137]. Several prospective studies on the role of BAL in assessing prognosis in sarcoidosis have been done, with conflicting results. Keogh et al [138] stratified patients on the basis of high-intensity alveolitis (arbitrarily defined as > 28% lymphocytes on BAL and a positive gallium 67 scan result) or low-intensity alveolitis (defined as < 28% lymphocytes or a negative gallium scan result) and noted a much higher rate of functional deterioration among patients with high-intensity alveolitis as compared with low-intensity alveolitis even though clinical features were similar between groups at the outset. Hollinger et al [124] noted that pretreatment BAL lymphocyte counts were a better predictor of corticosteroid responsiveness than clinical scores, PFTs, quantitative gallium scans, or SACE among 21 patients with pulmonary sarcoidosis. Lawrence et al [125] performed BAL before and after 6 weeks of corticosteroid therapy among 12 patients with recently diagnosed, symptomatic, pulmonary sarcoidosis. Striking reductions in the level of BAL IgG-secreting cells were noted following treatment, but changes in percent BAL lymphocytes were small and failed to correlate with the clinical course. In two separate studies, Buchalter et al [139] and Turner-Warwick et al [127] found that initial BAL cell counts were of no value in predicting evolution of disease or response to corticosteroid treatment. Similarly, Israel-Biet et al [140] prospectively followed 73 patients with stage 1 or 2 sarcoidosis for 2 years (none of whom were treated) and noted that initial BAL lymphocyte counts did not predict eventual outcome. However, persistence of BAL lymphocytosis at 12 months predicted a high rate of nonresolution at 24 months. Only 3 of 21 (13%) patients exhibiting BAL lymphocytosis at 12 months remitted by 24 months, compared with a recovery rate of 81% among 23 patients with normal BAL at 12 months. Bjemer et al [134] reported that initial BAL lymphocyte counts were increased in 77% of 45 patients with newly diagnosed sarcoidosis and bore no relationship to subsequent outcome. All of these studies assessed percent lymphocytes and did not analyze phenotypic markers. However, several investigators have found that quantifying BAL T-helper/inducer (T4) cells or T4/T8 ratio is a better reflection of disease activity than percent lymphocytes or T cells alone. Ceuppens et al [135] performed serial BAL in 12 patients with sarcoidosis (three treated, nine untreated) and found that the change in T4/T8 ratio mirrored disease activity in every case, even though changes in BAL lymphocytes were variable. Other investigators have confirmed the superiority of T4/T8 ratios as prognostic markers over lymphocyte counts without phenotype [131, 133, 141]. Costabel et al [133] reported that initial BAL T4/T8 ratios predicted subsequent functional deterioration better than PFTs, SACE, gallium scans, or BAL lymphocyte counts. Only 2 of 15 patients with normal T4/T8 ratios on initial BAL deteriorated, whereas 10 of 16 patients with high BAL T4/T8 ratios deteriorated. What conclusions can be drawn from these disparate studies? First, BAL lymphocyte counts are elevated in such a high percentage of patients with newly diagnosed sarcoidosis (70% to 85%) that the prognostic value is minimal. Quantitation of phenotypic markers (percent T-lymphocytes, T-helper cells, functional markers) may be a superior gauge of disease activity, but still cannot predict which course the disease will follow in individual patients. In a disease characterized by spontaneous remissions and relapses, no single parameter can be expected to reliably predict prognosis or responsiveness to therapy. High levels of T-helper cells and T4/T8 ratio on BAL may reflect active alveolar inflammation (alveolitis), but isolated values at a single point in time do not imply that functional or radiographic deterioration will inevitably occur. The type of clinical presentation also dictates to a large extent findings on BAL. For example, BAL lymphocytosis is often most pronounced among patients with an acute course associated with EN or acute uveitis; yet these patients virtually always remit spontaneously [128, 136]. In addition, some patients with clinically active disease but without BAL lymphocytosis have improved following initiation of corticosteroids, suggesting that lymphocyte markers are imperfect markers of disease activity [125, 127, 137, 139]. Thus, basing treatment on BAL, in the absence of clinical data, is inappropriate. If this technique is to be useful, sequential measurements assessing changes in lymphocyte populations (or other markers) over time would be of greatest benefit. However, due to the expense and invasive nature of bronchoscopy, performing serial BALs as a routine surveillance test is impractical. While we believe that BAL offers a more accurate assessment of the intensity of alveolitis compared with PFTs, chest radiography, and clinical scores, its predictive value is limited, and we do not advocate BAL in the routine staging or therapeutic strategy in sarcoidosis.

Angiotensin Converting Enzyme

Elevations in SACE occur commonly in active sarcoidosis, as granuloma macrophages release exaggerated amounts of this enzyme. This relationship was initially described by Lieberman [126] in 1975, who reported elevated SACE levels in 15 of 17 patients with active, untreated sarcoidosis, while the SACE level was normal in all 11 patients with inactive disease or on corticosteroids. Since Lieberman's original report, several investigators have reported elevated SACE levels in 30% to 80% of cases, with false-positive rates of only 1% to 5% [115, 123–125, 127, 131, 142]. Higher levels have been found in patients with clinically active disease and may decrease as the disease remits or in response to corticosteroid therapy [115, 124, 125]. Further, even in patients with normal SACE levels, decreases in the absolute level of SACE may occur in response to corticosteroids or with remission of the disease, suggesting that serial measurements may be useful even when values lie within the normal range [115, 123, 124]. However, elevated SACE levels may occur in other granulomatous disorders, such as acute histoplasmosis and talc granulomatous pneumonitis, so caution must be exercised in applying SACE as a specific diagnostic test. Disparate results between SACE, gallium scanning, and BAL have also been demonstrated [127, 142]. SACE appears to be less sensitive as an indicator of alveolitis as compared with BAL [142] and often fails to correlate with BAL lymphocytosis, gallium 67 scanning, or responsiveness to corticosteroids [127, 142]. The inability of SACE to reflect alveolar inflammation is perhaps not surprising, since SACE may reflect the total body granuloma burden rather than the intensity of inflammation at any single site. Thus, therapeutic decisions should not be based simply on SACE levels, as elevated SACE levels in asymptomatic patients would not warrant therapy. More importantly, normal SACE levels may be observed in patients with active disease (pulmonary or extrapulmonary) in whom treatment surely is required. Despite these limitations, SACE is an inexpensive and noninvasive test that provides adjunctive information to clinical data. Elevated SACE levels may identify patients with active disease or more likely to develop disease progression in whom activity of the disease is not clear based on clinical criteria. Similarly, declines in SACE level may be useful in following individual patients in whom clinical criteria are imprecise or difficult to interpret.

Pathogenesis

Sarcoidosis is characterized by an exaggerated immune response, with activated T-lymphocytes, T-helper cells, and mononuclear phagocytes at sites of disease activity [115]. Despite exhaustive investigations, the cause of sarcoidosis is not known. Sarcoidosis may be a manifestation of an exaggerated host response (possibly under genetic constraints) to inhaled antigen(s) or other exogenous or environmental factors. The pulmonary lesion in sarcoidosis begins as an alveolitis, with activated T cells and alveolar macrophages infiltrating the alveolar septae and spaces [115]. Interactions between these immune effector cells (T cells and AMs) are responsible for the induction, evolution, and immunoregulation of the granulomatous inflammatory process. The T-lymphocyte plays a key role in the granuloma formation by its ability to recruit, activate, and communicate with mononuclear phagocytes (blood monocytes and AMs), which are the precursors of the epithelioid and multinucleated giant cells and key structural elements of the granulomatous core. In addition, T-lymphocytes release interleukin-2, which stimulates T-cell replications and serves to perpetuate the T-cell alveolitis. The alveolar macrophage is a key cell in granuloma development by virtue of its potency as a secretory cell and its ability to interact with T-lymphocytes and other immune (and nonimmune) effector cells [3, 115]. AMs obtained from patients with active pulmonary sarcoidosis are activated, display enhanced antigen-presenting capacity, release increased amounts of oxygen radicals, and generate an array of monokines, which exert pleiotrophic effects on lymphocytes, fibroblasts, and possibly other cell types and may amplify and perpetuate the granulomatous process [115]. However, much additional work is required to delineate the factors that modulate and dictate the course of the inflammatory process.

Differential Diagnosis

Several features frequently found in sarcoidosis, including epidemiology (young age group, predominance in blacks), pronounced extrapulmonary and constitutional symptoms, and the tendency to relapse and remit spontaneously, may serve to differentiate this disorder from other ILD. Most importantly, symmetrical BHL can be demonstrated on chest radiography in most patients with sarcoidosis, but is virtually never seen in many other disorders that may be considered in the differential diagnosis, such as IPF, chronic eosinophilic pneumonia (CEP), pulmonary alveolar proteinosis (PAP), BOOP, eosinophilic granuloma (EG), etc. A relapsing or remitting course (even in the absence of therapy) is less specific for sarcoidosis, as a waxing and waning course may also occur with CEP, BOOP, PAP, and EG. Histological features, while characteristic, are not pathognomonic. For example, while noncaseating granulomata, the histologic hallmark of sarcoidosis, are not found in IPF or PAP, noncaseating granulomata may be observed in granulomatous infections (e.g., tuberculosis, mycoses), CEP, EG, HP, and granulomatous vasculitis (e.g., Wegener's granulomatosis). Thus, the diagnosis of sarcoidosis can be substantiated only when consistent clinical features are present and alternative etiologies capable of eliciting granuloma formation have been excluded.

Therapy

Treatment of sarcoidosis remains highly controversial. Corticosteroids are the cornerstone of therapy in patients with severe or progressive sarcoidosis and may be highly efficacious in inducing remissions. The long-term impact is less clear, however, as relapses may occur concomitant with discontinuation of therapy [15, 120, 143]. Owing to the high spontaneous remission rate observed in sarcoidosis and the toxicity of corticosteroids, corticosteroid therapy is not warranted in most cases, but should be reserved for patients with severe or progressive symptoms or organ dysfunction. Several retrospective studies have assessed the efficacy of corticosteroids in sarcoidosis [114, 116, 117]. Given the high rate of spontaneous remission observed in sarcoidosis and the lack of reliable parameters of disease activity, interpretation of the efficacy of corticosteroids has been difficult. In addition, treatment approaches reflect the bias of individual investigators, with wide differences in patient populations, parameters of disease activity, indications for therapy, dosage, and duration of therapy. Despite these limitations, however, favorable responses to systemic corticosteroids (as assessed by symptoms, PFTs, and chest radiography) have been demonstrated in 70% to 90% of cases with symptomatic pulmonary sarcoidosis [114–120]. Unfortunately, relapses occur in 20% to 50% of cases following discontinuation of therapy [114–120]. Thus, long-term therapy (sometimes for years) may be required in individual cases. Given these favorable short-term effects, several prospective studies have been performed to determine if early initiation of corticosteroids (even in asymptomatic or minimally symptomatic cases) may avert late complications, including pulmonary fibrosis. All of these studies have failed to show any favorable effects of corticosteroids on mortality or long-term prognosis [143–149]. In one early study, Israel et al [146] randomized 90 patients with pulmonary sarcoidosis to no therapy or prednisone, 15 mg daily for 3 months. At 3 months follow-up, there was greater improvement in PFTs in steroid-treated patients with stage 2 or 3 but not stage 1 disease, suggesting a favorable effect in at least subsets of patients. At 5 years, however, PFTs did not differ between groups. While this study has been interpreted as failing to support the long-term efficacy of corticosteroids, the lack of differences at prolonged follow-up may also be explained by the discontinuation of corticosteroids after only a brief course. Harkleroad et al [145] randomized 25 patients with pulmonary sarcoidosis and abnormal pulmonary function to receive either prednisone (for a minimum of 6 months) or no therapy on an alternate case basis. Improvement was noted among individuals in both groups, but PFTs did not differ between groups when evaluated at 6 months, 1, 2, 10, and 15 years. It should be emphasized, however, that the degree of pulmonary dysfunction was mild at the outset, and 4 of 13 corticosteroid-treated patients were asymptomatic on entry. Other investigators in Europe [143] and Japan [148] have also failed to demonstrate any beneficial long-term effects of corticosteroids on the course of sarcoidosis. Investigators in the Federal Republic of Germany initiated a long-term study in 1967 in which 172 patients with asymptomatic pulmonary sarcoidosis and normal pulmonary function (105 of whom had radiographic stage 2 or 3 disease) were randomized to either placebo or therapy with prednisone for 6 or 12 months [144]. Using this randomization scheme, two thirds of patients received prednisone, at an initial dose of 40 mg daily for 4 weeks, followed by weekly dose reductions of 5 mg until a maintenance dose of 10 mg was reached. Prednisone was discontinued, however, at 6 or 12 months among the treated patients. At the end of follow-up (mean of 8.9 years), chest radiographs had normalized in 83% of treated and 77% of untreated patients, a statistically insignificant difference. PFTs also did not differ between study groups. Reductions of DLCO below 70% of predicted values were present at completion of the study in only 11% of treated and 6% of untreated patients. A recently completed prospective study in the United States [149] randomized 183 patients to placebo or treatment with prednisone (40 mg daily for 3 months, with a taper to 20 mg daily for a 2-year course). At the end of follow-up at 2 years, no statistically significant differences were noted between groups in either chest radiography or PFTs. Together, these various studies support a conservative approach in the management of sarcoidosis. The routine use of corticosteroids in patients with normal PFTs or minimal or no symptoms is not warranted. Nonetheless, none of these studies address the role of therapy in symptomatic patients with progressive disease. It is precisely in this patient population that corticosteroids are most likely to be efficacious. Indications for corticosteroid therapy in sarcoidosis should be circumscribed and focused. Early therapy in asymptomatic or minimally symptomatic individuals has not been shown to improve pulmonary function or mortality and is not recommended. However, in some patients progression of the granulomatous and fibrotic process may lead to severe organ dysfunction and irreversible organ injury. Thus, in selected cases, aggressive treatment with corticosteroids or other immunosuppressive agents may be necessary to avert irreversible end-organ damage. While the precise indications and benefits of corticosteroids remain controversial, we believe that a trial of corticosteroid therapy is warranted for any patients with sarcoidosis involving the central nervous system, eye, myocardium, or with severe organ dysfunction or symptoms. Chronic hypercalcemia, which complicates sarcoidosis in 2% to 7% of cases, requires therapy as sustained hypercalcemia may lead to secondary complications including nephrolithiasis, nephrocalcinosis, and rarely, renal insufficiency [114–117]. The optimal dose and duration of corticosteroid therapy has not been defined; however, high doses for prolonged periods are rarely necessary. Response to moderate dose corticosteroid is often prompt and dramatic. Every other day prednisone (in a dose of 40 to 60 mg every other day) has been advocated as first-line therapy by some investigators and may be efficacious in patients with mild-to-moderate disease. For more severe disease when a prompt remission is desirable, we advise daily corticosteroids (the equivalent of 40 to 60 mg daily) for the first 4 to 6 weeks, with conversion to an alternate day dosing regimen at this point. We have often started at 60 mg daily prednisone for 1 to 2 weeks, with a taper to 50 mg for 1 to 2 weeks, 40 mg for 1 to 2 weeks, at which time the dose is converted to 60 mg every other day. This dose is maintained for 1 month, tapered to 50 mg every other day after 1 month, and then 40 mg every other day for 1 to 2 months. At this point, we usually taper to 30 mg every other day for 2 months, with dose reductions by 5 to 10 mg decrements every 2 months such that the corticosteroid can be discontinued altogether after a 12- to 18-month course of therapy. This regimen is arbitrary, and a variety of alternative approaches are reasonable. However, doses of corticosteroids necessary for control of sarcoidosis are typically much lower than those required for IPF and should be well tolerated in most instances. The rate of taper and duration of therapy needs to be modified according to the clinical response, activity and extent of disease, and side effects. As side effects are minimal when low-dose every other day corticosteroids are used, we often maintain low-dose steroids for prolonged periods (> 12 months) in patients with severe or chronic disease in order to sustain remissions and prevent relapse.

Inhaled corticosteroids have been considered as alternatives to systemic corticosteroids for the treatment of pulmonary sarcoidosis. While controlled data are lacking, European investigators found that inhaled budesonide administered to 10 patients was associated with radiographic improvement in 3 cases and abrogated the lymphocytic and macrophage alveolitis as assessed by BAL [150]. These data are intriguing, but additional prospective studies involving larger numbers of patients are required to assess the possible role of inhaled steroids in the therapy of sarcoidosis.

Other Therapeutic Agents in Sarcoidosis

Although corticosteroids remain the cornerstone of therapy, some patients with active sarcoidosis are refractory to corticosteroids or suffer serious side effects. In this context, a variety of anti-inflammatory agents and immunosuppressive/cytotoxic agents have been used, with anecdotal successes [117, 146–152]. Favorable responses have been reported with anti-inflammatory agents (phenylbutazone, indomethacin) but data are limited [147]. In uncontrolled studies, chloroquine has been reported to be effective in the treatment of cutaneous sarcoidosis and extrapulmonary complications associated with sarcoidosis, including hypercalcemia [153–155]. Immunosuppressive or cytotoxic agents including chlorambucil [147, 151], azathioprine [156], methotrexate [152, 157], cyclophosphamide [158], and cyclosporine A [159, 160] have also been tried in patients with severe or progressive disease refractory to corticosteroids or experiencing serious side effects from corticosteroids. No controlled studies have been done, however, so their relative potency and efficacy have not been clarified. Early experience with chlorambucil was favorable. In two separate studies, remissions were achieved in 8 of 10 [151] and four of eight [147] patients who had previously failed to respond to corticosteroids. Fewer data are available on cyclophosphamide, although favorable responses have been described [158]. Since alkylating agents such as chlorambucil and cyclophosphamide have serious potential toxicity including induction of neoplasia, we prefer less toxic agents such as azathioprine or methotrexate when an immunosuppressive agent other than corticosteroids is required. Oral low-dose methotrexate administered once weekly, 10 to 25 mg, may be efficacious in a variety of immune-mediated disorders including RA, psoriasis, and asthma. While controlled studies have not been done, favorable responses to methotrexate have been achieved in cutaneous, pulmonary, and multisystemic sarcoid [152, 158]. In one recent study, 12 of 14 patients exhibited objective improvement with oral methotrexate; five relapsed when therapy was discontinued and improved when methotrexate was reintroduced [152]. We currently use methotrexate as the preferred agent for those who fail to respond to corticosteroid. Potential serious toxicities of methotrexate include liver disease (including cirrhosis) and pneumonitis. This latter complication may be difficult to distinguish from recurrence of sarcoidosis, since granulomas may be a feature of methotrexate-induced pneumonitis. Prospective long-term trials are required to determine the efficacy and complications of methotrexate in the treatment of sarcoidosis. Cyclosporine A, a fungal decapeptide that inhibits T-cell proliferation, activation, and lymphokine release, has been remarkably effective in disorders characterized by T-cell activation, such as organ transplant rejection, uveitis, and psoriasis [161]. As activated T cells are critical in the immunopathogenesis of sarcoidosis, cyclosporine A has also been tried in refractory cases, with occasional responses [160]. However, cyclosporine has proved to be disappointing in clinical trials. In one recent study of 20 patients with active pulmonary sarcoidosis, cyclosporine A suppressed the release of interleukin-2 and monocyte chemotactic factor from sarcoid lung lymphocytes and inhibited T-cell proliferation in vitro [159]. In contrast to these favorable in vitro effects, oral cyclosporine administered for 6 months in eight patients failed to suppress T-cell alveolitis or lymphokine release in vivo or improve pulmonary function [159]. The poor response to cyclosporine A may reflect an intrinsically resistant patient population, but also raises the possibility that mechanisms other than T-cell activation need to be interrupted in order to control the disease. Cyclosporine is very expensive, and nephrotoxicity virtually always occurs with long-term use. Thus, the role of cyclosporine in the treatment of sarcoidosis has not been established, and its use should be restricted to investigators with experience with this agent for patients with disease refractory to corticosteroids.

Chronic Eosinophilic Pneumonia (CEP)

The association of peripheral blood eosinophilia and pulmonary parenchymal eosinophilia was recognized in 1952 by Reeder and Goodrich [162], who coined the phrase PIE syndrome to refer to this constellation of findings. Crofton and colleagues [163] published in that same year a classification scheme for pulmonary eosinophilia that recognized five separate pulmonary disorders associated with eosinophilia, which included both acute and chronic pneumonic processes.

CEP exhibits clinical and pathologic features that overlap with these other eosinophilic processes, but has distinctive features (e.g., radiographic findings, exquisite responsiveness to corticosteroids, lack of identifiable cause) that warrant classifying CEP as a separate disorder. The original description of CEP as a distinct disease entity is credited to Carrington and coworkers [164], who in 1969 reported nine women who presented with cough, dyspnea, fever, night sweats, and malaise, pulmonary and peripheral blood eosinophilia, and infiltrates on chest radiography. The duration of symptoms exceeded 2 weeks (to distinguish CEP from acute eosinophilic pneumonia or Loeffler's syndrome) and typically lasted several weeks or months [164]. The salient clinical, histologic, and radiologic features were further delineated by Liebow and Carrington [165] in a classic article that year. Since that time, several additional series of CEP have been reported, but the disorder is rare; only 19 patients with CEP were seen at two leading medical centers from 1973 to 1985, and slightly more than 100 published cases have been described [166]. Specific drugs have been reported to cause CEP (e.g., penicillin, sulfonamides, inhaled nickel), but most cases have no identifiable etiology [166]. CEP affects women twice as often as men; 82% of cases occur in adults over age 30, with most cases occurring in middle age [166]. The most common presenting symptoms are nonproductive cough and fever, which occur in approximately 90% of cases [164–166]. Dyspnea, often in association with wheezing, occurs in a majority of cases. Weight loss, sometimes exceeding 20 pounds, has been described in 60% of cases [164–166]. A chronic or subacute course is characteristic; in one recent review, symptoms were present for a mean of 7.7 months (range, 1 to 48) before the diagnosis of CEP [166]. A more rapid course, associated with severe respiratory insufficiency developing within several days, has also been described, but is rare [167]. A history of atopy (allergic rhinitis, drug allergies, asthma) antedating the onset of CEP can be elicited in one half of patients [166]. Asthma occurs in 40% to 50% of cases; asthmatic symptoms may precede the onset of CEP or develop at the onset or shortly following CEP [164–166]. Drenching night sweats occur in one quarter of patients and may erroneously suggest an infectious etiology [166]. Sinusitis and nasal polyposis have been described in 5% to 6% of cases [166]. Physical findings are usually not helpful, as the examination is often normal or may demonstrate only nonspecific findings of rhonchi, wheezes, or rales. Consolidation findings are uncommon, even in patients with extensive chest radiographic changes. Clubbing is not a feature of CEP. Except for atopic manifestations, asthma, and constitutional symptoms, extrapulmonary involvement does not occur in CEP.

Laboratory studies are often a clue to the diagnosis of CEP and may be helpful in monitoring the course of the disease. Peripheral blood leukocytosis occurs in nearly two thirds of patients [166]. However, the most consistent and useful laboratory abnormality is increases in the number and percent of blood eosinophils, which can be demonstrated in more than 85% of cases [164–166]. This blood eosinophilia can be striking, sometimes exceeding 80% eosinophils, although mean values of 20% to 30% are characteristic [164–166]. The erythrocyte sedimentation rate is increased in more than 90% of cases with active disease and decreases as the disease goes into remission [164–166]. Increases in serum IgE levels occur in approximately 50% of cases and may normalize as CEP remits [168]. The utility of IgE levels as markers of disease activity needs to be better defined, as limited data are available in this regard [166, 168]. Striking increases in serum IgE associated with pulmonary infiltrates, wheezing, and blood or tissue eosinophilia are also characteristic of allergic bronchopulmonary aspergillosis, a disorder that may complicate chronic asthma in up to 5% of cases [169]. Allergic bronchopulmonary aspergillosis also responds to corticosteroids, although the rate of response is rarely as rapid or complete as with CEP. Additional features that are uniformly present in allergic bronchopulmonary aspergillosis and differentiate this condition from CEP include immediate and delayed skin test reactivity to *Aspergillus* antigens, serum precipitins and IgE against *Aspergillus* species, and the recovery of *Aspergillus* in sputum, expectorated mucous plugs, or tissue [169]. It should also be emphasized that blood or tissue eosinophilia may occur in the context of specific etiologic disorders (such as sarcoidosis, vasculitis, tuberculosis, parasitic infections, etc.) so these disorders need to be excluded before affirming the diagnosis of CEP.

Chest Radiographic Changes

Peripheral, patchy, alveolar infiltrates, with ill-defined margins and relative sparing of the central portions of the lungs are characteristic [165, 166, 170, 171]. This distinctive pattern, termed the "photographic negative of pulmonary edema," has been considered by some investigators to be so distinctive that many authors believe that in the appropriate clinical setting the diagnosis of CEP can be established by the chest radiograph and presence of blood eosinophilia without resorting to lung biopsy [166, 170, 171]. These infiltrates more frequently involve the apical or axillary regions on chest radiography, and often spare the basilar segments. Infiltrates may be migratory and may spontaneously regress in one area while reappearing in different locations. In addition, relapses of CEP are frequently at the original sites of disease. While these radiographic features are highly suggestive of CEP, none of these findings are invariable or specific. Any segment or lobe can be involved, and one third of cases fail to display the peripheral location of radiographic infiltrates [166]. Further, the more classical photographic negative of pulmonary edema pattern can be appreciated in only about 25% of cases [166]. One radiographic feature of CEP that is rarely found in other ILDs is the rapidity with which radiographic clearing occurs with corticosteroid therapy. Following initiation of corticosteroids, resolution is typically dramatic, with rapid diminution of infiltrates within 24 to 48 hours and complete disappearance within 2 to 3 weeks (Fig. 11-13A to C). This rapid improvement is rarely seen to this degree with other steroid-responsive ILDs and may be a clue to the diagnosis, while awaiting the results of more substantive studies. Pleural effusions and cavitation have been described in 2% to 4% of cases, but are sufficiently unusual as to suggest an alternative diagnosis [166]. Hilar or mediastinal lymphadenopathy does not occur.

Pulmonary Function Tests

Reductions in VC, FEV_1, and expiratory flow rates occur in 60% to 80% of cases [166]. Impaired gas exchange, with hypoxemia and reduced DLCO, have been demonstrated in more than 90% of cases during acute flares of the disease [166]. The physiologic aberrations invariably improve or normalize with corticosteroid therapy. However, the obstructive defects may persist in some cases, particularly in patients with preexisting asthma or with a fixed obliterative bronchial component.

Lung Biopsy

Histologic features on lung biopsy demonstrate widespread collections of eosinophils and alveolar macrophages within alveolar spaces, interalveolar septae, interstitium, and bronchiolar structures [164–166]. Areas of necrotic eosinophils and eosinophilic fragments, termed eosinophilic abscesses, may be observed in areas of intense eosinophilic accumulation. A concomitant granulomatous component, with multinucleated Touton-type giant cells and large mononuclear phagocytes, often coexists (Fig. 11-13D). Many of these giant cells contain degenerating fragments of eosinophils, eosinophilic granules, and brightly colored Charcot-Leyden crystals. Foci of BO can be found in one quarter of cases [164–166]. Despite an intense inflammatory reaction, which may result in extensive consolidation of lung parenchyma and occlusion of bronchioles, parenchymal necrosis or fibrosis is minimal or

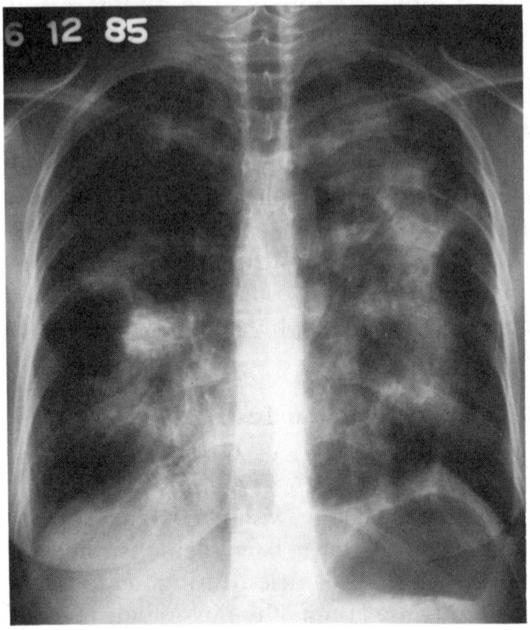
6 12 85

A

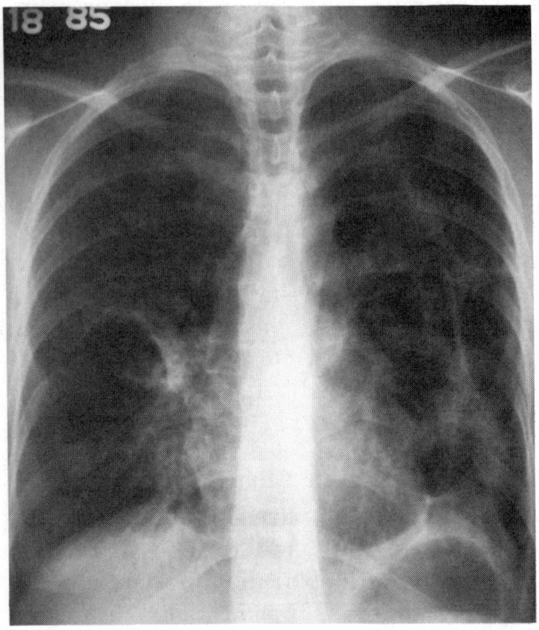
18 85

B

Fig. 11-13. (A) CEP. Chest radiograph of dense bilateral airspace disease with airbronchograms. BAL demonstrated 40% eosinophils and no infectious organisms were identified. Prednisone, 60 mg daily, was started, with prompt improvement. (B) CEP. Chest radiograph 6 days later exhibited marked resolution of pulmonary infiltrates. (C) CEP. Chest radiograph 1 month after initiation of prednisone therapy. The infiltrates had cleared completely and the patient was asymptomatic. (D) CEP. Photomicrograph of lung biopsy demonstrating multinucleated giant cells against a background of inflammatory cells, many of which are eosinophils (*arrows*).

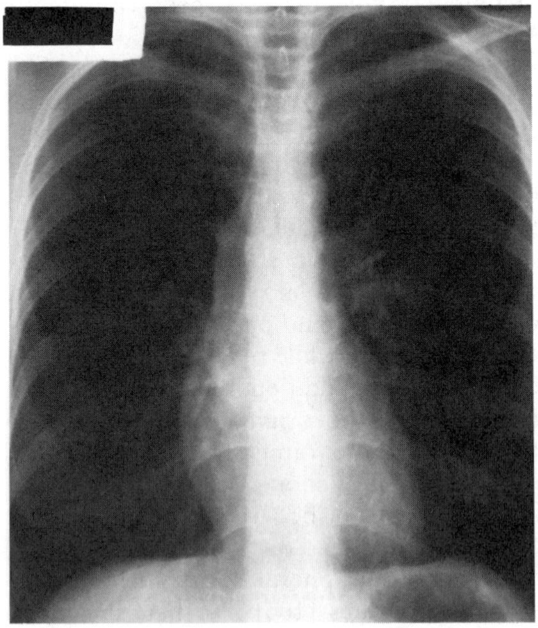

C

absent. Perivascular cuffing of small pulmonary vessels by eosinophils and mononuclear cells in areas contiguous to or within the parenchymal inflammatory infiltrates may occur, but vessel walls remain intact and are not necrotic. A primary vasculitis is not a feature of CEP and suggests an alternative diagnosis, such as Churg-Strauss syndrome (allergic angiitis and granulomatosis) [172]. While most of these histologic features have been elegantly described on the basis of open lung biopsy specimens, we believe that open lung

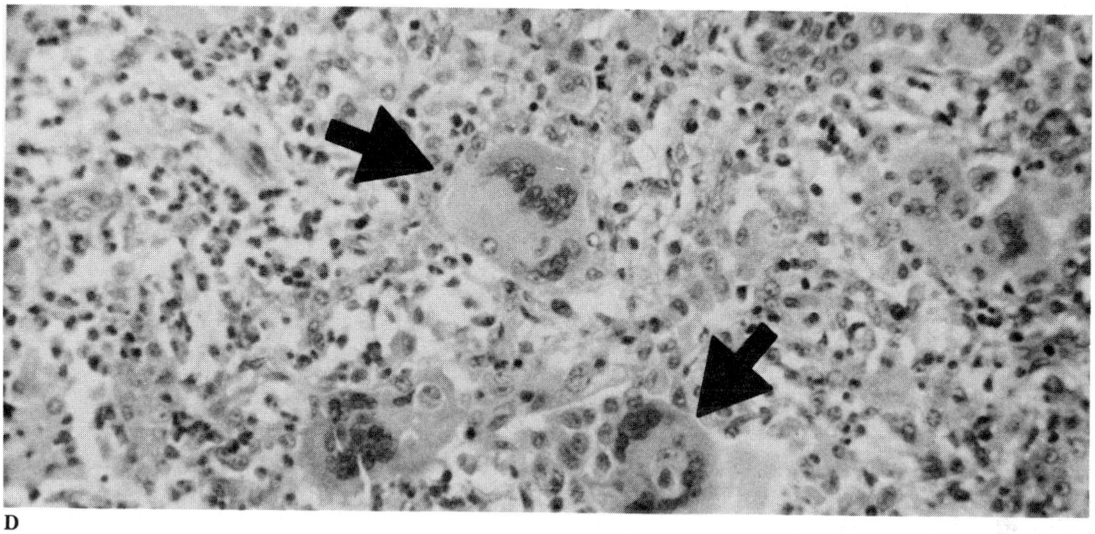

D

biopsy is rarely required in the diagnosis of CEP. Despite the small sample size and potential for sampling error, fiberoptic bronchoscopy with TBB and BAL are usually sufficient to substantiate the diagnosis of CEP. BAL cell differential counts may be helpful in suspecting the diagnosis in patients with new onset of ILD, even when blood eosinophilia is not present. Marked increases in BAL fluid eosinophils usually exceeding 20% are characteristic of CEP and have rarely been found in other conditions [173, 174]. Even when TBB is nondiagnostic, the presence of large numbers of eosinophils on BAL, together with compatible clinical, laboratory (blood eosinophilia, increased serum IgE), and radiographic findings, is sufficient to justify initiation of corticosteroid therapy. A prompt response to corticosteroid therapy, often within 24 to 72 hours may then substantiate the diagnosis. Open lung biopsy should be reserved for patients with atypical laboratory or radiographic features, or patients failing to respond to corticosteroids. However, in our experience, we have not required open lung biopsy to substantiate the diagnosis in over 15 cases within the past decade.

Pathogenesis

While the precise role of the eosinophil in the induction and modulation of the lung lesion of CEP has not been clarified, eosinophils and their secretory products appear to mediate the events leading to pulmonary injury. Eosinophils predominate in the histopathology of the lesion, and the extent of blood or tissue eosinophilia correlates with activity of the disease [166]. Corticosteroids the mainstay of therapy for this disorder, dramatically suppress eosinophilic number and function and have been shown to ablate eosinophilic alveolitis in CEP in vivo [166]. The eosinophil contains a variety of products such as major basic protein, eosinophilic-derived cationic protein, oxygen radicals, peroxidase, collagenase, neurotoxin, and other proinflammatory mediators that are capable of inducing lung damage [166]. In addition, eosinophils have been shown to be cytotoxic for lung parenchymal cells in vitro [166]. Interactions between eosinophils and mononuclear phagocytes (and possibly other immune effector cells) appear to be responsible for the evolution and modulation of the eosinophilic-granulomatous response. Intra-alveolar macrophages, multinucleated giant cells, a granulomatous component in the histopathology of CEP, and the observation that macrophages may ingest eosinophils and eosinophilic fragments support a role of the macrophage in the pathogenesis of the lesion [166, 168].

Treatment and Outcome

In the absence of treatment, the course of CEP may be protracted, with persistent cough, fever, dyspnea, and wheezing over many months; spontaneous remission occurs in fewer than 5% of cases [166]. Corticosteroids are dramatically effective in reversing the signs and symptoms of this disorder. Even in the context of acute respiratory failure requiring mechanical ventilation, fatalities and long-term sequelae are virtually nonexistent as long as treatment with corticosteroids is initiated [166, 167]. Owing to the rarity of this condition and the lack of prospective, controlled studies, the optimal dosage and duration of therapy has not been well defined and needs to be individualized. However, an initial dose of 0.5 to 1.0 mg/kg/d prednisone (or equivalent) is usually sufficient to induce a remission; lower dosages may be associated with a lower response rate [166]. The response to corticosteroids is often dramatic, with improvement in dyspnea, wheezing, malaise, and peripheral eosinophilia within 24 to 48 hours of initiation of therapy. Complete resolution of symptoms is achieved within 2 weeks in two thirds of patients and in over 90% by 4 weeks [166]. Improvement in the chest radiograph lags behind clinical improvement, but complete radiographic clearing typically occurs within 2 to 4 weeks. In one recent study, radiographic infiltrates had completely resolved within 2 weeks in 43 of 77 patients (55%), while a more gradual clearing was evident in the remaining cases [166]. Even in patients exhibiting dramatic responses to corticosteroids, chronic therapy (more than 12 months) is usually required, as relapses of CEP occur in 60% to 80% of cases when the steroid is tapered or discontinued [164–166, 171]. This tendency to relapse may persist over extended periods. In approximately one third of cases, life-long therapy may be required owing to predictable relapses each time the corticosteroid dose is tapered below a critical threshold value [166]. While exacerbations of disease promptly remit with reinitiation of high-dose corticosteroids, it is preferable (and less toxic) to maintain patients at low-dose steroids every other day to keep the disease in remission rather than repeatedly bolusing and tapering therapy due to multiple exacerbations. Our approach has been to initiate prednisone at a dose of 60 mg daily for the first 1 to 2 weeks, until the disease has been controlled. At that point, the dose is reduced by 10-mg decrements weekly and converted to 60 mg every other day after 4 to 6 weeks. Unless relapses occur, the dose is tapered by 10-mg decrements monthly for the next 3 months, followed by 5-mg decrements every 2 to 3 months thereafter. The dosage and rate of taper, however, may need to be modified according to clinical, laboratory, and chest radiographic parameters. Once the chest radiograph has cleared completely which is usually achieved within 2 to 6 weeks, follow-up radiography may not be required in the absence of clinical or laboratory relapse. Serial laboratory studies (complete blood count with differential count, total blood eosinophil counts, or serum IgE levels) at 6- to 12-week intervals have been helpful in predicting relapse, as increases in these parameters may occur in advance of clinical relapse. In cases where significant increases in serum IgE or eosinophils are demonstrable, modest increases in the dose of corticosteroids are appropriate and are usually efficacious in normalizing the laboratory parameters and preventing clinical relapse. When a dose of 15 mg every other day has been achieved, we slow the rate of taper to 1-mg decrements every 1 to 2 months. While some authors advocate tapering and discontinuing corticosteroid therapy over a 12-month period, we believe that the relapse rate is unacceptably high with this approach. Our approach has been to maintain the corticosteroid at the lowest every other day dose necessary to maintain a remission, which often requires long-term (more than 24 months) therapy at doses in the range of 8 to 15 mg every other day. This dosage is unlikely to be associated with either short- or long-term side effects and is preferable to allowing patients to relapse repeatedly, necessitating high-dose corticosteroids to induce remissions.

Acute Respiratory Failure

Recently, Allen et al [167] reported four patients with an acute febrile illness, hypoxemia, diffuse pulmonary infiltrates on chest radiography, and marked increase in percent eosinophils (mean, 42%; range, 28% to 50%) on BAL fluid, who exhibited dramatic responses to corticosteroids and erythromycin. Lung biopsies were not performed in these cases. This syndrome differed from CEP in the duration of symptoms (1 to 7 days), the severity of illness (two required mechanical ventilation), the diffuse rather than peripheral nature of radiographic infiltrates, and the lack of relapses despite the fact that corticosteroid therapy was discontinued in all cases within 10 days to 12 weeks. Thus, the authors suggested that this may represent an acute form of eosinophilic lung disease distinct from previously described syndromes, although we believe this may represent one end of the spectrum of CEP. Irrespective of whether this represents a distinct disease entity or not, several points can be made: BAL eosinophilia was present in every case even though blood eosinophilia was present in only one case and may be an invaluable diagnostic clue to the diagnosis; and the response to corticosteroids was dramatic, with defervescence in all cases within 24 hours and prompt improvement in hypoxemia and respiratory failure. In all cases, the chest radiograph had normalized within 4 weeks, and there were no sequelae of the disease. This underscores the value of prompt initiation of corticosteroid therapy empirically in patients with suspected eosinophilic pneumonia, when blood or BAL eosinophilia is present, while awaiting corroborating studies.

Eosinophilic Granuloma (EG)

Pulmonary eosinophilic granuloma or pulmonary histiocytosis X is a rare granulomatous disease of uncertain etiology that may present as ILD. EG can involve the lung as the sole or predominant site of disease or in the context of disseminated disease [175–178]. Most cases of EG occur in children less than 10 years old; osseous and extrapulmonary manifestations predominate [179–181]. By contrast, pulmonary EG typically affects adults between ages 20 and 50 [175–178]. Classical presenting features of childhood EG are related to single (unifocal) or multiple (multifocal) lytic lesions of bone: dissemination to lungs, viscera, kidney, liver, spleen, bone marrow, skin, gingiva, and other sites may also occur [179–181]. Common clinical manifestations of childhood EG include exophthalmos due to destruction of the orbital bones, chronic otitis media from destruction of the mastoid process of the temporal bone, and diabetes insipidus from involvement of the pituitary gland [179–181]. Extrapulmonary manifestations (particularly osteolytic bone lesions or diabetes insipidus) have been reported in only 15% to 20% of cases of pulmonary EG in adults [175–178]. It is possible that asymptomatic bone lesions may be present in a higher percentage of patients, however, as skeletal surveys have not been routinely performed in cases of pulmonary EG. When EG is limited to the lung, the prognosis is excellent, as stabilization or recovery occurs in 70% to 85% of cases [175–178]. However, when pulmonary EG occurs in the context of disseminated EG, as often happens in childhood cases, the prognosis is considerably worse [179–181]. The salient histopathologic features of EG include proliferations of atypical histiocytes (HX cells), lipid-containing histiocytes (foam cells), granulomatous inflammation, mononuclear and eosinophilic inflammatory cell infiltration, and fibrosis [175–181]. Over 300 cases of pulmonary EG have been reported, but the precise incidence is not known [175–178]. However, several studies suggest a prevalence of approximately 1 to 5 cases per million population [175–178]. EG is a rare cause of ILD, as EG accounted for only 3.4% of cases of ILD among 502 open lung biopsies reported by Gaensler and Carrington [5]. In one series of ILD that included 274 cases of sarcoidosis, only 15 cases of EG were detected [176]. Earlier studies suggested a male predominance, but more recent series have cited a female-to-male ratio of 3:2 [175, 177]. No familial or inheritable trait exists, but the disorder is almost exclusively seen in Caucasians, suggesting a genetic predisposition [175–178]. A history of cigarette smoking has been elicited in more than 80% of cases [175–178], suggesting that exogenous factors may be of critical importance in the pathogenesis.

The clinical manifestations of pulmonary EG are variable; 60% to 75% of patients have symptoms of cough or dyspnea, but 10% to 25% are asymptomatic, with incidental abnormalities on chest radiography [175–178]. Chest pain, due to pneumothorax or osteolytic rib lesions, occurs in nearly one quarter of patients. Less common symptoms include hemoptysis and wheezing, which occur in less than 5% of cases. Pulmonary symptoms are usually mild, but severe, even fatal, respiratory insufficiency may occur in up to 10% of cases [175, 176]. Constitutional symptoms such as weight loss, malaise, anorexia, and fever are present in 15% to 30% of cases [175–178]. The onset of symptoms is usually insidious, over several weeks or months; a rapidly progressive course is unusual. Physical findings are usually absent, but rales, rhonchi, wheezing, or diminished breath sounds may be present. Clubbing or changes consistent with pulmonary hypertension (an accentuated pulmonary second sound, right ventricular S_3 gallop or heave), although rare, may be present in far advanced disease. Laboratory studies (routine hematologic and serologic data, erythrocyte sedimentation rate) are usually normal and are not helpful in the initial diagnosis or assessing the extent or activity of the disease. In contrast to CEP, blood eosinophilia is not a feature of EG.

Chest Radiographic Findings

Abnormalities on chest radiography are present in virtually all cases. Diffuse reticular or reticulonodular infiltrates are usually present; in severe cases, extensive honeycombing, volume loss, and fibrosis may be evident. These changes are nonspecific and may be indistinguishable from other interstitial lung disorders. Several radiographic features, however, are sufficiently common in EG as to suggest the diagnosis. First, there is a predilection for mid and upper lung zones, with relative sparing of the basilar portions of the lungs [175–178]. Involvement of the costophrenic angles occurs in less than 20% of cases and has been associated with a worse prognosis [175–178]. Although the literature emphasizes the predominance disease in the mid and upper lung zones, this finding is not invariable, as lower lobe involvement was demonstrated in 74% of cases in one recent analysis of chest radiographs from 50 patients with pulmonary EG [182]. In that series, mid lung involvement was evident in virtually all cases, but upper lobes were involved in only 26% of cases. Another cardinal radiographic feature of pulmonary EG is the presence of multiple cystic radiolucencies, 5 to 15 mm in diameter, which reflect foci of honeycombing and emphysematous changes [175–178, 182]. More extensive emphysematous changes, with bullae, although rare, have been described. The nodular component of pulmonary EG is another radiographic hallmark [175–178, 182]. These nodules typically range in size from 1 to 5 mm, but may exceed 1.5 cm in diameter in some cases. Cavitation of larger nodules is rarely demonstrable by conventional radiography, although areas of cavitation were detected in 17% of cases on CT scanning [183]. Because the lesions of pulmonary EG have a predilection for the periphery of the lungs and may distend distal airways and alveolar spaces, rupture of subpleural blebs resulting in pneumothorax occurs in 5% to 20% of patients with EG and may be a presenting feature [175–178, 182] (Fig. 11-14A). Atypical radiographic findings that may rarely complicate EG include alveolar consolidation, atelectasis, and pleural effusions [175–178, 182]. Pleural thickening is uncommon, even in patients

Fig. 11-14. (A) EG. Chest radiograph demonstrating a left pneumothorax and extensive cystic changes in both lungs. There is a diffuse nodular component as well. These changes are characteristic of pulmonary EG. (B) Chest radiograph demonstrating diffuse infiltrates, nodules, and some airbronchograms. There is a slight upper lobe predominance. Open lung biopsy disclosed EG. (C and D) EG. Stellate fibrosis. See text for explanation.

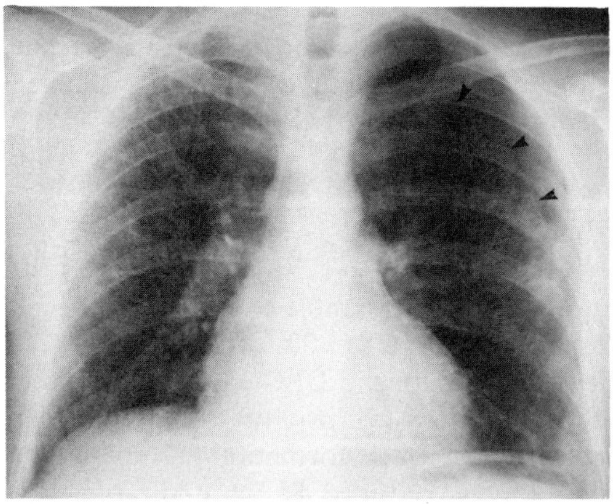
A

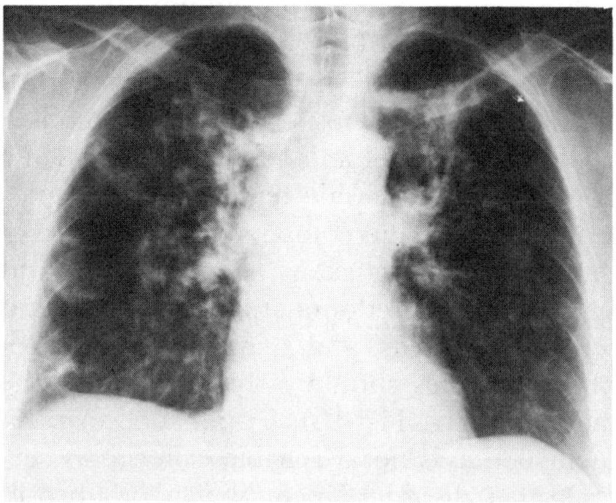
B

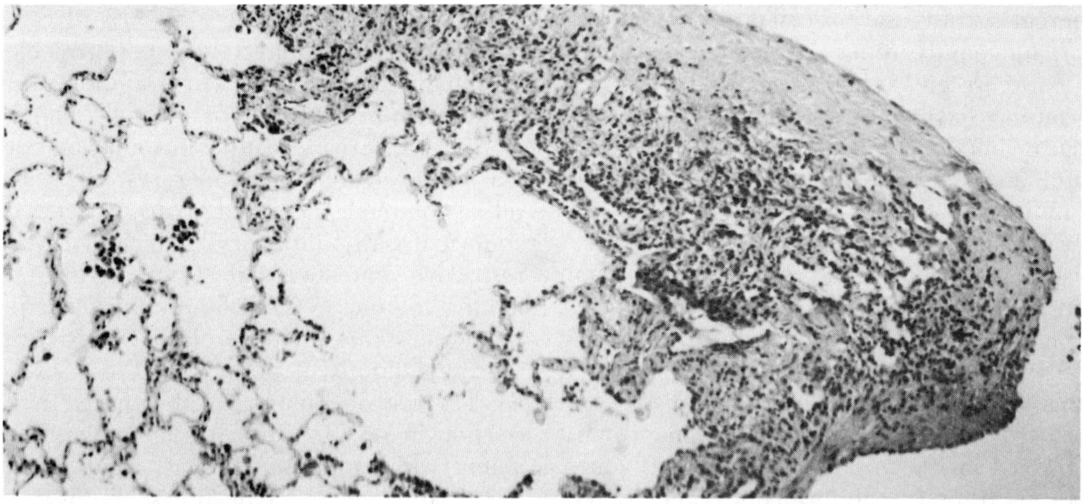
C

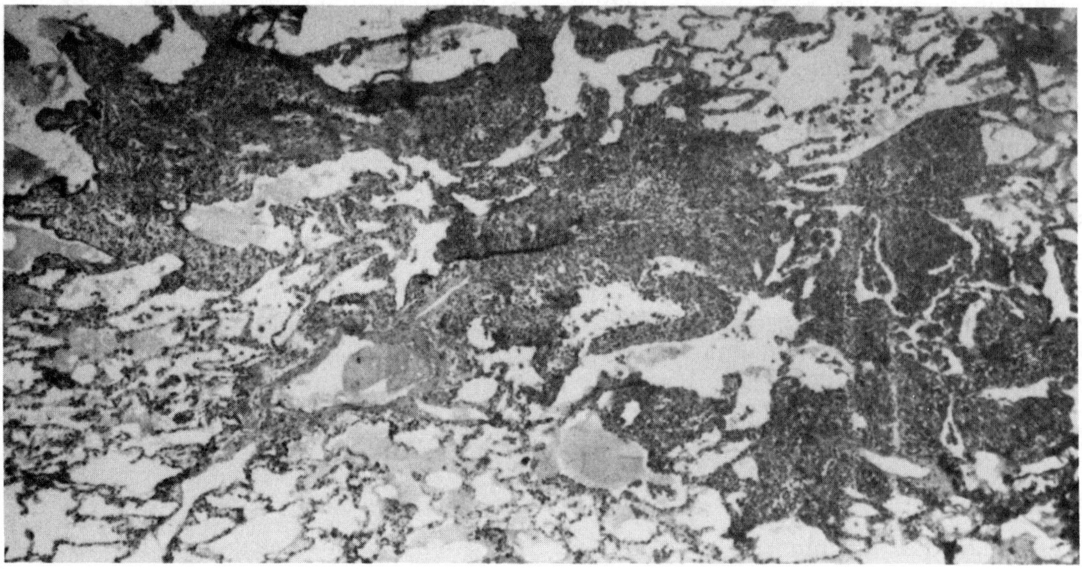
D

with a history of recurrent pneumothoraces. Hilar adenopathy has been described in less than 5% of cases [175–178, 182] and suggests an alternative diagnosis, such as sarcoidosis, silicosis, or granulomatous infection. While no single radiographic feature is pathognomonic for EG, the combination of pneumothorax, diffuse reticular, micronodular, and cystic changes predominating in the mid and upper lung fields, and sparing of the costophrenic angles should strongly suggest the diagnosis (Fig. 11-14B). Upper lobe involvement per se is not a reliable criteria, as several other disorders including cystic fibrosis, sarcoidosis, CEP, ankylosing spondylitis, tuberculosis, mycosis, and silicosis may exhibit predominantly upper lobe changes.

More recently, high-resolution chest CT scanning has been used to better define the nature and extent of the parenchymal lesions and assess disease progression [183, 184]. Findings on chest CT are similar to conventional chest radiography, but CT more accurately defines the extent and type of lesion and disease progression [183, 184]. Brauner et al [183] analyzed chest CT findings among 18 patients with pulmonary EG and noted that lesions were diffuse in 89% of cases, and that 50% of lesions were predominantly distributed in the upper and mid lung zones. A variety of CT abnormalities were noted, including thin-walled cysts (94%), nodules (78%), thick-walled cysts (39%), reticular shadows (22%), ground-glass opacities (22%), and cavitating nodules (17%). CT is more sensitive than conventional chest radiography in detecting small and large cysts and nodules; in addition, many lesions that appear reticular on chest radiography can be shown to have a cystic character on CT [184]. In addition, CT findings may correlate better with pulmonary function tests (e.g., diffusing capacity) than conventional radiography [184]. Notwithstanding the superiority of CT scanning as an imaging modality, its clinical application and role in the staging or management of pulmonary EG has not been defined. Because of the limited availability of thin-section CT scanning, its cost, and increased radiation exposure (particularly with serial studies) compared with conventional radiography, we do not believe that routine CT is necessary in the diagnosis or management of pulmonary EG.

Pulmonary Function Tests

Abnormalities on PFTs are evident in 75% to 90% of cases [175–178]. Reductions in VC and DLCO are the most common abnormalities, seen in 60% to 80% of cases [175–178]. Severe reductions in DLCO have been associated with a worse prognosis and correlate with radiologic cyst formation [175]. Obstructive defects (reduced FEV_1, expiratory flow rates, or increased residual volume) have been demonstrated in 30% to 60% of cases [175–178], which may reflect peribronchiolar inflammation, fibrosis, or granulomatous obliteration or distortion of airways. Changes in TLC are variable, as the TLC may be normal (or even increased) in cases where residual volume is increased. Thus, patterns of abnormality in pulmonary EG include a pure restrictive ventilatory defect, with reductions in lung volumes (VC, TLC) and normal expiratory flow rates, a pure obstructive defect, or combinations of both [175–178]. Severe airways obstruction associated with severe reduction in DLCO (physiologic changes consistent with emphysema) may occur in patients with severe bullous disease, but is rare. Stability of pulmonary function over time has been the rule in most cases, but spontaneous improvement or deterioration may occur [175–177]. The pattern of physiologic changes may also change as the disease evolves. For example, patients may present with a pure restrictive defect and then develop severe airways obstruction due to obliteration and destruction of bronchioles, alveolar ducts, and focal emphysematous and cystic changes. Serial pulmonary function studies are recommended to assess the course of the disease over time, but do not correlate either with radiographic changes or clinical symptoms [176].

Histopathology

On gross examination, numerous, firm subpleural nodules ranging from 2 mm to greater than 1 cm, scattered throughout the lung are characteristic [175–178]. The lesions are focal, interspersed by large areas of normal lung parenchyma and are located predominantly in interstitial and peribronchial areas. Varying degrees of fibrosis are also present. A distinctive feature on light microscopy at low power is a peculiar pattern of stellate fibrosis, characterized by dense central scarring surrounded by cellular peripheral tentacles, which has been demonstrated in over 80% of cases (Fig. 11-14C and D) [177]. These nodules contain a variety of histiocytes including atypical histiocytes (HX cells) (to be discussed in detail later), foamy macrophages, AM, and a variety of inflammatory cells (eosinophils, lymphocytes, plasma cells, polymorphonuclear leukocytes) [175–178]. Multinucleated giant cells, which represent the fusion product of histiocytes, may occasionally be found. Areas of central micronecrosis may be observed in up to 30% to 40% of cases. While eosinophils are often conspicuous, the number of eosinophils encountered is extremely variable and is not a reliable diagnostic criterion. While these nodules are organized and retain a granulomatous character, well-formed circumscribed sarcoid-like granulomata are uncommon. Perivascular infiltration may be observed in areas of intense inflammation, but a necrotizing vasculitis is not a feature of EG [176, 177]. A critical element to the histopathologic diagnosis of pulmonary EG is the presence of large numbers of atypical histiocytes (HX cells) in the alveolar interstitium, airspaces, and nodular lesions [175–178]. HX cells are derived from mononuclear phagocytes and play a key role in the evolution of the EG lesion. On light microscopy, these HX cells exhibit very characteristic cytologic features and should be easy to recognize on higher power magnification. HX cells are moderately large, ovoid histiocytic cells with pale eosinophilic cytoplasm, indistinct cell borders, oblong, clefted (indented) nuclei, with small or inconspicuous nucleoli [175–178]. HX cells have also been shown to contain distinctive rod-shaped, tubular, pentalaminar intracytoplasmic inclusions 42 nm in diameter (termed X bodies or Birbeck granules), which can be demonstrated by electron microscopy [175–178]. Because HX cells can usually be identified by light microscopic techniques, electron microscopy is usually not necessary to establish the diagnosis. On the basis of both ultrastructural and immunohistochemical characteristics, HX cells resemble Langerhans' cells found in normal epidermis and are believed to represent activated or reactive Langerhans' cells. While small numbers of HX cells (typically containing fewer X bodies) may be present in up to 10% to 15% of open lung biopsies from patients with other ILDs (including IPF) [185], large numbers of HX cells containing numerous X bodies are virtually diagnostic of EG [176, 186]. HX cells may also be detected in BAL fluid in patients with pulmonary EG, and are virtually pathognomonic for this disorder, as HX cells rarely are present in BAL in other conditions [187]. All histologic elements of the disease process (histiocytic proliferation, granulomatous inflammation, fibrosis, healing, and repair) may be observed in individual cases, but the disease appears to evolve in distinct phases. Early in the course of EG, histiocytic proliferation dominates. Later, granulomatous inflammation within the nodules and interstitium (with histiocytes, eosinophils, and mononuclear inflammatory cells) ensues. Finally, fibrosis represents the end result of the preceding cellular, inflammatory events. Fibrous tissue may replace these inflammatory nodules and may extend into the alveolar interstitium and bronchioles. Given the peribronchial location of many of the EG granulomatous nodules, destruction of bronchioles and alveolar ducts may lead to extensive cyst formation and focal emphysematous changes. Blebs, subpleural cysts, and adhesions along the visceral pleural may also be found. With long-standing pulmonary EG, the distinctive HX and inflammatory cells may no longer be evident, and the lung may be replaced by extensive fibrosis and honeycomb lung. At this point, it may be impossible to differentiate the histopathologic features from other end-stage ILDs. However, the presence of the characteristic stellate shape of scar tissue should suggest the diagnosis of EG, as this feature is rarely observed with other ILDs. It is important to recognize that some of the features that may be seen in pulmonary EG are nonspecific and may be observed in a variety of other ILDs, obscuring the diagnosis. For example, the presence of large numbers of eosinophils and granulomas may be observed in CEP. In that latter condition, however, interstitial nodules, HX cells, and fibrosis are not present. Focal intra-alveolar collections of macrophages, suggesting DIP, may also be found in pulmonary EG. The distinction between DIP and EG is not difficult as long as a sufficiently large biopsy specimen is obtained, as the major criteria for the diagnosis of pulmonary EG (HX cells, interstitial nodules, eosinophils) are not present in DIP. However, the diagnosis may be obscured when small biopsy specimens (such as TBB or percutaneous needle biopsies) are interpreted. Owing to the heterogeneity of histopathologic features of EG and the presence of many nonspecific features (such as fibrosis and eosinophilic infiltration), an open lung biopsy is usually required for a definitive diagnosis. However, TBB may be adequate in some cases, provided the clinical history is consistent and the characteristic HX cells are identified in large numbers either on the biopsy specimen or by BAL fluid.

Immunologic Techniques

More recently, immunohistochemical techniques have been shown to be helpful in the diagnosis of EG. Positive staining for S-100 protein and OKT6 antibody may identify the characteristic HX cells or Langerhans' cells and are far less expensive and time consuming than electron microscopy [186–190]. In this latter technique, there is potential for sampling error as individual cells must be examined. In EG, S-100 positive histiocytes, which display cytologic characteristics of Langerhans' cells, may be detected in clusters within stellate nodules and within the periphery of the lung [188]. While S-100 positive cells may be observed in other fibrotic pulmonary disorders, these are present in smaller numbers and are distributed more randomly throughout the lung parenchyma [188]. The relative number of S-100 positive cells is often sufficient to distinguish pulmonary EG from other conditions. In one series in which S-100 stains were applied to tissue from seven cases of pulmonary EG and 19 other pulmonary disorders, positive staining Langerhans' cells were identified in every case, but were quantitatively more abundant in EG [189]. Only EG had more than 75 S-100 positive cells per high power field whereas other lung disorders never exceeded 25 cells per high power field. In addition, active lesions of EG contained aggregates of contiguous S-100 staining cells; such aggregates were never seen in other conditions [189]. Other immunologic markers such as OKT6 common thymocyte antigen also stain in EG but require fresh or frozen tissue, whereas S-100 protein can be detected in routinely fixed and processed tissues. Chollet et al [187] analyzed BAL fluid for OKT6 reactive cells from 131 patients with a variety of pulmonary disorders, including 18 with pulmonary EG. OKT6 antibody reacts with 70% of human thymocytes, but not with circulating lymphocytes or monocytes [187]. All patients with pulmonary EG had positive OKT6 cells, comprising a mean of 5.6% of BAL cells; these cells had characteristics of Langerhans' cells on electron microscopy, with the typical irregular shape, indented nucleus, and Birbeck granules. By contrast, the mean number of positive OKT6 cells in other conditions was only 0.20% and in no case exceeded 2.8% [92]. Less than 1% of BAL cells displayed positive OKT6 among all 43 patients with sarcoidosis and 61 of 67 patients with miscellaneous pulmonary fibrotic disorders. Other monoclonal antibodies such as OKT4, OKT3, and OKT8 consistently failed to label HX cells. Thus, the demonstration of greater than 3% positive staining for OKT6 appears to be relatively specific for EG. It should be emphasized that neither immunohistochemical stains nor electron microscopy are required to substantiate the diagnosis of EG when the light microscopic changes are characteristic. However, in cases where light microscopic changes are not classical or sufficiently distinctive, these adjunctive techniques (particularly S-100 stains) may be diagnostic.

Pathogenesis

The pathogenesis of EG has not been clarified. The histiocyte (HX cell) appears to be the critical effector cell in the pathogenesis of the EG lesion, but whether the histiocytic proliferation in EG is reactive or neoplastic is not known. A primary neoplastic process is possible. Alternatively, an immune-mediated pathogenesis may be operative. Since HX cells are derived from mononuclear phagocytes and may have immune effector functions, it is possible that EG represents a hypersensitivity disorder in which Langerhans' (HX) cells are recruited and activated in response to an inhaled stimulus (or antigen). Circulating immune complexes, elevated IgG levels in BAL fluid, and granular deposits of immunoglobulin and complement in alveolar walls and blood vessels within the cellular nodular lesions of EG have been demonstrated in some cases [176, 177, 191], consistent with an immune-mediated pathogenesis, possibly in response to inhaled antigen(s). A striking association between pulmonary EG and cigarette smoking has been noted [175–178], suggesting that cigarette smoke may serve as an external irritant to initiate an alveolitis, stimulating the influx of macrophages and Langerhans' cells in the lower respiratory tract. HX cells have been shown to replicate in the alveolar structures, suggesting that alveolar proliferation of these cells may perpetuate or maintain the alveolitis [1, 176]. However, the factors that perpetuate (or abrogate) the inflammatory alveolitis have not been identified. The conspicuous infiltration of eosinophils throughout the lesion suggests an important role for the eosinophil in the immunopathogenesis of the lesion as well.

Prognosis and Clinical Course

The natural history and course of pulmonary EG is usually favorable, but is highly variable [175–178]. Rapid evolution of the disease is uncommon; symptoms usually develop insidiously over several weeks or months and then gradually remit within 6 to 24 months. Spontaneous resolution or stabilization of the process occurs in 65% to 85% of cases, but 5% to 15% of cases progress to fatal pulmonary insufficiency [175–178]. Widely discrepant results have been reported in the literature, which makes interpretation of the data difficult. One retrospective study analyzed 60 patients from multiple institutions who were followed for at least 6 months and noted that the prognosis for recovery or stabilization was excellent [177]. Sixteen patients who were asymptomatic at the time of diagnosis remained free of symptoms, and complete spontaneous remission of disease occurred in an additional 17 patients. Disease progression occurred in only five patients, with one fatality. Importantly, no patient presenting with isolated pulmonary EG developed disseminated disease. Only seven patients (12%) had moderate or severe pulmonary dysfunction. Overall, 55% were asymptomatic at time of last follow-up [177]. While this study analyzed both corticosteroid treated and untreated patients, there was no clear benefit of therapy as clinical outcome was excellent in both groups. In contrast to these generally favorable results, Basset et al [175] analyzed 67 patients with pulmonary EG from a variety of institutions in whom follow-up data was available, and reported a mortality of 25%. In that study, only nine (14%) improved, 27 (40%) remained stable, and 14 (21%) survivors exhibited functional deterioration. The differences in these studies may reflect heterogeneity in patient populations. For example, in the series reported by Basset et al, 10 of 67 patients had generalized, multisystemic disease before the detection of lung disease, and four children with Letterer-Siwe disease were included in the analysis [175]. By contrast, the series by Friedman et al [177] appears to be more representative of primary pulmonary EG in adults. In that latter series, which reviewed 100 cases of pulmonary EG, extrapulmonary involvement was infrequent; only four had bone lesions, five had diabetes insipidus, and three had disease in skin or lymph nodes. None had disseminated histiocytosis. Colby and Lombard [176] analyzed the course of 227 patients with pulmonary EG both treated and untreated, derived from 13 prior publications in whom follow-up data was available; this included both of the series previously alluded to [175, 177]. The course was usually favorable, as 155 cases (69%) had partial or complete resolution of disease or exhibited only minor stable deficits. However, a subset fared distinctly worse, as 37 (16%) died of the disease, and an additional 35 (15%) had disease progression or persistence of moderate-to-severe symptoms. The factors dictating prognosis have not been well defined, but disseminated multisystemic disease, severe reduction in DLCO, multiple pneumothoraces, extremes of age, extensive cystic changes or honeycombing on chest radiography, and extensive constitutional symptoms have been associated with a higher mortality [175, 176]. When the disease is confined to the lung, a favorable prognosis can be expected in 75% to 85% of cases, with mortality of 2% to 6% [175–178].

Therapy

Because of the fluctuating course and propensity of pulmonary EG to resolve spontaneously, the impact of therapy is not clear. Corticosteroids, vinca alkaloids (vinblastine or vincristine), and a variety of immunosuppressive and cytotoxic agents have been tried, with anecdotal claims for success. However, no prospective, controlled trials have been done, and no agent is of proven efficacy for control of the pulmonary lesion. Radiation therapy may provide excellent local control of painful bone lesions or diabetes insipidus complicating EG [179], but has no role in the pulmonary lesion. Prognosis for adults with limited organ involvement (lung, skin, or bone without visceral dissemination) has generally been excellent, so aggressive therapy has rarely been applied in this setting. Given the favorable prognosis in most cases of pulmonary EG and the potential for spontaneous remission, we believe that therapy should be considered only in patients exhibiting severe or progressive pulmonary symptoms or disseminated disease. In such cases, an empirical trial of corticosteroids, in doses similar to those used in IPF, for a 3- to 6-month trial, is reasonable. More prolonged therapy for 12 or more months may be warranted for patients exhibiting clear and objective improvement. When patients have severe, progressive disease refractory to corticosteroids, immunosuppressive, or cytotoxic agents including vinca alkaloids should be considered although limited data supporting their efficacy exist. Caution should be exercised in the use of cytotoxic or chemotherapeutic agents, however, as secondary malignancies including acute leukemias, have been described as late complications of therapy, typically in patients with multisystemic disease [179].

Pulmonary Alveolar Proteinosis

PAP is a rare syndrome originally described in 1958 by Rosen and colleagues [192] based on distinctive pathologic features noted in 27 cases (20 open lung biopsies, 7 necropsies) referred from across the world. In their original description, they noted that the alveolar spaces were filled with "granular and floccular acidophilic material . . . with minimal or no changes in the interalveolar septa." The pathologic features bore a striking resemblance to burnt-out *Pneumocystis carinii* pneumonitis although the interstitial mononuclear cell infiltration typical of *Pneumocystis* was lacking. Because of the apparent proteinaceous appearance of the intra-alveolar material, the term pulmonary alveolar proteinosis was applied. The biochemical characteristics of the intra-alveolar material has since been shown to contain predominantly phospholipids (including surfactant-like material) together with small amounts of protein [193]. In view of these characteristics, others have suggested that the term pulmonary alveolar phospholipoproteinosis is more appropriate [193]. Although the etiology for PAP is not known, a history of exposure to dust, chemicals, and a variety of solvents has been elicited in up to 50% of cases [193, 194]. Exposure to silica, fiberglass, volcanic ash, aluminum, cadmium, chlorinated resins, tin, asbestos, fluorescent tube dust, and inhalation of fumes from assorted solvents have all been reported to result in the PAP syndrome [193, 194]. Rare reports of PAP in siblings suggests that a genetic predisposition may also exist. While the precise incidence of PAP is not known, fewer than 300 cases have been reported, and a prevalence of one case per million adults has been suggested [193]. All ages can be affected, but most cases occur in the third and fourth decades. There is a male predominance of approximately 3:1. Morphologic findings identical to PAP have also been described in patients with other diseases, primarily in hematologic malignancies, but also in association with solid tumors, tuberculosis, and specific infections [195, 196]. Such cases have been termed secondary PAP or pseudoproteinosis to distinguish these cases from primary or idiopathic PAP [193, 195, 196]. Secondary PAP exhibits a much more focal and patchy involvement than PAP, and the pathogenic mechanisms are almost certainly different. The intra-alveolar process in secondary PAP may represent necrotic debris and exudate resulting from the disease process or attendant complications, rather than the surfactant phospholipid material responsible for primary PAP. Whole lung lavage, which has been highly efficacious as therapy for primary PAP, is of doubtful value in secondary PAP. In such cases, remission or relapse of the underlying disorder appears to be a more critical determinant of prognosis than the pulmonary lesion. This disorder is not further addressed in this chapter.

Clinical Features

The clinical presentation of PAP is similar to other ILD. The most characteristic symptoms are progressive dyspnea and cough, present in 60% to 80% of cases [193–202]. The cough is typically nonproductive, although occasional patients may expectorate plugs of grayish-yellow mucoid material. A sensation of chest heaviness and pleuritic chest pain have been described in up to one third of cases. Hemoptysis has been an uncommon symptom in most series, but was described in one quarter of patients in one recent series, usually as a complication by severe bouts of coughing [193]. A chronic course, with the insidious development of progressive cough or dyspnea over weeks or months, is characteristic. However, spontaneous remissions occur in 20% to 30% of cases, and a relapsing and remitting course has been described [192–202]. Fifteen percent to 30% of patients are asymptomatic and present only with an abnormal chest radiograph [193, 199]. Physical examination reveals inspiratory rales in 20% to 80% of patients; wheezing is unusual [193, 194]. Cyanosis and clubbing have been detected in 20% to 30% of cases [193, 194]. Constitutional symptoms (fever, weight loss, malaise, fatigue) are common, but extrapulmonary involvement does not occur. Routine hematologic and laboratory parameters are normal. However, elevations in the serum lactate dehydrogenase concentration, a feature first noted by Ramirez in 1963 [201], occur in approximately 80% of untreated patients and may be a useful diagnostic clue [202].

The presence of fever should be aggressively evaluated, as this often heralds the onset of infection. Untreated patients with PAP have a heightened susceptibility to infections that are normally eradicated by cell-mediated mechanisms such as *Nocardia,* invasive fungi, *mycobacteria,* and *staphylococci.* Before specific therapy for PAP was available, infections occurred in nearly 15% of cases and were responsible for significant mortality [192, 194]. Defects in AM chemotaxis, phagocytosis, and microbiocidal activity, and the presence of large amounts of intra-alveolar debris, which may be a culture medium for microorganisms, are responsible for this high incidence of infectious complications in untreated patients. Since the use of whole lung lavage as a therapeutic modality, the rate of infectious complications has declined dramatically, with most recent series reporting infection rates of less than 5% [193, 198–200]. This reduction in infection risk likely is related to restoration of AM macrophage function, as in vitro studies have demonstrated that AM defects in PAP can be reversed following whole lung lavage [203].

Chest Radiography

Chest radiography classically demonstrates symmetrical bilateral, perihilar alveolar infiltrates with sparing of the costophrenic sulci characteristic of a "bat wing" distribution (Fig. 11-15A) [193, 197, 198]. Radiographically, the differential diagnosis for diffuse alveolar infiltrates includes *Pneumocystis carinii,* pulmonary edema (both cardiac and noncardiac), alveolar hemorrhage syndromes, BOOP, DIP, and a wide gamut of ILD. Asymmetrical involvement may occur, and the disease is unilateral in up to 20% of cases (Fig. 11-15B). Patchy nodular infiltrates, combined alveolar-reticulonodular infiltrates, and pure interstitial (reticulonodular) patterns have also been described. Pleural effusions, cavitary lesions, and mediastinal or hilar adenopathy are not features of PAP and should suggest another etiology [193]. Although chest CT scans may more clearly delineate alveolar and interstitial components, we see no role for CT scans in the diagnosis or management of PAP.

Pulmonary Function Tests

The dominant physiologic aberrations in PAP are related to filling of the alveolar spaces with dense proteinaceous material, which inhibits gas exchange, leading to widened alveolar-arterial gradient, hypoxemia, severe intrapulmonary shunting, and reduced diffusing capacity [193, 197–200, 202]. While most of these aberrations are nonspecific, the demonstration of a large intrapulmonary shunt is highly suggestive of PAP, as hypoxemia seen in IPF or other ILD is due primarily to ventilation-perfusion inequality, with only minor degrees of shunting. The combination of a shunt fraction greater than 14% coupled with an elevation in the serum lactate dehydrogenase level is rarely seen in other ILD and strongly suggests PAP [202]. A mild-to-moderate restrictive ventilatory defect is characteristic, but lung volumes are less affected than measurements of gas exchange (DLCO, arterial blood gases). Airways obstruction does not occur as a manifestation of PAP, but may be observed in patients with a concomitant smoking history [193, 198, 200].

Histopathology

Gross pathology reveals patchy areas of dense consolidation that exude a whitish-yellowish substance on sectioning. Pleural involvement is not a feature. Microscopy of tissue sections reveals filling of alveoli and respiratory bronchioles with a granular acidophilic material and a paucity of AMs [192, 193, 200] (Fig. 11-15C and D). Classically, the alveolar structures remain intact and the interstitium is unaffected; however, occasional focal areas of mild inflammation or type II cell hyperplasia may be seen. Special stains are helpful to discern the nature of the alveolar filling process. This phospholipid material stains bright pink with periodic-acid Schiff reagent (PAS) and negative with alcian blue [193]. Positive immunoperoxidase staining of formalin-fixed lung tissue and BAL fluid using a specific antisurfactant apoprotein rabbit IgG antibody has also been demonstrated in PAP [204]. While immunohistochemical stains are rarely required to corroborate the diagnosis of PAP, they may be useful to distinguish primary from secondary (i.e., associated with hematologic malignancies) causes

Fig. 11-15. (A) PAP. Chest radiograph demonstrating bilateral airspace disease simulating pulmonary edema. Transbronchial lung biopsy demonstrated classical features of PAP. Following whole lung lavage, symptoms, chest radiographs, and blood gases improved dramatically. (B) PAP. Chest radiograph demonstrating asymmetrical alveolar infiltrates, with a distinct predominance to the left upper lobe and right lower lobe. Transbronchial lung biopsy was nondiagnostic (BAL was not performed). Open lung biopsy revealed PAP. The infiltrates cleared following whole lung lavage. (C) PAP. Photomicrograph demonstrating the alveolar spaces are filled with dense, proteinaceous debris. Note that there is no significant fibrosis, inflammation, or disruption of the alveolar architecture (hematoxylin-eosin, low power). (D) PAP. Photomicrograph demonstrating the alveolar spaces are completely filled with a dense proteinaceous exudate. The alveolar architecture is preserved and minimal inflammatory component is evident (hematoxylin-eosin, high power).

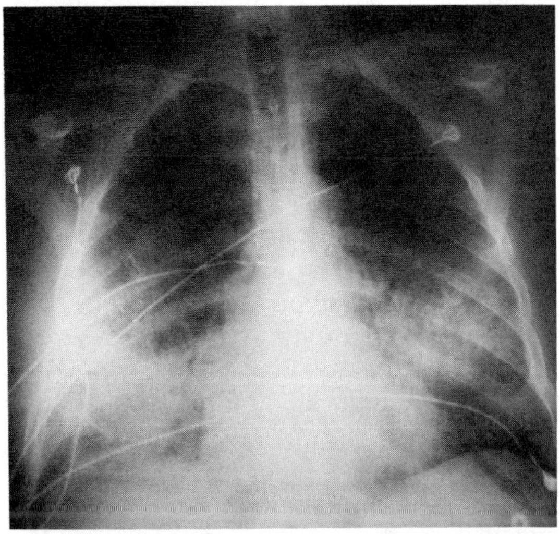
A

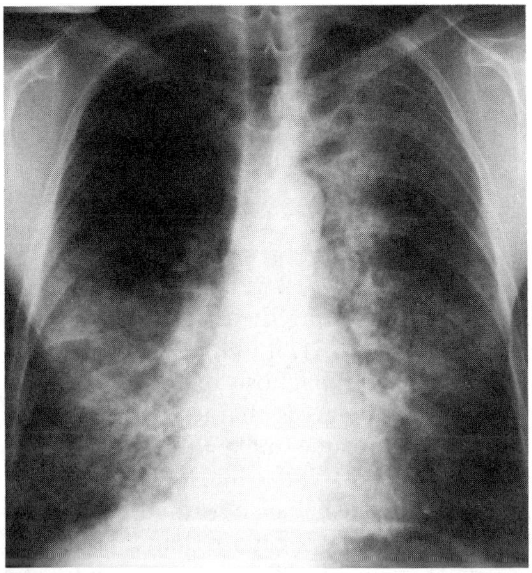
B

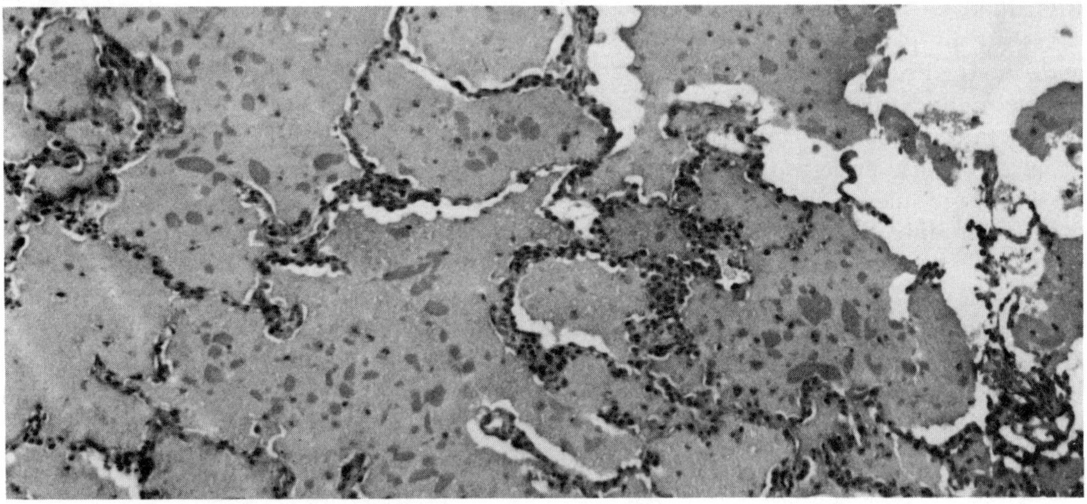
C

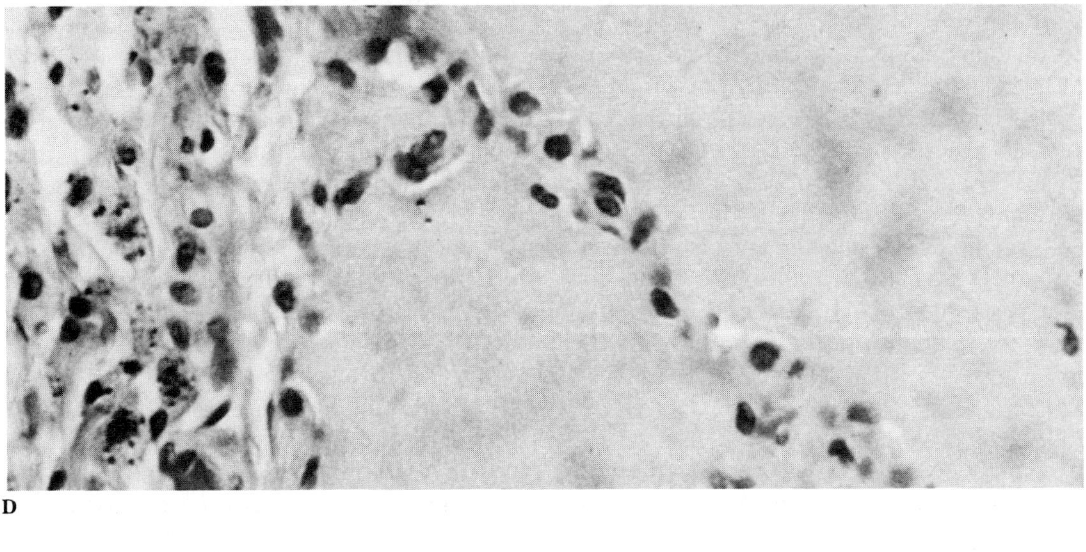
D

of PAP. Diffuse and uniform immunoperoxidase staining of lung tissue has been characteristic with primary PAP, whereas only focal staining has been demonstrated with secondary etiologies [204].

The diagnosis of PAP can often be established by fiberoptic bronchoscopy, provided the process is active. BAL may be particularly helpful in suggesting the diagnosis. We have found that the BAL findings may be so distinctive that the diagnosis of PAP can be established by the gross characteristics of BAL fluid. Thick, opaque, milky fluid with varying shades of yellow and white is characteristic and virtually never seen with other conditions. On standing for more than 20 minutes, layers of sediment may be observed. The BAL fluid is fixed, processed, and stained slides are prepared with hematoxylin-eosin and PAS (or PAS-alcian blue) stains. Characteristic findings include a large number of PAS-positive, eosinophilic, acellular bodies against a diffuse background of smaller eosinophilic granules (2 to 4 μm in size); AMs are few in number, but may contain granular, eosinophilic material within phagocytosomes or cytoplasm [193]. Transbronchial biopsy may establish the diagnosis if the typical PAS-positive, eosinophilic intra-alveolar filling process is evident. However, because of sampling error, TBB may not be sufficient particularly in patients with focal or limited disease. Open lung biopsy is warranted in all but unequivocal cases. Electron or transmission electron microscopy has also been performed on both tissue sections and BAL fluid [193]. Characteristic findings have included AMs engorged with phagolysosomes, complex inclusions, lamellar bodies, cholesterol inclusions, and lipid droplets [193]. Concentrically laminated lamellar bodies containing phospholipids, tubular myelin, and myelin structures may also be found free within alveolar spaces or in BAL fluid and, when present, are virtually pathognomonic for PAP [193].

Pathogenesis

The pathogenesis of PAP remains obscure. The massive accumulation of surfactant-like phospholipid components within the alveolar spaces suggests that the basic defect in PAP may relate to abnormal turnover of phospholipids, either by impaired clearance by AMs, excessive production by type II pneumocytes, or a combination of both [193, 197]. AMs from patients with PAP are engorged with surfactant-like phospholipids and exhibit defects in chemotaxis, antimicrobial function, phagolysosomal fusion, and growth in tissue culture; degenerating AMs have been detected within alveolar spaces, many of which contain substantial amounts of phospholipids within phagolysosomes [193, 197]. These defects may reverse following whole lung lavage, suggesting that defects in AM function noted in PAP are an acquired or secondary phenomenon, rather than a primary, intrinsic defect of phagocytes [203]. One may speculate that AMs are overwhelmed after engulfing large quantities of surfactant or surfactant breakdown products, leading to abnormal cellular function and premature cell death. Alternatively, it is possible that defective or abnormal macrophage function may be responsible for the PAP-like syndromes that may complicate patients with hematologic malignancies receiving chemotherapeutic agents [195–196]. In this context, decreased number of macrophages, together with defects in AM chemotaxis and phagocytosis, may result in impaired clearance of alveolar phospholipids and resultant secondary PAP. The exuberant intra-alveolar filling process in PAP may also reflect an unusual host response to a variety of toxic insults. It is of interest that pathologic processes similar to PAP have been elicited in experimental animals using a variety of inhalation and drug-induced models [193]. Exposure to silica, aluminum, nickel, bismuth, crushed fiberglass, volcanic ash, and a variety of dust particles may induce typical morphologic findings consistent with PAP [193]. In many of these models, instillation or inhalation of particulate matter results in an early influx of macrophages into the alveolar spaces, proliferation of type II pneumocytes, and increased accumulation of phospholipid in the surfactant pool. The demonstration of excessive lipoproteinaceous material filling the alveolar spaces and both intact and disintegrating AMs laden with phospholipid strikingly mimics PAP in humans. Ingestion of specific drugs (chlophentermine, amiodarone, iprindole, and others) may also induce morphologic changes consistent with PAP in animals [193]. These agents appear to act by causing accumulation of phospholipid lamellar inclusions, which are then taken up by AMs, and ultimately accumulate within the alveolar spaces. Whether a similar mechanism may operate in humans is not known, as no agent has been clearly implicated as a cause of PAP in humans.

Natural History and Treatment

The natural history of PAP is variable. Although progressive respiratory failure over weeks or months is characteristic, not all patients pursue a deteriorating course. Spontaneous remissions (often for prolonged periods) occur in 20% to 30% of patients so appropriate timing of therapeutic intervention needs to be individualized [192–194, 198–200]. Aggressive therapy may not always be required in the absence of significant symptoms or pulmonary dysfunction, but excessive delays in therapy may be deleterious and potentially life-threatening. Mortality of 30% and 32% was reported in two early series before the availability of specific therapy, with deaths due to respiratory failure or infectious complications [192, 194]. In early studies, a variety of therapeutic modalities including antibiotics, corticosteroids, and inhaled agents (trypsin, heparin, acetylcysteine) were tried but were without benefit [201]. In 1963, Ramirez et al [201] performed multiple segmental lung lavages using a polyethylene catheter inserted transtracheally in a patient with PAP and induced a sustained remission. They then developed a technique of whole lung lavage in 1965 [205], and modifications of this technique have been successfully applied by multiple investigators since that time [193, 198–200]. Whole lung lavage has markedly improved the prognosis of PAP, as fewer than 5% of patients now succumb to the disease or infectious complications [193, 198–200]. Additional techniques including lobar or segmental lavage using the fiberoptic bronchoscope or catheters have been developed [193], but we believe that whole lung lavage using a double-lumen endotracheal tube under general anesthesia is the safest and most efficacious therapy for this disorder. During this procedure, one lung is ventilated with 100% oxygen while the contralateral lung (typically the most severely affected) is allowed to deflate and is then repeatedly flooded and suctioned with 500 to 1000 mL aliquots of sterile saline at 37°C. Thick, viscid lipoproteinaceous material, in volumes nearly equivalent to the instilled saline, is then returned in the lavage effluent. This process is repeated until the effluent clears or markedly improves. This procedure usually requires 3 to 5 hours to complete and uses 15 to 30 L of normal saline on average. At the completion of lavage, the flooded lung is thoroughly suctioned, allowed to reexpand, and ventilated. The double lumen tube is then replaced with a single lumen tube and the patient is transferred to the recovery room and mechanically ventilated until acceptable oxygenation and spontaneous ventilation has been achieved. In most cases, extubation can be accomplished within 1 to 3 hours following completion of the procedure. Potential complications of whole lung lavage include worsening hypoxemia, hypotension, pneumothorax, displacement of the endotracheal tube, resulting in spillage of lavage fluid into the contralateral lung, and aspiration pneumonitis, but these untoward events can be minimized with proper airway and anesthetic techniques. Prognosis following lavage is variable. Within the first 24 hours of the procedure, cough, hypoxemia, and radiographic infiltrates may fail to improve or even worsen. However, gradual improvement typically follows, and normalization or improvement in symptoms, blood gases, PFTs, and chest radiographs occurs over the next 1 to 6 weeks. Most patients can be discharged from the hospital within 24 hours of the procedure. When bilateral disease is present, lavage of the opposite lung should be done at a later date. While the optimal timing of this has not been clarified, we usually wait for 3 to 6 weeks before lavaging the contralateral lung, because improvement may continue for several weeks following the initial lavage in some cases. When patients have more serious disease, lavage of the contralateral lung may be required within 5 to 10 days of the initial lavage. Favorable short-term responses to lung lavage have been achieved in 75% to 100% of cases [193, 198–200]. Recurrences of disease necessitating repeat lavage occur in 15% to 45% of cases within 1 to 5 years [193, 198–200], and occasional patients require 10 or more lavages over several years. Following completion of bilateral lung lavage, serial chest radiographs, oximetry (or arterial blood gases), serum lactate dihydrogenase levels, and clinical symptoms should be monitored at 4- to 6-week intervals for 3 to 6 months until stabilization or remission has been achieved. Beyond this point, consistent and prolonged follow-up visits (to include selected clinical, radiographic, and physiologic studies) every 6 to 12 months is recommended, even in asymptomatic patients, to identify recurrences. More frequent evaluation would of course be required for patients exhibiting persistent or progressive symptoms. Indications for whole lung lavage need to be individualized. However, repeated lavage should be considered when significant symptoms recur, together with deteriorating PFTs, arterial blood gases, or chest radiography.

Lymphangioleiomyomatosis

Lymphangioleiomyomatosis (LAM) is an extremely rare disease (fewer than 100 cases have been reported) that affects young women of childbearing age and may present as ILD of unknown etiology [206]. However, certain features that are commonly evident in LAM (such as pleural effusion, pneumothorax, hemoptysis) rarely manifest in other ILDs and may be clues to the diagnosis. The signs and symptoms of LAM are related to excessive proliferation of immature smooth muscle along peribronchial, venular, lymphatic, and alveolar structures [206]. Progressive obliteration and replacement of bronchioles and alveolar spaces by nodular masses of smooth muscle tissue may lead to fatal respiratory insufficiency, typically within 2 to 10 years of the onset of symptoms [206, 207]. Dyspnea is a cardinal symptom and is present in virtually all cases. Pneumothoraces complicate LAM in 40% of cases and may be the presenting or predominant features [206]. Chylous pleural effusions occur in 40% to 60% of cases [206] and in this context are virtually pathognomonic for LAM. Blood-streaked sputum or frank hemoptysis, due to obstruction of pulmonary veins and focal alveolar hemorrhage, have been described in up to 50% of cases [206, 207].

Although the etiology of LAM is poorly understood, estrogens clearly play a critical role in the pathogenesis of this disorder. LAM is only seen in premenopausal women and may be exacerbated by pregnancy, parturition, and the exogenous administration of estrogens, oral contraceptives, or gonadotropins [208, 209]. Both estrogen and progesterone receptors have been demonstrated in lung tissue from these patients (but not from normal individuals), and therapeutic regimens that ablate the effects of estrogen may reverse or stabilize the disease [207–209].

Chest Radiography

Chest radiography shows variable results [206]. Early in the course of the disease, chest radiographs may be normal or demonstrate only a pneumothorax, without evidence for interstitial disease. However, proliferation of the smooth muscle bundles along bronchovascular sheaths, interstitium, and alveolar walls leads to linear, reticular shadows, which are scattered throughout all lung fields in both central and subpleural locations. These reticular shadows may later coalesce as the disease progresses to form a micronodular or miliary pattern. Multiple cystic lesions, due to overdistention and destruction of the alveolar spaces, and honeycombing, may be the predominant findings late in the course of the disease. Obstruction of thoracic lymphatics results in fine, hazy, linear shadows (Kerley's B lines) or pleural effusions. While the clinical applicability of chest CT in the staging or diagnosis of LAM remains to be defined, high-resolution, thin-section CT may better demonstrate the thin-walled cystic and micronodular lesions, which typically range from 1 to 3 mm in diameter [210]. Mediastinal and periaortic lymphadenopathy may also be appreciated in nearly 50% of patients by CT scanning [210].

Pulmonary Function Tests

PFTs in LAM typically demonstrate an obstructive ventilatory defect, with reductions in forced vital capacity, $FEV_1\%$, expiratory flow rates, and air trapping (increased residual volume and functional residual capacity) [206]. A marked reduction in DLCO disproportionate to the degree of airways obstruction is characteristic of LAM. In contrast to most other ILDs, restriction is not found in LAM, and TLC is normal or increased.

Histologic Features

Owing to the rarity of this disease, most clinicians and pathologists may not be familiar with the salient clinical or pathologic features of the disease, and the diagnosis is missed. Proliferation of smooth muscle within alveolar structures frequently accompanies end-stage IPF or honeycomb lung, so the finding of nodular masses of smooth muscle characteristic of LAM may be mistaken for IPF. An open lung biopsy is usually required to substantiate the diagnosis, although compatible histologic features on TBB may be adequate in cases where clinical or radiographic features strongly support the diagnosis such as when chylous pleural effusion or ascites is present. The salient histopathologic feature on lung biopsy is the presence of multiple, focal hamartomatous collections of proliferating smooth muscle cells scattered in perivascular, perilymphatic, alveolar wall, and peribronchial locations [206]. Discrete masses or bundles of large or ovoid cells with hyperchromatic, spindle-shaped nuclei may be observed. The masses of smooth muscle may narrow or obliterate bronchioles and alveolar ducts and may lead to overdistention of alveoli, necrosis of the alveolar walls, and formation of microcysts and distal emphysematous changes. Recurrent pneumothoraces may result when these overdistended emphysematous cysts rupture. Obliteration of lymphatics may result in lymphatic engorgement, interstitial edema, and chylothorax. Occlusion of small pulmonary veins, foci of alveolar hemorrhage, and collections of hemosiderin-laden macrophages may also be observed. Receptors for progesterone and estrogen have been demonstrated by immunohistochemical staining in lung tissue of affected individuals, a finding not present in normal lung or other pathologic processes of the lung associated with smooth muscle proliferation [208]. While the dominant features are related to the pulmonary parenchymal involvement, foci of proliferating smooth muscle cells may also be found within thoracic, abdominal, and distant lymph nodes. Obliteration of abdominal lymphatics leading to chylous ascites is common, and lower extremity lymphedema may also occur.

Prognosis and Therapy

Unfortunately, the course of the disease is unrelenting and progressive in most cases, and most patients die within 10 years of the onset of symptoms [206, 207]. In view of the role of female hormones in the evolution of this disease, a variety of strategies to ablate estrogen effect including oophorectomy, tamoxifen (an estrogen inhibitor), progesterone, gonadotropin-releasing hormonal analogues, and oophorectomy combined with medical manipulation have been tried, with anecdotal successes [207]. Due to the rarity of this disorder, randomized prospective therapeutic trials have not been done, and optimal therapy has not been defined. Efficacy of therapy has been highly variable, with success rates ranging from 20% to 80% [207]. Failures may result from excessive delays in initiating therapy. In one recent report that analyzed outcome among patients treated with a variety of therapeutic regimens, stabilization or improvement in disease occurred in five of nine patients treated with oophorectomy, three of five treated with oophorectomy plus progesterone, and 7 of 13 treated with progesterone [207]. Favorable responses to tamoxifen were reported in only two of seven cases. Owing to the paucity of data on therapy, only tentative recommendations can be made. Clearly women must avoid pregnancy or any estrogen-containing compounds (such as oral contraceptives). We believe that either oophorectomy or progesterone usually in the form of monthly injections of medroxyprogesterone, 300 to 600 mg intramuscularly represent the logical first choice in therapy of this potentially fatal disorder. If monotherapy fails, combination therapy with progesterone and oophorectomy appears warranted. The role of alternative strategies, such as tamoxifen or gonadotropin hormone analogues, is not clear, but these agents should be considered in those patients who do not respond to therapy.

References

1. Crystal RG, Bitterman PB, Rennard SI, et al: Interstitial lung diseases of unknown cause: Disorders characterized by chronic inflammation of the lower respiratory tract. *N Engl J Med* 310:154–166, 1984
2. Daniele RP, Elias JA, Epstein PE, et al: Bronchoalveolar lavage: Role in the pathogenesis, diagnosis, and management of interstitial lung disease. *Ann Intern Med* 102:93–108, 1985
3. Hunninghake GW, Bedell GN: Interstitial lung disease. Concepts of pathogenesis. *Semin Respir Med* 6:31–39, 1984
4. Epler GR, McLoud TC, Gaensler EA, et al: Normal chest roentgenograms in chronic diffuse infiltrative lung disease. *N Engl J Med* 298:934–939, 1978
5. Gaensler EA, Carrington CB: Open biopsy for chronic diffuse infiltrative lung disease: Clinical, roentgenographic, and physiological correlations in 502 patients. *Ann Thorac Surg* 30:411–426, 1980
6. Crystal RG, Fulmer JD, Roberts WC, et al: Idiopathic pulmonary fibrosis. Clinical, histologic, radiographic, physiologic, scintigraphic, cytologic, and biochemical aspects. *Ann Intern Med* 85:769–788, 1976
7. Mathieson JR, Mayo JR, Staples CA, et al: Chronic diffuse infiltrative lung disease: Comparison of diagnostic accuracy of CT and chest radiography. *Radiology* 171:111–116, 1989
8. Mueller NI, Staples CA, Miller RR, et al: Disease activity in idiopathic pulmonary fibrosis: CT and pathologic correlation. *Radiology* 165:731–734, 1987
9. Swensen SJ, Aughenbaugh GL, Brown LR: High-resolution computed tomography of the lung. *Mayo Clin Proc* 64:1284–1294, 1989
10. Panos RJ, Mortenson R, Niccoli SA, et al: Clinical deterioration in patients with idiopathic pulmonary fibrosis. *Am J Med* 88: 396–404, 1990
11. Carrington CB, Gaensler EA, Coutu RE, et al: Natural history and treated course of usual and desquamative interstitial pneumonia. *N Engl J Med* 298:801–809, 1978
12. Haslam PL, Turton CWG, Lukosezek A, et al: Bronchoalveolar lavage fluid cell counts in cryptogenic fibrosing alveolitis and their relation to therapy. *Thorax* 35:328–339, 1980
13. Liebow AA, Steer A, Billingsley JG: Desquamative interstitial pneumonia. *Am J Med* 39:369–404, 1965
14. Rudd RM, Haslam PL, Turner-Warwick M: Cryptogenic fibrosing alveolitis: Relationships of pulmonary physiology and bronchoalveolar lavage to treatment and prognosis. *Am Rev Respir Dis* 124:1–8, 1981
15. Scadding JG, Hinston KFW: Diffuse fibrosing alveolitis (diffuse interstitial fibrosis of the lungs). Correlation of histology at biopsy with prognosis. *Thorax* 22:291–304, 1967
16. Stack BHR, Choo-Kang YFJ, Heard BE: The prognosis of cryptogenic fibrosing alveolitis. *Thorax* 27:535–542, 1972
17. Tukiainen P, Taskinen E, Hosti P, et al: Prognosis of cryptogenic fibrosing alveolitis. *Thorax* 38:349–355, 1983
18. Johnson MA, Kwan S, Snell MJC, et al: Randomized control trial comparing prednisolone alone with cyclophosphamide and low dose prednisolone in combination with cryptogenic fibrosing alveolitis. *Thorax* 44:280–288, 1989
19. Line BR, Fulmer JD, Reynolds HY, et al: Gallium-67 citrate scanning in the staging of idiopathic pulmonary fibrosis: Correlation with physiologic and morphologic features and bronchoalveolar lavage. *Am Rev Respir Dis* 118:355–365, 1978
20. Winterbauer RH, Hammar SP, Hallman KO, et al: Diffuse interstitial pneumonitis. Clinicopathologic correlations in 20 patients treated with prednisone/azathioprine. *Am J Med* 65:661–672, 1978
21. Watters LC, King TE, Schwarz MI, et al: A clinical, radiographic, and physiologic scoring system for the longitudinal assessment of patients with idiopathic pulmonary fibrosis. *Am Rev Respir Dis* 133:97–103, 1986
22. Dunn TL, Watters LC, Hendrix C, et al: Gas exchange at a given degree of volume restriction is different in sarcoidosis and idiopathic

pulmonary fibrosis. *Am J Med* 85:221–224, 1988
23. Turner-Warwick M: Bronchoalveolar lavage fluid cell counts in cryptogenic fibrosing alveolitis and their relation to therapy. *Thorax* 35:328–339, 1980
24. Weinberger SE, Kelman JA, Elson NA, et al: Bronchoalveolar lavage in interstitial lung disease. *Ann Intern Med* 89:459–466, 1978
25. Hallgren R, Bjermer L, Lundgren R, et al: The eosinophil component of the alveolitis in idiopathic pulmonary fibrosis. Signs of eosinophil activation in the lung are related to impaired lung function. *Am Rev Respir Dis* 139:373–377, 1989
26. Peterson MW, Monick M, Hunninghake GW: Prognostic role of eosinophils in pulmonary fibrosis. *Chest* 92:51–56, 1987
27. Turner-Warwick M, Haslam PL: The value of serial bronchoalveolar lavages in assessing the clinical progress of patients with cryptogenic fibrosing alveolitis. *Am Rev Respir Dis* 135:26–34, 1987
28. Dreisen RB, Schwarz MI, Theofilopoulos AN, et al: Circulating immune complexes in the idiopathic interstitial pneumonias. *N Engl J Med* 298:353–357, 1978
29. Gelb AF, Dreisen RB, Epstein JD, et al: Immune complexes, gallium lung scans, and bronchoalveolar lavage in idiopathic interstitial pneumonitis-fibrosis: A structure-function clinical study. *Chest* 84:148–153, 1983
30. Bogin RM, Buschman DS, Cherniack RM, et al: Gallium-67 lung scanning is not helpful in predicting the clinical course of patients with idiopathic pulmonary fibrosis. *Am Rev Respir Dis* (in press)
31. Watters LC, Schwarz MI, Cherniack RM, et al: Idiopathic pulmonary fibrosis. Pretreatment bronchoalveolar lavage cellular constituents and their relationships with lung histopathology and clinical response to therapy. *Am Rev Respir Dis* 135:696–704, 1987
32. Weese WC, Levine BW, Kazemi H: Interstitial lung disease resistant to corticosteroid therapy. Report of three cases treated with azathioprine or cyclophosphamide. *Chest* 67:57–60, 1975
33. Raghu G, DePaso WJ, Cain K, et al: Azathioprine combined with prednisone in the treatment of idiopathic pulmonary fibrosis: A prospective, double-blind, randomized, placebo-controlled clinical trial. *Am Rev Resp Dis* 144:291–296, 1991
34. Keogh BA, Bernardo J, Hunninghake GW, et al: Effect of intermittent high dose parenteral corticosteroids on the alveolitis of idiopathic pulmonary fibrosis. *Am Rev Respir Dis* 127:18–22, 1983
35. Toronto Lung Transplant Group: Unilateral lung transplantation for pulmonary fibrosis. *N Engl J Med* 314:1140–1145, 1986
36. Grossman RF, Frost A, Zamel N, et al: Results of single-lung transplantation for bilateral pulmonary fibrosis. *N Engl J Med* 322:727–732, 1990
37. Wiedeman HP, Matthay RA: Pulmonary manifestations of the collagen vascular diseases. *Clin Chest Med* 10:677–721, 1989
38. Zitnik RJ, Cooper JA Jr: Pulmonary disease due to antirheumatic agents. *Clin Chest Med* 11:139–150, 1990
39. Silver RM, Miller KS: Lung involvement in systemic sclerosis. *Rheum Dis Clin North Am* 16:199–216, 1990
40. Tazelaar HD, Viggiano RW, Pickersgill, et al: Interstitial lung disease in polymyositis and dermatomyositis. Clinical features and prognosis as correlated with histologic findings. *Am Rev Respir Dis* 141:727–733, 1990
41. Lakhanpal S, Lie JT, Conn DL, et al: Pulmonary disease in polymyositis/dermatomyositis: A clinicopathological analysis of 65 cases. *Ann Rheum Dis* 46:23–29, 1987
42. Roschmann RA, Rothenberg RJ: Pulmonary fibrosis in rheumatoid arthritis: A review of clinical features and therapy. *Semin Arthritis Rheum* 16:174–185, 1987
43. Walker WC, Wright V: Pulmonary lesions and rheumatoid arthritis. *Medicine* 47:501–520, 1968
44. Matthay RA, Schwarz MI, Petty TL, et al: Pulmonary manifestations of systemic lupus erythematosus: Review of twelve cases of acute lupus pneumonitis. *Medicine* 54:397–409, 1974
45. Sullivan WD, Hurst DJ, Harmon CE, et al: A prospective evaluation emphasizing pulmonary involvement in patients with mixed connective tissue disease. *Medicine* 63:92–107, 1984
46. Yousem SA, Colby TV, Carrington CB: Lung biopsy in rheumatoid arthritis. *Am Rev Respir Dis* 131:770–777, 1985
47. Wallaert B, Hatron P, Grosbois J, et al: Subclinical pulmonary involvement in collagen-vascular diseases assessed by bronchoalveolar lavage: Relationship between alveolitis and subsequent changes in lung function. *Am Rev Respir Dis* 133:574–580, 1986
48. Greene NB, Solinger AM, Baughman RP: Patients with collagen vascular disease and dyspnea. The value of gallium scanning and bronchoalveolar lavage in predicting response to steroid therapy and clinical outcome. *Chest* 91:698–703, 1987
49. Geddes DM, Corrin B, et al: Progressive airway obliteration in adults and its association with rheumatoid arthritis. *Q J Med* 184:427–444, 1977

50. Begin R, Masse S, Cantin A, et al: Airway disease in a subset of nonsmoking rheumatoid patients. Characterization of the disease and evidence of an autoimmune pathogenesis. *Am J Med* 72:743–750, 1982
51. Sostman HD, Matthay RA, Putnam CE: Methotrexate induced lung disease. *Medicine* 55:371–388, 1976
52. White DA, Rankin JA, Stover DE, et al: Methotrexate pneumonitis. Bronchoalveolar lavage findings suggest an immunologic disorder. *Am Rev Respir Dis* 139:18–21, 1989
53. Evans RB, Ettensohn DB, Fawaz-Estrup F, et al: Gold lung: Recent developments in pathogenesis, diagnosis, and therapy. *Semin Arthritis Rheum* 16:196–205, 1987
54. Hakala M: Poor prognosis in patients with rheumatoid arthritis hospitalized for interstitial lung fibrosis. *Chest* 93:114–118, 1988
55. Garcia JG, Parhami N, Killam D, et al: Bronchoalveolar lavage fluid evaluation in rheumatoid arthritis. *Am Rev Respir Dis* 133: 450–454, 1986
56. Garcia JG, James HL, Zinkgraf S, et al: Lower respiratory tract abnormalities in rheumatoid interstitial lung disease. Potential role for neutrophils in lung injury. *Am Rev Respir Dis* 136:811–817, 1987
57. Idell S, Garcia JG, Gonzalez K, et al: Fibrinopeptide A reactive peptides and procoagulant activity in bronchoalveolar lavage: Relationship to rheumatoid interstitial lung disease. *J Rheumatol* 16:592–598, 1989
58. Tishler M, Grief J, Fireman E, et al: Bronchoalveolar lavage: A sensitive tool for early diagnosis of pulmonary involvement in rheumatoid arthritis. *J Rheumatol* 13:547–550, 1986
59. Weiland JE, Garcia JG, Davis WB, et al: Neutrophil collagenase in rheumatoid interstitial lung disease. *J Appl Physiol* 62:628–633, 1987
60. Lomeo RM, Cornella RJ, Schabel SI, et al: Progressive systemic sclerosis sine scleroderma presenting as pulmonary interstitial fibrosis. *Am J Med* 87:525–527, 1989
61. Greenwald GI, Tashkin DP, Gong H, et al: Longitudinal changes in lung function and respiratory symptoms in progressive systemic sclerosis. Prospective study. *Am J Med* 83:83–91, 1987
62. Peters-Golden M, Wise WA, Schneider P, et al: Clinical and demographic predictors of loss of pulmonary function in systemic sclerosis. *Medicine* 63:221–231, 1984
63. Peters-Golden M, Wise RA, Hochberg MC, et al: Carbon monoxide diffusing capacity as predictor of outcome in systemic sclerosis. *Am J Med* 77:1027–1034, 1984
64. Steen VD, Owens GR, Fino GJ, et al: Pulmonary involvement in systemic sclerosis. *Arthritis Rheum* 28:759–767, 1985
65. Silver RM, Miller KS, Kinsella MB, et al: Evaluation and management of scleroderma lung disease using bronchoalveolar lavage. *Am J Med* 88:470–476, 1990
66. Miller KS, Smith EA, Kinsella M, et al: Lung disease associated with progressive systemic sclerosis. Assessment of interlobar variation by bronchoalveolar lavage and comparison with noninvasive evaluation of disease activity. *Am Rev Respir Dis* 141:301–306, 1990
67. Rossi GA, Bitterman PB, Rennard SI, et al: Evidence for chronic inflammation as a component of the interstitial lung disease associated with progressive systemic sclerosis. *Am Rev Respir Dis* 131:612–617, 1985
68. Silver RM, Metcalf JF, Stanley JH, et al: Interstitial lung disease in scleroderma. Analysis by bronchoalveolar lavage. *Arthritis Rheum* 27:1254–1262, 1984
69. Konig G, Ludenschmidt C, Hammer C, et al: Lung involvement in scleroderma. *Chest* 85:318–324, 1984
70. Edelson JD, Hyland RH, Ramsden M, et al: Lung inflammation in scleroderma: Clinical, radiographic, physiologic, and cytopathological features. *J Rheumatol* 12:957–963, 1985
71. Manoussakis MN, Constantopoulos SH, Gharavi AE, et al: Pulmonary involvement in systemic sclerosis. Association with anti-Scl 70 antibody and digital pitting. *Chest* 92:509–513, 1987
72. Furst DE, Clements PJ, Hillis S, et al: Immunosuppression with chlorambucil, versus placebo, for scleroderma. Results of a three-year, parallel, randomized double-blind study. *Arthritis Rheum* 32:584–593, 1989
73. deClerk LS, Desqueker J, Francx L, et al: D-penicillamine therapy and interstitial lung disease in scleroderma: Long-term follow-up study. *Arthritis Rheum* 3:643–650, 1987
74. Steen VD, Owen GR, Redmond C, et al: The effects of D-penicillamine on pulmonary findings in systemic sclerosis. *Arthritis Rheum* 28:882–888, 1985
75. Harrison NK, Glanville AR, Strickland B, et al: Pulmonary involvement in systemic sclerosis: The detection of early changes by thin section CT scan, bronchoalveolar lavage, and ^{99m}Tc-DPTA clearance. *Respir Med* 83:404–414, 1989
76. Sharp GE, Irving W, Tan E, et al: Mixed connective tissue disease. An apparently distinct rheumatic disease syndrome associated with a specific antibody to an extractable nuclear antigen (ENA). *Am J Med* 52:148–159, 1972

77. Lazaro MA, Maldonado Cocco JA, Catoggio LJ, et al: Clinical and serologic characteristics of patients with overlap syndrome: Is mixed connective tissue disease a distinct clinical entity? *Medicine* 68:58–65, 1989
78. Prakash V, Luthra H, Divertie M: Intrathoracic manifestations in mixed connective tissue disease. *Mayo Clin Proc* 60:813–821, 1985
79. Haupt HM, Moore GW, Hutchins GM: The lung in systemic lupus erythematosus. Analysis of the pathologic changes in 120 patients. *Am J Med* 71:791–798, 1981
80. Asura EL, Greenberg AS: Adverse impact of interstitial pulmonary fibrosis on prognosis in polymyositis and dermatomyositis. *Semin Arthritis Rheum* 18:29–37, 1988
81. Yoshida S, Akizuki M, Mimori T, et al: The precipitating antibody to an acidic nuclear protein antigen, the Jo-1, in connective tissue diseases: A marker for a subset of polymyositis with interstitial pulmonary fibrosis. *Arthritis Rheum* 26:604–611, 1983
82. Hochberg MC, Feldman D, Stevens MB, et al: Antibody to Jo-1 in polymyositis/dermatomyositis: Association with interstitial pulmonary disease. *J Rheumatol* 11:663–665, 1984
83. al-Janadi M, Smith CD, Karsh J: Cyclophosphamide treatment of interstitial pulmonary fibrosis in polymyositis/dermatomyositis. *J Rheumatol* 16:1592–1596, 1989
84. Cooper JAD Jr, White DA, Matthay RA: Drug-induced pulmonary disease: Part 1: Cytotoxic drugs. *Am Rev Respir Dis* 133: 321, 1986
85. Cooper JA Jr, White DA, Matthay RA: Drug induced pulmonary disease. Part 2. Noncytotoxic drugs. *Am Rev Respir Dis* 133:488–505, 1986
86. Rice KL: Pulmonary infiltrates associated with noncytotoxic drugs. *Semin Respir Infect* 3:229–239, 1988
87. Smith GJW: The histopathology of pulmonary reactions to drugs. *Clin Chest Med* 11:95–117, 1990
88. Holmberg L, Boman G, Bottiger IE, et al: Adverse reactions to nitrofurantoin. Analysis of 921 reports. *Am J Med* 69:733–738, 1980
89. Chandler DB: Possible mechanisms of bleomycin induced fibrosis. *Clin Chest Med* 11:21–39, 1990
90. White DA, Kris MG, Stover DE: Bronchoalveolar lavage cell populations in bleomycin lung toxicity. *Thorax* 42:551–552, 1987
91. Martin WJ II: Mechanisms of amiodarone pulmonary toxicity. *Clin Chest Med* 11:131–138, 1990
92. Martin WJ II, Rosenow EC III: Amiodarone pulmonary toxicity. Recognition and pathogenesis. *Chest* 93:1067–1075, 1242–1248, 1988
93. Adams GD, Kehoe R, Lesch M, et al: Amiodarone induced pneumonitis: Assessment of risk factors and possible risk reduction. *Chest* 92:254–263, 1988
94. Israel-Biet D, Venet A, Caubarrere I, et al: Bronchoalveolar lavage in amiadarone pneumonitis. Cellular abnormalities and their relevance to pathogenesis. *Chest* 91:214–221, 1987
95. Magro SA, Lawrence EC, Wheeler SH, et al: Amiodarone pulmonary toxicity: Prospective evaluation of serial pulmonary function tests. *J Am Coll Cardiol* 12:781–788, 1988
96. Zaher C, Hamer A, Peter T, et al: Low dose steroid therapy for prophylaxis of amiodarone induced pulmonary infiltrates. *N Engl J Med* 308:779, 1983
97. Epler GR, Colby TV, McLoud TC, et al: Bronchiolitis obliterans organizing pneumonia. *N Engl J Med* 312:152–158, 1985
98. Gosink BB, Friedman PJ, Liebow AA: Bronchiolitis obliterans: Roentgenologic-pathologic correlation. *Am J Roentgenol* 117:816–832, 1973
99. Guerry-Force ML, Muller NL, Wright JL, et al: A comparison of bronchiolitis obliterans with organizing pneumonia, usual interstitial pneumonia, and small airways disease. *Am Rev Respir Dis* 135:705–712, 1987
100. Katzenstein A, Myers J, Prophet W, et al: Bronchiolitis obliterans and usual interstitial pneumonia: A comparative clinicopathologic study. *Am J Surg Pathol* 10:373–381, 1986
101. King TE Jr: Bronchiolitis obliterans. *Lung* 167:69–93, 1989
102. Muller NL, Guerry-Force ML, Staples CA, et al: Differential diagnosis of bronchiolitis obliterans with organizing pneumonia and usual interstitial pneumonia: Clinical, functional, and radiologic findings. *Radiology* 162:151–156, 1987
103. Bartter T, Irwin RS, Nash G, et al: Idiopathic bronchiolitis obliterans organizing pneumonia with peripheral infiltrates on chest roentgenogram. *Arch Intern Med* 149:273–279, 1989
104. Cordier JF, Loire R, Brune J: Idiopathic bronchiolitis obliterans organizing pneumonia: Definition of characteristic clinical profiles in a series of 16 patients. *Chest* 96:999–1004, 1989
105. Turton CW, William G, Green M: Cryptogenic obliterative bronchiolitis in adults. *Thorax* 36:805–810, 1981
106. Kindt GC, Weiland JE, Davis WB, et al: Bronchiolitis in adults. A reversible cause of airway obstruction associated with airway

neutrophils and neutrophil products. *Am Rev Respir Dis* 140:483–492, 1989
107. Hakala M, Paakko P, Sutinen S, et al: Association of bronchiolitis with connective tissue disorders. *Ann Rheum Dis* 45:656–662, 1986
108. Chan CK, et al: Pulmonary complications of bone marrow transplantation. *Clin Chest Med* 11:323–332, 1990
109. Glanville AR, Baldwin JC, Burke CM, et al: Obliterative bronchiolitis after heart-lung transplantation: Apparent arrest by augmented immunosuppression. *Ann Intern Med* 107:300–304, 1987
110. Theodore J, Starnes VA, Lewiston NJ: Obliterative bronchiolitis. *Clin Chest Med* 11:309–321, 1990
111. Davison A, Heard B, McAllister W, et al: Cryptogenic organizing pneumonitis. *QJ Med* 207:382–394, 1983
112. Dorinsky PM, Davis WB, Lucas JG, et al: Adult bronchiolitis. Evaluation by bronchoalveolar lavage and response to prednisone therapy. *Chest* 88:58–63, 1985
113. Muller NL, Staples CA, Miller RA: Bronchiolitis obliterans oganizing pneumonia: CT features in 14 patients. *Am J Roentgenol* 154:983–987, 1990
114. Mayock RL, Bertrand P, Morrison CE, et al: Manifestations of sarcoidosis: Analysis of 145 patients with a review of nine series selected from the literature. *Am J Med* 35:67–89, 1963
115. Thomas PD, Hunninghake GW: Current concepts of the pathogenesis of sarcoidosis. *Am Rev Respir Dis* 135:747–760, 1987
116. Siltzach LE, James DG, Neville E, et al: Course and prognosis of sarcoidosis around the world. *Am J Med* 57:847–852, 1974
117. Siltzbach LE: Sarcoidosis: Clinical features and management. *Med Clin North Am* 51:483–502, 1967
118. Reich JM, Johnson RE: Course and prognosis of sarcoidosis in a nonreferral setting: Analysis of 86 patients observed for 10 years. *Am J Med* 89:61–66, 1985
119. Romer FK: Presentation of sarcoidosis and outcome of pulmonary changes. A review of 243 patients followed for up to 10 years. *Dan Med Bull* 29:27–32, 1982
120. Scadding JG: Prognosis of intrathoracic sarcoidosis in England. A review of 136 cases after five years observation. *Br Med J* 1165–1172, 1961
121. Hillerdal G, Nou E, Osterman K, et al: Sarcoidosis: Epidemiology and prognosis. A 15 year European study. *Am Rev Respir Dis* 130:29–32, 1984
122. Winterbauer RH, Belic N, Moores KD: A clinical interpretation of bilateral hilar adenopathy. *Ann Intern Med* 78:65–71, 1973
123. DeRemee RA, Rohrbach MS: Serum angiotensin-converting enzyme activity in evaluating the clinical course of sarcoidosis. *Ann Intern Med* 92:361–365, 1980
124. Hollinger WM, Staton GW, Fajman WA, et al: Prediction of therapeutic response in steroid-treated pulmonary sarcoidosis. Evaluation of clinical parameters, bronchoalveolar lavage, gallium-67 scanning, and serum angiotensin-converting enzyme levels. *Am Rev Respir Dis* 132:65–69, 1985
125. Lawrence EC, Teague RB, Gottlieb MS, et al: Serial changes in markers of disease activity with corticosteroid treatment in sarcoidosis. *Am J Med* 74:747–756, 1983
126. Lieberman J: Elevation of serum angiotensin converting enzyme (ACE) level in sarcoidosis. *Am J Med* 59:365–372, 1975
127. Turner-Warwick M, McAllister W, Lawrence R, et al: Corticosteroid treatment in sarcoidosis: Do serial lavage lymphocyte counts, serum angiotensin converting enzyme measurements and gallium-67 scans help management? *Thorax* 41:903–913, 1986
128. Valeyre D, Aumon G, Bladier D, et al: The relationship between non-invasive exploration in pulmonary sarcoidosis of recent origin as shown by bronchoalveolar lavages, serum angiotensin converting enzyme and pulmonary function tests. *Am Rev Respir Dis* 126:41–45, 1982
129. Betchel JJ, Starr T, Dantzker DR, et al: Airway hyperreactivity in patients with sarcoidosis. *Am Rev Respir Dis* 124:759–761, 1981
130. Line BR, Hunninghake GW, Keogh BA, et al: Gallium-67 scanning to stage the alveolitis of sarcoidosis: Correlation with clinical studies, pulmonary function studies, and bronchoalveolar lavage. *Am Rev Respir Dis* 123:440–446, 1981
131. Baughman RP, Fernandez M, Bosken CH, et al: Comparison of gallium-67 scanning, bronchoalveolar lavage, and serum angiotensin-converting enzyme levels in pulmonary sarcoidosis. Predicting response to therapy. *Am Rev Respir Dis* 129:676–681, 1984
132. Beaumont D, Herry JY, Sapene M, et al: Gallium-67 in the evaluation of sarcoidosis: Correlations with serum angiotensin-converting enzyme and bronchoalveolar lavage. *Thorax* 37:11–18, 1982
133. Costabel U, Bross KJ, Guzman J, et al: Predictive value of bronchoalveolar T cell subsets for the course of pulmonary sarcoidosis. *Ann NY Acad Sci* 465:418–426, 1986
134. Bjermer L, Rosenhall L, Angstrom T, et al: Predictive value of bronchoalveolar lavage cell analysis in sarcoidosis. *Thorax* 43:284–288, 1988
135. Ceuppens JL, Ludovicus M, Lacquet GM,

et al: Alveolar T cell subsets in pulmonary sarcoidosis: Correlation with disease activity and effect of steroid treatment. *Am Rev Respir Dis* 129:563–569, 1984
136. Ward K, O'Connor C, Odlum C, et al: Prognostic value of bronchoalveolar lavage in sarcoidosis: The critical influence of disease presentation. *Thorax* 44:6–12, 1989
137. Arnoux A, Marsac J, Stanislas-Leguern G, et al: Bronchoalveolar lavage in sarcoidosis. Correlation between alveolar lymphocytosis and clinical data. *Pathol Res Pract* 175:62–79, 1982
138. Keogh BA, Hunninghake GW, Line BR, et al: The alveolitis of pulmonary sarcoidosis. Evaluation of natural history and alveolitis-dependent changes in lung function. *Am Rev Respir Dis* 128:256–265, 1983
139. Buchalter S, App W, Jackson L, et al: Bronchoalveolar lavage cell analysis in sarcoidosis: A comparison of lymphocyte counts and clinical course. *Ann NY Acad Sci* 465:679–684, 1986
140. Israel-Biet D, Venet A, Chretien J: Persistent high alveolar lymphocytosis as predictive criterion of chronic pulmonary sarcoidosis. *Ann NY Acad Sci* 465:395–406, 1986
141. Bauer W, Gorny MK, Baumann HR, et al: T-lymphocyte subsets and immunoglobulin concentrations in bronchoalveolar lavage of patients with sarcoidosis and high and low intensity alveolitis. *Am Rev Respir Dis* 132: 1060–1065, 1985
142. Rossman MD, Dauber JM, Cardillo ME, et al: Pulmonary sarcoidosis: Correlation of serum angiotensin-converting enzyme with blood and bronchoalveolar lymphocytes. *Am Rev Respir Dis* 125:366–369, 1982
143. Selroos O, Sellergren TL: Corticosteroid therapy of pulmonary sarcoidosis. A prospective evaluation of alternate day and daily dosage in stage II disease. *Scand J Respir Dis* 60:215–221, 1979
144. Eule H, Weinecke A, Roth I: The possible influence of corticosteroid therapy on the natural course of sarcoidosis. *Ann NY Acad Sci* 465:695–701, 1986
145. Harkleroad LE, Young RL, Savage PJ, et al: Pulmonary sarcoidosis: Long-term follow-up of the effects of steroid therapy. *Chest* 82:84–87, 1982
146. Israel HL, Fouts DW, Beggs RA: A controlled trial of prednisone treatment of sarcoidosis. *Am Rev Respir Dis* 107:609–614, 1973
147. James DG, Carstairs LS, Trowell J, et al: Treatment of sarcoidosis: Report of a controlled therapeutic trial. *Lancet* 2:526–528, 1967
148. Yamamoto M, Saito N, Tachibana T, et al: Effects of an 18 month corticosteroid therapy to stage I and stage II sarcoidosis patients (a control trial). *In* Chretien J, Marsac J, Saltiel JC (eds): Sarcoidosis and Other Granulomatous Disorders. Paris, Pergamon Press, 1980, pp 470–474
149. Zaki MH, Lyons HA, Leilop L, et al: Corticosteroid therapy in sarcoidosis. A five-year controlled follow-up study. *NY State J Med* 87:496–499, 1987
150. Spiteri MA, Newman SP, Clarke SW, et al: Inhaled corticosteroids can modulate the immunopathogenesis of pulmonary sarcoidosis. *Eur Respir J* 2:218–224, 1989
151. Kataria YP: Chlorambucil in sarcoidosis. *Chest* 78:36–43, 1980
152. Lower EE, Baughman RP: The use of low dose methotrexate in refractory sarcoidosis. *Am J Med Sci* 299:153–157, 1990
153. Siltzbach LE, Teirstein AS: Chloroquine therapy in 43 patients with intrathoracic and cutaneous sarcoidosis. *Acta Med Scand* 425 (suppl): 302–308, 1964
154. British Tuberculosis Association: Chloroquine in the treatment of sarcoidosis. *Tubercle* 48:257–272, 1967
155. Adams JS, MM Diz, Sharma OP: Effective reduction in the serum 1,25-dihydroxyvitamin D and calcium concentration in sarcoidosis-associated hypercalcemia with short-course chloroquine therapy. *Ann Intern Med* 111:437–438, 1989
156. Sharma O, Hughes DTD, Geraint-James D, et al: Immunosuppressive therapy with azathioprine in sarcoidosis. *In* Levinsky L, Macholda F (eds): Fifth International Conference on Sarcoidosis. Prague, Universita Karlova, 1971, pp 635–637.
157. Toews GB, Lynch JP III: Methotrexate in sarcoidosis. *Am J Med Sci* 299:33–36, 1990
158. Demeter SL: Myocardial sarcoidosis unresponsive to steroids. Treatment with cyclophosphamide. *Chest* 94:202–203, 1988
159. Martinet Yves, Pinkston P, Saltini C, et al: Examination of the in vitro and in vivo effects of cyclosporine on the lung T-lymphocyte alveolitis of active pulmonary sarcoidosis. *Am Rev Respir Dis* 138:1242–1248, 1988
160. Rebuck AS, Stiller CR, Braude AC, et al: Cyclosporin (CyA) in the treatment of pulmonary sarcoidosis. *In* Schindler R (ed): Cyclosporin in Autoimmune Diseases. Berlin, Springer-Verlag, 1985, pp 193–196
161. Kahan BD: Cyclosporine. *N Engl J Med* 321:1725–1738, 1989
162. Reeder WH, Goodrich BE: Pulmonary infiltration with eosinophilia (PIE syndrome). *Ann Intern Med* 36:1217–1240, 1952
163. Crofton JW, Livingstone JL, Oswald NC,

et al: Pulmonary eosinophilia. *Thorax* 7:1–35, 1952
164. Carrington CB, Addington WW, Goff AM, et al: Chronic eosinophilic pneumonia. *N Engl J Med* 280:787–798, 1969
165. Liebow AA, Carrington CB: The eosinophilic pneumonias. *Medicine* (Baltimore) 48:251–285, 1969
166. Jederlinic PJ, Sicilian L, Gaensler EA: Chronic eosinophilic pneumonia. A report of 19 cases and a review of the literature. *Medicine* 67:154–161, 1988
167. Allen JN, Pacht ER, Gadek JE, et al: Acute eosinophilic pneumonia as a reversible cause of noninfectious respiratory failure. *N Engl J Med* 321:569–574, 1989
168. McEvoy JD, Donald KJ, Edwards RL: Immunoglobulin levels and electron microscopy in eosinophilic pneumonia. *Am J Med* 64: 529–536, 1978
169. Greenberger P: Allergic bronchopulmonary aspergillosis and fungosis. *Clin Chest Med* 9:599–608, 1988
170. Gaensler E, Carrington CB: Peripheral opacities in chronic eosinophilic pneumonia: The photographic negative of pulmonary edema. *Am J Radiol* 128:1–13, 1977
171. Pearson DJ, Rosenow EC III: Chronic eosinophilic pneumonia (Carrington's): A follow-up study. *Mayo Clin Proc* 53:73–78, 1978
172. Lanham JG, Elkon KB, Pusey CD, et al: Systemic vasculitis with asthma and eosinophilia: A clinical approach to the Churg-Strauss syndrome. *Medicine* (Baltimore) 63:65–81, 1984
173. Dejaegher P, Demedts M: Bronchoalveolar lavage in eosinophilic pneumonia before and after corticosteroid therapy. *Am Rev Respir Dis* 129:631–632, 1984
174. Grief J, Struhar D, Kivity S, et al: Bronchoalveolar lavage: A useful tool in the diagnosis of eosinophilic pneumonia. *Isr J Med Sci* 22:479–480, 1986
175. Basset F, Corrin B, Spencer H, et al: Pulmonary histiocytosis X. *Am Rev Respir Dis* 118:811–820, 1978
176. Colby TV, Lombard C: Histiocytosis X in the lung. *Hum Pathol* 14:847–856, 1983
177. Friedman P, Liebow A, Sokoloff J: Eosinophilic granuloma of lung. *Medicine* 60:385–396, 1981
178. Marcy TW, Reynolds HY: Pulmonary histiocytosis X. *Lung* 163:129–150, 1985
179. Greenberger JS, Crocker AC, Vawter G: Results of treatment of 127 patients with systemic histiocytosis (Letterer-Siwe syndrome, Schuller-Christian syndrome and multifocal eosinophilic granuloma). *Medicine* 60:311–338, 1981
180. Lieberman PH, Jones CR, Dargeon HWK, et al: A reappraisal of eosinophilic granuloma of bone, Hand-Schuller-Christian syndrome, and Letterer-Siwe syndrome. *Medicine* 48:375–400, 1969
181. Zinkham WH: Multifocal eosinophilic granuloma. Natural history, etiology, and management. *Am J Med* 60:457–463, 1976
182. Lacronique J, Roth C, Battesti JP, et al: Chest radiological features of pulmonary histiocytosis X: A report based on 50 adult cases. *Thorax* 37:104–109, 1982
183. Brauner MW, Grenier P, Mouelhi MM, et al: Pulmonary histiocytosis X: Evaluation with high-resolution CT. *Radiology* 172:255–258, 1989
184. Moore AD, Bodwin JD, Muller NL, et al: Pulmonary histiocytosis X: Comparison of radiographic and CT findings. *Radiology* 172:249–254, 1989
185. Kawanami O, Basset F, Ferrans VJ, et al: Pulmonary Langerhans's cells in patients with fibrotic lung disorders. *Lab Invest* 44:227–233, 1981
186. Soler P, Chollet S, Jacque C, et al: Immunocytochemical characterization of pulmonary histiocytosis X cells in lung biopsies. *Am J Pathol* 118:439–451, 1985
187. Chollet S, Soler P, Dournovo P, et al: Diagnosis of pulmonary histiocytosis X by immunodetection of Langerhans cells in bronchoalveolar lavage fluid. *Am J Pathol* 115: 225–232, 1984
188. Cagle P, Mattioli C, Truong L, et al: Immunohistochemical diagnosis of pulmonary eosinophilic granuloma on lung biopsy. *Chest* 94:1133–1137, 1988
189. Flint A, Lloyd RV, Colby TV, et al: Pulmonary histiocytosis X. Immunoperoxidase staining for HLA-DR antigen and S100 protein. *Arch Pathol Lab Med* 110:930–933, 1986
190. Webber D, Tron V, Askin F, et al: S-100 staining in the diagnosis of eosinophilic granuloma of lung. *Am J Clin Pathol* 84:447–453, 1985
191. King TE Jr, Schwartz MI, Dreisin RE, et al: Circulating immune complexes in pulmonary eosinophilic granuloma. *Ann Intern Med* 91:397–399, 1979
192. Rosen SH, Castleman B, Liebow AA: Pulmonary alveolar proteinosis. *N Engl J Med* 258:1123–1142, 1958
193. Prakash UB, Barham SS, Carpenter HA, et al: Pulmonary alveolar phospholipoproteinosis: Experience with 34 cases and a review. *Mayo Clin Proc* 62:499–518, 1987
194. Davidson JM, MacLeod WM: Pulmonary alveolar proteinosis. *Br J Dis Chest* 63:13–28, 1969

195. Bedrossian CWM, Lunda MA, Conklin RH, et al: Alveolar proteinosis as a consequence of immunosuppression: A hypothesis based on clinical and pathological observations. *Hum Pathol* II (suppl):527–535, 1980
196. Carnovale R, Zornoza J, Goldman AM, et al: Pulmonary alveolar proteinosis: Its association with hematologic malignancy and lymphoma. *Radiology* 122:303–306, 1977
197. Claypool WD, Rogers RM, Matuschak GM: Update on the clinical diagnosis, management, and pathogenesis of pulmonary alveolar proteinosis (phospholipidosis). *Chest* 85: 550–558, 1984
198. DuBois RM, McAllister WAC, Branthwaite MA: Alveolar proteinosis: Diagnosis and treatment over a 10-year period. *Thorax* 38:360–363, 1983
199. Kariman K, Kylstra JA, Spock A: Pulmonary alveolar proteinosis: Prospective clinical experience in 23 patients for 15 years. *Lung* 162:223–231, 1984
200. Selecky PA, Wasserman K, Benfield JR, et al: The clinical and physiological effect of whole-lung lavage in pulmonary alveolar proteinosis: A ten-year experience. *Ann Thorac Surg* 24:451–460, 1977
201. Ramirez RJ, Schultz RB, Dutton RE: Pulmonary alveolar proteinosis: A new technique and rationale for treatment. *Arch Intern Med* 112:419–424, 1963
202. Martin RJ, Rogers RM, Myers NM: Pulmonary alveolar proteinosis: Shunt fraction and lactic acid dehydrogenase concentrations as aids to diagnosis. *Am Rev Respir Dis* 117: 1059–1062, 1978
203. Hoffman RM, Dauber JH, Roger RM: Improvement in alveolar macrophage migration after therapeutic whole lung lavage in pulmonary alveolar proteinosis. *Am Rev Respir Dis* 139:1030–1032, 1989
204. Singh G, Katyal SL, Bedrossian CWM, et al: Pulmonary alveolar proteinosis. Staining for surfactant apoprotein in alveolar proteinosis and in conditions simulating it. Chest 83: 82–86, 1983
205. Ramirez RJ, Kieffer RF Jr, Ball WC Jr: Bronchoalveolar lavage in man. *Ann Intern Med* 63:819–828, 1965
206. Carrington CB, Cugell DW, Gaensler EA, et al: Lymphangioleiomyomatosis: Physiologic-pathologic-radiologic correlation. *Am Rev Respir Dis* 116:977–995, 1977
207. Eliasson AH, Phillips YY, Tenholder MF: Treatment of lymphangioleiomyomatosis: A meta-analysis. *Chest* 196:1352–1355, 1989
208. Berger U, Khaghani A, Pomerance A, et al: Pulmonary lymphangioleiomyomatosis and steroid receptor. *Am J Clin Pathol* 93:937–940, 1990
209. Shen A, Iseman MD, Waldron JA, et al: Exacerbation of pulmonary lymphangioleiomyomatosis by exogenous estrogens. *Chest* 91:782–785, 1987
210. Sherrier RH, Chiles C, Roggler V: Pulmonary lymphangioleiomyomatosis: CT findings. *Am J Roentgenol* 153:937–940, 1989

12

Restrictive Lung Diseases of Extrapulmonary Origin

Barry Lesser, John Haapaniemi, and Ernest L. Yoder

Primary care physicians are seeing more patients with restriction of the lungs and chest wall as the population ages. The term *restrictive lung disease* is confusing because it covers many different disorders. Most clinicians are quite comfortable dealing with obstructive lung disease as there is a defined therapeutic end point with bronchodilators that can be determined clinically and via spirometry. In contrast, the restrictive lung diseases are a varied group of disorders (Table 12-1) characterized by a reduction in lung volumes. A knowledge of the distinct pathophysiology is required in order to direct therapy. These disorders may be either extrapulmonary or pulmonary in origin. Parenchymal lung disorders that result in restrictive diseases are discussed in Chapter 11. Extrapulmonary disorders are addressed here and include disorders of the chest wall and neuromuscular apparatus.

Pulmonary Function Seen In Restrictive Lung Disease

The hallmark of restrictive lung disease is a reduction in the vital capacity. However, a reduced vital capacity may also be seen in obstructive ventilatory disorders, and therefore it is necessary to rule out the presence of underlying airway obstruction. Generally, all lung volumes are reduced, but the total lung capacity is affected in particular. Measurements of static lung volumes are necessary to document restrictive lung disease. Although flow rates are reduced, they are reduced proportionately to the volume. Therefore, the normal forced expiratory volume in 1 second (FEV_1) to forced vital capacity (FVC) ratio is preserved [1]. The maximal voluntary ventilation is usually normal except in the presence of neuromuscular disorders. Oxygenation is usually preserved while at rest; however, in parenchymal lung disorders desaturation occurs with exercise.

Diseases of the Chest Wall

All components of the chest wall including the sternum, ribs, and vertebrae may be involved in the development of restrictive lung disease either by themselves or in combination. In this section we discuss the unique problems associated with disorders of each of these structures.

Disorders of the Sternum

Exclusive of mild reductions in vital capacity, abnormalities of the sternum are usually not associated with any significant clinical or pulmonary function abnormality. Pectus excavatum is usually asymptomatic. Some patients may complain of chest wall pain and limitation of exercise tolerance, which is attributed to an increase in oxygen uptake and a higher workload [2, 3]. Pulmonary function studies are usually normal, but a slight restrictive defect may be detected as indicated by the reduction in vital capacity.

Pectus excavatum is frequently associated with connective tissue disorders including Marfan's syndrome and is identified by an abnormal depression of the sternum (Fig. 12-1). Pectus carinatum may be associated with congenital heart disease and is identified by an abnormally protuberant sternum. Most patients require no specific therapy except for correction of any cosmetic deformities.

Table 12-1. Common Extrapulmonary Causes of Restrictive Lung Disease

Diseases of the Chest Wall	Neuromuscular Diseases
Disorders of the sternum	Disorders of the spinal cord
Pectus excavatum	Trauma
Pectus carinatum	Space occupying lesion
Abnormalities of the ribs	Amyotrophic lateral sclerosis
Simple rib fracture	Post polio syndrome
Flail chest	Poliomyelitis
Thoracoplasty	Disorders of the nerve roots
Disorders of the vertebral column	Gullain-Barré syndrome
Kyphoscoliosis	Trauma
Ankylosing spondylitis	Peripheral neuropathies
Extrathoracic disorders	Disorders of the neuromuscular junction
Obesity	Myasthenia gravis
Ascites	Eaton-Lambert syndrome
Pregnancy	Botulism
	Antibiotics
Diseases of the Diaphragm	Organophosphate poisoning
	Disorders of the muscle unit
	Muscular dystrophies
	Myopathies

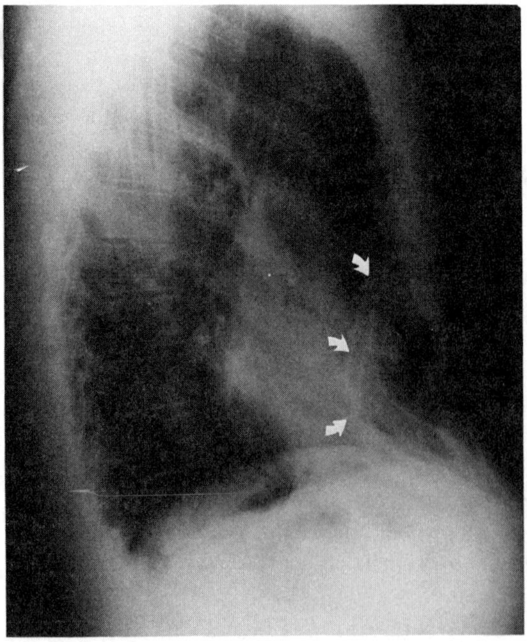

Fig. 12-1. Lateral chest roentgenogram showing pectus excavatum deformity (*arrow*).

Abnormalities of the Ribs

Instability of the chest wall may be seen with either simple fractures or those resulting in flail chest (see Chapter 19). In those patients with simple rib fractures splinting and volume reduction occurs as a result of the associated pain. In response to the reduction in tidal volume there is a compensatory increase in the respiratory rate to maintain minute ventilation. Secondarily, the cough reflex is voluntarily subdued, which may lead to impaired clearance of secretions and subsequent infection. These changes are more commonly observed in the elderly population but may occur in younger individuals depending on the degree of injury. Progression to acute respiratory failure has been seen as ventilation-perfusion mismatching worsens. Chest binders previously used in conjunction with analgesics further compounded the problem of cough and reduction in respiratory effort. It has since been shown that analgesics alone are effective in reducing pain and muscle splinting [4]. In those patients with more severe fractures intercostal nerve block may be beneficial.

Flail chest may occur secondary to multiple trauma or surgery including rib resection and thoracoplasty. Clinically there is paradoxical motion of the affected chest wall, and as pleural pressure changes during the respiratory cycle the unsupported chest wall moves opposite to the supported chest wall. Therefore, during inspiration the flail portion of the chest wall is sucked into the thorax, with associated mediastinal shift away from the affected side of the chest [5].

Despite the instability of the chest wall most of the respiratory problems are secondary to splinting and chest pain as seen in simple rib fractures. Again, retained secretions, atelectasis, and inflammatory changes with possible pneumonia are seen and may lead to respiratory insufficiency. Underlying pulmonary contusion is perhaps the most serious consequence of flail chest and prior to the 1970s was frequently overlooked [4]. Internal pneumatic stabilization with a volume cycled ventilator was considered the treatment of choice, but has since been found to be unnecessary if no other injury or complications warrant mechanical ventilation [4, 6]. Recent advances in patients with flail chest are due to recognition of the underlying pulmonary injury and attention given to providing good pulmonary toilet. The goal of therapy is prevention of atelectasis, ensuring adequate oxygenation, fluid restriction, and proper analgesia. Intercostal and epidural nerve blocks may be beneficial in extreme cases. In critically ill patients with respiratory failure, mechanical ventilation may be required until stabilization is achieved.

Kyphoscoliosis

Kyphoscoliosis is characterized by excessive angulation of the spinal column producing fixed abnormalities in the chest wall. Lateral angulation or curvature of the spine is known as scoliosis while the posterior curvature is known as kyphosis. Lateral or posterior angulation may occur separately or in combination. Kyphoscoliosis may be associated with a more severe respiratory impairment. The abnormality may be caused by defects in the vertebral bodies themselves, the connective tissue that encompasses the vertebrae, or the neuromuscular apparatus supporting the spinal column. The majority of cases of kyphoscoliosis are idiopathic while hereditary factors may play a minor role. A further list of disorders causing kyphoscoliosis are listed in Table 12-2.

As these patients age, the degree of spinal deformity worsens and symptoms of dyspnea and exercise intolerance tend to occur. Eventually these patients develop repeated respiratory infections and, depending on the degree of their deformity, may progress to ventilatory failure. Physical examination is remarkable for the gross deformity of the chest cage (Fig. 12-2a & b). The chest roentgenogram is difficult to interpret, owing to the severe chest wall abnormality (Fig. 12c). The presence of infiltrates, mass lesions, or pleural effusions may go undetected. Pulmonary arterial hypertension and cor pulmonale are late consequences of these earlier events.

Significant lung impairment resulting in ventilatory failure is directly attributed to the degree of kyphosis or scoliosis. The most commonly used method to measure the angulation of the spine has been described by Cobb [7]. Bergofsky et al [8] have suggested that patients with scoliosis greater than 100

Table 12-2. Kyphoscoliosis

Vertebral Disease
Osteoporosis
Osteomalacia
Neurofibromatosis
Connective Tissue Disorder
Marfan's syndrome
Ehlers-Danlos syndrome
Neuromuscular Disease
Muscular dystrophy
Poliomyelitis
Cerebral palsy
Thoracic Cage Abnormalities
Thoracoplasty
Idiopathic

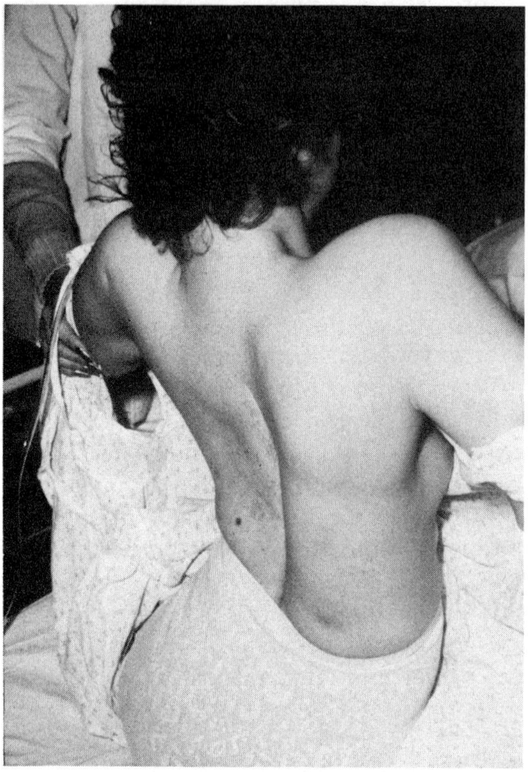

Fig. 12-2A. Back of patient with severe scoliosis secondary to poliomyelitis in her youth. Note significant rightward spinal curvature.

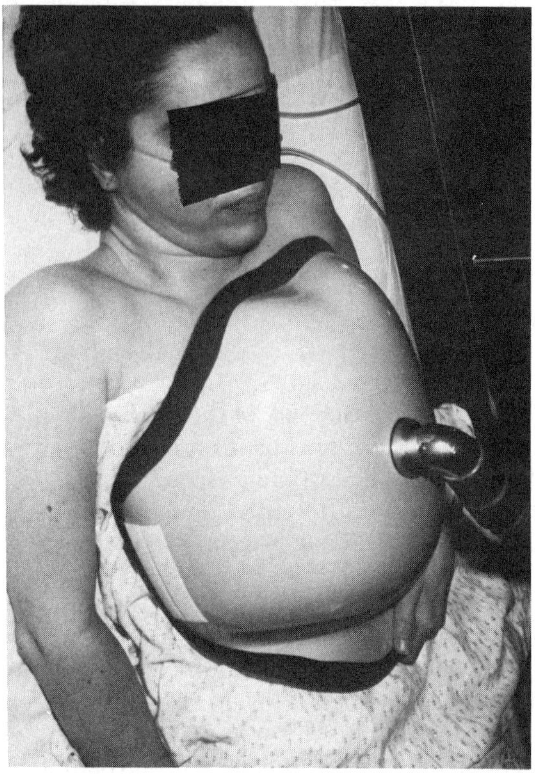

Fig. 12-2B. Same patient in cuirass type supplemental ventilator.

degrees are more likely to develop respiratory failure. They have also demonstrated an additive affect of scoliosis and kyphosis in producing ventilatory failure.

Pulmonary function typically shows a restrictive defect with reduction of FVC and FEV_1 and preservation of the normal FEV_1/FVC ratio. Lung volumes are uniformly reduced in relation to the severity of the thoracic cage abnormality [9]. Inspiratory muscle function is also reduced and probably contributes to the development of respiratory failure in some patients [10]. Ventilation-perfusion mismatching occurs as a result of hypoventilation and leads to hypoxemia with eventual hypercapnea. Hypoxemia is further influenced by a reduction in diffusing capacity [9].

The treatment for patients with kyphoscoliosis depends on the age, the patient, and the degree of deformity. Young patients with a

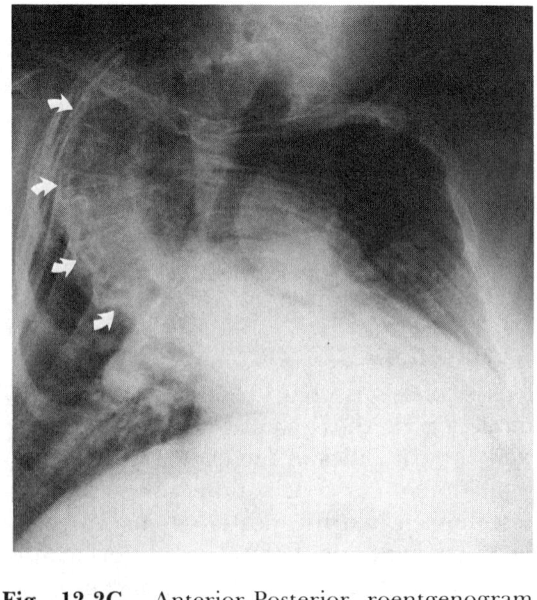

Fig. 12-2C. Anterior-Posterior roentgenogram of another patient showing severe kyphoscoliosis. Arrows outline angulation of vertebral bodies.

thoracic scoliosis of less than 100 degrees probably do not require any specific therapy for pulmonary symptoms. Surgical treatment involving placement of a metal rod results in spinal fixation and prevents progressing further spinal deformity. However, operative intervention is somewhat controversial as a method for improving pulmonary function. Swank et al [11], in a study of 222 patients over the age of 20, has shown that there was no improvement in vital capacity, FEV_1, or resting arterial PO_2. They further showed that there was approximately a 50% complication rate. This is in contrast to surgical correction in children and adolescents where early intervention may yield some benefit. Shannon et al [12] have shown improvement in gas exchange following surgery although lung perfusion remained abnormal, suggesting that permanent pulmonary vascular damage occurred before surgical correction.

Because surgical therapy in the adult is controversial, management is largely preventative. Avoidance of infection is imperative and may be accomplished by ensuring adequate immunization, early use of antibiotics for upper respiratory tract infection, maintaining adequate hydration, and proper use of supplemental oxygen. Intermittent positive pressure ventilation may improve lung mechanics. Sinha and Bergofsky [13] showed that intermittent positive pressure ventilation produced a 12 mm Hg reduction in the arterial PCO_2 and a 50% reduction in the work of breathing. These improvements lasted for up to 3 hours after each treatment. Several studies have shown nocturnal ventilation to be beneficial in diminishing the symptoms of dyspnea and the findings of cor pulmonale [14–16]. There was also an improvement in arterial oxygenation as well as a reduction in arterial PCO_2.

Ankylosing Spondylitis

Ankylosing spondylitis (AS) is a seronegative spondyloarthropathy that is associated with the HLA-B27 histocompatibility antigen. It is characterized by fibrosis and ossification of the ligamentous structures of the spine and rib cage. Although the term *ankylos* means bent or crooked, few patients actually progress to developing the classic bent spine. Primary AS usually develops during the second and third decade although a juvenile variant also occurs.

The clinical criteria for diagnosing AS include chronic low back pain, morning stiffness, limitation of chest wall expansion, and radiographic evidence of sacroiliitis (Fig. 12-3). Progressive ossification of the spine may result in the development of the classically described "bamboo" spine; however, this is seen in less than 1% of patients (Fig. 12-3). Systemic manifestations of AS include aortic insufficiency, heart block, iritis or conjunctivitis, and peripheral arthritis [17].

Pulmonary manifestations of AS are uncommon and include fibrobullous disease, which primarily affects the upper lobes, pleural thickening, pleural effusions, which are typically small and fleeting, and spontaneous pneumothoraces [18]. Fibrotic pulmonary disease, which occurs in approximately 1% of patients, is the msot common pulmonary manifestation of AS. It is usually seen in men

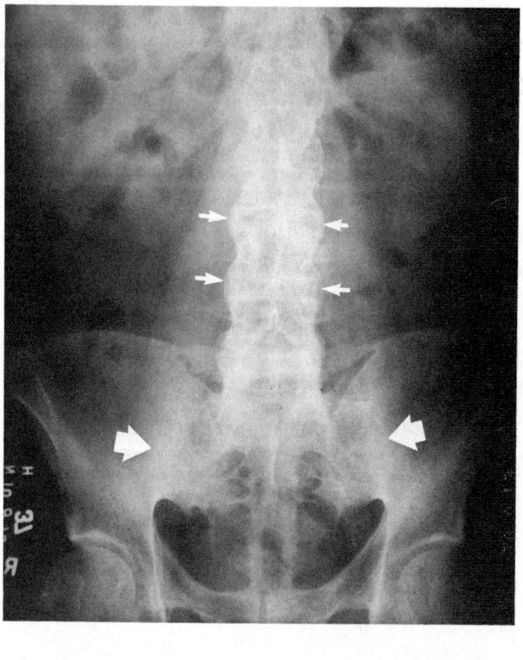

Fig. 12-3. Roentgenogram demonstrating classic bamboo spine (*small arrow*) and sacroiliitis (*large arrow*) of AS.

who have had the disease for more than 15 years and presents as a nonspecific chronic inflammation of the upper lobes, with resultant fibrosis. Because it radiographically mimics tuberculosis patients need to be worked up appropriately. As the disease progresses, cavitation may occur with secondary colonization by *Aspergillus* or other atypical organisms. Because of the extensive nature of the bullous changes, spontaneous pneumothoraces have been reported.

Pulmonary function studies usually show only a mild restrictive defect in spite of the severely restricted motion of the rib cage [18–20]. This is due in part to the fact that the diaphragm is usually uninvolved and can descend normally. Ventilatory failure is quite uncommon unless there is associated underlying lung disease or impairment of the diaphragmatic function. Static lung volumes usually reveal a reduction in vital capacity and total lung capacity; however, both the functional residual capacity and the residual volume tend to be increased because the chest cage tends to be frozen in the inspiratory position. Respiratory muscle weakness has also been demonstrated with reduction seen in maximal inspiratory and expiratory pressures [21].

The treatment of AS includes nonsteroidal anti-inflammatory medication, and an exercise program including extension exercises aimed at maintaining erect posture and normal height. Surgical therapy is occasionally advised for correction of the spinal deformities. Patients who develop massive hemoptysis as a result of their cavitary lung disease may require lung resection. However, primary surgery for the fibrobullous disease is contraindicated because of a high complication rate due to the development of bronchopleural fistula and empyema [18]. Despite these complications of AS disease, most individuals enjoy a normal lifestyle and social existence.

Thoracoplasty

Although not commonly performed today, there are many survivors of the pre-antituberculous chemotherapy era who underwent collapse therapy with thoracoplasty. The resultant chest wall abnormality may be quite extensive. Although a pure restrictive defect would be expected, most patients have a mixed obstructive and restrictive pattern seen on pulmonary function studies [22]. The obstructive component may be related to previous tuberculosis and underlying bronchiectasis, emphysema, and cigarette smoking, although the latter was not confirmed by Phillips et al [23]. There appears to be no significant correlation between the extent of the thoracoplasty and the observed pulmonary function [22]. The effect of an extensive thoracoplasty on pulmonary function is similar to that observed with pneumonectomy. The collapsed lung contributes very little to overall pulmonary function [24]. Exercise tolerance has been found to be limited as a result of reduced ventilatory capacity as measured by a reduction in lung volumes and respiratory frequency [25]. Pulmonary fibrosis from tuberculosis and lung compression from the surgery is most likely responsible for the restrictive defect. Cigarette smoking probably plays a role in the degree of obstruction seen in association with prior tuberculosis [23].

Long-term preservation of acceptable lung function is usually seen. However, patients need to be monitored for early recognition of respiratory failure. If ventilatory failure develops, mechanical ventilation may be required. Although positive pressure ventilators are usually required for acute stabilization, patients can often be maintained for long periods with negative pressure ventilators or mask continuous positive airway pressure devices [26, 27].

Diseases of the Diaphragm

Unilateral or bilateral paralysis of the diaphragm can lead to symptoms of dyspnea, especially when occurring in combination with other neuromuscular diseases. Unilateral paralysis usually occurs as a result of trauma, but manipulation of the phrenic nerve or lesions that may impair phrenic nerve conduction may result in paralysis. This is commonly seen following cardiac surgery and is attributed to hypothermia and stretching. Bilateral paralysis usually results from similar causes as those seen for unilateral paralysis, but the symptoms of dyspnea are more severe and may lead to serious morbidity [28].

The diagnosis of unilateral paralysis is often made incidentally when evaluating the chest roentgenogram. Paralysis can be confirmed by performing a sniff test under fluoroscopy, which would detect paradoxical diaphragmatic motion [29]. Bilateral diaphragmatic paralysis is perhaps easier to diagnose as the symptoms of dyspnea are more severe and exaggerated in the supine position. The physical examination reveals paradoxical motion of the abdomen and chest wall during inspiration. Fluoroscopy again confirms abnormal diaphragmatic excursions.

Pulmonary function studies show varying degrees of restriction depending on the severity of paralysis and whether it is unilateral or bilateral [30, 31]. Respiratory muscle function has been shown to be worse in patients with associated lung disease [32].

Therapy depends on the degree of paralysis and whether there is unilateral or bilateral involvement. In unilateral paralysis observation is usually all that is required, whereas in bilateral paralysis mechanical support of ventilation is usually required until the patient is stabilized. Negative pressure ventilators or rocking beds may be useful, allowing patients freedom from positive pressure ventilators. If the phrenic nerves are intact, phrenic nerve pacing may be beneficial. However, in most patients with bilateral diaphragmatic paralysis the phrenic nerves are nonfunctional.

Neuromuscular Disease

Neuromuscular diseases are responsible for a significant number of patients who develop restrictive lung disease. Prompt diagnosis is imperative before the onset of respiratory muscle fatigue in order to prevent or delay the associated complications, which include atelectasis, pneumonia, and respiratory failure [33, 34, 34a]. Unfortunately a number of patients present in acute respiratory failure, and neuromuscular disease may only be recognized on failing to wean from the ventilator.

The diagnosis is dependent on evaluation of the neuromuscular apparatus. Physical examination will detect affected muscle groups, presence of fasciculations, and presence of upper or lower motoneuron disease. Most patients have evidence of limb muscle weakness but in certain circumstances the respiratory unit may be most affected. Respiratory muscle weakness should be suspected if dyspnea is present. If dyspnea is exaggerated in the supine position, diaphragmatic weakness should also be suspected. If the muscles of the pharynx or larynx are involved, the patient may develop hoarseness, difficulty swallowing, and obstructive sleep apnea from muscle relaxation in the hypopharynx. Biochemical analysis including muscle enzymes and dystrophin will identify dystrophies and myopathies. Electromyelography (EMG) and nerve conduction studies distinguish between neuropathies, dystrophies, and myopathic processes while muscle biopsies further distinguish myopathies from dystrophies. Pharmacologic testing with edrophonium chloride (Tensilon) evaluates the neuromuscular junction. Evaluation of the respiratory apparatus is nonspecific for diagnostic purposes, but it is imperative for early interventional therapy to avoid acute ventilatory failure.

In patients with obvious neuromuscular disease, assessment of the respiratory apparatus is essential. Early in their course, patients may be asymptomatic, but pulmonary function studies may detect subtle abnormalities. Reductions in vital capacity and maximal voluntary ventilation are usually the earliest abnormalities seen. Respiratory muscle weakness alone does not account for the reduction in vital capacity. The majority of this decrement occurs as a result of reduced compliance secondary to microatelectasis and impaired chest expansion [35, 36]. Arterial blood gases usually are not helpful early in the patient's course, but if hypercapnea is detected, prompt action is required. Plum [37] and Walley [38] have demonstrated that when the vital capacity is reduced to 1 L or approximately 25% to 30% of the predicted normal for the patient, mechanical ventilatory support is usually required. Vital capacity can be easily determined at the bedside with a Wright spirometer. Measuring the vital capacity in the upright as well as the supine position is also quite helpful. If the vital capacity decreases significantly in the supine position, severe diaphragmatic weakness or paralysis is likely. Measurement of maximum static inspiratory pressures is easily performed at the bedside and is an excellent method of determining weakness or fatigue (Fig. 12-4). A normal inspiratory pressure ranges from −65 to −124 cm of water depending on age and sex [39, 40]. It must be pointed out, however, that this measurement is effort dependent and a low result may not necessarily indicate respiratory muscle weakness. However, it is safe to assume that if the inspiratory force exceeds −80 cm of water, the likelihood of clinical muscle weakness is remote.

Fig. 12-4. Inspiratory force meter adapted for use in an ambulatory patient.

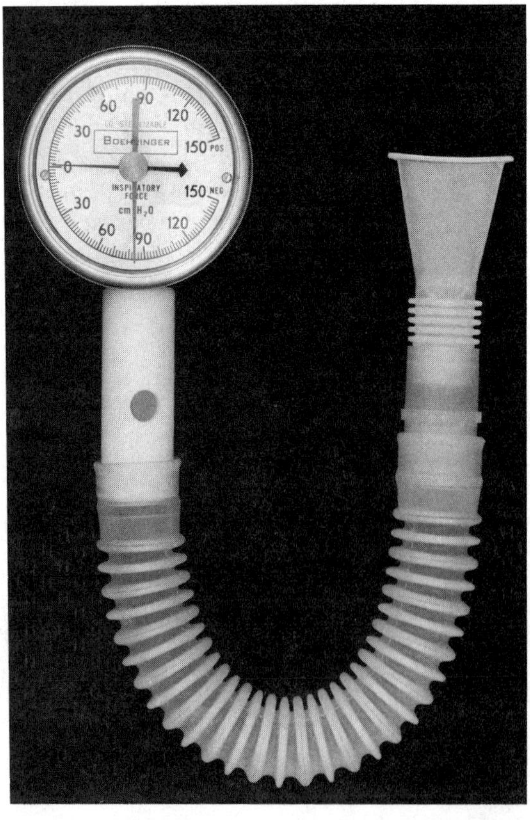

Other studies that may be necessary include assessment of phrenic nerve function and EMGs to specifically look at diaphragmatic function and transdiaphragmatic pressure measurements. Shochina et al [41] demonstrated phrenic nerve involvement in 14 of 26 patients with neuromuscular disease. Pulmonary function studies and fluoroscopy were normal in five of these patients despite symptoms of dyspnea, suggesting that phrenic nerve assessment should be performed in all patients with neuromuscular disease. In the usual patient with neuromuscular disease, the diagnosis is quite evident and assessment of respiratory muscle involvement can be easily accomplished with simple spirometry and inspiratory pressure measurements. Further assessment as mentioned may be helpful in planning an appropriate treatment program.

Because of the extreme impact on the patient's lifestyle, a timely diagnosis is important. A high index of suspicion in the proper clinical setting should suggest the presence of neuromuscular disease. Early diagnosis will help delay and prevent the eventual complications, including pneumonia, aspiration, and respiratory arrest. In the next section we discuss several distinct diseases that have the development of respiratory muscle weakness in common.

Spinal Cord Disorders

Spinal Cord Injuries

Spinal cord injuries usually result from accidents occurring in the workplace, associated with motor vehicles, or during various forms of recreation [42]. These injuries are frequently quite devastating, resulting in significant changes in lifestyle. It has been estimated that spinal cord injuries occur at a rate of 28 to 50 injuries per million persons per year [43]. Most deaths in these patients are directly attributable to pulmonary complications, usually pneumonia. Functional impairment, treatment modalities, and complications can differ, depending on location of the spinal cord injury.

Cervical cord injuries may be classified into high cervical injuries and mid or low cervical injuries. The eventual deficit seen in patients is based on direct mechanical injury and ischemia, which may lead to cord necrosis. Because of the traumatic nature of the injury and resultant ischemia irregular lesions of the cord may occur, leading to incomplete spinal lesions [42]. However, depending on the level of injury certain functional, prognostic, and therapeutic statements can be made.

High cervical spinal cord injuries (C1, C2) may affect both voluntary and involuntary respiratory function. Traumatic injury usually affects the cortical spinal pathways, resulting in near total respiratory muscle paralysis. However, the phrenic nerve apparatus is spared and phrenic nerve pacing may be effective.

Clinically these patients are dyspneic and cannot handle secretions due to an ineffective cough mechanism. Inspiratory efforts are characterized by contraction of the sternocleidomastoid and trapezius muscles with resultant muscle hypertrophy. In addition, other neck muscles may also be recruited, with the net effect of pulling the sternum cephalad, expanding the upper rib cage, and paradoxical inward displacement of the lateral walls of the rib cage [44].

There is a paucity of literature regarding pulmonary function in high cervical cord injuries. The total lung capacity is severely reduced and the tidal volume is variable. It has been shown that glossopharyngeal breathing, a technique of forcing small boluses of air into the trachea, may increase expiratory flow rate, thus improving speech and cough [45].

Patients with injuries to the mid or lower cervical cord make up the majority of patients with quadriplegia. Midcervical lesions affecting C3, C4, and C5 involve the phrenic nerves. These patients have secondary diaphragmatic paralysis that is unresponsive to phrenic nerve pacing. Lower cervical cord injuries involving C7 and C8 as well as the upper thoracic cord involving T1 through T6, have no significant effect on respiration. However, these patients do have involvement of the intercostal and abdominal musculature, which may lead to impairment in the patient's ability to cough.

Pulmonary function studies show a typical restrictive pattern [46, 47]. Vital capacity normally changes with position, decreasing going from the upright to the supine position. However, in quadriplegic patients the vital capacity actually increases in the supine position, probably due to the effect of gravity on the abdominal contents, causing a reduction in residual volume [48]. This has clinical implications as demonstrated by Goldman et al [49]. By preventing the gravitational forces on the abdomen through use of a binder, vital capacity may be improved in the sitting position. The compliance of the lungs has been shown to be reduced, but when compared with lung volumes, compliance is normal [50].

Patients with mid or low cervical cord injuries tend to have partial spontaneous recovery of pulmonary function during the first 12 months after injury. This improvement is related to the development of muscle spasticity once the initial phase of spinal shock and muscle flaccidity resolve [40]. Vital capacity may nearly double after 3 to 6 months, [51–53]. Forced inspiratory and expiratory flow rates showed a similar improvement. Further improvement in muscle function can be accomplished by various training regimens using inspiratory and expiratory resistances [46].

Therapy of patients with cervical spinal cord injuries varies depending on the level of involvement. High cord injuries initially require mechanical ventilation. However, since the phrenic nerves are spared, phrenic and diaphragmatic electrophrenic stimulation has been quite effective, allowing patients to be maintained off mechanical ventilation. Glossopharyngeal breathing may be helpful in the short-term. Electrophrenic pacing requires a period of muscle training directed at the diaphragm as significant atrophy may have occurred. Overstimulation may cause severe myopathic damage once the diaphragm is trained. One hemidiaphragm may be paced for up to 6 to 12 hours, which allows patients significant freedom from mechanical support.

For those patients who require long-term mechanical ventilation and do not have an intact phrenic nerve–diaphragmatic axis, special considerations apply, based on the level of cord injury. Those patients with lower cervical cord injuries often can be weaned from mechanical ventilation due to the spontaneous recovery of muscle function in association with respiratory muscle training [54]. However, some patients are unable to be successfully weaned and require either partial mechanical support, nocturnal ventilation, or around the clock continuous mechanical support. Special attention needs to be given to preventing pulmonary complications, specifically infections. A rigid program addressing pulmonary toilet must be stressed.

Amyotrophic Lateral Sclerosis

Amyotrophic lateral sclerosis (ALS) is a disease of uncertain etiology affecting the anterior horn cells of the motoneurons. Typically this is most marked in the cervical, lumbosacral, and lower thoracic spinal segments. Weakness with associated segmental atrophy is the usual, initial manifestation. Twenty-five percent of patients present with bulbar palsy and tend to develop respiratory complications early in their course, usually as a result of repeated aspiration. In those patients who present with spinal muscle atrophy, there is a delay in the onset of respiratory complications. Symptoms usually occur once bulbar paralysis is manifested or paralysis of the intercostal muscles develops. Rarely, dyspnea is a presenting feature. There have been case reports documenting neuromuscular disease, specifically ALS, as being the sole cause of acute respiratory failure without a previous neurologic diagnosis [55]. Most patients with ALS suffer progressive deterioration in neurologic function, with a life expectancy of approximately 3.6 years after the diagnosis is made [56, 57].

Pulmonary function studies consistently demonstrate a reduction in maximum voluntary ventilation (MVV). The initial forced vital capacity is low, with a mean of 80% of predicted [57]. Reductions in the MVV and FVC were most reliable in the cases of early pulmonary involvement in neuromuscular disease, specifically ALS [57]. Clinically, reductions in FVC and MVV by as much as 50% may be missed, emphasizing the importance of early evaluation with spirometry. The most reliable measurements to determine respiratory muscle weakness are maximal inspiratory (PI_{max}) and maximum expiratory pressures (PE_{max}) [58].

The residual volume may also be elevated in a significant number of patients with ALS and other neuromuscular diseases. There may also be associated discoordination of expiratory muscles, frequently the earliest indicator of neurologic involvement of the respiratory unit. Abnormalities of flow seen during expiration are most commonly seen in patients with bulbar signs, especially dysphagia. When looking at the flow/volume loop, the patients with discoordination on expiration may have a discontinuation of flow, suggesting abnormalities in the pharyngeal muscles with premature closure of the glottis or vocal cords (Fig. 12-5).

The treatment of ALS is beyond the scope of this chapter; however, when it pertains to

Fig. 12-5. Diagrammatic representation of flow/volume loop showing erratic expiratory efforts in patient with bulbar ALS.

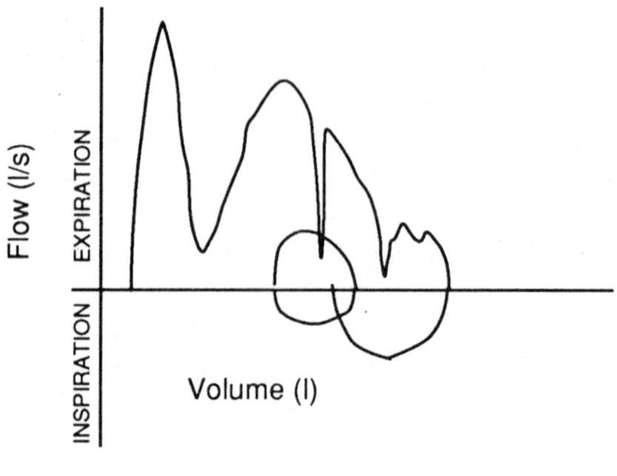
Flow (l/s)
EXPIRATION
INSPIRATION
Volume (l)

ventilation several tenets apply. It must be recognized that the course is progressive and eventually fatal as a result of ventilatory failure. Unless one intervenes with mechanical ventilatory support, the patients succumb to the disease. With this in mind, serial pulmonary function studies may be helpful to document deterioration in respiratory function and also serve as a guide for patient counseling. It is prudent to discuss the overall prognosis with the patient once a diagnosis is made, thus allowing time for the patient and his or her family to consider all the options.

Postpolio Syndrome

Poliomyelitis has become an uncommon disorder since the introduction of vaccinations in 1961. Postpolio syndrome is a recently described syndrome occurring in approximately 22% of these patients, causing neuromuscular weakness. Onset is typically 30 to 40 years after recovering from their acute episode of paralytic poliomyelitis [59]. The syndrome is heralded by the progression of muscle weakness in previously involved muscles, muscle atrophy, and the development of muscle fasciculations in previously weakened muscles. Symptoms seen in approximately 60% to 70% of patients include fatigue, weakness, and pain [60, 61]. The pain usually affects muscles as well as joints. Dyspnea with progressive respiratory insufficiency may occur and appears to be due to denervation of previously reinnervated muscles [59, 61]. Sleep disordered breathing suggestive of sleep apnea has also been noted [59, 62]. Patients who are suspected of having postpolio syndrome must be thoroughly evaluated to rule out other sources of weakness such as ALS. The diagnosis is made based on the clinical picture, historical information, and a characteristic EMG showing collateral reinnervation and an enlarged motor unit.

Pulmonary function studies demonstrate a reduction in vital capacity that is greater than what would have been expected from the muscle weakness alone [36]. This reduction is attributed in large part to reduced lung and chest wall compliance [36, 63]. The loss of lung compliance can be directly related to widespread microatelectasis as seen in other neuromuscular diseases [36].

Once confirmed, treatable conditions need to be sought such as obesity, compartment syndromes from using braces and other orthopedic devices, and muscle pain from fibrocytis or myocytis. Nonsteroidal anti-inflammatory agents are useful for muscle and joint pains. Replacing and updating orthotic devices on a periodic basis to relieve symptoms from peripheral nerve compression is advised. Pyridostigmine, an anticholinesterase agent, has been used in low doses to reduce fatigue and may be beneficial in as many as 50% of patients, although it does not appear to be effective in improving the weakness. Exercise in this group of patients is very controversial. It has been suggested that if the EMG is compatible with disuse atrophy, strength and exercise is usually helpful. However, if weakness is due to postpolio syndrome, any exercise program that is used should be nonfatiguing. The use of appropriate orthotic devices and/or wheelchairs in association with exercise is preferred. The goal of physical therapy should be to prevent disuse atrophy and muscle fatigue [64, 65]. Once respiratory failure is observed, mechanical ventilatory support may be required either on an intermittent or continuous basis to maintain stable respiratory mechanics. This can be accomplished as in other neuromuscular diseases with various types of mechanical support [66–68]. However, it must be realized that this is a progressive disease despite these interventions, and patients need to be counseled appropriately.

Sleep apnea has been observed in patients with postpolio syndrome and is distinctly less common in other neuromuscular diseases. The typical onset of sleep apnea occurs several years after recovery from the acute episode of poliomyelitis. Although central apnea would be expected, most oxygen desaturation occurs during obstructive and mixed apneas. However, the most severe episodes of hypoxia were caused by central hypopneas, defined by Hill et al [62], as a reduction in esophageal pressure swings. It has been suggested that brain stem damage occurring during the acute illness in conjunction with the mechanical abnormalities affecting the chest wall and respiratory muscles is responsible for the late development of sleep apnea. Cor pulmonale and respiratory failure may be reversed with oxygen therapy [62]. Snoring and daytime sleepiness are typical symptoms in patients with obstructive sleep apnea and suggest the need for polysomnography.

Guillain-Barré Syndrome

Guillain-Barré syndrome is an acute demyelinating neuropathy causing areflexic paralysis, usually progressive in an ascending fashion [69]. The most common clinical feature is weakness, commonly beginning in the lower extremities, with rapid ascent to the upper extremities, trunk, and occasionally the cranial muscles. Involvement of the respiratory muscles is the most serious sequela and may lead to respiratory failure and death if not recognized early. Involvement of the respiratory musculature occurs in approximately one third of patients [70].

The etiology of Guillain-Barré syndrome is uncertain but there is usually a preceding upper respiratory or gastrointestinal viral illness suggesting an autoimmune response. Cytomegalovirus and Epstein-Barr virus have been most commonly implicated. The diagnosis is made by clinical and laboratory features. Examination of the cerebrospinal fluid typically reveals an increased protein level with no inflammatory cells. EMG usually demonstrates a primary peripheral nerve system demyelination.

The prognosis is usually good, with most patients making a full recovery. Patients usually require supportive therapy, but close monitoring of both respiratory and cardiovascular systems is imperative. Serial measurements of vital capacity and inspiratory pressures are easily performed and detect early respiratory involvement. Continuous monitoring of the electrocardiogram will detect arrythmias that result from autonomic neuropathy. Plasmapheresis has been shown to accelerate recovery and is recommended early in acute disease. Steroids have not been shown to be beneficial. Those patients who progress to respiratory failure and require mechanical ventilation usually have prolonged courses and are difficult to wean from the ventilator until respiratory muscle weakness resolves [71]. With proper supportive treatment, most patients recover with minimal complications.

Myasthenia Gravis

Myasthenia gravis is an autoimmune disorder that affects the acetylcholine receptor of the motor end plate. It commonly affects both limb and respiratory muscles; however, it may be limited to ocular and bulbar muscles. The hallmark of this disease is muscle weakness and fatigability that is elicited by repetitive muscular contractions. As in the other neuromuscular diseases, the most serious complication is respiratory failure [72].

The most common initial symptoms are diplopia and ptosis secondary to ocular muscle weakness. Bulbar findings are common, manifested by dysphagia and dysarthria. Limb and respiratory muscle weakness may also occur in an asymmetric distribution. Although respiratory muscle weakness is uncommon, when present, it may herald ventilatory failure. Abnormalities of the thymus are common in myasthenia. Thymomas are seen in approximately 10% of patients. Thymic hyperplasia is seen more commonly, especially in younger patients.

The actual defect in myasthenia results from the presence of circulating antibodies directed at the acetylcholine receptor. There also appear to be morphologic changes at the neuromuscular junction, with loss of functional acetylcholine receptor sites. These abnormalities result in impairment of the postjunctional membrane, making it less sensitive to the application of cholinergic drugs. The diagnosis is confirmed by appropriate clinical features demonstrating muscle fatigability on repetitive tasks, a positive Tensilon test demonstrating recovery of muscle weakness, a characteristic EMG showing a decreased amplitude with repetitive stimulation, and detection of acetylcholine receptor antibodies [72, 73].

Aminoglycosides, which decrease acetylcholine release at the presynaptic junction, may impair neuromuscular transmission, resulting in progressive respiratory muscle weakness and subsequent respiratory failure. Symptoms of myasthenia may also be elicited by environmental, emotional, and physical factors including sunlight, stress, and illness [72].

Pulmonary function is similar to that seen in other neuromuscular diseases, with reduction in both vital capacity and total lung capacity and an increase in residual volume as the muscle weakness progresses. In myasthenic patients, there is a significant improvement in vital capacity, peak expiratory flow, and maximal inspiratory flow after administration of pyridostigmine [74]. Thymectomy in those patients with more severe disease resulted in a significant improvement in vital capacity [73].

Treatment reverses most if not all evidence of weakness by restoring function of the postjunctional membrane. This is accomplished by treatment with anticholinesterase agents such as neostigmine or pyridostigmine, which increase the viable acetylcholine concentration. Immunosuppressive therapy with azathioprine and corticosteroids are effective in patients with severe myasthenia [75]. Plasmapheresis may be helpful in removing the IgG autoantibody, but long-term benefits of plasmapheresis have yet to be determined. This form of treatment is useful in the early stage of therapy. Thymectomy is recommended for all young patients with generalized myasthenia and those patients with thymoma. Significant improvement is seen in approximately 85% of patients who undergo thymectomy [72, 73].

Eaton-Lambert Syndrome

The Eaton-Lambert syndrome is a paraneoplastic disorder usually associated with oat cell carcinoma of the lung. Pathologically there is impaired release of the acetylcholine at the nerve terminals. Most patients are diagnosed when prolonged apnea is seen after being given curare for elective surgery. The diagnosis is confirmed by a typical response to repetitive stimulation, which causes the amplitude potential to increase rather than decrease as it does in myasthenia gravis. Treatment requires the administration of guanidine, which promotes the release of the acetylcholine. Steroid therapy and plasmapheresis may be beneficial, but an exhaustive search for an underlying tumor needs to be undertaken. Proper treatment of the primary malignancy is usually curative of Eaton-Lambert syndrome [76].

Muscular Dystrophy

The muscular dystrophies are inherited progressive degenerative myopathies causing profound muscle weakness. In their late stages, death is usually due to ventilatory failure. The diagnosis is confirmed by history, electroneuromyography, elevated muscle enzymes, and histologic evidence of a diffuse myopathy. Recently, a protein product coined dystrophin has been identified in normal myogenic cells, which appears to be lacking in patients with Duchenne type muscular dystrophy. Patients with Becker's muscular dystrophy have either altered size or quantity of dystrophin [77]. The presence or absence of dystrophin and any alterations can be detected by Western blot and immunochemistry.

Duchenne type muscular dystrophy begins in childhood, with the development of proximal muscle weakness. It is manifested by a waddling gait and a classic mode of rising from the ground by "climbing up themselves" (Gower's sign). The genetic defect has been identified, demonstrating a deletion of the short arm of the X chromosome [77]. As weakness progresses, involvement of the thoracic muscles leads to lordosis and a protuberant abdomen. Scoliosis is seen in the late stages, which is partially attributed to prolonged sitting. As a result of the scoliosis and the respiratory muscle weakness, patients begin to develop dyspnea and are at increased risk for infections due to poor cough and associated weakness.

The other forms of muscular dystrophy, including limb dystrophy and facioscapulohumeral, differ in their age of onset and progressive nature. Becker's and Emery-Dreifuss dystrophies both have their onset in early childhood. Becker's dystrophy may also be quite devastating, but the progression of disease appears to be more variable. Emery-Dreifuss tends to be a more benign form of dystrophy; however, sudden death may occur due to cardiac standstill.

As in other neuromuscular diseases, ventilatory responsiveness is affected primarily because of muscle weakness as opposed to a depressed response to hypercapnia, hypoxia, or hyperoxia. It appears that both the peripheral and central chemoreceptors and the respiratory system function normally and that the increased respiratory frequency seen in muscular dystrophy occurs as a result of a smaller tidal volume [78]. Maximum inspiratory pressures are one of the earliest parameters used to detect respiratory muscle weakness. Perhaps more importantly, the maximal expiratory pressures are lower than the inspiratory pressures, which have profound effects on the cough mechanism [58]. As the disease progresses, there is a steady decline in these pressures.

Once respiratory failure is evident, mechanical support of ventilation is necessary [78a]. As in other progressive degenerative diseases, the institution of long-term mechanical support needs to be considered on an individual basis with proper psychosocial counseling [79].

Although it is hoped that effective drug treatment is on the horizon now that the defective gene locus has been identified, and the protein product dystrophin has been characterized, no specific therapy is yet available. Because of the progressive unrelenting nature of the muscular dystrophies and lack of an appropriate therapy, the best treatment is preventative. Genetic counseling, fetal blood sampling, and chromosomal analysis should be employed in families who are at risk for developing muscular dystrophy.

Obesity

Obesity is a common medical problem affecting over 50 million Americans [80]. The Framingham study showed that an increased risk of medical problems is seen when actual body weight is greater than 120% of ideal body weight. Although not often appreciated, morbid obesity may have profound effects on respiratory function.

The metabolic demands in obese patients are increased [80]. This is confirmed by measuring an increased oxygen consumption and carbon dioxide production at rest and with exercise. Minute ventilation is higher in order to maintain a eucapnic state, thus indicating an increased work of breathing. Ventilation-perfusion abnormalities have also been observed, which tend to be exaggerated in the supine position and account for the hypoxemia that is commonly seen in these patients.

It has been well documented that chest mechanics are altered as a result of obesity. Chest wall compliance is reduced mostly due to the deposition of adipose tissue [81]. The most consistent abnormality seen on pulmonary function studies is a reduction in expiratory reserve volume [81, 82]. This reduction in expiratory reserve volume is most marked in the supine position when the combination of the increased chest wall weight and the ascent of the diaphragm into the thorax is seen. In massively obese patients vital capacity and total lung capacity is significantly reduced. In 29 patients followed by Ray et al [81], before and after weight reduction, expiratory reserve volume was significantly increased after weight reduction. Since pulmonary function is relatively well maintained except in the massively obese, significant changes in pulmonary function may suggest parenchymal lung disease and possibly other concomitant disease processes.

As ventilatory efficiency decreases and ventilation-perfusion abnormalities worsen, hypoxemia with resultant pulmonary hypertension occurs. Weight reduction, although difficult to achieve, will reverse the respiratory complications seen as a consequence of obesity.

Management

Although we have spoken about several disease processes detailing specific diagnostic and therapeutic interventions, certain generalities can be made. In patients who develop severe restrictive lung disease with resultant respiratory muscle weakness, mechanical control of ventilation will eventually be necessary. Before the initiation of mechanical devices, care must be given to prevent the respiratory complications of the disease. Pulmonary toilet with cough and deep breathing exercises may be helpful initially and may be quite effective in association with incentive spirometry or intermittent positive pressure breathing. However, it is vital during this time period that respiratory mechanics be monitored as previously mentioned. Elective initiation of mechanical ventilation is based on clinical judgment. Once the vital capacity falls below 1 L or 25% to 30% of predicted, mechanical support is usually indicated [37, 38]. During the grace period before the development of severe respiratory muscle fatigue, several alternatives exist. Intermittent positive pressure breathing devices used several times a day may prevent atelectasis and help to mobilize the secretions. Patients who develop hypercarbia and respiratory muscle weakness may benefit from nocturnal ventilation either with negative pressure ventilators (tank ventilators, Pulmowrap by Lifecare [Boulder, CO], or body curaiss or shell) or positive pressure devices administered via a mouthpiece or nasal or face mask [83–88]. Most patients with fairly stable or slowly progressive disease benefit significantly from nocturnal ventilation, with reasonable maintenance of normal gas exchange. As the patient's disease progresses, tracheostomy and conventional positive pressure ventilation will eventually be required. However, this needs to be assessed individually, and some patients may benefit from intermittent use of conventional positive pressure ventilation in combination with a body ventilator, either negative or positive pressure device. Although any patient with neuromuscular or chest wall disease could benefit from negative pressure ventilators, especially early in the course, positive pressure devices may be more comfortable. In the patients with severe scoliosis, negative pressure devices may be extremely uncomfortable and poorly tolerated [89, 90].

A thorough understanding of the long-term prognosis is critical before any decisions regarding mechanical ventilation are made [91]. Counseling patients and their families early is mandatory in order to deliver proper medical care in conjunction with the patient's wishes. The decision to be placed on mechanical ventilation should be made when the patient is clinically stable and before the development of respiratory distress. Although most patients see this as a chance to extend their life, they quickly realize that the quality of their life has indeed suffered. As was pointed out by Sivak et al [92], those patients who chose mechanical ventilation had an unrealistic expectation of their eventual prognosis. The patient must also understand the financial and psychological burden placed on family members or other health care providers. Therefore, all decisions should be made in conjunction with family members, clergy, medical personnel, and other persons close to the patient. By using this team approach, with proper education of the patient and family, unnecessary intervention and obstacles can be avoided [91].

If the patient chooses to be placed on mechanical support several issues need to be addressed. The patient must realize that once mechanical ventilatory support is initiated, he or she will be maintained on this for the rest of his or her life. Therefore, an adequate assessment of the home or other viable options such as nursing home placement, etc., need to be considered with the patient before the decision to accept ventilatory support is made. Although patients may do very well at home from both a technical and physiological standpoint, the psychological aspects of chronic home ventilation rapidly become the overriding concern [91, 93]. Although patients can adapt to home ventilation with varying degrees of mobility, most patients with progressive neuromuscular disease eventually require continuous ventilation. This predisposes them to complications such as infections. None of the patients in the Sivak study recognized the full impact of their disease. With this in mind, it is imperative that the patient be allowed to make decisions regarding discontinuing ventilatory support should the patient find that the quality of his or her life and other factors make continuation of this form of therapy inappropriate. Unfortunately, this is a societal issue that has been taken out of the home and placed in the courts for ultimate decision making. These problems can be avoided with proper counseling and education; however, until this issue of life support can be handled more appropriately, patients who choose long-term mechanical support may in fact become prisoners of their own disease.

References

1. West JB: Restrictive diseases. *In* Pulmonary Pathophysiology—The Essentials, ed 2. Baltimore, Williams & Wilkins, 1982, pp 92–111
2. Mead J, Sly P, LeSouef P, et al: Rib cage mobility in pectus excavatum. *Am Rev Respir Dis* 132:1223–1228, 1985
3. Castile RG, Staats BA, Westbrook PR: Symptomatic pectus deformities of the chest. *Am Rev Respir Dis* 126:564–588, 1982
4. Richardson JD, Adams L, Flint LM: Selective management of flail chest and pulmonary contusion. *Ann Surg* 20:481–487, 1982
5. Webb AK: Flail chest—Management and complications. *Br J Hosp Med* 20:406–411, 1978
6. Trinkle JK, Richardson JD, Franz JL, et al: Management of flail chest without mechanical ventilation. *Ann Thorac Surg* 19:355–363, 1975
7. Edmonson AS: Scoliosis. *In* Crenshaw AH (ed): Campbell's Operative Orthopaedics, ed 7, vol 4. St. Louis, CV Mosby, 1987, p 3175
8. Bergofsky F, Turino G, Fishman A: Cardiorespiratory failure in kyphoscoliosis. *Medicine* 38:263–317, 1959
9. Weber B, Smith J, Briscoe W, et al: Pulmonary function in symptomatic adolescents with idiopathic scoliosis. *Am Rev Respir Dis* 111:389–397, 1975
10. Lisboa C, Moreno R, Fava M, et al: Inspiratory muscle function in patients with severe kyphoscoliosis. *Am Rev Respir Dis* 132:48–52, 1985
11. Swank S, Lonstein J, Moe J, et al: Surgical treatment of adult scoliosis. *J Bone Joint Surg* 63:268–287, 1981
12. Shannon D, Riseborough E, Kazemi H: Ventilation perfusion relationships following correction of kyphoscoliosis. *JAMA* 217:579–584, 1971
13. Sinha R, Bergofsky E: Prolonged alteration of lung motion. *Am Rev Respir Dis* 106:47–57, 1972
14. Hoeppner V, Crockcroft D, Dosman J, et al: Nighttime ventilation improves respiratory failure in secondary kyphoscoliosis. *Am Rev Respir Dis* 129:240–243, 1984
15. Fulkerson WJ, Wilkins JK, Eskenshade AM, et al: Life threatening hypoventilation in kyphoscoliosis: Successful treatment with a molded body brace-ventilator. *Am Rev Respir Dis* 129:185–187, 1984
16. Kirby GR, Mayer LS, Pingleton SK: Nocturnal positive pressure ventilation via nasal face mask. *Am Rev Respir Dis* 135:738–740, 1987
17. Shah BC, Khan MA: Review of ankylosing spondylitis. *Comp Ther* 13:52–59, 1987
18. Rosenow E, Strimlan C, Muhm J, et al: Pleuropulmonary manifestations of ankylosing spondylitis. *Mayo Clin Proc* 52:641–649, 1977
19. Gracad G, Hamosh P: The lung in ankylosing spondylitis. *Am Rev Respir Dis* 107:286–289, 1973
20. Feltelius N, Hedenstrom H, Hillerdal G, et al: Pulmonary involvement in ankylosing spondylitis. *Ann Rheum Dis* 45:736–740, 1986
21. Vanderschueren D, DeCramer M, Vandendaele P, et al: Pulmonary function and maximal transrespiratory pressures in ankylosing spondylitis. *Ann Rheum Dis* 48:632–635, 1989
22. Bredin CP: Pulmonary function in long-term survivors of thoracoplasty. *Chest* 95:18–20, 1989
23. Phillips MS, Miller MR, Kinnear WJ: Importance of air flow obstruction after thoracoplasty. *Thorax* 42:348–352, 1987
24. Westermann CJ: Pulmonary function in long-term survivors of thoracoplasty. (Communications to the editor). *Chest* 978:512, 1990
25. Phillips MS, Kinnear WJ, Shaw D, et al: Exercise responses in patients treated for pulmonary tuberculosis by thoracoplasty. *Thorax* 44:268–274, 1989
26. Phillips MS, Kinnear WJ, Shneerson JM: Late sequelae of pulmonary tuberculosis treated by thoracoplasty. *Thorax* 42:445–451, 1987
27. Sawicka EH, Branthwaite MA, Spencer GT: Respiratory failure after thoracoplasty: Treatment by intermittent negative-pressure ventilation. *Thorax* 38:433–435, 1983
28. Riley EA: Idiopathic diaphragmatic paralysis: A report of eight cases. *Am J Med* 32:404–416, 1962
29. Mier A: Sniff transdiaphragmatic pressure in the assessment of respiratory muscle function. *Prax Klin Pneumol* 42:812–813, 1988

30. Ridyard JB, Stewart RM: Regional lung function in unilateral diaphragmatic paralysis. *Thorax* 31:438–442, 1976
31. McCredie M, Lovejoy F, Kaltreider NL: Pulmonary function in diaphragmatic paralysis. *Thorax* 17:213–217, 1962
32. Lisboa C, Pare PD, Pertuze J, et al: Inspiratory muscle function in unilateral diaphragmatic paralysis. *Am Rev Respir Dis* 134:488–492, 1986
33. Schmidt-Nowara WW, Altman AR: Atelectasis and neuromuscular respiratory failure. *Chest* 85:792–795, 1984
34. Harrison DW, Collins JV, Brown GE, et al: Respiratory failure in neuromuscular diseases. *Thorax* 26:579, 1971
34a. Kelly BJ, Luce JM: The diagnosis and management of neuromuscular diseases causing respiratory failure. *Chest* 99:1485–1494, 1991
35. Ferris BG Jr, Mead J, Whittenberger JL, et al: Pulmonary function in convalescent poliomyelitis patients. *N Engl J Med* 247:390–393, 1952
36. DeTroyer A, Borenstein S, Cordier R: Analysis of lung volume restriction in patients with respiratory muscle weakness. *Thorax* 35:603–610, 1980
37. Plum F: Monographs in Medicine, series 1. Baltimore, Williams & Wilkins, 1952, p 225
38. Walley RV: Assessment of respiratory failure poliomyelitis. *Br Med J* 2:82, 1959
39. Black LF, Hyatt RE: Maximal respiratory pressures: Normal values and relationship to age and sex. *Am Rev Respir Dis* 99:696–702, 1969
40. Black LF, Hyatt RE: Maximal static respiratory pressures in generalized neuromuscular disease. *Am Rev Respir Dis* 103:641–650, 1971
41. Shochina M, Ferber J, Wolf E: Evaluation of the phrenic nerve in patients with neuromuscular disorders. *Int J Rehabil Res* 6:455–459, 1983
42. Mansel JK, Norman JR: Respiratory complications and management of spinal cord injuries. *Chest* 97:1446–1452, 1990
43. Kraus JF: Epidemiological aspects of acute spinal cord injury: A review of incidence, prevalence, causes, and outcome. *In* Becker DP, Povlishock JT (eds): Central Nervous System Trauma Status Report—1985. Bethesda, MD, National Institute of Neurological and Communicative Disorders and Stroke, National Institutes of Health, 1985, pp 313–322
44. DeTroyer A, Estenne M, Vincken W: Rib cage motion and muscle use in high tetraplegics. *Am Rev Respir Dis* 133:1115–1119, 1986
45. James WS III, Minh V, Minteer MA, et al: Cervical accessory respiratory muscle function in a patient with a high cervical cord lesion. *Chest* 71:59–64, 1977
46. Bergofsky EH: Mechanism for respiratory insufficiency after cervical cord injury. *Ann Intern Med* 61:435–447, 1964
47. Huldtgren AC, Fugl-Meyer AR, Jonasson E, et al: Ventilatory dysfunction and respiratory rehabilitation in post-traumatic quadriplegia. *Eur J Respir Dis* 61:347–356, 1980
48. Estenne M, DeTroyer A: Mechanisms of the postural dependence of vital capacity in tetraplegic subjects. *Am Rev Respir Dis* 135:367–371, 1987
49. Goldman JM, Rose LS, Williams SJ, et al: Effect of abdominal binders on breathing in tetraplegic patients. *Thorax* 41:940–945, 1986
50. DeTroyer A, Heilporn A: Respiratory mechanics in quadriplegia. The respiratory function of the intercostal muscles. *Am Rev Respir Dis* 122:591–600, 1980
51. Ledsome JR, Sharp JM: Pulmonary function in acute cervical cord injury. *Am Rev Respir Dis* 124:41–44, 1981
52. McMichan JC, Michel L, Westbrook PR: Pulmonary dysfunction following traumatic quadriplegia. *JAMA* 243:528–531, 1980
53. Pichurko B, McCool FD, Scanlon P, et al: Factors related to respiratory function recovery following acute quadriplegia. *Am Rev Respir Dis* 131:A337, 1985
54. Wicks AB, Menter RR: Long-term outlook in quadriplegic patients with initial ventilator dependency. *Chest* 90:406–410, 1986
55. Fromm GB, Wisdom PJ, Block AJ: Amyotrophic lateral sclerosis presenting with respiratory failure. Diaphragmatic paralysis and dependence on mechanical ventilation in two patients. *Chest* 71:5, 1977
56. Nakano KK, Bass H, Tyler HR, et al: Amyotrophic lateral sclerosis: A study of pulmonary function. *Diseases of the Nervous System* 37:32–35, 1976
57. Fallat RJ, Jewit B, Bass M, et al: Spirometry in amyotrophic lateral sclerosis. *Arch Neurol* 36:74–80, 1979
58. Inkley SR, Oldenburg FC, Vignos PJ Jr: Pulmonary function in Duchenne muscular dystrophy related to stage of disease. *Am J Med* 56:297–306, 1974
59. Codd MB, Mulder DW, Kurland LT, et al: Poliomyelitis in Rochester, Minnesota, 1935–1955: Epidemiology and long term sequelae: A preliminary report. *In* Halstead LS, Wiechers DO (eds): Late Effects of Poliomyelitis. Miami Symposia Foundation, 1985, pp 121–134
60. Halstead LS, Wiechers DO (eds): Late Effects of Poliomyelitis. Miami, FL, Symposia Foundation, 1985
61. Cashman NR, Maselli R, Wollmann RL, et al: Late denervation in patients with antecedent paralytic poliomyelitis. *N Engl J Med* 317:7–12, 1987

62. Hill R, Robbins AW, Messing R, et al: Sleep apnea syndrome after poliomyelitis. *Am Rev Respir Dis* 127:129–131, 1983
63. Brody AW, O'Halloran PS, Connolly JJ Jr, et al: Ventilatory mechanics and strength in subjects paralyzed after poliomyelitis. *Dis Chest* 46:263–275, 1964
64. Streib EW: Post polio syndrome: A common condition in need of recognition. *Iowa Medicine* 115–119, 1989
65. Salazar-Grueso EF, Siegel I, Roos RP: The post polio syndrome: Evaluation and treatment. *Comp Ther* 16:24–30, 1990
66. Guillenminault C, Motta J: Sleep apnea syndrome as a long-term sequela of poliomyelitis. Kroc Foundation Series. New York, Alan R. Liss, 1978, pp 308–315
67. Bach JR, Alba AS, Bohatiuk G, et al: Mouth intermittent positive pressure ventilation in the management of postpolio respiratory insufficiency. *Chest* 91:859–864, 1987
68. Ellis ER, Bye P, Bruderer JW, et al: Treatment of respiratory failure during sleep in patients with neuromuscular disease. Positive-pressure ventilation through a nose mask. *Am Rev Respir Dis* 135:148–152, 1987
69. Horowitz SH: The idiopathic polyradiculoneuropathies: A historical guide to an understanding of the clinical syndromes. *Acta Neurol Scand* 80:369–386, 1989
70. England JD: Guillain-Barre syndrome. *Annu Rev Med* 41:1–6, 1990
71. Gracey DR, McMichan JC, Divertie MB, et al: Respiratory failure in Guillain-Barre syndrome: A 6-year experience. *Mayo Clin Proc* 57:742–746, 1982
72. Seybold ME: Myasthenia gravis: A clinical and basic science review. *JAMA* 250:2516–2521, 1983
73. Herrmann C Jr, Lindstrom JM, Keesey JC, et al: Myasthenia gravis—Current concepts. Interdepartmental Conference, University of California, Los Angeles (Specialty Conference). *West J Med* 142:797–809, 1985
74. DeTroyer A, Borenstein S: Acute changes in respiratory mechanics after pyridostigmine injection in patients with myasthenia gravis. *Am Rev Respir Dis* 121:629–638, 1980
75. Toyka KV: Neuromuscular junction and muscle disease. *Current Therapy in Neurologic Disease* 3:385–391, 1990
76. Lange DJ: The Eaton-Lambert syndrome: Current concepts of pathogenesis and treatment. *Neurol Neurosurg Update* 4:1, 1983
77. Beggs AH, Kunkel LM: Improved diagnosis of Duchenne/Becker muscular dystrophy. *J Clin Invest* 84:613–619, 1990
78. Begin R, Bureau MA, Lupien L, et al: Control of breathing in Duchenne's muscular dystrophy. *Am J Med* 69:227–234, 1980
78a. Bayour A, Gilgoff I, Prentice W, et al: Decline in respiratory function and experience with long-term assisted ventilation in advanced Duchenne's muscular dystrophy. *Chest* 97:884–889, 1990
79. Smith PEM, Calverley PMA, Edwards RHT, et al: Practical problems in the respiratory care of patients with muscular dystrophy. *N Engl J Med* 316:1197–1205, 1987
80. Luce JM: Respiratory complications of obesity. *Chest* 78:626–631, 1980
81. Ray CS, Sue DY, Bray G, et al: Effects of obesity on respiratory function. *Am Rev Respir Dis* 128:501–506, 1983
82. Bedell GN, Wilson WR, Seebohm PM: Pulmonary function in obese persons. *J Clin Invest* 37:1049–1061, 1958
83. Garay SM, Turino GM, Goldring RM: Sustained reversal of chronic hypercapnia in patients with alveolar hypoventilation syndromes: Long-term maintenance with noninvasive nocturnal mechanical ventilation. *Am J Med* 70:269–274, 1981
84. Curran FJ: Night ventilation by body respirators for patients in chronic respiratory failure due to late stage Duchenne muscular dystrophy. *Am Rev Respir Dis* 125(suppl):139, 1982
85. Hill NS: Clinical applications of body ventilators. *Chest* 90:897–905, 1986
86. Bach JR, Alba A, Mosher R, et al: Intermittent positive pressure ventilation via nasal access in the management of respiratory insufficiency. *Chest* 92:168–170, 1987
87. Heckmatt JZ, Loh L, Dubowitz V: Night-time nasal ventilation in neuromuscular disease. *Lancet* 10:335:579–582, 1990
88. Elliott MW, Steven MH, Phillips GD, et al: Non-invasive mechanical ventilation for acute respiratory failure. *Br Med J* 300:358–360, 1990
89. Carrey Z, Gottfried SB, Levy RD: Ventilatory muscle support in respiratory failure with nasal positive pressure ventilation. *Chest* 97: 150–158, 1990
90. Leger P, Jennequin J, Gerard M, et al: Home positive pressure ventilation via nasal mask for patients with neuromusculoskeletal disorders. *Eur Respir J* 2(suppl 7):640–645, 1989
91. Plummer AL, O'Donohue WJ, Petty TL: Consensus conference on problems in home mechanical ventilation. *Am Rev Respir Dis* 140: 555–560, 1989
92. Sivak ED, Gipson WT, Hanson MR: Long-term management of respiratory failure in amyotrophic lateral sclerosis. *Ann Neurol* 12: 18–23, 1982
93. Peters SG, Viggiano RW: Subspecialty clinics: Critical care medicine. Home mechanical ventilation. *Mayo Clin Proc* 63:1208–1213, 1988

13

Pleural and Diaphragmatic Diseases

Robert Sharon, Angela DeSantis, and Lyle D. Victor

Pathophysiology of Pleural Effusions

A pleural effusion is a collection of fluid in the pleural space (Fig. 13-1), most often caused by cardiopulmonary disease. Pleural fluid develops when rates of entry and exit for fluid and protein are in disequilibrium due to an imbalance in the forces regulating fluid exchange or disease process at the pleural surface [1]. A pleural effusion collects in the space surrounded by the visceral and parietal pleura (Figure 13-1). The visceral pleura surrounds the lung itself while the parietal pleura envelopes the surface of the chest wall, diaphragm and mediastinum. The two pleural surfaces become continuous at the hilum. The visceral pleura has many lymphatic vessels, few pain fibers and a blood supply primarily from the pulmonary arterial circulation with a minor contribution from the bronchial arteries. The pulmonary veins drain the visceral pleura. Unlike the visceral pleura, the parietal pleura contains many pain fibers, a blood supply from systemic arteries and the venous drainage occurs through the azygous and hemiazygous veins [2]. The pleural space normally accommodates between 3 and 15 ml of fluid. However, 650 ml to 10 L of fluid may move through the pleural space within a 24 hour period [3]. A small amount of fluid exists between the parietal and visceral pleural layers enabling them to slide over each other. Visceral pleural capillaries and pleural lymphatics absorb fluid leaking from the parietal pleural capillaries. Pleural lymphatics absorb protein in addition to up to 20% of the fluid moving across the membranes [4].

Three physiologic phenomena influence pleural fluid dynamics; capillary hydrostatic pressure, colloid osmotic pressure and pleural pressure. Starling's law of transcapillary exchange influences the movement of fluid across the pleural space as described in the following formula

$$F = K\,(P_C - P_{PL}) - (\pi_C - \pi_{PL})$$

where F refers to movement of fluid from the capillaries to pleura space, K refers to the filtration coefficient, P_C refers to capillary hydrostatic pressure, P_{PL} refers to pleural space pressure, π_C refers to plasma oncotic pressure and π_{PL} refers to pleural fluid oncotic pressure. The hydrostatic pressure gradient is $(P_C - P_{PL})$ while the oncotic pressure gradient is $(\pi_C - \pi_{PL})$ [5].

Most of the pleural fluid absorption occurs via pleural lymphatics and microscopic openings on the pleural surface called stomata [6]. The pleural fluid filtration gradient begins in the parietal pleura (Fig. 13-1) where the intercostal arteries are responsible for generating systemic pressures in the microvasculature. Hydrostatic forces in the parietal pleura are responsible for fluid movement. Parietal pleural hydrostatic pressure is approximately 30 cm H_2O and the pleural pressure itself is about -5 cm H_2O. Therefore the net hydrostatic pressure is $30 - (-5) = 35$ cm H_2O resulting in movement of fluid from parietal pleural capillaries into the pleural space. In opposition to the hydrostatic pressure gradient is the plasma oncotic pressure, which is about 34 cm H_2O. The small amount of pleural fluid normally present has an oncotic pressure of about 5 cm H_2O [7]. Therefore the net oncotic pressure gradient is $34 - 5 = 29$ cm H_2O. The net gradient for fluid distribution therefore is $35 - 29 = 6$ cm H_2O and causes the movement of fluid from

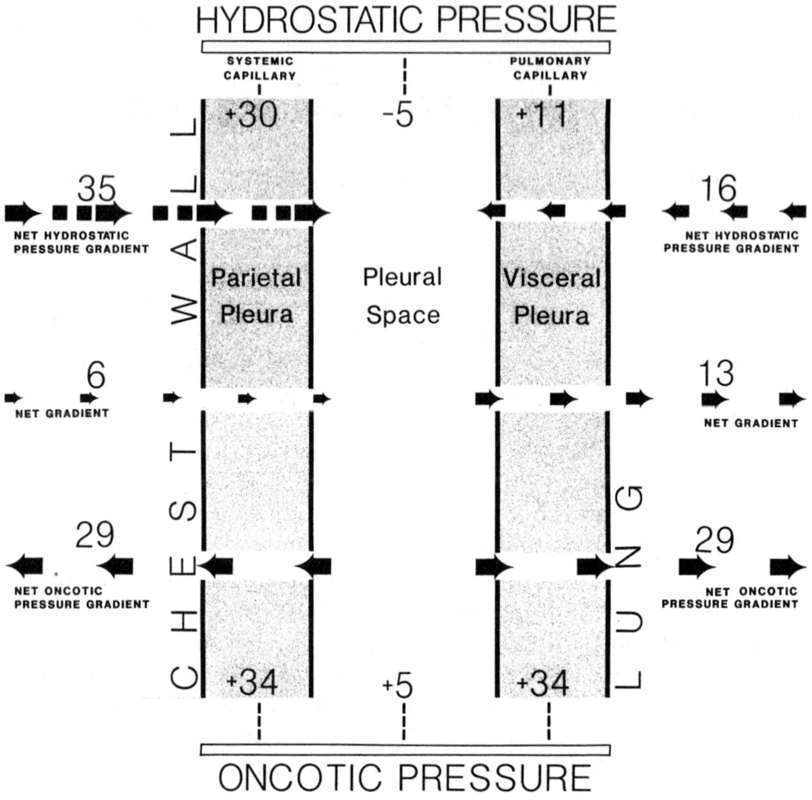
HYDROSTATIC PRESSURE
SYSTEMIC CAPILLARY
PULMONARY CAPILLARY
+30
-5
+11
35
16
NET HYDROSTATIC PRESSURE GRADIENT
NET HYDROSTATIC PRESSURE GRADIENT
Parietal Pleura
Pleural Space
Visceral Pleura
6
13
NET GRADIENT
NET GRADIENT
29
29
NET ONCOTIC PRESSURE GRADIENT
NET ONCOTIC PRESSURE GRADIENT
CHEST WALL
LUNG
+34
+5
+34
ONCOTIC PRESSURE

Fig. 13-1. Stylized drawing of chest wall, parietal pleura, pleural cavity, and visceral pleura showing how hydrostatic pressure and oncotic pressure influence net flow of pleural fluid in and out of the pleural space. Size of arrow reflects level of depicted pressure.

parietal pleural capillaries into the pleural space [8].

Fluid movement from the visceral pleura varies from that of the parietal pleura because the hydrostatic pressure of the visceral pleura is from the pulmonary capillaries instead of the systemic capillaries. Since the pulmonary capillary pressure is approximately 11 cm H_2O, the net hydrostatic pressure gradient across the visceral pleura is $11 - (-5) = 16$ cm H_2O. The oncotic pressure gradient of the visceral pleura equals the parietal pleural gradient of 29 cm H_2O. Therefore the net gradient for fluid exchange is $16 - 29 = -13$ cm H_2O. The negative sign demonstrates the fluid moves from the pleural space into the visceral pleural capillaries. This follows Starling's law of transcapillary exchange [8].

A low oncotic pressure may cause interstitial edema according to the Starling's equation. As a practical matter, however, pleural effusion or anasarca is not usually seen unless the serum protein is less than 1.5 g/dL.

There are other physiologic causes for pleural fluid collection besides oncotic and hydrostatic forces. For example, a reduced pressure in the pleural space such as from lung collapse or atelectasis may decrease pleural pressure and increase the interstitial pleural pressure gradient, encouraging pleural fluid collection [9]. Another cause for pleural fluid formation is inflammation, which encourages effusion formation by increasing microvascular circulation. Reduced lymphatic drainage, which may be seen in neoplasm or fibrosis, may be another physiologic cause of pleural effusion. Pleural effusions associated with peritoneal dialysis may be caused by movement of fluid collected in the abdominal cavity through defects in the diaphragm [10].

Transudate versus Exudate

Pleural fluid may be classified as a transudate or an exudate, depending on the specific gravity and the amount of protein and lactic dehydrogenase (LDH) contained in the fluid. It is useful to decide if a pleural fluid is transudative or exudative because of the great influence this information has on subsequent diagnosis and treatment.

A transudate is formed when hydrostatic and oncotic phenomena are responsible for fluid formation and the pleural surfaces are not pathologically involved. Transudates may be formed from either a reduction in plasma colloid oncotic pressure or an elevated hydrostatic pressure in the systemic and pulmonary circulation. For example, nephrotic syndrome and liver cirrhosis are two conditions that cause a decrease in plasma colloid-oncotic pressure because of a reduction in plasma proteins. The intravascular space has a reduced ability to contain free fluid under these conditions, thereby causing fluid to collect in the pleural space. The other major cause of transudative effusion is elevation of the hydrostatic pressure as may be seen in congestive heart failure or obstruction of the azygous vein or superior vena cava. However, these conditions do not always lead to the development of pleural effusions because significant disease usually must be present before pleural fluid collects.

Exudates, on the other hand, are caused by actual pathology at the pleural surface. There are two mechanisms involved in this process. First is from the increased capillary permeability allowing transfer of larger molecules such as protein as, may be seen in patients with pulmonary infections and neoplasm. A second mechanism causing an exudative effusion is obstruction of pulmonary lymphatics as might be encountered in lymphoma [11, 12].

For patient management, a distinction must be made between a transudate and an exudate. If the effusion is a transudate, the diagnostic possibilities are limited to congestive heart failure or conditions that reduce plasma oncotic pressure such as nephrotic syndrome or malnutrition. Further diagnostic procedures in these situations are unnecessary, and therapy is directed toward the underlying disease process. In contrast, if the effusion is an exudate, more extensive diagnostic procedures are needed because of the many causative factors and treatment choices.

Laboratory criteria are available to help distinguish a transudate from an exudate. A transudate is defined as a clear, serous fluid that is low in total protein, LDH and number of cells [13]. In transudative pleural effusions, there is an imbalance between hydrostatic and oncotic pressures, forming a low protein pleural fluid, without alteration in membrane permeability at the pleural surfaces. In contrast, an exudate is usually clear to turbid fluid, with a higher total protein and LDH, and a variable cell count. Localized vessel wall disease may cause an exudative pleural effusion by allowing movement of fluid and cells into the pleural space resulting in an effusion high in LDH and protein [13]. Transudative and exudative pleural effusions may be distinguished by simultaneously measuring LDH and protein. The laboratory criteria for this may be found in Table 13-1. One investigator used the ratio of pleural fluid protein to serum protein, pleural fluid LDH to serum LDH, and the absolute value of the pleural fluid LDH to differentiate a transudate from an exudate. All three criteria for a transudate must be present to make the determination of a transudative pleural effusion. However, only one of the three criteria need to be met to confirm the diagnosis of an exudative pleural effusion [11]. Exudative pleural effusions have many causes and therefore may require more extensive test-

Table 13-1. Laboratory Test Criteria to Differentiate a Transudate from an Exudate

Laboratory test	*Transudate*	*Exudate*
Fluid protein/serum protein	<0.5	>0.5
Fluid LDH/serum LDH	<0.6	>0.6
Fluid LDH	<⅔ upper limit of normal for assay used	>⅔ upper limit of normal for assay used

ing. A more specific laboratory method of separating transudates from exudates has been recently described [14]. Using a serum-effusion albumin gradient of 1.2 g/dL or less to suggest an exudate and greater than 1.2 g/dL to suggest a transudate, 57 of 59 effusions were correctly classified.

Pleural effusions may also be bloody, empyemic and chylous. A serosanguinous effusion may result from only 1 ml of blood in 500 ml of pleural fluid. A hemothorax is defined by a hematocrit that is 50% of the peripheral blood hematocrit. An empyema is a purulent exudative effusion with a white blood cell count of usually greater than 20,000 per mm [15]. Chylous effusions appear milky as a result from fluid leakage out of the thoracic duct.

Signs and Symptoms of Pleural Effusions

Shortness of breath is the most common symptom associated with pleural effusion. Although the exact pathophysiologic cause of the dyspnea is uncertain, underlying intrinsic lung disease, restriction of lung volume by accumulated fluid, or rapidity of fluid collection may play a role [16]. In the patient with pleuritic pain there may be dyspnea caused by splinting of the chest to avoid the pain. Massive pleural effusion may cause a "tension hydrothorax," with significant respiratory distress and acute right ventricular dysfunction [17]. Arterial hemoglobin desaturation may occur in the lateral decubitus position when the affected hemithorax is dependent [18].

Pleuritic pain is another symptom associated with pleural effusion. Pain is generated by the parietal pleura since only this surface is innervated by pain fibers. Pain is usually limited to the focus of pleural irritation. However, irritation of the central part of the diaphragm may cause referred pain to the ipsilateral shoulder. This is because the central portion of the diaphragm has afferent nerve pathways via the phrenic nerve that enter the spinal cord through the third, fourth, and fifth dorsal roots, which also supply pain fibers to the shoulder. The pain of a pleural effusion is most severe early in its formation when the visceral and parietal surfaces are able to rub against each other [19]. The pain is usually transient, often mild, but may be severe and pleuritic being described as sharp or knife-like with the intensity increasing with inspiration and decreasing with expiration [20].

A nonproductive cough may be present in moderately sized pleural effusions. The etiology of the cough is not well understood but may be related to compression by the fluid, bringing opposite bronchial walls into contact and mechanically stimulating cough reflex [20].

Some pleural effusions are characteristically asymptomatic. Approximately 67% of new mothers had asymptomatic pleural effusion after vaginal delivery in one study [21]. Other disorders that are often associated with asymptomatic pleural effusion include post-operative abdominal surgery, benign asbestos effusion (see Chap. 14), uremia, malignancy, and tuberculosis.

On physical examination patients will typically have reduced breath sounds and dullness to percussion at the lung bases. When

Table 13-2. Causes of Pleural Effusions

Transudates	*Exudates*
Cardiovascular	Primary tumors of the pleura
Congestive heart failure	Malignant mesothelioma
Constrictive pericarditis	Bronchiogenic carcinoma
Superior vena cava obstruction	Metastatic malignancies
Overexpanded fluid volume	Infections
Hypoalbuminemia	Tuberculosis
Intra-abdominal disease	Parapneumonic effusions
Hepatic hydrothorax (cirrhosis)	Empyema
Peritoneal dialysis	Fungi
	Viruses and mycoplasma
	Parasites
	Pulmonary embolism
	Connective tissue diseases
	Systemic lupus erythematosus
	Rheumatoid arthritis
	Sjögren's syndrome
	Wegener's granulomatosis
	Postmyocardial infarction syndrome (Dressler's syndrome)
	Myxedema
	Intra-abdominal causes
	Pancreatitis
	Abdominal surgery
	Hepatitis
	Trauma
	Hemothorax
	Chylothorax

a massive effusion is present there may be enlargement of one hemithorax.

Causes of Transudates

Cardiovascular

Congestive Heart Failure

One of the most common causes of transudative or exudative pleural effusion is congestive heart failure (Table 13-2). A study of chest roentgenograms and autopsy results showed that pleural effusions were present in about 40% of patients with ventricular failure [22]. Heart failure is probably underestimated in most reports of pleural effusion since cardiac congestion seldom presents diagnostic difficulties, and patients with pleural effusions do not receive the same attention as others with effusions of unknown cause. Many patients with congestive heart failure have bilateral pleural effusions. In those with only a unilateral effusion, right sided fluid occurs more commonly. One possible reason is the inclination for the right recumbent position to be assumed by patients with congestive heart failure, increasing the venous pressure in parts of the right lung [23].

Pathophysiology of Fluid Collection in Congestive Heart Failure A systemic hydrostatic pressure increase will theoretically increase the rate of formation of pleural fluid while an increase in pulmonary hydrostatic pressure will theoretically cause a decrease in pleural fluid formation. These two phenomena may act in concert to increase the formation and movement of fluid from the visceral pleura into the pleural cavity. It appears that, from a theoretical point of view, either right sided or left sided heart failure may result in pleural effusion. High systemic venous pressure appears to be the most influential cause of pleural fluid collection. Elevated pressures in this system may hinder the drainage of pleural lymphatic vessels into the systemic circulation [24]. Another series that showed elevated pulmonary capillary wedge pressures in patients with congestive heart failure suggests that pulmonary venous hypertension is important in the generation of abnormal pleural fluid [25]. Pleural effusion may be seen in patients with isolated left ventricular failure or biventricular failure, but are rarely encountered in isolated right ventricular failure. From a clinical standpoint isolated pulmonary arterial hypertension such as might be seen in chronic obstructive pulmonary disease is rarely associated with pleural effusion formation.

Clinical Manifestations of Congestive Heart Failure Pleural effusions in congestive heart failure are usually associated with the typical clinical presentation of the disease including dyspnea on exertion, orthopnea and paroxysmal nocturnal dyspnea. Interestingly, the degree of dyspnea does not necessarily correlate with the size of the pleural effusion. Physical signs of CHF include jugular venous distention and peripheral edema. A pleural effusion may cause a shift of the cardiac apex medially or laterally and cause difficulty in cardiac percussion and reduced accuracy in determining cardiac size clinically. Advanced heart failure may show signs of both right-sided heart failure, with distended neck veins, and peripheral edema, in addition to signs of left-sided heart failure with rales, an S_3 ventricular gallop, and physical signs of pleural effusion. Other signs of heart failure such as tachycardia, and ascites also may be present.

Diagnosis of Congestive Heart Failure The chest roentgenogram in congestive heart failure may show an enlarged heart and bilateral pleural effusions. One of the earliest roentgenographic signs of CHF is increased perihilar vascular markings. On occasion, fluid will localize in an interlobar fissure and, when viewed en face, will mimic tumor [26]. These so called "pseudo tumors" abate or totally disappear with treatment for the heart failure [27].

Congestive heart failure is the most common cause of bilateral pleural effusions. Physicians often treat patients with congestive heart failure and pleural effusion and wait to see if the effusion goes away. If the pleural effusion does not resolve, then a diagnostic thoracentesis may be considered. The problem with this approach is that with treatment the protein concentration in the fluid may increase such that the fluid appears to be an exudate when it originally was a transudate [28]. Therefore, one must be careful not to attribute the pleural effusion to congestive heart failure when it has another cause. In clinical situations where an enlarged heart is not present, other causes of pleural effusion should be sought, such as malignancy [23]. One series showed greater than 25% of patients with pleural effusion associated with heart failure had additional causes such as pulmonary emboli and pneumonia at autopsy [29]. When to do a thoracentesis for bilateral pleural effusions is a clinical challenge. Clinicians tend to use a diagnostic thoracentesis in situations of a hemithorax with a massive effusion, pleuritic chest pain, and/or fever, suggesting an underlying inflammatory process is present, or when hypoxemia occurs out of proportion to the degree of pulmonary edema [10]. Isolated left-sided effusions usually require a diagnostic pleural tap unless the clinical situation suggests an obvious etiology such as the postoperative state or acute pancreatitis.

The pleural fluid in CHF is usually a straw colored transudate with a protein level of less than 3.5 g/dl. Pleural fluid cell counts show a predominance of polymorphonuclear cells and other mononuclear cells such as small lymphocytes [30]. If the above criteria are met in a patient with an enlarged heart and bilateral pleural effusions, one may attribute the fluid collections to CHF. If the criteria for a transudate are not clear, or the patient has an exudate, further diagnostic studies are needed which may include cytological examination, pleural biopsy or CAT scanning.

Treatment Treatment of CHF will usually resolve the pleural effusion. Shortness of breath will improve, although the degree of dyspnea is not necessarily related to the size of the pleural effusion. Thoracentesis may transiently improve the dyspnea but, in our experience, effusions usually recur unless the underlying hydrostatic abnormality is treated.

Constrictive Pericarditis and Superior Vena Cava Obstruction

Elevations in hydrostatic pressure may occur in other disorders besides CHF. Constrictive pericarditis and superior vena caval syndrome (SVC) may cause pleural effusion by elevating hydrostatic pressures. In one study of 35 patients with constrictive pericarditis, 60% had radiologically demonstrable pleural effusions. The effusion was bilateral in 57% and right sided in the remaining 43% of these patients [31]. Other series show a left-sided preponderance of fluid [32]. Patients with superior vena cava obstruction only rarely have pleural effusion. A study by Perez and coworkers found a relatively small number of cases of superior vena cava syndrome associated with pleural effusion. In all cases, it was the tumor involvement of the pleura rather than the superior vena cava syndrome that was felt to be responsible for the pleural effusion [33]. Other explanations should be investigated in cases where there is a pleural effusion found in association with the superior vena cava syndrome.

Overexpanded Fluid Volume

Hypoalbuminemia

Patients with nephrotic syndrome, malabsorption syndromes or volume overload, may have significant hypoalbuminemia and decreased plasma oncotic pressure. Ascites, peripheral edema and pleural effusions, both unilateral and bilateral, may result. These effusions are most commonly bilateral since hypoalbuminemia is a systemic process. Proteinuria will accompany a pleural effusion caused from the nephrotic syndrome. A thoracentesis may be done to confirm a transudate if clinical diagnosis is not clear or effusions persist.

Diuretics and salt restriction is the usual treatment for edema and fluid due to reduced plasma protein concentration and oncotic pressures. The goal of therapy is to correct the hydrostatic and oncotic abnormalities so that less fluid will collect in the pleural space. Multiple thoracenteses are generally not effective in permanently inhibiting fluid formation in these disorders although in certain cases a tetracycline pleurodesis may be attempted [34].

Intra-Abdominal Disease

Hepatic Hydrothorax

Pleural effusions are seen in 5% to 6% patients with cirrhosis [35], especially when ascites are present. These hydrothoraces are more commonly located on the right side (67%), although they may present left sided (16%) or bilateral (16%) [36]. Pleural effusions are rarely seen in cirrhosis patients without ascites [37].

Pathophysiology and Clinical Manifestations

It is interesting to note that cirrhotic patients with a decrease in plasma oncotic pressure uncommonly have pleural effusion [38]. This is especially true if there is no accompanying ascites. One series of cirrhosis patients without ascites reported an absence of pleural effusions even if the serum albumin levels were below 2.5 gm/dl [35]. On the other hand, patients with cirrhosis and ascites may have large effusions causing dyspnea [39].

Pleural fluid may form in patients with cirrhosis and ascites through different mechanisms. Some authors conclude that pleural fluid accumulates because of transport of ascitic fluid from lymph vessels [35], while others have suggested that the ascitic fluid passes directly from the peritoneal cavity to the pleural cavity through defects in the diaphragm [36].

Diagnosis Pleural effusions associated with cirrhosis and ascites may be more precisely diagnosed by performing a dual paracentesis and thoracentesis. If both are transudates, cirrhosis as a cause is confirmed. The pleural fluid protein level is usually below 3.0 gm dl and is often higher than the ascitic protein level. The LDH level is low [36]. The pleural fluid may be serosanguinous because of clotting abnormalities often seen in cirrhotic patients. As there is a higher risk of pancreatitis and malignancy of the liver in these patients one should also perform amylase and cytological examinations on the fluid.

Treatment As the pleural effusions associated with cirrhosis are likely an extension of the peritoneal fluid collection, treatment of the pleural fluid is the same as the treatment for ascites. This includes diuretics and salt restriction. Refractory patients may require pleurodesis or shunt placement [40]. Multiple thoracenteses to control pleural fluid collection are ill advised because of the resultant protein depletion. Fluid recollects rapidly in this situation because the underlying cause is not adequately treated.

Dialysis Acute hydrothorax sometimes occurs during peritoneal dialysis [41]. Although they occur most frequently on the right, there have been case reports of effusions on the left as well [42]. It is thought that the pathogenesis of the hydrothorax in this condition is similar to that with ascites and pleural effusion. The introduction of large amounts of fluid into the abdomen during dialysis may stretch the diaphragm and lead to the development of diaphragmatic defects, allowing the dialysate into the pleural space. The pleural effusion is usually detected in the first 48 hours after starting the dialysis [38]. The dyspneic patient may require a diagnostic and therapeutic thoracentesis. Pleural fluid analysis reveals a remarkably low protein, often <1.0 g/dL, and an elevated glucose concentration [10]. Pleural effusions secondary to peritoneal dialysis may require discontinuation of the dialysis as the pleural effusion usually recurs when the peritoneal dialysis is again started [41]. Serosanguineous pleural effusions thought to be secondary to heparin use have been demonstrated during hemodialysis [43].

Causes of Exudative Pleural Effusions

Primary Tumors of the Pleura

Benign and Malignant Mesothelioma
Asbestos-related pleural effusion and mesothelioma are covered in Chap. 14.

Malignant Pleural Effusion
Malignancy is a common cause of pleural effusion, accounting for up to 40% of unilateral pleural effusions, and the older the patient group studied, the higher the percentage of malignant effusion [44]. Diagnosis is most often made from a positive pleural fluid cytology. Between 33% and 87% of malignant effusions have a positive cytology [45]. Occasionally a pleural biopsy is performed when malignant neoplasm is not initially shown on cytologic analysis. Rarely will a thoracoscopy (endoscopic biopsy) or an open thoracotomy be necessary for diagnosis. Effusions may be serous to frankly bloody and are most often exudates, although up to 10% may be transudates [46, 47]. Pleural fluid pH measurements may be helpful diagnostically as one third of malignant effusions have a pH level less than 7.30, carrying a poorer prognosis [48]. Pleural fluid glucose may be less than 60 mg/dL or even as low as levels seen in rheumatoid effusions.

Bronchogenic carcinoma and pleural effusions are generally regarded as inoperable, especially if malignant cells are recovered from the fluid [49]. On the other hand, about 5% of patients may have paramalignant effusions and may well qualify for surgical intervention [50]. Paramalignant effusions are those that are associated with thoracic carcinoma but without pleural malignancy. Possible causes for this phenomena include atelectasis, lymphatic obstruction, pneumonia, radiation pneumonitis, thromboembolic disease, and reduced plasma oncotic pressure.

Bronchogenic carcinoma is the most common neoplasm to cause pleural effusion, and adenocarcinoma is the most common cell type, possibly because of its more peripheral location [51].

Besides bronchogenic carcinoma there are other malignancies that metastasize to the pleural surfaces and cause pleural effusions. Carcinoma of the breast is the most common, followed by malignancy of the ovary, kidney, stomach, pancreas, and other sites within the abdomen. The liver is usually involved with metastases before lung involvement [52].

Pleural effusions may be associated with lymphomas. Mediastinal adenopathy may compromise lymphatic drainage in Hodgkin's disease as a cause of pleural fluid collection while direct pleural seeding is the main cause in non-Hodgkin's lymphoma [10]. Obstruction of the thoracic duct in lymphoma may be a cause of chylous effusion.

Collectively, metastatic malignancy produces about the same incidence of unilateral pleural effusion but causes more bilateral effusions than bronchogenic carcinoma. The size of the effusions are usually substantial and may be massive, involving a whole hemithorax. Effusion from metastatic malignancy may occur without roentgenographically discernible parenchymal involvement: in these instances the effusion probably results from isolated implants on the visceral pleural surface or is of paraneoplastic origin. Computed tomography scanning may be useful in identifying pleural involvement with malignancy.

Pleural metastases and effusion generally carry a poor prognosis, especially in the setting of bronchogenic carcinoma. In one series of 96 patients with malignant effusion, 86% were dead within 6 months [51]. Malignant effusion secondary to carcinoma of the breast may carry a better prognosis as there may be a response to chemotherapy [53]. Small, asymptomatic pleural effusions may be observed clinically while dyspneic patients need therapeutic thoracenteses for relief. If the effusion recurs rapidly after thoracentesis and is associated with significant disability, insertion of a chest tube and installation of tetracycline or other sclerosing agents to effect a pleurodesis may abate recurrence. In situations where effusion returns or there is a thick malignant rind of tissue entrapping the lung, open pleurectomy is very effective, although at a cost of some morbidity and mortality. We have used this option only rarely because many patients with malignant effusion have advanced disease with short life expectancies.

Pleural effusions have been reported in association with radiation therapy. In one series, the effusions were noted within 6 months of the radiation and tended to be persistent [54].

Benign pelvic tumors have been associated with pleural effusion [55]. Subsequent to this report a number of benign and malignant pelvic tumors have been reported to be associated with hydrothorax, including adenocarcinoma [56]. The development of pleural effusion under these circumstances may be related more to tumor size than histology.

Infections as a Cause of Pleural Effusion

Infections of the pleural space usually cause exudative pleural effusions. Aerobic, anaerobic, and tubercle bacilli are the most common infectious agents causing pleural fluid collection.

Tuberculosis

The presence of very few *Mycobacterium tuberculosis* organisms may cause a chronic, exudative pleural effusion. The generation of the pleural reaction and effusion is thought to be secondary to a hypersensitivity reaction to tuberculoprotein. The process may be initiated by the rupture of a subpleural area of tuberculous caseation [57]. Pyogenic infections, on the other hand, cause fluid to develop because of the intense inflammatory reaction generated by the heavy load of micro-organisms.

Many patients with tubercular effusions have a nonproductive cough and pleuritic chest pain, hence the appellation *tuberculous pleurisy with effusion.* Patients may or may not be febrile. Tuberculous pleurisy with effusion is usually unilateral and may be large enough to occupy an entire hemithorax [58]. Chest radiography usually shows only the pleural fluid, but about one third of patients have parenchymal infiltrates [58].

Diagnosis The diagnosis of tuberculous pleuritis depends on the demonstration of *Mycobacterium tuberculosis* in the sputum, pleural fluid, or pleural biopsy specimen. Caseating granulomas on histologic examination of pleural biopsy also may be used as presumptive evidence of tuberculosis.

Patients with unexplained exudative pleural effusions should have tuberculin skin testing remembering that an occasional anergic patient with disease may give a false negative result. Pleural biopsy may be necessary yielding caseating granulomas on the initial biopsy in approximately 60% of patients. If one obtains three pleural biopsies, the yield increases to about 80% and will increase to about 90% if culture of a sample of pleura is performed [59]. Even without identifiable organisms or caseating granulomas, a presumptive diagnosis may be assumed when the patient has a positive purified protein derivative skin test and a lymphocytic predominance in the pleural fluid [60]. Treatment for tuberculous pleurisy and effusion is covered in Chap. 18.

Parapneumonic Effusions and Empyema
Pneumonia is a common illness, occurring in up to 3 million people annually [61]. Pleural effusions will be found in almost 40% of patients with bacterial pneumonia [62]. A parapneumonic effusion is defined as any pleural effusion associated with bacterial pneumonia, bronchiectasis or lung abscess [63]. Some parapneumonic effusions may be frankly purulent and are then called empyemas. Most parapneumonic effusions resolve with treatment of the underlying disorder. Empyematous fluids, however, have traditionally been more difficult to manage because of the necessity of closed tube drainage or even open surgical intervention. The challenge for the clinician is to decide when drainage procedures are needed in the setting of a parapneumonic effusion.

Two groups of investigators have written extensively on effusions associated with pneumonia [62, 64]. These authors have divided parapneumonic effusions into two groups for therapeutic purposes. The first group, the uncomplicated, is effusions associated with pneumonia and is self-limited, responding to the treatment of the underlying inflammatory process. The second group is the complicated parapneumonic effusions needing some type of invasive drainage procedure. Frank pus or visible bacteria on gram stain denote a complicated parapneumonic effusion. Pleural fluid pH, LDH, and glucose concentration also separate the complicated from uncomplicated effusions. A thoracentesis fluid pH less than 7.10, LDH greater than 1000 U/L, and a glucose of less than 40 mg/dL suggest a complicated effusion [10, 62, 64] that will need to be drained.

Untreated parapneumonic effusions may progress from initially uncomplicated to later stages that are complicated. The first stage merely represents inflammatory exudate, with a polymorphonuclear leukocyte predominance, pH greater than 7.30, and a glucose equivalent to the patient's blood glucose [10, 62, 64]. This uncomplicated stage usually responds to intravenous antibiotics. The untreated patient however, may suffer invasion of the pleural space with micro-organisms that may cause collagen deposits and the formation of locules of fluid, fibrin, and pus. This so-called loculated stage is associated with reduced pH and glucose levels [10, 62, 64] and requires large-bore chest tube drainage for the patient to defervese. The final, organizational stage is associated with a fibrinopurulent rind that envelops and entraps the lung. Chest tube drainage may be ineffective and surgical decortication (removal of the thickened encasing inflammation and scarring) or an open drainage procedure may be necessary.

Organisms frequently responsible for complicated effusions and empyema are *Staphylococcus* and *Streptococcus* sp and gram-negative organisms. Anaerobic infections are also common causes of empyema in the community hospital setting and are seen in patients who may have aspirated. Patients with a history of alcoholism or loss of consciousness [65] or those with poor dentition who aspirate are most susceptible. Other clinical situations associated with empyema include ruptured esophagus (vide infra) after thoracic surgery and trauma.

Esophageal Rupture

Esophageal rupture may cause complicated pleural effusions and empyema. Early diagnosis may be life-saving because if not treated quickly the mortality approaches 100% [66].

Endoscopic examination and manipulation of the esophagus may be the most common cause of esophageal perforation. For example perforation may be associated with esophageal dilatation or foreign body removal [67]. Esophageal carcinomas, gastric intubation, chest trauma, and chest operations are also common causes of esophageal perforation. Boerhaave's syndrome is esophageal rupture occurring as a complication of vomiting.

The esophageal perforation enters the mediastinum, causing contamination with oropharyngeal contents and mediastinitis. Rupture of the mediastinal pleura may result in pleural effusion, pneumothorax, and subcutaneous emphysema and empyema. Effusions are most often left sided. The treatment of choice is surgical repair, which must be done within 24 hours to avoid gross contamination [66]. Conservative treatment with tube drainage and antibiotics may be the only alternative treatment in late rupture. There will likely be increased morbidity from mediastinal infection due to bacterial contamination [67].

Fungal, Viral, Mycoplasmal, and Parasitic Effusions

Fungal, viral, mycoplasmal, and parasitic effusions are uncommon. Discussions of these disorders may be found in other sources [10, 45].

Pulmonary Embolism

Up to half of patients with documented pulmonary embolus have an associated pleural effusion [68]. Yet, when considering a large series, embolization may account for fewer than 5% of the pleural effusions [69]. Pleural effusion may be the only manifestation of the disease in some cases [23]. The exact pathophysiologic mechanism for fluid formation is not clear. Most fluids are exudates, but about 20% may be transudates [68]. The effusions are most often unilateral and small. Occasionally the effusion may be associated with an infiltrate, suggesting associated pulmonary infarction. A peripheral, pie-shaped density is sometimes called a Hampton's hump [70].

Pleural fluid findings in pulmonary embolus are variable. Both embolus and infarction may cause a bloody effusion. Chest pain is common in patients who have pulmonary embolus and effusion [68].

Connective Tissue Diseases

Systemic Lupus Erythematosus and Rheumatoid Arthritis

Pleural effusions may be associated with systemic lupus erythematosus and rheumatoid arthritis. In systemic lupus erythematosus there may be a pleuritis and pleural thickening. Approximately 40% of patients in one autopsy series had fibrinous pleuritis [71]. Clinical signs and symptoms frequently include pleuritic chest pain, pleural friction rub, cough and shortness of breath, and fever [10, 72]. Half or more of patients with systemic lupus erythematosus have pleural effusions, which may be variable in size and bilateral or unilateral. There may be cardiomegaly either from associated myocardial disease or pericardial effusion. Basilar alveolar infiltrates and atelectasis also may be seen [73]. The finding of low complement levels is useful in the diagnosis of lupus pleuritis [74], while the finding of lupus erythematosus cells in the pleural fluid is diagnostic [75]. Patients with active disease should be treated with corticosteroids. A syndrome identical to lupus pleuritis may be induced by several commonly used drugs including chlorpromazine

(Thorazine), hydralazine (Apresoline), isoniazid (INH), phenytoin (Dilantin), procainamide (Procan, Pronestyl), and quinidine [10]. The medications of patients with pleural disease should be thoroughly evaluated.

Pleural effusions are less common in rheumatoid arthritis, occurring unilaterally in 2% to 5% of patients [76]. Most rheumatoid pleurisy disease occurs in men, though rheumatoid arthritis is more common in women. Rheumatoid pleurisy most often occurs in middle-aged men and may even appear before the onset of articular disease.

The pleural fluid may be turbid and greenish-yellow in color, or simply clear yellow [76]. A very low glucose concentration is a unique finding characteristic of rheumatoid pleural effusions [77]. A glucose level as low as 20 mg/dl, or even undetectable, is virtually diagnostic of a rheumatoid pleural effusion. However, one may encounter an occasional malignant pleural effusion with a low glucose level [78]. Rheumatoid factor may be found in the pleural fluid, but this finding is not specific. Complement levels in the effusion, as in lupus pleuritis, may be reduced. Rheumatoid effusions tend to persist for months or even years. Patients with rheumatoid arthritis tend to be on immunosuppressive drugs and are likely to suffer increased morbidity from associated rheumatoid pleuritis such as from empyema [79, 80].

Pleural effusion is not commonly seen as the direct result of disease activity in other collagen vascular and immunologic disorders such as Sjögren's syndrome, progressive systemic sclerosis, and dermatomyositis [45]. Pleural effusion has been reported in Wegener's granulomatosis [81, 82].

Postpericardiectomy/Postmyoarction Syndrome (Dressler's Syndrome)

This syndrome occurs in approximately 3% of patients following myocardial infarction [83] and in about 30% of patients after cardiac surgery [84]. Symptoms typically begin within weeks of the pericardial or cardiac insult. Patients may have fever with pericarditis and pleuritis and associated pain and friction rubs. It may recur over several years. Small pleural effusions located in the left hemithorax are seen in approximately 85% of patients. Pleural effusions may appear in the absence of pericarditis [85].

The pathogenesis of this syndrome is poorly understood but may be immunologic in origin. Anti-inflammatory agents may be used to treat symptoms although the disorder is self-limiting. Adrenocortical steroids may be used if symptoms are severe [85].

Intra-abdominal Causes

Pancreatitis

Fifteen to 55 percent of patients with acute pancreatitis or with pancreatic pseudo-cyst demonstrate pleuropulmonary abnormalities on chest radiography [86] including; elevated hemidiaphragm, basilar atelectasis, pleural effusion and pleural reaction. Pleural effusions from pancreatitis have been reported between 3% and 17% of cases. They are more common on the left side and a fraction of effusions are bilateral [87]. The pleural effusions are small and form early in the disease. A high concentration of amylase, increased out of proportion to the serum amylase, is a key diagnostic feature. Pleural effusions from pancreatitis do not require specific therapy because they usually resolve as the acute process abates. They tend to recur after thoracentesis [88].

Abdominal Surgery

Pleural fluid collections are often seen after abdominal surgery. Almost half the patients in one large series had a pleural effusion during the postoperative period [89]. Most of the pleural effusions were small. Fluid tended to be ipsilateral following upper abdominal surgery and more often encountered when there was postoperative atelectasis or free abdominal fluid present. Postoperative pleural effusion is usually a self-limited process, not requiring a diagnostic thoracentesis unless infection is suspected [34].

Chylothorax

Chylothorax refers to a pleural effusion that has a characteristic milky appearance with a high lipid content. The fluid, or chyle, has a milky appearance because its content of emulsified fat has light-scattering properties. Chyle has more fat than plasma [90], having a triglyceride concentration higher than 110 mg/dL and showing a chylomicron band in the lipoprotein electrophoresis [91]. The term *chyliform effusion* is confusing; it refers to a fluid resulting from pleural fluid cell degeneration, as might be seen in malignancy. *Pseudochylus* effusion may be seen in tuberculosis or nephrotic syndrome and is thought to be secondary to cholesterol crystals [45]. True chylothorax has important clinical implications. Chylothorax is caused by leakage of thoracic duct lymph or chyle into a pleural space. About 50% of the cases are due to some type of traumatic damage to the thoracic duct. However, many cases of chylothorax are due to tumor such as a lymphoma or involvement of the mediastinum with bronchogenic carcinoma. Chylothorax has been reported as a complication of coronary bypass surgery [92] and is commonly seen in the rare disorder, lymphangioleiomyomatosis. Chylothorax has been described in acute cervical hyperextension injuries [10]. Idiopathic spontaneous chylothorax occurs in approximately a third of cases [93]. The diagnosis of chylothorax may be suspected during thoracentesis if pleural fluid has a milky white appearance and, when allowed to settle, a creamy top layer develops. In only half the cases is the gross appearance of the fluid suggestive of chylothorax [94] because in some malnourished individuals the fluid is serous and in other patients it may be bloody.

Regardless of the cause of chylothorax, it will usually recur soon after initial drainage. Conservative management with repeated aspiration of fluid or thoracostomy tube drainage may be attempted in the hope of spontaneous resolution. However, loss of fat and protein may cause malnutrition, limiting the utility of long-term drainage procedures. Thoracic duct ligation may be necessary in selected cases. Radiation therapy results in adequate control of chylothorax in over 50% of patients with lymphoma or metastatic carcinoma. In the remainder of cases thoracic surgery and possible thoracic duct ligation may be necessary [95].

Disorders of the Diaphragm

The diaphragm is the principal muscle controlling respiration and is almost completely responsible for inspiration during quiet breathing. The structure and function of the diaphragm is unlike any other muscle in the body. Disorders of the diaphragm, which occur often, may be overlooked because the clinical manifestations are not apparent. The following discussion outlines the basic anatomy and physiology, functional disturbances, infections, and tumors of the diaphragm.

Anatomy and Physiology

The diaphragm is a musculotendinous sheet composed of bands of skeletal muscle fibers. The peripheral part has attachments to the back of the xiphoid process, the lower six ribs and their costal cartilages, and the lumbar vertebral bodies. The diaphragm has three major openings: aortic, esophageal, and vena caval. The muscle fibers of the diaphragm also form clefts or potential spaces that may develop anteriorly (foramina of Morgagni) and posteriorly (foramina of Bochdalek) [96].

Although the diaphragm is a single muscular structure, the right and left sides have separate embryologic origins and innervations. Motor fibers of the diaphragm are supplied by the phrenic nerve, which is formed from the C3, C4, and C5 nerve roots. Sensory fibers are supplied by the phrenic nerve and the lower six intercostal nerves. Under normal circumstances, the anterior horn cells of the phrenic nerve are under control of the respiratory center in the dorsal medulla [97].

The diaphragm is a vital pump for the respiratory system, differing from other skeletal muscles because life depends on its function. Inspiration is an active process that results from an increase in intrathoracic volume. On quiet inspiration the diaphragm may provide 75% of this increase in volume. The dome shape of the diaphragm and its attachments allows it to function in two different ways. First, contraction causes descent of the diaphragm and movement of the anterior abdominal wall outward. The second action of the diaphragm is to lift and expand the rib cage [98, 99]. Functional disturbances in diaphragmatic structure may cause severe hypoventilation and respiratory failure.

Functional Disturbances

Hiccup

Hiccup (singultus) results from sudden uncoordinated diaphragmatic and intercostal muscle contractions. The sound is generated from reflex glottic closure. Hiccups have been reported in association with many diseases and disorders. Organic causes include central nervous system dysfunction such as strokes, tumors, neurosyphilis, skull fractures, anesthesia, and encephalitis; neck tumors; and cardiothoracic lesions such as aneurysms, tumors, myocardial infarction, pericarditis, pneumonia, and lung abscess. More commonly, hiccup is caused by intra-abdominal conditions and functional digestive disturbances such as gallbladder disease, pancreatitis, gastritis, and peptic ulcer. Even gastric dilatation, hunger, and alcoholism may result in hiccup [99, 100].

Evaluation of the patient with hiccup involves identifying the underlying cause and may include the following studies: electrocardiography, chest radiography, abdominal radiography, and upper gastrointestinal series. Fluoroscopy may be useful in identifying which part of the diaphragm is involved.

Intractable hiccup can be very debilitating. While various treatment remedies have been proposed, few have been consistently effective. Swallowing ice water, breath holding with closed glottis (Valsalva maneuver), traction on the tongue, and rebreathing air in a paper bag can sometimes break the cycle. Major tranquilizers such as thioridazine (Thorazine) may suppress some central etiologies. The use of local anesthetic spray on the skin of the neck overlying the phrenic nerve may work in cases of unilateral hiccup. Stimulating the pharynx with a nasal catheter has also been reported to have high success rates in curing hiccups [100]. Ultimately, when all medical treatments fail, surgery on the phrenic nerve may be required to eliminate the hiccup [100].

Diaphragmatic Flutter

Diaphragmatic flutter was first reported in 1723 by Leeuwenhoek and is also known as respiratory myoclonus and Leeuwenhoek's disease [101]. Diaphragmatic flutter is due to rapid wave-like contractions that range from 35 to 480 beats per minute [102]. The cause usually is unknown, but a search for any irritative focus of the diaphragm or phrenic nerve should be carried out. Patients with diaphragmatic flutter may complain of palpitations of their upper abdomen or lower chest. On occasion this flutter may simulate angina, myocardial infarction, or pericarditis. Fluoroscopy establishes the diagnosis. Blockade of the phrenic nerve, quinidine, corticosteroids, and phenytoin (Dilantin) have sometimes been used to correct the flutter [102].

Eventration of the Diaphragm

Eventration describes a diaphragm that is thin and has been displaced upward in the thorax by the liver and viscera [103]. This displacement may be caused by a congenital abnormality that is uncommon or it may be acquired due to paralysis of the diaphragm [100]. Congenital eventration consists of a thick membranous sheet that replaces the normal diaphragmatic musculature that has not developed [104]. Eventrations appearing in childhood are most likely to be on the right side, while those in adulthood are usually on the left side [103]. Large eventrations are more likely to cause symptoms of respiratory insufficiency and are more common in children. Adults with eventration develop symptoms only if other pulmonary diseases have decreased their respiratory reserves [100].

Diaphragmatic Hernias

Hiatal Hernia Approximately 75% of diaphragmatic hernias occur through the esophageal hiatus. They are caused by an acquired widening of the esophageal hiatus by increased intra-abdominal pressure in older persons, especially those who are obese. The sliding hiatal hernias are much more common than the paraesophageal type. With sliding hernias, the cardioesophageal junction of the stomach slides upward into the posterior mediastinum. At least 50% of patients with sliding hernias are asymptomatic, while others may have symptoms of reflux or vague upper abdominal discomfort. Changes in posture such as recumbency, stooping, or squatting may exacerbate the symptoms. In paraesophageal hernias, the gastroesophageal junction is not displaced [105]. Occasionally, the hernia is large enough such that incarceration or volvulus of the stomach occurs [106]. Routine chest radiography sometimes shows a fixed hiatal hernia by an air–fluid level behind the cardiac shadow on the lateral view. More definitive diagnosis is usually made by a barium study, esophagoscopy, or esophageal motility study [103]. Most symptomatic patients respond to conservative medical treatment such as weight loss, elevation of the head of the bed, and antireflux dietary measures. Surgical repair is usually reserved for those few patients who do not respond to medical therapy alone.

Hernias Through the Foramina of Bochdalek and Morgagni Bochdalek hernia is a common cause of respiratory distress in the newborn, usually within the first 24 hours after birth. This is a neonatal thoracoabdominal emergency and requires prompt surgical repair. It is caused by a congenital posterolateral defect in the diaphragm and results in visceral herniation into the thorax. Over 90% of the hernias are left sided [107]. Bochdalek hernias in adults are usually detected as an asymptomatic posterior mediastinal mass on chest radiography [103].

Morgagni hernia in the retrosternal region typically appears in adults. It is usually associated with obesity, trauma, or increased intraabdominal pressure. Morgagni hernia is most often right sided and usually contains omentum and transverse colon. The importance of Morgagni hernias comes when they resemble intrathoracic tumors or cysts, and exploration is needed to determine the nature of the mass [103].

Traumatic hernia and rupture are covered in Chap. 19.

Diaphragmatic Paralysis

Paralysis of the diaphragm has many causes. In the newborn it may be caused by birth trauma. In older patients, the causes of paralysis are infectious, malignant, or iatrogenic. Older children and adults tolerate unilateral paralysis of the diaphragm and are often asymptomatic as only a 20% loss in lung ventilation and perfusion occurs [103]. In our experience, diaphragmatic dysfunction in association with even mild pulmonary parenchymal disease such as emphysema may be quite symptomatic, especially in the elderly.

Paralysis of the diaphragm has been reported in association with various viral syndromes such as herpes zoster and poliomyelitis. It also may occur as a complication of serum sickness from tetanus and diphtheria antitoxin. However, the most common cause of unilateral diaphragmatic paralysis is involvement of the phrenic nerve by tumor, either metastatic or primary. When bronchogenic carcinoma or mediastinal metastasis causes diaphragmatic paralysis, the disease is presumed inoperable. Patients are said to have idiopathic diaphragmatic paralysis when there is no satisfactory explanation or cause determined. This accounts for the second largest number of causes of unilateral diaphragmatic paralysis [100].

Bilateral diaphragmatic paralysis is most likely seen with chronic neuromuscular disease or spinal cord transection. Guillain-Barré syndrome is the most common cause of respiratory failure among the neuromuscular diseases [108]. Respiratory failure may occur when there is severe spinal cord involvement in multiple sclerosis. In amyotrophic lateral sclerosis respiratory failure from muscular inadequacy is the most common cause of death [109]. Traumatic damage to the spinal cord above C3 results in complete paralysis of the diaphragm and intercostal muscles. Before the development of the phrenic nerve pacer, these patients were permanently dependent on a mechanical ventilator [110]. Phrenic nerve palsy following cardiac surgery has been frequently reported in the literature. The phrenic nerve is positioned anatomically so that it is exposed to severe prolonged hypothermia with topical cooling of the heart during coronary bypass surgery. As the bag of ice is packed around the heart, it is applied to the nerve, with subsequent nerve injury. Paralysis also may occur without the use of topical cardiac hypothermia and the left phrenic nerve is more at risk. Unilateral paresis may result in minor symptoms, but bilateral paresis can result in chronic ventilatory insufficiency [111–113]. Paralysis of the right hemidiaphragm may be asymptomatic, but in left-sided paralysis the upward displacement of the stomach may cause gastrointestinal symptoms. Patients with diaphragmatic paralysis become breathless when they lie down. The chest wall motion is different in patients with diaphragmatic paralysis. In bilateral paralysis there is intercostal muscle retraction and paradoxical movement of the anterior abdominal wall inward during inspiration [98, 100]. These abnormalities may be even more pronounced during rapid eye movement sleep when there is generalized striated muscle paralysis. Diagnosis of diaphragmatic paralysis may be confirmed by fluoroscopy, electromyelography of the phrenic nerve, and measurement of transdiaphragmatic pressures [99].

Diaphragmatic Fatigue

Diaphragmatic fatigue is a recognized entity in which the diaphragm cannot maintain the work required for adequate ventilation. As with any muscle, fatigue occurs when the energy demand of the respiratory muscle exceeds the energy supply. There are many conditions that may result in diaphragmatic fatigue and should be considered in the differential diagnosis of diaphragmatic paralysis and weakness [114].

The energy supply to the diaphragm may be reduced in states of low cardiac output, hypoxemia, anemia, or malnutrition. The work of the diaphragm may be increased in conditions of airway obstruction such as occurs in asthma, chronic bronchitis, and emphysema. Hyperinflated pulmonary conditions also increase the work of breathing by causing shortening of the muscle fibers of the diaphragm and decreasing their maximal strength [103]. Usually there are several interrelated causes of diaphragmatic fatigue present in the same patient.

Various systemic disorders may involve the diaphragm and result in fatigue. Respiratory muscle weakness is part of the clinical criteria that define polymyositis and dermatomyositis [115]. Weakness also may contribute to the dyspnea present in scleroderma. Diaphragmatic fatigue and respiratory failure may be the first manifestation of myasthenia gravis [116]. Respiratory muscle weakness also may be a prominent feature of both hyperthyroidism and myxedema. Although the pathogenesis of respiratory failure in myxedema is multifactorial, there have been reports of phrenic nerve dysfunction in some of these patients [117].

Respiratory fatigue and failure have also been reported secondary to certain medications. The mechanism is thought to be due to neuromuscular blockade. Trimethadione (Tridione), neomycin sulfate (Neobiotic Sulfate), streptomycin (Streptomycin), polymyxin B (Aerosporin), and polymyxin E (Colistin) are among some of the drugs implicated [100]. The aminoglycosides and clindamycin can produce clinically significant neuromuscular paralysis and may enhance the action of other blocking agents. The mechanism appears to involve both an inhibition of the presynaptic release of acetylcholine and blocking of the postsynaptic receptor sites for acetylcholine. The neuromuscular paralysis caused by aminoglycosides usually results from rapid infusion of a bolus or a very high concentration of drug and can sometimes be reversed by prompt administration of calcium [118].

Acute respiratory failure has also been reported in association with hypophosphatemia. The respiratory system as a whole is especially susceptible to three hematologic complications of hypophosphatemia. These complications include hemolytic anemia, an increase in oxyhemoglobin affinity, and leukocyte dysfunction. Muscle contraction is also well known to require adenosine triphosphate a high energy phosphate containing compound. Patients with significant hypophosphatemia may develop ventilatory collapse because of impaired energy production and diphragmatic function and require mechanical ventilation [119].

Untreated respiratory fatigue can progress to respiratory failure. The radiologic evaluation of diaphragmatic fatigue includes plain film of the chest, electromyelography, and fluoroscopy. These studies can often aid in distinguishing diaphragmatic fatigue, weakness, and paralysis. Treatment of diaphragmatic fatigue generally requires ventilatory support that rests the respiratory muscles [100].

Infections of the Diaphragm

Infections of the diaphragm are rarely recognized despite the diaphragm being involved in infections of the pleural and peritoneal spaces. The diaphragm also may be involved in various parasitic infections. Of these infections, those involving intra-abdominal processes are most important.

Subdiaphragmatic Abscess

Subphrenic abscess is still a significant problem that complicates various surgical procedures. Although different definitions have been proposed for what constitutes the subphrenic space, for practical purposes it is defined as the region bounded by the diaphragm above and the transverse colon and mesocolon below. A subphrenic abscess is a collection of pus directly beneath the diaphragm. Several years ago, abdominal abscesses were commonly caused by intraperitoneal spread from a perforated viscus. Common primary diseases that may result in perforation include appendicitis, diverticulitis, cholecystitis, pelvic abscess, and peptic ulcer disease [120]. Today, there is a significant increase in the incidence of subphrenic abscess due to abdominal surgery or trauma [121].

Subphrenic abscesses should be considered as a thoracoabdominal clinical complex. Through radioactive cell-tagged studies a clear-cut pathway of lymphatic spread has been shown [119]. This is presumed to explain localization of infection below the diaphragm and spread through the diaphragm and into the thorax in advanced and untreated cases.

Subdiaphragmatic abscesses on the right side predominate. Clinical series have shown that biliary tract surgery was the most common cause for abscess on the right side. This was followed by gastric and duodenal surgery and right colon carcinoma resection [122]. Splenectomy was the most common procedure found to cause left-sided subphrenic abscesses. Gastric surgery, resection of left colon carcinoma, and hiatal hernia repair were also shown to result in left subphrenic abscess in descending order [120].

Thoracic symptoms referable to the diaphragm, including shoulder pain, hiccups, and pleurisy, should suggest the possibility of infection below the diaphragm. Pleuritic chest pain and fever were consistent findings in most patients with subphrenic abscess. Abdominal pain, nausea, vomiting, and ileus are often present and suggest some intra-abdominal process. Most abscesses cultured more than one organism. *Escherichia coli,* streptococci, and staphylococci are still the most common organisms. However, there has alos been an increase in gram-negative bacteria such as *Klebsiella, Aerobacter, Proteus,* and *Pseudomonas* [120].

Several radiographic studies may be useful in proving a subdiaphragmatic abscess. Plain films of the chest may reveal pleural effusion, consolidation, elevation of one hemidiaphragm, and air–fluid levels. Ultrasound is also effective in showing fluid-filled cavities. These cavities appear as complex fluid collections with debris and septae. Computed tomographic scanning shows the exact anatomic location and extent of the abscess and helps in planning the approach for drainage [122].

Subphrenic abscess is like an abscess elsewhere in the body and surgical or computed tomographic guided drainage is the treatment of choice. The use of antibiotics may cloud the clinical picture and has increased the number of cases that are subacute or chronic [121]. Also, in subacute or chronic walled off abscesses, the antibiotics may not reach the abscess cavity in concentrations high enough to destroy the bacteria.

Parasitic Infections

The diaphragm also may be involved in various parasitic infections. These include paragonimiasis, amebiasis, and trichinosis. *Entamoeba histolytica* is a protozoan that causes deep infections in the bowel wall. Diaphragmatic amebiasis is usually secondary to contiguous involvement from hepatic amebiasis. Paragonimus is a lung fluke that may penetrate the diaphragm as it tunnels through the lung [123].

Trichinosis is the only parasitic infection in which major diaphragmatic involvement occurs. The disease develops from ingesting undercooked meat, usually pork or bear, that contains the larvae of *Trichinella spiralis*. By hematogenous spread the larvae are deposited in muscles throughout the body. The larvae may become concentrated in the diaphragm and intercostal muscles, resulting in progressive weakness of these muscles. A severe enough infection may result in profound muscle weakness, myopathy, and acute respiratory failure, requiring ventilatory support. There is no satisfactory treatment for trichinosis. When a patient is known to have ingested the infected meat within 24 hours, thiabendazole or mebendazole should be given for 1 week. These drugs have little effect on the muscle larvae and have not been shown to alter the overall course of established infections. Severe symptoms can sometimes be controlled with bed rest, salicylates, and corticosteroids [124].

Tumors of the Diaphragm

Diaphragmatic tumors are rare. Most of the time, irregularities in the contour of the diaphragm represent local weakness or eventration. Of the reported primary tumors of the diaphragm, malignant neoplasms are slightly more common than benign ones [125]. Of the benign tumors, lipomas are the most common [126]. Other types include fibromas, angiofibromas, neurofibromas, and neurilemmomas. Most are asymptomatic and discovered only on chest radiography or at postmortem examination [127].

Primary malignant tumors of the diaphragm are all sarcomas and most frequently fibrosarcomas. Most patients are symptomatic, with referred diaphragmatic pain to the neck, shoulder, upper abdomen, or back. They also may complain of pleuritic chest pain. Pleural effusion frequently accompanies diaphragmatic malignancies. Metastatic tumors of the diaphragm are most often due to direct extension from adjacent organs. Direct spread is from tumors of the lung, stomach, pancreas, adrenal, kidney, colon, and liver. Lymphomas and breast tumors also may involve the diaphragm [128]. Computed tomographic scan is the most helpful radiographic technique for evaluating diaphragmatic masses. However, because the benign or malignant nature of the tumor cannot be established without histology, all diaphragmatic tumors must be removed by thoracotomy [103].

Cystic and inflammatory lesions may be included in a discussion of diaphragmatic masses. Cystic lesions may be congenital or acquired. Congenital cysts are mesothelial or bronchogenic in origin, while acquired cysts may develop from a posttraumatic hematoma [129] or from chronic inflammation in tuberculosis and hydatid disease [130]. Rarely, endometriosis in women may cause diaphragmatic defects or tumors. Although endometriosis of the diaphragm cannot be seen by radiography, there have been several case reports of recurrent pneumothorax in association with endometrial deposits [131].

Pleural and diaphragmatic diseases are common disorders seen in the primary care practice. They must be considered in the differential diagnosis of any patient who complains of chest symptoms. The causes are many and treatments vary. This chapter has clarified many of these problems from a primary care perspective.

References

1. Broaddus C, Staub NC: Pleural liquid and protein turnover in health and disease. *Semin Respir Med* 9:7–12, 1987
2. Siefkin A, Hirasuna J: Evaluation of the pleural effusion. *Medical Rounds* 2:54, 1988
3. Tattersall MHN: Intracavitary treatment of malignant pleural effusions. *Chemioterapia* 1:288–292, 1982
4. Leff A, Hopewell PC, Costello J: Pleural effusion from malignancy. *Ann Intern Med* 88:532–537, 1978
5. Agostoni E, Taglietti A, Setnikar I: Absorption force of the capillaries of the visceral pleura in determination of the intrapleural pressure. *Am J Physiol* 191:277–282, 1957
6. Wang NS: The preformed stomas connecting the pleural cavity and the lymphatics in the parietal pleura. *Am Rev Respir Dis* 111:12–20, 1975
7. Miserocchi G, Agostoni E: Contents of the pleural space. *J Appl Physiol* 30:208–213, 1971
8. Light RW: Physiology of the pleural space. *In* Pleural Diseases. Philadelphia, Lea & Febiger, 1990, pp 9–19
9. Sahn S: Pleural Disease, Eighth national ACCP pulmonary board review course, Infromedix, Garden Grove, CA, 1990
10. Sahn SA: The pleura. *Am Rev Respir Dis* 138:184–234, 1988
11. Light RW: Pleural effusions. *Med Clin North Am* 61:1341–1342, 1977
12. Vladutiu AO: Pleural Effusion. New York, *Futura,* 1986, p 9
13. Siefkin A, Hirasuna J: Evaluation of the pleural effusion. *Medical Rounds* 1:59–64, 1988
14. Roth BJ, O'Mhara TF, Cragun WH: The serum-effusion albumin gradient in the evaluation of pleural effusions. *Chest* 98:546–549, 1990
15. Black LF: The pleural space and pleural fluid. *Mayo Clin Proc* 47:493–506, 1972
16. Ream CR: Pleural effusions. A review of some basic facts and pertinent clinical remarks. *Journal of the Medical Society of New Jersey* 60:375, 1963
17. DeSouza R, Lipsett N, Spagnolo SV: Mediastinal compression due to tension hydrothorax. *Chest* 72:782, 1977
18. Neagley SR, Zwillich CW: The effect of positional changes on oxygenation in patients with pleural effusions. *Chest* 88:714, 1985
19. Sahebjami H, Loudon RG: Pleural effusions: pathophysiology and clinical features. *Semin Roetgenol* 12:269–275, 1977
20. Lowell JR: Pleural effusions. Baltimore, University Park Press, 1977, pp 15–17
21. Hughson WG, Friedman PJ, Feign DS, et al: Postpartum pleural effusion: A common radiologic finding. *Ann Intern Med* 97:856–858, 1982
22. Bedford DE, Lovibond JL: Hydrothorax in heart failure. *Br Heart J* 3:93, 1941
23. Rabin CB, Blackman NS: Bilateral pleural effusion; its significance in association with a heart of normal size. *J Mt Sinai Hosp* 24: 45–53, 1957
24. Mellins RB, Levine OR, Fishman AP: Effect of systemic and pulmonary venous hypertension on pleural and pericardial fluid accumulation. *J Appl Physiol* 29:564–569, 1970
25. Wiener-Kronich JP, Matthay MA, Callen PW, et al: Relationship of pleural effusions to pulmonary hemodynamics in patients with congestive heart failure. *Am Rev Respir Dis* 132:1253–1256, 1985
26. Laufer ST: Interlobar effusion associated with heart disease. *Nova Scotia Med Bull* 25:299–304, 1965
27. Millard CE: Vanishing or phantom tumor of the lung: Localized interlobar effusion in congestive heart failure. *Chest* 59:675–677, 1971
28. Pillay VKG: Total proteins in serous fluids in cardiac failure. *S Afr Med J* 39:142–143, 1965
29. Race GA, Scheifley CH, Edwards JE: Hydrothorax in congestive heart failure. *Am J Med* 22:83–89, 1957
30. Light RW, Erozan YS, Ball WC: Cells in pleural fluid: Their value in differential diagnosis. *Arch Intern Med* 132:854–860, 1973
31. Plum GE, Bruwer AJ, Clagett OT: Chronic constrictive pericarditis; Roentgenologic findings in 35 surgically proved cases. *Proc Mayo Clin* 32:555–556, 1957
32. Weiss JM, Spodick DH: Association of left pleural effusions with pericardial disease. *N Engl J Med* 309:13, 1983
33. Perez CA, Presant CA, Van Amburg AL III: Management of superior vena cava syndrome. *Semin Oncol* 5:123–143, 1978
34. Light RW: *Pleural Diseases.* Philadelphia, Lea & Febiger, 1983
35. Johnston RF, Loo RV: Hepatic hydrothorax; studies to determine the source of the fluid and report of thirteen cases. *Ann Intern Med* 61:385–401, 1964
36. Lieberman FL, Hidemura R, Peters RL, et al: Pathogenesis and treatment of hydrothorax complicating cirrhosis with ascites. *Ann Intern Med* 64:341–351, 1966
37. Frazer IH, Lichtenstein M, Andrews JT:

Pleuroperitoneal effusion without ascites. *Med J Aust* 2:520, 1983
38. Case records of the Massachusetts General Hospital (Case 10-1963). *N Engl J Med* 268: 320–325, 1963
39. Islam N, Ali S, Kabir H: Hepatic hydrothorax. *Br J Dis Chest* 59:222–227, 1965
40. Falchuk KR, Jacoby I, Colucci WS, et al: Tetracycline-induced pleural symphysis for recurrent hydrothorax complicating cirrhosis. *Gastroenterology* 72:319–321, 1977
41. Rudnick MR, Coyle JF, Beck LH, et al: Acute massive hydrothorax complicating dialysis. Report of 2 cases and a review of the literature. *Clin Nephrol* 12:38–44, 1979
42. Nassberger L: Left-sided pleural effusion secondary to continuous ambulatory peritoneal dialysis. *Acta Med Scand* 211:219–220, 1982
43. Calen MA, Steinberg SM, Lowrie EG, et al: Uremic pleural effusion—A study in 14 patients on chronic dialysis. *Ann Intern Med* 82:359, 1975
44. Chernow B, Sahn SA: Carcinomatous involvement of the pleura. *Am J Med* 63: 695, 1977
45. Fraser RG, Paré JA, Paré PD, et al (eds): The Pleura in Diagnosis of Diseases of the Chest. Philadelphia, W.B. Saunders, 1991, p 2728
46. Sahn S: Malignant pleural effusions. *Semin Respir Med* 9:43–53, 1987
47. Clarkson B: Relationship between cell type, glucose concentration and response to treatment in neoplastic effusions. *Cancer* 17: 914–928, 1964
48. Sahn SA, Good JT Jr: Pleural fluid pH in malignant effusions. Diagnostic, prognostic and therapeutic implications. *Ann Intern Med* 108:345–349, 1988
49. Brinkman GL: The significance of pleural effusion complicating otherwise operable bronchogenic carcinoma. *Dis Chest* 36:152, 1959
50. Decker DA, Dines DE, Payne WS, et al: The significance of cytologically negative pleural effusion in bronchogenic carcinoma. *Chest* 74:640–642, 1978
51. Chernow B, Sahn SA: Carcinomatous involvement of the pleura: Analysis of 96 patients. *Am J Med* 63:695–702, 1977
52. Meyer PC: Metastatic carcinoma of the pleura. *Thorax* 21:437–43, 1966
53. Fentiman IS, Millis R, Sexton S, et al: Pleural effusions in breast cancer: A review of 105 cases. *Cancer* 47:2087–2092, 1981
54. Bachman AL, Macken K: Pleural effusions following supervoltage radiation for breast carcinoma. *Radiology* 72:699–709, 1959
55. Meigs JV, Cass JW: Fibroma of the ovary with ascites and hydrothorax. With a report of seven cases. *Am J Obstet Gynecol* 33:249, 1937
56. Mokrohisky JF: So-called "Meigs's syndrome" associated with benign and malignant ovarian tumors. *Radiology* 70:578, 1958
57. Stead WW, Eichenholz A, Stauss HK: Operative and pathologic findings in twenty-four patients with syndrome of idiopathic pleurisy with effusion, presumably tuberculous. *Am Rev Respir Dis* 71:473, 1955
58. Berger HW, Mejia E: Tuberculous pleurisy. *Chest* 63:88–92, 1973
59. Levine H, Metzger W, Lacera D, et al: Diagnosis of tuberculous pleurisy by culture of pleural biopsy specimen. *Arch Intern Med* 126:269–271, 1970
60. Leslie WK, Kinasewitz GT: Clinical characteristics of the patient with nonspecific pleuritis. *Chest* 94:603, 1988
61. Donowitz GR, Mandell FL: Acute pneumonia. *In* Mandell GL, Douglas RG Jr, Bennett JE (eds): Principles and Practice of Infectious Disease, ed 3. New York, Churchill Livingstone, 1990, pp 540–555
62. Light RW, Girard WM, Jenkinson SG, et al: Parapneumonic effusions. *Am J Med* 69: 985–986, 1980
63. Light RW, MacGregor MI, Ball WC Jr, et al: Diagnostic significance of pleural fluid pH and PCO_2. *Chest* 64:591–596, 1973
64. Potts DE, Levin DC, Sahn SA: Pleural fluid pH in parapneumonic effusions. *Chest* 70: 328–331, 1976
65. Bartlett JG, Finegold SM: Anaerobic infections of the lung and pleural space. *Am Rev Respir Dis* 10:56–77, 1974
66. Micel L, Grillo HC, Malt RA: Operative and non-operative management of esophageal perforations. *Ann Surg* 194:57–63, 1981
67. Keszler P, Buzna E: Surgical and conservative management of esophageal perforation. *Chest* 80:158–162, 1981
68. Bynum LJ, Wilson JE III. Radiographic features of pleural effusions in pulmonary embolism. *Am Rev Respir Dis* 117:829–834, 1978
69. Storey DD, Dines DE, Coles DT: Pleural effusion: A diagnostic dilemma. *JAMA* 236: 2183–2186, 1976
70. Hampton AO, Castleman B: Correlation of postmortem chest teleroentgenograms with autopsy finding, with special reference to pulmonary embolism and infarction. *Am J Roentgenol Radium Ther Nucl Med* 43:305, 1940
71. Purnell DC, Baggenstoss AH, Olsen AM: Pulmonary lesions in disseminated lupus erythematosus. *Ann Intern Med* 42:619–620, 1955

72. Good JT Jr, King TE, Anthony VB, et al: Lupus pleuritis: Clinical features and pleural fluid characteristics with special reference to pleural fluid antinuclear antibody titers. *Chest* 84:714–718, 1983
73. Gould DM, Dayes ML: Roentgenologic findings in systemic lupus erythematosus. *J Chronic Dis* 2:136–145, 1955
74. Halla JT, Schrohenloher RE, Volankis JE: Immune complexes and other laboratory features of pleural effusions. *Ann Intern Med* 92:748–752, 1980
75. Good JT Jr, King TE, Anthony VB, et al: Lupus pleuritis: Clinical features and pleural fluid characteristics with special reference to pleural fluid antinuclear antibody titers. *Chest* 84:714–718, 1983
76. Carr DT, Mayne JG: Pleurisy with effusion in rheumatoid arthritis, with reference to the low concentration of glucose in pleural fluid. *Am Rev Respir Dis* 85:345, 1962
77. Carr DT, McGuckin WF: Pleural fluid glucose. *Am Rev Respir Dis* 97:302–305, 1968
78. Light RW, Ball WC Jr: Glucose and amylase in pleural effusions. *JAMA* 225:257, 1973
79. Jones FL, Blodgett RC: Empyema in rheumatoid pleuro-pulmonary disease. *Ann Intern Med* 74:665–671, 1971
80. Sahn SA, Lakshminarayan S, Char DC: "Silent" empyemas in patients on corticosteroids. *Am Rev Respir Dis* 107:873–876, 1973
81. Andrews BS, Arora NS, Shadforth MF, et al: The role of immune complexes in the pathogenesis of pleural effusions. *Am Rev Respir Dis* 124:115–120, 1981
82. Hunninghake GW, Fauci AS: Pulmonary involvement in the collagen vascular diseases. *Am Rev Respir Dis* 119:471–503, 1979
83. Dressler W: The post-myocardial infarction syndrome. *Arch Intern Med* 103:28, 1959
84. Kaminsky ME, Rodan BA, Osborne DR, et al: Post-pericardiotomy syndrome. *AJR* 138: 503–508, 1982
85. Domby WR, Whitcomb ME: Pleural effusion as a manifestation of Dressler's syndrome in the distant post-infarction period. *Am Heart J* 96:243, 1978
86. Kaye MD: Pleuropulmonary complications of pancreatitis. *Thorax* 23:297–305, 1968
87. Hammarsten JF, Honska WL Jr, Lines BJ: Pleural fluid amylase in pancreatitis and other diseases. *Am Rev Tuberculosis* 79:606, 1959
88. Cameron JL: Chronic pancreatic ascites and pancreatic pleural effusions. *Gastroenterology* 74:134–140, 1978
89. Light RW, George RB: Incidence and significance of pleural effusion after abdominal surgery. *Chest* 69:621–626, 1976
90. Nix JT, Albert M, Dugas JE, et al: Chylothorax and chylous ascites: A study of 302 selective cases. *Am J Gastroenterol* 28:40–55, 1957
91. Seriff NS, Cohen ML, Samuel P, et al: Chylothorax: Diagnosis by lipoprotein electrophoresis of serum and pleural fluid. *Thorax* 32:98–100, 1977
92. Zakhour BJ, Drucker MH, Franco AA: Chylothorax as a complication of aortocoronary bypass. Two case reports and a review of the literature. *Scand J Thorac Cardiovasc Surg* 22:95, 1988
93. Schmidt A: Chylothorax. Review of 5 year's cases in the literature and report of a case. *Acta Chir Scand* 118:5, 1959
94. Saats BA, Ellefson RD, Budahn LL, et al: The lipoprotein profile of chylous and non chylous pleural effusions. *Mayo Clin Proc 55:700, 1980*
95. Michel L, Grillo HC, Malt RA: Operative and non-operative management of esophageal perforations. *Ann Surg* 194:57–63, 1981
96. Leak LV: Gross and ultrastructural morphologic features of the diaphragm. *Am Rev Respir Dis* 119:3–21, 1979
97. Nochomovitz ML, Peterson DK, Stellato TA, et al: Electrical activation of the diaphragm. *Clin Chest Med* 9:349–358, 1988
98. Derenne JP, Macklem PT, Roussol CL: The respiratory muscles: mechanics, control, and pathophysiology, Part I. *Am Rev Respir Dis* 118:119–133, 1978
99. Loh L, Goldman M, Davis JN: The assessment of diaphragm function. *Medicine* 56: 165–169, 1977
100. Derenne JP, Macklem PT, Roussos CL: The respiratory muscles: Mechanics, control and pathophysiology, Part III. *Am Rev Respir Dis* 118:581–601, 1978
101. Phillips JR, Eldridge FL: Respiratory myoclonus (Leeuwenhoek's disease). *N Engl J Med* 289:1390, 1973
102. Rigatto M, DeMederos NP: Diaphragmatic flutter. Report of a case and review of the literature. *Am J Med* 32:103, 1962
103. Tarver RD, Godwin JD, Putman CE: The diaphragm. *Radiol Clin North Am* 22:615–631, 1984
104. Laxdal OE, McDonald HA, Mellin GW: Congenital eventration of the diaphragm. *N Engl J Med* 250:401, 1954
105. Ellis FH: Esophageal hiatal hernia. *N Engl J Med* 287:646, 1972
106. Pearson FG, Cooper JD, Ilves R, et al: Massive hiatal hernia with incarceration: A report of 53 cases. *Ann Thorac Surg* 35:45–51, 1983
107. Naeye RL, Shochat SJ, Whitman V, et al: Unsuspected pulmonary abnormalities associ-

ated with diaphragmatic hernia. *Pediatrics* 58:902–906, 1976
108. O'Donohue WJ, Baker JP, Bell GM, et al: Respiratory failure in neuromuscular disease: Management in a respiratory intensive care unit. *JAMA* 235:733, 1976
109. Fromm GB, Wisdom PJ, Block AJ: Amyotrophic lateral sclerosis presenting with respiratory failure. *Chest* 71:612, 1977
110. Nochomovitz ML, Peterson DK, Stellato TA, et al: Electrical activation of the diaphragm. *Clin Chest Med* 9:349–358, 1988
111. Curtis JJ, Nawarawong W, Walls JT, et al: Elevated hemidiaphragm after cardiac operations: Incidence, prognosis, and relationship to the use of topical ice slush. *Ann Thorac Surg* 48:764–768, 1989
112. Chandler KW, Rozas CJ, et al: Bilateral diaphragmatic paralysis complicating local cardiac hypothermia during open heart surgery. *Am J Med* 77:243–249, 1984
113. Kohorst WR, Schonfeld SA, Altman M: Bilateral diaphragmatic paralysis following topical cardiac hypothermia. *Chest* 85:65–68, 1984
114. Roussos C, Macklem PT: The respiratory muscles. *N Engl J Med* 307:786–797, 1982
115. Bolian A, Peter JB: Polymyositis and dermatomyositis. *N Engl J Med* 292:344, 1975
116. Selecky PA, Ziment I: Prolonged respirator support for the treatment of intractable myasthenia gravis. *Chest* 65:207–209, 1974
117. Domm BM, Vassallo CL: Myxedema como with respiratory failure. *Am Rev Respir Dis* 107:842–845, 1973
118. Pittinger CB, Adamson R: Antibiotic blockade of neuromuscular function. *Annu Rev Pharmacol* 12:169, 1972
119. Newman JH, Neff TA, Ziporin P: Acute respiratory failure associated with hypophosphatemia. *N Engl J Med* 296:1101–1105, 1977
120. Roberts EAB, Nealon TF: Subphrenic abscess: Comparison between operative and antibiotic management. *Ann Surg* 180:209, 1974
121. Carter R, Brewer LA: Subphrenic abscess: A thoracoabdominal clinical complex. *Am J Surg* 108:165–174, 1964
122. Connell TR, Stephens DH, Carlson HC, et al: Upper abdominal abscess: A continuing and deadly problem. *AJR* 134:759–765, 1980
123. Roberts PP: Parasitic infections of the pleural space. *Semin Respir Infect* 3:362–382, 1988
124. Brashear RE, Martin RR, Glover JL: Trichinosis and respiratory failure. *Am Rev Respir Dis* 104:245, 1971
125. Schwartz EE, Wechsler RJ: Diaphragmatic and paradiaphragmatic tumors and pseudotumors. *J Thorac Imaging* 4:19–28, 1989
126. Ferguson DD, Westcott JL: Lipoma of the diaphragm. *Radiology* 118:527–528, 1976
127. Anderson LS, Forrest JV: Tumors of the diaphragm. *Am J Roent Rad Ther* 119:259–265, 1973
128. Olafsson G, Rausing A, Holen O: Primary tumors of the diaphragm. *Chest* 59:568–570, 1971
129. Juvara I, Priseu A: Primary congenital diaphragmatic tumors. *Surgery* 60:255–259, 1966
130. Talana JA: Thoracic hydatid echinococcosis: diagnosis and treatment. *Dis Chest* 49:8–14, 1966
131. Davies R: Recurring spontaneous pneumothorax concomitant with menstruation. *Thorax* 23:370–373, 1968

Occupational Lung Disease

Walter J. Talamonti and William H. Heckman

Occupational diseases, particularly those of the lungs, have been recognized with increasing frequency over the past several decades as more has become known about exposure to specific agents. Unfortunately, the manifestations of this exposure are usually not recognized until a significant amount of time has elapsed and the disease has progressed.

Early recognition of occupational exposure requires a good occupational history from the patient. Coupled with a thorough understanding of the more common occupational hazards, the patient history will help the primary care physician develop a differential diagnosis. From here, he or she can make judicious use of laboratory tests to obtain the exact diagnosis. Some of the more common occupational exposures relevant to a primary care practice are discussed in this chapter.

Carbon Monoxide

Carbon monoxide (CO) is an odorless, invisible, tasteless gas that is the product of incomplete combustion of carbon-containing materials. Exposure can be from three sources: the surrounding environment, occupational exposure, and smoking.

Occupational exposure is significant in the following processes: catalytic crackers in petroleum refining, iron foundries, basic oxygen furnaces, sintering of blast furnace feed in steel mills, Kraft recovery furnaces in Kraft paper mills, and coke ovens [1]. Fire fighters, automotive mechanics, miners, welders, tunnel construction workers, and traffic controllers also may be exposed to CO. The environmental exposure occurs mainly from automobiles, with the gasoline powered internal combustion engine accounting for half of the total CO produced in 1968 [2]. The environmental exposure in urban areas exhibits a bifid pattern. This is greatest during the rush hour commute, usually 7 to 9 AM and 4 to 6 PM [3]. Smoking includes not only those individuals who smoke cigars, pipes, and cigarettes, but also those who are in confined spaces with smokers [4].

The severe exposure problem for CO is created by the great affinity for the substance to combine with hemoglobin. It has 240 times the affinity for hemoglobin than oxygen according to Haldane [5]. Due to this high affinity, small percentages of CO can result in high percentages of carboxyhemoglobin. Cigarette smokers can have carboxyhemoglobin levels of 5% to 7% or higher. Levels as low as 10% may produce headaches in most adults. Increasing concentrations produce giddiness, weakness, nausea, coma, and ultimately death with levels greater than 50%. Carboxyhemoglobin levels and their corresponding symptoms are listed in Table 14-1.

Carbon monoxide changes the configuration of hemoglobin so as to increase its affinity for oxygen. This results in impaired oxygen release to metabolizing cells at the tissue level. Cardiac output must increase to maintain adequate oxygen transport. Patients with occult cardiac disease may be prone to lethal cardiac levels less than that normally considered to cause a fatality because of these increased demands. The increased heart rate and cardiac output in CO poisoning along with diminished coronary circulation results in myocardial ischemia, which in turn may precipitate arrhythmias [6]. A recent study noted that the number and complexity of ventricular arrhythmias increased significantly during exercise with carboxyhemoglobin levels of 6% [6a].

Subacute or chronic exposure can result in

Table 14-1. Carboxyhemoglobin Levels and Their Symptoms

Levels of Carboxyhemoglobin (%)	*Symptoms*
10	Headache
10–20	Giddiness and tinnitus
20–30	Weakness and nausea
About 30	Clouding of mental capacity
35–45	Collapse and coma
> 50	Death in young adults [2]

"flu-like" symptoms and chronic headache. Also, excessive sweating, fever, hepatomegaly, skin lesions, leukocytosis, albuminuria, and glucosuria have been noted [7].

Treatment

Treatment requires removal from exposure and then use of pure oxygen by face mask. This will decrease the normal half-life of CO from 4 hours at room temperature to about 60 to 90 minutes. Half-life may be shortened further with the use of a ventilator and 100% oxygen [8, 9]. When a patient is comatose or has cardiac dysfunction, hyperbaric oxygen may be helpful [10]. To decrease oxygen demand, the patient should be kept absolutely quiet.

Hydrogen Cyanide

Hydrogen cyanide is a colorless, flammable, and explosive gas or liquid that has the smell of bitter almonds. It has many uses in industry, including use in the synthesis of acrylates and nitrites, as a fumigant, in electroplating, and in the extraction of gold and silver from ores. Some of the workers exposed to cyanide include jewelers, fumigant workers, electroplaters, coke oven workers, blast furnace workers, and acrylate makers [11].

Hydrogen cyanide is a potent and rapid acting poison. As little as 50 to 200 mg can be lethal. Inhalation is the quickest method of absorption, resulting in death within minutes. When ingested, death may take several hours [7].

Cyanide works by inhibiting oxidative phosphorylation at cytochrome oxidase (Fig. 14-1). This prevents oxygen from reoxidizing reduced cytochrome a_3, thereby inhibiting electron transport, mitochondrial oxygen utilization, and cellular respiration.

Acute cyanide poisoning is manifested by a headache, giddiness, sense of sinking, palpitations, dyspnea with inadequate ventilation, and ultimately unconsciousness. If convulsions occur, they are usually associated with brain hypoxia related to terminal respiratory arrest.

Headache, dyspnea, epigastric burning, vertigo, tinnitus, nausea, vomiting, tremor,

Fig. 14-1. Hydrogen cyanide inhibits electron transport at the cytochrome a–cytochrome a_3 step. From: Casarett & Doull, Toxicology, 2nd ed., p. 325. © 1980 McGraw-Hill. Reprinted with permission.

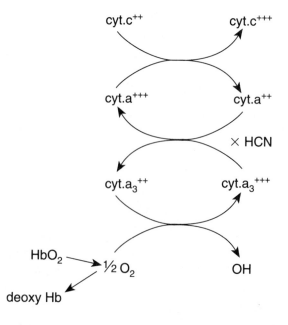

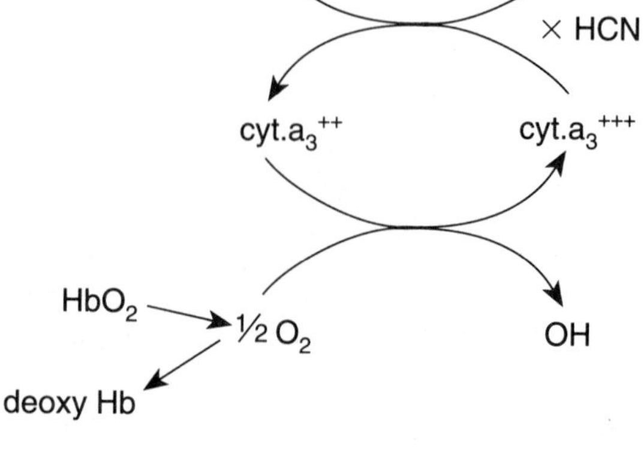
cyt.c++
cyt.c+++
cyt.a+++
cyt.a++
× HCN
cyt.a3++
cyt.a3+++
HbO2
½ O2
OH
deoxy Hb

and precordial pain were noted to be a true syndrome of chronic cyanide exposure by Colle [11]. Contact with the skin can cause an allergic type dermatitis, with longer exposures and solution strengths causing caustic burns [12–14].

Treatment

After acute cyanide exposure, treatment must begin immediately, usually with a cyanide antidote kit. If the victim had skin contact, the clothing must be removed and the skin washed to reduce absorption. Amyl nitrite is administered by inhalation using a new ampul every 3 minutes. This will produce about a 5% methemoglobinemia. It is followed by intravenous injection of 10–15 mL of a 3% solution of sodium nitrite over a 2- to 4-minute interval. Dosing is based on body weight and age to produce a 25% methemoglobin concentration.

Since cyanide has a high affinity for iron in the ferric state, it binds to the ferric form of cytochrome oxidase. Nitrites oxodize hemoglobin to methemoglobin, which competes with cytochrome oxidase for the cyanide ion.

$$Hb - Fe^{+2} + NaNO_2 \rightarrow Hb - Fe^{+3} + HNO_2$$

Cytochrome oxidase is returned to its normal state and cyanmethemoglobin is formed [15].

The level of methemoglobin must be monitored so as to not exceed 35% to 40%. High levels of methemoglobin may be treated with 1 to 2 mg/kg of methylene blue given intravenously. In vivo, the methylene blue is reduced to leukomethylene blue which reduces methemoglobin to hemoglobin.

To remove the cyanide from the body, an injection of 50 mL of a 25% solution of sodium thiosulfate is given slowly over 10 to 20 minutes. This drug causes the cyanide to be converted to thiocyanate by the enzyme rhodanase.

$$CN^- + S_2O_3^{-2} \xrightarrow{\text{RHODANESE}} CNS^- + SO_3^{-2}$$

Thiocyanate is relatively innocuous and is excreted in the urine.

All patients who require use of the antidote kit should be hospitalized and observed in a monitored bed since cardiac arrhythmias can occur. Pulmonary edema and lactic acidosis are other potential complications [16].

Hydrogen Sulfide

Hydrogen sulfide is a colorless, poisonous gas that is heavier than air. It has an extremely offensive odor of rotten eggs; however, the odor cannot be used as a reliable warning of toxicity. This is due to the olfactory nerve becoming rapidly fatigued at concentrations above 100 ppm [17]. Its toxicity is due to the reversible inhibition of cytochrome oxidase, which inhibits tissue respiration [18].

Hydrogen sulfide occurs in natural as well as industrial settings. It is a product of bacterial decomposition of protein as well as occurring in sulfur springs and volcanic gases [19]. Since it can occur in natural gas and petroleum deposits and in coal, lead sulfide, gypsum, and sulfur mines, it can also be a hazard in related processing operations [17]. It also occurs in sewage pools and manure piles and is released when the piles are disturbed [20, 21].

Symptoms associated with hydrogen sulfide exposure include headaches occurring at low concentrations, but may not be considered an early warning signal [17, 20]. Giddiness, increased mucus secretions, and pharyngeal soreness can also be seen [22]. Bronchitis, pneumonia, and pulmonary edema can also occur, sometimes with a delayed onset. This is why hospitalization and observation are important because the delay may be up to 72 hours [23, 24]. Transient hematuria, proteinuria, and abnormal liver function may be observed [22]. At concentrations of 15 ppm or less with fewer than 8 hours exposure, hydrogen sulfide can cause painful conjunctivitis associated with corneal erosion and spasm of the eyelids [17, 24, 25].

Treatment

As with hydrogen cyanide, treatment of hydrogen sulfide poisoning must be immediate. The amyl nitrite and sodium nitrite in the cyanide antidote kit are used, but not the sodium thiosulfate [26]. The patients must also use oxygen until the sulfmethemoglobin that is produced is metabolized [21]. Hospitalization is important due to the possibility of delayed pulmonary edema.

Hypersensitivity Pneumonitis

Hypersensitivity pneumonitis is an immunologic pulmonary disease that may present in many forms. The form is dependent on the immune response of the host and the nature and duration of exposure to the offending dusts. Usually this type of reaction affects the respiratory bronchioles and alveoli and is not related to atopy. There are many sources of occupational exposure to these agents. A partial list of the offending etiologic agents, their sources, and the condition caused is found in Table 14-2.

Clinical Findings

Acute Form

In the acute form of hypersensitivity pneumonitis symptoms occur 4 to 6 hours after exposure. These include fever up to 106°F, chills, malaise, cough, dyspnea, and headache. These symptoms may persist for 12 to 18 hours, with spontaneous recovery of the patient. Auscultation may reveal bibasilar and inspiratory rales, while a complete blood count may show leukocytosis with left shift. Eosinophilia of up to 10% may be present. Chest radiography may show fine nodules, a reticular pattern, and general coarseness of bronchovascular markings [22]. Lung biopsy is rarely necessary but if done may show infiltration of alveolar walls with plasma cells, monocytes, histiocytes, and lymphocytes [27, 28]. Noncaseating sarcoid-like granulomas with giant cells of both Langhan's and foreign body types may be found with lymphoid infiltrates [29].

Pulmonary function testing done 4 to 6 hours after exposure shows a decrease in forced vital capacity (FVC) and forced expiratory volume in 1 second (FEV_1) with minimal change in FVC/FEV_1. Sometimes, there is a decrease in FEV_1 and FVC immediately after exposure, which reverts to normal within an hour. This is followed in 4 to 6 hours by the late response, described above.

Treatment in the early acute phase is responsive to bronchodilators. The late phase is responsive only to corticosteroids or avoidance of exposure.

Chronic Form

The chronic form of hypersensitivity pneumonitis occurs over a period of several months and causes irreversible pulmonary damage. There is development of a progressive dyspnea that is associated with cough, weakness, weight loss, and general lethargy.

Auscultation may reveal crepitations in the lower lung fields, while cyanosis and clubbing may be present in the extremities. Chest radiography may show chronic interstitial fibrosis rather than evidence of pneumonitis. Pulmonary function testing may show the development of a restrictive ventilatory defect, with a decrease in diffusion capacity.

Pneumoconioses

Pneumoconiosis is literally defined as dust in the lungs. For purposes of occupational disease, it is defined as deposition of dust in the lungs and the tissue reaction to it [29]. Originally this definition included only inorganic dusts but has been broadened in some texts to include some aerosols and hypersensitivity diseases [22].

These dusts have to get into the lung in order to react and this requires them to become airborne. These airborne dusts or particulate matter range from 0.001 μm to greater than 1000 μm in diameter.

Particle Deposition

How and where particles are deposited in the lungs is determined primarily by three factors. The first is gravitational sedimentation, which states larger and denser particles settle out faster than smaller, less dense particles. The second factor is inertial impaction. This means a particle will continue in its original direction of travel even if the airstream in which it is suspended changes direction. It usually will impact the airway wall at a bifur-

Table 14-2. Etiologic Agents

Offending Agent	*Source and Condition*
Thermophilic actinomycetes	Moldy compost Causes malt workers' lung
Alternaria	Wood pulp Causes wood pulp workers' disease
Actinobifida dichotomica	Compost dust Causes mushroom workers' lung
Micropolyspora faene, Thermoactinomyces vulgaris, T. Candidus	Contaminated forced air Causes ventilation pneumonitis
Cryptostroma corticale	Moldy bark dust Causes maple bark strippers' lung
Aspergillus	Moldy malt Causes malt workers' lung
Penicillium	Cork dust Causes wood workers' lung
Pellularia	Redwood dust Causes sequoiosis
Aureobasidium pullulans	Contaminated steam Causes sauna-takers' disease
Fish proteins	Fish meal dust Causes fish meal workers' lung
Pig or ox protein	Therapeutic snuff Causes pituitary snuff-takers' lung
Diisocyanate	Chemical fumes Causes chemical workers' lung
Pyrethrum	Insecticide aerosol Causes pyrethrum alveolitis

cation. The third factor is Brownian diffusion. Particles are in random motion due to their bombardment by gas molecules and diffuse to the walls of the air passages. A fourth factor sometimes mentioned is interception, which is important only when discussing fibers. Fibers usually align themselves with the airstream in which they are traveling and therefore can get into the peripheral airways. It is thought that turbulence causes the fiber to change direction and intercept the airway walls since its length is now greater than the airway width.

Sedimentation and impaction account for the most particle deposition during breathing, with impaction being responsible for deposition of particles in the bifurcations of the lower airways [1]. These factors are responsible for most particles greater than 1 μm in diameter. Brownian motion plays a part in particles less than 1 μm in diameter. Brownian deposition is lowest where airway radii are large or air velocities are increased.

Most particles greater than 10 μm are deposited out in the nose and upper airways. Smaller particles make their way into the lower airways, with those between 0.5 and 5.0 μm being the most important in the causation of pneumoconioses [1].

Pneumoconioses may be classified into four types according to Nagelschmidt [30]: (1) diffuse interstitial fibrosis, (2) hyaline-nodular fibrosis or silicosis; (3) coalworkers' pneumoconiosis (CWP); and (4) mixed dust pneumoconiosis.

Diffuse Interstitial Fibrosis

There are many pneumoconioses that produce diffuse interstitial fibrosis. Some of the more common include aluminosis, asbestosis, and beryllosis. Asbestosis is the most common and is discussed in the following sections.

Asbestosis

Asbestos is a fibrous mineral that has been used for several thousand years before the birth of Christ. The term asbestos is derived from the Greek word meaning *unquenchable* in reference to its use as wicks in lamps in ancient times [31]. It is found in nature in two major types: amphibole and serpentine. Although they have the same formula, they differ in chemical structure and therefore have different properties. They are both considered fibers, being at least three times as long as they are wide [22]. Greater than 90% of the commercial use of asbestos in the United States involves crysotile, which is a serpentine type and is composed of curved fibers. The amphibole group, on the other hand, is composed primarily of straight fibers of various diameters. This group includes crocidolite, amotite, anthophyllite, actinolite, and tremolite.

The physical properties of asbestos include thermal resistance, high tensile strength, the ability of being spun into a fiber, incombustibility, and flexibility. Those properties make this mineral useful in a host of different products, including heat resistant clothing, heat and sound insulation, gaskets, brake linings, flooring, and electrical insulation [22].

Increased use of asbestos over the past 50 years has caused serious exposure to those individuals with repeated contact. The greatest risk is to those persons who are in asbestos mining, milling, and manufacturing processes. Exposure is also increased in those individuals in building and demolition, shipbuilding, and brake maintenance.

The inhalation of asbestos fibers results in a diffuse interstitial fibrosis of the lung parenchyma, usually accompanied by thickening of the parietal pleura. The severity of the fibrosis and its temporal appearance appear to be related to the intensity and duration of exposure. However, any exposure may result in some pleural thickening and/or fibrosis.

Asbestos fibers become lodged in terminal bronchioles and alveoli. These fibers then become engulfed by macrophages, which results in the death of the cells. This in turn attracts a reticulin fiber network. Activation of fibroblasts occurs resulting in collagen deposition and ultimately leading to the initial lesion of asbestosis, peribronchiolar fibrosis. This fibrosis then extends into surrounding tissue and alveolar septal fibrosis occurs. Normal airspaces are lost as fibrosis continues and eventually can result in a cystic or honeycomb appearance to the lung.

In addition to the fibrosis, asbestosis bodies or ferruginous bodies may be found. These form within macrophages that have engulfed an asbestos fiber. An iron-rich protein and polysaccharide matrix is secreted that surrounds the fiber and causes it to assume a dumbbell or beaded appearance (Fig.14-2). The fibers turn yellow-brown when stained with hematoxylin-eosin. Asbestos bodies can also be found in the sputum, pleura, pleural effusions, and other body organs. The appearance of asbestos bodies indicates previous exposure to asbestos, but does not indicate the presence or severity of asbestosis [32].

The signs and symptoms associated with as-

Fig. 14-2. Dumbbell-shaped asbestos bodies (arrows). From L. Victor & W. Talamont: Asbestos lung disease. *Hospital Practice* April 15, 1986, p. 265. Reprinted with permission.

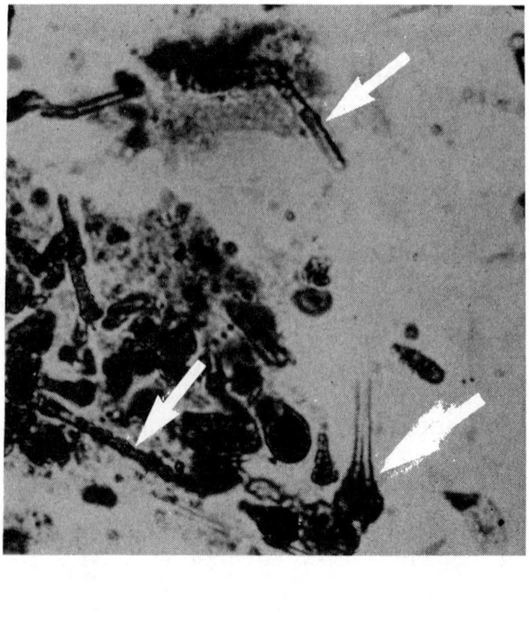

bestosis are unfortunately not specific to this form of diffuse interstitial pulmonary fibrosis. Also, symptomatology can be insidious, with a considerable lag time between exposure and the development of symptoms.

One of the earliest symptoms may be the development of dyspnea on exertion. The presentation is variable but usually follows a progressively worsening course. Cough is a late manifestation of asbestosis; usually of a nonproductive nature [33]. Other symptoms may include transient chest tightness or sharp chest pains. These are a result of strained intercostal muscles in the dyspneic patient. Fatigue may be found later in the disease.

Physical examination often reveals crepitations or high pitched rales. This is considered the most important physical finding and their presence is thought to be related to the duration of asbestos exposure [34]. These are dry, end-inspiratory, crackling rales that can be found in the posterior basilar portions of the lung fields.

Clubbing of the fingers and toes can sometimes be found (see Chapter 3). This may be associated with cyanosis of the digits as well. It is more often seen in advanced disease and may or may not advance in severity as the disease progresses.

Asbestos Pleural Effusions Asbestos exposure may result in the formation of pleural effusions. The fluid usually consists of a sterile exudate and often is blood tinged. It occurs within the first or second decade after initial asbestos exposure in about 20% of exposed individuals and can be bilateral and recurrent [35]. These effusions are often associated with significant chest pain.

Diagnosis

Pulmonary function testing is valuable in investigating the patient with asbestosis. It is helpful in establishing a diagnosis and also provides a means of following the progress of the disease.

The pulmonary functions are characterized by a restrictive impairment. There is a reduction in both FVC and total lung capacity. A reduction in diffusion capacity may also be found. The FVC is often decreased before any radiographic findings and is a more useful parameter than diffusion capacity for following the progress of the disease [22]. The FEV_1 may be decreased in advanced disease but the FEV_1/FVC percentage remains normal or slightly greater than normal. If other causes of restrictive airways disease can be eliminated, a decline in the FVC and vital capacity, greater than that expected with normal aging, together with a normal FEV_1/FVC is a good indicator of the progression of the fibrosis [34].

The ability of asbestosis to cause an obstructive form of lung disease is controversial. Some studies have shown decreased flows at low lung volumes, lower midexpiratory flow rates, and diminished closing volume in asbestos workers. This is suggestive of small airways disease [36–38]. These changes persisted after adjustments for smoking history were made. However, it has been shown that measurement of midexpiratory flow rates, closing volume, and decreased flow volumes is variable [39]. In addition, an increased prevalence of clinically significant airway obstruction reflected in decreased FEV_1/FVC unrelated to smoking has not been shown on a consistent basis in the individuals with asbestos exposure, [36, 40]. The incidence of obstructive lung defects in the asbestos-exposed individual seems then to be related to a high prevalence of smoking rather than to asbestos exposure itself [41, 42].

Radiographically, asbestosis may present early with very subtle features. The abnormalities are predominantly found in the lower one half to two thirds of the lung fields. An increase in what appear to be vessel opacities that may give the appearance of extensive vascular markings are among the earliest signs. These tend to become thicker with progression of the disease. In addition, small rounded opacities can also be seen. When these opacities become diffuse they can be seen obscuring the cardiac and diaphragmatic borders. These can give the "shaggy heart" appearance that is sometimes seen in asbestosis [43]. Pericardiac and lower lobe fibrosis are typical features of advanced asbestosis. Removal from asbestos exposure does not alter the progress of fibrosis seen roentgenographically.

In addition to the pulmonary radiographic findings there may also be pleural thickening and calcification. These are characteristics of asbestos related lung disease but, in themselves do not confirm a diagnosis of asbestosis. It can occur in the absence of parenchymal abnormalities as either diffuse or circumscribed lesions. The pleural plaques are fibrotic elevations of the parietal pleura. Visceral pleural thickening are found less often. The plaques themselves are thought to result from fibers that have not undergone phagocytosis and have migrated out of the lung into the pleural space. Here they cause a fibrotic reaction, resulting in the formation of collagen fibers separated by irregular spacings. Asbestos fibers can sometimes be seen in the pleural plaques.

Asbestos-Related Neoplasms Aside from the development of pulmonary fibrosis, asbestos exposure has been associated with the development of several types of cancer. These include diffuse malignant mesothelioma, lung cancer, cancer of the buccal mucosa, pharynx, larynx, gastrointestinal tract, and kidney [32]. The asbestos-related mortality for men who smoked more than a pack per day was found to be 2.8 times higher than the asbestos-related mortality of men who did not regularly smoke [44–46].

Diffuse malignant mesothelioma is a connective tissue neoplasm most commonly involving the pleura or peritoneum. There is consistent epidemiologic data identifying the development of this tumor in asbestos-exposed individuals in a variety of occupations [47–49]. There appears to be an increased risk for developing mesothelioma based on the fiber type. Crocidolite poses the greatest risk and amosite the next greatest. Anthophyllite and chrysotile pose less risk [50–53].

Clinically, mesothelioma presents with complaints of chest and shortness of breath. The pain frequently has a dull aching pleuritic nature. It may either be generalized or localized, often related to bone or nerve involvement [54]. Dyspnea is related to lung compression from accompanying pleural effusions and restriction of respiratory movements by the tumor. Findings associated with mesothelioma include weight loss, cough, clubbing, the syndrome of inappropriate antidiuretic hormone secretion, arthralgias, thrombocytosis, and fever [22].

Physical examination consistent with the presence of a pleural effusion may be seen in up to 80% of patients [23]. Tumor can also be seen growing through the chest wall and presenting as subcutaneous lumps. This may be seen as a sequelae to pleural aspiration or thoracotomy [31]. There is rarely evidence of metastasis to distant organs although local invasion may be seen. This can be manifested as enlarged supraclavicular lymph nodes, rib tumors, superior vena caval obstruction, and cardiac tamponade. The involvement of the peritoneum by mesothelioma usually presents as an abdominal mass with ascites. This tumor can directly spread into the pleural cavities, resulting in bilateral pleural effusions. Mesothelioma is a rapidly growing tumor and can be seen to progressively encase the lung.

The pleural mesothelioma may radiographically show a pleural effusion or nodular pleural thickening. Often both lesions are present. Mesothelioma is usually unilateral, although later stages can spread across the mediastinum. Rib crowding, elevation of the hemidiaphragm, or a shift of the mediastinum to the ipsilateral hemithorax can be seen [55].

The diagnosis of mesothelioma is often difficult to establish. Pleural fluid analysis and closed pleural biopsy have a low diagnostic yield. Thoracotomy is often necessary to obtain the diagnosis. Other cancers, including lung, stomach, colon, breast, pancreas, and ovary, can produce pleural metastasis that may mimic mesothelioma. Special histochemical testing along with gross pathology and microscopic study is necessary to firmly establish the diagnosis.

Histologic patterns associated with mesothelioma are epithelial, mesenchymal, and mixed. Treatment has included chemotherapy, radiation, and pleurectomy, although survival beyond 1 year is rare. The development of the tumor does not appear to be related to the degree of duration of asbestos exposure and can even be seen in individuals with only casual exposure.

The diagnosis of asbestosis can be a difficult problem for many reasons. Diffuse interstitial pulmonary fibrosis can be caused by a number of different agents. Pleural plagues and thickening often associated with asbestos exposure, are not diagnostic of asbestosis unless there is associated pulmonary parenclynal disease. Plaques and thickening may be due to distant infection as well. In addition the long duration between exposure and the development of significant lung disease, sometimes decades later, coupled with the lack of specific physical, clinical, and radiographic findings can perplex the clinician. A careful occupational history showing an exposure to asbestos coupled with appropriate clinical and radiographic findings can help make the diagnosis once other causes of pulmonary fibrosis have been eliminated.

Silicosis

Silicon and oxygen combine to form silicon dioxide, which is called silica. It may be in its free state or in combination with other elements. The free crystalline silica is the most common form that causes silicosis. Pure forms of free crystalline silica are rarely encountered and are usually seen with combinations of other rock products. When the proportion of free silica to the total is relatively high, nodular silicosis may occur. Mixed dust fibrosis is said to occur when the proportion is lower [34].

In nature, free silica consists of quartz, flint, tridymite, cristabolite, and rarely chert. Since the earth's crust consists of large amounts of silica, mining, quarrying, and tunneling expose workers to a high silicosis hazard. Manufacture of abrasives and sandblasting can also place the worker at high risk for silicosis. Less risky occupations include the manufacture of glass and ceramics and the production of fillers used in paints and rubber.

Silicosis may generally be divided into two forms: chronic, which occurs with exposure over a relatively long period of time, usually measured in years, and acute, which is rare and can occur with as little as a few weeks exposure. Chronic silicosis may be divided into three stages—slight, moderate, and severe—each with different but progressive clinical and radiographic findings. Table 14-3 helps to explain these findings.

Acute silicosis is a rare variant usually occurring after intense exposure to free silica varying from a few weeks to several years. It is most common in sandblasters working without adequate respiratory protection in enclosed spaces [58]. Other workers at risk include ceramic workers, open-cast coal miners, and silica flour workers.

Clinical findings include progressive dyspnea, which ultimately occurs at rest. Auscultation may reveal bronchial breath sounds and other signs of consolidation. Chest radiography shows large areas of consolidation,

Table 14-3. Clinical and Radiographic Findings of Chronic Silicosis

Slight	Mild dyspnea with exertion Slight and unproductive cough May have slight and diminished expansion on examination No or minimal work impairment Chest radiograph shows discrete nodular shadows
Moderate	Worsening dyspnea end cough Examination reveals diminished expansion of the chest Patchy dullness, and occasional bronchial breath sounds [56] Work capacity is impaired On radiography, both lung fields show nodular shadows
Severe	Respirations are labored May use accessory muscles, and visual retractions may be present May be right-sided cardiac hypertrophy leading to heart failure Unable to work Chest radiograph shows massive consolidation [57]

usually in the middle and lower zones. Spontaneous pneumothoraces may occur.

Acute silicosis is usually fatal, sometimes within a few months. Prognosis is dependent of the amount of retained dust within the lungs before the worker is removed from exposure [59]. The disease usually progresses despite treatment, although temporary relief of symptoms may be obtained with steroid use [60].

Symptoms not seen with silicosis include chest pain and wheezing. If a patient exhibits wheezing, their silicosis is usually accompanied by asthma or bronchitis. Hemoptysis and weight loss are not seen unless the patient has an accompanying disease such as tuberculosis.

It has long been thought that silicosis predisposes to tuberculosis [61]. The more advanced the silicosis, the greater the likelihood of contracting active tuberculosis [62].

Coal Worker's Pneumoconiosis (CWP)

CWP is secondary to the deposition of coal dust in the lung and the resulting reaction of the lung tissue to the dust. In the workplace, the term black lung is synonymous with CWP, although it is a legislatively defined term that includes chronic obstructive pulmonary diseases besides chronic diseases of miners [22].

Anyone within the mine can be exposed to coal dust, although those at the coal face have the highest exposure. At highest risk are the cutting machine operator and his or her helper, roof bolter, continuous miner operator, loading machine operator, and shot firer [31].

CWP may be divided into two forms: simple and complicated, which is also known as progressive massive fibrosis. Diagnosis and classification are based on the number and size of opacities present on the chest radiography. In simple CWP, opacities are small and rounded and found mostly in the upper lobes. Opacities greater than 1 cm in diameter occurring bilaterally in the upper and posterior regions of the lung makes a diagnosis of progressive massive fibrosis [31].

Simple CWP occurs from inhaling coal dust and has few symptoms, one of which is a slight cough productive of blackish sputum. Miners have minimal nondisabling shortness of breath, especially in absence of obstructive pulmonary disease. In pulmonary function studies, Motley et al [63, 64] were unable to show a relationshiop between FVC, FEV_1, and radiographic category. The findings of Motley et al are important to consider during evaluation for pulmonary disability.

Progressive massive fibrosis is the development of large nodules greater than 1 cm in diameter up to 2 to 10 cm in diameter. The masses represent large amounts of coal dust within macrophages and between reticulin and collagen fibers. Occasionally, one of these masses may rupture and the miner may cough up large quantities of black material called melanoptysis. Rarely the miner may aspirate this material and die.

PFTs show a restrictive defect and reduction in diffusion. There may be obstructive disease as well. In some cases ventilatory impairment may be severe and result in early death [65, 66]. The large masses are undetectable clinically and do not always progress and do not necessarily decrease life expectancy.

Reactive Airways Dysfunction Syndrome

Reactive Airways Dysfunction Syndrome (RADS) was described as an asthma-like illness after a single exposure to high levels of an irritating aerosol, vapor, fume or smoke [67]. RADS is characterized by onset of symptoms in a previously symptom-free person within 24 hours of exposure and persistence of bronchial hyperresponsiveness for at least 3 months. Many patients may have symptoms for years after the single high exposure. Pulmonary function studies may show airflow obstruction and methacholine challenge test is positive. Treatment involves symptomatic relief using bronchodilators and then reducing or eliminating subsequent exposures to the provocative agent.

Conclusion

This chapter is an overview of the more common occupational diseases that the primary care physician might confront. Attentiveness to the occupational history may help document a workplace exposure that otherwise might be missed on routine examination. Early recognition and treatment not only increases the patient's quality of life, but decreases the cost to society should that patient become disabled.

References

1. National Institute for Occupational Safety and Health: Occupational Diseases: A Guide to their Recognition. DHEW Publication No. (NIOSH) 77-181, 1977. Washington, DC, US Government Printing Office, 1977
2. National Institute for Occupational Safety and Health: Occupational Exposure to Carbon Monoxide. DHEW Publication No. (NIOSH) 73-11000, 1972. Washington, DC, US Government Printing Office, 1972
3. Environmental Protection Agency Environmental Assessment and Criteria Office: Air quality criteria for carbon monoxide. April 1979
4. Department of Health, Education and Welfare. Research on Smoking Behavior (NIDA Monograph 17). DHEW Publication No. (ADM) 78-581, December 1977. Washington, DC, US Government Printing Office, 1977
5. Haldane J: The action of carbonic oxide on man. *J Physiol* (Lond) 18:430, 1895
6. Ayres SM, et al: Systemic and myocardial hemodynamic responses to relatively small concentrations of carboxyhemoglobin (COHb). *Arch Environ Health* 18:699–704, 1969

6a. Sheps DS, Herbst MC, Hinderliter AL, et al: Production of arrhythmias by elevated carboxyhemoglobin in patients with coronary artery disease. *Ann Intern Med* 113:343–351, 1990

7. Braunwald E, Isselbacher KH, Petersdorf RG, et al: Harrison's Principles of Internal Medicine, ed 11. New York, McGraw-Hill, 1987
8. Forbes WH, Sargent F, Roughton FJW: The rate of carbon monoxide uptake by normal men. *Am J Physiol* 143:594, 1945
9. Stewart RD, Fisher TN, Hosko MJ, et al: Experimental human exposure to carbon monoxide. *Arch Environ Health* 21:154, 1970
10. Smith G, Sharp GR: Treatment of carbon monoxide poisoning with oxygen under pressure. *Lancet* 2:905–906, 1960
11. Colle R: Chronic hydrogen cyanide poisoning. *Maroc Med* 50:750–757, 1972
12. International Labour Office: Cyanogen and its compounds. *In* Occupation and Health: Encyclopedia of Hygiene, Pathology and Social Welfare, vol 1. Geneva, Noerclerc et Feuetrier SA, 1930, pp 553–560
13. Tovo S: Poisoning due to KCN absorbed through skin. *Minerva Med* 75:158–161, 1955
14. Dermatitis in the manufacture and use of alkalis. *In* Skin Hazards in American Industry, Part II, Public Health Bulletin 229. Washington, DC, US Public Health Service, 1936, pp 69–75
15. Gilman AG, Goodman LS, Gilman A: The Pharmacological Basis of Therapeutics, ed 6. New York, Macmillan, 1980, p 1651
16. Graham DL, Taman D, Theodore J, et al: Acute cyanide poisoning complicated by lactic acidosis and pulmonary edema. *Arch Intern Med* 137:1051, 1977
17. National Institute for Occupational Safety and Health: Occupational exposure to hydrogen sulfide. DHEW Publication No. (NIOSH) 77-158, 1977. Washington, DC, US Government Printing Office, 1977
18. McCormack MF: Sewer fume poisoning. *Journal of the American College of Emergency Physicians* 4:141–142, 1975
19. Macaluso P: Hydrogen sulfide. *In* Encyclopedia of Chemical Technology, ed 2, vol 19. New York, Interscience Publishers, 1969, pp 375–389
20. Donham KJ, Knapp LW, Monson R, et al: Acute toxic exposure to gases from liquid manure. *J Occup Med* 24:142, 1982
21. Osbern LN, Crapo RD: Dung lung: A report of toxic exposure to liquid manure. *Ann Intern Med* 95:312, 1981
22. Rom WN: Environmental and Occupational Medicine. Boston, Little, Brown and Company, 1983
23. Thoman M: Sewer gas: Hydrogen sulfide intoxication. *Chemical Toxicology* 2:383, 1969
24. Beasley RWR: The eye and hydrogen sulfide. *Br J Ind Med* 20:32–34, 1963
25. Michal FV: Eye lesions caused by hydrogen sulfide. *Cesk Oftalmol* 6:5–8, 1950
26. Stine RJ, Slosaberg B, Beecham BE: Hydrogen sulfide intoxication: A case report and discussion of treatment. *Ann Intern Med* 85:756, 1976
27. Seal RME, Hapler EJ, Thomas GO, et al: The pathology of the acute and chronic stages of farmer's lung. *Thorax* 23:469, 1968
28. Emanuel DA, Wengel FJ, Bowerman CI, et al: Farmer's lung. Clinical, pathologic and immunologic study of 24 patients. *Am J Med* 37:392, 1964
29. International Labour Office: The definition of pneumoconiosis. *In* Encyclopedia of Occupational Health and Safety, vol II, appendix VII. New York, McGraw-Hill, 1972, p 1558
30. Nagelschmidt G: The relation between lung

dust and lung pathology in pneumoconiosis. *Br J Ind Med* 17:247, 1960
31. Morgan WKC, Seaton A: Occupational Lung Diseases, ed 2. Philadelphia, WB Saunders, 1984
32. Victor LD, Talamonti WJ: Asbestos lung disease. *Hosp Pract* 21:257–268, 1986
33. Parkes WR: Asbestos-related disorders. *Br J Dis Chest* 67:261, 1973
34. Parkes WR: Occupational Lung Disorders, ed 2. Stoneham, MA, Butterworths, 1983
35. Kipen HM: Asbestos-related disease. *NJ Med* 85:915–918, 1988
36. Becklake MR, Ernst P: Asbestos exposure and airway response. *In* Gee JB (ed): Occupational Lung Disease. Contemporary Issues in Pulmonary Disease, vol 2. New York, Churchill Livingstone, 1984
37. Begin R, Cantin A, Berthiaume Y, et al: Airway function in lifetime-nonsmoking older asbestos workers. *Am J Med* 75:631–638, 1983
38. Mohsenifar Z, Jasper AJ, Mahrer T, et al: Asbestos and airflow limitation. *J Occup Med* 28:817–820, 1986
39. Cochrane GM, Prieto F, Clark TJH: Intrasubject variability of maximal expiratory flow volume curve. *Thorax* 32:171–176, 1977
40. Lerman Y, Seidman H, Gelb S, et al: Spirometric abnormalities among asbestos insulation workers. *J Occup Med* 30:228–233, 1988
41. Delcros L, Buffer PA, Greenberg DS, et al: Asbestos-associated disease: A review. *Tex Med* 85:50–59, 1989
42. Becklake MR: Asbestos-related disease of the lung and other organs: Their epidemiology and implications for clinical practice. *Am Rev Respir Dis* 144:187–227, 1976
43. Pregor L: Asbestos-Related Disease. New York, Grune & Stratton, 1978
44. Selikoff IJ, Hammond EC: Asbestos and smoking (editorial). *JAMA* 242:458, 1979
45. Selikoff IJ, Hammond EC, Churg J: Asbestos exposure, smoking, and neoplasia. *JAMA* 204:106, 1968
46. Hammond EC, Selikoff IJ, Seidman H: Asbestos exposure, cigarette smoking and death rates. *Ann NY Acad Sci* 330:473, 1979
47. National Research Council US, Committee on Nonoccupational Health Risks of Asbestiform Fibers: Asbestiform Fibers: Nonoccupational Health Risks. Board of Toxicology and Environmental Health Hazards, Commission on Life Sciences, National Research Council, Washington, DC, National Academy Press, 1984
48. US Department of Labor Occupational Exposure to Asbestos, Tremolite, Anthophyllite and Actinolite; final rules. *Fed Reg* 15:22612–22790, 1986
49. Greenberg M, Davies TA: Mesothelioma register 1967–68. *Br J Med* 31:91–104, 1974
50. McDonald AD, McDonald JC: Malignant mesothelioma in North America. *Cancer* 46: 1650–1656, 1980
51. Newhouse ML, Berry G, Skidmore JW: A mortality study of workers manufacturing friction materials with chrysotile asbestos. *Ann Occup Hyg* 26:899–909, 1982
52. McDonald AD: Mineral fibre content of lung in mesothelioma tumours; preliminary report. *IARC Sci Publ* 30:681–685, 1980
53. McDonald AD, McDonald JC: Mesothelioma after crocidolite exposure during gas mask manufacture. *Environ Res* 17:340–346, 1978
54. Elmes PC, Simpson MJC: The clinical aspects of mesothelioma. *Q J Med* 45:427, 1976
55. Dunn MM: Asbestos and the lung. *Chest* 95:6, 1989
56. Corn JK: Historical aspects of industrial hygiene—11. Silicosis. *Am Ind Hyg Assoc J* 41:125–133, 1980
57. Hunter D: The Diseases of Occupations, ed 6. London, Hodder and Stoughton, 1978, p 942
58. Buechner HA, Ansari A: Acute silico-proteinosis. *Dis Chest* 55:174, 1969
59. Raffle PAB, et al (eds): Hunter's Diseases of the Occupations. London, Hodder and Stoughton, 1987, p 646
60. Ziskind M, Jones RN, Weill H: State of the art—Silicosis. *Am Rev Respir Dis* 113:643, 1976
61. Gardner LU: The significance of the silicotic problem. *In* the 3rd Saranac Symposium on Silicosis. Trudeau Sch. Tuberc, Saranac Lake, NY, 1937
62. Chatgidakis CF: Silicosis in South African white gold miners. *Med Proc* 9:383–392, 1963
63. Motley HL, Lang LP, Gordon B: Pulmonary emphysema and ventilation measurement in one hundred anthracite coal miners with respiratory complaints. *American Review of Tuberculosis* 59:270, 1949
64. Motley HL, Lang LP, Gordon B: Studies on the respiration gas exchange in one hundred anthracite coal miners with pulmonary complaints. *American Review of Tuberculosis* 61: 201, 1950
65. Ortmeyer CE, Costello J, Morgan WKC, et al: The mortality of Appalachian coal miners, 1963 to 1971. *Arch Environ Health* 29:67, 1974
66. Oldham PD, Rossiter CE: Mortality in coal-worker's pneumoconiosis related to lung function: A prospective study. *Br J Ind Med* 22:93, 1965
67. Brooks SM, Weiss MA, Bernstein IL: Reactive airways dysfunction syndrome (RADS) persistent asthma syndrome after high level irritant exposures. *Chest* 88:376–84, 1985

15

Pulmonary Rehabilitation

Willane Krell

Goals of Pulmonary Rehabilitation

The major focus of pulmonary rehabilitation must be to assist patients in improving their general state of well-being. To this end, there are many facets of general health care and education that need to be presented to each patient. Too often, persons suffering with crippling dyspnea think they must learn to live with their symptoms. Certainly they must live with the disease, but symptoms and daily functioning can be improved.

Educating the patient and family as to the nature of the pulmonary disease is important for several reasons. Education helps improve compliance with medical recommendations [1]. Learning about their basic disease process relieves anxieties of the patient and family and allows them to better cope with the often chronic illness. As an added benefit, an educated patient can often learn to handle minor complications on his or her own and will be less likely to tax the medical care delivery system with phone calls and excessive emergency or office visits.

Education includes instructing patients in the proper use of medications, providing information about diet, and an individualized exercise program. Sessions with the patient can also be used to teach specific techniques (such as effective breathing patterns or postural drainage for secretions) to alleviate their symptoms.

The overall goal is to improve morbidity related to lung disease and allow the patient to function at his or her best possible level. Ultimately, improvement in terms of decreased hospitalizations or even decreased mortality in these patients is the desired result of pulmonary rehabilitation.

Patient and Family Education

The most common pulmonary disease to be considered is chronic obstructive pulmonary disease. Patients with asthma, pulmonary fibrosis, bronchiectasis, chest wall diseases (deformities, neurologic or neuromuscular dysfunction), and so on can also benefit from increased knowledge of their medical problem.

A number of pharmaceutical companies or home therapy companies provide physicians or other medical personnel with posters or charts illustrating pulmonary diseases. Additionally, there are commercial videotapes, slide-sound lectures, pamphlets, etc. available, often free, from the local Lung Association. Depending on time and resource limitations, simply sitting down with a pencil and paper may be of benefit to the patient. The information presented need not be technical or involved. Simply describing or showing what bronchospasm is and what triggers it, explaining where secretions come from, and so forth, will help the patient make sense of symptoms and better understand the rationale for the use of needed medications.

The importance of proper nutrition and hydration should be emphasized. Obviously, being overweight taxes an already overburdened respiratory system. Recent studies also stress that being underweight leads to increased morbidity and mortality [2–4]. Simple discussions about appropriate caloric intake and the four basic food groups are all that is needed in most cases. Hydration should not be neglected in discussions, either. Patients with concomitant cardiac disease or right-sided heart failure should be instructed in the use of diuretics (if applicable) and signs of insipient edema. The majority of patients tend to be underhydrated due to increased respiratory water loss or inadequate intake. As poor hydration can lead to problems with mucus viscosity, stressing the importance of proper fluid intake is important.

It is helpful to have the family present at patient education sessions. Often, the family member provides meals or helps with medications. Also, the family's assistance is invaluable, if not absolutely necessary, in instituting home respiratory therapy maneuvers such as postural drainage or chest physiotherapy (chest clapping). The family, rather than the patient, may bring up problems that the patient has not discussed with the physician. Airing anxieties and problems will help both the patient and the family. For example, sexual dysfunction related to dyspnea or other respiratory symptoms is common, yet infrequently brought up by the patient. Answering questions or offering solutions to these problems in daily living will assist the whole family unit in functioning well.

Smoking Cessation

Nowhere can the physician have greater impact than in the area of smoking cessation. In the majority of pulmonary patients, smoking is responsible for their disease and must be stopped to prevent further deterioration. For anyone, not just those people with lung disease, quitting smoking has great impact on health—respiratory, cardiovascular, gastrointestinal, or virtually any organ system named.

Group or individual sessions can be equally effective for smoking cessation. It has been shown that simply having the physician tell the patient they need to quit smoking is often successful [5]. Physicians who have received information on helping patients to quit and have altered their practice to emphasize smoking cessation are highly successful in achieving this goal [6, 7]. Educating the patient to the well-known effects of smoking on the lungs and heart can be helpful. One particularly effective strategy is to point out that smoking accelerates facial wrinkling [8]. The lines around the eyes and deep grooves around the mouth may be the result of decreased blood flow to the skin or just due to grimacing when getting a faceful of smoke; but, in either case, vanity about appearance is almost universal and (particularly for the rising number of young female smokers) this may be an effective deterrent to smoking.

Support groups or repeated counseling may be needed to successfully keep patients from smoking. Most patients do want to quit and may have already tried one or several of the heavily advertised products or devices that promise a magical cure from smoke addiction. It may be helpful to suggest that expensive devices are not as useful as a true desire to quit. Sympathy for "withdrawal" symptoms and the difficulty of the task are in order.

Recently, some pharmacologic aids to assist in controlling problems with withdrawal have been made available. Use of these drugs should be on an individual basis only. Nicorette Gum is a nicotine delivery system in a gum base. Nicotine is released as the gum is chewed. In order to select appropriate candidates for this medication, a history of the patient's smoking behavior should be obtained. The gum is most likely to be useful when the patient describes behaviors related to nicotine addiction: waking from sleep with a craving for cigarettes and smoking immediately on awakening [9]. It is less useful for the "nervous" or habit smoker. Generally, after 3 or 4 months of nonsmoking, the gum is gradually withdrawn (see Chap. 28).

Transdermal nicotine patches have very recently become available. As the patches have been advertised in the public media, demand for this product by patients has been very high. Use of the transdermal delivery system does bypass some of the major complaints of users to the nicotine gum, such as problems with dental work, local oral irritation and gastroesophageal symptoms, thus compliance with the therapeutic regimen may be improved. The manufacturers recommended a 10-week program in using the patches for smoking cessation. Prescriptions are written for two-week intervals. For the first 6 weeks, a patch containing 21 mg of nicotine is applied daily by the patient. This is followed by two weeks using a 14 mg patch daily, then two weeks using a 7 mg patch. Local irritation at the site of the patch can be minimized by placing the patches on the trunk rather than the extremities and by rotating the sites of patch application. Initial results with this transdermal system are encouraging, but as with all smoking cessation programs, ensuring long term smoking cessation is difficult. The physician must continue to play a supportive and encouraging role for patients who have quit smoking with this system.

Clonidine in the transdermal form has been successful in treating withdrawal symptoms from a wide variety of substances [10] and may also be useful in alleviating the anxiety, tension, and nervousness seen in tobacco withdrawal. A 0.2-mg patch applied to the trunk once weekly has been found helpful [11].

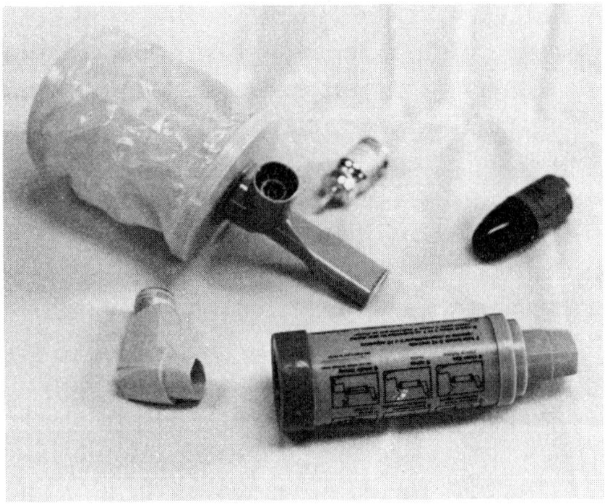

Fig. 15-1. Various available spacer devices for use with metered dose inhalers are shown. Delivery of aerosol medication can be improved with the use of such devices.

Compliance with Medications

As inhaled medications, in particular inhaled β_2-agonists, are a mainstay of therapy, it is imperative that each patient be personally instructed in proper use of their inhalation devices. Metered dose inhalers or nebulizers are valuable pharmacologic tools only if they can be used properly. Unfortunately, it has been shown that in many cases neither patients [12] nor physicians [13] possess the knowledge necessary to properly use inhalers.

For proper use of the metered dose inhaler, the patient should be instructed to dispense the inhalant at the end of a normal breath, then immediately inhale a complete breath (i.e., to total lung capacity) and hold the breath for up to 10 seconds if possible [14]. As many patients have difficulty coordinating the medication and their breathing, several simple alternative delivery systems have been developed. A wide variety of so-called spacer devices exist, ranging from simple tubes to elaborate bellows systems (Fig. 15-1). If expense is an issue, the cardboard tube from paper towels or toilet tissue can be used. The purpose of the spacer is to create a reservoir of sprayed medication that the patient can inhale at will, rather than in coordination with the spray. In children as well as in adults, spacers can improve delivery of aerosol medications [15–17]. Recently, a simple device that delivers powdered medication rather than a pressurized aerosol has become available. It allows patient-controlled inhalation of powdered albuterol, and as the particle size is comparable to that of an aerosol, there is little problem with irritation or bronchospasm. Patients simply inhale deeply from the container at their own speed, which eliminates "hand-inhalation" coordination problems [18].

Nebulizers can be obtained for use in patients' homes should there be problems with using the metered dose inhalers, with or without spacers. Although there is no superiority in delivery of medication [19, 20], some patients subjectively feel more relief when using one of these aerosol delivery systems. Particularly in patients with severe obstruction, this device may be easier to use. Both the patient and supporting family members should be instructed in the proper use of the machine and correct medication dosage.

For the variety of oral medications potentially used in chronic lung disease, information on their effects on disease and symptoms, as well as potential side effects and toxicity, should be reviewed with the patient and family. This information is important for many reasons, not the least of which is improving compliance with the medical regimen. Additionally, because many of the drugs used have the potential for side effects, toxicity (theophylline preparations), or interaction with other medications (theophylline, digoxin preparations, Coumadin [warfarin] and derivatives, and so on), the patient should be alerted to the potential problems. Reviews of scheduling of medications may help the patient adapt needed medications to his or her life-style. With some medications, such as corticosteroids, a discussion of complicated dose tapering regimens helps clarify matters for the patient.

Along with education on medications, time should be allowed for the patient to raise questions about the medications. If the patient has problems related to side effects, providing a means to mitigate these problems (by scheduling changes, taking pills with food, etc.) is useful in ensuring compliance. Anxiety related to medication effects should be alleviated.

Infection Control

A major cause of morbidity and mortality in patients with chronic lung disease is related to viral or bacterial infections in the airway: upper airway, bronchitis, and pneumonia. Prevention of infections must be a priority in caring for these patients. The role of bronchodilators and pulmonary toilet should be stressed.

Pneumovax is recommended for people with chronic lung disease. Although there have been questions raised as to its effectiveness in this population of patients [21, 22], it is recommended to prevent common community-acquired infections [23, 24].

Influenza vaccination yearly is also recommended for this population [25]. Over and above the effects of influenza itself, the injury to the airways caused by viral infections can lead to increased susceptibility to secondary bacterial infection. As the viral serotype changes from year to year, it is necessary to repeat immunization with each change in the vaccine. A standing order for a yearly vaccination placed in the patient's chart will improve delivery of the vaccine [26].

Amantadine is a useful but generally neglected means of prophylaxis for influenza. In high-risk populations (nursing homes, debilitated patients) or during epidemics of influenza, daily oral prophylaxis can decrease the incidence of infections. Further, when given early in the course of infection at therapeutic doses, amantadine can lessen the duration and severity of the infection [27, 28].

Early use of antibiotics in chronic lung disease patients was, until recently, somewhat controversial. Recent studies have indicated that when signs of exacerbation of underlying lung disease exist (increase in dyspnea, chest heaviness or congestion, change in mucus color or consistency), use of a broad-spectrum oral antibiotic decreases the severity of the exacerbation, reduces the number of days in the hospital, and generally decreases morbidity [29]. If outpatient oral antibiotics fail to resolve symptoms or if there is chest radiographic evidence of pneumonia, persistent fever, etc., hospitalization may be required.

Exercise Regimens and Breathing Retraining

The type of regimen prescribed depends in large part on the condition of the patient. Initial assessment of pulmonary function tests, oximetry at rest and with walking, as well as consideration of formal exercise testing, will provide a baseline assessment of the patient's physical condition. Listening to the patient is also a valuable aid in assessing his or her ability to function in daily life. Their descriptions of activities that provoke symptoms are valuable in customizing a training regimen [30].

Breathing Retraining

Simple observation of the patient's breathing pattern can suggest strategies to alleviate respiratory symptoms through breathing retraining. There is a tendency for patients to adapt inefficient breathing strategies (increased respiratory rate at the expense of tidal volume, use of less efficient nondiaphragmatic respiratory muscles) when dyspneic. Sometimes, merely pointing out the maladaptive breathing pattern is of help, but in many cases, working with the patient to teach specific maneuvers to assist in achieving more efficient use of the respiratory system is necessary.

One strategy that a large number of patients adopt on their own is pursed lip breathing. The mechanism by which retarding expiration via narrowing of the expiratory orifice (pursed lips) relieves respiratory symptoms is not entirely clear. Oxygen saturation can be demonstrably improved during pursed lip breathing [31, 32]. This phenomenon may be related to the increase in functional residual capacity (and thus oxygen stores/reserves) caused by back-pressure of the respiratory system during prolonged expiration. The relief of dyspnea noted by patients may relate to the improved oxygenation, but may also relate to some effect of the back-pressure on chest wall or diaphragm position, reducing feedback signals that led to the sensation of dyspnea (see Chapter 4). For those patients who have not taught themselves this maneuver, a simple demonstration of blowing out while the lips are held in a whistling position may suffice.

Diaphragmatic breathing might be the next breathing strategy taught to patients [33]. While the patient is using pursed lip breathing, have the patient press inward on their abdomen during expiration. This necessitates outward movement of the abdominal wall during inspiration, hence use of the diaphragm. The patient is then instructed to practice using diaphragmatic breathing when comfortable at rest. When exertion or other stresses occur, it is hoped the patient will be able to use both pursed lip and diaphragmatic breathing to alleviate respiratory symptoms.

Exercise and Conditioning

Depending on the initial condition of the patient, breathing exercises may be all that is tolerated. The goal, even in these patients, is to work toward a general conditioning program that stresses endurance over strength [30].

Walking is one of the best general conditioning exercises [34]. Initial exercise prescription might be gentle walking on level grade for a few minutes daily. Oximetric evaluation [35] or full cardiopulmonary exercise testing in some cases (particularly in those patients who have both cardiac and pulmonary disease) during walking may help in deciding on the safe level of activity for each patient.

Objective evaluation of a patient is useful not only for the data base it provides, but it may also help in addressing any fears the patient may have about ill effects of respiratory symptoms on the body with exertion. Often, there is an element of deconditioning in patients with lung disease because they have gradually curtailed their activities to avoid unpleasant, if not dangerous, respiratory symptoms. "Proving" to them that they can tolerate a given level of activity will help them comply with a prescribed regimen.

As the patient gradually learns to increase walking on level grade, other exercises can be added to the regimen. Two approaches (alone or in combination) are used. The first would be helping patients use their own activities of daily living as respiratory conditioning exercises. For example, stair climbing is often reported to be difficult. Teaching the patient to expire through pursed lips while stepping up, then resting and inspiring before beginning the next step, incorporates learned breathing techniques with exertion and allows the patient to expand abilities without increased dyspnea. Patients also often report difficulty with activities involving pushing or pulling (vacuuming, lawn work, etc.). Again, teaching them to use the specialized breathing techniques during activities will increase their exercise capacity.

The second approach is to use specific conditioning exercise programs, particularly involving the upper body. Cardiac and pulmonary patients often report dyspnea disproportionate to tasks involving arm exertion [36]. An upper extremity ergometer (Fig.

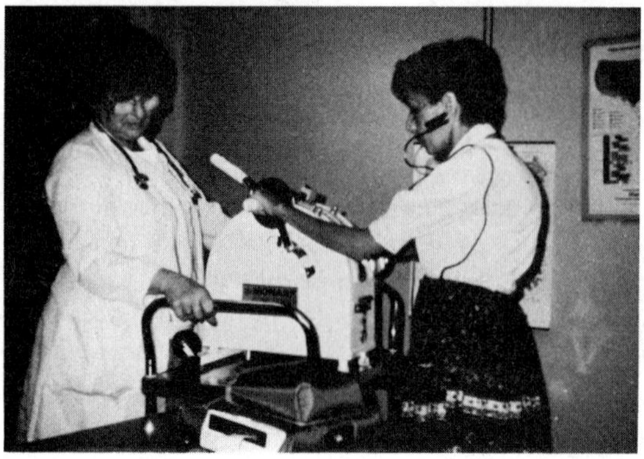

Fig. 15-2. Arm ergometer used for upper extremity work assessment is used while the patient is monitored by oximetry in the presence of a respiratory therapist.

15-2) used while monitoring oxygen saturation can provide safe upper extremity exercising. Arm calisthenics, sometimes with small weights, can be used as the patient progresses.

The ultimate goal to keep in mind when designing and implementing an exercise program for a patient is that the activities should be designed to improve overall physical condition to better deal with daily life. Specific techniques to strengthen respiratory muscles (inspiratory resistive training and the like) have produced limited results. The greatest improvement in the function of patients is seen with general conditioning regimens [37–39]. Increased confidence in their abilities develops as functional capacity is increased, with no increase, or perhaps a decrease, in respiratory symptoms.

Respiratory Therapy Modalities

This section deals primarily with modalities that improve pulmonary toilet and problems with secretions. Delivery of aerosolized medications, which is certainly a part of respiratory therapy techniques, has been discussed in relation to medications.

Postural drainage involves using gravity to assist in mobilizing secretions. In teaching patients the techniques of postural drainage, advantage can be taken of the fact that most patients have already noticed that certain body positions cause an increase in the production of mucus. Gravity's redistribution of secretions causes symptoms such as difficulties with secretions at night when body position is shifted, or the common occurrence of a productive cough after arising in the morning. Using this as a starting point, the drainage positions can be demonstrated and the benefits of clearing secretions under patient control made clear [40]. Having a position chart to remind patients of proper body positioning while performing drainage maneuvers in the home (Fig. 15-3) is very useful, as is continued reinforcement and retraining.

Chest physiotherapy, or chest percussion or chest clapping, may or may not be required in addition to postural drainage. The presence of a willing family member or friend to assist patients with this therapeutic modality is almost a must. Properly instructed, chest clapping by family members in the home is a very useful adjuvant to medical therapies. Recently, a number of small mechanical percussors have become available

Fig. 15-3. Sample of a patient handout demonstrating positions to be used to achieve successful postural drainage.

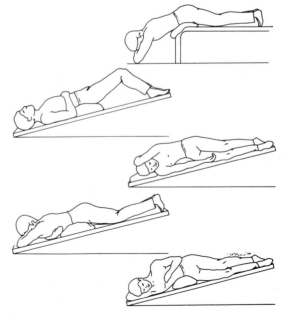

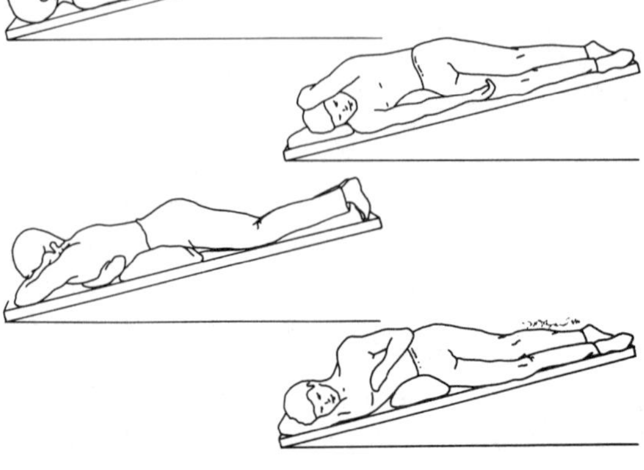

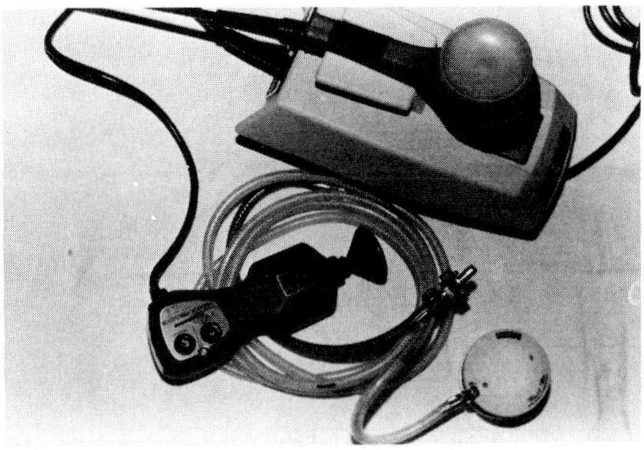

Fig. 15-4. Home percussor that can be used by the patient or family for home chest physiotherapy.

for use by therapists or in the home after instruction (Fig. 15-4). As the devices may not be covered by insurance, it is worthwhile to evaluate the device with consultation and demonstration involving the therapist, patient, and family for judging its potential usefulness before investing.

Interestingly, many patients have difficulty with cough. Some will force coughing, believing that the maneuver will relieve respiratory symptoms. The coughing actually produces airway irritation, potentially leading to bronchospasm or increased "need" to cough. These persons need to be instructed to control habit coughing. Others are unable to effectively cough, due to fear, pain, excessive sputum production with coughing, or inability to cough due to poor ventilatory capacity. These patients can be shown how to cough properly using diaphragmatic breathing techniques or by assisting the cough with arm or abdominal maneuvers.

Home Oxygen Therapy

With progression of underlying lung disease, the use of home oxygen therapy is considered. The basic guidelines for the institution of home oxygen therapy are (1) a PaO_2 of less than 55 mm Hg after 1 month of adequate medical therapy; (2) oxygen saturation by oximetry of less than 89% after 1 month of adequate medical therapy; and (3) signs of secondary organ damage related to hypoxemia, such as erythrocytosis (secondary polycythemia), right ventricular hypertrophy or cor pulmonale, and possibly sociointellectual deterioration [41]. Oxygen may also be prescribed for special circumstances, such as documented oxygen desaturation with exertion or exercise or sleep-related deoxygenation even in the absence of sleep apnea syndrome.

Air travel for patients with chronic lung disease deserves special note. Older planes, such as 707s or DC-9s, have a wider differential variation in cabin pressure than newer or larger planes. Even in these newer planes, there is a drop in pressure compared with sea level [42]. Patients who require oxygen on the ground will obviously still require oxygen when flying. For the patient who has borderline oxygenation, the question as to whether supplemental oxygen will be needed is more difficult to answer. Generally, airlines charge approximately $50 per leg of flight for oxygen, so the question of whether to use oxygen in these borderline patients has a financial impact as well as a medical impact on the patient. At this point, there are not enough data to predict who will require oxygen in flight, so firm recommendations cannot be made [43].

The choice of oxygen delivery system is dictated by the requirements of the individual patient. The use of oxygen tanks in the home, with incumbent problems of bulkiness, need for frequent deliveries, etc., has in general been superceded by the use of oxygen concentrators or liquid oxygen systems. Oxygen concentrators provide an inspired oxygen tension of up to 40%. Liquid oxygen systems are expensive but can provide for higher FIO_2 and flow rates. If the patient requiring oxygen is ambulatory, a portable oxygen system should be prescribed so patient activities are not limited by tethers to a tank or concentrator. Small tanks on carts or "backpack" type systems are shown in Fig. 15-5.

The familiar nasal cannula can be used for oxygen flow rates up to about 4 or 5 L/s. At higher flow rates, there is too much nasal irri-

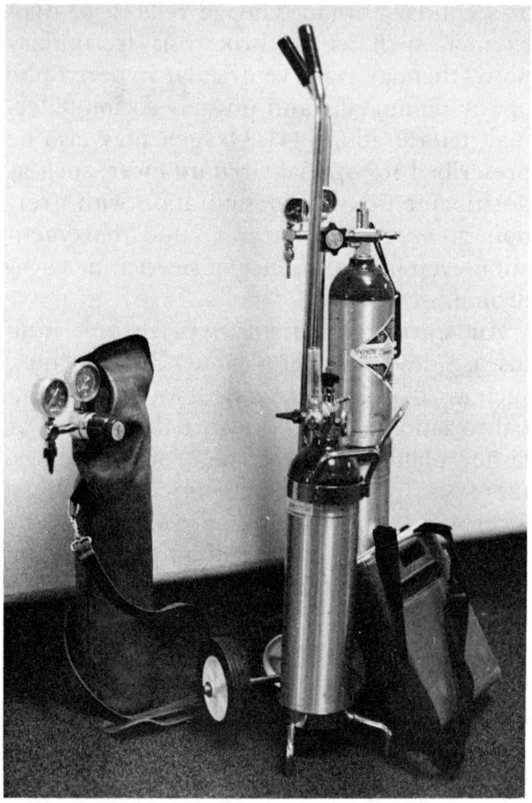

Fig. 15-5. Portable oxygen units available to allow patient greater mobility while on oxygen.

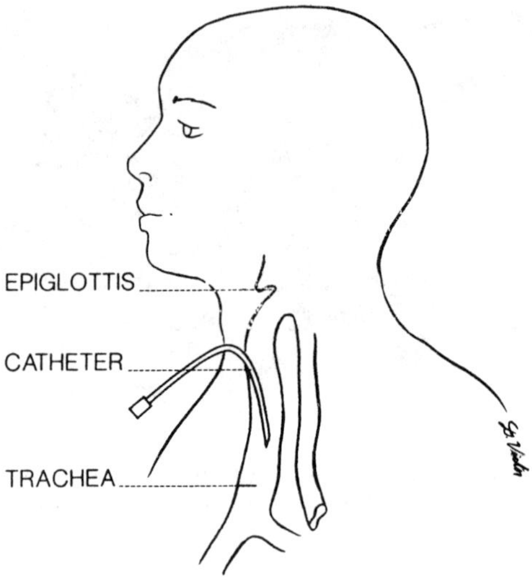
EPIGLOTTIS
CATHETER
TRACHEA

Fig. 15-6. Transtracheal oxygen catheter in position in the trachea for delivery of oxygen.

tation from the nasal jet of oxygen, so masks are used.

Transtracheal oxygen is a new modality that is well accepted by patients. Via a simple outpatient procedure, a cannula is inserted percutaneously into the trachea. Problems with nasal irritation or irritation around the ears from the plastic of the nasal cannula on the face are eliminated (Fig. 15-6). In many patients, sensitivity about their appearance in public while wearing oxygen devices leads to decreased compliance with the prescribed regimen. With transtracheal oxygen, the catheter can easily be hidden with a high collar. The importance of this admittedly cosmetic reason for considering transtracheal oxygen should not be undervalued in attempting to ensure patient compliance. As an added benefit, oxygen flow rates can usually be reduced by about half when oxygen is administered directly into the trachea [44, 45]. The expense of oxygen is reduced. Additionally, small portable tanks last about twice as long with the lower flow rates, allowing patients greater mobility.

Benefits of oxygen in qualifying patients have been demonstrated in terms of both morbidity and mortality. The Nocturnal Oxygen Therapy Trial [46] showed increased survival of patients using nighttime oxygen in comparison with patients not using oxygen (Fig. 15-7). The Continuous Oxygen Therapy Trial [47] demonstrated that continuous oxygen therapy produced additional benefits in terms of survival over nocturnal or "part-time" oxygen use (Fig. 15-8). Based on these results, compliance with use of needed oxygen must be stressed to each patient.

Home Ventilation

There are difficult moral and ethical questions to be discussed and answered with patients when considering the use of home mechanical ventilation. Additionally, the presence or absence of home support systems to sustain a patient outside the hospital on a ventilator need to be carefully evaluated.

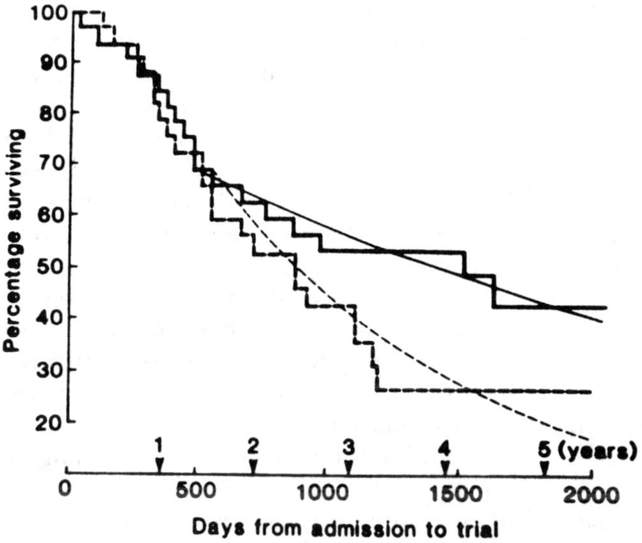
Percentage surviving
100
90
80
70
60
50
40
30
20
1
2
3
4
5 (years)
0
500
1000
1500
2000
Days from admission to trial

Fig. 15-7. NOTT results, which demonstrate improved survival of patients using nocturnal oxygen (solid line) versus patients not on oxygen (dotted line). (From N.R. Anthonisen. Long-term oxygen therapy. *Ann Intern Med* 99:519–527, 1983; with permission.)

Fig. 15-8. COTT (American) results, demonstrating further improvement in survival when oxygen was used continuously (open circles) versus use only nocturnally (open squares). (*From* Nocturnal Oxygen Trial Group: Continuous or nocturnal oxygen therapy in hypoxemic chronic obstructive pulmonary disease. *Ann Intern Med* 93:391–398, 1980; with permission.)

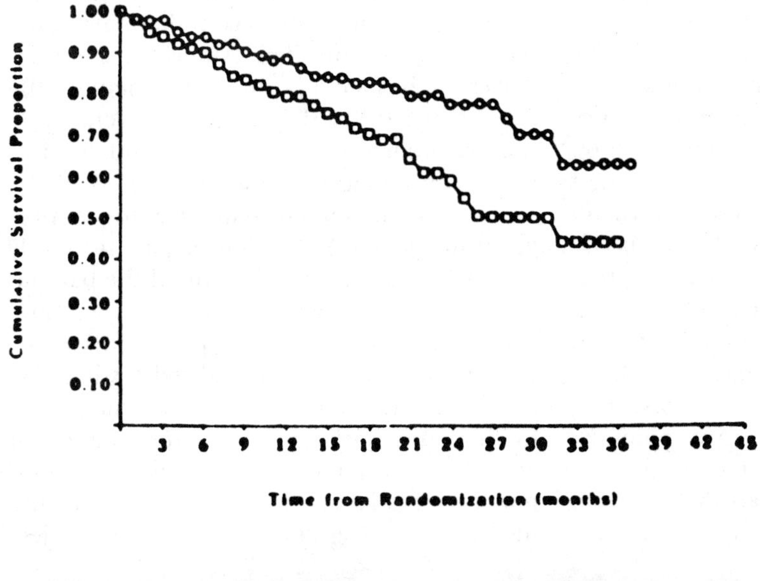
Cumulative Survival Proportion
1.00
0.90
0.80
0.70
0.60
0.50
0.40
0.30
0.20
0.10
3 6 9 12 15 18 21 24 27 30 33 36 39 42 45
Time from Randomization (months)

For patients with terminal disease, such as end-stage pulmonary fibrosis, malignancy, and progressive neuromuscular disease, such as amyotrophic lateral sclerosis, muscular dystrophy, chest wall deformities, and so on, the ethical questions regarding maintenance of ventilation must be thoroughly discussed with patients and families.

General indications for continuous home mechanical ventilation via tracheostomy as outlined here should be taken as guidelines rather than dogma, as the individual patient's wishes must be a primary concern. A first indication would be to "rescue" a patient with an acute problem who is expected to (eventually) recover the ability to ventilate on his or her own. A second indication might be patients with chronic stable respiratory failure who desire to continue life sustained by mechanical ventilation (spinal cord injuries, chest wall deformities, otherwise stable patients with end-stage lung disease) [48].

Consideration for part-time home ventilation is a viable option for some patients with borderline respiratory function, particularly if their functional abilities suggest they have not otherwise reached a terminal phase of their illness [49]. Several devices, other than the tracheostomy-ventilator unit, are available for this purpose. These devices act by creating negative pressure around the thorax, effectively pulling the chest wall outward and allowing assisted inspiration. The old iron lung, or whole body respirator, has been proved effective in maintaining ventilation [48], but the device is cumbersome. The cuirass type ventilators, which consist of a hard shell that is fitted over the anterior thorax, are somewhat less effective but are a bit easier to manipulate. In patients with chest wall deformities, the cuirass may be difficult to fit. The Pulmowrap® (Boulder, CO) is a newer device that consists of a small cage that is placed around the thorax, coupled with an airtight jacket. It is easy to fit patients and light enough that patients may be able to apply the device themselves. All these machines limit mobility, so they are generally used during nighttime. Daytime respiratory performance may be improved by nocturnal assistance alone [50] and declines in vital capacity may be reduced [51]. It is not clear at what stage such part-time ventilation is most beneficial. If long-term nocturnal ventilation is considered, upper airway collapse should be ruled out by clinical observation or a sleep study should be performed to rule out airway obstruction, as moving of the chest wall in the face of obstruction will not alleviate ventilatory problems.

Home care using positive-pressure ventilation, via tracheostomy or endotracheal tubes, has been shown to be a safe, cost-effective means of managing patients with chronic respiratory failure outside the hospital [52, 53].

A period of time for in-hospital training of the patient and family in the use of whatever type of ventilator is prescribed is near mandatory. They must be alerted to the mechanics of the system used and how to "troubleshoot" the devices. Generally, a week or two of training is required. Arrangements for professional home follow-up should also be made, with regular visits by a respiratory therapist and/or nursing personnel. An excellent monograph covering most aspects of nonhospital ventilator management is available for those desiring more detailed information [54].

Design of an Outpatient Rehabilitation Program

A multidisciplinary approach, individualized to fit the needs of each patient, is required in designing a comprehensive pulmonary rehabilitation program. The American Thoracic Society published a position statement on the subject in 1981 [55]. The goals of rehabilitation, sequence of the program, and services to be included are outlined therein.

The recommended sequence for a program includes (1) selection of patients likely to benefit; (2) initial evaluation of the patient, including history and physical examination, chest radiography, baseline pulmonary function testing, and any specialized testing (exercise testing, blood gases, etc.) suggested by the basic evaluation; (3) determination of goals for each patient; (4) outlining the components of care for the patient; (5) assessing the patient's progress subjectively and objectively (pulmonary function testing); and (6) ensuring long-term follow-up for those patients with chronic disease.

The components of the program should include (1) general education of the patient and family on the disease, proper nutrition, avoidance of smoking; and prevention of infection; (2) education and instruction in the use of prescribed medications; (3) information and advice on the role of respiratory therapy techniques such as aerosol therapy, oxygen use, and home ventilation; (4) instruction in physical modalities that may benefit the individual patient (relaxation training, breathing retraining, chest percussion and postural drainage, cough techniques); (5) exercise conditioning, with endurance rather than strength the goal; and (6) evaluation of the patient's daily functioning and outlining maneuvers to alleviate symptoms during performance of daily activities [56, 57].

The ideal setup would be to have a respiratory therapist or nurse practitioner devoted to the rehabilitation program working with the physician. As this may not always be possible, routine office visits can be used to accomplish the outlined goals by use of charts, discussions, videotapes, or demonstrations. Having ancillary personnel available does, however, assist in providing follow-up visits to ensure that long-term compliance with the therapeutic regimen is maintained and that patients understand and retain what had been taught. A complete discussion of the components and goals of a pulmonary rehabilitation program can be found in the text by Hodgkin et al [58] (Table 15-1).

Table 15-1. Components of a Rehabilitation Program

Patient selection and evaluation
Patient and family education
Proper nutrition
Smoking cessation
Medication instructions
Respiratory therapy techniques
Breathing retraining
Infection control
Exercise rehabilitation

Benefits of a Rehabilitation Program

Pulmonary rehabilitation programs are relatively new. As such there are few studies of long enough duration to demonstrate increases in survival for patients enrolled in such programs. In terms of reducing morbidity and improving the quality of life, there are several studies that demonstrate the benefits of a comprehensive approach to patients with chronic pulmonary disease.

In several studies, reductions in the number of days hospitalized (up to a reduction of 20 days per year) have been reported [59–63]. This represents not only a reduction in patient morbidity, but a significant cost savings to the health care system.

Patients generally report a reduction in symptoms such as cough, sputum production, anxiety, and dyspnea. Improvement in the quality of life and functional abilities accompanies the improvement in symptomatology [64].

Close attention to medical needs and education of the patient and family, with subsequent relief of symptoms and reductions in morbidity associated with chronic lung disease, can be achieved with an effective pulmonary rehabilitation program. Patients can return to productive lives with an improved sense of well-being and significantly improved quality of life, coping with successfully with underlying chronic lung disease.

References

1. Mazzuca SA: Does patient education in chronic disease have therapeutic value? *J Chron Dis* 35:521–529, 1982
2. Hoch D, Murray D, Blalock J, et al: Nutritional status as an index of morbidity in chronic airflow limitation. *Chest* 85:668–675, 1984
3. Driver AG, McAlevy MT, Smith VL: Nutritional assessment of patients with chronic obstructive pulmonary disease and acute respiratory failure. *Chest* 82:568–571, 1988
4. Braur SR, Dixon RM, Keim NL, et al: Predictive clinical value of nutritional assessment factors in COPD. Chest 85:353–357, 1984
5. Bronson DL, Flynn BS, Solomon LJ, et al: Smoking cessation counseling during periodic

health examinations. *Arch Intern Med* 149: 1653–1656, 1989

6. Cohen SJ, Stookey GK, Katz BP, et al: Encouraging primary care physicians to help smokers quit: A randomized controlled trial. *Ann Intern Med* 119:648–652, 1989
7. Cummings SR, Coates TJ, Richard RJ, et al: Training physicians in counselling about smoking cessation: A randomized trial of the "Quit for Life" program. *Ann Intern Med* 110: 640–647, 1989
8. Model D: District General Hospital, Eastborn, England. Smoker's face: An underrated clinical sign? *Br Med J* 29:1760–1762, 1985
9. Blondal T: Controlled trial of nicotine polacrilex gum with supportive measures. *Arch Intern Med* 149:1818–1821, 1989
10. Gold MS, Pottash AC, Sweeney DR, et al: Opiate withdrawal using clonidine: A safe, effective, and rapid nonopiate treatment. *JAMA* 243:343–346, 1980
11. Ornish SA, Zisook S, McAdams LA: Effects of transdermal clonidine on withdrawal symptoms associated with smoking cessation. *Arch Intern Med* 148:2027–2031, 1988
12. DeBlaquiere P, Christensen DB, Carter WB, et al: Use and misuse of metered-dose inhalers by patients with chronic lung disease: A controlled randomized trial of two instruction methods. *Am Rev Respir Dis* 140:910–916, 1989
13. Kelling JS, Strohl KP, Smith RL, et al: Physician knowledge in the use of canister nebulizers. Chest 85:612–614, 1983
14. O'Loughlin JM: Pharmacologic therapy for bronchial asthma. *Postgrad Med* 82:231–238, 1987
15. Dolovich M, Eng P, Ruffin R, et al: Clinical evaluation of a simple demand inhalation MDI aerosol delivery device. *Chest* 84:36–41, 1983
16. Sackner MA, Kim CS: Auxiliary MDI aerosol delivery systems. *Chest* 88:161S–170S, 1985
17. Newman SP, Woodman G, Clarke SW, et al: Effect of InspirEase on the deposition of metered-dose aerosols in the human respiratory tract. *Chest* 89:551–556, 1986
18. McFadden ER, Mills R: Inhaled albuterol powder for the prevention of exercise-induced bronchospasm. *Immunol Allergy Prac* 8:199–203, 1986
19. Summer W, Elston R, Therpe L, et al: Aerosol bronchodilator delivery methods. Relative impact on pulmonary function and cost of respiratory care. *Arch Intern Med* 149:618–623, 1989
20. Jenkins SC, Heaton RW, Fulton TJ, et al: Comparison of domiciliary nebulized salbutamol and salbutamol from a metered-dose inhaler in stable chronic airflow limitation. *Chest* 91:804–807, 1987
21. Williams JH, Moser KM: Pneumococcal vaccine and patients with chronic lung disease. *Ann Intern Med* 104:106–109, 1986
22. Simberkoff MS, Cross AP, Al-Ibrahim M, et al: Efficacy of pneumococcal vaccine in high-risk patients. Results of a Veterans Administration cooperative study. *N Engl J Med* 315:1318–1327, 1986
23. Bolan G, Broome CV, Facklam RR, et al: Pneumococcal vaccine efficacy in selected populations in the United States. *Ann Intern Med* 104:1–6, 1986
24. Sims RV, Steinmann WC, McConville JH, et al: The clinical effectiveness of pneumococcal vaccine in the elderly. *Ann Intern Med* 108: 653–657, 1988
25. Centers for Disease Control, Department of Health and Human Services: Recommendations for prevention and control of influenza. *Ann Intern Med* 105:399–404, 1986
26. Margolis KL, Lofgren RP, Korn JE: Organizational strategies to improve influenza vaccine delivery: A standing order in a general medical clinic. *Arch Intern Med* 148:2205–2207, 1988
27. Hermans PE, Cockerill FR: Antiviral agents. *Mayo Clin Proc* 62:1108–1115, 1987
28. Arden NH, Patriarca PA, Pasano MB, et al: The roles of vaccination and amantadine prophylaxis in controlling an outbreak of influenza A (H3N2) in a nursing home. *Arch Intern Med* 148:865–868, 1988
29. Anthonisen NR, Manfreda J, Warren CP, et al: Antibiotic therapy in exacerbations of chronic obstructive pulmonary disease. *Ann Intern Med* 106:196–204, 1987
30. Braun SR, Fregos RF, Reddan WG: Exercise training in patients with COPD. *Postgrad Med* 71:163–173, 1982
31. Mueller RE, Petty TL, Filley GF: Ventilation and arterial blood gas exchanges induced by pursed lip breathing. *J Appl Physiol* 41:508–516, 1970
32. Tiep BL, Burns M, Kao D, et al: Pursed lips breathing training using ear oximetry. *Chest* 90:218–221, 1986
33. Miller WF: A physiologic evaluation of the effects of diaphragmatic breathing training in patients with pulmonary emphysema. *Am J Med* 171:471–477, 1954
34. Ries AL, Moser KM: Comparison of isocapnic hyperventilation and walking exercise training at home in pulmonary rehabilitation. *Chest* 90:285–289, 1986
35. Zack MB, Palange AV: Oxygen supplemented exercise of ventilatory and nonventilatory muscles in pulmonary rehabilitation. *Chest* 88:669–675, 1985
36. Celli BR, Rassulo J, Make BJ: Dyssynchronous breathing during arm but not leg exercise in

patients with chronic airflow obstruction. *N Engl J Med* 314:1485–1490, 1986
37. Miller WF, Taylor HF: Exercise training in the rehabilitation of patients with severe respiratory insufficiency due to pulmonary emphysema: The role of oxygen breathing. *South Med J* 55:1216–1221, 1962
38. Pierce AK, Taylor HF, Archer RK, et al: Response to exercise training in patients with emphysema. *Arch Intern Med* 113:28–36, 1964
39. Nicholas JJ, Gilbert R, Gabe R, et al: Evaluation of an exercise therapy program for patients with chronic obstructive pulmonary disease. *Am Rev Respir Dis* 102:1–9, 1970
40. Kirilloff LH, Owens GR, Rogers RM, et al: Does chest physical therapy work? *Chest* 83: 436–444, 1985
41. Fulmer JD, Snider GL: American College of Chest Physicians (ACCP), National Heart, Lung and Blood Institute (NHLBI) Conference on Oxygen Therapy. *Arch Intern Med* 144:1645–1655, 1984
42. Aldrete JA, Aldrete LE: Oxygen concentrations in commercial aircraft flights. *South Med J* 76:12–14, 1983
43. Dillard TA, Berg BW, Rajagopal KR, et al: Hypoxemia during air travel in patients with chronic obstructive pulmonary disease. *Ann Intern Med* 111:362–367, 1989
44. Banner NR, Goven JR: Long term transtracheal oxygen delivery through microcatheter in patients with hypoxemia due to chronic obstructive airways disease. *Br Med J* 293:111, 1986
45. Christopher KL, Spofford B, McCarty DC, et al: Transtracheal oxygen therapy for refractory hypoxemia. *JAMA* 256:494–497, 1986
46. Medical Research Council Working Party: Long term domiciliary oxygen therapy in chronic hypoxic cor pulmonale complicating chronic bronchitis and emphysema. *Lancet* 1:681–686, 1981
47. Nocturnal Oxygen Therapy Trial Group: Continuous or nocturnal oxygen therapy in hypoxemic chronic obstructive pulmonary disease. Ann Intern Med 93:391–398, 1980
48. Bergofsky EH: Respiratory failure in disorders of the thoracic cage. *Am Rev Respir Dis* 119:643–669, 1979
49. Smith PEM, Calverley PMA, Edwards RHT, et al: Practical problems in the respiratory care of patients with muscular dystrophy. *N Engl J Med* 316:1197–1205, 1987
50. Curran FJ: Night ventilation by body respirators for patients in chronic respiratory failure due to late stage Duchenne muscular dystrophy. *Arch Phys Med Rehabil* 62:270–274, 1981
51. Rideau Y: Duchenne muscular dystrophy child: Care of wheelchair dependent patient: Death prevention (abstr). *Muscle Nerve 5* (suppl):86, 1986
52. Splaingard ML, Frats RC Jr, Harrison GM, et al: Home positive-pressure ventilation—Twenty years experience. *Chest* 84:376–382, 1983
53. Fischer DA, Prentice WS: Feasibility of home care for certain respiratory dependent restrictive or obstructive lung disease patients. *Chest* 82:739–743, 1982
54. O'Donohue WJ Jr, Giovanni RM, Goldberg AI, et al: Long-term Mechanical Ventilation: Guidelines for Management in the Home and at Alternate Community Sites. Report of a Subcommittee, Respiratory Care Section, American College of Chest Physicians. *Chest* 90:15–375, 1986
55. Pulmonary rehabilitation: Official American Thoracic Society Statement. *Am Rev Respir Dis* 124:663–666, 1981
56. Mahler DA, Weinberg DH, Wells CK, et al: The measurement of dyspnea: Contents, interobserver agreement and physiologic correlates of two new clinical indexes. *Chest* 85: 751–758, 1984
57. Mohsenifar Z, Horak D, Brown HV, et al: Sensitive indices of improvement in a pulmonary rehabilitation program. *Chest* 83:189–192, 1983
58. Hodgkin JE, Zorn EG, Connors GL (eds): Pulmonary Rehabilitation: Guidelines to Success. Stoneham, MA, Butterworths, 1984
59. Lertzman MM, Cherniack RM: Rehabilitation of patients with chronic obstructive pulmonary disease. *Am Rev Respir Dis* 114:1145–1165, 1976
60. Deflorio G, Johnson M, Tanzi F, et al: A prospective study of morbidity and cost/benefit outcomes for in-hospital pulmonary rehabilitation of patients with chronic obstructive lung disease. *Am Rev Respir Dis* 121:127, 1980
61. Johnson NR, Balchum O, Tanzi F, et al: Comprehensive pulmonary rehabilitation in severe chronic obstructive lung disease (COLD): Patient characteristics predictive of successful outcome in the Barlow Hospital study. *Chest* 76:356, 1979
62. Johnson NR, Tanzi F, Balchum OJ, et al: Inpatient comprehensive pulmonary rehabilitation in severe COPD: Barlow Hospital study. *Respiratory Therapy* 3:15–19, 1980
63. Hudson LD, Tyler ML, Petty TL: Hospitalization needs during an outpatient rehabilitation program for severe chronic airway obstruction. *Chest* 70:606–610, 1976
64. Petty T, Cherniak RM: Comprehensive care of COPD. *Clin Notes Resp Dis* 20:3–12, 1981

Pulmonary Infections: Upper Respiratory Tract Infections

Nancy M. McGuire

Upper respiratory tract infections can be quite similar in presentation, but quite diverse in terms of morbidity and mortality. One purpose of this chapter is to update the primary care practitioner on the current management of infections such as the common cold and to briefly explore new approaches to the long search for a cure in this leading cause of morbidity in the outpatient practice of medicine. The reader also is updated on the more serious infections of the upper respiratory tract such as laryngotracheobronchitis (croup), epiglottitis, and bacterial tracheitis that may initially present to a primary care practitioner in the outpatient setting. The clinician must be able to recognize these infections because, unlike the common cold, they may result in respiratory compromise and death. It is my purpose to alert the reader to the importance of diagnostic skills, management of the airway, and current antibiotic therapy.

The Common Cold

The common cold is an acute self-limited respiratory infection that is responsible for a significant amount of absenteeism from school and work in the United States. This infection rarely results in a significant complication. Upper respiratory tract infections, however, rank second to general medical examinations among principal ambulatory diagnoses [1].

The care nationwide for a cold has been estimated to cost more than $1.5 billion annually for medical care and diagnostic tests. The cost of prescription medications, over-the-counter medications, lozenges, and various rubs adds up to over 1 billion [2]. Many individuals with a common cold do not seek medical care, so this viral disease affects many more people than statistics indicate [2]. Despite the prevalence of this disease, it is somewhat perplexing that there has not been a significant amount of teaching either in medical schools or medical textbooks to train clinicians in the treatment of this very common illness [3]. Most practitioners, however, learn how to treat colds on their own and patients who do not seek medical advice usually resort to home remedies to self-treat.

Epidemiology

Research on the common cold began in the 1940s with assumptions as to the etiologic agent of the common cold [4]. Initially, researchers believed bacterial organisms were the prime candidates as etiologic agents [5]. Subsequently, other researchers began to look for a viral etiologic agent as technology improved the field of virology. Researchers had trouble growing the "cold" virus even though it was well known that a cold could be passed from the nose of one infected individual to another susceptible individual. More viruses were soon discovered with improvement in culture techniques. In fact, many new viruses were discovered to be the cause of the common cold.

Respiratory viruses were found to grow best in normal respiratory epithelium, human fetal tracheal, and nasal cells [6]. Today, the etiologic agents of the common cold consist of about six families of viruses that constitute about 100 types in total. They are RNA viruses. The rhinovirus constitutes about one third to one half of all the colds and the coronavirus constitutes about one fifth [7]. Other viruses known to be etiologic agents of the common cold include respiratory syncytial virus, parainfluenza virus, influenza, and adenovirus [8]. In about 35% of the cases, the cause is unknown.

Common colds occur worldwide. Increased incidence is usually associated with the cooler months in temperate areas and during the rainy season in tropical areas. This is usually because people are more likely to be found inside during winter and rainy weather, increasing the probability of transmission to susceptible individuals [8]. It has been found that damp, cold weather does not produce colds or susceptibility to colds. One study evaluated the risk factors of chilling volunteers in a draft and found no increase in the chance of acquiring a cold [9]. Furthermore, isolated antarctic explorers never experienced a cold unless they received a visitor or returned to civilization [10].

The average adult becomes ill with a cold two to four times a year, whereas children have 6 to 10 colds a year [11]. Women usually have more episodes of colds than men, and this may be due to their increased exposure to children. If a family member is ill there is usually a 40% chance of being infected if the exposure has been in the first 3 days of the illness [12]. Cigarette smokers have the same incidence of acquiring colds as nonsmokers. They may, however, have a more protracted course of coughing and wheezing [13]. Stress in daily life may also play a role in susceptibility to colds [13a].

Symptoms

The symptoms of the common cold are similar whether induced by rhinovirus or coronavirus [5]. There is usually a 2- to 3-day incubation period, with the illness usually lasting 1 week or occasionally 2 weeks or longer [14]. The predominant symptoms include nasal discharge, with subsequent obstruction, sneezing, sore throat, and cough. There may be associated systemic manifestations of fever, malaise, and tiredness. These symptoms are not as severe as those symptoms experienced with influenza.

Pathophysiology

Research on the common cold has primarily used rhinovirus as the infectious agent. Infection with the common cold begins with the deposition of the virus in the nasal mucosa. During the incubation period, the virus replicates, increasing the concentration of the virus. Symptomatic effects seem to be mediated by a host pathophysiologic response rather than any component of the virus [5]. The actual mechanisms, however, are still a mystery and not fully understood [3, 14].

During the symptomatic stage of a cold there is a reduction in the efficacy of the mucociliary transport system in the nose and throat. Cilia of the biopsied cells still beat with the normal frequency, but many cells lose substantial numbers of cilia [15]. Cells are shed, but there is little evidence of cell necrosis or mucosal damage. However, in influenza the epithelium is denuded down to the basement membrane. There is usually cellular infiltration by polymorphonucleocytes, plasma cells, and lymphocytes. Increased inflammatory mediators such as kinins have been found in affected areas [16]. Host responses may account for vascular engorgement, causing increased swelling and a decrease in the nasal passages, with increased permeability and transudation of serum proteins including IgA, IgG, and increased mucus production. Although colds simulate allergic rhinitis, with an increase in the mediators of allergic inflammation such as leukotrienes or histamine, none of these agents have been found in patients with the common cold [4]. However, nedocromil sodium, a mast cell degranulation inhibitor, diminished the severity of symptoms in a double-blind placebo-controlled trial on the coronavirus. Subsequently, recovery from the common cold may depend on production of interferon by the infected host.

Transmission

Susceptibility to the common cold may depend on many factors. Preexisting antibody such as serum neutralizing antibody in the host may play a significant part in susceptibility of the host to a cold [17, 18]. Nasal secretory antibody is also secreted locally and may be more protective against infection if specific for a particular cold virus. The half-life of this particular antibody, however, may limit effectiveness in protecting against future colds [17]. Although the mode of transmission of the common cold is still not completely known, some researchers believe the mechanism to be direct contact from a hand contaminated by nasal secretions to the hand of a susceptible host, who in turn inoculates the mucosa of the nose and conjunctiva [12, 17]. The rhinovirus can exist for hours on the hands and fomites, and contact with these items may also cause infection. Other researchers believe that transmission through the air by large and small particle aerosol generated by coughing and sneezing of inoculums of virus may be the predominant mode of spread [19].

Therapeutic Treatment

Various medications have been used by the majority of patients afflicted with the common cold. There are more than 800 oral nonprescription cold remedies that are currently on the market [3]. As with the testing of all medications, it is important to show efficacy and to prove no significant side effects by doing scientific studies. Unfortunately, studies on the treatment of the common cold have been difficult to do because the symptoms of a cold may be transient or very subjective. Studies need more concrete end points, such as the ability to collect nasal secretions and use patency studies. Some studies have also lacked suitable controls, with poor randomization or lack of follow-up of the patients [20, 21]. Thus, many studies of medications and treatment of the common cold may suffer bias.

The goal of symptomatic treatment should be to decrease symptoms associated with colds, such as headache, cough, and nasal stuffiness, and to increase functional status. Decreasing possible transmission to susceptible contacts should also be considered important. Most cough and cold medicines contain one or more sympathomimetic drugs and at least one antihistamine. Other drugs may be included in a cold preparation, such as analgesics, expectorants, antitussives, and belladonna alkaloids. Some of these over-the-counter medications have as many as eight ingredients, and for this reason antagonism and unwanted side effects may be unavoidable [3]. One of the most important principles in the treatment of the common cold should be to prescribe one medication at a time targeted at a specific symptom [3].

Antihistamines

Antihistamines block the H_1-receptor and have been used in the treatment of the common cold (Table 16-1). The histamine concentration in nasal sécretions does not increase in quantity during an infection with a cold. In contrast, a significant amount of histamine is produced in allergies [16, 21a]. Antihistamines, however, have been used in combinations to treat the symptoms of common cold. Controlled trials with alkylating type antihistamines such as chlorpheniramine and triprolidine have been found to reduce symptoms of natural colds [22, 23].

Oral chlorpheniramine also was found to cause a modest decrease in nasal discharge, sneezing, and nose blowing [24]. These agents have been known to cause increased drowsiness, and this sedating effect might alter the perception of symptoms. These agents may also alleviate nasal congestion and discharge because of the atropine-like action of antihistamines [25]. In controlled clinical trials of natural colds, however, there is little evidence that antihistamines provide clinically important benefits [14].

Sympathomimetics

Sympathomimetics are the most commonly used and advertised agents for the symptomatic treatment of the common cold. They can be administered systemically or topically by spray. Oral sympathomimetics usually have α-adrenergic properties that cause the constriction of the microvasculature of the nasal mucosa. This in turn relieves congestion by decreasing blood flow in a highly vascular mucosa and shrinking venous capacitance vessels in the turbinates. Phenylpropanol-

Table 16-1. Common Cold Medications and Their Components

	Decongestant	*Antihistamine*	*Analgesic*	*Antitussive*	*Alcohol*
Contact (Smith Kline Consumer Products)	75 mg phenylpropanolamine HCL	8 mg chlorpheniramine maleate	—	—	—
Dristan Caplets (Whitehall)	5 mg phenylephrine HCl	2 mg chlorpheniramine maleate	325 mg acetaminophen	—	—
Sudafed Plus Tablets (Burroughs-Wellcome)	60 mg pseudoephedrine	4 mg chlorpheniramine	—	—	—
Actifed Tablets (Burroughs-Wellcome)	60 mg pseudoephedrine	2.5 mg triprolidine HCl	—	—	—
Alka-Seltzer Plus Cold Medicine (Miles Inc.)	24.08 mg phenylpropanolamine biturate	2 mg chlorpheniramine maleate	325 mg aspirin	—	—
Vicks Nyquil Liquid (Richardson-Vicks Health Care)	60 mg pseudoephedrine HCL	7.5 mg doxylamine succinate	1000 mg acetaminophen	30 mg dextromethorphan hydrobromide	25%
Tylenol Cold Medication Liquid (McNeil Consumer Products)	60 mg pseudoephedrine HCL	4 mg chlorpheniramine maleate	650 mg acetaminophen	30 mg dextromethorphan hydrobromide	7%

amine and ephedrine are both α- and β-agonists and release norepinephrine from neuronal storage sites. They have direct effects on α-adrenergic receptors. Phenylpropanolamine and pseudoephedrine have been found to produce significant reductions of 35% to 55% in the nasal airflow resistance in the treatment of natural colds [26–28]. These medications usually peak in 1 hour and may last for 4 hours. However, sympathomimetics prescribed at these doses may cause vasoconstriction in other vascular beds that may potentiate high blood pressure. There is a greater risk of hypertension with the use of phenlypropanolamine than pseudoephedrine [29]. This may be a low risk in an otherwise healthy person. Topically applied nasal sympathomimetic agents may increase nasal patency, thereby causing subjective relief. Tachyphylaxis and rebound hyperemia may result after 3 or 4 days of use, so these agents cannot be used for long periods.

Anticholinergics

Activation of the parasympathetic nervous system may be important in the production of rhinorrhea and perhaps other cold symptoms. Medications such as the quaternary cholinergic antagonist, ipratropium bromide, have been used in the treatment of the common cold [30]. However, the overall value of anticholinergics in treatment remains to be determined [14]. Also, there may be side effects with oral anticholinergics, such as constipation, blurred vision, urinary retention, and dry mouth.

Nonsteroidal Anti-inflammatory Agents

Nonsteroidal anti-inflammatory agents such as aspirin and acetaminophen are widely used as effective analgesic and antipyretic agents. High fever, however, is not a major manifestation of the common cold. Aspirin and acetaminophen may provide significant relief of headache and sore throat. In one study, aspirin at a dose of 600 mg three times a day during the incubation period in rhinoviral infection was found to be of modest clinical benefit by increased viral shedding [31]. Aspirin was also found to decrease mucociliary clearance in the pharynx, trachea, and lung and may potentially interfere with viral mechanisms [32].

Cough Medicine

The cough reflex is a very complex series of events that serves to expel secretions and foreign material from the airways. There are cough receptors throughout the respiratory system [33]. A cough suppressant is indicated when a cough is nonproductive, disrupts sleep and work, or causes complications such as nausea, vomiting, and rupture of subconjunctival vessels [3]. There are three types of cough medications: (1) antitussives, (2) expectorants, and (3) mucolytics. Antitussives usually contain narcotics such as codeine, the standard agent, or dextromethorphan, which is very similar to codeine but has fewer side effects [34]. These agents act on the medullary cough center. These agents may have adverse side effects and cause gastrointestinal upset and drowsiness and may also release histamine, which may in turn trigger bronchospasm. Peripherally acting antitussive agents have been routinely used. Lozenges, syrups, cough drops, water, mist, and alcohol may have efficacy as local cough receptor suppressants. Expectorants decrease sputum viscosity and help remove secretions from respiratory airways. Guaifenesin is most frequently prescribed but is no more efficacious than placebo [35]. The best expectorants are actually good hydration, humidification of the airways with steam inhalation or oral liquids. In general, patients with colds do not need an expectorant or mucolytic agent because tenacious lower respiratory tract secretions are seldom present.

Vitamin C

Vitamin C has received a lot of attention as a preventative and treatment agent for the common cold. There has been no consistent evidence in the literature that vitamin C is an effective preventative or therapeutic agent. The long-term effects of high doses include potentiation of diarrhea, precipitation of oxalate or urate renal stones, hyperglycemia, and inhibition of the anticoagulant effect of warfarin [36].

Antibiotics

Occasionally patients ask their physicians for antibiotics or take old antibiotics stored in their medicine cabinets. Antibiotics have no place in the treatment of the common cold. Rarely, complications such as sinusitis or otitis media occur. Antibiotics are of benefit only in these unusual cases.

Antiviral Therapy

The study of antiviral therapy in the treatment of the common cold has been an active area of research. Early antiviral therapy may potentially provide symptom benefit if viral replication is ongoing. Amantadine has been an effective antiviral in the prevention of influenza A by interfering in the early stages of infection during viral uncoating. Its discovery encouraged belief that specific antiviral drugs aimed at the common cold could be developed [37]. Thus, much work has been done to test drugs that interfere with viral replication. Additionally, agents that inhibit the action of host inflammatory mediators have also been studied in an attempt to prevent the symptoms of the common cold [14].

The present goals of effective viral therapy are to develop an agent that (1) is without significant toxicity or side effects, (2) achieves effective concentrations in the nasal secretions following oral administration, (3) is effective in ameliorating illness, and (4) may prevent spread of disease to others (Table 16-2). However, by the time respiratory disease is obvious, the virus replication is probably complete and may not be modified by an antiviral agent.

Table 16-2. The Optimal Antiviral Agent for the Common Cold

High antiviral activity
Broad spectrum
Low toxicity and side effects
High concentration in nasal secretions

Enviroxime was discovered as the benchmark compound for treatment of the common cold. It was found to have weak activity in preventing and treating rhinovirus, but has no useful effect against natural colds [38, 39]. Another agent, dichloroflavan, has activity against some rhinoviruses by acting as a capsid-binding agent, but unfortunately did not achieve effective concentrations in the ciliated epithelium so it did not effectively prevent rhinovirus infection [39a]. Chalone, which also acts as a capsid-binding agent, has high antirhinovirus activity but did not prevent the common cold when given orally [40, 41]. Chalone did not work intranasally, either. A promising antiviral compound, R 61837, has been shown to be effective in decreasing the clinical signs and symptoms of a cold in about 75% of the serotypes, and clinical studies are currently in progress [42]. Unfortunately, clinical trials on the whole have indicated the discrepancies between in vivo and in vitro antiviral activity [14]. Currently, there are no antiviral agents for use in the treatment of the common cold [4].

Zinc has also been used to inhibit in vitro replication of the rhinovirus by acting to inhibit viral polypeptide cleavage [43, 44]. Zinc lozenges have been shown to decrease the duration of cold symptoms, but caused significant side effects of unpleasant taste and sores in the oral mucosa, and these agents cannot be recommended for treatment at this time.

Monoclonal antibodies have also been studied to block the host cell receptor site through which the rhinovirus attaches and enters the cells [45]. A preliminary report has suggested a reduction in infection when given as an intranasal spray to volunteers.

Interferon

Interferon is a naturally produced antiviral protein with a very broad spectrum of antiviral activity that inhibits translation of viral messenger RNA to a peptide [46]. Interferon has not been entirely effective for the treatment of the common cold; however, prophylactic studies have been done and are encouraging. Initially, the use of crude human interferon as an intranasal spray was found to prevent infection and illness produced by rhinovirus [47]. Purified recombinant interferon-α given prophylactically as a nasal spray also reduced 70% to 80% of the rhinovirus colds in families in which an individual with rhinovirus was introduced [9, 48, 49]. There were 40% fewer colds overall using prophylactic interferon spray. However, there may be temporary adverse side effects such as nasal inflammation, stuffiness, and bleeding with continued use of interferon. Leukocyte-derived human interferon did not seem to work when begun 40 hours after viral inoculation [50].

Vaccines

The prospects for a common cold vaccine seem limited at the present time, since there are so many different viruses that can cause colds. An intranasal vaccine that would elicit local broad-spectrum antibody production would be an ideal agent [3].

Complications

Complications of the common cold are exceedingly rare. There may be a 0.5% bacterial superinfection of the sinuses [51]. Middle ear infections may also be a problem in 2% of those infected with a cold. Antibiotics such as ceftin, ceclor, and augmentin may be useful in treating these bacterial infections particularly if *Staphylococcus aureus, Streptococcus pnemoniae,* β-lactamase producing *Hemophilus influenzae* and *Moraxella catarrhalis* are suspected. There may also be exacerbations of asthma, chronic bronchitis, and emphysema seen after infection with a cold [52]. Abnormalities in pulmonary function tests have been observed, such as decreased lung diffusing capacity and decreased expiratory airflow rates. Bronchial hyperactivity has been observed and may last for 3 to 12 weeks [53–56].

Symptomatic Treatment

Since there is no effective cure of the common cold, the best advice to give a patient is sensible self-care. It is important to rest and, if the cold is severe enough, to stay in bed. Sipping hot liquids may be of benefit. In fact, one study by Saketkoo et al [57] reported that chicken soup was more effective than sipping hot or cold water in mobilizing nasal secretions, the first line of host defense. A Viralizer (Viral Response Systems, Greenwich, CT) has also been used for symptomatic treatment. It is a heated nebulizer device that blows heated air or antiseptic decongestant and can be purchased for about $30 to $40 in a drug store. However, there have been no published studies that show evidence that it relieves symptoms or cures common colds [58]. If symptoms persist, a physician should be contacted.

It is important to note that patients can participate in breaking the transmission cycle of infection. While the natural mechanism of transmission is not fully determined with certainty, hand to hand, autoinoculation of mucosa and conjunctiva, or prolonged exposure to aerosols may be sufficient to transmit virus to a majority of exposed and susceptible individuals. Tissues that have been impregnated with citric/malic acid and sodium lauryl sulfate have been reviewed in two randomized, controlled, double-blinded trials and have been found to cause a modest reduction in secondary colds, but these results were not statistically significant [59, 60]. Those infected with colds can decrease transmission to others by washing hands, throwing away tissues that have been used, and decontaminating fomites with agents such as ethyl alcohol, lysol, or hydrogen peroxide.

Epiglottitis

Epidemiology and Clinical Presentation

Epiglottitis has been more commonly seen in the pediatric population as a very acute and aggressive inflammation of the epiglottis, resulting in acute airway obstruction and potential hypoxic brain injury and death. Successful outcome depends on accurate diagnostic skills and treatment. Sinclair [61] first described this entity in 1941 as a form of laryngitis caused by *Hemophilus influenzae* type B. Subsequently, Miller [62] described the features of acute epiglottitis in 1949 and emphasized the distinction between supraglottic and subglottic types of laryngeal inflammation associated with acute airway obstruction. The disease not only affects the epiglottis but also the supraglottic laryngeal and contiguous tissues from the vallecula to the arytenoids [62, 63].

Epiglottitis is a true medical emergency in children. The disease most commonly affects the age group between 8 months and 16 years, with the majority in the 2 to 4 year age group [64]. Epiglottitis has also been described as occurring more frequently in adults [65–67]. The average age of the adult patients has been in the early 40s [66, 67]. This disease is of very acute onset in both children and adults. Some of the patients in one series had been examined by their physicians within 48 hours before their admission to a hospital, and 21% were given antibiotics as outpatients and subsequently admitted to the hospital with impending respiratory failure [67]. However, the disease can follow two courses: benign and very life threatening [63].

Clinical Features

The presenting symptoms of epiglottitis are sore throat, dysphagia, hoarseness, drooling, and upper airway obstruction [64, 66–68]. Adult patients may also have anterior neck cellulitis, cervical lymphadenopathy, or associated tenderness, and this should alert the clinician to the possibility of epiglottitis [66]. The patient may be seen in the sitting position leaning forward and will resist any attempt to be placed in the supine position [68]. This is an attempt to maximize the opening of the airway because lying supine may obstruct the airway by the edematous epiglottis, especially in children.

The initial presentation of epiglottitis in children may be confused with croup (Table 16-3). In a study of children by Mauro et al [69] an attempt was made to differentiate epiglottitis from croup. Absence of spontaneous cough was the most sensitive predictor of acute epiglottitis [69]. Drooling was the most specific indicator of acute epiglottitis [69]. Agitation was also noted to be a predictor of epiglottitis. High fever is commonly seen, but

Table 16-3. Differences Between Laryngotracheobronchitis, Epiglottitis, and Bacterial Tracheitis

	Laryngotracheobronchitis	*Epiglottitis*	*Bacterial Tracheitis*
Clinical onset	Coryzal illness, several days	Acute	Following short prodromal illness unresponsive to treatment
Age range	3 months to 3 years	2–7 years Adults in 40s	Children <5 years
Fever	Minimal	High	High
Dysphagia	None	Yes; absence of cough	None
White blood count	Usually not increased	Increased	May be increased
Radiography	Narrowing in subglottic area, "hour-glass steeple sign"	Edematous epiglottis	Subglottic narrowing pseudomembrane
Predominant etiologic agent	Parainfluenza virus	*H. influenzae*	*S aureus, H influenzae*
Diagnosis	Exclusion of other diagnoses	Cherry red epiglottis in children; mild erythematous subglottic area in adults	Copious pus aspirated
Treatment	Cool mist; racemic epinephrine	Prophylactic airway in children; prophylactic airway; adults with respiratory difficulty; 2nd, 3rd generation cephalosporin	Nasotracheal airway, 2nd generation cephalosporin, repeated bronchoscopy
Complications	Respiratory failure; cardiac failure	Respiratory arrest; anoxic brain injury	Respiratory arrest, pneumonia; toxic shock

in one study 40% of the patients did not have fever [64]. Tachycardia may also be seen and may be a finding of hypoxia and impending airway obstruction [64].

Patients with a presentation suggesting epiglottitis should undergo indirect laryngoscopy. The examination should be done only by those clinicians who are experienced in intubation. This is especially important in children. The examination has not precipitated airway crisis in adults because they have larger airways [67]. The examination should be done only when it is possible to establish an artificial airway in the operating room or the emergency room.

The epiglottis on laryngoscopic examination has been described as being cherry red in children with *Hemophilus influenzae* infection. This may be different in adults as the epiglottis may appear to be mildly erythematous on direct visual examination [66, 70]. The epiglottic, vallecula, and base of the tongue tissues may appear in general to be swollen and inflamed and the term supraglottitis may be a more descriptive term [63, 70].

Lateral neck radiographs have been helpful in making the diagnosis of epiglottitis [63, 71]. Radiography may suggest the diagnosis in the majority of patients, but may miss a significant group of patients who may not have any evident swelling of the epiglottis or thickening of the aryepiglottic folds and were subsequently found to have epiglottitis by indirect laryngscopy [64, 67, 72]. Radiography may be useful in those patients whose clinical presentation is to some extent confusing, if the diagnosis is in doubt, or if the examination of the oral pharynx cannot be easily completed [64]. These radiologic examinations should not be done on the patient in respiratory distress. If for any reason a radiograph is to be obtained on a patient in minimal respiratory distress, it is imperative that a physician skilled at intubation should accompany the patient to the radiology department [64]. The patient should be in a sitting position for the examination. Again, caution and good judgment should be the mainstays of diagnosis. The diagnosis in most cases of epiglottitis, however, is confirmed by direct visualization of the epiglottis.

Etiology

Most cases of epiglottitis in children are caused by *Hemophilus influenzae* type B [67a]. In adults, *Hemophilus influenzae* has also been identified as the most frequent cause of severe epiglottitis [66, 67]. *Streptococcus pyogenes, Hemophilus parainfluenzae, Streptococcus pneumoniae,* and *Staphylococcus aureus* have also been significant pathogens in this disease process. Blood cultures are positive for bacterial organisms in up to 70%, with *Hemophilus influenzae* being the predominant isolate [66, 67]. *Streptococcus pneumoniae* has been isolated in patients with plasma cell dyscrasias and other malignancies [66, 68]. Some of these patients may be at risk because of chemotherapy or neutropenia. Pneumococcal epiglottitis may develop because of the potential mucosal damage secondary to chemotherapy or deficient production of opsonins [68].

Blood cultures are important and are helpful in guiding antibiotic therapy in patients. It should be noted that in children venipuncture may precipitate respiratory arrest so the airway should be established before drawing blood cultures [73]. Throat cultures have also been obtained, but this should be done only in patients with an established airway. Attempts to culture the throat have been occasionally negative for pathogens, and this may suggest that surface cultures may not reflect deep tissue infection [70]. The white blood count is usually elevated in patients with epiglottitis, but a minority of patients may have normal count [64].

Treatment

Airway

Maintaining the airway is the most important modality in the successful treatment of epiglottitis. This is true for adults as well as children. In one study, death occurred in adults before or within 6 hours of admission to a hospital [67]. Patients with epiglottitis may be seen in an office setting. If epiglottitis is suspected, the patient should be promptly transferred via ambulance with personnel skilled at intubation and tracheostomy.

Prophylactic airway placement reduces the mortality in children from 6% to under 1%, with nasotracheal intubation having lower rates of complication [74]. Tracheostomy was the most common form of airway control before 1976 [64]. In most cases, tracheostomy is much more invasive and may extend the hospital stay. Currently, nasotracheal tubes are now being used in the majority of pediatric patients. Patients are usually taken to the operating room for elective intubation [64]. In one study, however, not all the children were intubated [64]. The authors believed strongly that children under the age of 6 years should be prophylactically intubated because of their smaller airways and increased chance of obstruction. In this study, children older than 6 years without any respiratory compromise (26%) were considered for observation in a closely monitored setting with airway support readily available. The decision was made by an otolaryngologist in association with an intensivist only after very careful clinical assessment. These children were noted to have dysphagia without evidence of drooling, were oriented, had a mild tachycardia, and had good air entry on auscultation of the lungs [64]. Generally, in most cases of pediatric epiglottitis, children should have placement of a prophylactic airway. A nasotracheal tube may be removed when toxic manifestations resolve, a normal temperature is attained, and the tracheal secretions become clear [73].

The role of prophylactic airway in adult patients is more controversial. The authors of one study concluded that an airway should be established at the time of presentation to the emergency facility when the diagnosis of epiglottitis is suspected [67]. Other authors, however, advocate prophylactic airway in adult patients with significant respiratory compromise [63, 66, 70]. Adults with epiglottitis not requiring immediate intubation may be observed in the intensive care unit, with airway support readily available should it be necessary [70]. If there is any question about respiratory compromise, an airway should be placed.

Antibiotics

Since a majority of the cases of epiglottitis in children and adults have been due to *Hemophilus influenzae,* the antibiotic regimen should be tailored to this pathogen. Initially, treatment in children included drugs such as ampicillin and chloramphenicol. Initially ampicillin was the drug of choice for *Hemophilus influenzae,* but since this organism began to produce a β-lactamase, chloramphenicol was subsequently added for extended coverage [64]. However, some isolates of *Hemophilus influenzae* developed resistance to chloramphenicol. The current practice has been to use antibiotics such as cefuroxime, cefotaxime, ceftriaxone, or ampicillin sulbactam in children and adults with epiglottitis. These antibiotics are effective against the β-lactamase producing isolates of *Hemophilus influenzae.* If the organism is found to be β-lactamase negative then ampicillin can be used for treatment [70]. The patient is usually treated with parenteral therapy until stable and then may be switched to oral therapy for 10 to 14 days [70].

Steroids

Steroids have been occasionally used to treat the edema associated with epiglottitis. Since there have been no known randomized studies of the treatment of epiglottitis with steroids, the role of these agents is uncertain at this time [68, 70].

Complications

Epiglottitis is a life-threatening illness in both children and adults. Patients without respiratory difficulties survive, but in one series airway obstruction ensued in 18.3% of adult patients with some respiratory difficulty [66]. The overall mortality in this group of patients was 17.6%, while the mortality in those patients who underwent tracheostomy or endotracheal intubations was 6.4%. An overall mortality of 7.1% was seen in a series of patients reviewed by Mayo Smith [67], with no deaths occurring in patients who were intubated. A 4.6% death rate was seen in those patients who did not receive an airway [67]. These particular studies suggested a higher mortality in adults than in children.

Most patients who required an airway or who died had positive blood cultures for *Hemophilus influenzae.* Bacteremia may therefore suggest more fulminant disease [67]. Patients have also been noted to have epiglottic abscesses, and this should be suspected when there is delayed resolution of swelling [66, 67]. Patients with abscess formation may subsequently need incision and drainage [66, 67]. Patients with associated bacteremia may rarely develop metastatic infections such as pneumonia or meningitis [66, 67].

Laryngotracheobronchitis or Croup

Epidemiology and Clinical Presentation

Laryngotracheobronchitis (more commonly known as croup) is a very common respiratory illness in children between the ages of 6 months to 6 years. It is the most common form of airway obstruction in this age group and in some instances may be potentially life threatening [73]. This disease process seems to have a male predominance and is usually caused by a viral infection, most commonly parainfluenza I [75–77]. Other viruses such as parainfluenza II, III, influenza A, and respiratory syncytial virus are also etiologic agents. Adenovirus, rhinovirus, and measles may be infrequent causes of larynogtracheobronchitis. Bacterial infections have been described as very unlikely causes of this entity. This disease has a seasonal variation and viruses endemic in the community are prevalent. Parainfluenza peaks in fall and early winter, while respiratory syncytial virus peaks in midwinter and spring. The symptoms of croup are very gradual in onset and often occur after coryzal illness. Attacks usually occur at night, with the child initially developing hoarseness and then a barking cough. As airway obstruction increases, the child may begin to develop inspiratory stridor.

There is some speculation in the literature that there may be two types of croup: spasmodic recurrent croup and layngotracheitis. Spasmodic recurrent croup usually precedes an upper respiratory infection and occurs at night. It can worsen rapidly over a period of an hour and usually improves without treatment. This may in fact be due to an allergic reaction to viral antigens rather than true infection [78]. Laryngotracheitis occurs at night but is very abrupt in onset.

Laryngotracheobronchitis may result when the subglottic region becomes infected with the various viral agents. Edema and inflammation may result, which may in turn cause a narrowing in the subglottic area. Increased respiratory work is necessary because of obstruction and causes the patient to become increasingly exhausted and hypoxic. This disease presentation may also be seen in patients with epiglottitis, aspiration of a foreign body, or retropharyngeal abscess. In most cases, history and physical examination distinguish croup from epiglottitis. About 1.5% to 15% of children with croup need admission to the hospital for close observation. In 1% to 5% of the cases, the child may have such significant airway obstruction that intubation is necessary [75, 79, 80].

On physical examination a child with croup may have minimal dyspnea, fever, inspiratory stridor, and retractions of the intercostal and suprasternal areas. The lungs are usually clear, but in some cases wheezing may be heard on auscultation. The vast majority of cases of croup resolve with conservative management.

Treatment

There has been no generalized consensus about the optimal medical management of croup. Mist tents, humidified oxygen, corticosteroids, and racemic epinephrine have all been used [80a]. Most children are better by the time they are seen by a physician and usually can be sent home to be treated with cool mist. Nevertheless, some children have severe symptoms and need treatment in the hospital. The most important goal for the clinician is to make the correct diagnosis and to proceed with the appropriate therapy [80a]. Most studies addressing treatment have evaluated this particular patient population needing hospitalization [80a]. It is critical to ensure continuous observation as well as attempting to avoid disturbing the child with severe croup.

Humidified air has helped children with croup by moistening the secretions and decreasing edema in the inflamed areas of the larynx. There have been two studies that evaluated moist air and found no benefit [81, 82]. The use of oxygen has likewise been controversial, and there has been no controlled trial using oxygen that found it to be of benefit. There is some theoretical value to the use of oxygen as these children with croup may become hypoxic. It is not unreasonable to use a mist tent as long as it is tolerated by the child [80a].

Epinephrine with or without intermittent positive-pressure breathing was first introduced by Adair [79] in 1971 in the treatment of laryngotracheobronchitis. It is an α-adrenergic agent that can cause mucosal vasoconstriction and decrease edema in an inflamed subglottic region. There have been five prospective, double-blinded, and placebo-controlled studies that evaluated treatment with epinephrine. Four of the five studies were found to decrease airway obstruction with epinephrine [80a]. Epinephrine decreases the amount of airway obstruction in about 10 to 30 minutes after the administration and returns to baseline by 2 hours. A nebulizer rather than intermittent positive-pressure breathing is usually better tolerated as children do not tolerate a mask. If racemic epinephrine (0.25 mL of 2.25% racemic epinephrine in 3.5 mL of normal saline nebulizer) is used, the child should be admitted to the hospital because of the short time of drug activity and the tendency to develop respiratory problems after the drug wears off.

The use of steroids in the treatment of croup has been controversial. This modality has been used with the hope that it may decrease subglottic edema by suppressing inflammation. These studies have been difficult to accomplish because it is difficult to establish diagnostic criteria and an adequate steroid dose. Some trials have demonstrated a benefit of steroids. Dexamethasone, 0.6 mg/kg by intramuscular administration as a one-time dose, may decrease respiratory symptoms [73, 81a].

The most important challenge to the physician in the treatment of laryngotracheobronchitis is to exclude diagnoses such as epiglottitis, tracheitis, and retropharyngeal abscesses, which are caused by bacterial pathogens and subsequently respond to antibiotic therapy [80a]. Laryngotracheobronchitis is caused by viruses and therefore antibiotics are of no benefit in this disease and should not be used. Superinfection seems to be nonexistent in laryngotracheobronchitis.

Complications

Croup can be managed safely at home using a steam mist, but if the child is unresponsive, treatment in an emergency room may be necessary [73]. The key is to provide minimal disturbance and anxiety for the child [75, 79, 80, 83]. Between 1% and 5% of patients may have respiratory insufficiency requiring intubation. Obtaining arterial blood gases in some children may be anxiety provoking. Increases in both the respiratory rate and the pulse seem to correlate well with decreasing oxygen tension [84, 85]. However, hypercapnia is difficult to detect clinically. Arterial blood gases with minimal disturbance should be done if respiratory function is deteriorating. Indications for intubation include increased retractions of the chest wall, increasing tachycardia, increasing tachypnea, retention of sputum, and obvious fatigue. The duration of intubation is much longer in children with croup than with epiglottitis. Extubation may be accomplished in 2 to 4 days if an air leak develops around the tube, the secretions become thin and watery, and temperature returns to normal.

Children who have had croup may be at risk for developing abnormalities in the lung that may result in altered pulmonary function or hyperactivity of the airway later in life [86].

Bacterial Tracheitis

Epidemiology and Clinical Presentation

Bacterial tracheitis was first described in the literature as nondiphtheric laryngitis before the 1940s [87]. Subsequently, it was not seen again or written about until 1979 [88, 89]. It is a distinct clinical entity that is difficult to diagnose and may be associated with a high morbidity and mortality [90]. The disease was initially described as a very severe bacterial tracheitis that was associated with life-threatening airway obstruction of the trachea and very thick secretions that form adherent membranes within the tracheal lumen [90]. It was thought that the bacteria superinfect a primary viral upper respiratory illness caused by agents such as parainfluenza viruses I, II, III, and influenza. In some cases, however, viral cultures have been negative.

The predominant bacterial pathogen is *Staphylococcus aureus,* with *Hemophilus influenzae* being the second most common pathogen [87]. Other bacterial pathogens that have been cultured are *Streoptococcus pyogenes, Streptococcus pneumoniae,* and *Moraxella catarrhalis* [90]. It is not known whether viral infection causes mucosal damage, allowing bacterial superinfection [87].

Bacterial tracheitis has usually been described to occur in children less than 5 years of age, with the majority being less than 3 years old [87]. It does, however, occur in older children [87, 91]. There seems to be a male predominance similar to what is seen with laryngotracheobronchitis [87]. The occurrence of this disease is seasonal and has been predominantly seen from October through March [88, 90]. The presentation of this disease is similar to epiglottitis and croup. The child may have hoarseness and dyspnea. An unproductive cough and sore throat may also be manifestations of this disease. Wheezing may be heard on examination of the chest. Stridor may develop over a few hours following a short prodromal illness. There is usually no history of drooling or dysphagia, which is commonly seen in the presentation of epiglottitis. The patient with tracheitis usually has a high fever with associated leukocytosis, unlike croup.

The diagnosis should be considered when a child with respiratory obstruction is initially treated with racemic epinephrine, intravenous steroids, and antibiotics and there is no improvement [90, 92]. The child subsequently develops severe respiratory distress requiring intubation. The physician can usually make the diagnosis by laryngoscopy. Edema and moderate inflammation of the vocal cords and subglottic area may be seen. Copious mucus and purulent material may be aspirated from the tube. About one half of the patients may have pneumonia on chest radiography [87, 93]. A lateral neck film may suggest a prominent subglottic narrowing secondary to a pseudomembrane throughout the trachea. There may also be mucosal irregularity, which is usually due to ulceration [90, 91]. A white blood count may range from 4000 to 29,000. It must be remembered there is no laboratory test or radiography that can distinguish this disease from croup [93].

Management

Tracheitis should be suspected in any young patient being treated for presumed croup, epiglottitis, or a pharyngeal infection that is atypical and unresponsive to treatment [90]. An intraveous line should be established and direct laryngoscopy should be done under anesthesia. The diagnosis should be confirmed with a gram stain and culture and sensitivity of the purulent secretions aspirated. Rarely, blood cultures may be positive [87]. A nasotracheal tube should be inserted, and the patient should be monitored in an intensive care setting [87, 90, 93]. Continuous positive airway pressure and oxygen therapy should be monitored. A broad-spectrum antibiotic such as cefuroxime should be initiated. This is effective against organisms such as methicillin-sensitive *Staphylococcus aureus* and β-lactamase producing organisms such as *Hemophilus influenzae* and *Moraxella catarrhalis*. If the organism is found to be *Staphylococcus aureus*, the antibiotic may be switched to nafcillin or oxacillin if the patient has no allergy to pencillin. Antibiotics should be continued for at least 10 to 14 days. Some authors suggest that daily bronchoscopy should be done to remove secretions and purulent material [90]. Patients begin to heal 5 to 9 days after the initiation of therapy [90]. The nasotracheal tube may be removed once the patient becomes afebrile and a leak develops around the tube [90]. Decrease in the amount and viscosity of the secretions is also important in determining when to remove the tube. It has been noted that the majority of patients have required intubation and that 7.6 days is usually the mean duration of time for tube placement [90].

Complications

Morbidity in bacterial tracheitis is significantly high and is usually secondary to respiratory arrest, with 85% of the patients requiring endotracheal intubation and ventilatory support [88, 90, 93, 94]. If airway obstruction is severe, cardiopulmonary arrest may result with subsequent neurologic deficits and death [87]. Some patients have also died after extubation [87, 95]. Toxic shock syndrome has also been seen in this disease [90, 96]. In some cases the diagnosis is made only at autopsy [90]. The most common organism, *Staphylococcus aureus*, seems to suggest a worse prognosis than nonstaphylococcal disease.

Conclusion

The information that has been presented in this chapter is an attempt to familiarize the practitioner with potential problems of infections of the upper respiratory tract. These infections can be seen commonly in outpatient practice, and it is hoped that the clinician may think about these potential life-threatening diseases, attempt to diagnose them, and above all, be concerned about airway problems. The common cold is also seen quite often in the practice of medicine and although there is still no cure, it is a significant infectious respiratory disease that affects many patients.

References

1. Schneeweiss R, Rosenblatt RA, Cherkin DC, et al: Diagnosis clusters: A tool for analyzing the content of ambulatory medical care. *Med Care* 21:105–116, 1983
2. Couch RM: Common cold: Control. *J Infect Dis* 150:167–173, 1984
3. Lowenstein SR, Parrino TA: Management of the common cold. *Adv Intern Med* 32:207–234, 1987
4. Tyrrell DAJ: The common cold. My favorite infection. The eighteenth Marjory Stephenson Memorial Lecture. *J Gen Virol* 68:2053–2061, 1987
5. Tyrrell DAJ: Hot news on the common cold. *Ann Rev Micro* 42:35–47, 1988
6. Hoorn B, Tyrrell DAJ: On the growth of certain "newer" respiratory viruses in organ culture. *Br J Exp Pathol* 46:109–118, 1965
7. Larson HE, Reed SE, Tyrrell DAJ: Isolation of rhinovirus and coronavirus in adults. *J Med Virol* 5:221–229, 1980
8. Gwaltney JM: The common cold. *In* Mandell GL, Douglas RG, Bennett JE (eds): Principles and Practice of Infectious Diseases. New York, Churchill Livingstone, 1990, pp 489–493
9. Douglas RM, Lindren KM, Couch RB: Exposure to cold environment and rhinovirus common cold. *N Engl J Med* 279:742–747, 1968
10. Dick EC, Jennings LC, Neschevits CK, et al: Possible modifications of normal winter fly in respiratory disease outbreak at Mc Murdo Station. *Antarctic Journal of the United States* 15:173–174, 1980
11. Gwaltney JM, Hendley JO, Simon G, et al: Rhinovirus infections in an industrial population: The occurrence of illness. *N Engl J Med* 275:1261–1268, 1966
12. Gwaltney JM: Epidemiology of common cold. *Ann NY Acad Sci* 353:54–60, 1980
13. Aronson MD, Weiss ST, Ben RL, et al: Association between cigarette smoking and acute respiratory tract illness in young adults. *JAMA* 248:181–183, 1982

13a. Cohen S, Tyrrell DAJ, Smith AP: Psychological stress and susceptibility to the common cold. *N Engl J Med* 325:606–612, 1991

14. Sperber SJ, Hayden FG: Minireview: Chemotherapy of rhinovirus colds. *Antimicrob Agents Chemother* 32:409–419, 1988
15. Wilson R, Alton E, Rutman A, et al: Upper respiratory tract infection and mucociliary clearance. *Eur J Respir Dis* 70:272–279, 1987
16. Naclerio RM, Proud M, Lichtenstein LM, et al: Kinins are generated during experimental rhinovirus cold. *J Infect Dis* 157:133–142, 1988
17. Gwaltney JM: Rhinovirus. *Yale J Biol Med* 48: 17–45, 1975
18. Hendley JO: Rhinovirus colds: Immunology and pathogenesis. *Eur J Respir Dis* 64:340–343, 1983
19. Dick EC, Jennings LC, Mink KA, et al: Aerosol transmission of rhinovirus colds. *J Infect Dis* 156:442–448, 1987
20. Lambert RP, Robinson DS, Soyka LF: A critical look at oral decongestants. *Pediatrics* 55: 550–552, 1974
21. West S, Brandon B, Stolley D, et al: A review of antihistamines and the common cold. *Pediatrics* 56:100–107, 1975

21a. Eggleston PA, Hendley JO, Gwaltney JM: Mediators of immediate hypersensitivity in nasal secretions during natural colds and rhinovirus infection. *Acta Otolaryngol Suppl* 413: 25–35, 1984

22. Bye CE, Cooper J, Gupey DE, et al: Effects of pseudoephedrine and tripolidine, alone and in combination, on symptoms of common cold. *Br Med J* 281:189–190, 1980
23. Cruther JE, Kanter TR: The effectiveness of antihistamines in the common cold. *J Clin Pharmacol* 21:9–15, 1981
24. Howard JC, Kanter TR, Lilienfield LS, et al: Effectiveness of antihistamines in symptomatic management of the common cold. *JAMA* 242:2414–2417, 1979
25. Oral cold remedies. *Med Lett Drugs Ther* 22: 89–92, 1975
26. Dressler WE, Eyers T, Rankell AS: A system of rhinomanometry in the clinical evaluation of nasal decongestants. *Ann Otol Rhinol Laryngol* 86:310–317, 1977
27. Lea P: A double-blinded controlled evaluation of the nasal decongestant effect of the day nurse in the common cold. *J Int Med Res* 12: 124–127, 1984
28. Roth RP, Cantekin EI, Welch RM, et al: Nasal decongestant activity of pseudoephedrine. *Ann Otol Rhinol Laryngol* 86:235–241, 1977
29. Pentel P: Toxicity of over the counter stimulants. *JAMA* 252:1893–1903, 1984
30. Borum P, Olsen L, Winther B, et al: Ipratropium nasal spray: A new treatment for rhinorrhea in the common cold. *Am Rev Respir Dis* 123:418, 1981
31. Stanley ED, Jackson GG, Panusarn C: Increased viral shedding with aspirin treatment of rhinovirus infection. *JAMA* 231:1248–1251, 1975
32. Gerrity TR, Cotromanes E, Garrard CS, et al: Effect of aspirin on lung mucociliary clearance. *N Engl J Med* 308:139–141, 1983
33. Irwin RS, Rosen MJ, Braman SS: Cough: A

comprehensive review. *Arch Intern Med* 137: 1186–1191, 1977
34. Mathys H, Bleicher B, Bleicher U: Dextromethorphan and codeine: Objective assessment of antitussive activity in patients with chronic cough. *J Int Med Res* 11:92–100, 1983
35. Kuhn JJ, Hendley JO, Adams KF, et al: Antitussive effect of guaifenesin in young adults with natural colds. *Chest* 82:713–718, 1982
36. Dykes DM, Meier P: Ascorbic acid and the common cold. Evaluation of efficacy and toxicity. *JAMA* 231:1073–1079, 1975
37. Galbraith A: Influenza: Recent developments in prophylaxis and treatment. *Br Med Bull* 41: 381–385, 1985
38. Hayden FG, Gwaltney JM: Prophylactic activity of intranasal enviroxime against experimentally induced rhinovirus type 39 infection. *Antimicrob Agents Chemother* 21:892–917, 1982
39. Levandowski RA, Pachucki CT, Rubenis M, et al: Topical enviroxime against rhinovirus infection. *Antimicrob Agents Chemother* 22: 1004–1007, 1982
39a. Phillpotts, RJ, Wallace J, Tyrrell DAJ et al: Failure of oral 4′6′ dichloroflavan to prevent against rhinovirus infection in man. *Arch Virol* 75:115–121, 1983
40. Ishitsuka H, Ninomiya Y, Ohsawa C, et al: Direct and specific inactivation of rhinovirus by chalone RO 09-0410. *J Antimicrob Agents Chemother* 22:617–621, 1982
41. Phillpotts RJ, Higgins PG, Willman JS, et al: Evaluation of antirhinovirus chalone RO 09-0415 given orally to volunteer. *J Antimicrob Agents Chemother* 14:403–409, 1984.
42. Al-Nakib W, Tyrrell DAJ: A "new" generation of more potent synthetic antirhinovirus compounds: Comparisons of their MICs and their synergistic interactions. *Antiviral Res* 8: 179–188, 1987
43. Korant BD, Kaller JC, Butterworth BE: Zinc ion inhibit replication rhinovirus. *Nature* 248: 580–590, 1974
44. Korant BD, Butterworth BE: Inhibition by zinc of rhinovirus protein cleavage: Interaction of zinc with capsid polypeptides. *J Virol* 18:298–306, 1976
45. Tomassini JE, Colonno RT: Isolation of a receptor protein involved in the attachment to human rhinoviruses. *J Virol* 58:290–295, 1986
46. Ho M: Interferon for the treatment of infections. *Ann Rev Med* 38:51–57, 1987
47. Merigan TC, Reed SE, Hall TS, et al: Inhibition of respiratory virus infection by locally applied interferon. *Lancet*:563–567, 1975
48. Hayden FG, Albrecht JK, Kaiser DL, et al: Prevention of natural colds by contact prophylaxis with intranasal alpha 2 interferon. *N Engl J Med* 314:71–75, 1986
49. Monto AS, Shope TC, Schwartz SA, et al: Intranasal interferon alpha 2b for seasonal prophylaxis of respiratory infection. *J Infect Dis* 154:128–133, 1986
50. Phillpotts RJ, Tyrrell DAJ: Rhinovirus colds. *Br Med Bull* 41:386–390, 1985
51. Dingle JH, Badger GF, Jordan WS: Illness in the home: Study of 25,000 illnesses in a group of Cleveland families. Cleveland, The Press of Western Reserve University, 1964, p 1
52. Gregg I: Provocation of airflow limitation by viral infection: Implication for treatment. *Eur J Respir Dis* 64:369–379, 1983
53. Empey DW, Laitinen LA, Jacobs L, et al: Mechanisms of bronchial hyperactivity in normal subjects after upper respiratory tract infections. *Am Rev Respir Dis* 113:131–139, 1976
54. Hall WJ, Douglas RG: Pulmonary function during and after common respiratory infections. *Ann Rev Med* 31:233–238, 1980
55. Halperin SA, Eggleston PA, Hendley JO, et al: Pathogenesis of lower respiratory tract symptoms in experimental rhinovirus infection. *Am Rev Respir Dis* 128:806–810, 1983
56. McHardy VU, Ingus JM, Calder MA, et al: A study of infective and other factors in exacerbations of chronic bronchitis. *Br J Dis Chest* 74:228–238, 1980
57. Saketkoo K, Januszkiewicz A, Sackner MA: Effects of drinking hot water and chicken soup on nasal mucous velocity and airflow resistance. *Chest* 74:408–410, 1978
58. Viralizer. *Med Lett Drugs Ther* 31:8, 1989
59. Farr BM, Hendley JO, Kaiser DL: Two randomized controlled trials of virucidal nasal tissues in the prevention of natural upper respiratory infections. *Am J Epidemiol* 128:1162–1172, 1988
60. Longini IM, Monto AS: Efficacy of virucidal nasal tissues in interrupting familial transmission of respiratory agents. *Am J Epidemiol* 128:639–644, 1988
61. Sinclair SE: *Haemophilus influenzae* type B in acute laryngitis with bacteremia. *JAMA* 117: 170–173, 1941
62. Miller AH: Acute epiglottitis: Acute obstructive supraglottic laryngitis in small children caused by *Hemophilus influenzae* type B. *Trans Acad Opthalmol* 53:519–526, 1949
63. Shapiro J, Eavey RD, Baker AS: Adult supraglottitis: A prospective analysis. *JAMA* 259: 563–567, 1988
64. Sendi K, Crysdale WS: Acute epiglottitis. Decade of change. A 10 year experience with 242 children. *J Otolaryngol* 16:196–202, 1987
65. Gorfinkel JA, Brown R, Kabins S: Acute infectious epiglottitis in adults. *Ann Intern Med* 70:289–294, 1969

66. Khilinani V, Khatib R: Acute epiglottitis in adults. *Am J Med Sci* 287:65–70, 1984
67. Mayo Smith MF, Hirsch RJ, Wodzinski SF, et al: Acute epiglottitis in adults: An eight year experience in the state of Rhode Island. *N Engl J Med* 314:1133–1139, 1986
67a. Dajani AD, Asmar B1, Thirumoothia MC: Systemic *Haemophilus influenzae* disease: an overview. *J Pediatr* 94: 355–364, 1975
68. Lederman MM, Lowder J, Lerner PI: Bacteremic pneumococcal epiglottitis in adults with malignancy. *Am Rev Respir Dis* 125:117–118, 1982
69. Mauro RD, Poole SR, Lockhart CHL: Differentiation of epiglottitis from laryngotracheitis in a child with stridor. *Am J Dis Child* 142: 679–682, 1988
70. Baker AS, Eavey RD: Adult supraglottitis (epiglottitis) (editorial). *N Engl J Med* 314: 1185–1186, 1986
71. Mustoe T, Strome A: Adult epiglottitis. *Am J Otolaryngol* 4:393–399, 1983
72. Stenkiewicz JA, Bowes AK: Croup and epiglottitis. *Am J Otolaryngol* 4:393–399, 1983
73. Barker GA: Current management of croup and epiglottitis. *Pediatr Clin North Am* 26: 565–579, 1979
74. Cantrell RW, Bell RA, Morioka WT: Acute epiglottitis: Intubation versus tracheostomy. *Laryngoscope* 88:994–1005, 1978
75. Baugh R, Gillmore BB: Infectious croup: A critical review. *Otolaryngology* 95:40–46, 1986
76. Glezen WP, Loda FA, Clyde WA, et al: Epidemiologic patterns of acute lower respiratory disease of children in a pediatric group practice. *J Pediatr* 78:397, 1971
77. Williams HE, Pheland PD: Respiratory illness in children. Oxford, Blackwell Scientific, 1975, pp 26–37
78. Couriel JA: Management of croup. *Arch Dis Child* 63:1305–1308, 1988
79. Adair JC: Ten year experience with IPPB in treatment of acute laryngotracheobronchitis. *Anesth Analg* 50:649, 1979
80. Freelands AP: Acute laryngeal infections in childhood. *In* Kerr AG, Scott E (eds): *Browns' Otolaryngology*, ed 5. Stoneham, MA, Butterworth, 1987
80a. Skolnick NS: Treatment of croup: a critical review. *Am J Dis Child* 143:1045–1049, 1989
81. Lenney W, Milner AD: Treatment of viral croup. *Arch Dis Child* 53:704–706, 1978
82. Bourchier D, Fergusson DM: Humidification in viral croup: A controlled trial. *Aust Paediatr* 20:289–291, 1984
83. Wagener JS, Landau LI, Olinsky A, et al: Management of children hospitalized for laryngotracheobronchitis. *Pediatr Pulmonol* 2: 159–162, 1986
84. Newth CJL, Levison H, Bryan AC: The respiratory status of children with croup. *J Pediatr* 81:1068–1073, 1972
85. Taussig L, Castro O, Beaudry PH: Treatment of laryngotracheobronchitis. *Am J Dis Child* 129:790, 1975
86. Gurwitz D, Corey M, Levison H: Pulmonary function and bronchial reactivity in children after croup. *Am Rev Respir Dis* 122:95–99, 1980
87. Donnelly BW, McMillan JA, Weiner LB: Bacterial tracheitis: Report of eight new cases and review. *J Infect Dis* 12:729–735, 1990
88. Jones R, Santos J, Overall JL: Bacterial tracheitis. *JAMA* 242:721–726, 1979
89. Han BK, Dunbar JS, Striker TW: Membranous layngotracheobronchitis (membranous croup). *Am J Roentgenol* 133:53–58, 1979
90. Kasian GF, Bingham WT, Steinberg J, et al: Bacterial tracheitis in children. *Can Med Assoc J* 140:46–50, 1989
91. Ruddy J: Bacterial tracheititis in a young girl. *J Laryngol Otol* 102:656–657, 1988
92. Davidson S, Barzilay Z, Yahan J, et al: Bacterial tracheitis—A true entity? *J Laryngol Otol* 96:173–175, 1982
93. Liston SL, Gehrz RC, Jarvis CW: Bacterial tracheitis. *Arch Otolaryngol* 107:561–564, 1981
94. Freedman EM, Jorgensen K, Healy GB, et al: Bacterial tracheitis: two year experience. *Laryngoscope* 95:19–21, 1985
95. Liston SL, Gehrz RC, Siegel LG, et al: Bacterial tracheitis. *Am J Dis Child* 137:764–767, 1983
96. Surh L, Read SE: Staphylococcal tracheitis and toxic shock syndrome in a young child. *J Pediatr* 105:585–587, 1984

17

Community-Acquired Pneumonia

Nicholas J. Lekas

The diagnosis and management of acute pulmonary infections remains a challenge to the clinician despite major advances in medicine during recent decades. Nearly 3 million adults develop pneumonia each year in the United States, of whom more than 500,000 will require hospitalization [1–4]. Increasing emphasis on ambulatory care and restriction on hospitalization represent a challenge to the clinician whose primary goal must be the provision of high-quality patient care. Recognizing that many patients with pneumonia can be managed in the outpatient setting, the clinician must approach the diagnosis and management of each patient in a rational fashion to ensure the best therapy and its provision in the most cost-effective environment.

This chapter reviews important pathogenetic and epidemiologic concepts of pneumonia in general and addresses current thinking concerning the diagnosis and management of community-acquired pneumonia. Emphasis is placed on recognition of specific syndromes in the spectrum of community-acquired pneumonia. Unique features of pulmonary parenchymal infections in special groups of patients are discussed. These latter groups include the elderly, patients at risk for aspiration, and patients infected with the human immunodeficiency virus (HIV).

Pulmonary Defense Mechanisms

The respiratory tract is protected from microbial invasion by both mechanical and immunologic mechanisms (Table 17-1). The upper respiratory tract and oropharynx are heavily colonized with bacteria, representing over 200 species [5]. Bacterial agents and particulate matter are often inhaled or ingested, yet the infraglottic tracheobronchial tree and alveolar spaces are sterile in the majority of normal individuals. Studies of transtracheal aspiration performed on volunteers have found a few nonpathogenic organisms in up to 20% of normal individuals [5]. Upper airways and major bronchi rely on mechanical barriers and mucociliary clearance to trap and remove larger particles. Respiratory secretions containing mucous and secretory immunoglobulin A (IgA), as well as an effective cough reflex, enhance removal of pathogens [6]. In the terminal bronchioles, as the respiratory epithelium changes its character from a conduit of gases to a membrane designed for oxygen transport, mucociliary and mechanical means of protection are no longer effective. Particles less than 3 μm are inactivated or destroyed by the combined activity of opsonins, including immunoglobulins, complement, surfactant, and glycoproteins such as fibronectin, and cellular immune activity via T-lymphocytes, alveolar macrophages, and polymorphonuclear leukocytes [6]. These complicated respiratory host defenses may be altered at a number of points by external factors as well as underlying disease (Table 17-2) [1, 6–8].

Pathogenesis

Pneumonia occurs uncommonly in otherwise healthy adults. Parenchymal pulmonary infection results from an imbalance between microbial virulence, microbial inoculum, and host defense factors. As noted in the previous section, numerous conditions can adversely affect the multifaceted mechanisms of host defense; indeed, defects in host defense are

Table 17-1. Pulmonary Defense Mechanisms

Mechanical defenses
Filtration and humidification
Epiglottic function
Competent larynx allowing effective cough
Ciliary action of respiratory epithelial cells
Mucus blanket
Surfactant preventing alveolar atelectasis
Glycoproteins (fibronectin)
Immune defenses
Immunoglobulins, predominantly IgA and IgG
Complement factors, classic and alternate
Cellular defenses (alveolar level)
Alveolar macrophages and T-lymphocytes
Polymorphonuclear leukocytes

most often responsible for the development of pneumonia, either community-acquired or nosocomial [8].

The major mechanisms by which pathogens reach the lower respiratory tract are via aspiration, inhalation, or hematogenous seeding from another primary infective site [9]. Aspiration of oropharyngeal secretions or gastric contents occurs frequently; indeed, most people aspirate small amounts of oropharyngeal secretions during sleep [6, 10]. Continuous mucociliary transport and the normal cough reflex (while awake) effectively prevent infection most of the time. When such protective mechanisms are impaired as in alcohol intoxication, stroke, or with prior viral infection, pneumonia may develop. When the aspirated material contains large amounts of bacteria as occurs in patients with severe periodontal disease or following aspiration of gastric contents in achlorhydric patients, local defenses may not be sufficient to prevent the establishment of infection. Particulate material contained in the aspirate may produce areas of bronchiolar obstruction, thus facilitating anaerobiosis distally and predisposing to anaerobic pulmonary infection.

Colonization of the pharynx with potential pathogens is a major contributing factor to the development of serious pneumonia in elderly or compromised patients [11–14]. Valenti et al [15] demonstrated clearly that gram-negative pharyngeal colonization in elderly patients varied from 9% in independent apartment residents to 60% of patients in acute hospital wards. Such colonizing gram-negative bacteria probably arise by retrograde spread from the patients' own gastrointestinal tract [14]. In the hospital or nursing home, cross contamination from other patients on the hands of health care workers may also occur [9]. During severe stress, increased levels of salivary proteases lead to a loss of the mucosal glycoprotein fibronectin, which acts as an adhesive, maintaining normal gram-positive colonization of the pharyngeal mucosa. Gram-negative bacteria fill the bacteriologic void that is created and thereby colonize the pharynx [9]. This pathogenetic mechanism is responsible for many gram-negative nosocomial pneumonias and for the increased incidence of community-acquired gram-negative pneumonias in the elderly [14, 16, 17].

Inhalation of pathogens most often occurs with organisms that can be carried to the alveolus in droplet nuclei of less than 3 μm in diameter. At that location, defects in opsonization increase the risk of infection with encapsulated bacteria such as *Streptococcus pneumoniae* and *Hemophilus influenzae* [17a]. Cellular immune deficiencies manifesting as the inability of T-lymphocytes to effectively activate alveolar macrophages by the production of soluble lymphokines may predispose to mycobacterial or *Legionella* infection [6, 17b]. Intrinsic impairment of macrophage function due to concurrent infection with HIV, cytomegalovirus, or herpes simplex virus may predispose to *Pneumocystis carinii* pneumonia or other pulmonary fungal infections [18].

Hematogenously seeded pathogens may produce pneumonia, which is often focal and bilateral in appearance. Frequently, the pulmonary infective process is overshadowed by signs and symptoms referable to the primary site of infection. However, defective local pulmonary immunity as outlined previously may allow pulmonary infection to advance even as the primary site is responding to local defenses or antimicrobial treatment.

Patients with preexisting chronic broncho-

Table 17-2. Factors Predisposing to Pneumonia (Primary or Recurrent)

Mechanical factors
- Aspiration of oropharyngeal or gastric contents
  - Neurologic defects, seizure, stroke
  - Alcohol or drug intoxication
  - Anesthesia, endotracheal intubation
  - Normal sleep
- Obstruction of airways
  - Intrinsic airway obstruction, tumors or foreign body
  - Extrinsic airway obstruction, lymphadenopathy, tumors
- Abnormal ciliary function
  - Acquired
    - Toxic gases, tobacco smoke, hypoxemia
    - Infection, i.e., influenza and mycoplasma
    - Acidosis, uremia, pulmonary edema, malnutrition
  - Congenital
    - Immotile cilia syndrome
    - Kartagener's syndrome, Young's syndrome
- Surfactant/fibronectin deficiency
  - Acute lung injury, advanced age, malnutrition
- Miscellaneous mechanical factors
  - Neuromuscular dysfunction
  - Cystic fibrosis

Immunologic factors
- Deficient or abnormal immunoglobulins
  - IgG deficiency, especially IgG subclass deficiency
  - IgA deficiency
  - Chronic lymphatic leukemia, lymphoma
  - Multiple myeloma
- Complement deficiency
  - Alternate pathway, especially C3 and C5 components
- Abnormal cellular immunity
  - AIDS
  - Malnutrition, chronic steroid therapy
  - Advanced age
  - Antecedent viral illness
- Abnormal leukocyte number or function
  - Normal aging
  - Congenital disorders
  - Diabetes mellitus
  - Malnutrition
  - Leukemia
  - Hypothermia
  - Hypophosphatemia
  - Immunosuppression
  - Corticosteroid therapy

pulmonary disease are at significant risk for community-acquired pneumonia due to colonization of upper airways with potentially pathogenic organisms and due to defective mucociliary and cough clearance mechanisms [12, 19, 20]. Defects of alveolar immune function seen in such patients may reflect underlying immunoglobulin deficiency (IgA, IgG, or IgG subclass deficiency), corticosteroid therapy, or nutritional deficiency [6]. Preventative immunization with influenza vaccine and polyvalent pneumococcal vaccine is of great importance in enhancing effective clearance of potential pathogens [21, 22, 22a, 22b].

Pneumonia is the single most important infectious cause of death in the elderly [23, 24]. Multiple pathogenic factors are responsible for this increased risk. These include alterations in immune function, significant underlying diseases, and age-related changes in pulmonary function and local defense mechanism efficiency. Immunologic factors include reduction in polymorphonuclear leukocyte chemotaxis, reduction in cellular immune defenses, notably T-cell response to specific mitogens, and reduced cytokine production [7]. Reduced antibody response to specific antigens after vaccination may reflect defective T- and B-cell interaction, a qualitative B-cell defect, or a T-cell dependent reduction in cytokine production [7]. Local factors include aging of the respiratory tract, with impared elastic recoil of the lung, reduced cough and mucociliary efficiency, and a reduction of alveolar surface area. Serious chronic underlying diseases may favor gram-negative colonization of the pharynx, placing the patient at greater risk for aspiration pneumonia. Nutritional deficiency can compound all of these adverse factors and delays or hinders recovery from lower respiratory tract infection of all types [8].

Etiologic Agents and Epidemiology

Numerous microbial agents have been implicated as responsible pathogens in community-acquired lower respiratory tract infections (Table 17-3) [1]. Only a few micro-

Table 17-3. Important Etiologic Agents in Community-Acquired Pneumonia

- Bacterial
  - Common
    - *Streptococcus pneumoniae*
    - *Staphylococcus aureus*
    - *Hemophilus influenzae*
    - Mixed anaerobic bacteria (aspiration syndrome)
    - Gram-negative bacteria
      - *Escherichia coli*
      - *Klebsiella pneumoniae*
      - *Pseudomonas aeruginosa*
      - *Legionella* sp
  - Less common
    - *Actinomyces* sp
    - *Branhamella catarrhalis**
    - *Streptococcus pyogenes*
- Viral (adults)
  - Common
    - Influenza A and B viruses
    - Adenovirus types 3, 4, and 7
  - Uncommon
    - Rhinovirus
    - Adenovirus types 1, 2, and 5
    - Enteroviruses
    - Epstein-Barr virus
    - Cytomegalovirus
    - Respiratory syncytial virus
    - Varicella-zoster virus
    - Parainfluenza virus
    - Measles virus
    - Herpes simplex virus
- Fungal
  - Uncommon
    - *Aspergillus*
    - *Coccidioides immitis*
    - *Cryptococcus neoformans*
    - *Histoplasma capsulatum*
- Rickettsial
  - *Coxiella burnetii*
  - *Rickettsia rickettsiae*
- Bacteria-like organisms
  - *Mycoplasma pneumoniae*
  - *Chlamydia* sp
    - *C. psittaci*
    - *C. pneumoniae* (TWAR)
    - *C. trachomatis* (infants)
- Mycobacterial
  - *Mycobacterium tuberculosis*
- Parasitic
  - *Pneumocystis carinii*
  - *Strongyloides stercoralis*
  - *Ascaris lumbricoides*

Adapted from Mandel GL, Douglas RG Jr, Bennett JE (eds): Principles and Practice of Infectious Diseases, ed 3. New York, Churchill Livingstone, 1990.

*Official nomenclature: *Moraxella (Branhamella) catarrhalis;* current preferred usage is *Branhamella catarrhalis* [23a].

organisms are encountered frequently, whereas many others produce disease under special epidemiologic circumstances or situations.

As noted previously, respiratory tract infections occur commonly in the general population. Estimates of frequency in the United States include two to three upper respiratory tract infections per adult per year, 18 million episodes of bronchitis, and 3 to 4.5 million cases of pneumonia in ambulatory patients each year [25, 26]. Costs of these infections have been estimated at $15 billion per year for treatment and $9 billion per year in lost wages. In addition, the cost of hospitalization for the 500,000 cases of lower respiratory tract infection requiring admission are increasing steadily [3, 4]. Mortality from a community-acquired pneumonia ranges from less than 5% in young adults to 30% to 40% in the elderly or patients with underlying diseases [2, 24, 27].

Epidemiologic as well as clinical principles must be considered when evaluating patients with acute respiratory tract illnesses, as approximately 3% have pneumonia. Indeed, among those who self-select by visiting emergency rooms with such illnesses, 18% to 28% have pulmonary infiltrates [29]. Several important questions should be asked at the onset: Who is the patient? Where did he or she come from? What are his or her underlying diseases and allergies? What has he or she been doing recently? Answers to these questions allow the clinician to place the patient's illness in a clinical context that accounts for underlying illness, possible host defense defects, and likely exposures.

In the context of community-acquired pneumonia, several important risk categories or groups can be defined and etiologic agents can often be predicted based on accurate placement of the individual into a specific risk category (Table 17-4). Note that in all categories, elderly patients are at greater risk of pneumonia as discussed previously.

An understanding of the risk category also assists decision making regarding the advisability of antimicrobial therapy, drug route, and dose, as well as decisions regarding potential hospitalization. Obviously, patients may belong to more than one risk category, e.g., the young patient with Hodgkin's disease who is neutropenic postchemotherapy, drinks alcohol, and smokes heavily. Predicting the etiologic agent in such a patient is most difficult; initial therapy must be broad and fine-tuned by the results of diagnostic studies, which are reviewed in subsequent sections of this chapter.

Clinical Presentation

The patient with new respiratory tract symptoms and complaints suggestive of infection represents an important diagnostic challenge to the clinician. Several questions must be foremost in the physician's mind. Is pneumonia present or are respiratory symptoms explained by noninfectious cardiopulmonary disease? Does the patient have underlying risk factors that suggest a responsible pathogen or predispose to a poor outcome? Will the patient require hospitalization? What, if any, antibiotic should be chosen? Critical initial decisions are based on clinical and epidemiologic information since accurate microbiologic data may be unobtainable or may take days to obtain.

As noted in the previous section, risk categories may help predict the causative pathogen in patients with community-acquired pneumonia. In addition, recognition of certain important clinical syndromes may have relevance in answering the previously mentioned questions. These syndromes are (1) the typical or classic pneumonia syndrome, (2) atypical pneumonia, (3) the aspiration syndrome, and (4) pneumonia in the compromised host. Each syndrome is reviewed here, with emphasis on community-acquired pneumonia rather than nosocomial pneumonia. The discussion of compromised host pneumonias focuses on patients infected with HIV.

Typical Acute Community-Acquired Pneumonia (Classic)

The typical acute pneumonia syndrome usually presents with a rapid or sudden onset

Table 17-4. Pathogen Prediction by Risk Category

Risk Group or Category	*Pulmonary Pathogen or Syndrome*
Healthy adult	Atypical pneumonia syndrome *Mycoplasma, Chlamydia,* etc. Pneumococcal pneumonia
Chronic lung disease	Pneumococcal pneumonia *Hemophilus influenzae* *Branhamella catarrhalis*
Epidemic setting, crowding, military barracks	Viral pneumonia, influenza, adenovirus Postviral bacterial infections *S. aureus,* pneumococcus Atypical pneumonia syndrome
Nursing home resident	Aspiration pneumonia syndrome Gram-negative pathogens, *Klebsiella, E. coli, S. aureus,* pneumococcus Anaerobes
Loss of consciousness, alcoholism, seizure disorder, postoperative	Aspiration pneumonia syndrome Anaerobes, gram-negative pathogens, lung abscess
Immunocompromised patient	
Post chemotherapy	Bacterial pneumonia; gram-negative pathogens, *S. aureus*
Humoral deficiency	Pneumococcal pneumonia, *Hemophilus ifluenzae*
Cellular deficiency and AIDS	*Pneumocystis carinii,* fungal, pneumococcal, tuberculosis
Intravenous drug abuse	*S. aureus* (often resistant to oxacillin) Aspiration syndrome Septic pulmonary embolism
Nosocomial pneumonias	Gram-negative pathogens *S. aureus* *Legionella* Aspiration syndrome

of symptoms of fever, often heralded by a shaking chill, productive cough, pleuritic chest pain, and malaise. Most patients are over 40 years of age, and become ill in midwinter or early spring [1]. Nearly 80% of patients have one or more underlying diseases such as chronic pulmonary or cardiovascular disease, diabetes mellitus, or alcoholism. A history of antecedent viral respiratory tract infection can be elicited 36% to 50% of the time [1]. Recent loss of consciousness, dental work, or seizure leads to suspicion of the aspiration syndrome (see following). Elderly patients, especially those from nursing homes, are less likely to complain of cough, fever, chills, headache, sore throat, myalgia, or arthralgias than those admitted from the community [16, 17]. Such patients may present with unexplained deterioration of an otherwise stable underlying disease or an acute change in performance status. Symptoms in other organ systems such as abdominal pain or diarrhea may dominate the clinical picture.

Physical examination reveals fever (in most patients), tachypnea, tachycardia, and localized pulmonary findings of crackles, rhonchi, and consolidation, especially as the disease progresses. Confusion is a relatively common finding, occurring in 30% of all patients in a recent large study and in 48% of those patients admitted from nursing homes [23].

Nonspecific laboratory findings may be helpful in placing the patient's illness in perspective and confirming the likelihood of acute pneumonia. Leukocytosis is most common, with a white blood cell count of 15,000 to 30,000/mm^3; leukopenia may be present and is considered a poor prognostic sign [1].

Chest radiography usually demonstrates a localized infiltrate that may take several forms. Bronchopneumonia is most common; lobar consolidation, pleural effusion, and cavitation may also be seen. Lobar infiltrates are said to be typical of pneumococcal disease and may cavitate on occasion, especially when the infecting agent is *Streptococcus pneumoniae* type III. *Klebsiella pneumoniae* often produces a dense lobar infiltrate, which may cause outward bowing of adjacent fissures due to edema and fluid content. Cavitation signifies destruction of alveolar septae and is a feature of necrotizing pneumonias; hence, it is most common with *Staphylococcus aureus,* highly virulent pneumococci, anaerobes, gram-negative aerobic bacteria, and mycobacteria.

Arterial blood gases often demonstrate mild respiratory alkalosis with variable hypoxemia due to ventilation-perfusion abnormalities. The sputum is usually purulent or rust-colored and gram stain may be helpful (see following).

An accurate microbiologic diagnosis is often very difficult, if not impossible, to obtain in the typical pneumonia syndrome due to contaminating microflora on cultures or inadequate specimen collection without the use of invasive measures [5]. In a recent large review [27] of community-acquired pneumonia, an accurate microbiologic diagnosis was not possible in 49.8% of 719 patients seen over a 5-year period. Others have been unsuccessful in from 3% to 52% of patients studied [27]. In spite of this diagnostic uncertainty, certain important pathogens responsible for the typical or classic pneumonia syndrome should be discussed.

Streptococcus pneumoniae continues to be the most commonly responsible pathogen, accounting for 8.5% to 76% of cases and a significant incidence of bacteremia (20% to 25% of cases) [2, 4, 5, 17a]. Underlying conditions such as chronic lung disease, advanced age, cigarette smoking, dementia, and seizures are often present. More severe disease may be seen in patients with prior splenectomy and in those patients who have deficient opsonizing antibody production. Respiratory failure is not uncommon and was seen in 27.8% of cases in a recent series [27]. Mortality is significant, ranging from 2% to 40% in spite of advances in supportive care and highly effective antimicrobial therapy.

Hemophilus influenzae is an important pathogen in up to 20% of patients with community-acquired pneumonia [30]. Generally nontypable strains are responsible in adults and most commonly affect patients with preexisting chronic obstructive pulmonary disease. Chronic colonization with the *Pneumococcus* and *Hemophilus influenzae* in patients with chronic obstructive pulmonary disease may confuse the interpretation of culture findings in such patients [2, 31, 32].

Staphylococcus aureus may be responsible for up to 10% of community-acquired pneumonia, especially in the elderly and in patients recovering from influenza or other viral respiratory infections. Patients with postinfluenza staphylococcal or pneumococcal pneumonia often have a biphasic illness with the sudden onset of acute respiratory symptoms during convalesence [1]. Mortality of *S. aureus* pneumonia is high, reported at 54.6% in a recent study from Pittsburgh [33].

Legionella species, especially *Legionella pneumophila,* are important community-acquired pathogens although their incidence varies dramatically by geographic areas and institution. The patients are often smokers or have underlying cardiovascular disease and may have prominent associated gastrointestinal symptomatology. *Legionella* may progress rapidly to consolidation and effusion production or may be responsible for the atypical pneumonia syndrome (see following) [17b, 34–36].

Aerobic gram-negative bacilli are important pathogens in debilitated patients and those living in nursing homes [37]. Such organisms are also major responsible pathogens in nosocomial pneumonia. Community-acquired gram-negative pneumonia is most commonly caused by *Klebsiella pneumoniae*

[38] and *Escherichia coli.* Mortality is significant and relates greatly to the underlying disease of the host.

Branhamella catarrhalis has recently gained recognition as a pathogen responsible for the typical community-acquired pneumonia syndrome. This organism has undergone a number of name changes; the current official terminology is *Moraxella (Branhamella) catarrhalis;* however, the term *Branhamella catarrhalis* continues as the most popular name and will be used herein [23a]. It is seen most often in patients with preexisting chronic lung disease and may cause disease by itself or complicate therapy of *Hemophilus* or pneumococcal pneumonia by production of β-lactamases, which can interfere with antibiotic action. Mortality is considered to be low, but its inci-

Table 17-5. Unusual and Community-Acquired Pneumonias: Historical and Environmental Clues

		Pneumonia Presentation		
Disease	***Environmental and Exposure History***	***Typical***	***Atypical***	*1°/2°**
Anthrax	Cattle, horses, swine, goat hair, wool; wool carders, butchers, tanners	+ +		1°
Brucellosis	Cattle, swine, goats, raw milk; abattoir worker, veterinarian, farm worker		+ +	2°
Melioidosis	Travel to southeast Asia, Australia, South and Central America, Guam; military personnel	+ +	+ +	1°
Plague	Ground squirrels, prairie dogs, rabbits; hunter, camper, farm worker (Western United States)	+ +	+	2°
Tularemia	Tissue of squirrels, rabbits, foxes; bites of infected flies or ticks, handling infected meat		+ +	2°
Psittacosis	Bird exposure (budgerigars, cockatoos, parrots, parakeets, pigeons, turkeys)		+ +	1°
Legionellosis	Contaminated aerosols from air coolers, water supply; maintenance workers, hospitalized patients	+ +	+	1°
Coccidioidomycosis	Travel in San Joaquin Valley, southern California, southwest Texas, New Mexico, Arizona; farm and construction workers	+	+ +	1°
Histoplasmosis	Bat and chicken droppings; Ohio and Mississippi river valley; farm and construction workers, spelunkers		+ +	1°
Q fever	Cattle, sheep, or goat milk, placentas, or feces; farm workers	+	+ +	1°
Leptospirosis	Wild rodents, dogs, cats, cattle, or water contaminated with infected urine		+	1°
Cryptococcosis	Pigeon droppings, HIV, AIDS	+	+ +	1°
Sporotrichosis	Rose thorns; gardeners, florists		+ +	1°

*1°, lung is a primary site of infection; 2°, lung is involved secondarily.
+ +, Most common presentation of pulmonary involvement; +, less common presentation of pulmonary involvement.

dence is probably underestimated due to its position as a common upper respiratory tract colonizer [23a, 39, 40].

Certain epidemiologic considerations may be helpful in selecting appropriate therapy given the difficulty in establishing a causative diagnosis in the typical community-acquired pneumonia syndrome. Chronically debilitated patients or those with cardiovascular or pulmonary disease or diabetes mellitus have a higher incidence of *S. aureus*, gram-negative rods, and *H. influenzae*. Patients from nursing homes have a higher incidence of gram-negative pneumonia due to alteration in mucosal colonization. Splenectomized patients have an increased risk and incidence of infection with encapsulated organisms such as *S pneumoniae* or *H influenzae*. These organisms are also more likely if sinusitis, otitis, or meningitis coexist along with pneumonia.

An accurate environmental and travel history may disclose exposure to unusual pathogens as noted in Table 17-5. Some of these agents may present with the typical pneumonia syndrome although an atypical and slowly progressive illness is most commonly seen with these agents. Diagnosis requires a high index of suspicion and direct communication with the microbiology or serodiagnostic laboratory for advice on the appropriate specimen(s) needed to confirm the diagnosis.

The Atypical Pneumonia Syndrome

The atypical pneumonia syndrome is generally less severe than other forms of pneumonia that present with more acute onset of symptoms (Table 17-6). Often termed *walking pneumonia,* patients with this syndrome may continue to attend school or work yet are troubled by low-grade fever, a nonproductive cough, and often prominent extrapulmonary symptoms. The latter include one or more of the following: headache, diarrhea, abdominal pain, earache, myalgias, arthralgias, or mild pharyngitis [33a, 34, 35, 41]. A history of close contact with family members or dormitory roommates with similar illnesses is often obtained. Other useful epidemiologic historical questions should be asked as illustrated in Table 17-5. Atypical pneumonias are more commonly seen in the young and previously healthy, although they do occur in elderly or debilitated patients.

Physical findings of patients with the atypical pneumonia syndrome are variable and often scanty. A skin rash of erythema multi-

Table 17-6. Community-Acquired Pneumonia: Distinguishing Clinical Factors

Characteristics	*Typical Pneumonia*	*Atypical Pneumonia*
Onset	Acute	Subacute
Cough	Productive	Nonproductive
Extrapulmonary manifestations	Uncommon	Common
Headache		
Diarrhea		
Abdominal pain		
Pleuritic chest pain	Frequent	Uncommon
Chest radiography	Usually localized disease	Infiltrates, often patchy or diffuse
Chest examination findings	Consistent with radiography	Often do not correlate with radiographic findings
Pleural effusions	Common	Uncommon
Sputum smear	Polymorphonuclear leukocytes and predominant pathogen may be seen	Polymorphonuclear leukocytes, no predominant pathogen seen
Sputum culture	Pathogen often present	Negative or normal flora

forme may be seen in *Mycoplasma pneumoniae* infection, a pretibial rash can be seen in legionnaire's disease, and faint erythematous macular lesions on the thorax (Horder's spots) may be seen in patients with psittacosis. Some patients have a mild nonexudative pharyngitis as seen in mycoplasma, psittacosis, and *Chlamydia pneumoniae* infection (TWAR). Raynaud's phenomenon may be seen in patients with *Mycoplasma pneumoniae* infection, especially if cold agglutinin titers are high. Hemoptysis is occasionally noted in legionnaire's disease or psittacosis. Physical findings in the chest are variable and may be less impressive than radiographic findings. Lobar consolidation occurs occasionally. Patients with *Mycoplasma* and psittacosis may have involvement of other organ systems such as myocarditis, heart block, or pericarditis, and patients with Q fever may develop concomitant culture-negative bacterial endocarditis. Splenomegaly is commonly seen in psittacosis.

On general laboratory examination 80% of patients with atypical pneumonia have a white blood cell count of less than 10,000/mm^3. Hyponatremia may be seen in *Legionella* infection [1].

Considerable overlap of clinical signs and symptoms exists among the various causes of the atypical pneumonia syndrome. Because these infections are common in primary care practice, major causative pathogens and their clinical presentation are reviewed in detail.

Mycoplasma Pneumoniae

The most common atypical pathogen, *M. pneumoniae,* accounts for up to 20% of all cases of pneumonia [33a, 35]. Mycoplasma is a widely distributed organism, causing disease most commonly in temperate climatic zones. It is transmitted from person to person by aerosolization and requires close contact. Outbreaks are seen in families, schools, dormitories, and military barracks; its long incubation period of approximately 3 weeks and prolonged convalescence leads to a smoldering endemic behavior. The greatest incidence of *Mycoplasma* is seen in older children and young adults, though infection in younger children and the elderly is also recognized. *M. pneumoniae* is a mucosal pathogen, binding to respiratory epithelium, causing ciliary dysfunction, and inducing a local inflammatory response. The host response accounts for most of the manifestations of the clinical illness. The organism is shed for 2 to 8 days before symptoms and can be cultured from respiratory secretions for up to 10 to 14 weeks after the onset of disease, although its contagiousness declines rapidly after symptoms develop [42].

Clinical signs and symptoms of *Mycoplasma* include the primary constitutional symptoms of fever, headache, malaise, and a syndrome of pharyngitis, tracheobronchitis, or pneumonia. The pharyngitis due to *Mycoplasma* is indistinguishable on clinical grounds from that caused by group A streptococci or viruses. Tracheobronchitis is seen in 70% to 80% of patients, with the mildest manifestations of disease found in those less than 5 years of age. Pneumonia is recognized in 5% to 33% [42]. Cough develops 2 to 4 days after the constitutional symptoms and is usually nonproductive or yields purulent sputum containing mononuclear cells, polymorphonuclear leukocytes, and no predominant organisms. Patients without a cough probably do not have *Mycoplasma* pneumonia. Retrosternal chest pain of a nonpleuritic nature is common. Fever may reach 104°F but shaking chills are rare. Ear pain is seen frequently and frank myringitis is found on examination in 15% of patients. Bullous myringitis is occasionally seen and may become hemorrhagic. Chest examination reveals wheezes, rhonchi, rales, or signs of consolidation, but may also be negative. A skin rash may be seen in 15% of patients, and varies from a maculopapular to vesicular to vesiculobullous eruption [41]. In spite of a high incidence of infection and demonstrable pneumonia, less than 5% of patients with *Mycoplasma* are ill enough to require hospitalization [43]. Radiography reveals bronchopneumonic infiltrates in one or more lobes, usually in the lower lung fields.

The diagnosis of *Mycoplasma* pneumonia is made on clinical grounds in view of the difficulty with which the organism is isolated.

Cold agglutinin titers representing IgM antibody to the I antigen on the red blood cell membrane are seen in 50% of patients and seem to occur more commonly with severe illness [42].

The clinical course of untreated *Mycoplasma* pneumonia includes fever for from 2 days to 2 weeks, malaise, cough, and chest radiographic abnormalities for 2 to 6 weeks. Complications include respiratory failure, clinical relapse after 2 to 3 weeks, clinically inapparent sinsusitis, and several nonrespiratory syndromes such as intravascular hemolysis due to high cold agglutinin titers, skin rash progression to Stevens-Johnson syndrome, or neurologic symptoms, which are seen in 10% of hospitalized patients. Neurologic complications include encephalitis, aseptic meningitis, meningoencephalitis, and mononeuropathy or polyneuropathy. All of these neurologic symptoms appear to be secondary to immunologic reactions triggered or initiated by the *Mycoplasma pneumoniae* infection rather than by invasion of the organism itself [33a, 34, 43].

Legionella pneumophila

Like *Mycoplasma, Legionella* are responsible for a wide spectrum of clinical syndromes; however, *Legionella pneumophila* also often causes typical acute pneumonia as discussed previously. The incidence of community-acquired pneumonia due to *Legionella pneumophila* varies widely and ranges from 1% to 15% [1, 17b, 36]. It may also cause nosocomial pneumonia with an incidence of 1% to 4%, depending on the institution [1]. Two major clinical syndromes have been recognized: Pontiac fever and legionnaire's disease. The former is an acute febrile flu-like illness without pneumonia, with an incubation period of 24 to 48 hours and an attack rate of nearly 90%. Nonproductive cough may be seen, but chest radiography is invariably negative and all patients recover in 1 week without symptoms. Pneumonia syndromes termed legionnaire's disease may be acute and indistinguishable on clinical grounds from pneumococcal pneumonia [44] or may be more insidious, hence presenting as an atypical pneumonia. Following an incubation period of 2 to 10 days, the patient develops constitutional symptoms of fever, malaise, and headache. Diarrhea is seen in 25% to 50% of cases and is usually watery [35]. Other gastrointestinal symptoms such as nausea, vomiting, and abdominal pain are seen in 10% to 20% of patients. A recent comparative study found that these symptoms are equally common in other types of pneumonia; however, hyponatremia is more commonly seen in legionnaire's disease [1, 35]. Legionnaire's disease is usually seen in adults and is very rare in children. Most patients have underlying chronic illness or a history of smoking, alcohol abuse, or liver disease. A seasonal distribution may be seen in summer and early fall and exposure to some source of stagnant water may be identified. When cough develops it is productive of a small amount of mucoid sputum. Pleuritic chest pain is present in 30% to 40% of patients as opposed to *Mycoplasma* pneumonia in which pleuritic chest pain is quite rare. Mild hemoptysis may be seen in 20% to 40% of patients and headache is seen in 20% to 30%, with mental confusion in 30% of patients. On physical examination patients with *Legionella* pneumonia may have bradycardia, and the physical examination may be more impressive than the chest radiograph in contrast to the situation as seen in *Mycoplasma.* Hypophosphatemia is also more commonly seen than in other atypical pneumonias and mild-to-moderate elevations of liver function studies are also found [35]. The peripheral white blood cell count is usually elevated, and patients may have hematuria. Radiographic examination reveals abnormal infiltrates by the third day that may be unilateral and may progress over several days to involve more than one lobe, in spite of therapy, which is ultimately effective. Pleural effusions are seen in 24% to 63% of patients [35]. The extent of the radiographic infiltrates does not correlate with the severity of the illness or the outcome; however, sputum examination and culture for *Legionella pneumophila* are more likely to be positive when large infiltrates are present [17b, 43]. Ultimate clearing of infiltrates may require up to 6 months, depending on the extent of underlying pulmonary disease.

Chlamydia psittaci

Psittacosis is a zoonosis caused by *C. psittaci*. Birds of all species may serve as hosts for this organism, which is generally transmitted to humans by inhalation of aerosols of dried excreta containing the pathogen [33a, 45]. Psittacosis is a relatively uncommon infection, yet remains an important occupational hazard of pet shop owners, pigeon farmers, veterinarians, and workers in poultry processing plants. The organism may be contained in blood and tissues as well as excreta. Person-to-person transmission is very rare. Avian-to-human transmission may require only brief contact and may explain the 20% of human cases in which no history of known bird contact can be elicited [45].

C. psittaci is an obligate intracellular pathogen and produces a systemic illness after invasion via the respiratory tract and infection of the reticuloendothelial system. Clinical manifestations of the disease are generally confined to the respiratory tract, although the heart, pericardium, brain, meninges, and adrenals occasionally are involved.

Following an incubation period of 7 to 15 days, psittacosis may present abruptly with fever and chills or may begin more gradually over 2 to 4 days with headache and malaise. Headache is a most prominent and consistent clinical feature and may overshadow respiratory symptoms, which develop a few days after the onset of the headache. A persistent dry hacking cough is characteristic of all cases, occasionally productive of mucoid or blood-streaked sputum. Pleuritic chest pain is rare and respiratory failure may develop as a result of extensive pulmonary involvement [46]. Mental status changes are generally attributed to hypoxemia rather than to primary central nervous system involvement.

Physical examination of the chest rarely identifies consolidation; however, fine rales in the lower lung fields are common. Occasionally pleural or pericardial rubs are found. Hepatosplenomegaly is common and palpable splenomegaly is found in 10% to 70% of patients and should alert the clinician to consider psittacosis in the differential diagnosis [34]. Relative bradycardia is also common as in other infections caused by intracellular pathogens such as typhoid fever and brucellosis. Laboratory findings are of little assistance; although the peripheral white blood cell count is usually normal, mild leukopenia or anemia may develop. Hepatomegaly is not accompanied by abnormal liver function studies and the cerebrospinal fluid is normal in spite of signs of meningismus and severe headache. Sputum examination shows no organisms and few leukocytes. Chest radiographic findings are variable and include soft patchy lower lobe infiltrates, small miliary infiltrates, or nodules. Occasionally lobar consolidation is found. Since isolation of *C. psittaci* is hazardous and uncommonly performed, serology must be relied on [45]. The diagnosis rests on a high index of suspicion and a careful history eliciting bird contact in 80% of patients. Psittacosis should also be considered in patients with pneumonia that is unresponsive to usual antibiotics associated with high fevers, myalgias, relative bradycardia, and especially if splenomegaly is seen [45].

Chlamydia pneumoniae (TWAR)

The TWAR strain of *Chlamydia* recently officially named *Chlamydia pneumoniae* is now recognized as a common cause of acute respiratory tract infection and pneumonia [47]. The agent is distinct from *Chlamydia trachomatis* and *C. psittaci*. Humans are the only known natural host as no animal reservoirs have been found. The mode of transmission of *C. pneumoniae*, its infectiousness, incubation period, and pathogenesis are unknown. Serologic surveys demonstrate a rising incidence of seropositivity through life, beginning in the teenage years, with an adult seroprevalence of 25% to greater than 50%. The infection has a worldwide distribution and reinfection appears to be common. Some epidemics in military recruits have been identified [47].

C. pneumoniae (TWAR) infections are usually mild or asymptomatic. Clinical syndromes attributed to this agent include pharyngitis, sinusitis, bronchitis, and pneumonia. In comparative studies of TWAR, *Mycoplasma*, and viral acute respiratory illness reviewed by Grayson et al [47], hoarseness was found significantly more often (30%) in TWAR infections than in either *Mycoplasma* (3%) or viral respiratory infections (4%). Abnormal breath sounds were found in 85% of patients with TWAR versus only 10% of virally infected patients. On the other hand, fever was less common in TWAR infections (10%) compared with an incidence of 34% in *Mycoplasma* and 44% in acute viral respiratory infections. Grayson et al further noted that 5% of isolated sinusitis in young adults may be attributed to TWAR, and sinusitis accompanies lower respiratory tract infections due to this organism in at least 5% of cases.

Serologic surveys have demonstrated that approximately 10% of pneumonia in ambulatory patients and hospitalized patients may be due to *C. pneumoniae* (TWAR) [47, 48]. Generally these pneumonias are mild and present with a single subsegmental infiltrate. Patients with TWAR pneumonia often have prolonged mild illness with a persistent cough. More severe disease has been documented in compromised or elderly patients. This organism is estimated to be responsible for approximately 4% of bronchitis in young people and may result in prolonged residual bronchial inflammation following recovery from pneumonia. *C. pneumoniae* infection may manifest as a mild fever of unknown origin although this is more common with *C. psittaci* infection.

Laboratory findings in patients with *C. pneumoniae* infection do not distinguish it from other agents responsible for the atypical pneumonia syndrome. Peripheral white blood cell count is normal in greater than 90% of patients and no other more specific findings are available. Culture techniques remain a research tool and serology using a microimmunofluorescence test for IgM and IgG antibodies have been used to diagnose this infection. IgM antibody persists for approximately 2 to 6 months after infection, whereas IgG antibody persists for life. Periodic increases in titer of IgG antibody seen later in life suggest that reinfection is common [33a, 47, 49]. *Chlamydia* complement fixation antibodies cross react with *C. psittaci, C. pneumoniae,* and *C. trachomatis,* so some cases thought to be due to psittacosis may be due to *C. pneumoniae.* Complement fixation antibodies usually increase during the first infection but do not increase during subsequent infections [49].

Q Fever

Q fever is an unusual zoonosis caused by the rickettsial organism *Coxiella burnetii.* Although many species of animals may become infected with this organism, camels, sheep, and goats are the primary animal reservoirs. Human infection results from inhalation of aerosols contaminated with these desiccation-resistant organisms. Following an incubation period of 20 days (14 to 39) patients present with an acute or subacute illness characterized by fever, headache, malaise, chills, and myalgias. Although *C. burnetii* is an intracellular parasite similar to other rickettsial organisms, no rash is seen in infected patients. Following inhalation of organisms and proliferation in the lungs, rickettsemia occurs and a variety of clinical syndromes may develop. These include a self-limited febrile illness (2 to 14 days), pneumonia, endocarditis, hepatitis, osteomyelitis, or neurologic illness including encephalitis, aseptic meningitis, toxic confusional state, dementia, extrapyramidal disease, or manic psychosis [50].

Q fever pneumonia may present as an atypical pneumonia, rapidly progressive pneumonia, or an asymptomatic pneumonia as part of another Q fever syndrome. The atypical pneumonia is characterized by a dry nonproductive cough with negative blood and sputum cultures. Indeed cough may be seen in only 28% of patients with radiographic evidence of pneumonia. Fever occurs in all patients and severe headache is seen in 75%. Pleuritic chest pain is seen in 28%, with nausea in nearly half the patients and diarrhea in 21% [50]. Nausea and diarrhea may be presenting patient complaints.

Physical examination of the chest may reveal a few basilar crackles or signs of consolidation. Splenomegaly is seen in 5% of patients and patients with Q fever do not demonstrate a skin rash as seen in other rickettsial diseases.

Chest radiographic findings demonstrate subsegmental or segmental pleural-based densities in most patients with pneumonic involvement. In addition 35% of patients have small pleural effusions. Resolution of chest radiographic changes ranges from 10 to 70 days, with a mean of 30 days. Pathologically the infiltrates noted on chest radiography represent nodular peribronchial consolidation, with interstitial infiltrates composed of lymphocytes. Serology is the mainstay of diagnosis of Q fever. Complement fixation is most commonly used and has no cross-reactivity with other rickettsial diseases. IgM antibodies alone cannot be relied on to diagnose acute disease since they may persist for up to 678 days, and in 3% of patients in one large study IgM antibodies were present in significant titers after 1 year [50].

Viral Agents

Viral agents may be responsible for the atypical pneumonia syndrome in adults [1, 41]. Influenza A and B and adenovirus types III, IV, and VII are most commonly seen. Occasionally, other viruses may be associated with primary viral pneumonia in adults, including respiratory syncytial virus, rhinovirus, parainfluenza virus, and enterovirus, although infiltrates seen in association with these viral pathogens may be due to bacterial superinfection of damaged respiratory epithelium [51, 51a].

Influenza most often presents with fever, malaise, myalgias, mild sore throat, arthralgias, and later a prominent cough, which is usually nonproductive. Primary viral pneumonia has been seen frequently during large epidemics. It produces a diffuse hemorrhagic pneumonitis with severe tracheitis and bronchitis and carries a high mortality. Secondary bacterial pneumonia may also develop in patients with underlying cardiac, pulmonary, or metabolic disease or in debilitated elderly people. Secondary bacterial pneumonia usually occurs during convalescence from acute influenza. The acute or subacute onset of cough and sputum production heralds secondary infection with such pathogens as the *Pneumococcus, S. aureus,* or *H. influenzae.* A mixed viral and bacterial superinfection may also be seen. Pneumonic syndromes in association with influenza usually affect people with preexistent chronic illness [52].

Adenovirus types III, IV, and VII are not uncommon causes of the atypical pneumonia syndrome. Patients living in crowded conditions, such as military recruits, may develop an acute flu-like illness with cough, fever, sore throat, and rhinorrhea in conjunction with pharyngitis and abnormal chest findings on physical examination. Chest radiography demonstrates patchy interstitial infiltrate in the lower lung fields. Some authors have suggested that nearly 40% of all atypical pneumonias are due to adenovirus in some population groups. This illness is most often self-limited with little risk of superinfection and rare mortality [51].

Aspiration Pneumonia

As noted previously, aspiration of oropharyngeal contents is a major pathogenic factor in the development of pneumonia. When aspirated secretions or material containing large numbers of anaerobic bacteria are inadequately removed by cough and mucociliary defenses, anaerobic pleuropulmonary infection may develop. Such bacteria generally originate in the mouth or contain periodontal secretions, which may contain 10^{12} anaerobic bacteria per milliliter [5]. Factors that predispose to such infection include alcoholism, seizure disorders, dysphagia, cerebrovascular accidents, and general anesthesia [10]. Poor oral hygiene and significant periodontal disease are major secondary risk factors.

Once aspiration has occurred and anaerobic bacteria have become established, several syndromes may ensue, depending on the virulence of the microbial agents. It is important to note that nearly all such infections are caused by a mixture of anaerobic bacteria and a few aerobes as well. Anaerobic pneumonia may present in an acute or subacute fashion, usually acting similar to pneumococcal pneumonia, but presenting with foul-smelling and -tasting sputum and often with hemoptysis. Pleural effusion and empyema may develop as the organisms make their way to the pleural surface. Lung abscesses form as pulmonary parenchyma is destroyed and should be thought of as pneumonia with cavitation. Patients often present with a slowly progressive illness, with associated weight loss, night sweats, and prominent foul sputum. The differential diagnosis includes cancer with superimposed infection, pulmonary tuberculosis, and pathogenic fungal infection. Ten percent to 30% of patients with lung abscess have lung cancer. Pure infection is more likely if patients have a good history for an aspiration episode, fever, and leukocytosis [53].

Laboratory findings in anaerobic pleuropulmonary infection include moderately elevated white blood cell counts, usually greater than 11,000/mm^3, and signs of chronic infection, including a normochromic normocytic anemia and hypoalbuminemia. The chest radiographic findings suggestive of anaerobic infection include cavitary lesions, necrotizing pneumonia, and pleural effusions, especially if an air–fluid level is seen in the pleural space or within a cavitary lesion. Most such anaerobic pulmonary infections are seen in the dependent portions of the lungs, with the right lung involved 75% of the time [53]. Posterior basal segments or superior segments of the lower lobes are most commonly affected. Although staphylococcal and gram-negative pneumonia may involve the same segments of the lung and are often acquired by aspiration, anaerobic infection is more indolent in its presentation in comparison with the acute presentations of these more typical aerobic pathogens.

Pulmonary Manifestations of AIDS

The recognition of HIV infection in the early 1980s and the epidemic spread of this disease have led to its recognition as a major and complex medical illness with which all practitioners must be familiar. Depending on the nature and location of practice, the primary care physician will undoubtedly encounter patients infected with this virus. Not uncommonly, such infection is unsuspected, either due to failure to recognize risk factors in the individual patient or due to subtle or atypical presenting complaints of symptomatic HIV infection.

Infection with the HIV virus results in profound defects in host immune defenses [18]. HIV infection causes gradual and ultimately severe depletion of T-helper lymphocytes. This cell plays a central role in regulation of the immune system by the production of cytokines that regulate T- and B-lymphocytes, natural killer cells, macrophages, mononuclear cells, and granulocytes. Defects in cell-mediated immunity, humoral immunity, and granulocyte function result; HIV-infected patients have heightened susceptibility to a variety of infections and opportunistic neoplasms [18].

Patients with HIV infection frequently suffer from opportunistic pulmonary infection and neoplasms. The most common opportunistic pulmonary infection in the United States in such patients is *Pneumocystis carinii,* accounting for nearly 65% of AIDS defining diagnoses [18, 54, 55]. Other etiologic agents responsible for acute and chronic pulmonary infections in AIDS patients are listed in Table 17-7. Patients with HIV infection and respiratory complaints require careful and thorough evaluation to facilitate a speedy diagnosis in view of the severe immune deficiency and potentially lethal nature of opportunistic infections in such patients [56, 56a].

In contrast to its often fulminant presentation in cancer patients, *Pneumocystis carinii* pneumonia in AIDS patients is usually insidious in its onset [57]. Patients complain of low-grade fever, malaise, nonproductive cough, and slowly progressive dyspnea, not unlike the atypical pneumonia syndrome discussed previously. Eighty percent of patients have a dry cough, although 5% to 10% deny respiratory complaints altogether. In one study the median duration of symptoms before diagnosis was 21 days. Longer prodromes may correlate with better host response [18].

Community-acquired bacterial pneumonia in HIV-positive patients is usually due to *S. pneumoniae* or *H. influenzae* in view of the defects noted in antibody production in such patients. The presentation of pneumococcal pneumonia is similar to non-AIDS patients in that the onset is usually acute, with symptoms lasting fewer than 5 days [18, 56a]. Chest radiography demonstrates characteristic lobar or segmental infiltrates and treatment is similar. AIDS patients, however, may respond more slowly and, according to some reports, as many as 80% are bacteremic [18, 58]. *H. influenzae* pneumonia also presents similarly to that seen in non-HIV positive patients, i.e., with the acute onset of pulmonary symptoms. However, pulmonary infiltrates may present with a diffuse interstitial pattern and mimic *P. carinii* pneumonia. Twenty-five percent of AIDS patients with *H. influenzae* pneumonia are bacteremic [18]. Some studies have suggested that AIDS patients with bacterial pneumonia are predisposed to relapses or recurrent episodes [16, 58] in spite of appropriate antimicrobial therapy. Pleuritic chest pain in AIDS patients is much more commonly seen in bacterial pneumonia than in *P. carinii* pneumonia. Other important pulmonary processes in HIV-positive patients include tuberculosis, which may present with an accelerated clinical course and disseminate early [58a, 58b], and pulmonary Kaposi's sarcoma, which usually occurs in patients with extensive disease elsewhere and often presents with pleural effusion.

Physical examination of the chest in AIDS patients is of limited value in defining underlying infectious pathology. The evaluation of AIDS patients with pulmonary complaints requires a careful algorithmic approach to avoid the pitfalls of underdiagnosis. It is useful to separate chest radiographic findings in such patients into normal, focal, effusions/cavitation, hilar adenopathy, and interstitial infiltrates. This classification, as illustrated in Table 17-7, helps direct further investigations. *P. carinii* pneumonia may present with a negative chest radiograph in 5% to 10% of patients; however, it usually presents with diffuse or perihilar interstitial infiltrates, which are seen in 48% to 94% of cases [59, 60]. Katz et al [59] demonstrated that HIV-positive patients with acute respiratory complaints could be stratified according to risk of *Pneumocystis* pneumonia based on chest radiographic findings (diffuse or perihilar infiltrates), mouth lesions, lactate dehydrogenase more than 220 μ/L, and erythrocyte sedimentation rate greater than 50 mm/h. In spite of normal chest radiography, the presence of two or three of these factors conferred a risk of *Pneumocystis carinii* pneumonia of 47% in their study. If interstitial infiltrates are seen, diagnostic studies such as sputum induction, bronchoscopy with lavage, or bronchoscopy with biopsy should be performed as soon as possible to confirm the diagnosis of *Pneumocystis.* Other useful tests to rule out *Pneumocystis* include alveolar-arterial O_2 difference on exertion, which should increase in patients with interstitial pneumonia, diffusing capacity, which will also be abnormal in interstitial disease, and gallium scanning [60]. Gallium citrate scanning of the chest is usually abnormal in *Pneumocystis carinii* pneumonia even when chest radiography is normal, but again is a nonspecific feature, which if positive would justify further, more invasive studies to confirm a diagnosis and support therapeutic options. Sputum induction with inhaled 3% saline and careful laboratory examination in experienced hands can be up to 80% sensitive for *Pneumocystis carinii* [18]. Of course, routine studies including gram stain and culture, acid-fast bacilli smear and cultures, and fungal smear and cultures should also be obtained. When *Pneumocystis carinii* pneumonia is suspected, therapy should be initiated even before the diagnostic work-up is complete.

Laboratory Diagnosis of Community-Acquired Pneumonia

As discussed in previous sections of this chapter, community-acquired pneumonia may be caused by a number of different pathogens. Knowledge of the specific etiologic agent can greatly simplify the management of patients with lower respiratory tract infections. As a

Table 17-7. Pulmonary Disease in AIDS

	Radiographic Pattern				
Pathogenic Process	*Normal*	*Focal Infiltrate*	*Pleural Effusion*	*Mediastinal Adenopathy*	*Interstitial*
Protozoa					
Pneumocystis carinii	+	+			
Bacterial					
Streptococcus pneumoniae		+	+		+
Hemophilus influenzae		+	+		+
Mycobacterium tuberculosis		+	+	+	+
Mycobacterium avium				+	
Legionella			+	+	
Fungi					
Cryptococcus neoformans		+		+	
Histoplasma capsulatum	+	+		+	+
Coccidioides immitis		+		+	+
Candida albicans		+			
Virus					
Cytomegalovirus					+
Adenovirus					+
Tumor					
Kaposi's sarcoma		+	+	+	
Non-Hodgkin's lymphoma				+	
Nonspecific pneumonitis (idiopathic)					+

first step, an understanding of the clinical setting may help predict the etiologic agent, especially when unusual epidemiologic information is available. However, such clinical clues are frequently inaccurate, as illustrated by Farr et al [61], who could predict pneumococcus, mycoplasma, or an undetermined pathogen correctly only 42% of the time using discriminate analysis in a large series of 441 adults. Confirmation of a probable pathogen requires laboratory testing. Unfortunately, cultures of sputum are subject to oropharyngeal contamination with normal flora or colonizing potential pathogens, which may not be responsible for lower respiratory infection. Adult oropharyngeal colonization rates cited by Bartlett [5] include *S. pneumoniae,* 15% to 50%; *H. influenzae,* 25% to 70% (type B, 5% to 6%); *S. aureus,* 5% to 10%; group A streptococci, 5% to 10%; and Enterobacteriaceae, 2% to 70%, depending on culture methods and host status. Certain organisms are nearly always pathologic if found, including *Legionella, Mycobacterium tuberculosis, Mycoplasma pneumoniae,* pathogenic fungi such as histoplasma, coccidioides, cryptococcus, and viruses [5]. To complicate matters, cultures of expectorated sputum in community-acquired pneumonia reveal a likely pathogen in only 15% to 30% of all cases, with the highest yields of 30% to 60% in patients who are hospitalized [5, 61, 63]. In 30% to 50% of cases, no pathogen is identified. Standard methods such as sputum gram stains and culture often lack sensitivity and specificity and are now being supplemented by newer diagnostic techniques. This section reviews current clinical and diagnostic methods that may assist the clinician.

Smears

Although much maligned and often discarded, direct examination of a carefully collected expectorated sputum sample can

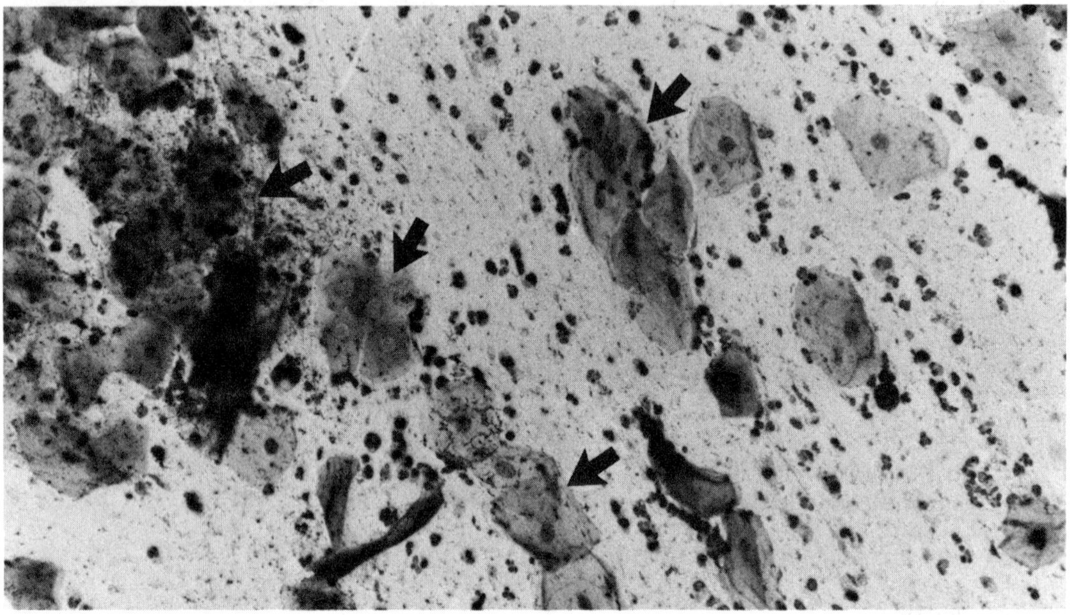

Fig. 17-1. Sputum with oropharyngeal contamination (> 25 epithelial cells per low power field).

provide valuable clues to the clinician and laboratory regarding causative pathogens [5, 9, 62, 64–66]. To obtain the most useful sample, the patient should be well hydrated and the mouth should be rinsed before sample collection. Examination of the gram stain under low power for evidence of oropharyngeal contamination (squamous epithelial cells) and leukocytes will assist in determining its value (Fig. 17-1). Samples can be graded by examination under low power for the relative numbers of leukocytes and epithelial cells. Using the strictest criteria, i.e., greater than 25 leukocytes per 10× field and less than 10 epithelial cells for 10× field, 74% of submitted samples were considered unsuitable for culture due to contamination in one study [62]. Examination of gram stains of purulent samples, those containing more than 25 leukocytes per 10× field, however, can provide useful information to aid the clinician and assist in directing microbiologic examination. Several important pathogens can be suspected by typical morphologic appearance on gram stain. These include the following: gram-positive diplococci (probably pneumococcus) (Fig. 17-2; see color plate), gram-positive cocci in pairs and groups (staphylococci) (Fig. 17-3; see color plate), gram-positive cocci in chains (streptococci), gram-negative diplococci, gram-negative coccobacilli (probably hemophilus) (Fig. 17-4; see color plate), gram-negative diplococci (probably branhamella) (Fig. 17-5; see color plate), gram-negative bacilli (Fig. 17-6; see color plate), or mixed bacteria, in which various morphologic types of bacteria are seen with no predominant organism. The presence of yeast in sputum gram stains (Fig. 17-7; see color plate) is of uncertain significance, most often representing oropharyngeal or tracheal colonization. Many patients, especially those with the atypical pneumonia syndrome, have scanty or purulent sputum with few microorganisms and no apparent predominant pathogen.

Direct examination of the sputum in patients with suspected *P. carinii* pneumonia and tuberculosis can yield a diagnosis with reasonable specificity and sensitivity [5, 9]. Induction of sputum by the inhalation of 3% to 5% saline by ultrasonic nebulizer over 20 minutes [67] can produce suitable sputum samples for examination by Geimsa stain for pneumocystis or auramine rhodamine stains for mycobacteria. The diagnostic yield for *P. carinii* is 55% on direct examination of the induced sample and may be increased to 78% if the sample is liquified and centrifuged in an experienced laboratory. Bronchoscopy and bronchoalveolar lavage can increase the sensitivity of identification of pneumocystis to nearly 100% (Fig. 17-8; see color plate) [18].

Cultures

Culture examination of expectorated sputum or samples obtained via more invasive techniques such as transtracheal aspiration or transthoracic needle aspiration can yield useful results [68]. As noted previously, samples such as expectorated sputum, nasopharyngeal aspirates, tracheostomy aspirates, and bronchoscopy aspirates are often contaminated with oropharyngeal flora, whereas transtracheal aspirates, pleural fluid, and transthoracic aspirates are generally not contaminated by extraneous bacteria. In all types of samples, infecting pathogens tend to be present in larger numbers and when quantitated, are usually present in 10^5 or more bacteria per milliliter of exudate, or per gram of tissue [5]. Prior antibiotic therapy may significantly impair the ability to culture common pathogens, especially *S. pneumoniae* and *H. influenzae.* In carefully done studies reviewed by Bartlett [5], pneumococcus and hemophilus were frequently found in pretherapy samples, but rapidly disappeared from sputum samples obtained after therapy had been initiated. This may also be true for anaerobic bacteria when samples are obtained via transtracheal aspiration. Posttherapy cultures not uncommonly grow gram-negative bacteria that, as noted previously, fill the bacteriologic void in the respiratory tract; yet, these bacteria are generally of little significance unless found in sputum in association with new pulmonary infiltrates and other evidence of infection. *Branhamella catarrhalis,* an important pathogen in patients with preexisting lung disease, is not recognized as such by many microbiologic laboratories [5]. Its presence may be highly suspected by the appearance of the gram-stained smear (Fig. 17-5), and careful cultures on selected media usually identify it. Culture of respiratory secretions for *Legionella* is quite valuable, with a sensitivity of 50% to 80% and a specificity of 100%. Results are usually available within 2 to 5 days [43].

Immunologic Methods

Limitations of traditional methods such as gram stain and culture have led to the development of methods of detection of microbial antigens as well as new serologic and immunologic-based techniques to identify pathogens in respiratory infections. These methods are particularly valuable in the diagnosis of agents responsible for the atypical pneumonia syndrome. Pneumococcal antigen can be readily detected in sputum and is a reliable diagnostic method, with a sensitivity of 89% in an experimental setting [63]. A variety of methods have been studied, including latex agglutination, counterimmunoelectrophoresis, enzyme-linked immunosorbent assay (ELISA), and more recently, DNA probes. A commercial kit is available for the detection of *H. influenzae* type B antigen in sputum, but is not widely used. In the case of pneumococcus and hemophilus, such testing methods may not differentiate colonization from infection and should be used to complement rather than replace culture techniques [63].

Of the 22 known species of *Legionella,* nine have been implicated in pneumonia and only two are relatively frequent, namely, *L. pneumophila,* which accounts for nearly 85% of cases, and *L. micdadei,* which accounts for 5% to 10%. In addition to respiratory secretions, various serologic, direct fluorescent antibody stains and antigen assays have been studied. Serology is confirmatory with a fourfold increase in serum antibody titer to 1:128 or higher or a single titer of 1:256 in an appropriate clinical syndrome [43]. Such serologic information is often delayed and is of limited value in the acute situation. The best method to establish the diagnosis of *Legionella* infection is with direct fluorescent antibody staining of pulmonary secretions. This test requires highly competent laboratory personnel and has a significant false-negative rate of 30% to 70% [63]. The combination of expectorated sputum culture and direct fluorescent antibody stain is currently the most useful method for the identification of *Legionella*. In the future, the detection of *Legionella* antigen in the urine may prove more useful than sputum detection methods [63a] and DNA probes for the identification of this organism may also be available soon [63].

Mycoplasma pneumoniae is uncommonly cultured because of the specialized techniques required to identify this organism in the routine microbiology laboratory. Most cases are confirmed by retrospective serologic studies, which are available after the acute phase of illness. An increase in antibody titer from acute to convalescent (fourfold) is generally seen, and antibody may persist at elevated levels for many years. As noted previously, cold agglutinin titers may be elevated, with a minimum positive titer of 1:32. New diagnostic techniques include antibody detection techniques by ELISA. Antigen detection techniques are under investigation, but are currently unreliable. The most promising such method is a DNA probe, which is expected to have high sensitivity and specificity [63].

Although rapid methods are currently available for the detection of *Chlamydia trachomatis* antigen by ELISA methods, the chlamydial agents *C. psittaci* and *C. pneumoniae*, which invade the lung in adults, are not so easily identified. Serologic studies are available but are not genus specific. Experimental techniques using microimmunofluorescence for *C. pneumoniae* are very reliable and specific, but not generally available [47, 63]. As noted previously, *Coxiella burnetii* can be cultured but may be dangerous and therefore, serology is the safest method for making the diagnosis. New techniques such as microagglutination and ELISA are becoming available [50].

Virology

Few viruses colonize the respiratory tract; therefore, a positive viral culture from any part of the respiratory epithelium is generally considered pathogenic and if found in association with pulmonary infiltrates, would likely be the cause of such infiltrates. ELISA testing for respiratory syncytial virus antigen is available and allows the rapid institution of appropriate specific antimicrobial therapy for this agent. The influenza, parainfluenza, and adenoviruses may be detected by the use of cell culture, as well as direct examination of respiratory samples by immunofluorescence or ELISA techniques. These techniques are not readily available and require use of reference laboratories [51].

Two important viral agents, namely herpes simplex virus and cytomegalovirus, may colonize the repiratory tract, and cause clinical disease. Herpes simplex may be found in secretions in normal patients, as well as in immunocompromised hosts, including patients infected with HIV. However, herpes simplex is uncommonly associated with lower respiratory tract infections. Cytomegalovirus is commonly found in secretions of AIDS patients and does cause pneumonia [69]. Histologic as well as virologic and serologic evidence should be sought to support a diagnosis of pneumonia due to either herpes simplex or cytomegalovirus. If both cytomegalovirus culture and tracheobronchial cytology are positive, infection can be considered likely. However, if cytomegalovirus cytology is negative with a positive culture, further direct tissue examination would be necessary to confirm infection [69]. Specific antimicrobial therapy may be toxic, especially in compromised hosts, and therefore, its use in this setting requires confirmatory histology.

Radiography

It is difficult to diagnose and manage patients with pneumonia without radiographic examination of the chest. Under most circumstances, the diagnosis of pneumonia depends on demonstration of a pulmonary infiltrate by radiography to confirm a clinical suspicion. The pattern of the initial infiltrate seen may be less useful in helping to predict the etiologic agent [70]. In general, lobar infiltrates may be caused by the pneumococcus, *Legionella*, and some gram-negative bacteria, in particular, *Klebsiella.* Bronchopneumonic infiltrates are characteristic of *H. influenzae, Branhamella,* staphylococci, and *Mycoplasma.* Interstitial infiltrates may be seen in *Mycoplasma, Chlamydia,* and viruses. Abscess cavities, pneumatoceles, or multiple lucencies within a pulmonary infiltrate suggest necrotizing infection due to *S. aureus,* virulent pneumococci, *Legionella,* anaerobes, gram-negative bacilli, or tuberculosis. Radiography may also reveal pleural effusions in a significant percentage of typical pneumonias, and in some atypical pneumonias as well [70, 73]. Multilobar disease can be identified and the course of the illness can be followed.

Pulmonary infiltrates associated with acute pneumonia usually resolve eventually, leaving no residual radiographic abnormalities or scarring of various degrees. When infiltrates do not resolve with what seems to be appropriate therapy, consideration of concomitant infection with unusual or particularly virulent pathogens or a noninfectious process should be considered. Noninfectious processes may include inflammatory conditions such as vasculitis, lipoid pneumonia due to aspiration of oil, a foreign body, or neoplasm, primary or metastatic. Unusual infections can include tuberculosis (typical or atypical), nocardiosis, actinomycosis, and other deep fungi.

Radiographic resolution of common pneumonias was reviewed carefully by MacFarlane et al [74], who noted several interesting findings. Patients with bacteremic pneumococcal pneumonia or legionnaire's disease usually deteriorate radiographically before signs of clearing are seen. The time to radiographic clearing in pneumococcal pneumonia was 3 to 5 months for bacteremic cases and 1 to 3 months for nonbacteremic cases. *Legionella* pneumonia regularly required 2 to 6 months to clear completely, whereas *Mycoplasma* pneumonia cleared completely in 2 weeks to 2 months and psittacosis in 1 to 3 months. Residual pulmonary scarring was noted in 25% to 35% of cases of bacteremic pneumococcal disease and was rarely seen in nonbacteremic disease. Scarring was also seen in 10% to 25% of patients with legionnaire's disease and 10% to 20% of patients with psittacosis. Others have noted delayed resolution in pneumococcal pneumonia according to the age of the patient, with those over 50 years requiring 12 weeks versus those under 50 years requiring 4 weeks. Underlying chronic obstructive pulmonary disease may slow healing and lead to slower clearing of infiltrates [75, 76].

Management

As illustrated in previous sections of this chapter, community-acquired pneumonias represent a wide spectrum of disease, from mild self-limited infections to severe life threatening illnesses. Mortality of community-acquired pneumonia is significant, with an overall mortality of 18% to 21% in two recent important studies [3, 50]. Factors contributing to increased mortality include increased age, increased number of lobes involved in the infectious process, mental status changes, concomitant neoplastic or other comorbid illnesses, and high-risk infections such as staphylococcal, gram-negative, aspiration, or postobstructive pneumonias [3].

Once the initial clinical and basic laboratory evaluation has been undertaken, the physician must make a determination as to what form of management is appropriate for the given patient. Several factors must be considered, including the degree of illness of the patient, his or her overall health status, the setting in which the patient has become infected and in which the patient lives, and the potential pathogens. The recognition of several risk factor categories as noted previously is important and may assist the clinician in management decisions. In addition to a consideration of antibiotics of choice for empiric and definitive therapy, this chapter also addresses the decision to hospitalize as well as adjunctive measures and preventive issues. Table 17-8 delineates specific criteria that can be used to assist the clinician in determining whether hospitalization is appropriate and whether a complicated course can be anticipated. This work is taken from a recent, careful article by Fine et al [26]. Patients who are

Table 17-8. Community-Acquired Pneumonia: Hospital Admission Criteria

A. Appropriateness Evaluation Protocol Criteria
  1. Severe vital sign abnormality
    a. Heart rate > 140/min
    b. Systolic blood pressure < 90 mm Hg
    c. Respiratory rate > 30/min
  2. Altered mental status
  3. Arterial hypoxemia ($PO_2 < 60$ mm Hg)
  4. Extrapulmonary suppurative infection (i.e., septic arthritis, meningitis)
  5. Severe acute electrolyte, hematologic, or metabolic abnormality
    a. Blood urea nitrogen > 50 mg/dL, creatinine > 2.5 mg/dL
    b. Na < 130 mEq/L
    c. Hematocrit < 30%
    d. Polymorphonuclear leukocytes < 1000/mm^3
B. Additional independent predictors of a complicated course
  1. Age > 65 years
  2. Comorbid illness
    a. Prior history of diabetes mellitus, renal insufficiency, or congestive failure
    b. Hospitalization within past year
  3. Temperature > 38.3°C (101°F)
  4. Immunosuppression
    a. Use of systemic corticosteroids or systemic chemotherapy for malignant neoplasm within prior 6 months
  5. High-risk etiology
    a. Staphylococcal, gram-negative, or aspiration pneumonia
    b. Postobstructive pneumonia

One or more criteria increase the risk of complicated course from 40% (1) to 100% (4 or more).
Adapted from Fine MJ, Smith DN, Singer DE: Hospitalization decision in patients with community-acquired pneumonia: A prospective cohort study. *Am J Med* 89:713, 1990

severely ill, as defined by the appropriateness evaluation protocol criteria, clearly require hospitalization and this decision is made easily in this group of patients. However, consideration should be given to the additional independent predictors of a complicated course as denoted under B in Table 17-8, which can be used to help support a physician's decision to hospitalize a patient who might otherwise not appear to meet specific criteria. Note that only one of the criteria addresses the infectious etiology of the pneumonia itself and most of the risk factors relate to age, underlying disease, and degree of illness.

Antibiotic Therapy

The choice of antibiotics is relatively simple if the etiologic agent has been identified; however, such is usually not the case when the patient presents to the physician and a decision regarding antimicrobial therapy must be made urgently. A "diagnostic" sputum gram stain may help narrow down etiologic possibilities; however, as noted earlier, sputum is often unavailable or nondiagnostic [9, 68, 77]. In addition, sputum cultures may be of little additional benefit and invariably the results arrive too late to affect the initial antimicrobial choice [5, 28, 78]. When selecting empiric antimicrobial therapy, it is useful to consider the classification that we have used elsewhere in this chapter, namely, typical, atypical, aspiration, and compromised host categories. Additional variables must be considered as well, including age, underlying disease, degree of the illness, and whether or not hospitalization is being considered. Empiric antimicrobial regimens are outlined in Table 17-9.

Specific Pathogens

Important points referable to specific microbial pathogens are reviewed to expand on the

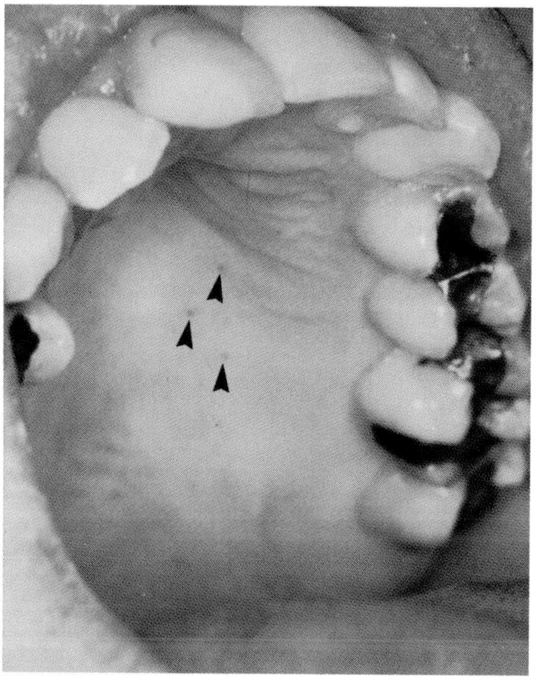

Figure 6-1

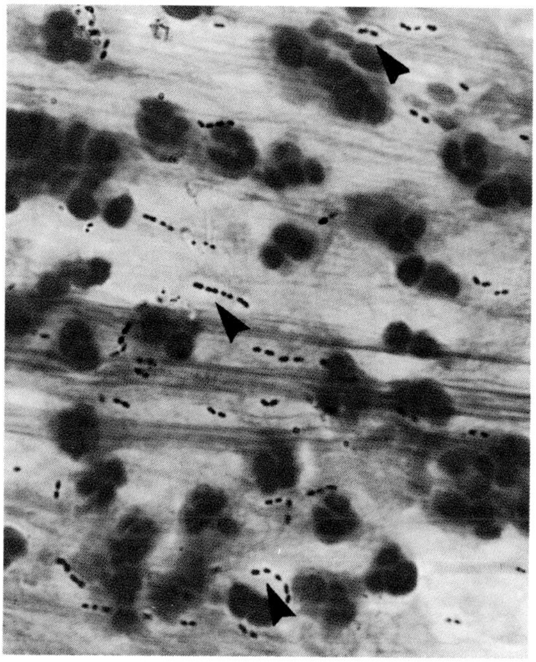

Figure 17-2

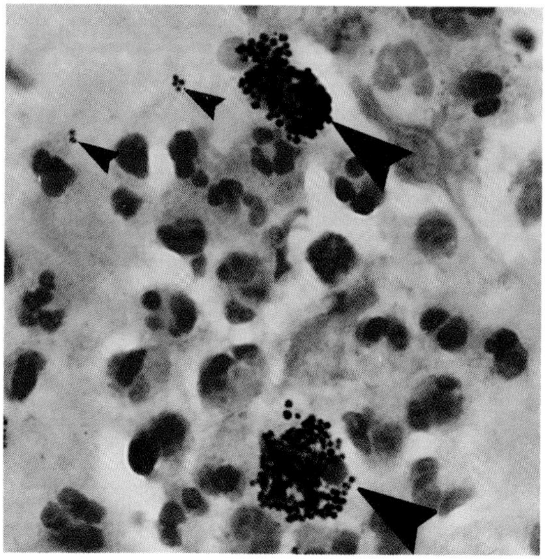

Figure 17-3

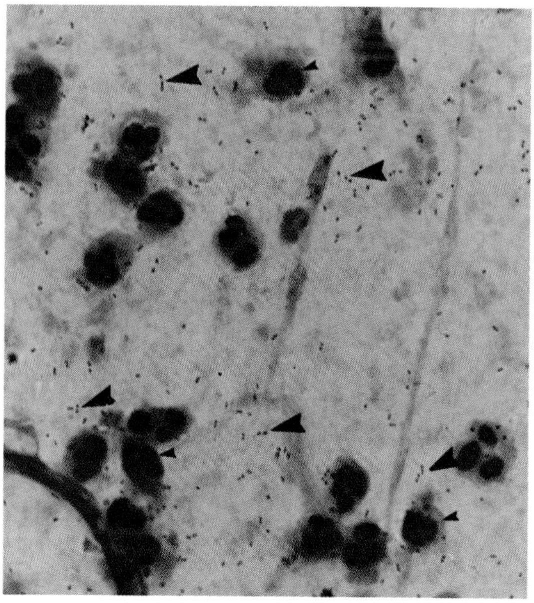

Figure 17-4

Fig. 6-1. Telangiectasias on hard palate (arrows) in a patient with Osler-Weber-Rendu disease.

Fig. 17-2. Sputum with numerous gram-positive diplococci consistent with *S. pneumoniae* (gram stain, 1000×).

Fig. 17-3. Sputum with gram-positive cocci in clumps and intracellularly consistent with *S. aureus* (gram stain, 1000×).

Fig. 17-4. Sputum with leukocytes and numerous gram-negative diplococci consistent with *H. influenzae* (gram stain, 1000×).

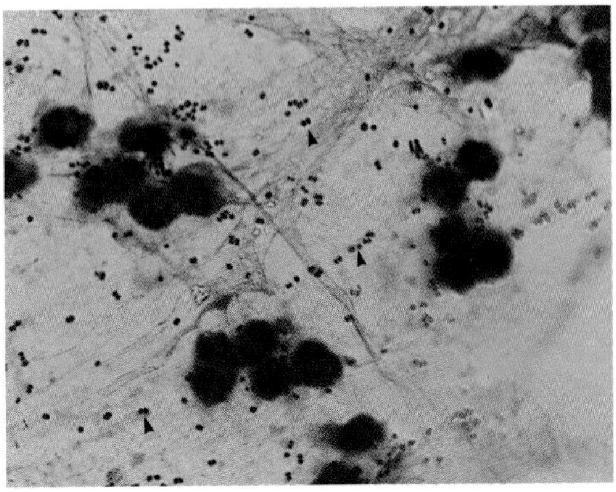

Figure 17-5

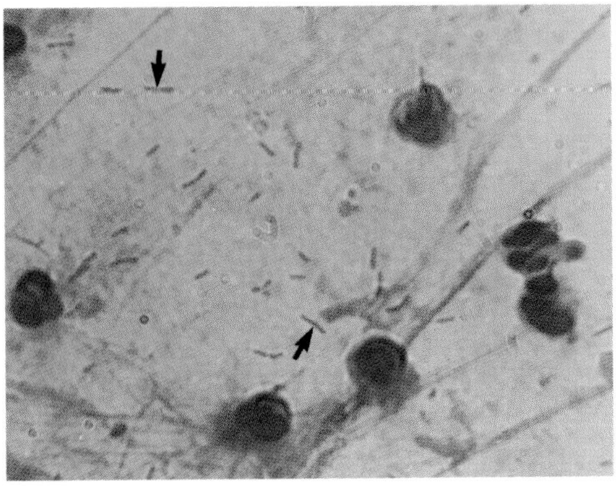

Figure 17-6

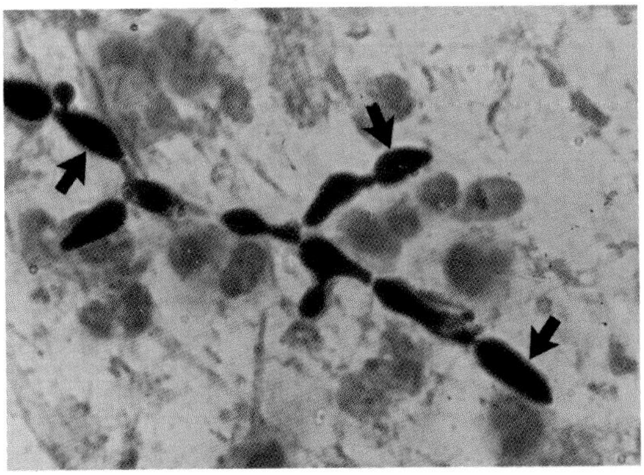

Figure 17-7

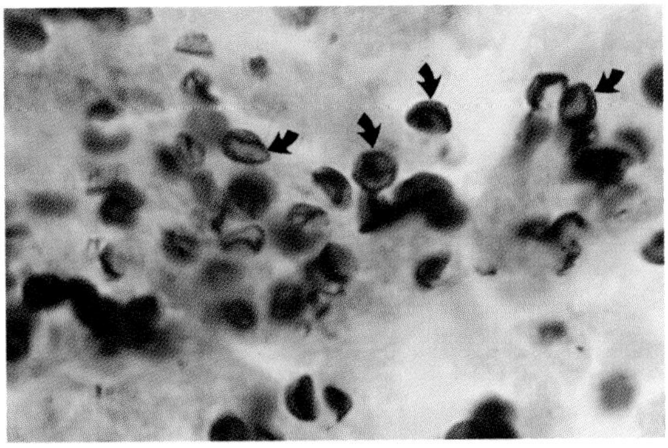

Figure 17-8

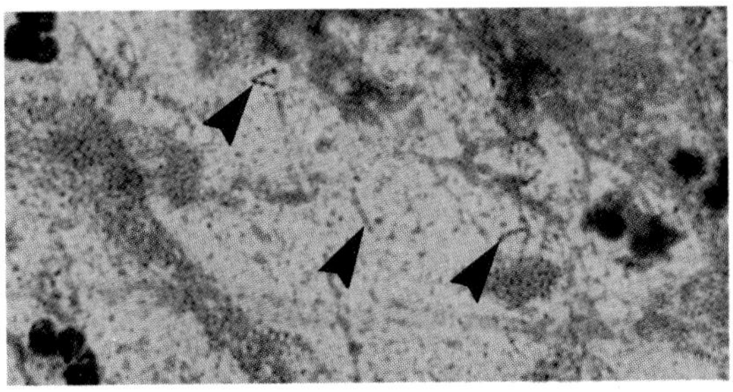

Figure 18-10

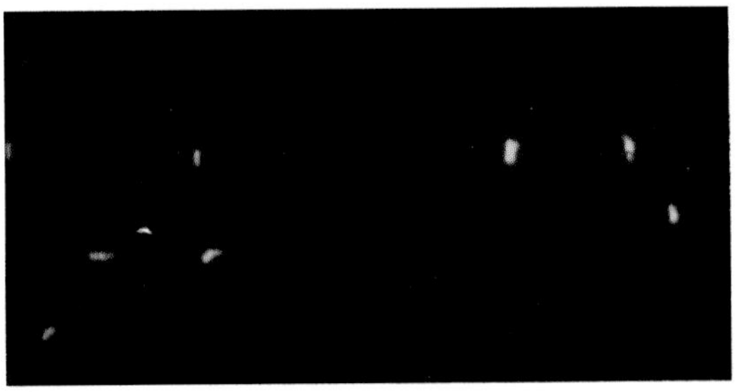

Figure 18-11

Fig. 17-5. Sputum with numerous darkly staining gram-negative diplococci consistent with *Branhamella* sp (gram stain, 1000×).

Fig. 17-6. Sputum with leukocytes and numerous gram-negative rods. Note that gram-negative bacilli cannot reliably be distinguished from one another by this method, though long, slender bacteria such as these are consistent with *Pseudomonas* sp (gram stain, 1000×).

Fig. 17-7. Yeast with pseudohyphae and gram-negative rods in the respiratory secretions of a severely ill hospitalized patient. Clinical significance of the yeast cannot be determined on this basis alone (gram stain, 1000×).

Fig. 17-8. *Pneumocystis carinii* cysts in alveolus (Gomori's methenamine silver stain, 1000×). Bronchoalveolar lavage and even induced sputum can readily retrieve cysts in view of their abundance within alveoli.

Fig. 18-10. Acid-fast stain, bright field microscopy. Acid-fast organisms appear red.

Fig. 18-11. Acid-fast stain, fluorescent microscopy, auramine-rhodamine stain. The acid-fast organisms appear bright yellow.

Table 17-9. Empiric Antimicrobial Therapy Community-Acquired Pneumonia

Group	*Characteristics*	*Presentation*	*Etiology*	*Therapy*	*Duration*
A	Mild illness, age < 40	Typical/acute	Pneumococcus	Penicillin Erythromycin	7 d
	No cigarette abuse, no underlying lung disease	Atypical	*Mycoplasma* *Chylamydia* Viral	Erythromycin [1] or doxycycline or ofloxacin	10–14 d
B	Mild illness, smoker, underlying lung disease	Typical	Pneumococcus *H. influenzae* Branhamella	Cephalosporin (2nd or 3rd generation) Trimethoprim sulfa Amoxicillin/ clavulanate*	7 d 14 d 10 d
		Atypical	*H. influenzae* *Branhamella*	Trimethoprim/ sulfamethoxazole Amoxicillin/ clavulanate Doxycycline*	10–14d
C	Seriously ill, age > 60, underlying disease	Typical	Pneumococcus *H influenzae* *S aureus* Gram-negative *Legionella*	Cephalosporin (2nd or 3rd generation) + Erythromycin if *Legionella* considered	2–3 wk
D	Aspiration syndrome Community: cerebrovascular accidents, syncope, alcoholism, drug abuse, seizure		Pneumococcus Anaerobes Gram-negative pathogens	Clindamycin + gentamicin* Cefoxitin, ceftriaxone Ampicillin/sulbactam Ticarcillin/clavulanate	10–21 d
	Nursing home/ hospital		Gram-negative pathogens *Staph aureus* *Pseudomonas*	Ticarcillin/piperacillin and tobramycin and vancomycin/ nafcillin if *Staph* suspected or ticarcillin/clavulanate and tobramycin	10–21 d

*clarithromycin/azithromycin
**clindamycin with or without gentamicin if pure anaerobic infection suspected clindamycin alone is sufficient.

information included in the table concerning initial empiric therapy.

Streptococcus pneumoniae This organism is exquisitely sensitive to penicillin, which can be dosed orally for mild disease or very effectively at parenteral doses of 600,000 units every 12 hours. Rare cases of penicillin resistance have been reported throughout the world, and most laboratories perform a screening susceptibility to ensure that all pneumococci are still sensitive to penicillin. Erythromycin or clindamycin are alternatives for the penicillin-allergic patient.

Hemophilus influenzae Approximately 20% of *H. influenzae* isolated from adult patients are resistant to ampicillin by virtue of β-lactamase production; therefore, empiric therapy should account for this susceptibility pattern until the results of laboratory testing are available. An agent effective against β-lactamase producing organisms is generally chosen, including trimethoprim/sulfamethoxazole or a second- or third-generation cephalosporin. These medications can be used intravenously or orally, depending on the degree of illness in the patient. The new macrolide antibiotics, clarithromycin and azithromycin, have broad activity for respiratory pathogens including β-lactamase producing *H. influenzae* and will become very useful members of our oral antibiotic armamentarium [78a]. The newer quinolones have demonstrated effective activity against *H. influenzae;* however, they are not as active against the pneumococcus [32]. Duration of therapy for *H. influenzae* bronchitis or bronchopneumonia should be 2 weeks in view of the frequently slow response of this pathogen.

Branhamella catarrhalis This organism also frequently produces β-lactamase; therefore, empiric antibiotic therapy when this pathogen is considered should include either erythromycin, clarithromycin, azithromycin, or amoxicillin/clavulanic acid. Doxycycline is also effective and certainly, if the organism is β-lactamase negative, ampicillin or amoxicillin would be a reasonable alternative as well [39].

Legionella pneumophila Most patients with legionnaire's disease have underlying illnesses and are usually hospitalized. Intravenous erythromycin at doses of 2 to 4 g/d for 3 weeks is the indicated antibiotic. Patients who respond rapidly can complete their course with oral erythromcyin or clarithromycin. Patients who are severely ill with legionnaire's disease may benefit from the addition of oral or intravenous rifampin as adjunctive and possibly synergistic therapy. Intravenous doxycycline may replace erythromycin in patients who are intolerant to this antibiotic. Studies are underway investigating the role of newer quinolone antibiotics in patients with *Legionella* infection [34, 43].

Staphylococcus aureus Staphylococcal pneumonia is best treated with a semisynthetic penicillin, such as nafcillin or oxacillin, at doses of 9 to 12 g/d or a first-generation cephalosporin such as cefazolin at doses of 6 to 8 g/d for 2 to 3 weeks. A previous history of nursing home residence, prolonged hospitalization, or intravenous drug abuse should lead to an initial choice of vancomycin in view of the high risk of colonization and infection with β-lactam resistant staphylococci among patients with these epidemiologic histories. Once susceptibility data are available, therapy can be switched if indicated. Intravenous trimethoprim/sulfamethoxazole is also effective in treating *S. aureus* infections, including those that are resistant to the β-lactam antibiotics [32].

Anaerobes Patients with aspiration pneumonia due to anaerobic bacteria originating in the oral cavity will often respond to high-dose intravenous penicillin therapy at doses of 2,000,000 units every 4 hours intravenously. This traditional therapy is most appropriate for those patients without recent hospitalization or recent antibiotic therapy, who presumably are infected with organisms that continue to be highly penicillin sensitive, as is the case with most mouth anaerobes. Patients who are compromised by virtue of significant underlying disease, residence in nursing homes, or those with a history of recent antibiotic therapy are best treated with antibiotics that have activity against more resistant anaerobes, which may colonize the oral cavity in such situations [5]. Clindamycin is the drug of choice in this setting, as it has excellent activity against resistant anaerobes; some authors consider it the primary drug of choice for anaerobic pneumonia [78b]. In addition, drugs such as ampicillin/sulbactam, amoxicillin/clavulanic acid, and ticarcillin/clavulanic acid would also be appropriate in treating such anaerobic pathogens, as resistance to penicillin among anaerobes is usually mediated by β-lactamase production. Duration of therapy in anaerobic pleuropulmonary infections depends on the chronicity of the infection. Anaerobic aspiration pneumonia can be treated with a shorter course of 7 to 10 days, whereas established lung abscesses and empyemas require prolonged therapy from 3 to 6 weeks, with combined intravenous and subsequently oral antibiotics [78b, 79, 80]. Oral clindamycin is a useful drug in such patients and carries no greater risk of diarrhea than other oral antimicrobials, although patients should always be cautioned regarding the possibility of developing serious diarrhea while taking any broad-spectrum oral antimicrobial agent.

Gram Negative Pathogens *Klebsiella pneumoniae* and *Escherichia coli* are important gram-negative pathogens that may be responsible for community-acquired pneumonia in compromised and elderly patients [15, 16]. Therapy of first choice in such patients should include a third-generation cephalosporin (ceftriaxone, cefotaxime, ceftizoxime, or cefoperazone), with the addition of an aminoglycoside (preferably gentamicin), until the patient has a significant clinical response [2]. The duration of therapy is usually 2 to 3 weeks; the aminoglycoside need not be given for the entire duration of therapy, since most isolates of *Klebsiella, E. coli,* and many other gram-negative pathogens are highly susceptible to these new cephalosporins. Alternative therapy includes extended spectrum penicillins, such as piperacillin or mezlocillin, or trimethoprim/sulfamethoxazole; when these agents are chosen, concomitant aminoglycoside therapy should be given for the majority of the therapeutic course [1].

Mycoplasma pneumoniae Pneumonia due to *Mycoplasma* can be effectively treated with either oral erythromycin (500 mg every 6 hours), clarithromycin, azithromycin or oral doxycycline (100 mg every 12 hours). Each of these agents has excellent activity and yields good clinical response, although laboratory testing would suggest that the macrolide antibiotics have a much higher degree of activity in vitro [78a, 81]. Intravenous therapy with either erythromycin or doxycycline is also effective in patients who are ill enough to require hospitalization. The newer quinolones, particularly ofloxacin, are currently under study and appear to have good activity against *Mycoplasma* and *Chlamydia* [82, 83].

Chlamydia pneumoniae Patients infected with *C. pneumoniae* are generally not ill enough to require hospitalization, but may require specific antimicrobial therapy. The drugs of choice in this infection are also erythromycin and doxycycline, both of which appear to be effective [43]. In addition, the new macrolides and quinolones such as ofloxacin have also demonstrated efficacy in the treatment of these infections [82]. Patients with *Mycoplasma* or *C. pneumoniae* infections require therapy for 10 to 14 days.

Other Atypical Pathogens
Psittacosis, Q fever, and *Chlamydia trachomatis* infections are effectively treated with tetracycline as a first agent of choice. Chloramphenicol, rather than erythromycin, has been recommended as an alternative in patients with psittacosis and Q fever who are unable to tolerate tetracycline [35, 43].

Pneumocystis carinii The management of *P. carinii* pneumonia in AIDS patients and other immunocompromised patients has undergone considerable study. Current recommendations for therapy include the initiation of intravenous trimethoprim/sulfamethoxazole as a primary therapeutic agent in all patients who are not known to be allergic to sulfa. The dosage regimen is trimethoprim, 20 mg/kg/d plus sulfamethoxazole, 100 mg/kg/d, given intravenously or orally for a total duration of 14 to 21 days. Sixty-five percent of AIDS patients experience an adverse reaction, primarily rash and neutropenia, and many require an alternative regimen (35% to 45%). Twenty percent to 30% of patients fail to respond to trimethoprim/sulfamethoxazole therapy. Effective alternative antimicrobials include intravenous pentamidine (4 mg/kg/d), which may itself require a change to an alternate agent in 45% of cases due to adverse reactions or nonresponse. Adverse reactions to pentamidine include neutropenia, anemia, renal insufficiency, abnormal liver function studies, and hyponatremia. Pancreatitis and abnormal serum glucose levels are also significant adverse reactions. Aerosolized pentamidine has been used for therapy of mild cases as well as for prophylaxis. An important additional well-studied regimen for *P. carinii* pneumonia is the combination of dapsone, 100 mg/d, plus trimethoprim, 20 mg/kg/d. This regimen has shown promise as an oral therapy for mild disease and to complete therapy in patients who have responded rapidly to intravenous regimens. Cross-reactivity of dapsone (a sulfone) with sulfa drugs is not well established. Other regimens are under study and will no doubt provide alternatives to current therapy for this kind of problem [84].

Three important studies were published in 1990 reporting trials of the use of adjunctive corticosteroids for the management of *P. carinii* pneumonia in patients with AIDS. Each trial demonstrated the efficacy of concomitant corticosteroid therapy in patients with moderate-to-severe disease, including significant reductions in morbidity (e.g., respiratory failure) and mortality in treated groups. On the basis of this evidence, a panel from the National Institutes of Health recommended that patients older than 13 years of age with documented or suspected *P. carinii* pneumonia with moderate-to-severe pulmonary dysfunction (defined as a $PO_2 < 70$ mm Hg or an arterial-alveolar gradient > 35 mm Hg) be started on adjunctive corticosteroid therapy as early as possible during the course of their illness. Greatest efficacy was demonstrated when the steroids were begun within 72 hours of beginning anti-*Pneumocystis* therapy. Although the optimal dosage has not yet been determined, a reasonable regimen is as follows: oral or parenteral prednisone, 40 mg twice daily for 5 days, then 40 mg daily for 5 days, followed by 20 mg daily for the duration of the anti-*Pneumocystis* therapy. No adverse reactions were identified in patients receiving such therapy in spite of severe underlying immunosuppression [85–87].

Patient Compliance

Issues related to patient compliance with therapeutic regimens should be addressed in any discussion of serious infections such as pneumonia. Patients who are ill enough to require hospitalization generally are obligated to comply by virtue of the presence of nurses, who usually administer medications as recommended by the attending physician. Patients who are cared for in the ambulatory setting, however, represent a challenge to the physician who must strive for safe and effective therapy that will result in a satisfactory clinical response, avoiding ultimate hospitalization. Factors that discourage patient compliance include the necessity to take multiple drugs, often including regular medications in addition to those needed for the management of pneumonia. Oral antibiotics may be associated with adverse reactions or side effects and dosing schedules may be inconvenient. When a physician-patient relationship has not been well established, the patient may not comply with the full course of therapy, risking complications due to incomplete therapy. New agents with better pharmacokinetic and therapeutic profiles should enhance patient compliance, yet their high cost may be prohibitive. Factors that may encourage patient compliance with antibiotic therapy include an uncomplicated therapeutic regimen prescribed by a physician, who is able to provide the patient with continuity of care by virtue of a long-standing relationship. Frequent follow-up visits are appropriate in the management of ambulatory pneumonia since adjunctive therapy such as bronchodilators or expectorants may be necessary and patient compliance with the full course of therapy must be assured. A concerned and caring attitude by the physician is perhaps the most important component of the therapeutic regimen [88].

Prevention of Community-Acquired Pneumonia

Although modern medicine has provided highly effective antimicrobial therapy, rapid diagnostic methods, and advanced supportive care, pneumonia remains a major cause of mortality (especially among the elderly), morbidity, and economic cost to society. Long before effective therapy became available, public health measures and more recently, hospital infection control procedures, have had a major impact on the incidence of infections of all types. Prophylaxis and preventative activities directed at populations with high risk for community-acquired pneumonia may also have significant impact in reducing the morbidity, mortality, and cost of community-acquired pneumonias. This section reviews immunizations and other means of preventing community-acquired pneumonia.

Immunization

Available vaccines that have demonstrated efficacy in the prevention of respiratory infection in adults include the influenza virus vaccine, and the polyvalent pneumococcal polysaccharide vaccine. Both the influenza virus vaccine and the pneumococcal vaccine are intended primarily for use in high-risk populations. Table 17-10 details current recommendations for the use of these agents.

Influenza Virus Vaccine

The influenza vaccine is prepared annually from inactivated virus representing the influenza A and B strains most likely to circulate during the anticipated influenza season. The efficacy of this vaccine is excellent when it is directed against the appropriate strain. Current vaccines are 60% to 80% effective in the general population. In nursing home patients, the efficacy of preventing disease has been lower (20% to 30%), but complications of influenza such as pneumonia have been reduced by 60% and death by 85% [22].

Influenza vaccine is well tolerated and is frequently administered in vaccination campaigns in senior citizen centers, nursing homes, and hospitals. Those individuals who may not have had previous exposure to the current circulating influenza strain should receive two doses separated by 4-weeks. The Guillain-Barré syndrome seen following the swine flu vaccine program in 1976 has not been reported with subsequent vaccine preparations. Anaphylactic hypersensitivity to eggs is considered a contraindication to the use of this vaccine.

Influenza vaccine is usually administered in the fall, yet may be efficacious when given along with a prophylactic amantadine to high-risk patients during the course of an influenza outbreak, such as in a nursing home or chronic care facility [22].

Table 17-10. Influenza and Pneumococcal Vaccination Recommended for High-Risk Groups [22]

	Influenza Vaccine		
Category	*1st Priority*	*2nd Priority*	*Pneumococcal Vaccine*
Chronic cardiovascular disease	X		X
Chronic pulmonary disease	X		X
Nursing home residents	X		
Healthy people > 65 years			X
Chronic metabolic disease (including diabetes mellitus)		X	
Renal failure		X	
Chronic anemia		X	X
Immunosuppressive including HIV		X	X
Children on long-term aspirin		X	
Health care workers with patient contact		X	
Splenic dysfunction (e.g., sickle cell)			X
Hodgkin's disease			X
Multiple myeloma			X
Cirrhosis			X
Alcoholism			X
Chronic cerebrospinal fluid leak			X

Pneumococcal Vaccine

The pneumococcal polysaccharide vaccine is highly antigenic and has been available commercially in the United States since 1979. The current vaccine contains capsular antigen representing the 23 types of pneumococci which account for 85% of all bacteremic pneumococcal disease in the United States. Eighty percent to 95% of vaccinated individuals will develop a satisfactory antibody response [22]. Efficacy of 60% to 80% has been demonstrated in healthy, high risk young people, i.e., military recruits and South African gold miners, in prevention of bacteremic pneumococcal disease. The diagnostic difficulties reviewed earlier have hampered research efforts to prove the efficacy of pneumococcal vaccine in other high risk populations. However, a recent case control study of over 1000 episodes of invasive pneumococcal infection has clearly confirmed the efficacy of this vaccine in the prevention of invasive disease in immunocompetent patients [22b]. An additional study has also confirmed the cost-effectiveness of vaccination of large populations of high risk individuals [22a].

Given these very supportive data regarding efficacy and cost-effectiveness, it seems prudent to vaccinate high-risk populations as outlined in Table 17-10. The vaccine is well tolerated and redosing is not generally recommended. Revaccination is appropriate in particularly high risk groups, who have received either the 14 valent vaccine or for whom more than 6 years has elapsed since their original vaccination. Patients who lose antibody rapidly, such as those with nephrotic syndrome, may also benefit from booster injections [22].

Vaccination in HIV-Positive Patients

Limited studies have failed to demonstrate adverse effects from the administration of inactivated or live virus vaccines in persons infected with HIV. Although antibody response may be suboptimal, it is recommended that all vaccinations be updated in HIV-positive persons. With the exception of oral polio vaccine, HIV-infected persons should be vaccinated in the same manner as normal individuals. Measles, mumps, and rubella vaccine can be given; however, oral polio vaccine should be replaced with an inactivated polio virus vaccine. Pneumococcal and influenza vaccine not usually considered for normal young people should be administered to patients who are HIV-positive in spite of potentially suboptimal antibody response [22].

Other Preventative Measures

Vaccine administration may prevent invasion of certain virulent pathogens; however, numerous important pulmonary pathogens are not "covered" by currently available vaccines. Most literature pertaining to the prevention of pneumonia relates to hospital-acquired pneumonias, which carry a high mortality. Such methods include careful compliance with infection control procedures such as handwashing, maintenance of universal precautions, and extreme care to prevent contamination of respiratory therapy equipment. Vigorous suctioning and pulmonary toilet, including mobilization, is also important. Indeed, this latter principle can be applied to the prevention of community-acquired pneumonia, especially in compromised patients who may not cough, deep breathe, or ambulate adequately.

Host immune or mechanical defects may represent a major risk factor in the development of community-acquired pneumonia. Such defects include those caused by medication, including immunosuppressive therapy and steroids, which may reduce the host immune response, H_2-blockers and antacids, which may be associated with increased colonization of the stomach and pharynx with potential pathogens, and sedatives, which may impair the cough reflex. In addition, antibiotics may promote colonization with potential pathogens as well. Nutritional deficiency may impair the T-cell and macrophage function and also reduce fibronectin synthesis, which can again affect colonization of the pharynx [9]. Adverse nutritional factors may also affect the efficiency of the cough reflex. Chronic foci of infection in the head and neck such as periodontal and chronic sinus infections may serve as sources of bacterial contamination of the respiratory tract and predispose patients to aspiration pneumonia [21].

Antibiotic prophylaxis for community-acquired pneumonias is generally not recommended, as routine antibiotic therapy may serve only to increase the risk of colonization of the pharynx with new potential pathogens. *P. carinii* prophylaxis has, however, demonstrated clear benefit in HIV-positive patients and in some immunocompromised children in institutions with a high incidence of this complication. HIV-positive patients with a history of a previous episode of *P. carinii* pneumonia or those patients with CD_4 cell counts of less than 200/mm^3 or CD_4 cells representing less than 20% of the total lymphocyte count can be very effectively prophylaxed with trimethoprim/sulfamethoxazole, one double strength tablet once or twice daily, aerosolized pentamidine, 300 mg every 4 weeks, or other regimens such as dapsone, 100 mg every day, or sulfadoxine/pyrimethamine (Fansidar), 1 tablet weekly [84].

Community-acquired pneumonia is a common illness affecting millions of Americans annually. It is associated with significant morbidity, mortality, and cost to society. This chapter has reviewed the epidemiology, etiology, clinical features, diagnosis, complications, management, and prevention of a wide spectrum of community-acquired pneumonias affecting the adult population. Emphasis has been placed on the recognition of diagnostically useful risk factors and the identification of the various clinical syndromes with which community-acquired pneumonia may present. An increased emphasis on prevention can affect the incidence of this syndrome, especially among the elderly. Current research efforts directed at rapid identification of pathogens and improved oral and parenteral therapy will clearly help clinicians provide more cost-effective care in the most appropriate clinical setting.

References

1. Donowitz GR, Mandell GL: Acute pneumonia. *In* Mandell GL, Douglas RG Jr, Bennett JE (eds): Principles and Practice of Infectious Diseases, ed 3. New York, Churchill Livingstone, 1990, pp 540–555
2. McHenry MC: Community-acquired pneumonias. *In* Cunha BA (ed): Infectious Diseases in the Elderly. Chicago, Year Book Medical, 1988, pp 116–143
3. Fine MJ, Orloff JJ, Arisumi D, et al: Prognosis of patients hospitalized with community-acquired pneumonia. *Am J Med* 88:5–1N, 1990
4. Lynch JP III, Chavis A, Streiter RM: Bacterial pneumonia in the community: Evolving concepts. *Intern Med* 10:53, 1989
5. Bartlett JG: Diagnosis of bacterial infections of the lung. *Clin Chest Med* 8:119, 1987
6. Reynolds HY: Host defense impairments that may lead to respiratory infections. *Clin Chest Med* 8:339, 1987
7. Delafuente JC: Immunosenescence: Clinical and pharmacologic considerations. *Med Clin North Am* 69:475, 1985
8. Plewa MC: Altered host response and special infections in the elderly. *Emer Med Clin North Am* 8:193, 1990
9. Lekas NJ: Clinical microbiology: Nosocomial infections and microbiologic procedures. *In* Victor LD (ed): Manual of Critical Care Procedures. Rockville, MD, Aspen, 1989, pp 187–205
10. Huxley EJ, Viroslav J, Gray WR, et al: Pharyngeal aspiration in normal subjects and patients with depressed consciousness. *Am J Med* 64:564, 1978
11. Johanson WB, Woods DE, Chaudhuri T: Association of respiratory tract colonization with adherence of gram-negative bacilli to epithelial cells. *J Infect Dis* 139:669, 1979
12. Irwin RS, Erickson AD, Pratter MR, et al: Prediction of tracheobronchial colonization in current cigarette smokers with chronic obstructive bronchitis. *J Infect Dis* 145:234, 1982
13. Irwin RS, Whitaker S, Pratter MR, et al: The transiency of oropharyngeal colonization with gram-negative bacilli in residents of a skilled nursing facility. *Chest* 81:31, 1982
14. Palmer LB: Bacterial colonization: Pathogenesis and clinical significance. *Clin Chest Med* 8:455, 1987
15. Valenti WM, Trudell RG, Bentley DW: Factors predisposing to oropharyngeal colonization with gram-negative bacilli in the aged. *N Engl J Med* 298:1108, 1979
16. Raju L, Khan F: Pneumonia in the elderly: A review. *Geriatrics* 43:51, 1988
17. Gleckman RA, Bergman MM: Bacterial pneumonia: Specific diagnosis and treatment in the elderly. *Geriatrics* 42:29, 1987

17a. Musher DM: Infections caused by *Streptococcus pneumoniae:* Clinical spectrum, pathogenesis, immunity, and treatment. *Clin Infect Dis* 14:801, 1992

17b. Nguyen MH, Stout JE, Yu VL: Legionellosis. *Infect Dis Clin North Am* 5:561, 1991

18. Chaisson RE, Volberding PA: Clinical manifestations of HIV infection. *In* Mandell GL, Douglas RG Jr, Bennett JE (eds): Principles and Practice of Infectious Disease, ed 3. New York, Churchill Livingstone, 1990, pp 1059–1091

19. Gump JW, Phillips CA, Forsyth BR, et al: Role of infection in chronic bronchitis. *Am Rev Respir Dis* 113:465, 1976

20. Marcy TW, Merrill WW: Cigarette smoking and respiratory tract infection. *Clin Chest Med* 8:381, 1987

21. Niederman MS: Strategies for the prevention of pneumonia. *Clin Chest Med* 8:543, 1987

22. Hinman AR, Orenstein WA, Bart KJ, et al: Immunization. *In* Mandell GL, Douglas RG Jr, Bennett JE (eds): Principles and Practice of Infectious Diseases, ed 3. New York, Churchill Livingstone, 1990, pp 2320–2333

22a. Gable CB, Holzer SS, Engelhart L, et al: Pneumococcal vaccine: Efficacy and associated cost savings. *JAMA* 264:2910, 1990

22b. Shapiro ED, Berg AT, Austrian R, et al: The protective efficacy of polyvalent pneumococcal polysaccharide vaccine. *N Engl J Med* 325:1453, 1991

23. Sims RV: Bacterial pneumonia in the elderly. *Emerg Med Clin North Am* 8:207, 1990

23a. Verghese A, Berk SL: *Moraxella (Branhamella) catarrhalis. Infect Dis Clin North Am* 5:523, 1991

24. Centers for Disease Control: Mortality trends—United States, 1986–1988. *MMWR* 38:117, 1989

25. Chavis A, Streiter RM, Lynch JP III: Community-acquired pneumonia: The atypical pneumonia syndrome. *Intern Med* 10: 51, 1989

26. Fine MJ, Smith DN, Singer DE. Hospitalization decision in patients with community-acquired pneumonia: A prospective cohort study. *Am J Med* 89:713, 1990

27. Marrie TJ, Durant H, Yates L: Community-acquired pneumonia requiring hospitalization: 5-year prospective study. *Rev Infect Dis* 11:586, 1989

28. Singal BM, Hedges JR, Radack KL: Decision rules and clinical prediction of pneumonia: Evaluation of low yield criteria. *Ann Emerg Med* 18:13, 1989

29. Heckerling PS, Tape TG, Wigton RS, et al: Clinical prediction rule for pulmonary infiltrates. *Ann Intern Med* 113:664, 1990

30. Parker RH: *Hemophilus influenzae* respiratory infection in adults. *Postgrad Med* 73:179, 1983

31. Yoo OH, Donath J, Desmond E, et al: The problem of diagnosing bacterial pneumonia in patients with chronic bronchitis. *Mt Sinai J Med* 55:395, 1988

32. Bartlett JG: Community-acquired bacterial infections. *Current Opinion in Infectious Diseases* 2:521, 1989

33. Kaye MG, Fox MJ, Bartlett JB, et al: The clinical spectrum of *Staphylococcus aureus* pulmonary infection. *Chest* 97:788, 1990

33a. Martin RE, Bates JH: Atypical pneumonia. *Infect Dis Clin North Am* 5:585, 1991

34. Glynn JR, Jones AC: Atypical respiratory infections, including chlamydia TWAR infection and legionella infection. *Current Opinion in Infectious Diseases* 3:169, 1990

35. Cotton EM, Strampter MJ, Cunha BA: Legionella and mycoplasma pneumonia—A community hospital experience with atypical pneumonias. *Clin Chest Med* 8:441, 1987

36. Rudin JE, Wing EJ: Prospective study of pneumonia: Unexpected incidence of Legionellosis. *South Med J* 79:418, 1986

37. Marrie TJ, Durant H, Kwan C: Nursing home-acquired pneumonia. *J Am Geriatr Soc* 34:697, 1986

38. Carpenter JL: Klebsiella pulmonary infections: Occurrence at one medical center and review. *Rev Infect Dis* 12:672, 1990

39. McGowan JE: Respiratory tract infections due to *Branhamella catarrhalis* and *Neisseria* species. *In* Remington JS, Schwartz MN (eds): *Current Clinical Topics in Infectious Diseases.* New York, McGraw-Hill, 1987, pp 181–203

40. Slevin NJ, Aitken J, Thornley PE: Clinical and microbiologic features of *Branhamella catarrhalis* bronchopulmonary infections. *Lancet* 1:782, 1984

41. Gobbo PN, Cunha BA: Atypical pneumonias. *In* Cunha BA (ed): Infectious Diseases in the Elderly. Chicago, Year Book Medical, 1988, pp 93–115

42. Couch RB: *Mycoplasma pneumoniae* (primary atypical pneumonia). *In* Mandell GL, Douglas RG Jr, Bennett JE (eds): Principles and Practice of Infectious Diseases, ed 3. New York, Churchill Livingstone, 1990, pp 1446–1457

43. Bartlett JB: Atypical and *Legionella* infections. *Current Opinion in Infectious Diseases* 2:526, 1989

44. Granados A, Podzamczer D, Gudiol F, et al: Pneumonia due to *Legionella* pneumophila and pneumococcal pneumonia: Similarities and differences on presentation. *Eur Respir J* 2:130, 1989

45. Scheffner W: *Chlamydia psittaci* (psittacosis).

In Mandell GL, Douglas RG Jr, Bennett JE (eds): Principles and Practice of Infectious Diseases, ed 3. New York, Churchill Livingstone, 1990, pp 1440–1442

46. Wainwright AP, Beaumont AC, Kox WJ: Psittacosis: Diagnosis and management of severe pneumonia and multi organ failure. *Intensive Care Med* 13:419, 1987
47. Grayson JT, Campbell LA, Kuo CC, et al: A new respiratory tract pathogen: *Chlamydia pneumoniae* strain TWAR. *J Infect Dis* 161: 618, 1990
48. Grayston JT, Diwan VK, Cooney M, et al: Community and hospital-acquired pneumonia associated with *Chlamydia* TWAR infection demonstrated serologically. *Arch Intern Med* 149:169, 1989
49. Scheffner W: TWAR. *In* Mandell GL, Douglas RG Jr, Bennett JE (eds): Principles and Practice of Infectious Diseases, ed 3. New York, Churchill Livingstone, 1990, pp 1443–1444
50. Marrie TJ: *Coxiella Burnetii* (Q fever). *In* Mandell GL, Douglas RG Jr, Bennett JE (eds): Principles and Practice of Infectious Diseases, ed 3. New York, Churchill Livingstone, 1990, pp 1472–1475
51. Rose RM, Pinkston P, O'Donnell C, et al: Viral infection of the lower respiratory tract. *Clin Chest Med* 8:405, 1987
51a. Greenberg SB: Viral pneumonia. *Infect Dis Clin North Am* 5:603, 1991
52. Betts RF, Douglas RG Jr: Influenza virus. *In* Mandell GL, Douglas RG Jr, Bennett JE (eds): Principles and Practice of Infectious Diseases, ed 3. New York, Churchill Livingstone, 1990, pp 1306–1325
53. Toews GB: Approach to the patient with suspected pneumonia. *In* Kelly WN (ed): Textbook of Internal Medicine. Philadelphia, JB Lippincott, 1989, pp 2076–2082
54. Walzer PD: Diagnosis of *Pneumocystis carinii* pneumonia. *J Infect Dis* 157:629, 1988
55. Hopewell PC: *Pneumocystis carinii* pneumonia: Diagnosis. *J Infect Dis* 157:1115, 1988
56. Luce JM, Clement MJ: Pulmonary diagnostic evaluation in patients suspected of having a HIV-related disease. *Semin Respir Infect* 4:93, 1989
56a. Cohn DL: Bacterial pneumonia in the HIV infected patient. *Infect Dis Clin North Am* 5:485, 1991
57. Masur H, Kovacs JA: Treatment and prophylaxis of *Pneumocystis carinii* pneumonia. *In* Sande MA, Volberding PA (eds): The Medical Management of AIDS. Philadelphia, W.B. Saunders, 1988, pp 181–192
58. Fels AOS: Bacterial and fungal pneumonias. *Clin Chest Med* 9:449, 1988
58a. Barnes PF, Block AB, Davidson PT, et al: Tuberculosis in patients with human immunodeficiency virus infection. *N Engl J Med* 324:1644, 1991
58b. White K: HIV and tuberculosis: An old plague returns with added fury. *AIDS Patient Care* 4:16, 1990
59. Katz MH, Baron RB, Grady D: Risk stratification of ambulatory patients suspected of *Pneumocystis* pneumonia. *Arch Intern Med* 151:105, 1991
60. Levine SJ, White DA: *Pneumocystis carinii*. *Clin Chest Med* 9:395, 1988
61. Farr BM, Kaiser DL, Harrison BD, et al: Prediction of microbial aetiology at admission to hospital for pneumonia from the presenting clinical features. *Thorax* 44:1031, 1989
62. Manresa F: Rapid clinical diagnostic methods in respiratory infections. *Current Opinion in Infectious Disease* 2:536, 1989
63. Ausina V: Rapid laboratory diagnostic methods in respiratory infections. *Current Opinion in Infectious Disease* 2:541, 1989
63a. Shurmann RB, Horbach D, et al: Prevalence and diagnosis of Legionella pneumonia: A 3 year prospective study with emphasis on application of urinary antigen detection. *J Infect Dis* 162:1341, 1990
64. Gleckman R, DeVita J, Hibert D, et al: Sputum gram's stain assessment in community-acquired bacteremia pneumonia. *J Clin Microbiol* 26:846, 1988
65. Peterson LR: Using the microbiology laboratory in the diagnosis of pneumonia. *Semin Respir Infect* 3:106, 1988
66. Perlino CA: Laboratory diagnosis of pneumonia due to *Streptococcus pneumoniae*. *J Infect Dis* 150:139, 1984
67. Zaman MK, White DA: The techniques of sputum induction. *Journal of Critical Illness* 5:763, 1990
68. Geckler RW, McAllister K, Germillion DH, et al: Clinical value of paired sputum and transtracheal aspirates in the initial management of pneumonia. *Chest* 87:631, 1985
69. Jacobsen MA, Mills J: Cytomegalovirus infection. *Clin Chest Med* 9:443, 1988
70. Wollschlager CM, Khan FA, Khan A: Utility of radiography and clinical features in the diagnosis of community-acquired pneumonia. *Clin Chest Med* 8:393, 1987
71. Kerttula Y, Leinonen M, Koskela M, et al: The aetiology of pneumonia. Application of bacterial serology and basic laboratory methods. *J Infect* 14:21, 1987
72. Martin SJ, Hoganson DA, Thomas ET: Detection of *Streptococcus pneumoniae* and *Hemophilus influenzae* type b antigens in acute nonbacteremic pneumonia. *J Clin Microbiol* 25:248, 1987
73. Golden JA, Sollitto RA: The radiology of

pulmonary disease: Chest radiography, computed tomography and gallium scanning. *Clin Chest Med* 9:481, 1988

74. MacFarlane JT, Miller AC, Smith WH: Comparative radiographic features of community-acquired Legionnaire's disease, pneumococcal pneumonia, Mycoplasma pneumonia, and psittacosis. *Thorax* 39:28, 1984
75. Breitenbucher RB, Peterson PK: Infections in the elderly. *In* Mandell GL, Douglas RG Jr, Bennett JE (eds): Principles and Practice of Infectious Diseases, ed 3. New York, Churchill Livingstone, 1990, pp 2315–2320
76. Jay SJ, Johanson WJ, Pierce AK: The radiographic resolution of *Streptococcus pneumoniae* pneumonia. *N Engl J Med* 293:798, 1975
77. Tobin MJ: Diagnosis of pneumonia: Techniques and problems. *Clin Chest Med* 8:513, 1987
78. Lentino JR, Lucks DA: Nonvalue of sputum culture in the management of lower respiratory tract infections. *J Clin Microbiol* 25:758, 1987

78a. Bryan JP: New macrolides. *Current Opinion in Infectious Diseases* 4:722, 1991

78b. Gudiol F, Manresa F, Pallares R, et al: Clindamycin vs. penicillin for anaerobic lung infections: High rate of penicillin failures associated with penicillin resistant *Bacteroides melaninogenicus. Arch Intern Med* 150:2525, 1990

79. Dorca J: Bacterial respiratory infections and pneumonia. *Current Opinion in Infectious Diseases* 3:176, 1990
80. Sanford JP: Guide to Antimicrobial Therapy 1990. West Bethesda, Antimicrobial Therapy, 1990
81. Kenny GE, Cartwright FD; Susceptibility of *Mycoplasma pneumoniae* to several new quinolones, tetracycline and erythromycin. *Antimicrob Agents Chemother* 35:587, 1991
82. Lipsky BA, Tack KJ, Kuo C, et al: Ofloxacin treatment of *Chlamydia pneumoniae* (strain TWAR) lower respiratory tract infections. *Am J Med* 89:722, 1990
83. Stocks JM, Wallace RJ, Griffith DE, et al: Ofloxacin in community-acquired lower respiratory infections. *Am J Med* 87:6C-52S, 1989
84. Leoung GS, Hopewell PC: *Pneumocystis carinii* pneumonia: Therapy and prophylaxis. *In* Cohen PT, Sande MA, Vollberding PA (eds): The AIDS Knowledge Base. Waltham, MA, Thc Medical Publishing Grouping, 1990, pp 6.5.4:1–15
85. Montaner JSG, Lawson LM, Levitt N, et al: Corticosteroids prevent early deterioration in patients with moderately severe *Pneumocystis carinii* pneumonia and the acquired immunodeficiency syndrome (AIDS). *Ann Intern Med* 113:14, 1990
86. Bozzette SA, Sattler FR, Chiu J, et al: A controlled trial of early adjunctive treatment with corticosteroids for *Pneumocystis carinii* pneumonia in the acquired immunodeficiency syndrome. *N Engl J Med* 323:1451, 1990
87. Gagnon S, Boota AM, Fischl MA, et al: Corticosteroids as adjunctive therapy for severe *Pneumocystitis carinii* pneumonia in the acquired immunodeficiency syndrome. A double-blind, placebo-controlled trial. *N Engl J Med* 323:1444, 1990
88. Gantz N: Patient compliance in the management of adult respiratory infections. *Intern Med* 11:62, 1990

Tuberculosis

Dana G. Kissner

Historic Background

Tuberculosis, a technically curable and preventable disease, has afflicted humans since prehistoric times. In 1882, when Robert Koch announced his discovery of the tubercle bacillus, one seventh of all deaths in Europe were due to tuberculosis. Hopes for a cure were only briefly raised by Koch's suggestion in 1890 that a filtrate of cultured tubercle bacilli, later known as old tuberculin, had therapeutic value. Although this antigenic material was soon found to be useless as a cure, it subsequently proved successful in identifying infected individuals.

Once tuberculosis was established as an infectious disease with no known cure, measures for control became based on identifying and isolating cases. Tuberculosis patients and their physicians, who themselves were frequently former patients, were isolated in private sanitoriums, such as that established in 1884 by Trudeau, and in public tuberculosis hospitals, away from mainstream medicine. The prevention and treatment of tuberculosis became a public health issue. Organizations were formed, most notably the National Association for the Study and Prevention of Tuberculosis (now known as the American Lung Association), for the purposes of "not only the scientific study of the disease of tuberculosis, but a study of all its relations to man, social and economic, and all measures for its prevention, eradication and cure" [1]. By 1938 there were 732 tuberculosis hospitals in the United States. Rest and good nutrition were the mainstays of therapy. Active treatment consisted of surgical procedures to collapse the lung in an attempt to prevent the formation and promote the healing of cavities. Today we still see evidence of previous therapy with artifical pneumothorax (Fig. 18-1), artificial phrenic nerve paralysis (Fig. 18-2), plombage (Fig. 18-3), thoracoplasty (Fig. 18-4), and resection. Many of these patients now seek medical care because of symptoms due to respiratory insufficiency and cor pulmonale (see Chapter 12).

In 1944 Selman Waksman ushered in the modern era of chemotherapy for tuberculosis when he announced his isolation of streptomycin. Subsequent experimental work and clinical trials, including the first controlled randomized clinical trial of a drug, revealed its efficacy in the treatment of tuberculosis, as well as its toxicity [2]. It also became apparent that the development of drug resistance limited the ability of streptomycin to effect a cure. In 1946 Lehman reported that para-aminosalicylic acid was effective in treating tuberculosis. Subsequent cooperative trials showed that combining streptomycin and para-aminosalicylic acid prevented the emergence of resistance and established the basic principle, which remains true today, that treatment of tuberculosis should always consist of at least two effective drugs. The introduction of isoniazid in 1952 soon eliminated the need for injections necessary to administer streptomycin. However, prolonged therapy of 2 or more years was shown to be necessary if cure and prevention of relapse were to be achieved, especially in the case of cavitary disease [3]. Supervised intermittent therapy was shown to be an effective means of dealing with the problem of poor patient compliance [4]. In 1963 ethambutol became available and soon replaced the poorly tolerated para-aminosalicylic acid, which often had to be given in as large a quantity as 24 pills per day. Subsequent to the introduction of rifampin for clinical use in 1967, it was demonstrated that a 9-month course of isoniazid and rifampin could effect a cure and prevent relapse.

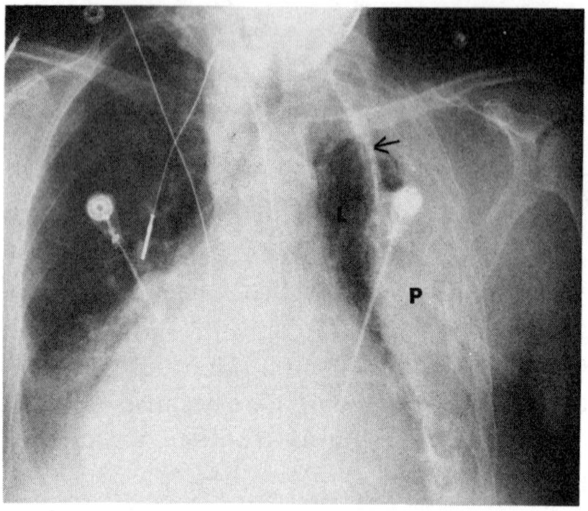
L
P

Fig. 18-1. Chest radiograph demonstrating late effects of induced pneumothorax. The pleura (*arrow*) is calcified. The pleural space (P) is filled with fibrous tissue. The underlying lung (L) has never reexpanded. The cardiac enlargement is due to right ventricular dilitation.

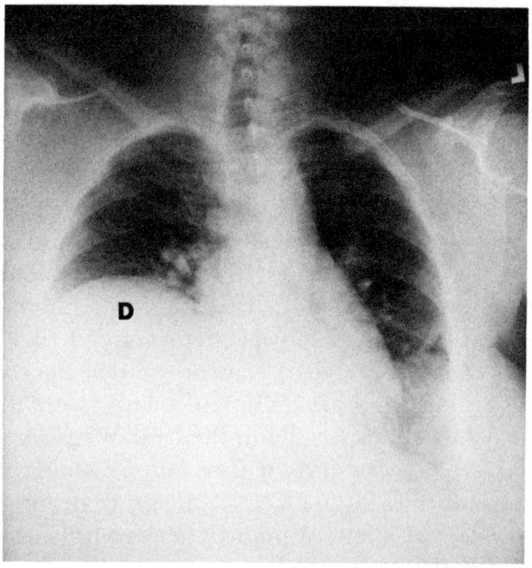
D

Fig. 18-2. Chest radiograph demonstrating late effects of artificial phrenic nerve paralysis. The marked elevation of the right hemidiaphragm (D) is the result of induced phrenic nerve paralysis.

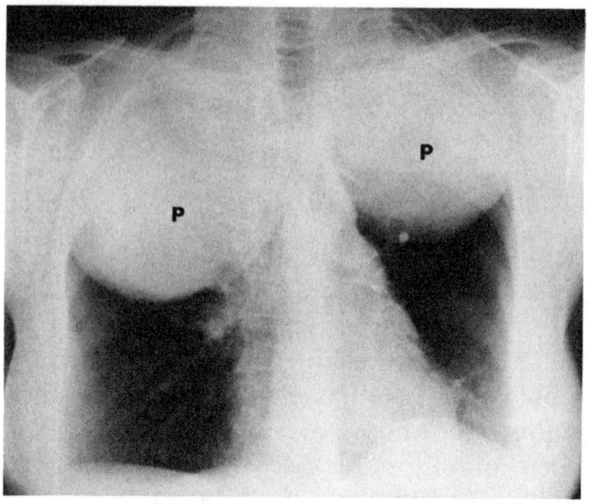
P
P

A

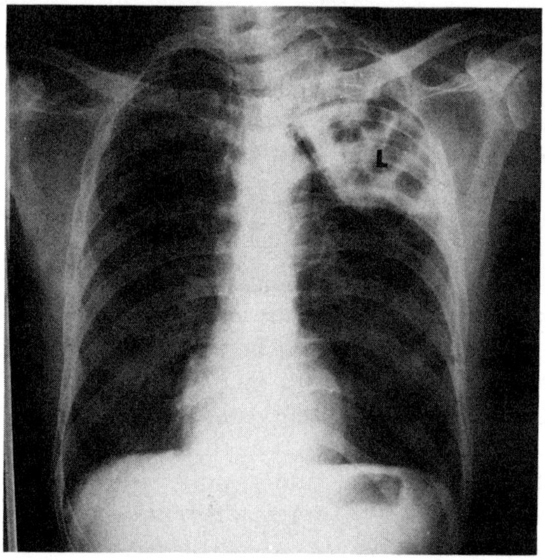
L

B

Fig. 18-3. Chest radiographs demonstrating plombage. Numerous materials were used as "plombs" in the space between the chest wall and the parietal pleura or between the ribs and periosteum in an attempt to collapse the lung. (A) Plombage with paraffin (P). (B) Plombage with hollow lucite balls (L). Erosion into adjacent structures, pyogenic infection, and even late tuberculosis have occurred with plombs left in place.

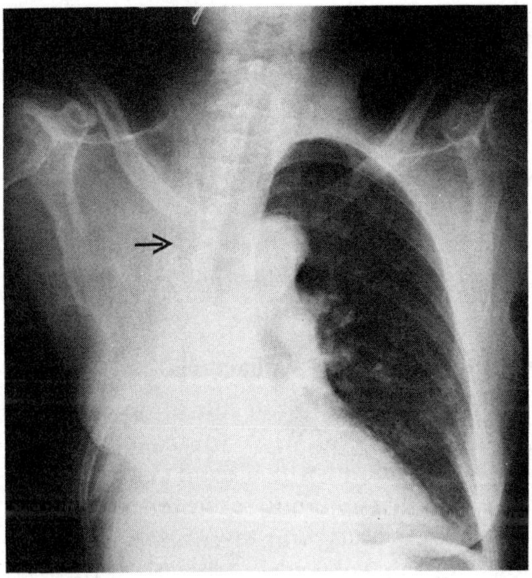

Fig. 18-4. Chest radiograph demonstrating thoracoplasty. Subperiosteal rib resections were performed in attempts to collapse and close cavities. The periosteum left in place regenerated ribs in a collapsed position (*arrow*).

Today, a lasting cure is possible after 6 months of isoniazid and rifampin, supplemented by an initial 2 months of pyrazinamide (PZA), and efforts are being made to shorten treatment time even further.

A clinical trial conducted in Madras, India, the results of which were published in 1959, demonstrated that patients could be as effectively treated at home as in a sanitorium, and that the number of household members with newly acquired disease did not increase with home therapy [5]. Other studies concluded that home therapy did not pose a risk of increased infection rates among household members [6, 7]. Thus, the basic tenet that rest is essential in tuberculosis therapy was disproved but not abandoned. It took time for enforced rest, segregation of patients in sanitoriums, and surgical procedures to close cavities to be abandoned. The closing of the Trudeau sanitorium in 1954 represented the demise of the age of the sanitorium. Between 1954 and 1967 the number of hospital beds for tuberculosis patients decreased from 111,715 to 43,069 [8].

Epidemiology

Tuberculosis death rates and, to a lesser extent, new case rates, which had fallen steadily in the United States even before the introduction of effective chemotherapy, decreased dramatically afterward. In 1959 the Arden House Conference on Tuberculosis took place, sponsored by the National Tuberculosis Association and the Public Health Service Tuberculosis Program. The conferees optimistically and prematurely agreed that "Eradication (or elimination) of tuberculosis is a perfectly feasible objective in the United States" [9]. However, with the reduction in tuberculosis incidence and the shift of treatment from specialized centers to the community, physician awareness of the disease and skill in diagnosis and treatment waned [10, 11]. Lack of patient compliance also contributed to the persistence of the disease [12]. Still, rates decreased, on average 5% per year, until 1984, when for the first time they plateaued. Between 1985 and 1990 the number of new cases of tuberculosis reported to the Centers for Disease Control rose for the first time, from 22,201 to 25,701, an increase of 15.8%. It has been estimated that this represents an excess of 28,000 cases over historic trends [13]. Infection with the human immunodeficiency virus (HIV), outbreaks among the homeless, and the continued influx of infected foreign-born persons are considered to be some of the reasons for the increase in tuberculosis incidence.

There is great variability in rates between regions of the United States and between racial and ethnic groups. Whereas tuberculosis has virtually been eliminated from some regions of the country, it has been increasing in others, especially in those areas with a high prevalence of HIV infection [14]. Two thirds of the reported cases occur in blacks, Hispanics, and Asian/Pacific Islanders and one fourth occur in foreign born people [15]. In both these groups the incidence is rising [13].

Other high incidence populations are persons infected with HIV, alcoholics, intravenous drug users, and residents of long-term residential facilities such as nursing homes, prisons and psychiatric institutions [16]. Worldwide, it is estimated that there are 10 to 30 million active cases, an annual incidence of 3.7 to 10 million new cases, and 1 to 3 million deaths per year due to this preventable and treatable disease [17]. Another "Stratregic Plan for the Elimination of Tuberculosis in the United States" has been developed by the Centers for Disease Control/ Department of Health and Human Services' Advisory Committee for Elimination of Tuberculosis and endorsed by many medical organizations. The goal is the elimination (< 1 per million population) of tuberculosis by the year 2010 [18]. It is yet to be seen whether or not this too will be an overly optimistic goal. Rene and Jean Dubos' statement made almost 40 years ago holds true today, "However desirable a goal, the complete elimination of tubercle bacilli is rendered impossible by economic and social factors" [19]. The goal of this chapter is to help remove one obstacle to the elimination of tuberculosis by providing a practical guide to the diagnosis and management of tuberculosis to physicians who may uncommonly see the disease and thus may be unfamiliar with its clinical presentation and the principles of diagnosis and treatment.

Microbiology

Tuberculosis is caused by *Mycobacterium tuberculosis,* one of many species of genus *Mycobacterium. M. tuberculosis* is a nonmotile, nonsporulating rod, with a cell wall rich in lipids. It is an obligatory aerobe, grows and metabolizes slowly, and can survive in macrophages. When the Ziehl-Neelsen and auramine (fluorescence) stains for acid fastness are used, dye enters the cell and binds to a component of the cell wall. Because of the characteristics of the cell wall, the dye is retained despite decolorization with strong acid or acid-alcohol. Gram staining results are variable. The organisms may be gram positive, but often do not stain and appear as ghost forms. Growth on culture medium is slow, taking 3 to 6 weeks to become apparent. Other mycobacteria included under the term tuberculosis complex are *M. bovis,* which can be transmitted to humans through the ingestion of milk from infected cows, *M. leprae,* which causes leprosy, and *M africanum,* which is found in Africa. These organisms, like *M. tuberculosis,* are strict pathogens.

Nontuberculous Mycobacteria

Included under the term nontuberculous myocobacteria (NTM) are more than 30 species, only some of which have clinical significance. Other frequently used terms for these organisms are atypical mycobacteria, anonymous, and mycobacteria other than tuberculosis. These mycobacteria may appear in clinical specimens such as sputum as a result of (1) disease, (2) colonization of the respiratory tract, especially in the presence of preexisting lung disease, and (3) contamination from water or soil (Table 18-1). Person-to-person spread of NTM is very rare. Water and soil are likely sources of infection.

Distinguishing between lung disease caused by NTM and preexisting lung disease with colonization by NTM can be very difficult. The most common species causing lung disease are *M. kansasii* and *M. avium* complex. Symptoms, such as cough, dyspnea, malaise and hemoptysis are nonspecific. A diagnosis of pulmonary disease caused by NTM can be made in a patient with a cavitary infiltrate on chest radiograph if the following conditions are met: 1) two or more sputums (or sputum plus bronchial washing) are acid-fast bacilli smear-positive and/or result in moderate growth of NTM on culture and 2) other possible etiologies are excluded. In patients with noncavitary infiltrates, a diagnosis of NTM lung disease can be made if conditions 1 and 2 above are met and the sputum cultures fail to convert to negative with bronchial hygiene or 2 weeks of antimycobacterial chemotherapy. If the organisms do clear with the above measures, observation for possible progression should be continued. If a lung biopsy is performed, yields the organism, and shows

Table 18-1. Species of Mycobacteria: Pathogenicity in Humans

Pathogenicity	*Species*	*Runyon Group or Rate of Growth*	*Drug Sensitivity**	*Type of Disease*
Always	*M. leprae*	Very slow		Leprosy
	M. tuberculosis	Slow		Tuberculosis
	M. bovis	Slow	+	Tuberculosis
	M. africanum	Slow	+	Tuberculosis
Sometimes	*M. avium* complex (*M. intracellulare*)	III	−	Pulmonary, extrapulmonary, disseminated
	M. kansasii	I	+	Pulmonary, extrapulmonary
	M. xenopi	II	+	Pulmonary (common water contaminant)
	M. scrofulaceum	II	−	Lymphadenitis, pulmonary
	M. szulgai	II	+	Pulmonary, extrapulmonary
	M. simiae	I		Pulmonary
	M. fortuitum chelonei complex	IV	−	Soft tissue and wound infection, cornea, pulmonary
	M. marinum	I	+	Cutaneous, swimming
	M. ulcerans	III	+	Cutaneous, buruli ulcer
Very rare	*M. terrae complex*	III		Cutaneous
	M. smegmatis	IV		Cutaneous
Never	*M. gordonae*	II		Common water contaminant
	M. gastri	III		
	M. triviale	III		
	M. flavescens	II		
	M. vaccae	IV		
	M. phlei	IV		

*Susceptible to commonly used antituberculosis drugs.

histopathologic changes consistent with mycobacterial disease (i.e., granulomatous inflammation), a diagnosis of NTM pulmonary disease can be made. Finally, this diagnosis can be established in cases where lung biopsy has negative culture results, but shows mycobacterial histologic changes, two sputums are culture positive, other causes of granulomatous disease have been excluded, and there is no prior history of granulomatous disease [20].

NTM may be classified by their rate of growth and pigmentation characteristics (Table 18-2). With the exception of *M. simiae,* pathogenic NTM do not produce niacin, whereas *M. tuberculosis* does. Some NTM are sensitive to antituberculous agents, whereas others are resistant. *M. avium* complex (also known as *M. avium intracellulare*), a drug-resistant organism, is the most common mycobacteria causing disease in patients with the acquired immunodeficiency syndrome (AIDS). It is frequently disseminated and a cause of death in this patient population.

Transmission and Pathogenesis of *Mycobacterium tuberculosis*

Tuberculosis is spread from person to person by airborne droplet nuclei. Very rarely there may be direct inoculation into injured skin. When a person with pulmonary tuberculosis coughs or sneezes he or she aerosolizes parti-

Table 18-2. Runyan Classification of Nontuberculous Mycocbacteria

Group I	Photochromogens	Slow growers, pigmented in light
Group II	Scotochromogens	Slow growers, pigmented in light and dark
Group III	Nonphotochromogens	Slow growers, nonpigmented
Group IV	Rapid growers	

cles containing varying quantities of *M. tuberculosis.* Droplet nuclei, which are 1 to 10 μm in size, remain airborne and can be inhaled by a susceptible person. Tuberculosis is not highly contagious. Only about 30% of close contacts and 15% of other contacts of an active case are found to be infected or diseased at the time of contact investigation [21]. Transmission usually requires close, frequent, or prolonged contact or the production of numerous droplet nuclei containing large numbers of viable organisms. Because fomites are not involved in the transmission of tuberculosis, special handling of clothing and linens, sterilization of dishes and utensils, and wearing of special caps and gowns are neither helpful nor indicated. Effective measures to control the spread of tuberculosis are listed in Table 18-3.

Once inhaled by a susceptible host, the tubercle bacilli may reach the alveoli where they are engulfed by alveolar macrophages. Initially the tubercle bacilli multipy within the macrophages and spread via the lymphatics to the regional lymph nodes and through the bloodstream to distant organs where they may remain quiescent but viable. The early inflammatory lesion in the lung, which may be in any location, together with the infected regional lymph nodes, is called the primary complex. When the primary focus in the lung fibroses and calcifies, it is referred to as the Ghon's lesion. Tissue damage is caused by the host's reaction to the tubercle bacillus, rather than by the organism itself. Within several weeks of infection, the host develops an immune response. This is manifested by a delayed hypersensitivity reaction to the intracutaneous injection of antigens derived from *M. tuberculosis* (a positive tuberculin skin test result). There is also relative, but not absolute, protection from exogenous reinfection [22]. In about 90% of cases the host's immune system limits the growth of the bacilli, allows for healing of the initial lesions, and permanently prevents disease from occurring. However, bacilli may remain dormant but viable within these individuals. In about 5% of cases there is early progression, within several years of exposure, to clinical disease, either in the lung, an extrapulmonary site, or in multiple sites. In another 5% there is initial healing of lesions and control of the growth of bacilli. However, after years or decades, the bacilli, which have remained quiescent, begin to multiply and cause clinical disease, again either in the lung, especially the apical and posterior segments of the upper lobes and superior segments of the lower lobes, or in nonpulmonary sites.

Table 18-3. Methods to Control the Transmission of Tuberculosis

Chemotherapy
Covering the nose and mouth of the patient with tuberculosis
Ventilating the room (20 air changes per hour) and exhausting the air to the outside rather than recirculating it
Ultraviolet irradiation of the air

Infection Versus Disease

A clear distinction must be made between tuberculosis infection and disease. In the former there is no clinical, radiologic, or bacteriologic evidence of disease, but the skin test response is significant. These people, although neither ill nor contagious, constitute the largest reservoir of tuberculosis cases in the United States. It is estimated that there are approximately 10 to 15 million infected people in the United States, and that over 90% of cases of active tuberculosis arise from this pool [23]. Even among people seroposi-

Table 18-4. Classification of Tuberculosis

0:	No exposure, no significant tuberculin skin test reaction
1:	Exposure, no significant tuberculin skin test reaction
2:	Infection, no clinical, radiologic, or bacteriologic evidence of disease, but skin test reaction is significant
3:	Tuberculosis, current disease
4:	Tuberculosis, no current direase, but there is a history or other evidence of previous disease
5:	Tuberculosis suspect, diagnosis pending

tive for HIV, it appears that most cases of active tuberculosis arise from those previously, rather than newly, infected with tuberculosis [14]. Whether or not an infected individual develops disease depends on the relationship between the tubercle bacillus and the host. Risk factors for the development of disease are discussed later in the section dealing with isoniazid prophylaxis.

In tuberculosis disease there is either confirmatory bacteriologic evidence, or there is both a significant skin test reaction *and* clinical and/or radiologic evidence of current disease. The American Thoracic Society's classification system is presented in Table 18-4.

The Tuberculin Skin Test

The tuberculin skin test is useful, but not 100% accurate, in identifying individuals infected with *M. tuberculosis.* Tuberculins are culture extracts of *M. tuberculosis* containing antigens to which the infected individual has become sensitized. When injected intracutaneously into the sensitized individual, tuberculin elicits a delayed (cellular) hypersensitivity reaction. This is characterized by the development of induration 24 to 72 hours after injection. There are two types of tuberculins available: old tuberculin, which is a crude nonstandardized product contaning extraneous antigens, and purified protein derivative (PPD), which is standardized and without sensitizing properties. In 1939 Florence Seibert, who first prepared PPD, made a single large lot, 49608, from a single strain of tubercle bacillus. Known as PPD-S, this has become the international standard. A standard test dose is 5 tuberculin units. To be licensed, commercial products must show biologic equivalence, meaning ability to elicit a similar size (±20%) skin test response in humans to 5 tuberculin units or 0.1 μg/0.1 mL of PPD-S. Commercial products labeled 1 and 250 tuberculin units are not bioassayed and are therefore not useful in diagnosing infection with tuberculosis.

There are two main methods of skin testing: the percutaneous multiple puncture method, which can be used with old tuberculin or PPD, and the intracutaneous Mantoux test for which only PPD is available. The multiple puncture technique is useful for screening, but because the size of the reaction elicited is not standardized, any reaction, with the exception of vesiculation, should be confirmed with the administration of a Mantoux test. The method of administering and measuring the response to the Mantoux test is demonstrated in Fig. 18-5. It is important that tuberculin be refrigerated, kept in the dark, and used as soon as possible after the syringe has been filled. Severe reactions to PPD, consisting of vesiculation and ulceration with regional lymphadenopathy and fever, occur, but are rare, random, and not related to a prior history of a positive reaction. Covering with a bland ointment is usually sufficient therapy [24].

Although the Mantoux PPD skin test is very useful in identifying those individuals infected with *M. tuberculosis,* it is not perfect. There are both false-positive and false-negative test results. In other words, not all skin test reactors have been infected with *M. tuberculosis* and not all nonreactors are uninfected. False-positive reactions may occur because individuals sensitized to cross-reacting antigens, in particular to those present in NTM, may react to tuberculin. Although these reactions are usually smaller than those due to hypersensitivity to *M. tuberculosis,* there is no clear demarcation between the two. The distribution of reaction sizes in populations with a high risk for *M. tuberculosis*

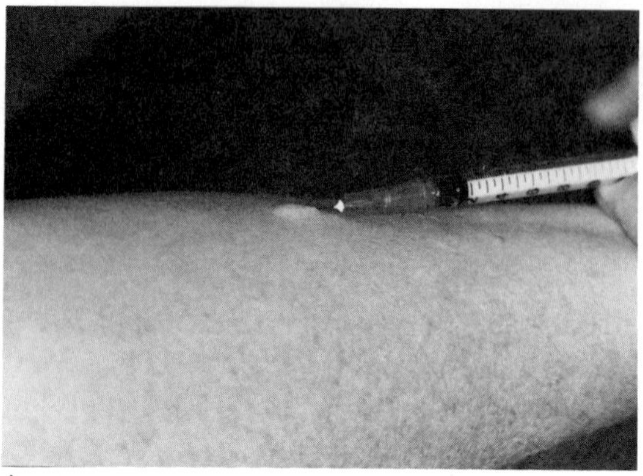

A

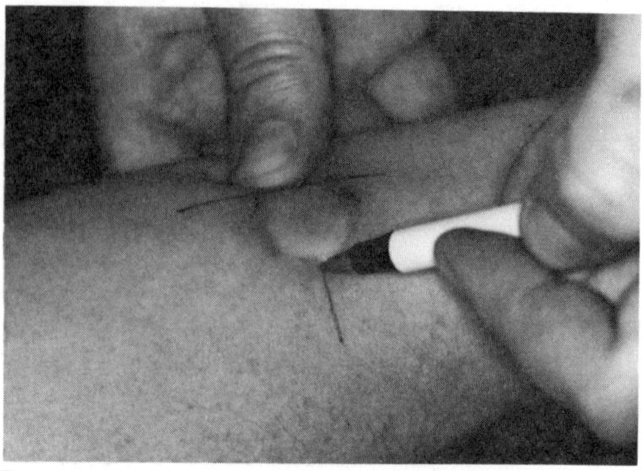

B

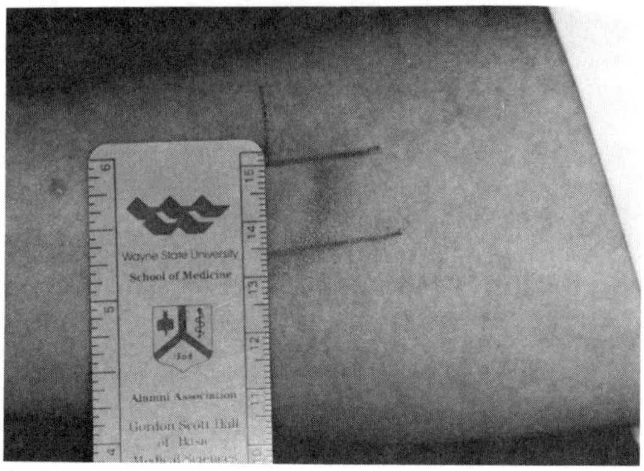
Wayne State University
School of Medicine
Alumni Association

C

Fig. 18-5. Mantoux skin test. (A) 0.1 mL of PPD is injected just under the skin of the volar surface of the forearm, resulting in the formation of a wheal. (B and C) Tests should be read 2 to 3 days after injection. The presence or absence of induration is determined by palpation and inspection. Erythema is unimportant and should not be considered. Measurement of the diameter of induration should be made transversely to the long axis of the forearm and recorded in millimeters. Drawing a line with a ballpoint pen toward the margin of the skin test reaction, putting traction on the skin if necessary, and stopping when resistance is felt allows for accurate measurement.

infection and low risk for infection with other mycobacteria, such as Alaskan Eskimos, is bimodal. One portion of these populations has reaction sizes less than 5 mm. The reaction size in the remainder of the population forms a normal distribution, or bell-shaped curve, similar to that found in patients with tuberculosis, ranging from about 5 mm to more than 26 mm, with a peak at 15 to 17 mm. The distribution of reaction sizes is very different in populations with little risk for *M. tuberculosis* infection, but significant risk for infection with NTM, such as residents of the southeastern United States who have had no contact with a tuberculosis case. In these populations there is a greater number of reactions that are 4 to 14 mm, and there is no bell-shaped curve. In these latter populations it is difficult to distinguish skin test reactions representing infection with *M. tuberculosis* from those representing cross-reactions. In order to properly interpret the skin test, other factors besides size must be taken into account. In general, interpreting a reaction size of 10 mm or greater as representing infection with *M. tuberculosis* identifies most cases of tuberculosis infection, while not falsely classifying too many cross-reactions. However, if one is dealing with patients who have had little opportunity to come into contact with cross-reacting antigens, or in whom the suspicion of tuberculosis infection is high, such as household contacts, or those with a compatible disease or chest radiography, a reaction size of 5 mm should be considered significant. Because it takes 2 to 10 weeks after the initial infection with *M. tuberculosis* for hypersensitivity to develop, the skin test result may be negative or small in size during this time. In addition, if the patient being tested has factors predisposing to false-negative skin tests, as is discussed in the next paragraph, it is probably safer to consider a smaller reaction as significant. For more detailed discussions of the scientific basis for interpreting tuberculin skin tests the reader is referred to several excellent reviews [24–27].

To complicate interpretation of the tuberculin skin test further are numerous factors, including errors of administration and storage, which may lead to a false-negative reaction in people truly infected with *M. tuberculosis*. Skin test reactions are dependent on the presence and proper functioning of specifically sensitized lymphocytes. The following conditions may lead to false-negative reactions: concurrent infections, recent or overwhelming infection with *M. tuberculosis*, live virus immunization, chronic illnesses such as renal failure, protein malnutrition, immunosuppressive drugs such as corticosteroids, diseases of the lymphoid organs including sarcoidosis and lymphoma, HIV infection, very young or old age, and severe stress. In some patients, especially the elderly, there may be waning of the delayed hypersensitivity to tuberculin, resulting in an apparently negative skin test response. In these individuals a second test, performed as early as 1 week after the first one, may result in a significant reaction. This is known as the booster effect. The first test has not sensitized the individual to tuberculin, but rather has boosted or increased the size of the reaction. Because of the booster phenomenon, a person should not be classified as a nonreactor on the basis of a single administration of tuberculin. Rather a second skin test should be performed. If the reaction to the second test is positive, it most likely represents a boosted reaction and the person should be classified as a tuberculin reactor. If the reaction to the second test is insignificant, the person should be classified as a nonreactor, and, any subsequent increase in the size of the reaction by 10 mm or more in a person under age 35, or 12–15 mm or more in one age 35 or over, should be considered a new infection or skin test conversion [27–29].

Further cautionary notes need to be raised for interpreting skin test results in elderly residents of chronic care facilities. In some of these patients a third dose of antigen is required to boost the reaction to a significant level [30, 31]. In addition, when skin test results in this population are read on both days 2 and 7, some will be positive on only day 2 and others only on day 7 [32]. Detailed recommendations for diagnosing and managing tuberculosis infection in long-term care facilities for the elderly have been published by the Advisory Committee for Elimination of Tuberculosis [28].

Table 18-5 lists indications for tuberculin skin testing and Table 18-6 lists guidelines for interpreting skin test results. It should always be kept in mind that these are guide-

Table 18-5. Indications for Tuberculin Skin Testing

1. Clinical or radiographic signs of TB
2. Close contacts of persons with or suspected of having TB
3. Persons with a chest radiograph suggestive of past TB
4. Persons with the following medical conditions that increase the risk of developing tuberculosis after infection:
   - silicosis
   - gastrectomy
   - jejunoileal bypass
   - weight 10% below ideal body weight
   - chronic renal failure
   - diabetes mellitus
   - immunosuppresive therapy including prolonged high-dose corticosteroid use
   - hematologic disorders such as leukemia, lymphomas
   - malignancies
   - HIV infection
5. Persons with risk factors for HIV infection in whom HIV infection status is unknown
6. Intravenous drug users
7. Foreign-born persons from countries with a high prevalence of TB
8. Residents and personnel of long-term-residential facilities such as nursing homes, prisons, psychiatric institutions
9. Health care personnel
10. Medically underserved, low-income populations including high incidence racial and ethnic minorities such as Blacks, Hispanics, Native Americans, and Asian/Pacific Islanders

Table 18-6. Interpretation of Tuberculin Skin Test Results: Criteria for Positive Reactions

Reaction size	*Population*
5 mm or more	Persons with HIV infection Persons with risk factors for HIV infection with unknown HIV status Close recent contacts of an infectious TB case Persons with chest radiographs consistent with TB
10 mm or more	Persons with other medical conditions that increase the risk of TB after infection: silicosis, gastrectomy, jejunoileal bypass, weight 10% below ideal body weight, chronic renal failure, diabetes mellitus, prolonged use of high dose corticosteroid therapy, use of other immunosuppressive therapy, hematologic disorders such as leukemias and lymphomas, and other malignancies Persons belonging to groups with a high incidence of TB: persons from foreign countries with a high prevalence of TB; medically underserved low income groups; certain ethnic and racial minorities such as Blacks, Hispanics, Native Americans, and Asian/Pacific Islanders; residents of long term care facilities such as nursing homes, prisons, psychiatric institutions Intravenous drug users known to be HIV seronegative
15 mm or more	All individuals not falling within the above categories

lines only. Skin testing may be indicated for other groups, and lower or higher cutoff points for identifying positive reactions may be indicated, depending on individual and local circumstances [16, 23, 27].

Diagnosis

The diagnosis of tuberculosis begins with a suspicion of the disease, usually based on compatible symptoms, an abnormal radiographic finding, a positive tuberculin skin test, or a history of exposure to an infectious case. Symptoms may include cough, hemoptysis, weight loss, fatigue, fever, night sweats, hoarseness, or pain. It needs to be emphasized that a completely asymptomatic patient may still have active tuberculosis. Patients with extrapulmonary tuberculosis usually have symptoms referable to the site of their disease without pulmonary symptoms, and early in the course of their disease patients with disseminated (miliary) tuberculosis may experience only malaise and weight loss. Tuberculosis is the cause of some cases of fever of unknown orign. It is important to remember that tuberculosis has protean manifestations, and suspicion for it must remain high.

Between 1963 and 1986 the number of reported cases of pulmonary tuberculosis in the United States decreased by about 5% per year while the number of extrapulmonary cases decreased by an average of 0.9% annually, resulting in an increase in the percentage of extrapulmonary cases. In 1986 17.5% of reported tuberculosis cases had a major extrapulmonary site [33]. Extrapulmonary tuberculosis is more common in persons with HIV infection than in those without, making it likely that the percentage of extrapulmonary cases will continue to increase. Forty percent to 60% of patients with concomitant HIV infection and tuberculosis have involvement of extrapulmonary sites as opposed to about 20% of those without HIV infection [34, 35].

The lymphatic system is the most common site for nonpleural extrapulmonary tuberculosis. About 30% of HIV-infected persons with tuberculosis have primarily lymph node involvement. Tuberculosis should be suspected in all patients with unexplained pleural effusions. The fluid is usually a clear yellow exudate, but can be bloody. White cell count is usually 300 to 3000, with lymphocytes, or less commonly polymorphonuclear cells, predominating. Glucose may be normal or low, and pH is less than 7.40 and may be very low. Empyema can result from rupture of a caseous focus into the pleural space, with formation of a bronchopleural fistula and a mixed tuberculous and nontuberculous infection. Chest tube drainage is required for such an empyema, but not for uncomplicated tuberculous effusions, which resolve either spontaneously or with chemotherapy. Unexplained urinary symptoms or the finding of sterile pyuria or hematuria should raise suspicion for genitourinary tuberculosis. Tuberculosis of the kidney (Fig. 18-6) can result in calyceal dilatation, parenchymal cavitation or calcification, papillary necrosis, "autonephrectomy" (complete destruction of the kidney), ureteral strictures, and contraction of the bladder. The pelvic organs in men and women may be affected. Tuberculous meningitis can be acute or chronic and can present with fevers, headache, and mental status changes. Nuchal rigidity occurs in the minority of patients. Cerebral spinal fluid protein is elevated, glucose low or normal, and white cell count modestly elevated. Tuberculomas present as mass lesions. Unexplained pericardial effusions and ascites should raise suspicion for tuberculosis. Tuberculosis should also be considered in the differential diagnosis of skeletal or joint pain. Unrecognized Pott's disease (Fig. 18-7), osteomyelitis of the vertebral bodies, may result in paraplegia. Abnormal liver function test results or jaundice may be due to hepatobiliary tuberculosis. Anemia, thrombocytopenia, leukopenia, leukocytosis, leukemoid reactions, and consumptive coagulopathy may all be due to tuberculosis. Bone marrow biopsies and cultures can be useful in establishing a diagnosis.

Although routine radiography to screen for tuberculosis is no longer recommended, those done for other purposes may suggest the diagnosis [36]. Chest radiographic manifestations of tuberculosis are varied and are listed in Table 18-7. Examples of cavitary and miliary tuberculosis are shown in Figs. 18-8 and 18-9. A point to be emphasized is that activity of disease cannot be determined by

Fig. 18-6. Tuberculosis of the kidney. Intravenous pyelogram demonstrates cavities (c) and infundibular stenosis (*arrow*).

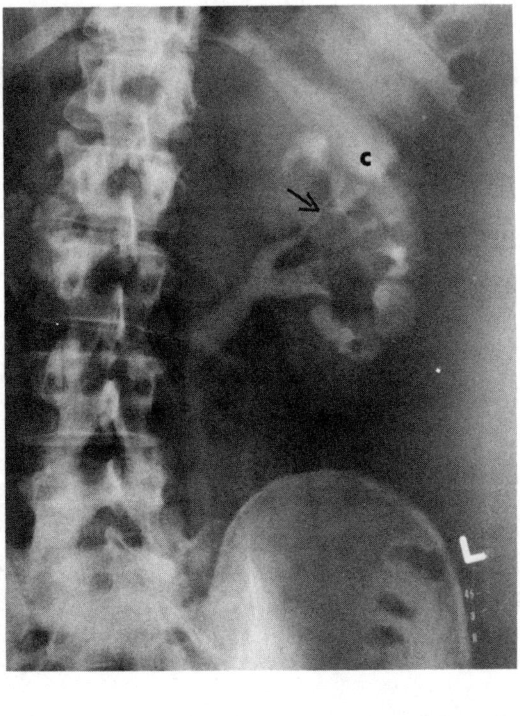
c
L

Fig. 18-7. Pott's disease (tuberculosis of the spine). Lumbar spine radiograph demonstrates destruction and loss of height of continguous vertebral bodies, narrowing of the intervertebral disk space, and gibbous formation (*arrow*).

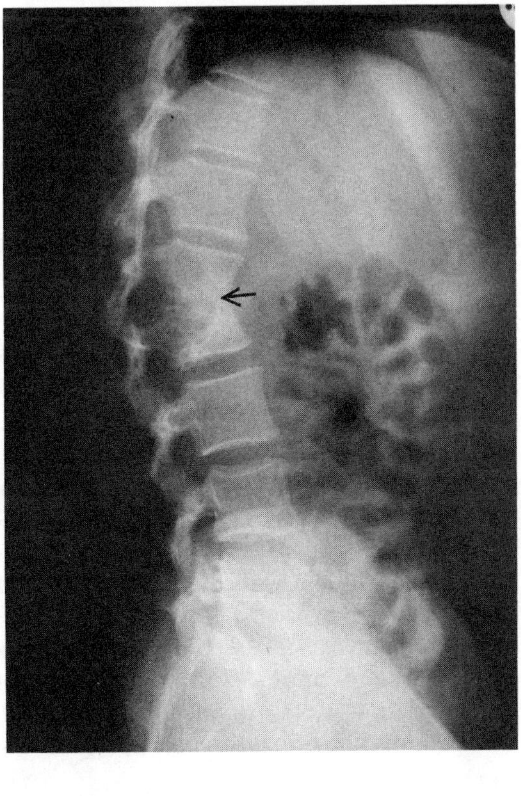

Table 18-7. Chest Radiographic Manifestations of Tuberculosis

Cavities with little fluid, often accompanied by disseminated nodular densities; most common in upper posterior lung fields (Fig. 18-8)
Small patchy areas of increased density, single or multiple
Apical densities, especially in the regions bound by the clavicle, first rib and sternum; lordotic views sometimes required to see these well
Retraction of the upper lobes, sometimes with pleural thickening and parenchymal densities
Symmetric or asymmetric hilar and/or mediastinal adenopathy, enlarged right paratracheal lymph nodes
Pleural effusion; may be minimal, very large, simple, or loculated
Enlarged cardiac shadow due to a pericardial effusion
Nodule or mass resembling neoplasm
Areas of consolidation
Segmental or lobar atelectasis due to endobronchial disease or bronchial stenosis
Parenchymal and/or mediastinal/hilar calcifications
Uniformly distributed nodules 2 to 3 mm in size throughout the lungs (miliary tuberculosis) (Fig. 18-9); early in the course of the disease these may be barely apparent

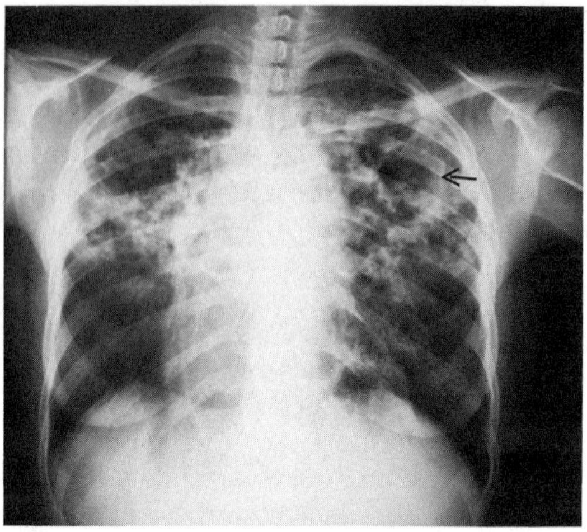

Fig. 18-8. Chest radiograph with changes typical of cavitary tuberculosis. The wall of a large cavity with no air–fluid level can be seen in the left upper lobe (*arrow*). There is retraction upward of both hila due to upper lobe volume loss and widespread nodular and small cavitary densities, most marked in the upper lobes.

Fig. 18-9. Chest radiograph with features typical of miliary tuberculosis. There are widespread uniformly distributed nodules of 2 to 3 mm, representing disseminated tuberculous lesions.

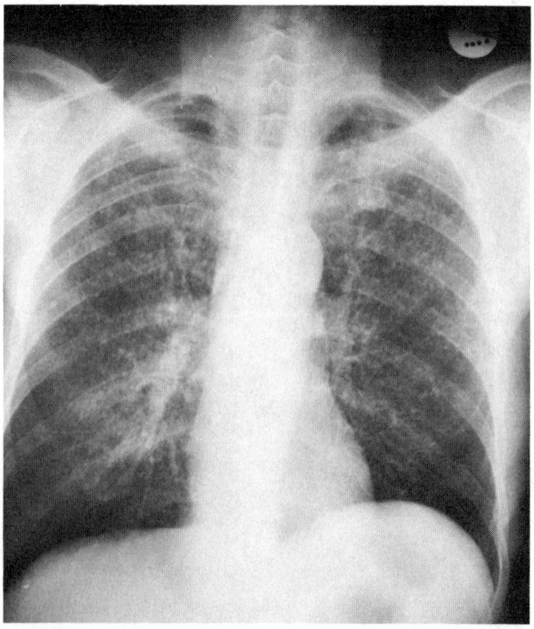

radiography alone. Even lesions that appear to be chronic and stable may harbor actively multiplying bacilli.

Once tuberculosis is suspected, skin testing is indicated. However, a negative skin test result does not rule out tuberculosis, and a positive skin test result only confirms infection. The size of the skin test response does not correlate with the probability of active disease, but rather with the likelihood that there was infection with *M. tuberculosis* rather than a cross-reaction [24]. Identification of tubercle bacilli in a clinical specimen is usually necessary to confirm disease. There are, however, circumstances where demonstration of the organism proves impossible. When tuberculosis is highly suspected, and there is subsequent radiologic and/or clinical improvement after initiation of treatment, a presumptive diagnosis may be appropriate [37]. The presence of granulomas, in particular those with caseation, in histologic specimens from patients suspected of having tuberculosis, especially when there is a history of exposure and/or a significant skin test reaction, may appropriately lead one to make a presumptive diagnosis.

The first step in identifying *M. tuberculosis* is to perform an acid-fast stain on appropriate clinical specimens. Final confirmation requires culturing the organism and differentiating it from other mycobacteria. The basis for the acid-fast stain has been described earlier. Acid-fast stains can be rapidly performed and can provide an estimate of the number of organisms being aerosolized and thus the infectiousness of the patient. However, they do not differentiate *M. tuberculosis* from other acid-fast organisms, and they are less sensitive than cultures. It has been estimated that at least 100 acid-fast bacilli per milliliter of sputum are required for detection by acid-fast stains. It takes 3 to 8 weeks to identify growth of *M. tuberculosis* using standard culture techniques. Newer techniques, such as the Bactec system (Johnston Laboratories, Inc., Cockeysville, MD) can detect growth of *M. tuberculosis* and differentiate it from other mycobacteria considerably more rapidly. However, this system cannot provide a colony count and cannot identify the species of NTM detected. Serologic tests based on enzyme-linked immunosorbent assays and radioimmunoassays have been developed [38, 39]. These tests are rapid and inexpensive, but problems of sensitivity and specificity exist. The exact role of these tests has not yet been defined.

Ideally, three to five consecutive early morning sputum samples should be obtained. Sputum production can be induced with a nebulized saline solution. The samples should be transported to the laboratory as soon as possible or refrigerated. They should not be pooled. Gastric aspiration can be performed, but is uncomfortable, must be done early in the morning, and must be processed within 4 hours, which excludes mailed-in specimens. Specimens obtained during and after bronchoscopy are useful in diagnosing tuberculosis when sputum cannot be obtained or when sputum culture results are negative. Three to five nonpooled first morning midstream urine samples in volumes of 50 to 100 mL are useful. Other appropriate specimens include pleural, pericardial, ascitic, joint, cerebral spinal, or abscess fluid. Pleural, pericardial, peritoneal, hepatic, lymph node, and pelvic organ tissue can be stained, cultured, and examined histologically, as can bone marrow aspirates.

Two main methods of performing acid-fast bacilli stains are employed. Bright-field microscopy, which includes the Ziehl-Neelsen and Kinyoun staining procedures, uses carbol-fuchsin, which stains mycobacteria red (Fig. 18-10; see color plate). The stained smears must be examined under a high-power oil objective, making this a more time-consuming procedure. Because this method requires little equipment or training, it can be performed by the clinician when it is thought this information is urgently needed. The Kinyoun method is described in Table 18-8. Fluorescent microscopy using auramine or auramine-rhodamine dyes is more sensitive and can be done more rapidly because

Table 18-8. Kinyoun (Cold Basic Fuchsin Acid-Fast Stain)

1. Spread drop of specimen over a 1 to 2 cm area on slide
2. Air dry
3. Place on slide warmer at 65° to 75°C for 15 minutes
4. Remove from warmer and flood slide with formalin for 15 minutes
5. Rinse with water
6. Flood with carbol fuchsin (Kinyoun formula) for 5 minutes
7. Rinse with water
8. Decolorize with acid-alcohol until no more color appears (about 2 minutes)
9. Rinse with water
10. Flood with methylene blue for 1 to 2 minutes
11. Rinse with water, drain, and air dry
12. Examine under oil immersion objective (1000 ×)

larger fields can be scanned using a 25 × objective. Organisms appear bright yellow (Fig. 18-11; see color plate). Disadvantages include the staining of nonviable organisms and a greater possibility of false-positive results. Acid-fast stains are reported as number of organisms per slide seen. The clinician must remember that a positive acid-fast bacilli stain does *not* establish the diagnosis of tuberculosis. Culture and identification of the organism must be performed. Cases of tuberculosis should be reported to the public health department.

Treatment

Once the diagnosis of tuberculosis has been suspected and appropriate specimens collected and submitted to the laboratory, treatment should be initiated. Again, it must be emphasized that sputum acid-fast bacilli stains may be negative and culture results may not be available for 3 to 8 weeks. Hospitalization for isolation purposes is not necessary. The decision to hospitalize a patient for diagnostic or therapeutic purposes should be based on the same factors as for any other disease. Antituberculosis drugs available in the United States, along with their available forms and recommended doses, are listed in Tables 18-9 and 18-10. Isoniazid, rifampin, streptomycin, and PZA are bactericidal drugs useful in initial treatment. Ethambutol is also a first-line drug, but is bacteriostatic and is most useful in preventing drug resistance and in cases where drug toxicity has occurred. The remaining drugs are less effective, more toxic, and should be reserved for treatment of multiple drug-resistant tuberculosis.

There are three main principles involved in the treatment of tuberculosis. The first is

Table 18-9. First-Line Antituberculosis Drugs

		Daily Dose		*Maximum Daily Dose*	*Twice Weekly Dose*	
Name	*Forms*	*Adult*	*Child*		*Adult*	*Child*
Isoniazid	Tablet:* 100 mg 300 mg Syrup: 50 mg/5 ml Vial: 1 g	5 mg/kg PO or IM	10–20 mg/kg PO or IM	300 mg	15 mg/kg, maximum 900 mg	20–40 mg/kg, maximum 900 mg
Rifampin	Capsule:* 150 mg 300 mg Syrup: 10 mg/mL	10 mg/kg PO	10–20 mg/kg PO	600 mg	Same as daily dose	Same as daily dose
Pyrazinamide	Tablet: 500 mg	15–30 mg/kg PO	15–30 mg/kg PO	2 g	50–70 mg/kg	50–70 mg/kg
Ethambutol	Tablet: 100 mg 400 mg	15–25 mg/kg PO	15–25 mg/kg PO	2.5 g	50 mg/kg	50 mg/kg
Streptomycin	Vial: 1 g 4 g	15† mg/kg IM	20–40 mg/kg IM	1 g‡	25–30 mg/kg IM	25–30 mg/kg IM

*A combination capsule is available containing 150 mg of isoniazid and 300 mg of rifampin.
†For persons over age 60 use 10 mg/kg.
‡For persons over age 60 the maximum dose should be 750 mg.
Abbreviations: PO, by mouth; IM, intramuscular.

Table 18-10. Second-Line Antituberculosis Drugs

Drug	*Form*	*Daily Dose in Children and Adults (mg/kg)*	*Maximum Dose in Children and Adults (g)*
Capreomycin	Vials: 1 g	15–30 IM	1
Kanamycin	Vials: 75 mg 500 mg 1 g	15–30 IM	1
Ethionamide	Tablets: 250 mg	15–20 PO	1
Para-aminosalicylic acid	Tablets: 500 mg 1 g	150 PO	12
Cycloserine	Capsules: 250 mg	15–20 PO	1

Abbreviations: IM, intramuscular; PO, by mouth.

that the numbers of tubercle bacilli in the body should be quickly reduced. Within several weeks of therapy the ability of most patients to infect others becomes negligible [40, 41]. Chemotherapy is the most effective method of preventing further spread of tuberculosis. Success is based on conversion of sputum cultures to negative. A therapeutic regimen is a failure if sputum has not converted within 5 to 6 months. This can be due to the selection of inappropriate drugs, noncompliance on the part of the patient, or drug resistance.

The second principle is that drug resistance must be prevented. It has been estimated that 1 out of every 10^6 tubercle bacilli will spontaneously mutate and develop resistance to one drug. Therefore, the more organisms there are, as in the case of cavitary tuberculosis, the higher the likelihood of resistance developing. If only that one drug is administered, these resistant organisms will multiply, while the sensitive ones are destroyed. Therefore, tuberculosis should always be treated with two or more drugs to which the organism is susceptible. Unfortunately, because it takes 3 to 8 weeks for culture results to become available, and several more weeks for drug susceptibility tests to be performed, treatment usually begins before susceptibility information is available. However, there are certain conditions under which resistance should be suspected: (1) a history of previous therapy for tuberculosis, (2) a history of exposure to a drug-resistant case, and (3) residence in, or origination from, a geographic area where resistance is common, such as southeast Asia, Central and South America, Africa, and selected regions of the United States. Resistance is most common to isoniazid and streptomycin and unusual to rifampin and ethambutol. In persons at high risk of having drug-resistant tuberculosis, the initial treatment regimen, where there has been prior therapy, should include two drugs that have not been previously employed, and in the cases where isoniazid resistance is suspected, two drugs in addition to isoniazid. In patients who fail to improve on therapy, at least two new drugs should be added. If the reason for failure to improve is resistance to one of the initial drugs, then the treatment has essentially been with only a single effective agent. The likelihood is then high that a spontaneous mutation has led to drug resistance to that single agent. If another single agent is then added, it too is the only effective drug and resistance to it can develop also. In order to prevent this disastrous situation where there may be no effective drug remaining it is important to remember: Never add a single agent to a failing regimen.

The third principle of treatment for tuberculosis is to prevent relapse by treating for a sufficient period of time. There is evidence that there are three populations of *M. tuberculosis*. The first is an actively growing extracellular one. It is from this population that resistant organisms are most likcly to emerge. Isoniazid, rifampin, and streptomycin are all very active against this group. The second consists of slow or intermittently growing intracellular organisms in an acid milieu. PZA is the most effective agent against this population.The third group is also slow or intermittently growing, but is extracellular and in the neutral pH environment of solid caseous areas. Rifampin is the most active drug against this population. The last two populations are the most persistent. Prolonged therapy is necessary to eradicate these persistent populations and prevent relapse. The exact duration of therapy necessary to prevent relapse depends on the drugs employed.

The following is a summary of treatment plans for non-HIV infected persons, based on the recommendations of the American Thoracic Society and the Centers for Disease Control [42]. In the absence of drug resistance and adverse reactions isoniazid should be used for the duration of therapy. Regimens of less than 6 months' duration should not be employed because of high rates of relapse. If isoniazid, rifampin, and PZA are given for 2 months, followed by isoniazid and rifampin for 4 months, to a compliant patient with fully susceptible organisms, then treatment can be completed after 6 months. Isoniazid and rifampin given for 9 months is equally effective, but sputum conversion occurs more slowly, and noncompliance rates are higher. In either of these regimens, medications can be given on a twice a week basis after an initial 2 months of daily therapy. Because it is feasible to directly supervise medications given twice a week, this is ideal for patients in whom compliance is a problem. If drug resistance is a possibility, ethambutol can be added initially to either of these regimens until drug susceptibility studies are available. If isoniazid cannot be used, or if there is documented isoniazid resistance, ethambutol and rifampin should be administered for 12 to 18 months. If rifampin cannot be used, isoniazid and ethambutol can be given for 12 to 18 months.

Treatment of extrapulmonary tuberculosis should be guided by the same principles as for pulmonary tuberculosis. Bone lesions, though usually treatable with chemotherapy alone, may require drainage and debridement [44]. In about one third of cases of lymph node tuberculosis, there is appearance of new lymph nodes, enlargement or persistence of existing ones, or fluctuation and sinus formation during or after otherwise successful antituberculous therapy [45]. These occurrences do not necessarily mandate a change or prolongation of therapy [46]. Treatment of pericardial disease may include drainage of fluid to prevent tamponade and pericardectomy to prevent or treat the late occurrence of constrictive pericarditis. Consideration should be given to the addition of a short course (several weeks) of corticosteroids for tuberculosis of the larynx, eye, central nervous system, mediastinal lymph nodes in children, pericardium, and peritoneum. They are sometimes useful in severely toxic patients with miliary tuberculosis. Tuberculosis can be associated with Addison's disease due to cortical destruction of the adrenal gland. Replacement doses of corticosteroids should be administered to patients with compatible signs and symptoms, after appropriate evaluation for adrenal insufficiency.

Because patient compliance largely influences the success of a treatment program [47], it is recommended that patients be seen at least monthly to monitor for signs of clinical improvement, proper drug usage, adverse drug effects, and to provide education and encouragement to complete a course of therapy. Sputum should be examined by acid-fast stain and cultured on a monthly basis until conversion and again at the completion of therapy. If a full treatment program has been adhered to, long-term follow-up after completion is not necessary [48, 49].

All drugs have the potential of causing adverse reactions, and physicians prescribing antituberculous medications must be familiar with their side effects, monitor patients for their development, and recognize and treat appropriately their occurrence.

Isoniazid

Isoniazid is rarely associated with peripheral neuropathy, probably as a result of its ability to increase urinary excretion of pyridoxine (vitamin B_6). Vitamin B_6 supplementation of approximately 50 mg/d is recommended for people at risk for neuropathy, such as those with diabetes, uremia, and alcoholism. In addition, supplementation is recommended for pregnant women, people with seizure disorders, and those with malnutrition. Central nervous system stimulation and depression and mood behavior changes have been reported. When isoniazid is taken with either phenytoin or carbamazepine the serum levels of both the isoniazid and the second medication increase.

The most common and well-publicized adverse reaction to isoniazid is hepatitis. About 10% to 20% of the people taking isoniazid have asymptomatic elevation in their serum liver function test levels. Overt hepatitis is much less common and was not even recognized in the US Public Health Service trials on isoniazid prophylaxis conducted between 1955 and 1968. However, because of reports linking isoniazid to hepatitis, and the development of 19 cases of clinical liver disease among 2321 employees on Capitol Hill taking isoniazid prophylaxis, a prospective study was initiated to monitor the incidence of liver disease among persons receiving isoniazid preventive therapy. A total of 13,838 persons in 21 cities were enrolled from 1971 to 1972. There appeared to be a relationship between age and the development of probable isoniazid-induced hepatitis, with no cases in persons under 20 years old, 3 cases per 1000 in those 20 to 34, 12 cases per 1000 in those 35 to 49, 23 cases per 1000 for those 50 to 64, and 8 cases per 1000 for those over 64. Most, but not all, cases occurred within the first 3 months of treatment [50]. Daily alcohol consumption appeared to increase the risk for hepatitis. It is now recommended that patients have baseline liver function tests performed before beginning isoniazid therapy. They should be instructed on what signs or symptoms of hepatitis to watch for and to report their occurrence at once. Repeat liver function tests should be performed when signs or symptoms of hepatitis occur. Routine monitoring of liver function tests should be reserved for older patients in whom the risk of isoniazid hepatitis is greater. Consideration for discontinuation of isoniazid should be made if the serum aminotransferase level exceeds three to five times the upper limit of normal. It should be discontinued if there is clinical evidence of liver disease and abnormal liver function results. Patients must be educated about the symptoms of hepatitis and given instructions to discontinue medications and seek medical advice when they occur.

Isoniazid has also been associated with hypersensitivity reactions leading to fever, rash, and a lupus-like syndrome and with a variety of hematologic abnormalities [51].

Rifampin

Rifampin colors secretions and urine orange and patients should be warned of this effect. One of the most significant effects of rifampin is to decrease the effectiveness of a large number of drugs: corticosteroids, digitoxin, cyclosporine, quinidine, propranolol, metoprolol, clofibrate, sulfonylureas, warfarin, and methadone. Women using birth control pills should be advised to use another form of birth control as rifampin may cause their pills to lose effectiveness. An important drug–drug interaction is that caused by isoniazid, rifampin, and ketoconazole. When taken together, as may frequently be recommended in patients with AIDS, they each lose effectiveness [52, 53].

Other reactions to rifampin include gastrointestinal upset, hepatitis, skin rashes, thrombocytopenia, pure red cell aplasia, and hemolytic anemia. Acute renal failure can occur in association with rifampin therapy, especially when the drug is used in high doses intermittently or when therapy is interrupted and then reinstituted.

Pyrazinamide

Although PZA can cause hepatotoxicity, it does so rarely in currently recommended doses and does not lead to an increase in adverse effects when used for the first 2 months of an isoniazid and rifampin containing regimen [43, 54]. High serum levels of uric acid can occur, but are usually asymptomatic and do not require therapy. Arthralgias and fever are rare side effects.

Streptomycin

Streptomycin must be given intramuscularly. About 2% to 3% of isolates of *M. tuberculosis* are resistant. The major toxic effect is ototoxicity, with vestibular manifestations being more common than hearing loss. These effects are related to dosage and duration of therapy and occur more frequently in elderly patients. In general, total dose should not exceed 120 g. Early signs of ototoxicity may be elicited by having patients turn 180 degrees while walking and observing for loss of balance. Nephrotoxicity is less of a problem than with other aminoglycosides. Hypersensitivity reactions and rash may occur.

Ethambutol

Unlike the first four drugs discussed, ethambutol is bacteriostatic rather than bactericidal. If either ethambutol or streptomycin is substituted for PZA in the initial phase, the effectiveness of the regimen is decreased [42]. The major toxicity, which is dose related, is optic neuritis. At doses of 15 mg/kg/d the incidence is less than 1%. The earliest symptom is loss of the ability to perceive the color green. Central scotomas and decreased visual acuity occur later. The dose of ethambutol must be reduced in the presence of renal insufficiency.

Second-Line Drugs

Kanamycin and capreomycin must be administered parenterally and may cause ototoxicity and nephrotoxicity. Para-aminosalicylic acid causes gastrointestinal upset, hypersensitivity reactions, hepatoxicity, and sodium overload. Ethionamide causes gastrointestinal upset, hepatotoxicity, and hypersensitivity reactions. Cycloserine frequently causes behavioral changes and can result in psychosis, convulsions, and rash.

Prevention of Tuberculosis

Tuberculosis is not only treatable, but preventable. There are two methods of prevention: vaccination and isoniazid preventive therapy. Bacille Calmette-Guérin (BCG) is a vaccine derived from an attenuated strain of *M. bovis*. Vaccination with BCG does not protect the individual from infection with *M. tuberculosis* and is useful only in those not previously infected. It enhances the host's immune response, thus protecting him or her from complications of the primary infection. Unfortunately, efficacy in clinical trials has ranged from 0% to 80% [42]. This may be due to differences in the potency of the various BCGs employed and to differences in the populations studied. In the United States, where most cases of tuberculosis derive from persons already infected, BCG has little role. Vaccination with BCG may sensitize an individual to tuberculin, making subsequent interpretation of skin tests difficult.

Many clinical trials have demonstrated the efficacy of isoniazid, taken daily for 12 months, in preventing tuberculosis among those already infected. When taken as directed for most of the year the effectiveness is close to 90%. Although maximal protection is achieved with 12 months of isoniazid chemoprophylaxis, substantial benefit is also gained with 6 months of therapy [55].

Isoniazid is not recommended as prophylactic therapy in all persons infected with *M. tuberculosis*. The benefit of the drug, both to the patient and society, must be weighed against the cost of administering it and the

Table 18-11. Groups at High Risk for Developing Tuberculosis and Indications for Isoniazid Preventive Therapy

1. Persons infected with HIV, or highly suspected of being infected with HIV and whose PPD reaction is 5 mm or more should receive 12 months of isoniazid
2. Close contacts of an infectious TB case whose PPD is 5 mm or more should receive isoniazid for 6–12 months. For children and adolescents, if PPD is less than 5 mm, isoniazid preventive treatment should be begun and the skin test repeated in 3 months. If it remains less than 5 mm isoniazid can be discontinued
3. Newly infected people. These are individuals whose skin test has converted to positive within the past 2 years. Isoniazid for 6–12 months should be considered for people under age 35 with a skin test reaction increase of 10 mm or more and for people over age 35 with an increase of 15 mm or more. The booster phenomenon must be taken into consideration when interpreting skin test conversions
4. People with a PPD reaction of 5 mm or more and a chest radiograph compatible with healed parenchymal tuberculosis should receive isoniazid for 12 months
5. People with a positive PPD of 10 mm or more and medical conditions that increase the risk for developing tuberculosis should receive 6–12 months of isoniazid:
   - silicosis
   - gastrectomy
   - jejunoileal bypass
   - weight 10% below ideal body weight
   - chronic renal failure
   - diabetes mellitus
   - immunosuppressive therapy including prolonged high-dose corticosteroid use
   - hematologic disorders such as leukemia, lymphomas
   - malignancies
   - intravenous drug users known to be seronegative for HIV
6. Persons under age 35 with a PPD reaction of 10 mm or more, and none of first five risk factors, but from one of the following high incidence groups, should be treated for 6–12 months with isoniazid:
   - People from foreign countries with a high prevalence of tuberculosis
   - High-risk ethnic groups such as Blacks, Hispanics, Asian/Pacific Islanders, and Native Americans
   - Medically underserved, low-income populations
   - Residents of long-term care facilities such as prisons, nursing homes, and psychiatric institutions
7. People under age 35, with no risk factors and from low-incidence groups, with a PPD reaction of 15 mm or more should be considered for 6–12 months of isoniazid therapy. However, the relative prevalence of *M. tuberculosis* infection versus cross-reactivity in the population being tested can be taken into account when determining at what size reaction to recommend isoniazid chemoprophylaxis

risk of side effects, namely hepatitis. Isoniazid chemoprophylaxis is recommended in those individuals in whom the risk of developing tuberculosis is high and outweighs the risk of developing hepatitis. Table 18-11 lists the groups at high risk of developing tuberculosis and defines the indications for isoniazid preventive therapy [16, 23, 27]. It should be recognized, however, that there is substantial controversy surrounding the recommendation to treat the young tuberculin reactor (at least as defined by a reaction size of 10 mm induration) with no other risk factor for developing tuberculosis) [56–58]. Contraindications to isoniazid preventive therapy include prior adequate therapy for tuberculosis, a major adverse reaction to the drug, and the presence of active, progressive tuberculosis. Patients should be educated regarding possible adverse reactions to isoniazid, and should be monitored monthly.

Recommendations for the prevention and control of tuberculosis have been published for the following specific settings: foreign-born persons entering the United States [59], long-term care facilities for the elderly [28], and health care facilities [60].

Human Immunodeficiency Virus Infection and Tuberculosis

The person with concomitant HIV and *M. tuberculosis* infections presents a special challenge to tuberculosis control programs. HIV infection is an important risk factor for the development of tuberculosis, and tuberculosis is unique as an opportunistic infection in the HIV-infected person because it is not only preventable and treatable, but also transmissible. Tuberculosis often precedes other opportunistic infections and the development of other signs of AIDS. Extrapulmonary tuberculosis in conjunction with a positive antibody to HIV fulfills the national surveillance case definition of AIDS. Blood cultures performed with the lysis-centrifugation system are positive for *M. tuberculosis* in 26% to 42% of patients with tuberculosis and HIV infection [61]. Because most cases of tuberculosis in HIV-infected persons arise from those previously infected with *M. tuberculosis* [14, 62], it is very important to identify via tuberculin skin tests and offer prophylactic therapy to those individuals with concomitant infections. However, because newly acquired tuberculosis infection in HIV-infected individuals can progress rapidly to active disease, it is also essential that HIV-infected persons exposed to an infectious case of tuberculosis be identified and also offered preventive therapy [63]. In addition, patients diagnosed as having tuberculosis should be offered HIV testing and counseling. Response to antituberculosis therapy in patients with HIV infection and tuberculosis appears to be good. However, current recommendations are to prolong therapy several months [61, 62]. Isoniazid, rifampin, and PZA are recommended for the first 2 months of treatment, with isoniazid and rifampin continued for 7 additional months, or for 6 months after culture results are negative, whichever is longer. In cases where isoniazid resistance is suspected, ethambutol can be added until susceptibility tests are available. If isoniazid cannot be used, or there is isoniazid resistance, rifampin and ethambutol can be administered for 18 months, or 12 months beyond the time that culture results are negative, whichever is longer. Finally, if rifampin cannot be used, the duration of therapy should be 18 to 24 months or 12 months beyond culture conversion.

It is yet to be seen whether or not the stepped-up efforts recommended by the Advisory Committee for the Elimination of Tuberculosis to eradicate tuberculosis by the year 2010 will succeed. Trends between 1985 and 1990 suggest otherwise. Poverty, homelessness, lack of access to medical care, insufficient resources, and the AIDS epidemic all are thwarting once again efforts to eliminate this curable and preventable ancient disease. Tuberculosis remains a serious problem for some population groups in the United States and for large numbers of people throughout the world. Physicians must be alert to the disease and remain knowledgeable about diagnosing, treating, and preventing it.

References

1. Dubos R, Dubos J: The white plague: Tuberculosis, man and society, ed 1. Boston, Little, Brown and Company, 1952, p 214
2. D'Esopo ND: Clinical trials in pulmonary tuberculosis. *Am Rev Respir Dis* 125:85–93, 1982
3. British Medical Research Council: Long-term chemotherapy in the treatment of chronic pulmonary tuberculosis with cavitation. A report to the Medical Research Council by the Tuberculosis Chemotherapy Trials Committee. *Tubercle* 43:201–267, 1962
4. Tuberculosis Chemotherapy Centre, Madras: Intermittent treatment of pulmonary tuberculosis. A concurrent comparison of twice-weekly isoniazid plus streptomycin and daily isoniazid plus p-aminosalicylic acid in domiciliary treatment. *Lancet* 1:1078–1080, 1963
5. Tuberculosis Chemotherapy Centre, Madras: A concurrent comparison of home and sanitorium treatment of pulmonary tuberculosis in South India. *Bull WHO* 21:51–144, 1959
6. Kamat SR, Dawson JJY, Devadatta S, et al: A controlled study of the influence of segregation of tuberculous patients for one year on the attack rate of tuberculosis in a 5 year period in close family contacts in South India. *Indian Journal of Tuberculosis* 4:11–23, 1966
7. Riley RL, Moodie AS: Infectivity of patients with pulmonary tuberculosis in inner city homes. *Am Rev Respir Dis* 110:810–812, 1974
8. Lowell AM: Tuberculosis morbidity and mortality and its control. *In* American Public Health Association Vital and Health Statistics Monographs. Tuberculosis. Cambridge MA, Harvard University Press, 1969, p 32
9. Tucker WB: Highlights of the conference. *In* The Arden House conference on tuberculosis: Sponsored by the National Tuberculosis Association and the US Public Health Service,

Tuberculosis Program, 1959, DHEW Publication no. (PHS) 784
10. Byrd RB, Horn BR, Solomon DA, et al: Treatment of tuberculosis by the nonpulmonary physician. *Ann Intern Med* 86:799–802, 1977
11. MacGregor RR: A year's experience with tuberculosis in a private urban teaching hospital in the postsanitorium era. *Am J Med* 58:221–228, 1975
12. Addington WW: Patient compliance: The most serious remaining problem in the control of tuberculosis in the United States. *Chest* 76(suppl):741–743, 1979
13. Jareb JA, Kelly GD, Dooley Jr SW, et al: Tuberculosis morbidity in the United States: final data, 1990. *In:* CDC Surveillance Summaries, December 1991. *MMWR* 40(No. SS-3): 23–27, 1991
14. Selwyn PA, Hartel D, Lewis VA, et al: A prospective study of the risk of tuberculosis among intravenous drug users with human immunodeficiency virus infection. *N Engl J Med* 320:545–550, 1989
15. Centers for Disease Control: Summary of notifiable diseases, United States, 1990. *MMWR* 39(No. 53):1–61, 1991
16. Centers for Disease Control: Screening for tuberculosis and tuberculous infection in high-risk populations: Recommendations of the Advisory Committee for Elimination of Tuberculosis. *MMWR* 39(No. RR 8):1–7, 1990
17. American Thoracic Society Committee on Priorities for Tuberculosis Research: ATS Conference on Tuberculosis Research: Future research in tuberculosis: Research initiatives in the immunology of tuberculosis. *Am Rev Respir Dis* 138:1327–1329, 1988
18. Centers for Disease Control: A strategic plan for the elimination of tuberculosis in the United States. *MMWR* 38(suppl 3):1–25, 1989
19. Dubos R, Dubos J: The white plague: Tuberculosis, Man and Society, ed 1. Boston, Little, Brown and Company, 1952, p 219
20. American Thoracic Society: Diagnosis and treatment of disease caused by nontuberculous mycobacteria. *Am Rev Respir Dis* 142: 940–953, 1990
21. Centers for Disease Control: Tuberculosis in the United States—1979. HHS Publication no. (CDC) 82-8322. Atlanta, GA, Center for Prevention Services, Tuberculosis Control Division, 1981
22. Nardell E, McInnis B, Thomas B, et al: Exogenous reinfection with tuberculosis in a shelter for the homeless. *N Engl J Med* 315:1570–1575, 1986
23. Centers for Disease Control: The use of preventive therapy for tuberculosis infection in the United States: Recommendations of the Advisory Committee for Elimination of Tuberculosis. *MMWR* 39(No. RR 8):9–12, 1990
24. Reichman LB: Tuberculin skin testing: The state of the art. *Chest* 76(suppl):764–770, 1979
25. Snider DE: The tuberculin skin test. *Am Rev Respir Dis* 125:108–118, 1982
26. American Thoracic Society: The tuberculin skin test. *Am Rev Respir Dis* 124:356–363, 1981
27. American Thoracic Society: Diagnostic standards and classification of tuberculosis. *Am Rev Respir Dis* 142:725–735, 1990
28. Centers for Disease Control: Prevention and control of tuberculosis in facilities providing long-term care to the elderly: Recommendations of the Advisory Committee for Elimination of Tuberculosis. *MMWR* 39(No. RR 10):7–20, 1990
29. Stead WW, To T: The significance of the tuberculin skin test in elderly persons. *Ann Intern Med* 107:837–842, 1987
30. Gordin FM, Perez-Stable EJ, Flaherty D, et al: Evaluation of a third sequential tuberculin skin test in a chronic care population. *Am Rev Respir Dis* 137:153–157, 1988
31. Burstin SJ, Muspratt JA, Rossing TH: The tuberculin test: Studies of the dynamics of reactivity to tuberculin and *Candida* antigen in institutionalized patients. *Am Rev Respir Dis* 134:1072–1074, 1986
32. Slutkin G, Perez-Stable EJ, Hopewell PC: Time course and boosting of tuberculin reactions in nursing home residents. *Am Rev Respir Dis* 134:1048–1051, 1986
33. Rieder HL, Snider DE, Cauthen GM: Extrapulmonary tuberculosis in the United States. *Am Rev Respir Dis* 141:347–351, 1990
34. Rieder HL, Couthen GM, Bloch AB, et al: Tuberculosis and acquired immunodeficiency syndrome—Florida. *Arch Intern Med* 149: 1268–1273, 1989.
35. Chaisson RE, Schecter GF, Theuer CP, et al: Tuberculosis in patients with the acquired immunodeficiency syndrome: Clinical features, response to therapy and survival. *Am Rev Respir Dis* 136:570–574, 1987
36. Kissner DG: Tuberculosis: Missed opportunities. *Arch Intern Med* 147:2037–2040, 1987
37. Gordin FM, Slutkin G, Schecter G, et al: Presumptive diagnosis and treatment of pulmonary tuberculosis based on radiographic findings. *Am Rev Respir Dis* 139:1090–1093, 1989
38. Good AC: Serologic methods for diagnosing tuberculosis. *Ann Intern Med* 110:97–98, 1989
39. Daniel TM, Debane SM: The serodiagnosis of tuberculosis and other mycobacterial diseases by enzyme-linked immunosorbent assay. *Am Rev Respir Dis* 135:1137–1151, 1987
40. Brooks SM, Lassiter NL, Younger EC: A pilot study concerning the infection risk of sputum positive tuberculosis patients on chemotherapy. *Am Rev Respir Dis* 108:799–804, 1973

41. Gunnels JJ, Bates JH, Swindoll H: Infectivity of sputum positive tuberculosis patients on chemotherapy. *Am Rev Respir Dis* 109:323–330, 1974
42. American Thoracic Society: Treatment of tuberculosis and tuberculosis infection in adults and children. *Am Rev Respir Dis* 134:355–363, 1986
43. Combs DL, O'Brien RJ, Geiter LJ: USPHS tuberculosis short-course chemotherapy trial 21: effectiveness, toxicity, and acceptability. *Ann Intern Med* 112:397–406, 1990
44. Dutt AK, Moers D, Stead WE: Short-course chemotherapy for extrapulmonary tuberculosis. *Ann Intern Med* 104:7–12, 1986
45. Campbell IA, Dyson AJ: Lymph node tuberculosis: A comparison of treatments 18 months after completion of chemotherapy. *Tubercle* 60:95–99, 1979
46. British Thoracic Society Research Committee: Short course chemotherapy for tuberculosis of lymph nodes: A controlled trial. *Br Med J* 290:1106–1109, 1985
47. Addington WW: Patient compliance: The most serious remaining problem in the control of tuberculosis in the United States. *Chest* 6(suppl):741–743, 1979
48. Edsall J, Collins G: Routine follow-up of inactive tuberculosis, a practice to be abandoned. *Am Rev Respir Dis* 107:851–853, 1973
49. Ad Hoc Committee on the Discharge of Patients from Medical Surveillance: Discharge of tuberculosis patients from medical surveillance. *Am Rev Respir Dis* 113:709–710, 1976
50. Kopanoff DE, Snider DE, Caras GJ: Isoniazid-related hepatitis: A U.S. Public Health Service Cooperative Surveillance Study. *Am Rev Respir Dis* 117:991–1001, 1978
51. Goldman AL, Braman SS: Isoniazid: A review with emphasis on adverse effects. *Chest* 62: 71–77, 1972
52. Engelhard D, Stutman HR, Marks MI: Interaction of ketaconazole with rifampin and isoniazid. *N Engl J Med* 311:1681–1682, 1984
53. Abadie-Kemmerly S, Pankey GA, Dalvisio JR: Failure of ketoconazole treatment of *Blastomyces dermatidis* due to interaction of isoniazid and rifampin. *Ann Intern Med* 109:844–845, 1988
54. Snider DE, Graczyk GE, Rogowski J: Supervised six-months treatment of newly diagnosed pulmonary tuberculosis using isoniazid, rifampin, and pyrazinamide with and without streptomycin. *Am Rev Respir Dis* 130:1091–1094, 1984
55. International Union Against Tuberculosis Committee on Prophylaxis: Efficacy of various durations of isoniazid preventive therapy for tuberculosis: Five years of follow-up in the IUAT Trial. *Bull WHO* 60:555–564, 1982
56. Taylor WC, Aronson MD, Delbanco TL: Should young adults with a positive tuberculin test take isoniazid? *Ann Intern Med* 94:808–813, 1981
57. Tsevat J, Taylor WC, Wong JB, et al: Isoniazid for the tuberculin reactor: Take it or leave it. *Am Rev Respir Dis* 137:215–220, 1988
58. Snider DE: Decision analysis for isoniazid preventive therapy: Take it or leave it? *Am Rev Respir Dis* 137:2–4, 1988
59. Centers for Disease Control: Tuberculosis among foreign-born persons entering the United States: Recommendations of the Advisory Committee for Elimination of Tuberculosis. *MMWR* 39(No. RR 18):1–21, 1990
60. Centers for Disease Control: Guidelines for preventing the transmission of tuberculosis in health-care settings, with special focus on HIV-related issues. *MMWR* 39(No. RR 17): 1–29, 1990
61. Barnes, PF, Bloch AB, Davidson PT, Snider DE: Tuberculosis in patients with human immunodeficiency virus infection. *N Engl J Med* 324:1644–1650, 1991
62. Centers for Disease Control: Tuberculosis and human immunodeficiency virus infection: Recommendations of the Advisory Committee for the Elimination of Tuberculosis (ACET). *MMWR* 38:236–250, 1989
63. Daley CL, Small PM, Schecter GF, et al: An outbreak of tuberculosis with accelerated progression among persons infected with the human immunodeficiency virus: An analysis using restriction-fragment-length polymorphisms. *N Engl J Med* 326:231–235, 1992

Blunt Chest Trauma

Thomas Siegel

Civilian injuries resulting in blunt chest trauma may be caused by falls, industrial accidents, acts of violence, and traffic accidents. More than 200,000 deaths are attributed to motor vehicle accidents per year, with 50,000 of these occurring in the United States alone. The severity of this trauma results in a mortality of 20 deaths per 100,000 population in this country, with 25% of these deaths due to thoracic injuries [7] (Table 19-1). In an additional 25% to 50% of deaths, thoracic trauma causes a significant comorbidity [7].

Morbidity or disability from thoracic trauma is more difficult to quantify. In 1985 there were 31,000 injuries per 100,000 people. Of these, the National Safety Council estimates as many as 6,200 disabilities per 100,000 may arise from chest trauma. Taking into account that "Collateral damage," arising from extremity and head and neck injuries account for most disabilities this figure may be high. However there can be no doubt that chest trauma accounts for significant disability, with inherent economic impact on the patient and on society.

This chapter discusses the types of thoracic injuries most often encountered by the primary care physician. These include injury to the bony thorax such as sternal fractures, uncomplicated rib fractures, and minor pulmonary and cardiac contusions.

Historic Perspective

Despite the constraints of a nascent discipline, and limited to reliance on experience alone, early physicians displayed a remarkable understanding of nonpenetrating chest trauma and developed diagnostic, prognostic, and treatment regimens for their patients. Hippocrates described the association of pleurisy and empyema with chest wall contusion and established the association of rib fracture and hemoptysis. His management included firm dressing of the chest with linen, which was to be changed every other day. Further, if hemoptysis was present, the course of treatment was to continue for 40 days, otherwise the dressing could be removed at 20 days. This remained the standard of care for centuries [6].

The physiology, diagnosis, and treatment of blunt chest trauma were slow to evolve. The advent of the high vacuum hot cathode x-ray tube by Coolidge made it possible to standardize penetration power and intensity of the roentgenogram. Examination of the bony thorax and lung parenchyma first became feasible during the second decade of this century. Great strides were made following this, with the contributions of Evarts Graham and Richard Bell of the Empyema Commission of World War I. Closed chest tube thoracostomy drainage followed. Quantum advances followed the discovery and availability of antibiotics, positive pressure ventilation, blood volume management, advanced diagnostic imaging, application of blood gas studies, close hemodynamic monitoring, and the advent of the intensive care environment.

Mechanisms of Thoracic Injury

Blunt chest trauma is caused by two mechanisms. The first and most common is the acceleration/deceleration injury most often seen in motor vehicle accidents. Injury results from the inertial lag in movement of thoracic visceral contents when compared with that of the thoracic bony skeleton at the time of im-

Table 19-1. Frequency of Various Injuries in Motor Vehicle Accidents

Location	%
Extremities	34
Head and neck	32
Chest	25
Abdomen	15

Adapted from LoCicero III J, Mattox KL: Epidemiology of Chest Trauma. *Surgical Clin NA* 69:1, 15–19, Feb 1989

pact. The second mechanism of injury is a result of compression of the thorax. In this situation the intrinsic strength of the bony skeleton to maintain its structural integrity is overcome by external force. This occurs in a fall or crush injury.

Inventory of Thoracic Injury

A review of 1500 patients with thoracic injuries was catalogued by Beeson and Saegesser [8] and culled from their experience from Lausanne, Switzerland between 1962 and 1972, showed that 71% of injuries were to the chest wall; 34% of these were classified as major and 24% as minor. Thirteen percent had flail chest, which is an unstable bony thoracic cage injury accompanied by paradoxical motion whereby the chest wall atypically caves inward instead of expanding outward on inspiration. Of interest is that 12% of their patients had thoracic visceral injury without evidence of skeletal injury. Those to the heart, esophagus, and diaphragm accounted for 7% each, and the aorta and great vessels sustained injury 4% of the time.

Table 19-2. Percentage of Specific Types of Thoracic Organ Injury in 1500 Patients from Switzerland

Type of Location	%
Chest wall	54
Flail chest	13
Pneumothorax	20
Hemothorax	21
Pulmonary	21
Miscellaneous	18

From LoCicero III J, Mattox KL: Epidemiology of Chest Trauma. *Surg Clin NA*, 69:1, 15–19, Feb 1989

Injury to the Bony Thorax

Sternal Fractures

Fracture of the sternum results most frequently from direct injury to the anterior chest. Although crush injury and forced hyperflexion have been reported to cause sternal fracture, the force of deceleration in motor vehicle accidents and steering wheel impact is the most common cause. Sternal fractures are more commonly seen in elderly patients and are uncommon in children and young adults, owing to elasticity of the costal cartilage and ribs. Midbody sternal fractures are most common, followed by the manubrium, the lower body, and the upper body (Table 19-3). Fractures of the xiphoid process rarely occur.

In a 5-year retrospective study, Wojcik and Morgan [5] reported a 53% incidence of associated injury (Table 19-4), reflecting the severity of force necessary to fracture the sternum.

Diagnosis of sternal fracture may be suspected by the characteristic posture of the alert patient. To reduce pain the patient splints the sternum by leaning forward, with shoulders rotated internally and the head bent forward by flexion of the neck. Inspection may reveal deformity, and gentle sternal compression may elicit fracture crepitance. However, undisplaced fracture is confirmed

Table 19-3. Localization of Sternal Fractures

Location	%
Midbody	74
Manubrium	12
Lower body	8
Upper body	6

From Wojcik JB, Morgan AS: Sternal Fractures—The Natural History, *Annals of Emergency Medicine*, 17(9): 912–914, 1988

Table 19-4. Injuries Associated with Sternal Fractures in Motor Vehicle Accidents

Injury	%
Rib fractures	38
Long bone fractures	25
Head injury	18
Myocardial contusion	15
Pneumothorax	8
Intra-abdominal injury	8
Maxillofacial fractures	5
Spinal cord injuries	5

From Wojcik JB, Morgan AS: Sternal Fractures—The Natural History, *Annals of Emergency Medicine,* 17(9): 912–914, 1988

on only a lateral or oblique chest roentgenogram. Because of the prevalence of associated injury, all patients should be thoroughly investigated for cardiac, pulmonary, and major vascular injury (Table 19-4).

Isolated undisplaced sternal fractures can usually be managed conservatively with analgesics. Occasionally, infiltration of the fracture site with a local anesthetic having a long half-life, such as bupivacaine (Marcaine), may be of help. In displaced sternal fractures the manubrium is not usually involved and owing to its fixation proximally, there may be anterior displacement and overriding of the distal fragment. Most often the posterior periosteum remains intact. Severely displaced fractures and those patients in whom pain cannot be relieved by conservative measures may require open reduction and internal fixation.

Sternal fracture has been reported to result from seat belt injury. A 5-year retrospective study by Trinca and Dooley [9] from Australia, where seat belt use is mandatory, showed an increase in minor thoracic trauma, but a decline in more life-threatening injuries. Other studies support this observation [10, 11].

Simple Rib Fractures

By definition simple rib fractures are those fractures that are not associated with other significant injuries such as pneumothorax, hemothorax, pulmonary contusion, and cardiac contusion. Because of the resiliency and elasticity of their cartilage, children rarely suffer rib fractures. Adults frequently fracture ribs as a result of sports injuries, road traffic accidents, and falls. Men predominate in a ratio of 2.7 : 1. Older adults may develop rib fractures from the forceful muscular contraction that may accompany paroxysms of coughing or from straining, particularly with osteoporosis. The male-to-female ratio in the elderly population is reported to be 1.2 : 1. Significantly, those patients over 65 years of age have a higher morbidity and mortality from blunt chest trauma than their younger counterparts [2, 12].

Rib fractures usually occur either at the site of impact or at the posterior angle, where the rib is weakest structurally. The ribs most frequently broken are the fifth through ninth. Lower rib fractures are often accompanied by liver or spleen injury. Interestingly, liver trauma is more frequent as a result of traffic accidents in Britain, and splenic injury is more common in the United States, owing to driving convention. The direction and the force of the impact, as well as the number of ribs fractured and their displacement, account for the magnitude of underlying injuries. Direct injury is likely to cause more damage by forcing rib fragments into the pleural space, resulting in pulmonary parenchymal trauma, as well as intercostal vessel injury, pneumothorax, and hemothorax. However, force applied in an anteroposterior projection and over a wide area causes the ribs to buckle outward, breaking at midshaft and sparing the parenchyma [3].

Diagnosis in the alert and oriented patient is usually straightforward. Typically the patient describes a pleuritic-like pain with inspiration that is localized to the site of fracture. Splinting on the affected side is common. Physical examination may disclose deformity on inspection. Gentle palpation may reveal a stepoff at the site of an overriding fracture fragment in a displaced fracture and will elicit point tenderness. Chest compression laterally or anteroposteriorly away from the fracture site will cause pain and may disclose crepitation, or grinding sensation, at the fracture site. Roentgenologic evaluation may be unsatisfactory, particularly in undisplaced fractures. Trunkey [13] reports 30% to 50% false-negative results. Callus formation on radiography 3 to 6 weeks later may disclose previously missed fractures. It is prudent to reevaluate patients with even the most uncomplicated fractured ribs 48 to 72 hours after injury to prevent late pulmonary complications.

Fractured ribs may be insidious and certainly have the potential to lead to serious complications. Splinting and suppression of cough may lead to retained secretions, atelectasis, carbon dioxide retention, hypoxia, increased work of breathing, and pneumonia. In the pediatric and geriatric patient in whom reserve may not be optimal, abscess, empyema, and even death can result.

The treatment should focus on aggressive pulmonary toilet. To achieve this adequate analgesia is the hallmark of supportive care. If oral or parenteral systemic medication fails to provide the necessary relief, the nerves supplying the fractured ribs as well as the nerves two levels above and two levels below should be blocked by injection of an anesthetic agent. As the intercostal nerves arise posteriorly, it is best to block the nerve posterior to the fracture site. The neurovascular bundle lies inferior to the rib margin; therefore, the site of injection should take this into account. A local anesthetic with a long half-life, such as bupivacaine 5%, is most advantageous. It may be necessary to repeat the blocks at intervals of 12 to 24 hours once or twice. In hospitalized patients continuous epidural fentanyl analgesia has been shown to be effective in improving ventilatory function and reducing pain [1]. External splinting with binders, adhesive taping, or rib belts is not advised. Because these measures limit pulmonary excursion they may contribute to progressive atelectasis and impede clearing of secretions. It is particularly unwise in patients with limited pulmonary reserve, in the elderly, or those with significant lung disease such as chronic obstructive pulmonary disease.

Traumatic Hernia and Rupture

Traumatic rupture of the diaphragm usually results from blunt trauma to the lower thorax or upper abdomen. The usual cause is a fall or automobile accident. Penetrating trauma is more common than blunt injury, although the latter results in a larger hernia [14]. Over 90% of the ruptures are left sided and involve the posterior and central portions of the diaphragm. Gunshot wounds damage both hemidiaphragms equally, but stab wounds tend to lacerate the left hemidiaphragm more than the right [15]. Symptoms of acute rupture may be nonspecific and include dyspnea, cyanosis, and shoulder pain [16]. Delayed herniation may occur years later through small defects and result in symptoms of incarceration and strangulation. The stomach is the most likely organ to herniate. The chest radiographic findings may include an abnormal diaphragmatic contour or abnormal air–fluid level in the lower thorax [17]. These lesions do not heal spontaneously and usually require prompt surgical repair.

Pulmonary Contusion

A pulmonary contusion is an injury to lung parenchyma, resulting in hemorrhage and edema. The mechanism of injury appears to be rapid deceleration analogous to blast injury, with a high pressure wave restricted by the closed confines of the thoracic cage. The energy of the high pressure wave is transmitted to the lung parenchyma. Two early physical signs of lung contusion may be found in patients with parenchymal injury following rib fracture. The first is hemoptysis, which is indicative of alveolar or bronchial injury. Even if the quantity is small, hemoptysis is a clear sign of pulmonary contusion or laceration. The second important early physical sign of pulmonary parenchymal injury is that of crepitus arising because of subcutaneous emphysema. Gentle palpation at or around the fracture site may elicit this sign, a sensation of crackling in the soft tissue just beneath the skin. It is evidence of a break in the integrity of the visceral and parietal pleura and may be associated with pneumothorax as well.

Routine chest radiography often fails to disclose contusion until well after the injury. Usually appearing 12 to 24 hours after trauma, the patchy infiltrates of pulmonary contusion may already be well on their way to producing respiratory failure. The most reliable clinically available diagnostic modality for evaluation of pulmonary parenchyma is the computed tomography scan. Early diagnosis of pulmonary contusion and follow-up studies to assess the progress of the injury can be made with computed tomography scans.

Treatment of minimal-to-moderate contusion consists of aggressive pulmonary toilet, supportive analgesia, including rib blocks, continuous epidural anesthesia where appropriate, and broad-spectrum antibiotics. Serial arterial blood gas monitoring may be useful in assessing respiratory gas exchange. Supplemental oxygen by mask or nasal cannula, and bronchodilators when there is evidence of bronchospasm, may also be needed.

Myocardial Contusion

Two entities have been described to separate cardiac injuries resulting from blunt thoracic trauma. Grouped together as myocardial contusion, cardiac concussion may be differentiated from cardiac contusion by the lack of cellular damage in concussion and the presence of myocardial necrosis in contusion. The clinical significance of cardiac contusion is the occurrence of arrhythmias such as premature atrial and ventricular contractions in the short-term as well as thromboembolism, valvular heart disease and failure, and acute congestive heart failure. Late sequelae may include ventricular aneurysm and restrictive pericarditis.

Diagnosis is often made initially by electrocardiography, which may show nonspecific S- and T-wave changes and even new q waves, but this is not specific for cardiac contusion. The serial determinations of creatine phosphokinase-MB isoenzyme and two-dimensional echocardiography are among the recent approaches to diagnosis.

The mainstay of management for cardiac contusion has been careful cardiac monitoring in the hospital as major cardiac complications may occur.

Conclusion

Outpatients frequently suffer chest trauma, with rib fractures, minor chest wall trauma, and pulmonary contusions most commonly encountered. Significant myocardial concussion and contusion are uncommon events in the ambulatory setting. Conservative approaches to management with rest and analgesia are most often used.

References

1. Mackersie RC, Shackford SR, Hoyt DB, Karagianes TG: Continuous Epidural Fentanyl Analgesia: Ventilatory Function Improvement with Routine Use in Treatment of Blunt Chest Injury. *The Journal of Trauma*, 27(11): 1207–1212, 1987
2. Shorr RM, et al: Blunt Chest Trauma in the Elderly. *The Journal of Trauma*, 29(2):234–237, 1989
3. Kirsh MM: Acute Thoracic Injuries in Trauma Emergency Surgery & Critical Care ed. John H Siegel, Churchill Livingstone, 1987
4. Mattox KL, ed.: Thoracic Trauma, in *Surgical Clinics of North America*, 69:1 Feb 1989
5. Wojcik JB, Morgan AS: Sternal Fractures—The Natural History, *Annals of Emergency Medicine*, 17(9):912–914, 1988
6. Wagner RB, Slivko B: Highlights of the History of Nonpenetrating Chest Trauma. *Surg Clin NA*, 69:1, 1–14, Feb 1989
7. LoCicero III J, Mattox KL: Epidemiology of Chest Trauma, *Surg Clin NA*, 69:1, 15–19, Feb 1989
8. Beeson A, Saegesser F: Color Atlas of Chest Trauma and Associated Injuries. Oradell, Medical Economics Books, 1983
9. Trinca GW, Dooley BJ: The effects of mandatory seat belt wearing on the mortality and pattern of injury of car occupants involved in motor vehicle crashes in Victoria. *Med J Aust*, 1:675–678, 1975

10. Hamilton JR, Dearden C, Rutherford WH: Myocardial contusion associated with fracture of the sternum: Important features of the seat belt syndrome. *Injury,* 16:155–156, 1974
11. Michelinakis E: Safety belt syndrome. *Practitioner,* 207:77–80, 1971
12. Pate JW: Chest Wall Injuries. *Surg Clin NA,* 69:1, 59–70, Feb 1989
13. Trunkey DD: In Blaisdell FW, Trunkey DD: Trauma management, Vol III: Cervicothoracic Trauma. New York, Thieme, 1986
14. Bekassy SM, Dave KS, Wooler GH, et al: "Spontaneous" and Traumatic Rupture of the Diaphragm. *Ann Surg,* 177:320–324, 1973
15. Estrera AS, Platt MR, Mills LT: Traumatic Injuries of the Diaphragm. *Chest,* 75:306–313, 1979
16. Wise L, Connors J, Hwang YH, et al: Traumatic Injuries to the Diaphragm. *J Trauma,* 13:946–950, 1973
17. Tarver RD, Godwin JD, Putman CE: The Diaphragm. *Radiol Clin N Amer,* 22:3, 615–631, 1984

Pulmonary and Mediastinal Neoplasms

Enrique Signori and Oscar Signori

Pulmonary neoplasms are among the most common cancers found in men and women. Early diagnosis and treatment of these disorders represent one of the great challenges of medicine. This chapter gives an overview of the epidemiology, etiology, diagnosis, and treatment of several kinds of pulmonary neoplasms and related disorders.

Epithelial lung cancer, or bronchogenic carcinoma, accounts for the overwhelming majority of pulmonary neoplasms. Bronchial adenomas, mesenchymal, and miscellaneous tumors represent only 5% to 7% of lung neoplasms [1] and therefore are not the focus of this discussion.

Epidemiology

There were an estimated 168,000 new lung cancers and approximately 146,000 deaths from this disease in 1991. Thirty-four percent of cancer deaths in men and 22% in women are due to lung cancer. This disease has long been the leading cause of cancer deaths in men and will soon surpass the number of deaths caused by breast cancer in women [2]. Patients with lung cancer have a poor prognosis, with a 5-year survival rate of only 11% in blacks and 13% in whites for all stages of the disease and 30% and 37%, respectively, for localized stages [2]. Further, survival trends have not shown major improvements over the years.

As tobacco is the leading cause of lung cancer, incidence and death rates have paralleled cigarette consumption. Consequently, women have suffered a rapid increase in the incidence of primary lung cancer. They tend to develop the disease at a younger age and after smoking for fewer years than men [3]. It is foreseen that current changes in the smoking habits of the general population such as fewer people starting to smoke, increased number of smokers quitting, and lower tar cigarettes will not translate to a substantial decline in lung cancer death rates until the first quarter of the twenty-first century [4].

Etiology

Tobacco was thought to be a cause of lung cancer early in the nineteenth century, but it was not until 1950 that the first conclusive epidemiologic evidence linking cigarette smoking with bronchogenic carcinoma was published [5]. Since then, a cause and effect relationship has been well established relating to the duration of smoking, the number of cigarettes smoked, depth of inhalation, tar and nicotine content in the cigarettes, as well as the age at the initiation of smoking [6]. The risk of male smokers developing lung cancer is nearly 20 times that of nonsmokers, and because there have been no compound variables that might affect the association between smoking and lung cancer, the cause and effect relationship is beyond question [7]. The risk of developing lung cancer declines after discontinuation of smoking and equals that of lifelong nonsmokers after 10 to 15 years of cessation [8].

Many carcinogens, mutagens, and tumor promoters have been identified in tobacco smoke [6], including nitrosamines, ammonia, formaldehyde, 2-naphthylamine, 4-aminobiphenyl, aniline, nickel, acrolein, benzene, cadmium, methane, nicotine, benzol(α)pyrene phenol, tar, acetylene, hydrogen cyanide, vinyl choloride, etc. [9]. The use of low tar, low nicotine cigarettes (the "low-yield" or oxymoronic "safe cigarette") decreases cancer risks [9, 10] by reducing the total amount of carcinogens in the smoke; but its use may prevent smokers from focusing on the paramount issue of cessation of smoking, with all its attendant benefits [11]. Cigarette smoking increases the risk of developing all histologic types of lung cancer, including adenocarcinoma. The risk increases faster for squamous cell carcinoma than for adenocarcinoma. The risk for developing neoplasm, however, declines faster for squamous cell carcinoma than for adenocarcinoma after cessation of smoking [12]. The risk for bronchogenic carcinoma cell cancer relates more to the duration of cigarette smoking than to the intensity of the smoking.

Passive smoking, or the inhalation of environmental tobacco smoke by the nonsmoker, has been reported to increase the risk of lung cancer among spouses of smokers. The overall increased risk of lung cancer in nonsmoking women married to smokers is about 30% higher than that of those women married to nonsmokers, while the increase in risk associated with heavy passive smoking is up to 70% higher [13].

The lung cancer epidemic that has afflicted us since the 1920s has a most preventable cause: cigarette smoking. As physicians we must dedicate our efforts to eradicating tobacco use. We can act in this regard in three arenas: (1) supporting the efforts of patients to stop smoking, and (2) lobbying for legislative measures targeted at curtailing tobacco product use and advertising, and (3) working to protect and enhance the rights of nonsmokers [5, 10].

In addition to tobacco smoke, there are other environmental pulmonary carcinogens that induce malignancy: asbestos [14], acrylonitrile [15], arsenic [16], beryllium [17], bischloromethyl ether, chloromethyl methyl ether [18], cadmium [19], chromium [16, 20], mustard gas [21], nickel [16], ionizing radiation [22], and vinyl chloride [23] are substances associated with a definite increased risk of lung cancer in humans [24].

These carcinogens very commonly have synergistic or multiplicative effects with cigarette smoking [25]. For example, asbestos exposure increases the risk of developing primary lung cancer three- to fivefold in nonsmokers; that risk increases up to 80 times in smokers [14]. Most of these exposures occur in the workplace. Considering that 47% of men and 38% of women holding blue collar jobs are smokers [26], and therefore, are at greater risk of developing lung cancer, elimination of occupational exposures coupled with an attack on nicotine addiction are not only medical matters, but financial and social needs as well.

The number of occupations in which workers could contact pulmonary carcinogens is innumerable (from foundry workers to fur dressers). In order to determine an occupational exposure to a potential pulmonary carcinogen, several facts must be determined before an opinion is given, namely, was there a reasonable probability of exposure? Was the exposure significant? Was the latency period consistent with the exposure in question? Was the histologic type of cancer consistent with the exposure in question? Were there any confounding variables that might have reduced the risk of carcinogenicity of the exposure in question? This information, once known, will allow a reasonable assessment of the probability that the lung cancer is the result of occupational factors [24].

Air pollution may be an important risk factor in the etiology of lung cancer [27]. Diesel exhaust emissions may produce some excess risks of lung cancer for those who work for long periods in high exposure occupations. These are very common occupations and therefore the population at risk may be large [28].

Silica exposure, although placing a worker at risk for a pneumoconiosis (silicosis) cannot be firmly implicated as a lung carcinogen [29, 30].

Epidemiologic evidence has been published in the last few years suggesting increased risk of cancer in patients with a deficient diet of vitamin A. Similar observations have been made with beta carotene, selenium, and vitamin E [31, 32]. These findings have served as rationales for the initiation of chemoprevention trials at the national level.

The clinician on an empiric basis may encourage patients to supplement their diets with vitamin A, vitamin E, and selenium if the patients' dietary habits are inadequate or are smokers and have an increased risk for developing a pulmonary neoplasm.

Radon is a ubiquitous and highly mobile gas found in the soil and atmosphere. It is a member of the radioactive decay chain of 238 uranium and 226 radium. Radon decays in a sequence of short-lived radionuclides that are known as radon decay products, radon daughters, or radon progeny [33]. These decay products are heavy metals (polonium and lead) and when airborne attach rapidly to particles. Human exposure to radon occurs mostly through the inhalation of these particles with attached radioactive decay products. The probability of inhaling them depends on the concentration of particulate matter in the inhaled air, e.g., particles of cigarette smoke or on very "dusty air" [33]. Studies have shown as early as the 1950s that underground miners exposed to radon in uranium mines are at higher risk of developing lung cancer than the general nonexposed population [34, 35].

Radon also emanates from the soil and building materials, accumulating in poorly ventilated structures. Radon enters a building through the flow of air from the soil pores and through "leakiness" in the structure of the house. Concentration of radon within the house depends on its contents in the soil, as well as the room in the house, e.g., higher concentration in the basement [36].

Indoor concentrations of radon average 1.5 pCi/L for US houses [37, 38], but it is possible that many homes have considerably higher concentrations than the average [36]. Extrapolating data from exposure and risk of lung cancer in uranium miners to the exposure in US homes has allowed estimation of the risk of contracting lung cancer due to indoor, nonoccupational radon exposure as a 0.5% risk over a lifetime [36]. This risk is considerably higher for smokers; of the 16,000 deaths per year associated with radon exposure, only 500 occur in nonsmokers [39]. The Environmental Protection Agency has shown great concern for this problem. This has resulted in (1) the issue of an advisory establishing the nature of the threat; (2) a recommendation to schools to test for radon and take remedial action if needed; (3) a recommendation that homes in the United States be surveyed for radon levels; and (4) The Indoor Radon Abatement Act, which passed into law in October 1988 [40].

Critics have argued that using miner studies to estimate the effect of low doses of radon might not be appropriate or valid. Others suggest that more emphasis should be placed on smoking cessation since smokers represent most of those who develop lung cancer after radon exposure.

Our recommendations for persons concerned about radon exposure include the following:

1. Contact the Environmental Protection Agency, which is the best source of information regarding monitoring service and control techniques.
2. Stop smoking.
3. Test the home for radon concentration if living in an endemic area.
4. If testing is necessary it should be done in the living space for at least a year: take remedial action if necessary.

Pathogenesis of Lung Cancer

A definite pathogenetic mechanism for the development of lung cancer is unclear, but the emerging evidence can be summarized as follows [41]. Epithelial lung cells under heavy and continuous carcinogen exposure, probably enhanced by a certain inherited metabolic phenotype, suffer a number of genetic changes that result in the activation of oncogenes, with the inactivation of recessive or tumor suppressor genes. Although many genetic changes are somatic in nature, epidemiologic evidence suggests that some of those changes are inherited in a Mendelian fashion. Parallel to and perhaps as a consequence of those genetic changes, autocrine and paracrine growth factors are produced by the bronchial epithelial cells. These growth factors cause the accumulation of individual cells with genetic lesions, helping their proliferation and transformation into malignant clones. In addition, they stimulate other epithelial cells in the bronchi to expand and further produce growth factors with similar effects.

Pathology

There are four major histologic types of bronchogenic carcinoma. Squamous cell carcinoma accounts for 30% to 35% of carcinoma and adenocarcinoma accounts for 30% to 33% of lung cancers. Small-cell carcinomas (SCC) make up 20% to 25% and large-cell carcinomas 15% to 20% of all lung cancers [42, 43]. For clinical reasons (more aggressive behavior, initial responsiveness to radiation and chemotherapy), small-cell carcinoma is considered as a class of its own, while the other three are grouped under the denomination of non–small-cell lung cancer.

Clinical Manifestations and Diagnosis

Fifteen percent of lung cancer patients are asymptomatic at the time of diagnosis; all others have symptoms due to the primary tumor, metastatic disease, paraneoplastic syndromes, or a combination [44].

Cough, hemoptysis, dyspnea, obstructive pneumonitis, and vague chest pains are common features. As the cancer spreads within the thorax, several complex clinical conditions can occur: hoarseness, superior vena cava syndrome, pleural and pericardial effusions, esophageal obstruction, Horner's syndrome, or superior sulcus syndrome.

Smokers should be suspected of having a malignancy if there is (1) new onset of cough; (2) change in the nature of a cough already present; (3) hemoptysis; (4) no improvement of an episode of acute bronchitis or pneumonia within 2 weeks of antibiotic treatment; and (5) progressive dyspnea. These patients should then be thoroughly investigated for the presence of malignancy since smaller tumors are expected to have better prognoses [45].

Metastatic disease outside the chest commonly involves lymph nodes, central nervous system, liver, bone, bone marrow, and adrenal glands. Causes of morbidity in lung cancer are paraneoplastic syndromes, particularly weight loss, anemia, thrombophlebitis, pericarditis, adrenocorticotropic hormone secretion, inappropriate antidiuretic hormone secretion, hypercalcemia, finger clubbing, hypertrophic pulmonary osteoarthropathy, and a variety of neurologic manifestations, e.g., myopathy, peripheral neuropathies, and subacute cerebellar degeneration [46].

Many diagnostic techniques are available for making the diagnosis of lung cancer. Chest radiography is the most important method for the detection of bronchogenic carcinoma [47]. Its usefulness as a screening method is controversial, although a yearly anteroposterior and lateral film of the chest for heavy smokers or smokers exposed to a carcinogen in the workplace may be reasonable.

Sputum cytology may diagnose up to 95% of lesions if the sample is adequately prepared and interpreted by an expert; a negative cytology result in a patient who is clinically suspicious should never be a reason to terminate the investigation [48].

Flexible fiberoptic bronchoscopy with bronchial washings, brushings, and forceps biopsies is helpful in the diagnosis of central lesions [49]. It is also used in the localization of occult lung cancer [50], with or without the application of fluorescent bronchoscopy [51].

Transbronchial needle aspiration of lesions in the lung parenchyma was found to be reliable in submucosal and peripheral lesions that are not within the reach of the bronchoscope [52, 53].

Percutaneous needle biopsy of the lung is becoming an accepted method for the diagnosis of peripheral lesions [54]. As with many other procedures, the experience of the radiologist and the cytopathologist is important to achieve accurate results and limit complications. Percutaneous needle aspiration biopsies of hilar and mediastinal masses have been purported to be a safe and accurate method for diagnosing metastatic carcinoma to the mediastinum [55], in spite of the definite risk of blood vessel puncture.

Pleural biopsy, coupled with thoracentesis, offers good results in patients with malignant pleural disease. Diagnostic yield may improve with the introduction of the flexible bronchoscope or thoracoscope into the pleural space (thoracoscopy) [56].

Anatomic Staging of Lung Cancer

Once the diagnosis of lung cancer is established by histopathology, it is important to determine the stage of the disease [57]. This has both prognostic and therapeutic implications [58]. Because of the different patterns of spread and velocity of growth, however, staging for non–small-cell carcinomas (NSCC) and small cell carcinomas SCC are different. In a NSCC, the major component is the intrathoracic assessment; whereas in SCC extrathoracic involvement plays a major role.

Non–Small-Cell Lung Cancer

Staging the three histologic types in this group is based on the TNM system. *T* indicates the size and extent of the primary tumor, *N*, regional lymph node status, and *M* refers to visceral metastasis [59, 60]. TNM worksheets are readily available, but not reproduced in this chapter [61]. When properly completed with all the pertinent information, they are an integral part of the patient's record. Determination of the tumor staging by the TNM system requires a careful thoracic and extrathoracic investigation. Key elements in the assessment of thoracic disease are conventional chest radiography, a computed tomography (CT) scan, and mediastinoscopy [62]. Chest radiography is the first study performed in a TNM evaluation. A CT scan represents the best single method available to carry out this staging, because the thorax can be seen in exquisite detail [63–65]. CT is also of great assistance for treatment planning in patients who are candidates for radiotherapy.

Magnetic resonance imaging (MRI) [66, 67] and gallium scanning [68, 69] may be valuable in the completion of TNM staging. Currently we do not include them routinely in our approach to thoracic staging.

Mediastinoscopy is a safe and reliable technique for staging and should be performed when a chest radiography and CT scan have not sufficiently clarified the TNM landscape. It is usually performed through a midline cervical incision and permits biopsy of ipsilateral and contralateral mediastinal lymph nodes; modifications of technique also facilitate assessment of both hilar and subaortic nodes. Mediastinoscopy is particularly useful in cases where a CT scan has not clearly determined unresectability. Complications inherent to all surgical procedures preclude the routine use of mediastinoscopy in every patient [65]. Transtracheal needle aspiration of the carina has been used with variable success depending on the experience of the operator and the availability of a committed cytopathologist. The procedure is especially useful in patients who are at higher risk for more invasive studies (e.g., mediastinoscopy or thoracotomy).

The extrathoracic evaluation of the TNM system in NSCC should be economical in the use of diagnostic procedures. Initial assessment includes a complete blood count, blood chemistries, and liver function studies. We do not routinely obtain radionuclide studies (liver, bone, brain) or metastatic bone survey radiography. These studies performed in asymptomatic individuals have a low yield [70–72]. The principal role of staging in NSCC is to provide a definitive answer to the question; is the patient a candidate for surgical resection and cure? Information derived from the TNM system allows the identification of surgically potentially curable patients. Mediastinal lymph node positivity generally supports a conservative treatment approach. In one series of 874 patients, 79% of those showing positive nodes die within 1 year. In contrast, 97% of the mediastinal node negative group were resectable and have a 25% 5-year survival [73, 74].

Small-Cell Carcinoma

The biology of SCC makes the TNM staging system clinically irrelevant, except in a small group of patients in whom surgery may be contemplated [75]. More than 80% of patients may have advanced disease [76] at the time of the initial diagnosis. The most commonly used staging system in SCC recognizes two large categories: limited and extensive disease [58, 77]. Limited staging describes disease confined to one hemithorax, including ipsilateral supraclavicular lymph nodes. Extensive disease represents disease found anywhere else.

The most appropriate way to assess thoracic disease in SCC is conventional chest radiography plus CT. These methods may provide information on the primary lesion and possible intrathoracic involvement. The CT scan will be of great assistance for radiation therapy treatment planning.

In contrast to NSCC, the extrathoracic evaluation of disease in SCC is extremely important because of the high probability of metastatic spread at the time of initial diagnosis [78]. In addition to the routine blood count, blood chemistries (especially those with prognostic value) [79], and liver function studies, an abdominal CT is required in view of the frequent visceral metastases with SCC. The liver and the adrenal glands are most often involved. The spleen, pancreas, and kidneys are additional targets for metastasis. A radionuclide bone scan [80] and bilateral bone marrow biopsies and aspirations [81] are an integral part of SCC staging as well. Knowledge of the bone marrow status is useful to find a baseline and ascertain myeloid reserve in preparation for chemotherapy. Metastatic disease also suggests poor prognosis [82] and a high risk for leptomeningeal involvement. New techniques, including flow cytometry, may help to detect early marrow involvement, resulting in improved staging and treatment planning [83]. A CT of the head is also part of the extrathoracic evaluation; central nervous system metastasis may be present initially in one quarter of patients and reach up to 80% as the disease progresses [84, 85]. At present, MRI of the brain is used when CT findings are equivocal, but the MRI is becoming the most important of the two because of its increased sensitivity.

In SCC, the staging is seldom concerned with determination of resectability, but provides invaluable information regarding overall prognosis, treatment planning, monitoring therapeutic successes and failures, and the identification of subsets with a special prognostic significance [86].

Biomarker Profiles

We use a baseline "battery" of new tumor markers in patients at the time of diagnosis as one of the tools to follow disease activity and results of treatment (Table 20-1). Their true place however, has not been established and they do not form part of the regular staging planning.

Immunosuppressive acid protein, neuron-specific enolase, and squamous cell carcinoma markers are still investigational and cannot be used alone for diagnostic purposes inasmuch as their total performance characteristics have not been established. Carcinoembryonic antigen and beta human chorionic gonadotropin are well known tumor markers. Lipid-associated sialic acid plasma measures total gangliosides and glycoproteins with a sensitivity ranging between 77% and 97%, depending on tumor type. Neuron-specific enolase may have particular value in small-cell carcinoma, with a sensitivity of over 70%. Immunosuppressive acidic protein is promising in adenocarcinoma of the lung with a greater than 80% sensitivity [87].

Flow Cytometry Analysis

Flow cytometric analysis of lung cancer samples has shown that patients with diploid squamous cell carcinoma survive significantly longer than those with aneuploid tumors. These findings do not apply to adenocarcinoma and are independent of stage, nodal status, nuclear grade and mitotic rate [88, 89].

Oncogenes

The finding of an activated K-RAS oncogene in adenocarcinoma of the lung indicates a poorer prognosis and shorter survival despite early stage and complete tumor excision [90].

Table 20-1. Tumor Markers

NSCC	
Adenocarcinoma	CEA, IAP and LASA-P
Squamous cell	CEA, LASA-P and SCCM
Large cell	CEA, IAP and LASA-P
SCC	CEA, LASA-P, NSE, B-HCG

Abbreviations: CEA, carcinoembryonic antigen; IAP, immunosuppressive acidic protein; LASA-P, lipid associated sialic acid plasma; NSE, neuron-specific enolase; SCCM, squamous cell carcinoma marker; B-HCG, beta human chorionic gonadotropin; SCC, small cell carcinoma.

Therapy

A detailed discussion of the therapy of primary lung cancer is beyond the scope of this chapter. It is reasonable to suggest that the decisions required for treating these patients are usually best made with the input of a surgeon and radiation and medical oncologist.

Surgery is the treatment of choice for patients with stage I (localized disease without lymph node involvement) and stage II (lymph node involvement limited to intrapulmonary or hilar nodes) disease. Stage III patients (larger tumors or significant nodal involvement) with involvement of adjacent structures, e.g., chest wall and main bronchus, may be candidates for resection under special circumstances.

Radiation therapy with curative intent is given to patients with non–small-cell lung cancer in two situations: (1) the disease is beyond the limits of resectability, but still within the confines of the chest; and (2) in early stages for patients who are not in clinical conditions to tolerate a thoracotomy and/or the removal of lung tissue. Preoperative radiotherapy has been effective for patients with superior sulcus tumors while postoperative treatment is better reserved for patients with large tumors or those with positive hilar of mediastinal lymph nodes.

Thoracic radiation therapy is a very important component in the management of limited stage, small-cell lung cancer.

Chemotherapy is the main treatment for small-cell lung cancer. Its role in the management of NSCC of the lung is still well within the realms of research. If a remission (usually partial) occurs with chemotherapy, palliation is occasionally accomplished. Patients with advanced lung cancer and bleeding or obstructing tumors of the main stem bronchii or the carinal area, but with identifiable lumen, may benefit from laser therapy. This is a palliative technique, very effective in controlling hemoptysis and relieving dyspnea, but does not change the outcome. Major complications of laser therapy include perforation, hemorrhage, acute respiratory failure, and death. Better techniques and equipment improvements have made complications less frequent [91]. Brachytherapy, the delivery of radiation to a tumor with interstitial sources, can be an alternative to the use of laser. It is effective in palliating recurrence even in previously irradiated bronchogenic carcinoma.

Follow-Up

Patients who have completed therapy and are in clinical remission probably should be followed every 3 to 4 months [92]. Chest roentgenography is of some value for detecting recurrence. The performance of scans routinely remains controversial. All patients with lung cancer should be advised to stop smoking, especially those in remission. The stress of the disease and its therapy is not a reason to perpetuate the habit (e.g., "hard to quit now") but the foundation on which to quit tobacco consumption.

An adequate intake of vitamin A should be ensured and revision of dietary habits implemented. It is obligatory for the physician caring for these patients to (1) observe carefully for the development of recurrence or a second primary (particularly lung, head, and neck) and (2) attend to the many medical problems caused not only by the lung cancer and its treatment, but to other common diseases afflicting this population of patients, e.g., coronary artery disease and chronic obstructive pulmonary disease.

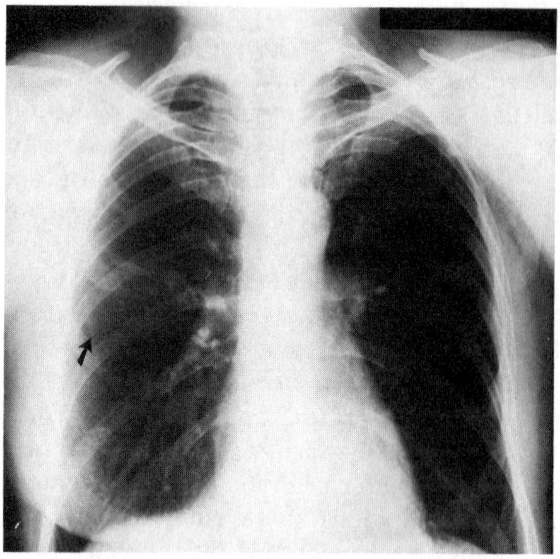

Figure 20-1. Chest radiogram depicting a small noncalcified nodule in the right mid-lung zone. The absence of the left breast suggests a metastatic lesion.

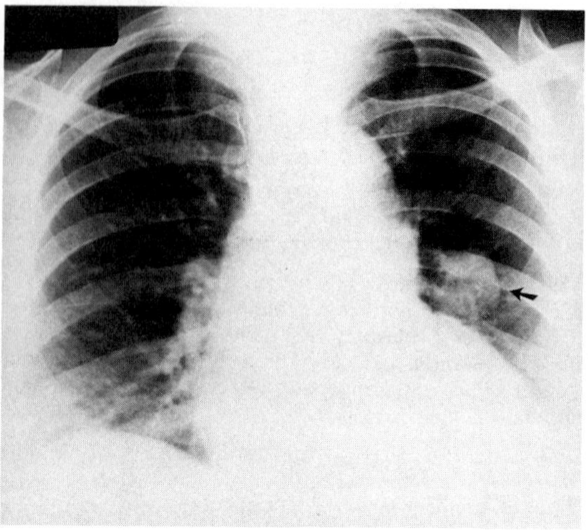

Figure 20-2. Chest radiogram of a left mid-lung nodule with "pepper-pot" calcifications representing a benign hamartoma (Courtesy of Lawrence F. Campbell, M.D. Oakwood Hospital).

Solitary Pulmonary Nodules

A solitary pulmonary nodule (SPN) is a lesion that usually measures less than 4 cm in diameter, is surrounded by normal pulmonary parenchyma, causes no symptoms, and is not associated with other abnormal radiographic findings such as lymphadenopathy, atelectasis, and/or pneumonia (Fig. 20-1, 20-2) [93].

The diagnosis of SPN may not be initially suspected by the clinical history or physical examination. Frequently SPNs are found by chance, and they may be seen in as many as 1 or 2 in every 1000 routine chest roentgenograms [94]. Nonetheless, it is relevant to know about smoking, occupational exposures, and the history of previous pulmonary diseases (pneumonia, tuberculosis, pneumoconiosis, or cancer). A SPN associated with a history of voice changes or dysphagia suggests a possible bronchogenic carcinoma [95]. In the physical examination, particular attention must be paid to primary or metastatic neoplasm (e.g., breast or renal masses, hepatomegaly, and lymphadenopathy). Approximately 31% of lung cancers present at onset as SPN [96] and more than 40% of all SPNs are malignant [94]. As such they represent an important medical challenge. The most important etiologies of SPN are shown in Table 20-2.

Differential Diagnosis

Important questions concerning the differential diagnosis of SPN include:

1. Is the lesion in the lung? A careful search for cutaneous or soft tissue masses and the use of radiographic surface markers may be helpful.

Table 20-2. Differential Diagnosis of Solitary Pulmonary Nodules

Malignant lesions
Bronchogenic carcinomas: all types
Metastases
Adenomas, carcinoids
Others
Benign lesions
Calcified granulomas (tuberculosis, fungal, others)
Hamartomas
Congenital (e.g., bronchopulmonary sequestration and cysts)
Miscellaneous

2. If the lesion is in the lung, is it a true SPN or something else (e.g., plaque, vascular malformations, or cysts must be considered)?
3. If it is a true SPN, is this a recent or an old finding? The patient's own history and the availability of old chest radiographs are important.
4. Is the SPN a benign or malignant lesion? The following two considerations are important.
   a. The patient's history is of value if it establishes a long-term presence of the lesion. Many patients are aware they have had abnormal chest radiography for many years.
   b. Recent or old chest roentgenograms may show the presence of specific patterns of calcification (diffuse, laminated, or a central nidus) in granulomas that suggest a benign lesion. The so-called pepper-pot calcifications, along or combined with fat, is typical of a hamartoma (Fig. 20-2) [97, 98]. However, occasionally malignant lesions may have calcifications. By far, the single most reliable sign suggesting a benign SPN is the careful study of comparative films showing a lesion unchanged or smaller over a period of 2 years or more [99]. It is important to recognize that benign lesions also may grow. These qualifications still leave us searching for new nonsurgical techniques that will be able to establish benignity in SPNs [96].
5. If the SPN is malignant, is it a primary or metastatic lesion? A careful history and physical examination may help to decide the previous existence of a history of malignancy or permit the identification of an extrapulmonary neoplasm.

Diagnostic Menu for Solitary Pulmonary Nodules

Chest roentgenography There are roentgenographic features that help separate malignant from benign lesions. Malignant SPNs tend to be more irregular with spiculated or lobulated perimeters in contrast to benign lesions that may have rounded borders. There may be significant exceptions, however, as in inflammatory pseudotumors that have spiculated margins [100, 101]. Recent data suggest that scanning equalization radiography may increase the ability to evaluate SPNs [102].

Computed Tomography of the Thorax CT is an important aid in assessing SPNs as it provides density and morphologic information. Using thin-section scans, for example, accurate detection of calcifications can be made by analysis of their pattern: malignant calcifications are usually eccentric, smaller, and scattered within the SPN [103]. Further, CT scans may reveal unsuspected calcifications in 20% to 25% of all SPNs [104, 105]. CT scans are even more helpful in determining the status of the mediastinum and the presence of more than one nodule than in diagnosing benignity in SPNs [106].

Magnetic Resonance Imaging (MRI) Lung tissue shows modest signal intensity on MRI with little normally being observed within the parenchyma, thereby allowing easy visibility of SPNs. Because of poorer spatial resolution, respiratory motion, and decreased SPN/lung parenchyma contrast, MRIs are less sensitive than CT scans, particularly for very small SPNs. This is also true for SPNs close to the diaphragm and chest wall. MRI, on the other hand, may be better for more central nodules. MRI is not very precise in determining the location of a SPN because the landmarks useful for this type of localization (fissures, vessels, etc.) are poorly seen. The present role of MRI can be defined as complementary to the CT scan. MRI should be selectively considered when CT scan findings are unclear or fail to provide definitive information, particularly if they can help to prevent an unnecessary, more radical intervention [107, 108].

Invasive Procedures

Fiberoptic Bronchoscopy Fiberoptic bronchoscopy (FOB) permits brushing, washing and transbronchial biopsy or aspiration. FOB is a very important tool in the evaluation and diagnosis of SPNs. It is particularly valuable in symptomatic patients complaining of cough, blood-tinged sputum, changes in voice, or difficulty in swallowing, and in those with a positive sputum cytology [104]. In these instances, a FOB may reveal a visible endobronchial lesion. FOB serves a dual function as a diagnostic and staging tool. The diagnostic accuracy ranges between 25% and 55% in those SPNs that are 2 to 4 cm in diameter. This may improve to almost 70% with a transbronchial needle aspiration. The main limitation of this technique is the high incidence of false-negative diagnoses [109]. FOB is safe and has little serious morbidity even in elderly patients [110].

Percutaneous Needle Biopsy Aspiration of the Lung Percutaneous needle biopsy aspiration has become an important resource [111, 112] in the diagnosis of SPNs. The morbidity of this procedure is low and often eliminates the need for surgery. The diagnostic yield may be very high in the hands of a dedicated radiologist and cytopathologist [113]. For a cytologic report to be acceptable, it has to prove a specific benign diagnosis. Reports that are vague or nondescriptive (e.g., "benign cellular elements") may lead to a false diagnosis of a negative SPN [114, 115], which is unacceptable.

Thoracoscopy Direct observation and biopsy of the pleural cavity through a small incision is a procedure that may be of value in situations where a patient has an undiagnosed pleural effusion. Thoracoscopy is not generally used in the evaluation of a SPN [116].

Summary of Diagnostic Techniques
In selecting from this diagnostic menu to evaluate a SPN, the most important issue is how many items are justifiable, prudent, and safe to use before a decision is made to proceed with a thoracotomy. All true SPNs are resectable, but should all of them be expediently resected [117]? Algorithmic solutions have been recommended to solve this dilemma by other authors [118].

In our practice, we follow a straightforward approach. We use a pathway that sequentially includes chest radiography (including search for old films), CT scan, fiberoptic bronchoscopy, and percutaneous needle biopsy of the lung. Selected resources, not a part of a main diagnostic stream, are the MRI and thoracoscopy. How far we go in this diagnostic pathway is dictated by how long it takes to meet our criteria for benignity as shown in Table 20-3. In patients who have reached the end of this pathway without establishing SPN benignity, we recommend conventional thoracotomy and resection, unless a major contraindication for surgery is present [119]. In this regard, local excision using yttrium aluminum garnet (YAG) laser or brachytherapy may be beneficial in high-risk and elderly patients [93].

Table 20-3. Criteria for Benignity of Solitary Pulmonary Nodules

Study	Benign Result
1. Chest radiography	"Benign" calcifications
CT scan	Size unchanged or smaller for 2 years +
2. FOB and percutaneous needle biopsy of the lung	Cytology with specific benign diagnosis
	Relative benignity factors
	Nonsmoker
	Less than 40 years old
	Long-standing history of "a spot in the lung"

Pulmonary Masses

Lung masses that are adjacent to the mediastinal or parietal pleura are not strictly considered SPNs. Masses adjacent to the pulmonary hilum and mediastinum may be particularly difficult to evaluate when small because they "silhouette" or blend with the central structures of the chest. The clinical evaluation of the more peripheral lesions is similar to that of an SPN. However, central masses tend to invade mediastinum and therefore a more ambitious use of fiberoptic bronchoscopy is warranted. FOB is especially useful because these lesions are often visible endobronchially. If the endoscopist does not see a visible lesion, transtracheal needle aspiration or fluoroscopically guided forceps biopsy through the bronchoscope has been shown to be useful.

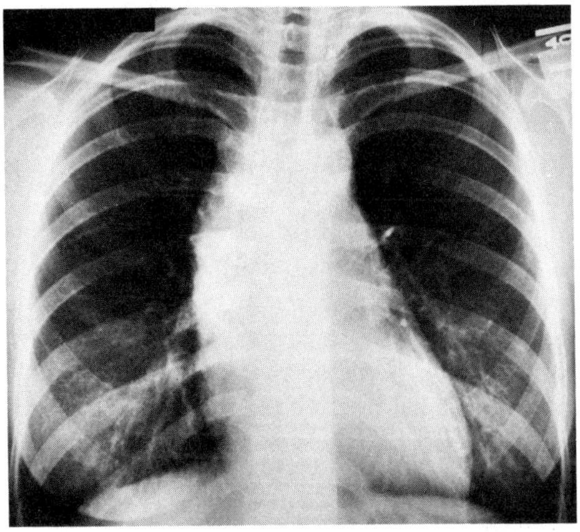

Figure 20-3. Chest radiogram of a large mediastinal mass in a patient with nodular sclerosis Hodgkin's lymphoma.

Mediastinal Neoplasms

The mediastinum is an anatomic space located between the spine posteriorly, the sternum anteriorly, and the mediastinal pleura laterally (see Fig. 26-3). For descriptive purposes, the mediastinum is divided in compartments—anterior, middle, and posterior [120]—and some authors use a superior mediastinum classification.

Mediastinal masses are often silent; yet when symptoms are present they relate to increased pressure by the tumor on nearby structures.

Masses located in the superior mediastinum may cause a superior vena cava syndrome (SVCS) (Fig. 20-3). Those in the middle mediastinum may cause hoarseness by compression of the recurrent laryngeal nerve, or hiccups, cough, and dyspnea. Those in the posterior mediastinum may trigger dysphagia and interscapular vertebral pain. Other less frequently noted symptoms are pains of the chest wall and arms, Horner's syndrome (ptosis, enophthalmus, and miosis), bilateral or hemilateral perspiration, and paralysis of the vagus nerve with tachycardia, cough, dyspnea, and on occasion, stridor.

The clinician is often confronted by the presence of a mediastinal mass detected on routine chest roentgenography. While proceeding with a work-up, it is helpful to remember that there is a certain correlation between the age of the patient, the location of the mass, and its histologic type. The initial work-up requires a chest roentgenogram in frontal and lateral projections with fluoroscopy; subsequent studies depend on the location of the mass, its mobility under fluoroscopy, as well as the presence and nature of the symptoms. Most patients should have a CT scan of the chest [121]. This aids in determining whether the mass is solid, vascular, cystic, fatty, or calcified. On occasion, angiography and esophagography may be needed, while MRI is used only in those cases in which CT scanning is not possible due to iodine contrast allergy.

Tissue diagnosis is required when the mediastinal mass is not fat, aneurysm, or a hiatal hernia or obviously benign process by CT (e.g., substernal thyroid). Frequently, a percutaneous needle biopsy with CT or fluoroscopic guidance will yield a diagnosis, although for lymphomas, larger samples are required and open thoracotomy is necessary. The proximity of major vessels or the absence of a skillful operator sometimes preclude a needle biopsy to avoid bleeding or complications.

The most common anterior mediastinal mass between the ages of 40 and 60 years are thymomas. In the younger age groups lymphomas and teratomas are seen. Goiters may present as a superior mediastinal mass at any age. The middle mediastinum, particularly in the lower portion, is a site for hiatal hernias, metastatic cancer, and sarcoidosis. The middle mediastinum is also the site of preference for aortic aneurysms and pericardial and bronchogenic cysts, while most of neurogenic tumors arise in the posterior mediastinum.

Superior Vena Cava Syndrome (SVCS)

SVCS results from compression or occlusion of the superior vena cava (SVC), impeding the venous return originated in the head, neck, upper extremities, and upper thorax to the right side of the heart.

The SVC is located in a reduced anatomic space between the innominate veins and the right atrium. Because of its thin walls and location, the SVC is particularly vulnerable to external compression, which is of a malignant origin in greater than 80% of patients. Bronchogenic carcinomas represent more than half of the cases, and the rest are accounted for by lymphomas and metastatic breast cancer [122]. Approximately 50% of benign mediastinal obstructions in one study were due to mediastinal fibrosis, probably secondary to histoplasmosis [123]. The recent increase in popularity of central venous lines and catheters have increased episodes of damage to the SVC. Catheter-induced thrombosis is one cause of benign SVC occlusion [124, 125, 126]. Direct invasion by tumor remains the most frequent cause of SVCS, however.

Diagnosis of Superior Vena Cava Syndrome

There are two important considerations in the diagnosis of SVC: (1) confirmation of obstruction, and (2) determination of a tissue diagnosis. SVCS is, when suspected, an easy clinical diagnosis. In a review of 86 cases from the Mayo Clinic [127], the most common complaints were fullness of the head (80%), dyspnea (63%), and cough (55%). In the same series, the most frequent physical findings included dilated neck veins (80%), chest wall venous collaterals (76%), and edema of the upper body (70%). These signs are illustrated in Fig. 20-4.

Two diagnostic modalities help determine obstruction. The chest radiograph may show a superior mediastinal widening or a right hilar mass. A normal chest radiograph, however, does not rule out a SVCS. This is especially true when there is evidence of SVC obstruction clinically. The other diagnostic

Figure 20-4. Superior vena cava syndrome resulting from complete obstruction of the superior vena cava by non-small cell bronchogenic carcinoma. The facial and upper chest swelling and collateral circulation are readily apparent.

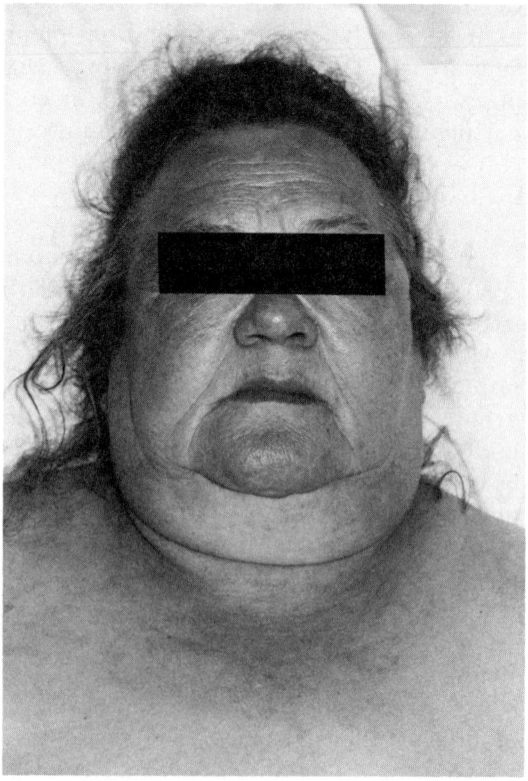

tool is the radionuclide superior vena cavagram. In our institution, this is done by injecting a bolus of technetium 99m sodium pertechnetate in the antecubital vein. This permits visualization, and functional evaluation with serialization of the axillary, subclavian, the innominate veins and the superior vena cava as it enters the right atrium [128] (Fig. 20-5).

We perform this study routinely when an SVC syndrome is suspected and find that it provides reliable information, not only on the site of obstruction, but also in treatment planning and follow-up. It may predict the results of therapy [129, 130].

Figure 20-6 illustrates a complete cutoff of the SVC secondary to encroachment by mediastinal Hodgkin's lymphoma. The presence of collateral circulation suggests long-standing obstruction and augurs fewer therapeutic benefits from radiation therapy [129].

In our experience, the ready performance and high accuracy of nuclide scanning obviates the need for contrast venography in most clinical situations.

Determining a tissue diagnosis in SVCS should be an exercise in pragmatism. According to a compilation of studies, sputum cytology should be obtained in most cases as

Figure 20-5. Normal radionuclide superior vena cavagram. There are normal and patent venous systems of the right upper extremity, axillary, subclavian, and innominate veins and superior vena cava (Courtesy of Reza Abghari, M.D. Oakwood Hospital).

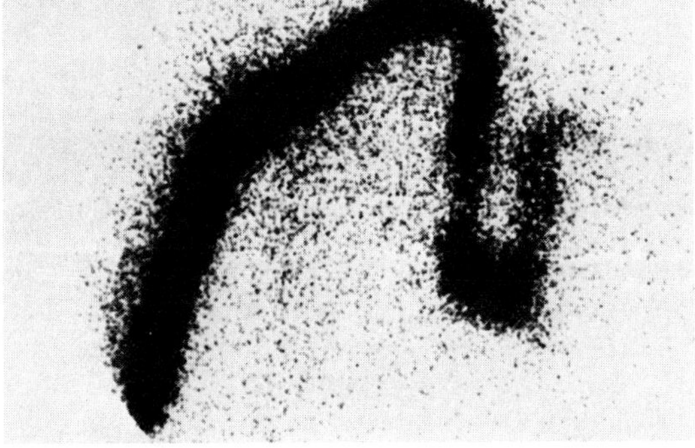

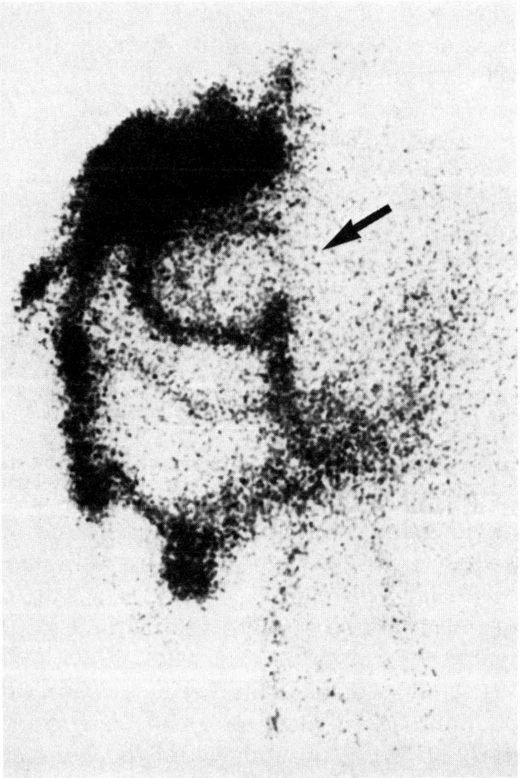

Figure 20-6. Radionuclide vena cavagram. There is non-visualization of the superior vena cava with extensive collateral flow surrounding the right subclavian vein consistent with an obstruction of the superior vena cava at the region of the right and left innominate vein junction (Courtesy of Reza Abghari, M.D. Oakwood Hospital).

it will be positive in about 49%. If a pleural effusion is present, the cytologic analysis will yield high positive rate for malignancy (73%). If an abnormal lymph node is palpable, the biopsy will be diagnostic in 67% of cases. FOB may help in about half of cases [131]. If the previously mentioned sequence fails to secure a tissue diagnosis, percutaneous needle biopsy of the lung is a safe procedure and offers a high diagnostic yield. We do not recommend mediastinoscopy because of a high rate of complications. Open minithoracotomies have the highest positive yield, but we resort to them only in those cases where less invasive procedures have failed.

Paradoxically, the diagnosis of a benign cause of SVCS may be more difficult. Difficulty in securing a causative factor suggests a possible benign origin. In benign conditions, symptoms are usually of longer duration and have a more gradual onset. A notable exception to this is the SVCS due to central venous lines.

Treatment

SVCS has traditionally been considered an oncologic emergency, which may necessitate therapy before determination of a tissue diagnosis. However, this policy has not been substantiated [123]. In most cases of SVCS, it is safe and prudent to clinically evaluate the presence and location of obstruction and to establish a tissue diagnosis before definitive treatment. This clinical evaluation will help formulate the type and aggressiveness of treatment.

In most nonmalignant SVCS, a conservative approach is justified. In the iatrogenic group of SVCS, the removal of the catheter plus anticoagulations is in order.

In malignant SVCS, irradiation initiated with high-dose fractionation is the treatment of choice for NSCCs and for the majority of other metastatic tumors [122].

Combination chemotherapy alone [132] or in combination with radiation therapy is indicated in small-cell bronchogenic carcinomas and non-Hodgkin's lymphomas [133].

Surgical treatment of SVCS has been attempted, but it is at best unconvincing [134]. The use of an intravascular stent has recently been found to have palliative value in persistent SVCS [135].

We find the use of intravenous dexamethasone of value for short-term improvement in patients with high-grade obstruction. Other supportive resources such as an elevated bed, diuretics, and oxygen are helpful.

The ultimate outcome of SVCS is related to the underlying etiology. Except for non-Hodgkin's lymphoma and testicular tumors, patients with malignant SVCSs have a short survival rate, measured in months. In contrast, patients with benign SVCSs may live for years. Unfortunately, malignant SVCSs greatly outnumber benign etiologies.

Conclusion

The specter of lung cancer is frightening to high-risk patients. Many current and ex-cigarette smokers avoid visits to their primary care physician until clear symptoms are evident. Often their lesions are not resectable at this point. This chapter has presented the epidemiology, etiology, and diagnostic evaluation in an effort to prevent or diagnose this often lethal disorder early. The primary care physician plays a pivotal role in this endeavor.

References

1. Robbins SL: *Basic Pathology*. 1976
2. Boring C, Squires T, et al: Cancer statistics, 1992. *Ca-A Cancer Journal for Clinicians* 42: 19–38, 1992
3. McDuffie HH, Kloassen DJ, Dosman JA: Female/male differences in patients with primary lung cancer. *Cancer* 59:1825–1830, 1987
4. Brown CC, Kessler LG: Projection of lung cancer mortality in the United States. *J Natl Cancer Inst* 80:43–51, 1988
5. Winder EL: Tobacco and health: A review of the history and suggestions for public health policy. *Public Health Rep* 103:8–18, 1988
6. Loeb LA, Ernster VL, Warner KE, et al: Smoking and lung cancer, an overview. *Cancer Res* 44:5940, 1984
7. Hammond EC: Smoking habits and air pollution in relation to lung cancer. *In* Lee DHK (ed): Environmental Factors in Respiratory Disease. New York, Academic Press, 1972, pp 177–198
8. Doll R, Hill AB: Mortality in relation to smoking: Ten year observations of British doctors. *Br Med J* 1:1399, 1964
9. Peto R, Doll R: Control of lung cancer. *In* Mizell M, Correa P (eds): Lung Cancer, Causes and Prevention. Deerfield Beach, FL, Verlaj, Chemie International 1984, pp 1–19
10. Wynder EL, Kabat GC: The effect of low yield cigarette smoking on lung cancer risk. *Cancer* 62:1223–1230, 1988
11. Cullen JW: Strategies to stop smoking. *Cancer Prevention* May 1989

12. Lubin JA, Blot WF: Assessment of lung cancer risk factors by histologic category. *J Natl Cancer Inst* 73:383–389, 1984
13. Blot WJ, Fraumeni JF Jr: Passive smoking and cancer. *Cancer Prevention* October 1–8, 1989
14. Craighead JE, Mossman BT: The pathogenesis of asbestos-related diseases. *N Engl J Med* 306:1446, 1982
15. O'Berg MT, Chen JL, Burke CA, et al: Epidemiologic study of workers exposed to acrylonitrile: An update. *J Occup Med* 27:835–840, 1985
16. Sunderman JW: A review of the carcinogenicities of nickel, chromium and arsenic compounds in men and animals. *Prev Med* 5:279–294, 1986
17. Infante PF, Wagoner JK, Sprince NL: Mortality patterns from lung cancer and non-neoplastic respiratory disease among white males in the beryllium case registry. *Environ Res* 21:15–34, 1980
18. Weiss W: Epidemic curve of respiratory cancer due to chloromethyl ethers. *J Nat Cancer Inst* 69:1265–1272, 1982
19. Elinder CG, Kjellstrom T, Hodgstedt C, et al: Cancer mortality of cadmium workers. *Br J Ind Med* 42:651–665, 1985.
20. Waterhouse JAH: Cancer among chromium platers. *Br J Cancer* 32:262, 1975
21. Frank AL: Occupational lung cancer. *In* Harry CC (ed): Pathogenesis and Therapy of Lung Cancer. New York, Marcel Dekker, 1978, pp 25–51
22. Archer VE: Occupational exposure to radiation as a cancer hazard. *Cancer* 39:1802–1806, 1977
23. Alderson M: *Occupational Cancer.* London, Butterworths, 1986
24. Cone JE: Occupational lung cancer. *Occupational Medicine* 2:273–295, 1987
25. Steenland K, Thun M: Interaction between tobacco smoking and occupational exposures in the causation of lung cancer. *J Occup Med* 28:110–118, 1986
26. LaRosa JH, Hines CM: A guide to heart and lung health at the workplace. Washington, DC, US National Institute of Health, Publication No. 86–2210, September 1986
27. Higgins IT: Air pollution and lung cancer, diesel exhaust, coal combustion. *Prev Med* 13:207–218, 1984
28. Fraser D. Lung cancer risk and diesel exhaust exposure. *Public Health Rev* 14:139–171, 1986
29. McDonald JC: Silica silicosis and lung cancer (editorial). *Br J Ind Med* 46:289–291, 1989
30. International Agency for Research on Cancer: Monographs on the evaluation of the carcinogenic risk of chemicals to humans, vol 42. Silica and some silicates. Lyon, *IARC,* 1987
31. Colditz GA, Sdempfer MJ, Willet WC: Diet and lung cancer: A review of the epidemiologic evidence in humans. *Arch Intern Med* 147:157–160, 1987
32. Hinds NW, Kolonel LN, Hankin JH, et al: Dietary vitamin A, carotene, vitamin C and risk of lung cancer in Hawaii. *Am J Epidemiol* 119:227–237, 1984
33. International Agency for Research in Cancer: Monographs on the Evaluation of Carcinogenic Risks to Humans. 43:173–259, 1988
34. Saccomanno G, Yale C, Dixon W, et al: An epidemiological analysis of the relationship between exposure to radon progeny, smoking, and bronchogenic carcinoma in the U-mining population of the Colorado Plateau 1960–1980. *Health Phys* 50:605–618, 1986
35. Howe GR, Nair RC, Newcomb HB, et al: Lung cancer mortality (1950–1980) in relation to radon daughter exposure in a cohort of workers at the Eldorado Beaverlodge Uranium Mine. *J Natl Cancer Inst* 77:3357–3362, 1986
36. Nero AV Jr: Indoor radon exposure and lung cancer. *Cancer Prevention* December 1989
37. Nero AV Jr, Schwehr MB, Nazaroff WW, et al: Distribution of airborne radon 222 concentrations in U.S. homes. *Science* 234:992, 1986
38. Cohen BL: A national survey of radon 222 in U.S. homes and correlating factors. *Health Phys* 51:175, 1986
39. Nazaroff WW, Teichman KY: Indoor radon, exploring policy options for controlling human exposures. Lawrence Berkeley Laboratory Report, LBL-27148, 1989
40. Tilyou SM: The debate over radon continues. *Newsline, The Journal of Nuclear Medicine,* 36:987–996, 1989
41. Minna JD, Pass H, Glatstein E, et al: Cancer of the lung. In Devita V, Hellman S, Rosenberg ES (eds): Cancer Principles and Practice of Oncology, ed 3. Philadelphia, JB Lippincott
42. Yesner R, Carter D: Pathology of carcinoma of the lung. Changing patterns. *Clin Chest Med* 3:257, 1982
43. Mathews MJ, Mackay B, Lukeman J: The pathology of non-small cell cancer of the lung. *Semin Oncol* 10:34, 1983
44. Cohen MH: Signs and symptoms of bronchogenic carcinoma. *Semin Oncol* 3:183, 1974
45. Early Lung Cancer Detection: Summary and conclusions. *Am Rev Respir Dis* 130:565, 1984

46. Spiro SG: Lung cancer diagnosis and staging. Recent Results *Cancer Res* 92:1984
47. MacMahon H, Courtney JV, Little AG: Diagnostic methods in lung cancer. *Semin Oncol* 10:20–33, 1983
48. Savage P, Donovan WN, Dellinger RP: Sputum cytology in the management of patients with lung cancer. *South Med J* 77:840, 1984
49. Martini N, McCormick PM: Assessment of endoscopically visible bronchial carcinomas. *Chest* 73:718, 1978
50. Sanderson DR, Fontana RS, Woolner LB, et al: Bronchoscopic localization of radiographically occult lung cancer. *Chest* 65:608, 1974
51. Doiron DR, Profio E, Vincent RG: Fluorescent bronchoscopy for detection of lung cancer. *Chest* 76:27, 1979
52. Shure D, Fedullo PF: Transbronchial needle aspiration in the diagnosis of submucosal and peribronchial bronchogenic carcinoma. *Chest* 88:49, 1985
53. Shure D, Fedullo PF: Transbronchial needle aspiration of peripheral masses. *Am Rev Respir Dis* 128:1090, 1983
54. Khouri NF, Stitik FP, Erozan YS, et al: Transthoracic needle aspiration biopsy of benign and malignant lung lesions. *Am J Roentgenol* 144:281, 1985
55. Williams RA, Haaga JR, Karagiannis E: CT guided paravertebral biopsy of the mediastinum. *JCAT* 8:575, 1984
56. Boutin C, Cargnino P, Viallet JR: Thoracoscopy in the early diagnosis of malignant pleural effusions. *Endoscopy* 12:155, 1980
57. Spiro SG: Diagnosis and staging. Recent Results *Cancer Res* 92:16–29, 1984
58. Zelen M: Keynote address on biostatistics and data retrieval. *Cancer Chem Rep* 4:31–41, 1973
59. Mountain CF: A new international staging system for lung cancer. *Chest* 89(suppl 4): 2256–2335, 1986
60. Beahrs OH, Henson DE, et al. (eds): Manual for Staging of Cancer, ed 3. Philadelphia, J.B. Lippincott Co, 1988, pp 6–10
61. Beahrs OH, Henson DE, et al (eds): Manual for Staging of Cancer, ed 3. Philadelphia, J.B. Lippincott Co, 1988, pp 115–121
62. Lähde S, Hyrynkangas K, Merikanto J, et al: Computed tomography and mediastinoscopy in the assessment of resectability of lung cancer. *Acta Radiol* 30:169–173, 1989
63. Chasen MH: Imaging primary lung cancers, pleural cancers and metastatic disease. *CA—A Cancer Journal for Clinicians* 37:194–210, 1987
64. Martin N, Heelan R, Wescott J, et al: Comparative methods of conventional, computed tomographic, and magnetic resonance imaging in assessing mediastinal involvement in surgically confined lung carcinoma. *J Thorac Cardiovasc Surg* 90:639–648, 1985
65. Unruh H, Chiu RC-J: Mediastinal assessment for staging and treatment of carcinomas of the lung. *Ann Thorac Surg* 41:224–229, 1986
66. Poon PY, Bronskill MJ, Henkelman RM, et al: Mediastinal lymph node metastases from bronchogenic carcinoma: Detection with MR imaging and CT. *Radiology* 651–656, 1987
67. Poon PY, Bronskill MJ, Henkelman RM, et al: Magnetic resonance imaging of the mediastinum. *J Can Assoc Radiol* 37:173–181, 1986
68. Milroy R, Smith ML, Faichney A, et al: Mediastinal imaging in lung cancer. *Q J Med* 60:715–723, 1986
69. Santiago S, Houston D, Ezer J, et al: Gallium scanning and tomography in the preoperative evaluation of lung cancer. *Cancer* 58: 341–343, 1986
70. Hooper RG, Beechler GR, Johnston MC: Radioisotope scanning in the initial staging of bronchogenic carcinomas. *Am Rev Respir Dis* 118:279–286, 1978
71. Williams SJ, Green M, Kerr IH: Detection of bone metastases in carcinoma of the bronchus. *Br Med J* 1:1004, 1977
72. Signori EE: The value of baseline bone and liver scans in the initial staging of primary breast cancer following mastectomy. *In* Proceedings, PS 11.1-2:4-7, part 282, XIII International Conference Chemotherapy, Vienna, Austria, 1983
73. Ashraf MH, Milsom PL, Walesby RK: Selection by mediastinoscopy and long term survival in bronchial carcinoma. *Ann Thorac Surg* 30:208–214, 1980
74. Mountain CF: Assessment of the role of surgery for control of lung cancer. *Ann Thorac Surg* 24:365–373, 1977
75. Baker RR, Ettinger DS, Ruckdeschel JD, et al: The role of surgery in the management of selected patients with small cell carcinoma of the lung. *J Clin Oncol* 5:697–702, 1987
76. Mountain CF, Hermes KE: Management implications of surgical staging studies. *In* Muggio F, Rozencweig M (eds): Lung Cancer: Progress in Therapeutic Research. New York, Raven Press, 1979, pp 233–242
77. Hansen HH, Dombernowsky P: Small cell anaplastic carcinoma of the lung: Staging. *In* Livingston RG (ed): Lung Cancer 1. The Hague, Martin Nijhoff, 1981, pp 157–168
78. Drings P, Konig R, Vogt-Moykopf: Diagnostic procedures in small cell lung carcinoma. Recent results. *Cancer Res* 97:87–106, 1985
79. Souhami RL, Bradbery I, Geddes DM, et al:

Prognostic significance of laboratory parameters measured at diagnosis in small cell carcinomas of the lung. *Cancer Res* 45:2878–2882, 1985
80. Pistenma DA, McDougall IR, Kriss JP: Screening for bone metastases. Are only scans necessary? *JAMA* 231:46–50, 1975
81. Hirsch RF, Hansen HH, Hainau B: Bilateral bone marrow examinations in small cell anaplastic carcinoma of the lung. *Acta Pathol Microbiol Scand* 87:59–62, 1979
82. Hirsch FR, Hansen HH: Bone marrow involvement in small cell anaplastic carcinoma of the lung. Prognosis and therapeutic aspects. *Cancer* 46:206–221, 1980
83. Bunn PA, Schlam M, Gazdar A: Comparison of cytology and DNA content analysis by flow cytometry in specimens from lung cancer patients (abstr). *Proc Am Soc Clin Oncol* 21:40, 1980
84. Bunn PA, Nugent J, Matthews MJ: Central nervous system metastases in small cell bronchogenic carcinoma. *Semin Oncol* 5:314–322, 1978
85. Hirsch FR, Paulson OB, Hansen HH, et al: Intracranial metastases in small cell carcinoma of the lung: Correlation of clinical and autopsy findings. *Cancer* 50:2433, 1982
86. Abrams J, Austin Doyle L, Aisner J: Staging prognostic factors and special considerations in small cell lung cancer. *Semin Oncol* 15: 261–277, 1988
87. Biomarker Profiles. Written communication. Dianon Systems, Inc., Stratford, CT 1986
88. Sahin AA, Ro JY, et al: Flow cytometric analysis of the DNA content of non-small cell lung cancer. *Cancer* 65:530–537, 1990
89. Isobe H, Miyamoto H, et al: Prognostic and therapeutic significance of the flow cytometric nuclear DNA content in non-small cell lung cancer. *Cancer* 65:1391–1395, 1990
90. Slebos RJC, Kibbelaar RE, et al: K-ras oncogene activation as a prognostic marker in adenocarcinoma of the lung. *N Engl J Med* 323(August 30):561–565, 1990
91. Van Trigt P, Wolfe GW: Laser therapy for palliation of bronchogenic and eosphageal carcinoma. *In* Roth, Ruck, Descher, et al (eds): *Thoracic Oncology*. 1989
92. Choi NC, Grillo HC, Huberman MS: Lung cancer. *In* Blake C (ed): Cancer Manual, ed. 17. American Cancer Society, Massachusetts Division, 1986
93. Moghissi K: Local excision of pulmonary nodular (coin) lesion with non-contact yttrium-aluminum garnet laser. *Thorac Cardiovasc Surg* 97:147–151, 1989
94. Godwin JD: The solitary nodule. *Radiol Clin North Am* 21:709–721, 1973
95. Heater K, MacMahon H, Vyborny CJ: Occult lung carcinoma presenting with dysphagia—the value of computed tomography. *Clinical Imaging* 13:122–126, 1989
96. Stoller JK, Ahmad M, Rice TW: Solitary pulmonary nodule. *Cleveland Clinic Med* 55: 68–74, 1988
97. Anderson RW, Arentzen CE: Carcinoma of the lung. *Surg Clin North Am* 60:793–814, 1980
98. Siegelman SS, Khouri NF, Scott WW Jr, et al: Pulmonary hamartomas: CT findings. *Radiology* 160:313–317, 1986
99. Good CA, Wilson TW: The solitary circumscribed pulmonary nodule: Study of seven hundred five cases encountered roentgenologically in a period of three and one-half years. *JAMA* 166:210–215, 1958
100. Geddes DM, Elliott M: The solitary pulmonary nodule. *Br Med J* 298:67–68, 1989
101. Ishida T, Oka T, Nishino T, et al: Inflammatory pseudo-tumor of the lung in adults: Radiographic and clinicopathological analysis. *Ann Thorac Surg* 48:90–95, 1989
102. Wandtke JC, Plewes DB, McFaul JA: Improved pulmonary nodule detection with scanning equalization radiography. *Radiology* 169:23–27, 1988
103. Zerhouni E: Computed tomography of the pulmonary parenchyma: An overview. *Chest* 95:901–907, 1989
104. Rohwedder JJ: The solitary pulmonary nodule. A new diagnostic agenda (editorial). *Chest* 93:1124–1125, 1988
105. Zerhouni EA, Stitik FP, Siegelman SS, et al: Computed tomography of the solitary pulmonary nodule. A national cooperative study. *Radiology* 160:319–327, 1986
106. Würsten HU, Vock P: Mediastinal infiltration of lung carcinoma (T4N0-1): The positive predictive value of computed tomography. *Thorac Cardiovasc Surg* 35:355–360, 1987
107. Webb WR: The role of magnetic resonance imaging in the assessment of patients with lung cancer: A comparison with computed tomography. *J Thorac Imaging* 4:65–75, 1989
108. Müller NL, Gamsu G, Webb WR: Pulmonary nodules: Detection using magnetic resonance and computed tomography. *Radiology* 155:687–690, 1985
109. Wagner ED, Ramzy I. Greenberg S, et al: Transbronchial fine-needle aspiration. Reliability and limitations. *Am J Clin Pathol* 92: 36–41, 1989
110. Knox AJ, Mascie-Taylor BH, Page RL: Fiberoptic bronchoscopy in the elderly: Four years' experience. *Br J Dis Chest* 82:290–293, 1988

111. Kealy WF, Hogan JM, Hurley MF: Percutaneous fine needle aspiration of pulmonary mass lesions—A critical examination of the accuracy of cell typing of malignant tumors. *Ir J Med Sci* 158:85–87, 1989
112. Caya JG, Clowry LJ, Wollenberg N, et al: Transthoracic fine needle aspiration cytology. *Am J Clin Pathol* 82:100–103, 1984
113. Dziura BR: Fine needle aspiration of the lung: A pathologist's perspective. *J Thorac Imaging* 2:49–51, 1987
114. Steen-Hansen E, Thommesen P: Clinical management of the benign cytological report in patients with solitary pulmonary nodules. *Rüntgen-Bl* 41:458–461, 1988
115. Penketh ARL, Robinson AA, Barker V, et al: Use of percutaneous needle biopsy in the investigation of solitary pulmonary nodules. *Thorax* 42:967–971, 1987
116. Page RD, Jeffrey RR, Donnelly RJ: Thoracoscopy: A review of 121 consecutive surgical procedures. *Ann Thorac Surg* 48:66–68, 1989
117. Hix WR, Aaron BL: Solitary pulmonary nodule. What should be included in the work up? *Postgrad Med* 86:57–58, 63–64, 1989
118. Cummings SR, Lillington GA, Richard RJ: Estimating the probability of malignancy in solitary pulmonary nodules. *Am Rev Respir Dis* 134:449–452, 453–460, 1986
119. Drings P: Preoperative assessment of lung cancer. *Chest* (suppl 96):42S–44S, 1989
120. Silverman NA, Sabiston DC: Mediastinal masses. *Surg Clin North Am* 60:757, 1980
121. Newell JD: Evaluation of pulmonary and mediastinal masses. *Med Clin North Am* 68: 1463, 1984
122. Perez CA, Presant CA, VanAmburg III AL: Management of superior vena cava syndrome. *Semin Oncol* 5:123–134, 1978
123. Schraufnagel DE, Hill R, Leech JA, et al: Superior vena cava obstruction—Is it a medical emergency? *Am J Med* 70:1169–1174, 1981
124. Sculier JP, Feld R: Superior vena cava obstruction syndrome: Recommendations for management. *Cancer Treat Rev* 12:209–218, 1985
125. Fritz T, Richeson JF, Fitzpatrick P, et al: Venous obstruction. A potential complication of transvenous pacemaker electrodes. *Chest* 83:534–539, 1983
126. Baiocchi L, Cohen A: Superior vena cava thrombosis following subclavian vein catheterization. *J Cardiovasc Surg* 22:190–193, 1981
127. Parish JM, Marschke RF Jr, Dines DE, et al: Etiologic considerations in SVCS. *Mayo Clinic Proc* 56:407–413, 1981
128. Gollub S, Hirose T, Klauber J: Scintigraphic sequelae of superior vena caval obstruction. *Clin Nucl Med* 5:89–93, 1980
129. Scrantino C, Salazar OM, Rubin P, et al: The optimum radiation schedule in treatment of superior vena caval obstruction: Importance of 99m Tc scintiangiograms. *Int J Radiol Oncol Biol Phys* 5:1987–1995, 1979
130. Struse TB: Demonstration of a progressive superior vena caval obstruction reversed following radiation therapy. *Clin Nucl Med* 1:247–250, 1976
131. Yahalom J: Superior vena cava syndrome. *In* DeVita VT Jr, Hellman S, Rosenberg SA (eds): Cancer Principles and Practice of Oncology, ed 3. Philadelphia, JB Lippincott 1989, pp 1971–1977
132. Spiro SG, Shah S, Harper PG, et al: Treatment of obstruction of the superior vena cava by combination chemotherapy with and without irradiation in small cell carcinoma of the bronchus. *Thorax* 38:501–505, 1983
133. Perez-Soler R, McLaughlin P, Velosquez WS, et al: Clinical features and results of management of superior vena cava syndrome secondary to lymphoma. *J Clin Oncol* 2:260–266, 1984
134. Dortevelle P, Chapelier A, Navajas M, et al: Replacement of the superior vena cava with polytetra fluoroethylene grafts combined with resection of mediastinal-pulmonary malignant tumors. *J Thorac Cardiovasc Surg* 94: 361–366, 1987
135. Soldes OS, Carrosco CH, Charnsangavej C, et al: Use of stents in superior vena caval obstruction secondary to neoplastic disease. *The Cancer Bulletin* 42:359–364, 1990

Normal Sleep and Biologic Rhythms

Sheldon Kapen

Although modern research into basic sleep mechanisms began almost 40 years ago, in the United States attention has been given to sleep disorders only in the last 15 years, and its dissemination in the medical community and introduction into medical school curricula has occurred only in the last decade. During that latter period the importance of the sleep-wake cycle as a factor in health and the pathophysiology of many diseases has become increasingly clear, as evidenced by the proliferation of certified sleep disorder centers throughout the nation. One area for which an awareness of sleep disorders is particularly important is pulmonary medicine, because sleep and biologic rhythms can have a direct effect on respiration. This chapter reviews the physiology and biochemistry of the sleep-wake cycle and the principles of biologic rhythms.

Normal Sleep Cycle: Physiologic Description of Sleep in the Adult

Sleep Architecture

The normal sleep cycle can be assessed in physiologic terms by polysomnography, which is the measurement of multiple biologic functions during sleep. Sleep is a dynamically changing process, with a distinct architecture characterized by temporal progression of the various sleep stages, which can be divided into rapid eye movement (REM) and nonrapid eye movement sleep (NREM) [1]. NREM sleep consists of stages 1 to 4, which demonstrate not only changes in the background electroencephalogram (EEG) but also show progressive elevations of the threshold for arousal by external stimuli (Fig. 21-1). The normal EEG background during relaxed waking with the eyes closed consists of an alpha rhythm, with a frequency of 8 to 12 cycles per second (cps) and a greater prominence over the posterior leads of the scalp (parietal and occipital regions). With the onset of stage 1, corresponding to drowsiness, there is a decrease in amplitude, desynchronization, and the elimination of the alpha rhythm, accompanied by slow rolling eye movements. Stage 2 is characterized by a predominant theta rhythm (4 to 7 cps) and the presence of spindles, which are brief transients with an internal frequency of 12 to 15 cps occurring at a rate of six to eight times per minute, with a duration of 1 to 2 seconds. K complexes, also present in stage 2 sleep, are biphasic transients of high amplitude and are seen best at the vertex of the skull (Fig. 21-1). The cerebral cortex undergoes transient inhibition during the spindles and transient facilitation during the K complexes [2]. The latter may occur spontaneously or in response to an external stimulus (e.g., a phone ringing). Frequently, spindles are seen at the onset or on the trailing edge of K complexes. Stages 3 and 4, the deepest stages of sleep, reveal the increasing presence of delta activity (1 to 3 cps) and a decrease of sleep spindles and K complexes. By convention, delta waves make up 20% to 50% of the background in stage 3 and over 50% of stage 4 [1].

On being aroused during the REM stage of sleep, a subject will report having a dream 70% of the time. REM dreams are bizarre, highly visual, divorced from normal temporal constraints and usual standards of credibility, and "single-minded" in the terminology of Rechtschaffen [3], by which he means the relentless pursuit of the goals of the dream, regardless of the implausibility or unlikelihood of their attainment. Freud alluded to these

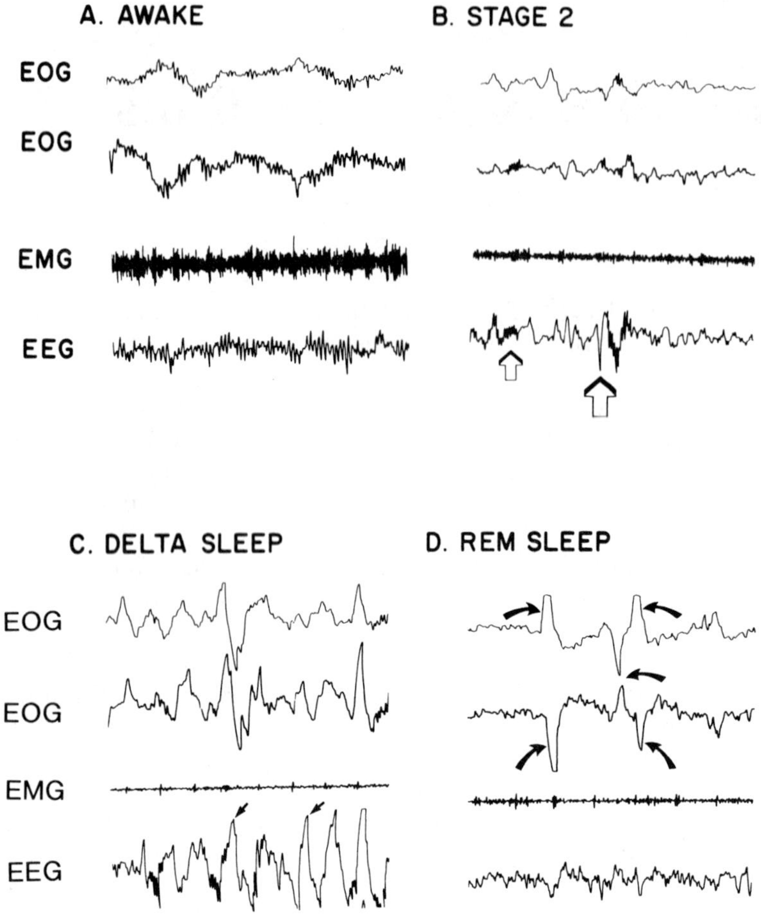
A. AWAKE
B. STAGE 2
EOG
EOG
EMG
EEG
C. DELTA SLEEP
D. REM SLEEP
EOG
EOG
EMG
EEG

Fig. 21-1. Sleep stages. (A) Awake. Relatively high EMG with a predominantly alpha rhythm in the EEG. (B) Stage 2 sleep. Note relative muscular relaxation as manifested by a lower amplitude EMG. Smaller arrow on the EEG channel points to a sleep spindle and the larger arrow to a K complex. (C) Delta or slow wave sleep. Note predominance of high voltage slow waves (small arrows) that also may be seen in the eye leads because delta waves are predominantly frontal in origin. (D) REM sleep. Note rapid eye movements (curved arrows), very low EMG suggestive of muscular atonia, and a low voltage, mixed frequency EEG pattern similar to stage 1 (drowsiness). EOG, electro-oculogram; EMG, electromyogram of mentalis muscles; EEG, electroencephalogram from a central lead.

thought patterns and termed them primary process, in contrast to secondary process thought patterns, which he described as the type occurring during rational waking activity.

REM sleep is recognized neurophysiologically by not only the EEG but by the characteristics of the electro-oculogram and the electromyogram of the mentalis muscles (Fig. 21-1). The EEG background is similar to that of stage 1. The electro-oculogram shows frequent, random REMs singly and in bursts. The electromyogram is at its lowest level and may fall to zero. Somatic musculature is inhibited during REM sleep except for the extraocular muscles and the diaphragm. During REM sleep, the brain is otherwise quite active and neurons in many central nervous system nuclei reach their highest frequency of firing. The autonomic nervous system undergoes great variability, particularly heart rate and arterial blood pressure, which increase and decrease randomly and seemingly chaotically [4]. The regulation of respiration is also different during REM sleep. While metabolic control (feedback by blood gases and pH) is dominant during NREM sleep, it is suppressed during REM sleep and is superseded by open-loop stimulation from higher centers, the behavioral mode of regulation [5]. The latter is responsible for the interruption of rhythmic respiration during wakefulness, so as to allow speech, swallowing, etc. All the autonomic changes are particularly evident during bursts of REMs while the interburst periods are associated with relative autonomic quiescence.

Penile erection (tumescence) is an important autonomic event associated with REM sleep [6]. Beginning in childhood and continuing until old age, tumescence appears with the onset of each REM period and subsides with its termination. However, the nightly duration of tumescence decreases in older people by about 50%. The ubiquity of REM-associated nocturnal penile tumescence and its reliability are useful in differentiating organic from psychogenic impotence. This is because nocturnal tumescence is decreased or eliminated when the cause of impotence is organic, while tumescence is unaffected by psychogenic impotence. Organic impotence is most commonly caused by diabetes; the side effects of medications, particularly antihypertensive drugs; and neurologic problems such as spinal cord damage.

The features of REM sleep may be divided into those that are tonic (i.e., relatively unchanged throughout the REM period) and those that are phasic (i.e., intermittent or paroxysmal) (Table 21-1) [7]. Tonic phenomena include EEG desynchronization, muscle atonia, and a theta rhythm in the hippocampus of subprimate mammals. REMs, singly and in bursts, are a prominent phasic event. Other phasic events include sawtooth waves on the EEG, muscle twitches superimposed on the inhibition, more profound transient muscle inhibition occurring during REMs, autonomic events, pontine-geniculate-occipital (PGO) spikes; and penile tumescence [8]. PGO spikes are biphasic potentials that can be recorded in experimental animals by means of electrodes implanted in the above areas of the visual system. They originate in the pons, from which they are disseminated to more rostral structures. PGO spikes are considered to represent pacemakers of the phasic events seen in REM sleep. They begin to appear during the last few moments of slow wave sleep and continue to be recorded singly and in bursts throughout the REM period. The differences in physiology between periods of phasic phenomena and those of quiescence are so profound as to almost justify two separate states of REM sleep—phasic and nonphasic.

For adults, stage 1 accounts for 5% to 10%

Table 21-1. Tonic and Phasic Features of REM Sleep

Tonic	*Phasic*
EEG desynchronization	REMs
Decreased or absent tone in somatic musculature	Intermittent enhanced inhibition of somatic musculature
Theta rhythm in hippocampus (in subprimates)	Myoclonic jerks
	Autonomic variability
	Pontine-geniculate-occipital (PGO) spikes
	Penile tumescence

of total sleep, stage 2 for 50%, stages 3 and 4 for 15% to 20%, and REM for 20% to 25% [9]. These figures that are normal for adults are quite different for newborns, young children, and older individuals (over age 65).

Sleep Continuity

Sleep continuity refers to the latency, sustainability, and persistence of sleep. Sleep onset or latency is usually expressed as the time that transpires from the moment of first reposing to the onset of the first 10 minutes of undisturbed sleep. Other measures include wakefulness after the onset of sleep, the number of awakenings 15 seconds or more in duration, the number of briefer arousals, and the number of stage changes. The percent of stage 1 is a good index of disrupted sleep and is usually elevated in patients with obstructive sleep apnea.

Rapid Eye Movement Measures

The normal sleep cycle begins with NREM sleep, which progressively increases in depth and continues for 90 to 100 minutes until the first REM period takes place. The time from sleep onset to the beginning of the first REM period is termed REM latency. Thereafter, REM periods occur approximately every 90 minutes. Successive REM periods tend to be longer in duration and the REM-NREM cycles tend to be shorter. REM latencies less than 60 minutes are considered abnormally short, as in the majority of cases of endogenous depression. The vast majority of narcoleptics have sleep-onset REM periods, defined as latencies less than 20 minutes.

Ontogeny of Sleep

Sleep in the Normal Infant

The EEG of newborns is immature and cannot be used for staging sleep by adult standards. For instance, sleep spindles and K complexes only appear by the age of 2 months, and a well-organized alpha rhythm is also absent at birth [10]. The overall frequencies of the EEG are also slower than in the adult. For these reasons, the terminology is different in the newborn and young infant; instead of NREM sleep, we recognize quiet sleep, and active sleep is analogous to REM sleep. Quiet sleep is characterized by a pattern known as *tracé alternans* until the age of 6 to 8 weeks. This pattern features periodic bursts of high amplitude slow waves alternating with periods of lower amplitude faster activity. Breathing is regular and there are no body movements. During active sleep, the EEG pattern is continuous; there are also irregular respiration and twitches of the trunk and extremities.

Until the age of approximately 10 months, sleep-onset REM periods are normal, although not necessarily dominant [10]. Furthermore, active sleep accounts for 45% to 50% of total sleep time at birth (the percent is even higher in premature babies). This decreases to about 30% at 1 year of life. Thus, with maturation, active sleep decreases and quiet sleep increases, a process that is perhaps consistent with the progressive development of inhibitory mechanisms within the brain. Young infants also have a more polycyclic pattern to their sleep-wake cycle, in that they have alternating periods of sleep and wakefulness throughout the 24 hours. With advancing age, sleep becomes more confined to the nocturnal hours except for residual daytime napping [10].

Sleep in the Aged

Although mild changes occur in sleep characteristics throughout the life span, aging traits become noticeable after age 50 and particularly after age 65. The most prominent change in the sleep pattern is the greater disruption caused by poor sleep maintenance [11]. Sleep latency is relatively preserved, but there are increased numbers of arousals and awakenings and an enhanced wakefulness after sleep onset. Along with these alterations in sleep continuity, there is a tendency for more daytime napping, which adds to the nocturnal sleep problem by impairing sleep hygiene and regularity. These features of aged sleep correlate with increasing complaints of insomnia in older people. In addition, numerous studies have documented a higher incidence of obstructive sleep apnea and nocturnal myoclonus in the senior population [12, 13]. Since these disorders may profoundly disrupt sleep, they may account for some of the sleep maintenance problems, although it is unclear to what extent they contribute.

Delta sleep is markedly decreased in the aged [14]. When amplitude and frequency criteria are both taken into account, some older subjects may have a complete absence of stages 3 and 4. This phenomenon has received much attention in the literature and indeed is as prominent as insomnia in distinguishing the sleep of elderly people. The total duration and percentage of REM sleep tend to be preserved. However, REM latency tends to decrease with age, although with wide variability [15].

Sleep Deprivation

Individuals vary widely in the daily amount of sleep they require [16]. This variability is also seen at different stages of a person's life and on a day-to-day basis, depending on environmental and physiologic influences. Thus, one person's shortfall is another person's normal allotment of sleep. Sleep deprivation, measured by an individual's own need, leads first and foremost to sleepiness and fatigue, which are accompanied by malaise, irritability, and impaired concentration and vigilance [17]. When recovery sleep takes place, there is a marked increase of delta sleep, both in quantity and intensity [17]. This corresponds with the general belief that stages 3 and 4 represent the restorative function of sleep, the lack of which leads to sleepiness and its accompanying symptoms.

Any serious study of partial or total sleep deprivation requires a method of quantifying sleepiness. There is a subjective scale, the Stanford Sleepiness Scale [18], which has proved useful in the past, but the gold standard is undoubtedly the Multiple Sleep Latency Test, first introduced by Richardson et al [19] and elaborated by Carskadon and Dement [20]. The subject is allowed five opportunities to sleep during the day, typically beginning at 10:00 AM. He or she is instructed to relax and try to doze off while being recorded with electrodes for sleep staging. Between naps, the subject is prevented from sleeping. The end point for each nap is the first appearance of stage 1 on the polysomnogram, and the mean of all the naps is an index of sleepiness. Normal individuals have a mean latency of about 15 minutes, while less than 10 minutes signifies sleepiness. In almost all subjects, the latency dips during the 2:00 PM nap. This is called the "postlunch dip," but it is really a result of an endogenous rhythm of alertness and drowsiness and not due to the ingestion of a meal.

The Multiple Sleep Latency Test is quite effective in measuring excessive sleepiness in normal individuals that results from insufficient sleep [21] or hypnotic administration [22]. As such, it can be used to follow the effects of jet lag and shift work (see following sections). Studies in adolescent [23] and aged subjects [24] have revealed widespread, previously unrecognized sleepiness resulting from an unmet sleep need or from pathophysiologic processes. The Multiple Sleep Latency Test has now become routine in clinical sleep laboratories in the work-up of patients with sleep disorders such as obstructive sleep apnea syndrome and narcolepsy.

Sleep as a Biologic Rhythm

Under normal circumstances, the hours when a person falls asleep and awakes are fairly constant from day to day. These events are entrained by the light-dark cycle and social influences. Most other functions of the body are entrained to the same cycle and are constantly phase related to each other, resulting in a condition known as internal synchronization, which is explained more fully in the section on The Suprachiasmatic Nucleus, below. This section addresses two fundamental questions regarding the control of the sleep-wake cycle.

Question number 1: What controls the normal alternation of sleep and wakefulness? Tonic wakefulness, attention, vigilance, and phasic arousal are dependent on the normal functioning of the ascending reticular activating system [25]. This encompasses a series of collections of cells, which occupy the tegmentum of the brain stem from the medulla to the midbrain. In 1949, Moruzzi and Magoun [25] found that stimulation of the reticular formation at high frequencies aroused drowsy or sleeping cats and desynchronized (activated) the electrocorticogram in a manner similar to that of natural wakefulness. Later, Lindsley et al [26] reported that destruction of the reticular core resulted in a hypersomnolent state, thus confirming that the reticular formation is tonically active.

The discovery of the area responsible for wakefulness suggested that sleep is a passive process secondary to deactivation of this area, the ascending reticular activating system. However, later work pointed to sleep as an active process precipitated by sleep-inducing centers. Three of these centers have been identified: the nucleus and tractus solitarius, located in the dorsolateral tegmentum of the medulla [27] (Figs. 21-2A and 2F); the raphe nuclei, part of the serotonergic system and located in the midline of the pons and midbrain [28] (Figs. 21-2C and 2E); and the basal forebrain, cholinergic structures found in the ventromedial parts of the forebrain near the basal ganglia and hypothalamus [29, 30] (Fig. 21-2D). Destruction of any one of these areas results in insomnia in experimental animals, whereas stimulation, particularly of the basal forebrain, leads to behavioral and EEG signs of sleep.

Question Number 2: What controls the REM-NREM cycle? The periodic appearance of REM sleep seems to be controlled by mechanisms located in the pontine area of the brain stem [31]. REM sleep is triggered by cholinergic systems scattered throughout the pontine tegmentum and is turned off by the noradrenergic nucleus, the locus coeruleus, located in the dorsolateral tegmentum of the pons [32] (Figs. 21-2B and 2F), and by the serotonergic cells of the raphe nuclei [33] (Figs. 21-2C and 2E). Reciprocal interrelationships between these areas have been demonstrated by numerous pharmacologic and neurophysiologic studies.

The Biologic Clock

The Suprachiasmatic Nucleus

Most, if not all, physiologic activities are periodic, in that they have peaks and nadirs within a 24-hour cycle set by the solar day of 24 hours [34]. This property is true for both complex behaviors and for subcellular functions. A set of environmental zeitgebers (literally, time givers) control and eventually entrain all the bodily rhythms. The most prominent of these are the light-dark cycle and the societal rhythm of rest and activity. The multitude of circadian rhythms (*circa,* about; *dian,* day) do not all have the same phases, but under normal conditions, they have a constant phase relationship to each other. For instance, the most prominent rhythms reach their nadirs during sleep and their peaks or acrophase (the time of the statistically derived highest amplitude of a rhythm) during the activity period. Characteristically, cortisol secretion is highest during the early morning hours [35]; REM sleep propensity is greatest during the latter part of sleep [36]; and body temperature reaches its acrophase in late afternoon [34]. Most performance rhythms follow that of body temperature rather closely, but a notable exception is memory function, which tends to peak during the late morning hours [37]. The end result is internal synchronization, a complicated temporal network of phase relationships, with distinct timing for specific rhythms [34].

When humans or experimental animals are isolated from all time cues, a process called free running takes place [34]. The rhythmic activities, freed from entrainment, have cycles that are approximately, but not exactly, 24 hours in length. The usual cycle length for humans is about 25 hours, while for nocturnal animals it generally is shorter than 24 hours [38]. The reorganization of circadian rhythms into a new steady state under free-running conditions proves that there is an internal biologic clock, or oscillator, that acts independently when freed from the constraints of entrainment [39]. Although inter-

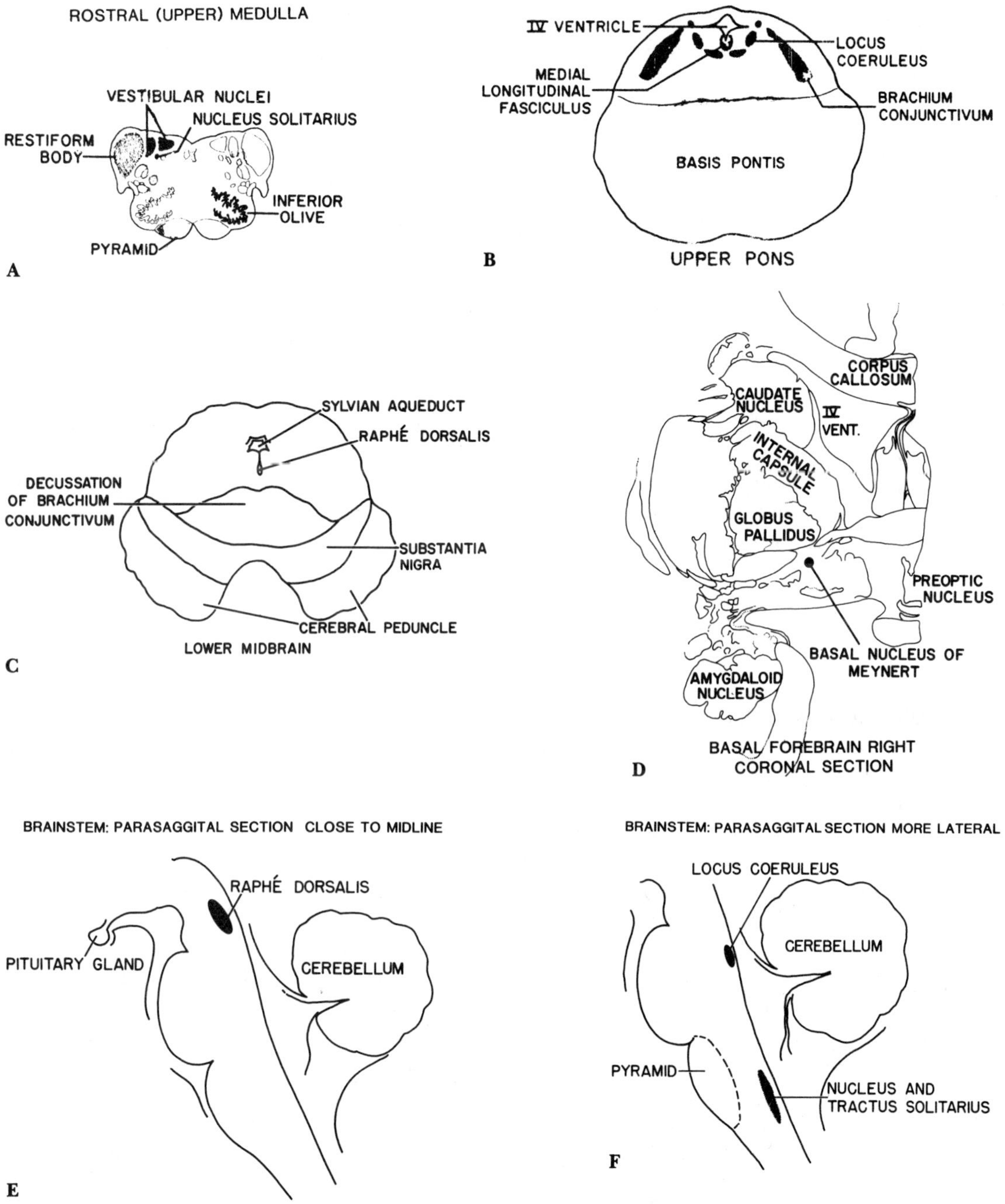
ROSTRAL (UPPER) MEDULLA
VESTIBULAR NUCLEI
NUCLEUS SOLITARIUS
RESTIFORM BODY
INFERIOR OLIVE
PYRAMID
A
IV VENTRICLE
LOCUS COERULEUS
MEDIAL LONGITUDINAL FASCICULUS
BRACHIUM CONJUNCTIVUM
BASIS PONTIS
B
UPPER PONS
SYLVIAN AQUEDUCT
RAPHÉ DORSALIS
DECUSSATION OF BRACHIUM CONJUNCTIVUM
SUBSTANTIA NIGRA
CEREBRAL PEDUNCLE
LOWER MIDBRAIN
C
CORPUS CALLOSUM
CAUDATE NUCLEUS
IV VENT.
INTERNAL CAPSULE
GLOBUS PALLIDUS
PREOPTIC NUCLEUS
BASAL NUCLEUS OF MEYNERT
AMYGDALOID NUCLEUS
BASAL FOREBRAIN RIGHT CORONAL SECTION
D
BRAINSTEM: PARASAGGITAL SECTION CLOSE TO MIDLINE
RAPHÉ DORSALIS
PITUITARY GLAND
CEREBELLUM
E
BRAINSTEM: PARASAGGITAL SECTION MORE LATERAL
LOCUS COERULEUS
CEREBELLUM
PYRAMID
NUCLEUS AND TRACTUS SOLITARIUS
F

Fig. 21-2. Schematic drawings of important sleep-inducing areas. (A) Cross-section of upper medulla showing nucleus solitarius. (B) Cross-section of upper pons showing locus coeruleus. (C) Cross-section of lower midbrain showing nucleus raphe dorsalis. (D) Cross-section at level of basal ganglia (right half) showing several important parts of the basal forebrain including the preoptic nucleus and the basal nucleus of Meynert. (E) Parasagittal cut of brainstem near midline showing nucleus raphe dorsalis. (F) More lateral parasagittal cut of brainstem showing locus coeruleus and nucleus and tractus solitarius.

nal synchronization is still the case in free-running organisms, phase relationships are different from those that are present under conditions of entrainment. For instance, the temperature rhythm advances so that the nadir occurs closer to sleep onset and likewise, REM latency becomes shorter than usual [39].

What are the principles governing circadian rhythms? How does the biologic clock respond to environmental perturbation? Light stimuli have received close attention in recent years. When a free-running experimental animal in constant darkness (termed DD) is exposed to a light pulse, the response depends on the relative timing of the pulse [38]. Most experiments have used locomotor activity cycles of rodents as an end point. Under constant conditions, the animals become active for part of the cycle and inactive for the remainder. The active phase is termed the subjective night since these are nocturnally active animals. When the experimental subject is exposed to a light pulse during the first part of the active phase, it responds with a delay in the onset and offset of the next period of activity [38]. On the other hand, a light pulse occurring during the latter part of the active phase and the first several hours of the subjective day results in an advance of these end points. A light pulse has no demonstrable effect during other phases of the rest-activity cycle. Plotting the effect of these pulses (delay or advance) against circadian time (the phase of the circadian cycle) leads to a phase-response curve, which represents the direction and magnitude of a phase shift in response to any particular stimulus [38]. These phase shifts are thought to represent the actual change in timing of the biologic clock.

Until recently, humans were thought to be impervious to the phase-shifting effects of light stimuli. However, several reports have documented responses to light stimuli quite similar to those in lower animals. Using the body temperature as a marker, Czeisler et al [40] described definite resetting effects of light in normal volunteers. The same researchers had previously reported a phase delay in sleep onset induced by evening bright light in an elderly woman suffering from insomnia [41]. Light stimuli were employed more recently to improve the adaptation of shift workers on a night work schedule [42]. Finally, various schedules of evening or morning bright light exposure have been successfully used for patients suffering from seasonal affective disorder, in whom winter depression is a presumed consequence of seasonally short daylight exposure [43].

Several other important properties of the biologic clock should be mentioned. When free running is carried out in constant darkness, it may go on indefinitely. If constant light is applied, the rest-activity cycle length (or tau) is usually longer than in constant darkness [34]. Furthermore, higher light intensities increase the tendency to disruption of the circadian rhythms and eventual arrhythmicity results, characterized by random episodes of rest and activity [39]. Another well-recognized phenomenon is that of splitting, in which the activity phase divides into two separate periods, each with its own cycle length [34], thus suggesting that there may be two oscillators instead of one. An analogous phenomenon in free-running humans is seen in about 25% of individuals. Approximately 2 weeks after the onset of free running, the sleep-wake cycle suddenly assumes a much longer cycle length, up to 45 to 50 hours, but the temperature cycle does not lengthen and indeed, actually shortens minimally, e.g., from 24.6 to 24.4 hours [39].

An effective method of explaining these events is to propose a dual oscillator model, in which an interaction between the oscillators occurs [39]. One of these oscillators may be the suprachiasmatic nucleus (SCN) [44], a small paired structure at the base of the brain on either side of the midline just above the optic chiasm. When the SCN is destroyed, the sleep-wake cycle and several other rhythmic processes become arrhythmic [45]. Cellular recording techniques and radioactive tracer metabolic studies have revealed enhanced activity within the SCN during daylight hours and reduced activity in the dark [46, 47]. These properties are those that would be expected if the SCN acted as a clock, and indeed the surgically isolated SCN continues to show circadian rhythms of cellular activity since, even when SCN tissue is removed from the brain and studied in culture, periodic cellular activity continues for many cycles [48].

The SCN is entrained by the light-dark cycle via a nerve bundle that branches off the optic nerve, called the retinohypothalamic tract [49]. The SCN controls the biologic rhythms of many target organs, including those of the pineal gland. It is well recognized that melatonin synthesis and secretion by the pineal gland occur mainly in the dark [50]. Thus, the pineal gland is an important timekeeper, measuring the length of the day and acting as a photoperiodic neural/humoral transducer.

Jet Lag

Rapid travel across time zones leads to a mismatch between the phase of the endogenous clock and that of the new environmental cycle. For instance, a flight to London from New York might leave at 9:00 PM New York time (3:00 AM London time) and arrive at 4:00 AM (10:00 AM). At 11:00 PM London time, the traveler's body time is 5:00 PM, an hour not conducive to sleep, despite the probable sleep deprivation the traveler suffered during the actual flight. Adaptation occurs at a rate of approximately 1 hour per day, meaning that it might take 1 week to adapt to a new time zone after an intercontinental flight [51]. Furthermore, different rhythms such as cortisol and body temperature adapt at different rates, leading to a syndrome of fatigue, malaise, dysphoria, and overall poor functioning that is commonly known as "jet lag" [51]. When traveling in a westward direction, coping mechanisms are more efficient, jet lag is less severe, and adaptation is more rapid than is the case when traveling eastward [52]. This is because the free-running endogenous cycle length is greater than 24 hours, and it is thus easier to delay rhythms, or put off going to bed (westward) than to advance them, or to try to go to sleep earlier (eastward) [34].

The effects of jet lag can be partially alleviated by behavioral approaches. For instance, for several days before the trip a traveller can manipulate his or her daily schedule to conform as much as possible to that of the destination. Thus, before the flight to London, one could retire several hours earlier than usual. A second approach involves the use of a short-acting benzodiazepine, such as triazolam [22] or midazolam, to enhance sleep onset and maintenance at circadian times that would otherwise not be conducive to sleep. There is evidence that these agents may also act to phase shift the biologic clock [53, 54], a feature that would add to their hypnotic properties. Also, melatonin, in pharmacologic doses, may have phase-shifting properties [55], and light stimuli may be useful, as is discussed in the next section on shift work [42].

Shift Work

About 20% to 25% of all workers in developed countries are employed in shift work [56], either on a rotating or permanent basis. When working on a night shift, an employee is expected to be in an active, alert state during a period when mental and physiologic processes governed by the biologic clock are usually at their nadirs. Furthermore, the majority of people are resting at that time, which adds social reinforcement to what the shift worker's body is telling him or her. To understand the impact of shift work on the individual and on his or her quality of work, several questions must be answered. The first is whether or not night shift workers are partially or fully adapted to their work routines, i.e., has there been an appropriate phase shift of the endogenous clock? If they have not adapted to their work routines, are there adverse consequences? And, if there are adverse consequences, can precautions or therapeutic means be adopted to alleviate them?

The literature suggests that in those night shift workers who are on a permanent work schedule, adaptation is not complete (Fig 21-3) [57]. Furthermore, most individuals revert to a day-active schedule on weekends because of personal preference, social pressures, and the difficulty of adhering to a routine that is

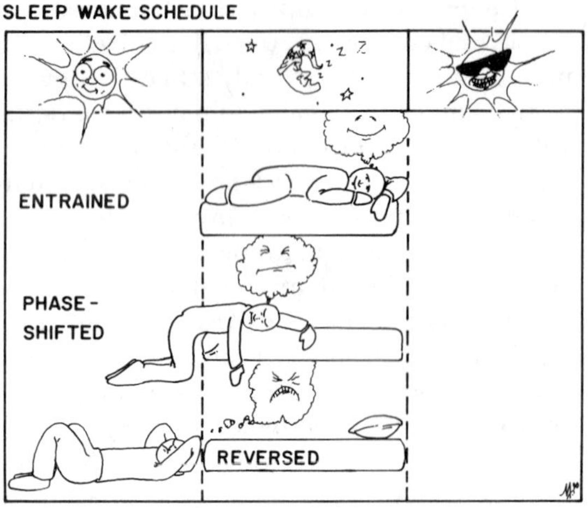
SLEEP WAKE SCHEDULE
ENTRAINED
PHASE-SHIFTED
REVERSED

Fig. 21-3. The problems associated with shift work are illustrated here. The top panel shows normal nocturnal sleep when the subject is on a regular day shift. When the subject is on a night shift, however, he must sleep during the daytime hours and will experience sleep disruption (lower two panels) because of the phase reversal between the sleep wake cycle and the biological clock.

different from family's, friends', and business associates'. Therefore, it is apparent that the night shift work schedule is desynchronized with the activity and alertness rhythms set by the entrained biologic clock and the schedules of most people in society. As for rotating shift work, it is even more unlikely that adaptation ever takes place, particularly for workers in occupations requiring very frequent shift changes such as airline pilots. Thus, shift workers are rarely if ever fully adapted to their work schedules.

There are adverse consequences to this lack of adaptation. Shift work leads to increased complaints of insomnia, gastrointestinal symptoms, and psychosomatic problems [58]. The rate of associated morbidity might be understated because enough long-term studies have not been performed; in addition, the issue of mortality has not been addressed. Job performance during the night shift can be impaired, as can be inferred from the increased rate of motor vehicle accidents between the hours of 2:00 and 4:00 AM [59]. Akerstedt [60] did ambulatory physiologic recordings in Swedish train engineers at night and reported many episodes of microsleeps that were associated with impairments in performance. It is thought that the Three Mile Island nuclear plant mishap, which occurred in the early hours of the morning, may have resulted from lapses of alertness at a time corresponding with a natural rhythmic peak of sleepiness [59].

Research on the management of shift work and treatment of the symptoms and complications stemming from it is still in its infancy. Proper sleep hygiene and counseling regarding time management should be included in any therapeutic regimen [61]. Perhaps safe and effective pharmacologic agents may be developed in the future. Attention should also be given to preselecting subjects who are more likely to have fewer difficulties adapting to night shifts. For instance, night people ("owls") adapt more readily to phase shifts than do day people ("larks") [62]. Owls are individuals who may have difficulty arising in the morning but increase their level of alertness throughout the day, frequently having their highest level of alertness around midnight or later. Owls have an increased capacity to sleep late in the morning and seem to function better than larks during times of irregular sleep/wake scheduling. Larks, on the other hand, are early risers with a high level of alertness early in the day while requiring an early bed time. They seem to function less well with irregular sleep/wake scheduling. People tend to become larks as they age. In addition, age is correlated with greater inflexibility of circadian rhythms [63].

What is the Purpose of Sleep

After many years of sleep research, a definitive answer to the role of sleep continues to elude us. Intuitively, however, it serves the functions of rest and recovery. Recent work seems to support a restorative theory for sleep, particularly for delta sleep [17]. Growth hormone is secreted during slow wave sleep [64]; and a reduction of glycolytic metabolism in the brain has been shown in studies using positron emission tomography [65]. Furthermore, the most striking effect of long-term sleep deprivation in rats is a precipitous terminal decline in core body temperature [66]. Immunomodulant substances such as interleukin-1 [67] are released in response to infection and have been shown to be very powerful delta sleep inducers. Thus, sleep may play an active role in recuperation from the effects of infectious disease, and it may be critical for the normal functioning of the immune system. Indeed, changes in delta sleep have been described in conditions in which there are perturbations of immunologic functions such as AIDS [68] and multiple sclerosis [69]. These avenues of research should be avidly pursued in the future.

References

1. Rechtschaffen A, Kales A: A Manual of Standardized Terminology, Techniques and Scoring System for Sleep Stages of Human Subjects. Los Angeles, UCLA Brain Information Service/Brain Research Institute, 1968
2. Erhart J, Erhart M, Muzet A, et al: K-complexes and sleep spindles before transient activation during sleep. Sleep 4:400, 1981
3. Rechtschaffen A: The single-mindedness and isolation of dreams. Sleep 1:97, 1978
4. Snyder F, Hobson JA, Morrison DF, et al: Changes in respiration, heart rate and systolic blood pressure in human sleep. J Appl Physiol 19:417, 1964
5. Kryger J: Breathing during sleep in normal subjects. Clin Chest Med 6:577, 1985
6. Karacan I: Evaluation of nocturnal penile tumescence and impotence. *In* Guilleminault C (ed): Sleeping and Waking Disorders: Indications and Techniques. Menlo Park, CA, Addison-Wesley, 1982, pp 343–371
7. Moruzzi G: The sleep-waking cycle. Ergeb Physiol 64:1, 1972
8. Mikiten T, Niebyl P, Hendley C: EEG desynchronization of behavioral sleep associated with spike discharges from the thalamus of the cat. Fed Proc 20:327, 1961
9. Williams RL, Karacan I, Hursch CJ: EEG of Human Sleep: Clinical Applications. New York, John Wiley and Sons, 1974
10. Ellingson RJ, Peters JF: Development of EEG and daytime sleep patterns in normal full-term infants during the first 3 months of life: Longitudinal observations. EEG Clin Neurophysiol 49:112, 1980
11. Dement WC, Miles LE, Carskadon MA: "White paper" on sleep and aging. J Am Geriat Soc 30:25, 1982
12. Carskadon MA, Dement WC: Respiration during sleep in the aged human. J Gerontol 36:420, 1981
13. Ancoli-Israel S, Kripke DF, Mason W, et al: Sleep apnea and nocturnal myoclonus in a senior population. Sleep 4:349, 1981
14. Feinberg I, Fein G, Floyd TC, et al: Delta (.5 Hz) EEG waveforms during sleep in young and elderly normal subjects. *In* Chase M, Weitzman ED (eds): Sleep Disorders: Basic and Clinical Research. New York, Spectrum Publications, 1983, pp 449–464
15. Hayashi Y, Endo S: All-night sleep polygraphic recordings of healthy aged persons: REM and slow-wave sleep. Sleep 5:277, 1982
16. Webb WB, Agnew HW: Are we chronically sleep deprived? Bull Psychom Soc 6:47, 1975
17. Horne JA: A review of the biological effects of total sleep deprivation in man. Biol Psychol 7:55, 1978
18. Hoddes E, Zarcone V, Smythe H, et al: Quantification of sleepiness: A new approach. Psychophysiology 10:431, 1973
19. Richardson GS, Carskadon MA, Flagg W, et al: Excessive daytime sleepiness in man: Multiple sleep latency measurement in narcoleptic and control subjects. EEG Clin Neurophysiol 45:621, 1978
20. Carskadon MA, Dement WC: The multiple sleep latency test: What does it mean? Sleep 5:567, 1982
21. Carskadon MA, Dement WC: Cumulative effects of sleep restriction on daytime sleepiness. Psychophysiology 18:107, 1981
22. Seidel WF, Roth T, Roehrs T, et al: Treatment of a 12-hour shift of sleep schedule with benzodiazepines. Science 224:1262, 1984
23. Carskadon MA, Harvey K, Duke P, et al: Pubertal changes in daytime sleepiness. Sleep 2:453, 1980
24. Carskadon MA, van den Hoed J, Dement WC: Sleep and daytime sleepiness in the elderly. J Geriatr Psychiatry 13:135, 1980
25. Moruzzi G, Magoun HW: Brain stem reticular formation and activation of the EEG. EEG Clin Neurophysiol 1:455, 1949
26. Lindsley DB, Bowden J, Magoun HW: Behavioral and EEG changes following chronic brain stem lesions in the cat. EEG Clin Neurophysiol 2:483, 1949
27. Magnes J, Moruzzi G, Pompeiano O: Synchronization of the EEG produced by low frequency electrical stimulation of the region of the solitary tract. Arch Ital Biol 99:33, 1961
28. Jouvet M: The role of monoamines and acetylcholine containing neurons in the regulation of the sleep-waking cycle. Ergeb Physiol 64:165, 1972
29. Sterman MB, Clemente CD: Forebrain inhibitory mechanisms: Cortical synchronization

induced by basal forebrain stimulation. Exp Neurol 6:91, 1967
30. Szymusiak R, McGinty D: Sleep suppression following kainic acid-induced lesions of the basal forebrain. Exp Neurol 94:598, 1986
31. Vertes RP: Brainstem control of the events of REM sleep. Progr Neurobiol 22:241, 1984
32. Hobson JA, McCarley RW, Wizinski PW: Sleep cycle oscillation: Reciprocal discharge by two brainstem neuronal groups. Science 189:55, 1975
33. McGinty D, Harper RM: Dorsal raphe neurons: Depression of firing during sleep in cats. Brain Res 101:569, 1976
34. Moore-Ede MC, Sulzman FM, Fuller CA: The Clocks That Time Us. Cambridge, MA, Harvard University Press, 1982
35. Weitzman ED, Fukushima DK, Nogeire C, et al: Twenty-four hour pattern of the episodic secretion of cortisol in normal subjects. J Clin Endocr Metab 33:114, 1971
36. Hauri P: The Sleep Disorders. Kalamazoo, MI, Upjohn, 1977
37. Monk TH, Weitzman ED, Fookson JE, et al: Task variables determine which biological clock controls circadian rhythms in human performance. Nature 304:543, 1983
38. Mistlberger R, Rusak B: Mechanisms and models of the circadian timekeeper system. *In* Kryger MH, Roth T, Dement WE (eds): Principles and Practice of Sleep Medicine. Philadelphia, Harcourt Brace Jovanovich, 1989, pp 141–152
39. Aschoff J, Wever R: Human circadian rhythms: A multioscillator system. Fed Proc 35:2326, 1976
40. Czeisler CA, Kronauer RE, Allen JS, et al: Bright light induction of strong (type O) resetting of the human circadian pacemaker. Science 244:1328, 1989
41. Czeisler CA, Allen JS, Strogatz SH, et al: Bright light resets the human circadian pacemaker independent of the timing of the sleep-wake cycle. Science 233:667, 1986
42. Czeisler CA, Johnson MP, Duffy JF, et al: Exposure to bright light and darkness to treat physiologic maladaptation to night work. N Engl J Med 322:1253, 1990
43. Terman M: On the question of mechanism in phototherapy for seasonal affective disorder: Considerations of clinical efficacy and epidemiology. J Biol Rhythms 3:155, 1988
44. Rusak B, Tucker I: Neural regulation of circadian rhythms. Physiol Rev 59:449, 1979
45. Stephan FK, Zucker I: Circadian rhythms in drinking behavior and locomotor activity of rats are eliminated by hypothalamic lesions. Proc Natl Acad Sci USA 69:1583, 1972
46. Inouye ST, Kawamura H: Persistence of circadian rhythmicity in a mammalian hypothalamic "island" containing the suprachiasmatic nucleus. Proc Natl Acad Sci USA 76:5962, 1979
47. Schwartz WJ, Davidson LC, Smith CB: In vivo metabolic activity of a putative circadian oscillator, the rat suprachiasmatic nucleus. J Comp Neurol 189:157, 1980
48. Green DS, Gillette R: Circadian rhythm of firing rate recorded from single cells in the rat suprachiasmatic brain slice. Brain Res 245: 198, 1982
49. Moore RY, Lenn NJ: A retinohypothalamic projection in the rat. J Comp Neurol 146:1, 1972
50. Klein DC: Photoneural regulation of the mammalian pineal gland. *In* Photoperiodism, Melatonin and the Pineal (CIBA Foundation Symposium 117). London, Pitman, 1985, pp 38–56
51. Arendt J, Marks V: Physiological changes underlying jet lag. Br Med J 284:144, 1982
52. Nicholson AN, Pascoe PA, Spencer MB, et al: Sleep after transmeridian flights. Lancet 2: 1205, 1986
53. Van Reeth O, Turek FW: Administering triazolam on a circadian basis entrains the activity rhythm of hamsters. Am J Physiol 256:R639, 1989
54. Wee BEF, Turek FW: Midazolam, a short-acting benzodiazepine, resets the circadian clock of the hamster. Pharmacol Biochem Behav 32:901, 1989
55. Petrie K, Conaglen JV, Thompson L, et al: Effect of melatonin on jet lag after long haul flights. Br Med J 298:705, 1989
56. Maurice M: Shift Work. Geneva, ILO, 1981
57. Folkard S, Monk TH, Lobban MC: Short and long term adjustment of circadian rhythms in "permanent" night nurses. Ergonomics 21:785, 1978
58. Reinberg A, Veux N, Andlauer P (eds): Night and Shift Work: Biological and Social Aspects. Oxford, Pergamon Press, 1981
59. Mitler MM, Carskadon MA, Czeisler CA, et al: Catastrophes, sleep, and public policy: Consensus report. Sleep 11:100, 1988
60. Akerstedt T: Sleepiness as a consequence of shift work. Sleep 11:17, 1988
61. Folkard S, Minors DS, Waterhouse JM: Chronobiology and shift work: Current issues and trends. Chronobiologia 12:31, 1985
62. Akerstedt T, Torsvall L: Shift work. Shift-dependent well-being and individual differences. Ergonomics 24:265, 1981
63. Foret J, Bensimon B, Benoit O, et al: Quality of sleep as a function of age and shift work. *In* Reinberg A, Vieux N, Andlauer P (eds): Night and Shift Work: Biological and Social Aspects. Oxford, Pergamon Press, 1981, pp 149–154

64. Sassin JF, Parker DC, Mace JW, et al: Human growth hormone release: Relation to slow-wave sleep and sleep-waking cycles. Science 165:513, 1969
65. Buchsbaum MS, Gillin JC, Wu J, et al: Regional cerebral glucose metabolic rate in human sleep assessed by positron emission tomography. Life Sci 45:1349, 1989
66. Bergmann BM, Everson CA, Kushida CA, et al: Sleep deprivation in the rat: V. Energy use and mediation. Sleep 12:31, 1989
67. Krueger JM, Walter J, Dinarello CA, et al: Sleep-promoting effects of endogenous pyrogen (interleukin-1). Am J Physiol 246:R994, 1984
68. Norman SE, Chediak AD, Kiel M, et al: Sleep disturbances in HIV-infected homosexual men. AIDS 4:775, 1990
69. Giancarlo T, Kapen S, Saad J, et al: Analysis of sleepiness and fatigue in multiple sclerosis. Ann Neurol 26:187, 1989

Clinical Evaluation of Excessive Daytime Sleepiness

Robert Wittig

The current nosology of sleep disorders identifies several conditions that may present with a chief complaint of excessive or inappropriate sleepiness [1, 2]. As with many other physical complaints the list of possible etiologies is long (Table 22-1), but the list of likely etiologies is much shorter. The first national cooperative study of 4698 consecutive patients presenting to sleep disorders centers around the United States [3] revealed excessive sleepiness was the most common presenting symptom (51%). Our experience suggests the proportion of patients presenting with a chief complaint of sleepiness between 1987 and 1989 was similar to the cooperative study of 1982, but the distribution of underlying causes identified was somewhat different (Table 22-2). Whether this reflects a change in diagnostic criteria, a change in patient population, or is a function of our local population is not clear. In any case, sleep apnea syndrome is the most common diagnosis of patients with excessive sleepiness.

The Chief Complaint

Sleepiness is a universal human experience. To be abnormally sleepy an individual must be falling asleep in circumstances that are considered unusual. The patient's concern typically increases as the situations in which he or she falls asleep become more embarrassing, inappropriate, or dangerous. Because people use different vocabularies to describe tiredness or sleepiness, the physician's first task is to determine whether the patient is describing sleepiness or fatigue, lethargy, or a lack of energy. Sleepy people actually fall asleep and are observed doing so by others. The clinical severity of sleepiness is judged according to the inappropriate times and places in which it occurs. The minister who falls asleep giving a sermon or the physician who falls asleep giving a presentation both exhibit more severe sleepiness than those who fall asleep listening to either. Similarly sleepiness while driving can be judged by the consistency with which it occurs. The patient who falls asleep waiting at a traffic light on the drive to work in the morning is more sleepy than the patient who is drowsy a few days per week on a 45-minute commute home at 5:00 PM.

The same degree of sleepiness can be pathologic or not depending on the circumstances or time of day. There is a circadian (daily) rhythm of sleepiness and alertness in all of us. We are most sleepy during that part of the day we customarily spend sleeping. There is a secondary period of sleepiness about midday, at least among those who ordinarily sleep at night (Fig. 22-1). In short, the physician must inquire about the timing and circumstances of the patient's sleepiness, its consistency and chronicity, as well as its magnitude to decide whether or not the patient is describing abnormal sleepiness.

Pathologic sleepiness of all etiologies manifests as falling asleep in sedentary situations. The sleepiest people manage to stay awake while physically active. Sedentary activities occupy a major portion of daily life, however, and include sitting at computer terminals, working, reading, watching television, attending meetings, classes, lectures, eating meals, and driving. The physician must inquire about daily sedentary activities of the patient to judge the severity of the complaint.

Table 22-1. Disorders of Excessive Somnolence

	ICD-9-CM Code
Dysomnias	
Intrinsic sleep disorders	
Narcolepsy	347
Recurrent hypersomnia	780.54-2
Idiopathic hypersomnia	780.54-7
Posttraumatic hypersomnia	780.54-8
Obstructive sleep apnea syndrome	780.53-0
Central sleep apnea syndrome	780.53-1
Periodic limb movement disorder	780.52-4
Restless legs syndrome	780.52-5
Intrinsic sleep disorder, not otherwise specified	780.52-9
Long sleeper	307.49
Subwakefulness syndrome	307.47-1
Extrinsic sleep disorders	
Inadequate sleep hygiene	307.41-1
Insufficient sleep syndrome	307.49-4
Hypnotic dependent sleep disorder	780.52-0
Stimulant dependent sleep disorder	780.52-6
Environmental sleep disorder	780.52-6
Extrinsic sleep disorder, not otherwise specified	780.52-9
Circadian rhythm disorders	
Time zone change (jet lag) syndrome	307.45-1
Shift work sleep disorder	307.45-1
Irregular sleep-wake pattern	307.45-3
Sleep disorders associated with medical/psychiatric disorders	
Associated with mental disorders	
Mood disorders	
Alcoholism	

From International Classification of Sleep Disorders: Diagnostic and Statistic Manual Produced by the Diagnostic Classification Steering Committee of the American Sleep Disorders Association, Rochester, MN, 1990; with permission.

Table 22-2. Disorders of Excessive Sleepiness

Diagnosis	*1982 National Cooperative Study*	*1987–1989 Henry Ford Hospital*
Sleep apnea syndromes	857 (43.2%)	545 (61%)
Narcolepsy	496 (25.0%)	68 (5.6%)
Idiopathic CNS hypersomnolence	175 (8.8%)	21 (1.7%)
No hypersomnia abnormality	108 (5.4%)	114 (9.4%)
Other hypersomnia	99 (5.0%)	42 (3.5%)
Insufficient sleep		158 (13%)
Psychiatric disorders	73 (3.7%)	6 (0.5%)
Periodic limb movement disorder	70 (3.5%)	13 (1.1%)
Medical, toxic, environmental	53 (2.7%)	34 (2.8%)
Drug and alcohol dependency	30 (1.5%)	11 (0.9%)
Psychophysiologic	22 (1.1%)	1 (0.1%)
Total	1983 (99.9%)	1013 (99.6%)

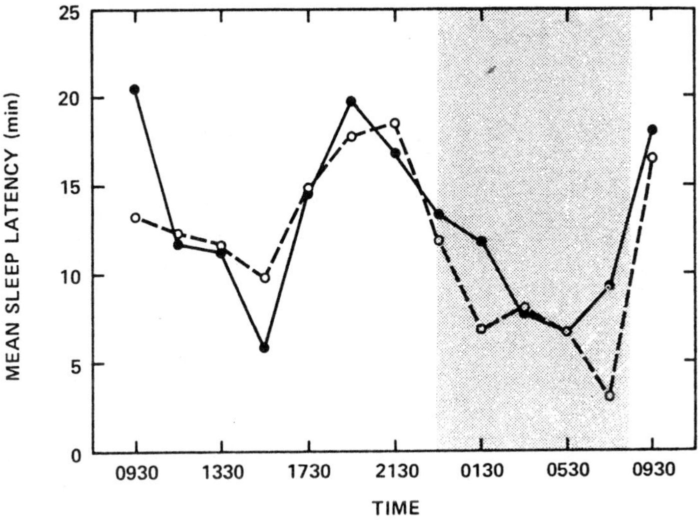

MEAN SLEEP LATENCY (min)
25
20
15
10
5
0
0930
1330
1730
2130
0130
0530
0930
TIME

Fig. 22-1. Mean sleep latency in minutes for young (open circles, n = 8) and old (filled circles, n = 10) subjects as a function of time of day. Shaded area demarks nocturnal sleep period. (*From* Richardson GS, Carskadon MA, Arav EJ, et al: Circadian variation of sleep tendency in elderly and young adult subjects. *Sleep* 5:S87, 1982; with permission)

Severity is judged by how pervasive the sleepiness is (i.e., in how many settings it occurs) and how quickly it becomes apparent once the patient begins the sedentary task. Sleepiness only at certain discrete times of day (e.g., midafternoon) would therefore not be as severe as sleepiness that is unremitting from the time the patient gets up to the time he or she returns to bed.

It should be apparent that the patient who is abnormally sleepy actually nods or dozes off in the vulnerable setting. Sleepiness that can be resisted and hidden successfully from others is of a much milder degree than that of patients overtly falling asleep in the same settings.

Onset of Symptoms

The duration of the patient's sleepiness can be helpful in clinically deducing its etiology. The only sleep disorder with a characteristic age of onset is narcolepsy, which typically begins in adolescence or early adulthood [4–6], most commonly between the ages of 15 and 25. If a 53-year-old patient dates the onset of sleepiness to his or her late 40s, narcolepsy is less likely than other etiologies. Narcolepsy is a specific disorder with characteristic laboratory findings, not a generic term for abnormal sleepiness.

One should inquire whether the sleepiness has progressively worsened since it was first noticed or whether it is intermittent. Patients with sleep apnea syndrome sometimes have noticed waxing and waning of their sleepiness. The history might further suggest a correlation with weight gain and loss. Often periods of abnormal sleepiness correlate with changes in work shift or lifestyle. The young adult working full time and attending night school or the person working two full-time jobs may have a protracted period of increased sleepiness such that he or she is falling asleep in many situations. The sleepiness would then remit when the patient is able to return to a schedule that permits regular, adequate nocturnal sleep. The adult who recalls periods of great sleepiness in the past may have had sleepiness of a different etiology from that with which he or she currently presents. The physician may only be able to speculate about the etiology of past bouts of sleepiness while focusing on the present problem.

The only recurring illnesses associated with hypersomnolence are bipolar affective disorder, in which the depressive phase may be associated with complaints of sleepiness (in which case a history of cyclic mood changes should also be elicited), or Kleine-Levin syndrome. Kleine-Levin syndrome is a rare cause of abnormal sleepiness. The history is one of recurrent periods of hypersomnolence in which the patient typically only wishes to eat and sleep. This disorder occurs predominantly (3 : 1) in males, and is often associated with hyperphagia and hypersexuality in the acutely ill stage [1, 2, 7]. Episodes of illness last 4 to 30 days and then remit. Between episodes there is no evidence of illness or personality disorder. The symptomatic periods can recur unpredictably for years. The interested reader is referred to the literature for more information on this rare disorder.

Sleep apnea syndrome can occur at any age. The diagnosis is suggested by ancillary symptoms of snoring and apneas observed during sleep. The patient's snoring and breathing during sleep are best described by a bed partner, family members, or other witness to behavior during sleep.

Sleepiness due to irregular and/or inadequate sleep times rarely begins before adolescence. It is most common in working age people, particularly those whose work schedule requires very early rising times or necessitates daytime sleep. Independent of age, this diagnosis (irregular, insufficient sleep) is suggested by a detailed history (see following). Even when another sleep disorder is suspected, the patient should be encouraged to get at least 7 hours of sleep on a daily basis because excessive sleepiness of any other etiology will be exacerbated by insufficient or irregular sleep habits. Because people take more medications as they age, sleepiness secondary to sedating medications becomes more likely.

Sleep History

Once the physician has assessed the severity and duration of the sleepiness it is important to determine whether or not the patient's habits are contributing to the problem. The physician should determine the usual working hours or daytime activities of the patient. Does the patient change shifts? If overtime is worked, how much and at what time? Work hours have a major influence on daily sleep times. Is the patient spending enough time in bed? Although no amount of sleep can be said to suffice for everyone, if one is sleeping less than 7 to 8 hours, which is normal for adults [8], insufficient daily sleep may be suspected. Daily sleep times are best assessed with a sleep log in which the patient records bedtimes, arising times, and perceived quantity and quality of daily sleep. Over 2 weeks this can be very useful to confirm suspected irregularities in sleep times and to determine average daily sleep times. If no symptoms are present to suggest other pathology (e.g., narcolepsy, sleep apnea, medication or drug effects), it is reasonable to suggest the patient increase nightly sleep time on a regular basis. This too can be followed with logs. If regular, adequate (e.g., 8 hours) nightly sleep resolves the sleepiness problem, laboratory evaluation may be unnecessary. Often, however, patients who are sleepy because they do not sleep enough resist changing the habit. Laboratory studies (clinical polysomnogram and Multiple Sleep Latency Test [MSLT] may be necessary to demonstrate findings consistent with chronically insufficient sleep and rule out other pathology to the patient's satisfaction [19].

Patients whose sleepiness derives from deteriorated quality of nocturnal sleep (e.g., obstructive sleep apnea syndrome or periodic leg movements associated with fragmented sleep) seldom describe their sleep as good quality. They generally are aware of at least occasional nocturnal awakenings, although not what is causing them. The pathologically sleepy patient is likely to return quickly to sleep and is unlikely to complain of long awakenings.

Patients with narcolepsy likewise seldom describe their night's sleep as of normal continuity. An occasional patient with narcolepsy is as concerned about sleep disturbance at night as about sleepiness during the day.

Even those who sleep relatively well and for a normal duration (e.g., 7 to 8 hours) usually are aware of more than one nightly awakening. If the narcoleptic patient remains in bed he or she is likely to be asleep again within a short time (< 30 minutes). If instead he or she leaves the bed and becomes active for a period of time (1 hour or more), a significant loss of nighttime sleep occurs and results in even worse daytime sleepiness.

In general, patients who sleep the most soundly with the fewest awakenings and have the greatest difficulty arising are the most likely to be those who are chronically sleep deprived.

Sleep apnea syndrome patients usually arouse easily at the desired time in response to alarm clocks, but often complain of tiredness on awakening, "like I haven't slept at all." Patients with narcolepsy likewise generally arouse easily, but then complain of the onset of sleepiness within 1 to 2 hours of getting up, sooner in severe cases.

One should also routinely inquire as to the adequacy of the sleep environment. Are there factors (heat, cold, noise, etc.) that could be disrupting sleep? Is there a bed partner the patient or physician can interrogate about the patient's behavior during sleep?

In addition to the principal sleep period it is necessary to ascertain how much the patient is sleeping at other times. Are naps taken regularly or not, and how long are they? Does the patient feel better, more alert, after naps or not? Patients with narcolepsy who are getting adequate nocturnal sleep (7 or more hours) are typically quite refreshed after surprisingly brief (5 to 20 minute) naps. Patients with other causes of sleepiness occasionally report short naps to be refreshing as well, though less often than do narcoleptic subjects. Patients with narcolepsy may find such short naps of no benefit if their sleep-wake schedules have become completely disorganized.

Those who ultimately meet historic and polysomnographic criteria for a diagnosis of idiopathic hypersomnolence [1] typically find even long naps of no help.

Often very sleepy people doze off in a family room for hours before retiring to bed. The quantity of sleep regularly obtained may thus be much greater than the time spent in bed. Careful enquiry of the patient or a cohabitant should give the physician a reasonably accurate picture of the patient's daily habits.

Ancillary Symptoms

Ancillary or accessary symptoms are commonly associated with disorders of excessive daytime sleepiness. The most common disorders and the accessory symptoms with which they are most often associated follow.

Sleep Apnea Syndrome

Sleep apnea syndrome is almost invariably associated with loud snoring. But snoring is common, afflicting 25% of men and 15% of women [9]. The incidence increases with age so that between the ages of 40 and 65, 65% of men and 40% of women are reported to be habitual snorers. Therefore, snoring is considerably more common than sleep apnea syndrome, which has been estimated to afflict 1% to 2% of the adult male population [10, 11]. Indeed, most men in the 40 to 65 age group who complain of excessive sleepiness also are habitual snorers, whether or not the sleepiness is related to the snoring.

The physician must interrogate family members or cohabitants as to the character of the patient's snoring. Irregularity should be of more concern than loudness. Anyone who spends a night near someone with sleep apnea syndrome is likely able to describe the interrupted breathing. The patient with this disease is likely to have hundreds of interruptions every night, each punctuated by loud gasps or snorts as breathing resumes [12]. The physician should try to determine how often and for how long observers have been concerned about the patient's breathing during sleep. The sleep apnea syndrome patient is seldom, if ever, aware of the extent of the breathing problems during sleep.

Adults with obstructive sleep apnea syndrome often experience nocturnal heartburn. The frequency of gastric reflux or heartburn may increase with worsening obstructive apnea. Some patients keep antacids or liquids at the bedside. The presumed mechanism is that the negative intrathoracic and intraesophageal pressure generated by the struggle to pull in air during total or partial upper airway obstruction overcomes the gastroesophageal sphincter pressure and literally sucks gastric contents into the thoracic esophagus. Gastroesophageal reflux of this nature resolves once the sleep-related upper airway obstruction is effectively treated.

About 32% of sleep apnea syndrome patients experience headaches on awakening [14]. The headache is most often bifrontal or bitemporal and is often described as a sinus headache. It usually passes quickly, but may persist for hours. Patients with this type of headache typically notice them 1 to 3 days per week. Such headaches should occur in the absence of known precipitants (e.g., alcohol, although alcohol may precipitate obstructive apnea) to be attributed to an intrinsic sleep disorder.

Patients with sleep apnea syndrome often complain of restless sleep because the repetitive brief arousals from sleep to resume breathing can be associated with body movements. Occasionally patients are found sleeping in bizarre positions, such as sitting up in bed, sitting on the side of the bed (threatening to topple), or kneeling on the floor with thorax prone on the bed and the head propped up. Such positions probably are the result of subconscious efforts to find a position that relieves the upper airway obstruction. While most obstructive sleep apnea patients are restless sleepers, only a few assume such unorthodox sleeping positions. The frequency with which these and other symptoms are associated with sleep apnea syndrome in our own patient population is shown in Table 22-3.

Narcolepsy

The accessory symptoms of narcolepsy (cataplexy, hypnogogic hallucinations, and sleep paralysis) can be interpreted as phenomena that are normal during REM sleep but are occurring at abnormal times. They are accessory to the primary complaint of excessive sleepiness, although occasionally a patient identifies an accessory symptom as the chief complaint.

Abnormal sleepiness is usually the first

Table 22-3. Accessory Symptoms

Symptom	*Apnea (No. = 417)*	*Narcolepsy (No. = 107)*	*Insufficient Sleep (No. = 59)*
Snoring	95%	51%	79%
Daytime sleepiness	90%	100%	100%
Memory lapses	53%	44%	—
Morning headaches	32%	—	—
Enuresis	6%	—	—
Cataplexy	—	81%	—
Hypnogogic hallucinations	—	65%	—
Sleep paralysis	—	61%	—
Nocturnal sleep disturbance	(High)	76%	(Low)
Reported weekday sleep time	—	7.5 hr	6.4 hr
Reported weekend sleep time	—	8.0 hr	8.5 hr
Age of onset	42 ± 8 yr	20 ± 9 yr	28 ± 14 yr
Percent male	98%	52%	57%

From references 6, 14, and 19.

symptom that develops [4–6], generally between the ages of 15 and 25, but in some individuals as early as age 6 [15–17]. The accessory symptoms may not be noticed until years later [4–6]. Cataplexy is the most characteristic symptom of narcolepsy occuring in 80% to 100% of patients, depending on whether cataplexy or polysomnographic criteria is required for the diagnosis [4, 6]. Cataplexy is a noticeable loss of muscle tone triggered by emotions. The severity of the weakness and the muscle groups affected vary from patient to patient, as can the nature of the emotional stimulus triggering the phenomenon. Laughter and anger are most commonly associated with cataplexy. The muscles most commonly affected are postural, such that the patient has a sensation that his or her knees are buckling. In the most severe case, the patient actually collapses. Less severely affected patients quickly assume a sitting position, if possible, or may catch hold of a table to prevent themselves from falling. The weakness is transient, typically lasting only seconds. The severity of cataplexy can vary over time in an individual patient. The same patient who found cataplexy to be only a minor annoyance for many years may find late in life that minor emotional stimuli precipitate a collapse. Cataplexy may well become the chief complaint of these individuals and may be more disabling than their sleepiness. Conversely, the patient whose cataplexy early in life is particularly severe may learn to modify its expression, perhaps through altered modulation of emotions. Such patients may not be bothered by cataplexy when they present even though they do sometimes experience it.

The occurrence of cataplexy can be difficult to elicit during history taking. The physician should be careful to use open-ended questions. The response to "When you laugh or become angry, does anything happen to you that does not seem to happen to other people?" is likely to be convincing if cataplexy is present. The response to "Have you ever laughed so hard you became weak in the knees?" is less likely to differentiate those with cataplexy from normal people. To distinguish cataplexy from weakness with extreme emotion or as a response to tickling, it should be triggered by minor stimuli, often enough to be considered remarkable. To have laughed so hard you were "rolling in the aisle" on a few occasions over several years does not mean one has cataplexy.

Hypnogogic hallucinations and sleep-onset paralysis are the other symptoms commonly associated with narcolepsy. Both can be interpreted as manifestations of phenomena that occur normally during REM sleep (dreams or hallucinations and muscle atonia or paralysis) occurring at an abnormal time, i.e., at sleep onset. A patient with the hypnogogic hallucinations of narcolepsy typically describes visual and auditory imagery when falling asleep in a nap or at the onset of the primary sleep period. The hallucinations are often frightening or threatening, something the patient hears and sees but is powerless to thwart. The hallucinations typically are accompanied by paralysis (the atonia of REM sleep). The entire episode is brief, lasting at most a few minutes, usually much less. The patient may twitch or mumble incoherently. The episode can usually be terminated by the touch of another or terminates spontaneously, perhaps as the result of the patient's strenuous efforts to rouse him- or herself. It is tempting to think the episodes that are recalled are frightening because if it doesn't distress you, you don't struggle so hard to wake up. If arousal and awakening ensue, the event is likely to be remembered. If the patient instead passes through the hypnogogic experience into prolonged sleep, there would be no memory trace.

Hallucinations and paralysis of the voluntary musculature are, of course, normal concomitants of REM sleep that occur approximately every 90 minutes after sleep onset. Three percent to 6% of normal sleeping adults experience sleep paralysis, but most often at sleep offset, usually after having been asleep more than 1 hour [1, 18]. It can occur with an abrupt awakening from REM sleep. The patient with narcolepsy, who is able to lapse directly from wakefulness into REM sleep without the normal 80 to 100 minute latency, is thus able to describe REM sleep phenomena at sleep onset, if able to awaken from them. Therefore, patients with narcolepsy are not aware of every instance in which they lapse directly into REM sleep at sleep onset. Some may have no awareness of it and therefore do not experience hypnogogic hallucinations or sleep-onset paralysis. Rarely are hypnogogic hallucinations or sleep paralysis identified as the chief complaint; their occurrence is most often found in the search for auxiliary symptoms to suggest the diagnosis of narcolepsy.

Finally, disturbed nocturnal sleep has been suggested by some to be a fourth accessory symptom of narcolepsy as 30% to 80% of narcoleptic patients complain of difficulty maintaining sleep as well as difficulty maintaining wakefulness [6, 20]. Indeed, a patient sometimes presents with insomnia (difficulty maintaining, not initiating sleep in these cases) and is found further in the history to be sleepy as well. The patient then may attribute the sleepiness to poor nocturnal sleep. An alert clinician who discovered the full extent of the patient's symptoms should guess the correct diagnosis before diagnostic sleep studies are performed.

Chronically Insufficient Sleep

Some of the symptoms associated with chronically insufficient sleep may properly be called ancillary symptoms. The magnitude of the sleepiness described by these patients is likely to be less than that of patients with narcolepsy or severe sleep apnea. They typically describe a sleepiness that is worse late in the day. The commute to work is often less troublesome than the return home later. These patients typically have sleep periods on work nights (e.g., 11:30 PM to 5:30 AM) that are 2 or more hours shorter than on days off work or when on vacation [19]. Nocturnal sleep, in contrast to that of sleep apnea or narcolepsy patients, is most often described as deep, with rare awakenings. It is often very difficult to arouse in the morning, making chronic tardiness for school or work a common chief complaint. Patients often complain of difficulty arousing to an alarm in the morning, again contrasting with what is usual in patients with narcolepsy and sleep apnea, and will use snooze alarms repeatedly to "ease the transition" to wakefulness. These characteristic complaints plus a history suggesting average nightly sleep times significantly shorter than is normal for adults (7 to 8 hours) suggest the diagnosis.

Idiopathic Hypersomnolence

This diagnosis is likely to be made only after laboratory study. It requires the demonstration of pathologic sleepiness despite seemingly adequate (often more than 8 hours) average nightly sleep time and no symptoms or laboratory signs of significant sleep abnormality. There are no accessory symptoms of narcolepsy (and no sleep-onset REM periods on laboratory study) or any other sleep disorder, no evidence of psychiatric disorder relevant to a diagnosis of sleepiness or relevant pharmacologic agents. Naps typically are longer than in patients with apnea or narcolepsy; short naps are unlikely to be refreshing. In the laboratory, pathologic sleepiness persists despite documented regular extension of nocturnal sleep to considerable length (> 9 hours), in marked contrast to the normalization that occurs in patients whose problem is behavioral.

Drug and Medication Effects on Sleepiness

No history of abnormal sleepiness is complete without detailed information about the use of relevant pharmacologic agents. Alcohol and caffeine are the two most commonly used drugs that affect daytime alertness. These, as well as drugs used illegally, can greatly confuse the clinical and polysomnographic evaluation of sleepiness if the clinician is unaware of the frequency and quantity of their use. Prescription drugs for allergies, hypertension, epilepsy, affective or psychotic disorders, anxiety, or pain can also complicate the sleepiness evaluation. The physician who is aware of the effects on sleep of commonly used drugs and medications can sometimes persuade the patient to change habits or can prescribe alternative medications and improve the symptoms. If diagnostic sleep studies are deferred until after this is done, the results are less likely to be ambiguous.

Alcohol

Alcohol has complex effects on sleep. Acutely, alcohol is likely to shorten sleep latencies (shorten the time it takes to fall asleep or increase sleepiness), but it can also cause fragmentation of ensuing sleep and contribute to a sleep maintenance insomnia (inability to stay asleep). Alcohol's acute effect on alertness is influenced by the subject's underlying level of sleepiness [21–23]. Whether the patient's complaint is one of sleepiness or insomnia, a detailed alcohol consumption history often helps the physician understand the patient's condition.

There is a circadian rhythm in sleepiness and alertness such that the greatest sleepiness occurs at night during the customary sleep period. Falling asleep at night in public may suggest no abnormal sleepiness. There is a secondary period of sleepiness that usually occurs about midday. Increasing sleepiness is likely to first become bothersome around midday. Alcohol with lunch exacerbates that sleepiness. Therefore, patients who complain of sleepiness should avoid alcohol entirely. If consumed in the evening, in addition to disturbing sleep, it will worsen snoring. It may also cause partial airway obstruction during sleep (snoring) to become total airway obstruction (worse snoring, obstructive apnea) [24]. In short, alcohol, even in moderation, only worsens sleepiness. The problem becomes one of persuading the patient that evening libations, though unchanged over the years, coupled with a significant weight gain, may now be the source of embarrassing or inappropriate sleepiness. If possible, it is best to withdraw the patient from alcohol and proceed with the evaluation.

Caffeine

Caffeine, if taken in unusually large amounts, can have a significant bearing on daytime sleepiness. It would seem paradoxical that a stimulant could worsen sleepiness, but it sometimes happens. At ordinary levels of intake (< 500 mg daily) caffeine is used by many to fight sleepiness. Occasionally a patient presents who is consuming huge doses (> 1000 mg daily) in beverage or tablet form [25]. Such patients can so disrupt their sleep schedules that the chief complaint is abnormal sleepiness instead of insomnia. Chronic partial sleep deprivation is offset by escalating daily doses of caffeine in an ultimately futile effort to keep functioning. The underlying sleep deprivation prevents the occurrence of insomnia. Eventually the stimulant dosage is raised to the point that nocturnal sleep, already short, is further compromised by the drug. Higher doses, once a remedy, further disrupt sleep and lead to even worse daytime functioning. Withdrawal of caffeine and increased nightly sleep may resolve the symptoms, without further diagnostic studies.

Excessive use of other stimulants can likewise lead to excessive sleepiness. The drug most likely encountered in current practice is cocaine. Withdrawal from cocaine at high doses can produce severe sleepiness and REM rebound, possibly including sleep-onset REM periods. Polysomnographic evaluation might then be misinterpreted to suggest narcolepsy if the physician, either by history or a urine toxicologic screen, failed to realize the patient's cocaine use.

Sedating Drugs

Sedating drugs (narcotics, barbiturates, analgesics) that are abused can also produce excessive sleepiness, but persons abusing these compounds seldom present to sleep disorders centers complaining of sleepiness. Urine toxicologic screens would be very helpful to avoid misdiagnoses in these cases as well.

Several classes of prescription medications produce sedation as an unwanted side effect. Patients taking one or more of these can become so symptomatic as to have difficulty functioning. Those medications most often implicated are antihistamines, antihypertensives, analgesics, anticonvulsants, antidepressants, and anxiolytics.

The H_1-blocking antihistamines are almost

all sedating [26]. Although sedation may be a desirable effect at bedtime, it is not during the hours of wakefulness. Except for terfenadine (Seldane) and astemizole (Hismanal), recently available nonsedating H_1-blockers, all other effective H_1-blockers produce some degree of sedation. Individuals vary widely in their susceptibility so it is difficult to specify which drugs are more or less troublesome. In general one should consider discontinuing a drug or substituting a nonsedating alternative early in the course of an evaluation of sleepiness. An alternative strategy is to prescribe a sedating H_1-blocking antihistamine at night and a stimulating decongestant, e.g., pseudoephedrine or phenylpropanolamine [15], during the daytime. Alternatives to decongestant-antihistamine regimens might include nasal steroids or cromolyn sodium for control of allergic symptoms, with the advice of an otorhinolaryngologist or allergist.

Antihypertensives

Several antihypertensive medications adversely affect sleep-wake function, either by disturbing nocturnal sleep, increasing drowsiness, or both. Those most likely to cause excessive sedation are the central and peripheral α-adrenergic agonists, clonidine (Catapres) and methyldopa (Aldomet) [27]. The incidence of daytime sleepiness is high enough (33% of patients taking methyldopa and an even greater number of patients taking clonidine [27, 28]) to justify consideration of alternative antihypertensive medications as an early step in the clinical evaluation of sleepiness.

β-Blockers have been associated with various complaints including sleepiness, tiredness, disturbed sleep, and an increased incidence of disturbing dreams. It has been suggested that the sleep complaints, whether of daytime drowsiness or of disturbed nocturnal sleep, are more common with the lipophilic β-blockers or with the β-blockers that possess sympathomimetic activity (Table 22-4) [29–34].

In general, if a patient taking a β-blocker complains of altered sleep-wake function, particularly one commonly associated with an increased incidence of sleep complaints (e.g., propranolol (Indernal), metaprolol (Lopressor), or pindolol (Visken)), it would not be unreasonable to switch to an alternative (e.g., atenolol (Tenormin)) with a lower incidence of sleep-related side effects.

Beyond the clinical effects of electrolyte abnormalities, the diuretics have not been implicated in sleep pathology. The newer classes of drugs (Angiotensin Converting

Table 22-4. Antihypertensives

	Incidence of Sedation	*Lipid Solubility Partition Coefficient*	*Sympathomimetic Activity*
α-Adrenergic agonists			
Methyldopa (Aldomet)	33%		
Clonidine (Catapres)	50%		
β-Adrenergic blockers			
Atenolol (Tenormin)		0.23 (low)	0
Nadolol (Corgard)		0.7	0
Pindolol (Visken)		1.75	+ +
Acebutolol (Sectral)		1.9	+
Timolol (Blocadren)		2.1	0
Metaprolol (Lopressor)		2.15	0
Propranolol (Inderal)		3.65 (highest)	0

Adapted from Gilman AG, Rall TW, Nies AS [26]; and Nicholson A, Bradley C, Pascoe P [27].

Enzyme [ACE] inhibitors, calcium channel blockers) have thus far not been found to cause alterations of sleep-wake function.

Anticonvulsants

Anticonvulsants all are sedating to varying degrees. Valproic acid may be the least sedating among this group of psychoactive agents. In general, the simpler the anticonvulsant regimen the less likely sedation will be a problem. The higher the doses required to control seizure activity, the more likely are decrements in cognitive functioning. The goal is satisfactory seizure control with the fewest side effects. The sleep clinician's role, beyond suggesting simplification of an anticonvulsant regimen or use of less sedating drugs, may be to rule out other conditions contributing to the sleepiness. This can often be done clinically by looking for concomitant symptoms of narcolepsy, sleep apnea syndrome, irregular and insufficient sleep habits, or possible exacerbating effects of medications the patient is taking for other reasons. Occasionally a patient presents whose cataplexy has been misdiagnosed as an epileptic disorder. Such patients sometimes are treated for years with anticonvulsant agents despite a lack of efficacy for their "seizures." It is easiest to suggest antiepileptic drugs be stopped when drug therapy has had little or no effect on the condition being treated. Anticonvulsants can also be stopped under supervision if the patient has been seizure free for years [35].

Tricyclic Antidepressants

A common side effect of tricyclic antidepressants, particularly amitriptyline (Elavil) and doxepin (Sinequan), is sedation. For patients with insomnia secondary to an affective disorder this is therapeutic, not a side effect. The tricyclics vary in the degree of sedation they cause, although most are to some degree sedating. These drugs, in addition to effects on alertness, all significantly affect sleep parameters when given in therapeutic doses. All suppress REM sleep, significantly prolonging REM latency and reducing REM sleep time. This effect in conjunction with the effects on alertness can modify polysomnographic findings enough to render the results uninterpretable. Withdrawal of these drugs might be considered if there are doubts as to the diagnosis of a major affective disorder or to the tricyclic's efficacy, or if the patient is adversely affected by the drug's side effects. In such cases the benefits to the evaluation of sleepiness may outweigh risks of discontinuation.

Although most of the tricyclic antidepressants are sedating, newer drugs being used to treat depression may actually be stimulating. Fluoxitine, for example, precipitates insomnia in many patients [36]. Its presence complicates the evaluation of sleep disorders by disrupting nocturnal sleep and increasing daytime alertness, again possibly rendering polysomnographic studies uninterpretable.

Anxiolytics

All available anxiolytics are sedating and therefore may cause or contribute to sleepiness. The benzodiazepines, used both as anxiolytics and hypnotics, are *all* sedating. The compounds of this drug class differ pharmacologically in rates of absorption, routes of metabolism and excretion, and durations of action. This means that an agent chosen as a hypnotic (e.g., flurazepam) administered at night to promote sleep may well last into or throughout the next day and the next and cause or exacerbate daytime sleepiness (Table 22-5). Patients with anxiety disorders usually do not complain of excessive sleepiness. Indeed, the ability to fall asleep in socially inappropriate, embarrassing situations would argue against the presence of pathologic anxiety.

A more common situation arises in the case of the moderately obese middle-aged adult, who has been prescribed a sedative (e.g., diazepam), a β-blocker, and perhaps other medications after a myocardial infarction. The patient continues to drink alcohol in moderation and perhaps gains more weight with time. Eventually the patient presents and the physician realizes that the patient is falling asleep inappropriately. The patient is likely to snore and may have irregular habits as well. The physician can begin by addressing

Table 22-5. Benzodiazepines: Hypnotics and Sedatives

Benzodiazepine	*Elimination Half-Life (hr)*
Triazolam (Halcion)	2–4
Oxazepam (Serax)	5–10
Chlordiazepoxide (Librium)	5–15
Alprazolam (Xanax)	10–14
Temazepam (Restoril)	10–17
Lorazepam (Ativan)	10–20
Diazepam (Valium)	30–60
Clorazepate (Tranxene)	50–80
Flurazepam (Dalmane)	50–100

Adapted from Gilman AG, Rall TW, Nies AS, et al: The Pharmacologic Basis of Therapeutics, ed 8. Elmsford, NY, Pergamon Press, 1990; with permission.

the possible iatrogenic components of the problem by discontinuing sedating medication, advising abstinence from alcohol, and modifying the cardiac regimen to eliminate cardiovascular drugs that may be contributing to the problem. The timing of polysomnographic studies would be dictated by the severity of symptoms and the response to changes in the medical regimen.

The cumulative effect of several potentially problematic medications frequently affects sleep. Medications that did not produce noticeable problems in the past over time and with the addition of new medications can set up a pathologic situation. The physician must then simplify the clinical situation to the point where diagnostic studies yield diagnostic results or the problem resolves and such studies become unnecessary.

Analgesics

In general, the nonsteroidal anti-inflammatory agents are not known to contribute to problems with inappropriate sleepiness. The narcotic and synthetic narcotic analgesics can cause sleep pathology. In a general medical practice, patients who require frequent narcotic (or synthetic narcotic) analgesics usually have medical problems that make sleepiness an unlikely chief complaint. Occasionally patients take these medications for questionable indications, in which case they should be discontinued early in the evaluation. Many of these agents are marketed as combination products with either a barbiturate or caffeine, or both, further complicating any assessment of sleep pathology if not discontinued.

The family of a patient requiring narcotics may observe signs (loud snoring, apneic episodes) in which a polysomnographic study might lead to changes in patient management, without a primary concern for sleepiness. The physician will have to decide when the benefits of these potent drugs are worth the risk of potential adverse effects on alertness, sleep, and respiration during sleep.

Antipsychotic Medications

Antipsychotic or neuroleptic medications also produce sedation. Patients for whom these drugs are prescribed usually require them for treatment of a major thought disorder associated with psychosis. Because of their diverse pharmacologic properties some of these medications (e.g., the phenothiazines) are often prescribed at low doses as antiemetics, antinauseants, or antihistamines. Used for these indications they can still precipitate or exacerbate sleepiness. As antipsychotics, the phenothiazines, thioxanthines, butyrophenones, and others vary in the degree of sedation that can be expected. If a patient complains of or seems oversedated on an agent, alone or in combination with other medications, a psychiatrist or pharmacologist familiar with available therapeutic choices and likely side effects should be consulted.

In conclusion, many classes of medications commonly affect alertness or increase sleepiness. Evaluation of the sleepiness requires detailed knowledge of the patient's use of legal and illegal psychotropics, over-the-counter medications, and all prescription medications. The sleep laboratory evaluation is best accomplished with as few complicating pharmacologic contributions as possible. In cases where simplification or modification of a drug regimen eliminates the problem, no further evaluation or treatment may be necessary. In cases that proceed to an objective evaluation, including an MSLT, interpretation and proper attribution of sleepiness will be greatly facilitated by prior elimination of confounding variables.

Daytime Sleepiness in the Pediatric Age Group

The evaluation of sleepiness in the pediatric age group (younger than 18 years) proceeds in much the same manner as in adults. Before school age, falling asleep in the daytime is unlikely to be seen as a problem in a child who otherwise is developmentally normal. Abnormal sleepiness will not likely be noticed until the child reaches an age at which he or she is expected to stay awake for prolonged periods. For most this is not until the school years. Early in schooling, nap times are often provided. It is the child who is falling asleep in settings where peers are not that will come to medical attention. When parents hear from the school that the child is falling asleep or is more tired, irritable, or less attentive than others, especially if this corroborates their own impressions, the pediatrician is likely to be consulted. Outside of school the sleepy child is likely to fall asleep in situations analogous to those in which sleepy adults fall asleep: riding in automobiles, watching television, trying to read, and in other physically inactive, sedentary situations.

A clinician evaluating sleepiness in children has to be familiar with the normal evolution of sleep times and sleeping behavior across the pediatric age range. Normal daily sleep times decrease from 16 hours at age 1 week to 11 hours by age 5, to 8 hours by age 18 [37]. Since children, like adults, can become sleepy with insufficient or disturbed nocturnal sleep, the clinician must take careful history of sleep habits and behavior. An advantage in evaluating children is that a parent is usually present, and questions about unusual behavior during sleep can be answered quickly.

There are few large case series of sleepiness in children, so the epidemiology and extent of the problem is unknown. Data from Stanford [38] (Table 22-6) suggest 50% of cases of pathologic sleepiness between the ages of 2 and 11 could be attributed to recognized neurologic disorders, e.g., epilepsy, or to medications taken for a recognized medical disorder. These children would be managed by optimal treatment of their known neurologic or medical condition. The remaining 50% of patients in this age group had obstructive sleep apnea syndrome or narcolepsy. Obstructive sleep apnea is associated not with obesity at this age but with tonsillar or adenoidal hypertrophy. Tonsil and adenoidectomy is curative in at least two thirds of cases [39–41]. In the remainder a spectrum of anatomic abnormalities of the upper airway may account for sleep-related upper airway obstruction. All pediatric cases of obstructive sleep apnea should be evaluated by a pediatric otorhinolaryngologist before attempting treatment.

Narcolepsy, though uncommon before puberty, does occur. In the early years there may be no accessory symptoms [5, 6]. Sleepiness most often is the first symptom to appear. Polysomnographic studies (a nocturnal polysomnogram and the Multiple Sleep Latency Test) are the only way to make the diagnosis at this age.

Thus, even in the 2 to 11 age range the available data suggest a large percentage of easily treatable abnormal sleepiness occurs in developmentally normal, otherwise well children.

The Stanford experience with 11 to 16 year olds suggests an even higher preponderance of obstructive sleep apnea syndrome and narcolepsy (Table 22-6) in a series of 153 children referred for pathologic sleepiness [38]. In this age group behavioral factors are becoming more important. Major neurologic and medical diagnoses are likely to have been made earlier and account for fewer diagnoses. Sedating medications (increased from 4% to 6% of patients) must be sought in the history.

The only other large pediatric series (115) is reported from Boston and is not broken down by age [42]. Seventy-eight percent of

Table 22-6. Complaints of Excessive Daytime Sleepiness in Children Seen at the Stanford Sleep Center, 1972 to 1984

Complaint	*No.*
Children 2–11 years of age (Tanner stage I)	
Neurologic problem with or without mental retardation	58
Neurologic problem with epilepsy	31
Obstructive sleep apnea syndrome	92
Narcolepsy	5
EDS related to medical treatment	4
EDS associated with medical disorders without secondary obstructive sleep apnea syndrome	5
EDS of unknown etiology	2
Total	197
Children 11–16 years of age (Tanner stage II)	
Neurologic problems with or without mental retardation or epilepsy	14
Obstructive sleep apnea syndrome	69
Narcolepsy	38
CNS hypersomnia	11
EDS related to medical treatment	6
EDS associated with medical disorders without secondary obstructive sleep apnea syndrome	5
EDS associated with delayed sleep phase syndrome	3 (19)*
EDS with periodic hypersomnia	4
EDS of unknown origin	3
Total	153

*Delayed sleep phase syndrome is common in teenagers, who generally complain of a combination of sleep-onset insomnia, difficulty waking up in the morning, and tiredness during the day. Nineteen patients had these complaints, but sleep-onset insomnia seemed most problematic to them.

Abbreviation: EDS, excessive daytime sleepiness.

From Guilleminault C: Sleep and its Disorders in Children. New York, Raven Press, 1987. Reprinted with permission.

patients referred for excessive sleepiness had sleep apnea syndrome or narcolepsy.

As pediatricians become more aware of the ease with which the differential diagnosis of abnormal daytime sleepiness can be made in children with appropriate clinical and laboratory evaluations, more children are likely to be diagnosed. As case series expand, better information on the epidemiology of sleepiness in children will become available. Abnormal sleepiness in children can have far-reaching negative consequences on educational attainment and psychosocial development; it is not a symptom to treat lightly. Even with today's knowledge most sleepy children can be effectively treated if correctly diagnosed.

Family History

Certain sleep disorders are known to be genetically influenced. Narcolepsy, which has an incidence between 3 and 16 per 10,000 [1, 4, 5], is strongly associated with the HLA-DR2 or DQw1 antigen. Within the families of narcoleptic patients, there is a reported eightfold increased risk compared with the general population. Sleep apnea syndrome has also been reported to have a familial pattern. When investigating a family history one needs to remember there are many causes of pathologic sleepiness and more than one can be found in many families. The incidence of obstructive sleep apnea syndrome, for example, may be as high as 1% to 2% of the adult male population [10, 11]. Thus, within the family of a narcoleptic patient there is a greater chance that other sleepy family members have sleep apnea syndrome than narcolepsy. Further, since the diagnosis of narcolepsy was made in the past without benefit of objective confirmation, in an era when physicians' knowledge of the differential diagnosis of sleepiness often included only one or two possibilities, old diagnoses may well have been in error. There is now data to suggest that abnormally sleepy relatives of patients with narcolepsy are in fact more likely to have sleepiness of other causes than narcolepsy [43]. Thus, one cannot assume that relatives of sleepy patients have the same disorder as the patient.

The Physical Examination For Daytime Sleepiness

The physical examination seldom provides diagnostic information helpful in the differential diagnosis of abnormal sleepiness. Patients with most etiologies of sleepiness have normal physical and neurologic examinations.

The cause of sleepiness most associated with specific findings on physical examination is sleep apnea syndrome. An assortment of abnormalities that result in a smaller than normal upper airway have been described. In the stereotypic patient, an obese, middle-aged man, these include large uvulae, low soft palates, and wide tonsillar pillars. Many patients also have vertical folds of redundant mucosa in the posterior oropharynx.

The first clue that the upper airway may be smaller than normal comes when one attempts to see the oropharynx. The oropharynx can rarely be seen even on phonation without use of a tongue blade in patients with sleep apnea. Often the gag reflex is so active the oropharynx can hardly be seen even with a tongue blade. This contrasts markedly with the visualization of an oropharynx of normal patency, although it is a nonspecific finding.

The obese adult man with this disease typically has a large neck as well (Fig. 22-2). In a case series of 56 consecutive sleep apnea syndrome patients (mean apnea index > 20) compared with 53 equally obese male patients without sleep apnea syndrome (apnea index < 5) we found the mean neck circumference of the sleep apnea syndrome patients to be 17.9 ± 1.6 versus 15.9 ± 1.0 in the nonapneic patients (unpublished data). Neck size was shown to be an important discriminating factor on physical examination.

A number of patients other than overweight men have this disease. A host of contributing abnormalities from the nasal cavity to the larynx have been described. Nasal deformities, septal deformities, turbinate enlargement, enlarged tonsils and adenoids (more common in pediatric cases), webbing of the vocal cords, vocal cord paresis, a large floppy epiglottis, etc. have all been associated with sleep apnea syndrome [44]. The skeletal structure of the skull and jaw may also contribute to a smaller than normal oropharyngeal airway. Patients with Down's syndrome, achondroplasia, congenitally small mandibles, and syndromes associated with craniofacial features that produce a smaller than normal nasal, oropharyngeal, or hypopharyngeal airway all are predisposed to developing sleep-related obstruction without obesity. Tumors of the neck, amyloidosis, acromegaly, and other conditions in which soft tissue structures compromise the cross-sectional area of the upper airway have been associated with sleep apnea syndrome [44]. The disease can therefore be seen as a final common pathway resulting from a wide array of factors that impinge on the normal patency of the upper airway. Because of normal changes in airway muscle tone that accompany sleep, symptoms of upper airway compromise are likely to occur first during sleep.

It is not unreasonable to question patients whose airways appear compromised about symptoms of sleep apnea. While the great majority of apnea patients have anatomic findings that may be implicated in the evolution of the disease, the reverse is not necessarily true. There are many patients with crowded throats, large tonsils, small jaws, or masses in the neck who lack any symptoms of the disease. The differences among these

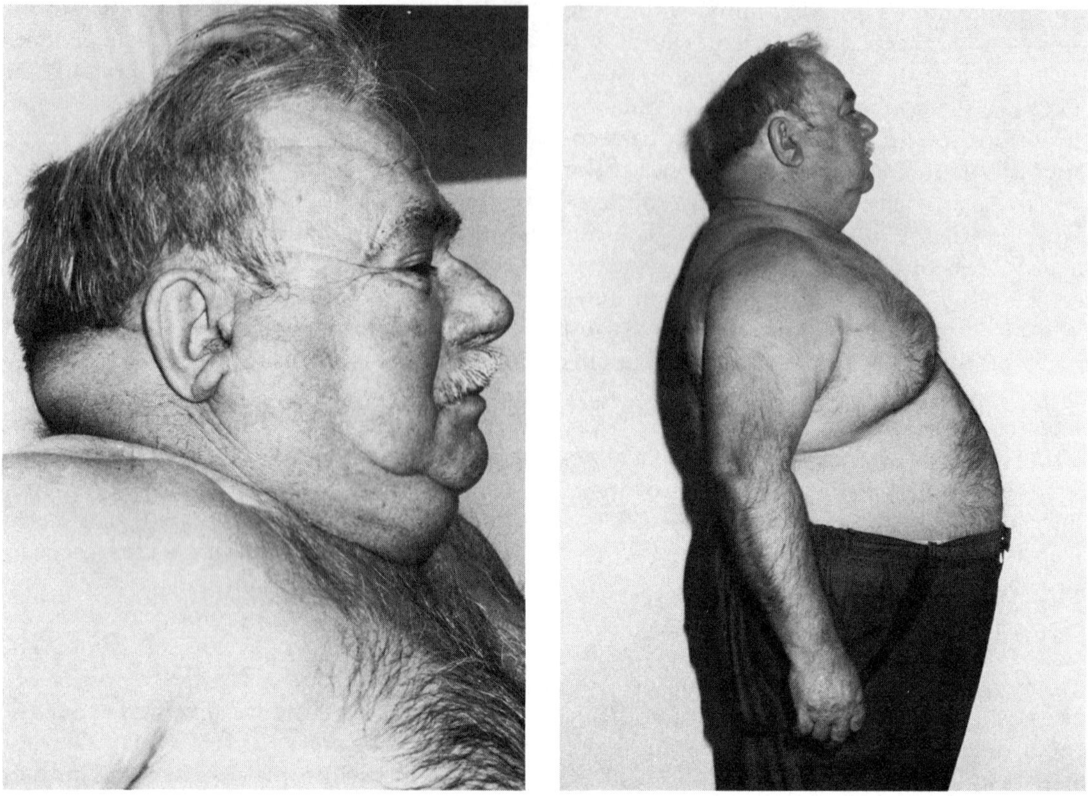

A B

Fig. 22-2. (A and B) Obstructive sleep apnea. Patient with severe obstructive sleep apnea. Note short, thick neck, receding jaw, and obesity.

patients may be in the summation of resistance across the entire upper airway, the presence of additional risk factors (e.g., alcohol, or sleep deprivation) that contribute to sleep-related airway obstruction, or subtle differences in the motor control of the upper airway during sleep. People with small airways who lack any symptoms of sleep apnea syndrome need not be investigated further. Those in whom symptoms are serendipitously discovered this way should be investigated.

An assortment of medical conditions with characteristic features on physical examination are associated with an increased incidence of sleep apnea. Among these are Cushing's disease [45], acromegaly [46], and hypothyroidism [47, 48].

The office cardiopulmonary examination should screen for hypertension, evidence of right- or left-sided heart failure, or compromised pulmonary status. Patients with heart failure have a high incidence of central type sleep apnea. Cardiac or pulmonary disease evident in the awake patient can usually be treated before performing sleep studies. If possible, sleep studies should be deferred until an acute illness has been treated. The central sleep apnea common in the patient in acute heart failure, for example, can obscure the importance of upper airway obstruction occurring in the same patient. Studies performed on acutely ill patients may have little impact on immediate management and have to be repeated after the clinical status improves.

Laboratory Investigation of Sleepiness

Laboratory studies in a sleep disorder center often are required to establish a diagnosis or to measure the severity of disease. Diagnostic sleep studies are an appropriate first course of action in symptomatic patients who have regular, adequate sleep habits, are not using psychotropic agents or medications that could be implicated as causes, and who require no immediate treatment of an acute medical condition.

Deciding when such costly diagnostic studies are warranted before eliminating contributing factors is a matter of clinical judgment. When there are doubts as to optimal management of a sleep evaluation, consultation should be sought with a specialist in sleep disorders medicine. It is embarrassing and wasteful to have performed such costly diagnostic studies only to achieve ambiguous or nondiagnostic results.

If the decision is made to proceed with sleep laboratory testing, attention should be given to several factors. The polysomnographic study should be timed to correspond to the patient's usual principal sleep period. In some cases this requires studies be done in the daytime to fit the work schedules of some patients. In general, the duration of a polysomnographic study should correspond to a normal adult nocturnal sleep period, typically 8 hours. Useful information on sleep efficiency and respiration during the longest REM periods (which can be expected toward the end of the study) will not be obtained if shorter studies are done. Timing the polysomnographic study to start at the time of the patient's usual sleep period increases the likelihood sleep quantity will approach or exceed that which is usual for the patient.

When regularity of sleep habits is an issue or likely to influence the diagnostic impression, the patient should complete sleep logs including bedtimes and arise times for 1 to 2 weeks before the study.

Instrumentation should be tailored to the purpose of the study. If by history and physical examination sleep apnea syndrome is highly unlikely, it may be well to omit use of the oximeter because this instrumentation is the most likely to be uncomfortable to the patient. In such patients sleep-related apnea will not be missed if nasal and oral airflow and respiratory effort are still monitored. The various methods of respiratory effort monitoring (thoracic and abdominal strain gauges, intercostal electromyography (EMG), inductive plethysmography, etc.) allow reasonably unobtrusive measurement of respiratory effort, while carefully placed thermistors or thermocouples can adequately detect the presence or absence of and relative changes in airflow to detect most apnea or hypopnea. More aggressive respiratory monitoring instrumentation requiring the use of masks or esophageal balloons is difficult for most patients to tolerate and may compromise the diagnostic utility of the study. The more unpleasant the instrumentation, the more it should be reserved for cases in which differential issues cannot be resolved any other way. In general, the less instrumentation the more likely the patient's laboratory sleep will resemble his or her usual sleep.

Polysomnography must nevertheless routinely include measurement of physiologic parameters adequate to define sleep. The methods for doing this are well presented elsewhere [49] as are standardized methods for the scoring of human sleep [50]. In addition to standard sleep scoring parameters (central electroencephalography, submental EMG, and electro-occulograms), studies routinely include single lead electrocardiography (to monitor cardiac rate and rhythm), respiratory monitoring to answer the relevant diagnostic questions, and bilateral anterior tibialis EMG monitoring (because of the frequency with which periodic limb movements during sleep occur, which are sometimes diagnostically significant).

Other parameters can be monitored if the differential diagnosis requires them. A more extensive electroencephalography montage than is customary to identify sleep stage parameters can be used if a seizure disorder is suspected. Videotape monitoring of the entire study can be useful either for suspected seizure activity or for cases in which other types of unusual behavior during sleep are suspected. Additional EMG leads may be useful if specific sleep-related movements are suspected. Esophogeal pH might be recorded if gastroesophogeal reflux is suspected during sleep. Core body temperature can be recorded and correlated with sleep when it might be useful to evaluate a circadian rhythm disorder. Sonography and body position monitoring can help evaluate position effects on snoring and respiration during sleep. Other physiologic parameters can be monitored as well. The principal requirement is that the parameter recorded have a bearing on the differential diagnosis being considered and the instrumentation involved should not be so obtrusive as to preclude an adequate sleep study.

Polysomnography of the patient's principal sleep period serves to document the quantity and quality, normal or abnormal, of the patient's sleep before the actual measurement of daytime sleepiness. Physiologic sleepiness can be quantified using the MSLT. The patient is kept in the laboratory the day after the nocturnal polysomnogram and given opportunities to nap every 2 hours beginning 1½ to 3 hours after arising. In between the nap opportunities the patient is to stay awake and out of bed. The environment is standardized; the patient must be comfortable, lying down in a quiet, dark room for the nap opportunities. The patient must not consume substances (e.g., caffeine, alcohol, nonprescription drugs) known to affect sleepiness one way or the other. The patient may take usual prescription medications. Complete guidelines for the consistent performance of the MSLT are published and should be followed by whomever is performing these tests [51].

On the day of the MSLT additional diagnostic testing may be done. This may include urine drug testing, other laboratory drug work, or psychometric screening.

The outcome of the MSLT, the sleep latencies across the day, the sequence and speed with which specific sleep stages are entered at different times of day, is often diagnostic. The MSLT gives an objective measure of the sleepiness that is the patient's chief complaint. In cases of narcolepsy it documents the occurrence not only of pathologic sleepiness but also the sleep-onset REM periods that are pathognomonic of that condition. In cases of sleepiness of other origins the objective severity of sleepiness can greatly influence management. A sleepy patient with 25 apneic episodes on average per hour of nocturnal sleep may be treated more aggressively if the mean daytime sleep latency is 3 minutes (severe sleepiness) than if it is 8 minutes (borderline normal).

After all the clinical and laboratory data have been interpreted, a plausible diagnosis and treatment plan should emerge. Often the explanation is simple as in cases of continuous obstructive apnea during sleep or classic cases of narcolepsy. At least as often, however, diagnosis requires integration of multiple medical and behavioral facets of the history plus the polysomnographic data to satisfactorily explain the patient's problems. The following case examples illustrate both situations.

Example 1

A 46-year-old man who has gained 50 lb since he quit smoking 5 years ago has become an increasingly loud snorer (Fig. 22-2). His wife began noticing interruptions in his breathing during sleep several years ago. She was so irritated by his snoring she began sleeping in a separate room 18 months ago. He presents because he has been caught sleeping at work and is threatened with disciplinary action. He is also concerned about increasing inability to stay awake while driving, though he has had no accidents he can attribute to sleepiness. His habits are regular. He seldom drinks alcohol and takes no medications.

Polysomnographic study revealed 427 mixed and obstructive type apnea in 6.8 hours of sleep (on an 8-hour study). The lowest oxyhemoglobin saturation was 71%, which occurred during REM sleep; he regularly desaturated to 83% in non-REM sleep. Saturation was below 85% for 11 minutes of each hour of sleep. The mean sleep latency was 3.5 minutes on a four nap MSLT, with no sleep-onset REM periods. Thyroid function testing was normal. There was no reason to suspect additional medical illness.

The diagnosis is obstructive sleep apnea syndrome. Effective treatments will be medical (nasal continuous positive airway pressure [CPAP mask]) or surgical (various options), coupled with efforts to lose weight and avoidance of drugs, alcohol, or medications known to worsen sleep apnea or daytime sleepiness.

Example 2

A similarly straightforward history and corroborative test results could be imagined for a case of narcolepsy. A 28-year-old laborer gives a 10-year history of excessive sleepiness despite regular (7 to 8 hours) nightly sleep times. He drinks no alcohol (he has never liked it) and has always been in good health. For 5 years he has felt that his knees might buckle in response to a good joke or associated with certain sporting activities. He has noticed it after hitting particularly well in baseball or on making an important catch, such that he might stumble briefly. He has not noticed hypnogogic hallucinations or sleep paralysis.

A nocturnal polysomnogram showed 6.9 hours of mildly fragmented sleep (out of 8 hours of study), without apnea, periodic movements, or a sleep-onset REM period. The sleep latency at night was 2.5 minutes. The MSLT showed a mean sleep latency of 4.0 minutes, with three sleep-onset REM periods. The suspected diagnosis of narcolepsy was confirmed.

Treatment is likely to consist of education about narcolepsy and how to cope with it best behaviorally, as well as appropriate pharmacologic therapy. Optimal pharmacotherapy will have to be tailored to the individual and is likely to require frequent contact (by phone or in person) before a satisfactory regimen is found.

Example 3

A 15-year-old high school junior gives a 2-year history of abnormal sleepiness. During the school year he is likely to fall asleep riding in cars or in his 11:00 AM to noon chemistry class. He has not fallen asleep in any other social settings or even while doing homework. During the school year he was going to bed between 10:30 and 11:30 PM and estimated 10 to 20 minutes to fall asleep. He awakened to an alarm at 5:30 AM, with some difficulty and feeling tired, for preschool choir practice. He would sometimes nap after school for 1 to 2 hours. The family is unaware of him snoring, but he sleeps in his own room. Nothing remarkable has been noted about his breathing during sleep when he naps in the living room, however. He denied any accessory symptoms of narcolepsy. There was no history of drug, alcohol, or medication use. He was seen during summer vacation when there was less evidence of daytime sleepiness. A 2-week sleep log (during summer vacation) showed nightly bedtimes to vary from midnight to 4:30 AM, and daily sleep time to vary from 2.5 to 12 hours, averaging 9.0 hours.

Since the patient was not complaining of inappropriate sleepiness while on summer vacation, and since there was no reason to suspect an intrinsic sleep disorder by history, the most likely cause of the patient's trouble during the school year was thought to be insufficient nightly sleep. He and his parents were instructed in the importance of regular, adequate nightly sleep, possibly meaning 8 to 9 hours in this patient's case. Polysomnographic study was deferred. The patient was advised to return if he had problems with sleepiness again.

Example 4

A 23-year-old man, vice president of his father's company, complained of 4 months of extreme sleepiness. He was falling asleep at his desk, in social settings, watching TV (after 10 minutes), and driving any distance greater than 20 miles. His snoring was awakening people on other floors of his house, and apneas were noticed. Despite sleeping 11 to 12 hours a night he was difficult to awaken in the morning. He denied any accessory symptoms of narcolepsy. He was taking no medications. He did admit to past use of marijuana but denied current use of illicit drugs. Alcohol usage was significant, amounting to 6 to 12 drinks 2 days per week. Past medical history was unremarkable.

He was 67 inches tall and weighed 236 lb. Blood pressure was 130/80 and his pulse was 108 and regular. Oropharyngeal examination revealed markedly enlarged tonsils separated by less than 1 cm. The space between was filled by a large uvula.

Polysomnography showed 69 obstructive apneas and hypopneas per hour of sleep. Sleep time was 7.6 of 8 hours in bed. Oxygen saturation dropped as low as 50%. The mean sleep latency on the MSLT was 4 minutes, with no sleep-onset REM periods.

Following tonsillectomy snoring and sleepiness were reported to resolve, but the patient did not return for postoperative sleep studies. He did return 3 years later complaining his symptoms had recurred 1 year after surgery. His weight had increased 11 lb. Alcohol consumption had increased as well, to 1 pint of liquor three days per week. A sleep log confirmed this, as well as daily sleep times varying from 3 to 14 hours, averaging 10 hours. He was advised to abstain from alcohol and to regularize his sleep habits. Subsequent polysomnography was remarkable. He slept 7.5 of 8 hours in bed (94% efficiency), with normal sleep architecture and only 9 apneas and hypopneas per hour of sleep (inadequate to explain his symptomatology). The MSLT showed a mean sleep latency of less than 1 minute and three sleep-onset REM periods. The patient was again questioned about accessory symptoms of narcolepsy. He had none. Blood was drawn for HLA typing and was negative for both the DR2 and DQw1 antigens. It was unclear what the correct diagnosis should be until the patient admitted he had been using up to 3 g of cocaine daily for years. Symptoms resolved after completion of a drug rehabilitation program.

Conclusion

As in most areas of medicine, the classic patients are not the typical cases encountered in practice. The skilled clinician will almost always deduce the correct diagnosis from a careful history and use laboratory studies to corroborate the clinical impression, determine the severity of disease, or resolve a differential diagnosis. The greatest skill is probably involved in the latter, setting up the clinical and laboratory evaluation so that the differential questions are indeed resolved and laboratory test results are not ambiguous. Accomplishing this efficiently requires a clinician with considerable breadth of experience in sleep disorders. It is my hope that this chapter will enable primary care physicians to better address the problem of sleepiness and manage many cases well enough to avoid referral to a specialized center. It is also my hope that these same physicians will be more aware of the intrinsic sleep disorders causing pathologic sleepiness and refer these cases, as well as the diagnostic dilemmas, for specialized care.

References

1. International Classification of Sleep Disorders: Diagnostic and Statistic Manual Produced by the Diagnostic Classification Steering Committee of the American Sleep Disorders Association. Rochester, MN, American Sleep Disorders Association, 1990
2. Diagnostic Classification of Sleep and Arousal Disorders. *Sleep* 2, 1979
3. Coleman R, Rofwarg H, Kennedy S., et al: Sleep-wake disorders based on a polysomnographic diagnosis: A National Cooperative Study. *JAMA* 247:997–1103, 1982
4. Aldrich M: Narcolepsy. *N Engl J Med* 323: 389–394, 1990
5. Kales A, Cadieux R, Soldatos C, et al: Narcolepsy-cataplexy I: Clinical and electrophysiologic characteristics. *Arch Neurol* 39: 164–168, 1982
6. Rosenthal L, Merlotti L, Young D, et al: Subjective and polysomnographic characteristics of patients diagnosed with narcolepsy. *Gen Hosp Psychiatry* 12:191–197, 1990
7. Smolk PR, Roth B: Kleine-Levin syndrome: Etiopathogenesis and treatment. ACTA Universitatis Carolinae, Monographia CXXVII,

Univerzita Karlova, Praha, Czechoslovakia, 1988
8. Williams RL, Karacan I, Hursch CJ: Electroencephalography of Human Sleep: Clinical Applications. New York, John Wiley and Sons, 1974
9. Lugaresi E, Cirignotta F, Coccagna G, et al: Some epidemiologic data on snoring and cardiocirculatory disturbances. *Sleep* 3:221–224, 1980
10. Lavie P: Sleep habits and sleep disturbances in industrial workers in Israel: Main findings and some characteristics of workers complaining of excessive daytime sleepiness. *Sleep* 4:147–158, 1981
11. Gislason T, Almquist M, Eriksson G, et al: Prevalence of sleep apnea syndrome among Swedish men—An epidemiological study. *J Clin Epidemiol* 41:571–576, 1988
12. He J, Kryger MH, Zorick FJ, et al: Mortality and apnea index in obstructive sleep apnea: Experience in 385 male patients. *Chest* 94: 9–14, 19
13. Roth T, Roehrs T, Kryger M: Mortality in Obstructive Sleep Apnea; Sleep and Respiration. New York, Wiley-Liss, 1990, pp 347–352
14. Roth T, Roehrs T, Conway WA: Behavioral morbidity of apnea. *Seminars in Respiratory Medicine* 9:554–559, 1988
15. Young D, Zorick F, Wittig R, et al: Narcolepsy in a pediatric population. *Am J Dis Child* 142: 210–213, 1988
16. Wittig R, Zorick F, Roehrs T, et al: Narcolepsy in a seven year old child. *J Pediatr* 102:725–727, 1983
17. Chisolm RC, Brook CJ, Harrison GF, et al: Prepubescent narcolepsy in a six yr old child. *Sleep Res* 15:113, 1985
18. Parkes JD: Sleep and its Disorders. Philadelphia, WB Saunders, 1985
19. Roehrs TA, Zorick FJ, Sicklesteel J, et al: Excessive sleepiness associated with insufficient sleep. *Sleep* 6:319–325, 1983
20. Wittig R, Zorick F, Piccione P, et al: Narcolepsy and disturbed nocturnal sleep. *Clin Electroencephalogr* 14:130–134, 1983
21. Roth T, Zorick F, Roehrs T: The interaction of daytime sleepiness and sedative properties of drugs. *Psychopharmacol Bull* 23:440–443, 1987
22. Zwyghuizen-Doorenboss A, Roehrs T, Lamphere J, et al: Increased daytime sleepiness enhances ethanol's sedative effects. *Neuropsychopharmacology* 1:279–286, 1988
23. Zwyghuizen-Doorenboss A, Roehrs T, Timms V, et al: Individual differences in the sedating effects of ethanol. *Alcoholism: Clinical and Experimental Research,* 14:400–404, 1990
24. Issa FG, Sullivan CE: Alcohol, snoring, and sleep apnea. *J Neurol Neurosurg Psychiatry* 45:353–359, 1982
25. Gilliland K, Bullock W: Caffeine: A potential drug of abuse. *Adv Alcohol Subst Abuse* 3:53–73, 1983/1984
26. Gilman AG, Rall TW, Nies AS, et al: The Pharmacologic Basis of Therapeutics, ed 8. Elmsford, NY, Pergamon Press, 1990
27. Nicholson A, Bradley C, Pascoe P: Medications: Effect on sleep and wakefulness. *In* Kryger M, Roth T, Dement W (eds): Principles and Practice of Sleep Disorders Medicine. Philadelphia, WB Saunders, 1989, pp 228–236
28. Carskadon M, Cavallo A, Rosekind M: Sleepiness and nap sleep following a morning dose of clonidine. *Sleep* 12:338–344, 1989
29. Rosen RC, Kostis JB, Taska LS, et al: Beta blocker effects on objective and subjective measures of sleep in normotensive male subjects. *Sleep Research* 15:42, 1986
30. Gengo FM, Huntoon L, McHugh WB: Lipid soluble and water soluble beta blockers: Comparison of the central nervous system depressant effect. Arch Intern Med 147:39–43, 1987
31. Drayer DE: Lipophilicity, hydrophilicity, and the central nervous side effects of beta blockers. *Pharmacotherapy* 7:87–91, 1987
32. Betts TA, Alford C: Beta blockers and sleep: A controlled trial. *Eur J Clin Pharmacol* 28: 65–68, 1985
33. Cove-Smith JR, Kirk CA: CNS related side effects with metaprolol and atenolol. *Eur J Clin Pharmacol* 28(suppl):69–72, 1985
34. Koella WP: CNS related (side) effects of beta blockers with special reference to mechanisms of action. *Eur J Clin Pharmacol* 28(suppl): 55–63, 1985
35. Callaghan N, Garrett A, Goggin T: Withdrawal of anticonvulsant in patients free of seizures for two years. *N Engl J Med* 318:942–946, 1988
36. The safety of fluoxitine—An update. *Br J Psychiatry* 153(suppl):77–86, 1988
37. Ferber R: Solve Your Child's Sleep Problems. New York, Simon and Schuster, 1985, p 19
38. Guilleminault C: Sleep and Its Disorders in Children. New York, Raven Press, 1987, pp 177–231
39. Guilleminault C, Winkle R: A review of 50 children with obstructive sleep apnea syndrome. *Lung* 159:275–287, 1981
40. Ferber R, Friedman E, Dietz W: Obstructive sleep apnea in childhood: 80 cases. *Sleep Research* 12:245, 1983
41. Yitzchak F, Cravath R, Pollak C, et al: Obstructive sleep apnea and its therapy: Clinical and polysomnographic manifestations. *Pediatrics* 71:737–742, 1983

42. Ferber R, Boyle P: Six year experience of a pediatric sleep disorders center. *Sleep Research* 15:120, 19
43. Guilleminault C: Genetic aspects of narcolepsy. Presented in Symposium: Narcolepsy: From Molecular Aspects to Human Studies. Assoc. Prof. Sleep Soc., 4th Annual Meeting, Minneapolis, MN, June 29, 1990
44. Fairbanks D, Fujita S, Ikematsu T, et al: Snoring and Obstructive Sleep Apnea. New York, Raven Press, 1987
45. Shipley J, Starkman M: EEG sleep in Cushing's disease. *Sleep Research* 19:102, 1990
46. Perks WH, Horrocks PM, Cooper RA, et al: Sleep apnea in acromegaly. *Br Med J* 280: 894–897, 1980
47. Rajagobal KR, Abbrecht PH, Derderias SS, et al: Obstructive sleep apnea in hypothyroidism. *Ann Intern Med* 101:491–494, 1984
48. Grunstein RR, Sullivan CE: Hypothyroidism and sleep apnoea: Mechanisms and management. *Aust N Z J Med* 16:635, 1986
49. Guilleminault C (ed): Sleeping and Waking Disorders: Indications and Techniques. Menlo Park, CA, Addison Wesley, 1982
50. Rechtschaffen A, Kales A: A Manual of Standardized Terminology, Techniques, and Scoring System for Sleep Stages of Human Subjects. Brain Information Service, Brain Research Institute, UCLA, 1968
51. Carskadon M: Guidelines for the multiple sleep latency test: A standard measure of sleepiness. *Sleep* 9:519–524, 1986

Sleep Disorders: Insomnia

Edward J. Stepanski

Insomnia is defined as the inability to initiate or maintain sleep and is a very common medical complaint. Recent epidemiologic survey data reveal that 35% of adult Americans have had difficulty sleeping at some time in the past year [1]. Half of this group (17% of the adult population) described this difficulty as serious. These estimates are similar to those cited in previous research, although there is variability depending on the definition used (Table 23-1). Another recent epidemiologic survey that used a very strict definition of insomnia reported that 10.2% of the community had insomnia [2]. To be considered positive for insomnia, respondents must have had difficulty sleeping for a 2-week period and have sought treatment or reported that the sleep problem interfered significantly with their life. In recognition of the prevalence of insomnia there have been many investigations aimed at understanding and treating this symptom. However, progress in the evaluation and treatment of insomnia has been very gradual. In part, this delay is due to the heterogeneity of patients presenting with this complaint. In the first nosologic system for sleep disorders published by the Association of Sleep Disorder Centers in 1979 [3], insomnia is described as being associated with some other disorder in all but two diagnostic categories. This system acknowledges that insomnia is a symptom common to many distinct medical, psychiatric, or behavioral disorders.

A National Institute of Mental Health Consensus Conference in 1983 agreed that symptomatic treatment with hypnotic medications is most appropriate for transient (duration of less than 1 week) and short-term (duration up to 1 month) insomnia [4]. In the case of chronic insomnia, however, treatment should be aimed at the specific factors precipitating the symptom. Therefore, an evaluation and diagnosis is needed for patients with chronic insomnia before rational treatment can be prescribed. The diagnosis should lead to specific treatment approaches aimed at the causative or precipitating factors in the insomnia. This chapter describes assessment procedures for and diagnostic categories of complaints of chronic insomnia.

A Model of Chronic Insomnia

While the focus over the past decade has been on the differences between subgroups of insomnia patients (precipitating factors), there are also similarities among patients presenting with insomnia (predisposing factors). It is likely that some individuals are more predisposed to insomnia than others, and this predisposition is elicited with exposure to a precipitant of poor sleep. Such a model could explain why only certain individuals with periodic leg movements complain of insomnia, while others remain asymptomatic or become excessively sleepy during the day [5].

A recent study has shown that some subjects, who are otherwise normal sleepers, consistently sleep more poorly in response to laboratory adaptation than do others [6]. The subjects who adapt poorly sleep as well as those who adapt well once they are adapted to the laboratory. One interpretation of this finding is that vulnerable subjects are predisposed toward transient insomnia in the presence of a precipitating factor (the stress of sleeping in the laboratory for the first time with electrodes attached to the face and head) even though they sleep well otherwise. The mechanism of this predisposition is not known, but one possibility is a tendency toward greater physiologic hyperarousal. Such

Table 23-1. Prevalence of Insomnia in Different Population Studies

Authors	*Country*	*Sample (no.)*	*Problem in Focus*	*Criteria*	*Age Range (yr)*	*Sex Distinction*	*Prevalence (M/F) (%)*
Bixler et al 1979 [84]	USA	1006	Insomnia	Current problem	>18	No	32.2
Bixler et al 1979 [84]	USA	1006	Trouble falling asleep	Current problem	>18	No	14.4
Bixler et al 1979 [84]	USA	1006	Nocturnal awakenings	Current problem	>18	No	22.9
Karacan et al 1976 [85]	USA	1645	Trouble with sleeping	Often or all the time	>18	Yes	10.9/15.4
Lugaresi et al 1983 [87]	San Marino	5713	Insomnia	Always or almost always	3–94	No	13.4
Partinen et al 1983 [88]	Finland	31,140	Difficulty falling asleep	Report	18–39 >60	Yes	18.8–19.6/20.3–16.5 31.1/42.5
Welstein et al 1983 [89]	USA	6340	Difficulty falling asleep	Complaint	6–103	Yes	11.9/15.3
Welstein et al 1983 [89]	USA	6340	Nocturnal awakenings	Complaint	6–103	Yes	12.0/18.6
Welstein et al 1983 [89]	USA	6340	Insomnia	Yes	6–103	Yes	3.2/5.0
Karacan et al 1983 [86]	USA	2347	Difficulty falling asleep	Often or always	>18	Yes	6.0/11.2
Karacan et al 1983 [86]	USA	2347	Difficulty maintaining sleep	Often or always	>18	Yes	12.9/17.4

From Liljenberg B, Almqvist M, Hetta J, et al: The prevalence of insomnia: The importance of operationally defined criteria. *Ann Clin Res* 20:393–398, 1988; with permission.

a tendency has been demonstrated in patients with chronic insomnia and in a group of poor sleepers [7–9]. For example, patients with insomnia have been shown to have higher heart rates at bedtime and while in bed at night, both during sleep and wakefulness [7, 9]. They also show greater responsivity of heart rate when a stressful reaction-time task is administered [7]. Further evidence of hyperarousal can be found when measuring daytime alertness in insomniac patients with the Multiple Sleep Latency Test [10]. Patients presenting with a complaint of chronic insomnia were found to be significantly more alert during the day than were normal sleepers, despite the fact that the insomniac group slept significantly less the previous night. However, much more research is needed before a predisposition to insomnia can be definitively described.

Evaluation of Insomnia

In nearly all cases, a complaint of insomnia is secondary to another primary condition. Only with an understanding of the underlying cause(s) of the insomnia can a rational treatment plan be devised. Precipitating factors may be medical or psychiatric illness, behavioral factors, medication effects, or primary sleep disorders. Careful assessment is needed for every patient presenting with a complaint of insomnia. For this reason, assessment of these patients is generally more

Table 23-2. Disorders of Initiating and Maintaining Sleep (Insomnias)

Diagnostic Category	*No.*	*%*	*Range/Center (%)*
Psychiatric disorders	424	34.9	3.9–66.8
Psychophysiologic	186	15.3	1.0–32.9
Drug and alcohol dependency	151	12.4	2.9–25.2
Sleep-related myoclonus and RLS	148	12.2	2.8–26.3
No insomnia abnormality	112	9.2	0.0–28.7
Sleep apnea syndromes	75	6.2	0.0–18.4
Other insomnia conditions	68	5.6	0.0–12.6
Medical, toxic, and environmental	46	3.8	0.0–12.6
Childhood onset insomnia	4	0.3	0.0–1.6
Total	1214	99.9	

From Coleman RM, et al: Sleep-wake disorders based on a polysomnographic diagnosis: A national cooperative study. *JAMA* 247:997–1003, 1982. Copyright 1982, American Medical Association. Reprinted by permission.

time consuming than assessment of other patients presenting in a clinical practice. The incidence of specific diagnoses for those patients presenting with insomnia varies markedly among different sleep centers (Table 23-2). To some extent this results because the department in which a sleep center is located accepts referrals of different patient types. Additionally, however, this variability in diagnosis results from bias related to the expertise of the sleep specialist, i.e., a psychiatrist will find more psychiatric insomnia, an internist will find more medical insomnia, and a psychologist will find more behavioral insomnia. A multidisciplinary evaluation, or at least a multidisciplinary review of all new cases, is essential for patients presenting with chronic insomnia.

Initial Interview

The initial interview should include a sleep history, medical history, psychiatric history, and at least a brief physical examination. Additional consultations, psychometric testing, or laboratory tests may be ordered as needed.

Sleep History

The sleep history should determine the following:

1. duration of the sleep problem,
2. severity of the insomnia,
3. daytime consequences the patient attributes to his or her poor sleep,
4. typical sleep-wake schedule (bedtimes and arising times) both during the week and on weekends,
5. type and location of presleep activities,
6. depth of sleep and timing of awakenings,
7. behavior during awakenings,
8. patterns of caffeine and alcohol use,
9. pattern of sleeping pill use,
10. napping behavior, and
11. characteristics of the sleep environment.

Ideally, the patient will have already completed 2 weeks of sleep logs before the initial interview so that the log can be reviewed at this time. Sleep logs consist of a diary of bedtimes, arising times, use of medications and alcohol, and napping. Behavioral monitoring of this type is important both during the evaluation phase and during treatment. For purposes of evaluation, sleep logs provide information regarding sleep habits that diverge from the patient's description or may uncover relations between sleep disturbance and specific behaviors of which the patient is unaware.

Medical and Medication History

The medical history should include both acute and chronic illnesses. Any condition associated with pain, decreased pulmonary function, chronic renal failure, or neurologic disorders is likely to affect sleep quality negatively (research on this topic is discussed in the following sections). Other disorders, such as hypertension or cardiac arrhythmias, may be important because of the medications used for treatment. A careful history of paroxysmal nocturnal dyspnea or orthopnea should be obtained.

Of particular significance in the evaluation of insomnia is the medication history. Many commonly prescribed medications have been shown to have an adverse effect on sleep. Much of the information in this area is related to patients' subjective reports of sleep quality or quantity. Studies that have obtained objective measures (electroencephalogram [EEG] recordings) are few and generally do not find as much evidence of sleep disturbance as is reported by patients. However, many drugs do cause disrupted sleep, and these results are discussed.

It is likely that certain predisposed patients experience more severe adverse effects on sleep quality and quantity from centrally acting medications even if many other patients do not. Usually the therapeutic benefit of using these medicines outweighs the side effects, and therefore the drug should not be discontinued. In some instances, however, the drug can be changed to another that may have fewer effects on sleep. Sleeplessness, as with most side effects, is more likely at higher dosages. Therefore, another strategy is to try a lower dosage that is still clinically effective but may have fewer effects on sleep. Alternatively, the timing of the dosages may be altered such that the patient is not taking a dose immediately before bedtime.

Psychiatric History

Knowledge of past episodes of psychiatric illness, in addition to current mental status, is necessary in all patients complaining of insomnia. A primary concern is the possibility of affective illness. The presence of an anxiety disorder must also be ruled out. Obsessive-compulsive behavior, phobias, or panic attacks may be important contributors to a complaint of poor sleep. More difficult to assess, but also important, is the possibility of a personality disorder. Borderline, obsessive-compulsive, and passive-aggressive personality disorders can lead to poor sleep because of intermittent episodes of intense tension and anxiety along with chronically elevated tension levels. Sleep may also be disturbed because of the behavioral abnormalities that often accompany these disorders (e.g., an irregular sleep-wake schedule, abuse of drugs). To assist in identifying patients with psychopathology, many sleep centers routinely administer psychometric tests, such as the Minnesota Multiphasic Personality Inventory, as part of an evaluation of a complaint of insomnia.

Careful scrutiny of potential use of illicit drugs or alcohol abuse is also necessary. Obviously acute use of alcohol can be expected to have profound deleterious effects on sleep quality, particularly at high dosages [11]. What is less well-known is that sleep abnormalities may be present in alcoholic patients even after 1 year of sobriety [12]. If drug use is suspected, then obtaining a urine drug screen as part of the evaluation is recommended. A drug screen is especially important at the time of polysomnography (PSG), if one is performed, since the presence of stimulants or hypnotics could have a profound influence on the interpretation of the recording.

Bed Partner Interview

Interviewing the patient's partner especially if they share a bedroom, can be helpful in several respects. First, information regarding the patient's snoring, stopped breathing episodes, or leg movements can be obtained. Second, the partner may be able to provide a more accurate view of how much time the patient is actually sleeping. This is helpful in judging to what extent the patient may tend to exaggerate the severity of his or her sleep difficulty. A spouse or other family member can also corroborate crucial aspects of the patient's history, including incidence of daytime naps, pattern of alcohol intake, use of sleeping pills, current situational stressors, or psychiatric history.

Physical Examination

The physical examination should be a standard component of the insomnia evaluation. The examination should include mental status assessment, a neurologic examination, an ear, nose, and throat examination, and evaluation of cardiopulmonary functioning. In the Insomnia Clinic at the Henry Ford Hospital Sleep Disorders and Research Center we have found previously undiagnosed cases of congestive heart failure, severe hypertension, and chronic obstructive pulmonary disease in patients seeking evaluation for insomnia. This occurred despite our policy of accepting only physician-referred patients. In these instances, we refer the patients for evaluation and treatment of their medical condition before proceeding with further evaluation of the sleep complaint.

Ongoing Monitoring

Even after collecting all this information, the cause of the insomnia may not be immediately clear. Multifactorial etiologies of insomnia are common in patients referred to sleep centers because those patients with obvious psychiatric insomnia or medical insomnia have often already been detected by the family physician and referred elsewhere. Determining which factors should be given primary consideration in treatment often involves ongoing monitoring. Changes in the patient's sleep-wake schedule, medication regimen, alcohol intake, or other behavior can be recommended following the initial interview. The patient's compliance and the impact of the changes can be monitored through the use of sleep logs and phone contacts and/or brief office visits. Weekly follow-up is essential (twice per week contact is optimal) as otherwise the patient will not continue behavior changes for more than a few days. Further changes and adjustments can be made based on the patient's progress. Some behavioral interventions made in this way (e.g., turning off the radio before sleep, delaying the bedtime) may entirely eliminate the poor sleep. Even when sleep does not improve as a result of these initial recommendations, diagnostic information is being obtained. By ruling out certain behavioral factors as contributing to the insomnia, another disorder may emerge (e.g., depression) as the primary problem and a diagnosis can be made. In other instances, further evaluation and/or treatment is needed as described in the following section.

Polysomnographic Procedures

At some point in the evaluation procedure, clinical PSG may be necessary to make a diagnosis. This procedure consists of all night recording of (minimally) the EEG, electrocardiogram, electro-oculogram, electromyogram (submental and anterior tibialis of both legs), and respiration. This test might be performed soon after the initial interview if there is reason to suspect a primary sleep disorder (e.g., bed partner reports stopped breathing episodes, patient complains of frequent leg twitches). In other instances the test might be ordered only after the patient has spent several weeks correcting behavioral components to his or her sleep problem without significant improvement in sleep. As many diagnostic hypotheses as possible should be ruled out before performing a sleep recording. If poor sleep hygiene, environmental factors, or medication effects are suspected in the etiology of an insomnia complaint, then these factors should be remediated before consideration of a PSG. When the contribution of these factors to the disturbed sleep has been attenuated or eliminated, and the patient still reports sleeping poorly, then the PSG can be more helpful. If the PSG is administered before addressing behavioral or medication issues, then its usefulness is diminished. The amount of sleep disturbance on a PSG due to arthritic pain, an irregular sleep-wake schedule, or use of a lipid-soluble β-blocker cannot be determined. Prior attempts to address these factors are needed before the PSG can be optimally helpful.

There is some controversy in the sleep field as to when a PSG is needed in the evaluation of insomnia. Some extreme opinions hold that a PSG is never indicated in the evaluation of insomnia. While it is not necessary on every patient, and it is not the first step of an evaluation, there is a definite role for the PSG in evaluating and diagnosing a complaint of insomnia. At a minimum the PSG is uniquely capable of providing certain diagnostic information. First, it will objectively document the degree of sleep disturbance. About 9.2% of patients presenting to sleep centers with a complaint of insomnia are found to have subjective insomnia [13]. This is defined as normal sleep quantity and quality in the presence of a subjective report of insomnia [14]. This diagnosis cannot be made without a PSG. Second, the PSG can determine the extent that sleep-disordered breathing or a movement disorder is contributing to disturbed sleep. Older patients complaining of insomnia are especially at risk for these events, and only a PSG will provide this information.

Additionally, it is likely that other information provided by a PSG will be helpful. The number and timing of wake periods, abnormal rapid eye movement (REM) sleep parameters, idiopathic arousals, and awakenings are all assessed by a PSG. PSG variables have been shown to vary as a function of the diagnostic subcategory of insomnia (Table 23-3).

A Multiple Sleep Latency Test is recommended in the evaluation of insomnia only for patients who also give a history of excessive daytime sleepiness. While most patients with insomnia report daytime tiredness, they do not typically complain of excessive sleepiness (tendency to actually fall asleep during the day). The sleepiness complaint needs to be objectively evaluated as it may provide diagnostic information or alter consideration of certain treatment approaches. For example, a patient with objective sleep disturbance secondary to medical illness who is also found to be excesssively sleepy during the day on the Multiple Sleep Latency Test would not be a candidate for sleep restriction therapy or long-acting hypnotics.

Diagnosis of Insomnia

Medical Illness

Many medical conditions can potentially cause short and/or disrupted sleep, especially in individuals with a history of prior episodes of insomnia. Some of the more common conditions are described in the following section.

Pulmonary Disease

Patients with chronic obstructive pulmonary disease often report that their sleep is fragmented by frequent awakenings, with difficulty returning to sleep [15]. PSG data have documented increased stage 1 sleep (the lightest stage of sleep), increased arousals, decreased REM sleep, and decreased total sleep time [15–17]. Presumably the sleep fragmentation in these patients is related to hypoxemia and/or hypercapnia during sleep, particularly during REM sleep. An additional complication is that most of these patients are taking medications that adversely affect sleep quality (e.g., theophylline). Patients with this type of insomnia may report sleeping better in an easy chair than in bed.

Although there are few objective sleep studies available, insomnia has also been reported in patients with interstitial lung disease [18]. In these patients, sleep disruption is probably related to hypoxemia and breathing dysrhythmias.

Rheumatologic Disease

Sleep abnormalities have been described in patients with the fibrositis syndrome [19]. These patients have been shown to complain of difficulty maintaining sleep and daytime fatigue [19]. PSG recordings exhibit alpha intrusions during non-REM sleep and alpha-delta activity [19]. Alpha waves have a frequency of 6 to 12 cycles per second and are usually confined to drowsy wakefulness. Alpha-delta refers to the mixture of delta waves (<2 cycles per second, activity associated with the deepest stages of sleep) and alpha waves during non-REM sleep. However, these sleep findings may not be specific to fibrositis patients since similar sleep abnor-

Table 23-3. Sleep Parameters in Patients with Complaints of Insomnia and in Normal Control Subjects

	Total Sleep Time (min)		*Percent Wake*		*Wake Before Sleep (min)*		*Wake During Sleep (min)*		*Wake After Sleep (min)*		*Percent Stage 1 Sleep*	
Category	***Mean***	***SD***	***Mean***	***SD***	***Mean***	***SD***	***Mean***	***SD***	***Mean***	***SD***	***Mean***	***SD***
Normal subjects (N = 20)	408.7	59.9*	17.6	10.5*	28.0	27.9	52.3	41.6	10.6	13.8*	14.3	4.9
Patients with psychophysiologic disorder (N = 5)	360.7	7.3	23.0	11.3	32.3	37.2	60.5	44.4	8.1	10.1	24.2	12.7†
Patients with psychiatric disorder (N = 12)	289.8	100.0†	38.6	21.0†	70.4	74.1	62.8	51.3	42.0	48.5†	12.8	6.2
Patients with disorder related to drug or alcohol use (N = 10)	319.4	127.6†	26.0	27.4	57.0	125.7	46.7	42.9	4.5	6.5	15.9	12.0
Patients with respiratory impairment (N = 6)	280.7	148.2†	30.3	29.8	39.5	78.2	55.7	40.0	9.1	12.6	25.5	11.0*,†
Patients with nocturnal myoclonus (N = 9)	406.4	55.3*	9.1	5.9*	12.7	11.4	23.5	15.0	2.3	6.5*	16.4	11.2
Patients with RLS (N = 9)	230.9	84.2†	51.6	15.7†	46.2	73.0	176.0	96.5*,†	11.2	12.9	15.3	7.0
Patients with disorder associated with medical diseases (N = 6)	308.8	106.8†	23.2	19.9	31.9	32.6	61.4	85.2	7.8	10.0	21.5	11.0
Patients with atypical PSG feature (N = 4)	393.3	54.5	18.7	10.9	21.6	19.7	64.6	41.2	6.1	6.7	13.8	10.0
Patients with subjective complaint without objective PSG findings (N = 16)	400.0	50.0*	10.5	6.2*	14.2	15.0*	28.5	24.4	4.7	9.1*	14.6	5.1
Patients with circadian rhythm disorder (N = 7)	468.5	70.3*	13.0	7.0*	30.9	26.0	32.0	26.2	5.1	4.4	13.6	3.5

*These values were significantly different from those for the patients with psychiatric disorder ($P < 0.05$, two-tailed t test).
†These values were significantly different from those for the normal control subjects ($P < 0.05$, two-tailed t test).
From Zorick F, Roth T, Hartse K, et al: Evaluation and diagnosis of persistent insomnia. *Am J Psychiatry* 138:769–773, 1981; with permission.

malities have been described in chronic pain patients not diagnosed with fibrositis [20]. Also, alpha intrusion occurs during non-REM sleep in patients with rheumatoid arthritis [21]. Another recent study found significantly greater sleep fragmentation in patients with rheumatoid arthritis than in age-matched control subjects [22]. An alpha-delta pattern in the sleep EEG was also noted in these patients.

Central Nervous System Dysfunction

Insomnia is a consequence of many different disorders of the nervous system. Patients with Alzheimer's disease have been shown to have decreased delta sleep, decreased REM sleep, and increased wakefulness during the night compared with age-matched normal controls [23]. These sleep changes were evident in patients with mild stages of Alzheimer's disease and became proportionately greater in Alzheimer's disease groups with more severe dementia. Decreased total sleep time and sleep stage abnormalities have also been documented in patients with dementia from other etiologies [24].

Parkinson's disease is associated with a long sleep-onset latency and decreased total sleep time [25]. Insomnia persists in these patients even with appropriate treatment of the disease [26].

Medication Effects

Obviously, any medication that acts as a central nervous system stimulant has the potential to interfere with sleep. Use of methylphenidate [27], pemoline [28], or amphetamine [29] at bedtime causes a significant reduction in total sleep time. Caffeine ingested close to bedtime has been shown to cause longer sleep-onset latencies and an increased number of awakenings during the first half of the night [30]. Medicines used as bronchodilators also can worsen sleep. Theophylline, albuterol, and terbutaline may lead to more frequent awakenings and shorter total sleep times, especially at high dosages. Theophylline has been shown to worsen sleep parameters in patients with nocturnal asthma even though their respiratory symptoms were improved [31]. In this study total sleep time was significantly decreased in the treatment group compared with placebo (a mean difference of 47 minutes). Contradictory findings have been reported in patients with chronic obstructive pulmonary disease. Decreased total sleep time while taking theophylline has been reported, but another study found no sleep changes with theophylline [32, 33].

Results of studies of the sleep effects of antihypertensive medications have been inconsistent. One study reports that propranolol, pindolol, and metoprolol all reduce sleep continuity in normotensive subjects [34]. Another study of propranalol, pindolol, metoprolol, and atenolol reports that only pindolol caused a significant increase in wakefulness [35]. Other investigations report that both metoprolol and clonidine significantly increased wake time across the night compared with placebo [36, 36a]. Fewer adverse sleep effects have been reported with atenolol, and this may be a better medication for those patients complaining of insomnia [37].

In trials of the antidepressant fluoxetine, patients reported having insomnia significantly more often than those patients taking either tricyclic antidepressants or placebo [38]. This effect was particularly pronounced at dosages above 20 mg.

Many over-the-counter medications also contribute to disturbed sleep. Decongestant medications, such as phenylpropanolamine or pseudoephedrine, may lead to complaints of insomnia in some patients. However, no study with objective measures of sleep have been performed on patients using these medications. Caffeine is added to some compounds and often the patient is unaware of this (Table 23-4).

Psychiatric Illness

Depression

Virtually all patients with major affective illnesses complain of disrupted sleep and daytime fatigue [39]. The single most common diagnosis for patients presenting to sleep centers complaining of insomnia is affective illness [13]. Patients with insomnia secondary to

Table 23-4. Caffeine Content in Nonprescription Drugs

Drug	*Caffeine (mg)*
Analgesics*	
Anacin Analgesic Coated	32
Aspirin Free Excedrin Analgesic	65
Excedrin Extra-Strength Analgesic	65
P-A-C Analgesic	32
Vanquish Analgesic	33
Stimulants*	
Vivarin	200
No-Doz	100
No-Doz Maximum Strength	200
Beverages	
Various Soft Drinks	36–54
Coffee (5 oz. cup)	
Brewed, drip method	115
Brewed, percolator	80
Instant	65
Decaffeinated	3
Tea (5 oz. cup)	
Brewed, major U.S. brands	40
Brewed, imported brands	60
Instant	30
Iced (12 oz. glass)	70

**From* Medical economics data. Physicians' Desk Reference for Nonprescription Drugs. Oradell, NJ: Medical Economics Company, 1991.

affective illness report frequent awakenings with difficulty returning to sleep, early morning awakenings without returning to sleep, and daytime fatigue [39]. These patients also have some of the other symptoms of depression, such as disturbed appetite, daytime lethargy, anhedonia, and decreased mood. However, depressed patients presenting to a sleep center are more likely to view their sleep disturbance as the primary problem that in turn causes the other symptoms. PSG shows many idiopathic arousals and awakenings, decreased total sleep time, decreased delta sleep, and abnormal REM parameters [40]. These include a shortened REM latency, a long first REM period, and increased REM density (a greater than normal number of rapid eye movements per minute of REM sleep).

Anxiety Disorders

Obsessive-compulsive disorder, generalized anxiety disorder, phobias, and posttraumatic stress disorder may all elicit insomnia. Anxiety states frequently precipitate difficulty initiating sleep, but poor sleep maintenance may also be a feature of these disorders. A patient may awaken in response to a nightmare, as in posttraumatic stress disorder, or may awaken for other reasons and be unable to return to sleep easily because of obsessive thinking or somatic manifestations of anxiety. The PSG findings for these patients show a nonspecific pattern of disrupted sleep consisting of a long sleep-onset latency, many idiopathic arousals and awakenings, increased percentage of stage 1 sleep, and a lowered sleep efficiency [41]. These patients can be differentiated from psychophysiologic insomnia patients based on their daytime function. Anxiety disorder patients have anxiety symptoms during the day and experience difficulty functioning in other areas of their lives (e.g., job, family, friends). Patients with psychophysiologic insomnia have anxiety and tension that surface primarily at bedtime and relate soley to their concerns regarding their sleep.

Many patients with anxiety disorders may also be taking anxiolytic medication and the pattern of drug use needs to be carefully monitored. These patients may be self-medicating at night.

Alcoholism

Acute use of alcohol shortens sleep-onset latency, decreases REM sleep, and disrupts sleep continuity, particularly in the second half of the night [42]. Although the effect depends on tolerance, a dose of about 0.6 mg/kg of body weight (four to five drinks) has been shown to reliably disrupt sleep. Sleep disruption is more severe in the instance of chronic alcoholism. Increased awakenings, increased stage 1 sleep, decreased delta sleep, and decreased total sleep time are found in the sleep of chronic alcoholics [11]. Sleep fragmentation also occurs during acute withdrawal from alcohol, and REM rebound is noted at this time [43]. Behavioral disruption of the sleep cycle has also been noted in the sleep of alcoholic subjects, both with use of alcohol and during withdrawal [44]. Short sleep periods, 3 to 4 hours in duration, are spread out over the 24 hours in this population.

Primary Sleep Disorders

Sleep-Related Breathing Disorders

Although most patients with obstructive sleep apnea syndrome present with a primary complaint of excessive daytime sleepiness, some of these patients also complain of insomnia [13]. Patients who present with a complaint of insomnia and are found to have sleep apnea are more likely to have significantly more central, rather than obstructive, apneas and fewer overall episodes than those patients with excessive daytime sleepiness [45]. Although only 6.2% of patients presenting to a sleep center with an insomnia are diagnosed as having sleep apnea, the risk of sleep-disordered breathing in older patients is much higher [5, 46]. Therefore, when evaluating a patient over 60 years of age, the possibility of sleep-disordered breathing as a contributor to the sleep complaint needs to be more seriously considered than in younger patients. At the same time, care should be taken not to overinterpret the importance of a small number of apneic events (<20 events per hour of sleep). Even though the presence of respiratory events (apneas and hypopneas) is more common in the elderly, this does not mean that they are always the primary cause of the insomnia.

The significance of abnormal respiration on a PSG for a patient complaining of insomnia must be considered in the context of the relevant sleep parameters. The degree to which increased wakefulness and stage 1 sleep is a consequence of the apnea and/or hypopnea (<50% airflow for >10 seconds) must be judged. As the respiratory event index (apnea + hypopnea/hours of sleep) becomes greater, so does the likelihood that abnormal respiration is the primary cause of poor sleep. Indexes of about 15 to 30 are usually the minimum necessary for apnea to be considered the primary cause of significant insomnia. The PSG of patients diagnosed with insomnia secondary to sleep-disordered breathing show decreased total sleep time, a long sleep-onset latency, increased stage 1 sleep, and frequent awakenings and arousals that follow respiratory events [47].

Movement Disorders

Periodic limb movement disorder (PLMD) consists of rhythmic twitches in the limb muscle occurring during sleep, which may lead to EEG arousals and/or awakenings. Most commonly, this disorder is characterized by periodic leg movements (PLMs) in one or both legs. The movements occur in series (about every 20 to 30 seconds) and may last several hours [48]. Presence of PLMs, even with several hundred movements, does not necessarily lead to a diagnosis of PLMD. A determination should be made as to the contribution of the PLMs to the objective sleep disturbance in each case. Two hundred PLMs that routinely lead to arousals and account for all of the patient's major awakenings in the absence of other pathology is convincing. In contrast, 300 PLMs that occur in the first 2 hours of sleep may produce little effect on the EEG. If this happens in a patient with increased time awake in the second half of the night then PLMD is not the proper diagnosis. In patients complaining of insomnia, this disorder is accompanied by increased wake during sleep and stage 1 sleep on a PSG [47].

Restless legs syndrome (RLS) is primarily characterized by unpleasant tingling sensations in the legs on lying down to sleep. This sensation is relieved by movement of the legs or may persist until the patient gets out of bed and walks around. This condition is usually also accompanied by PLMs, both during wakefulness and during sleep. However, RLS is marked by severe difficulty initiating persistent sleep, as opposed to the maintenance difficulties seen in PLMD. Patients with RLS often have their soundest sleep in the early morning (5 to 7 AM).

Various medical conditions and medications can cause PLMD or RLS. Iron deficiency, chronic uremia, neuropathy, rheumatoid arthritis, and CNS dysfunction have been associated with PLMs during sleep or RLS [22, 49–51]. Use of stimulant medications [52] or tricyclic antidepressants [53, 54] has also been reported to produce PLMs in certain patients. While it has been reported that periodic movements in sleep may also follow withdrawal from opiates, barbiturates, alcohol, benzodiazepines, and other hypnotic medications [3], there have been no controlled studies to support this claim. Idiopathic PLMD or RLS should be differentiated from these specific causes when feasible since this may aid in selecting a treatment approach.

Behavioral and Psychophysiologic Disorders

Inadequate Sleep Hygiene

This type of insomnia results from the practice of sleep habits that are not conducive to sound sleep. Habits that commonly contribute to this disorder include daytime napping, irregular sleep schedules, spending too much time in bed, using the bed for sleep-incompatible behaviors (e.g., watching TV, reading, eating, working) or engaging in physically or mentally demanding activities immediately before bedtime. On a PSG these patients may report sleeping better in the laboratory than at home, presumably because they are unable to engage in some of their bad sleep habits while in the laboratory.

Psychophysiologic Insomnia

This disorder is a conditioned insomnia that results from the interaction between high levels of physiologic arousal and a preoccupation with the inability to sleep. The patient learns to associate sleeplessness and/or heightened arousal with external stimuli (e.g., the sight of the clock on the nightstand) or with cognitions (e.g., "I'm tired and need to fall asleep quickly"). The patient is likely to obsess about the sleep problem and become increasingly tense as bedtime approaches. This condition is marked by a long sleep-onset latency, decreased sleep efficiency, and increased stage 1 sleep on the PSG [55].

Sleep State Misperception (Subjective Insomnia)

In this condition the patient complains of persistent insomnia, but is found to have sleep of normal duration and quality on a PSG. Subjective reports of poor sleep (long latency, short total sleep time, etc.) must be documented following the nighttime recording. Some patients with objectively normal sleep in the laboratory subjectively report that this sleep was better than at home. In this instance, a diagnosis of subjective insomnia is not made since the patient is able to accurately report the sleep quality. This diagnosis has previously been made in about 10% to 20% of patients presenting to sleep centers [13, 47]. However, the more precise criteria for this diagnosis provided in the new classification system may alter these prevalence rates (ICSD) [14].

Circadian Rhythm Disorders

Delayed Sleep-Phase Syndrome

In this condition, the patient complains of difficulty initiating sleep and difficulty arising in the morning. These patients are able to oversleep on weekends and typically do not have sleep maintenance problems. This condition occurs when the patients' desired sleep schedule begins earlier than their physiologic sleep rhythm and although their actual sleep times occur at the same time each day. On the PSG, sleep is normal, with the exception of a long sleep-onset latency [56].

Advanced Sleep-Phase Syndrome

As in delayed sleep-phase syndrome, this condition is a dissynchrony between the patients' environmental schedule and the internal sleep rhythm. In this case, they feel sleepy before their scheduled bedtime, fall asleep quickly, awaken early, and are unable to return to sleep. Sleep is normal if it is recorded beginning at the time of the patient's early evening sleepiness.

Irregular Sleep-Wake Pattern
This disorder represents an almost total loss of any circadian rhythmicity to the sleep-wake pattern. The patient is unable to sustain sleep at night, but also takes frequent naps during the day. Even the timing of these daytime naps is irregular, with sleep able to occur at any time of the day.

Treatment of Chronic Insomnia

As is clear from the process described previously, treating chronic insomnia often means treating another primary disorder. For example, in the case of insomnia secondary to an affective disorder, the appropriate treatment is psychotherapy and/or pharmacologic treatment for depression. However, there are many behavioral and pharmacologic treatments that have been developed specifically for sleep disorders. While it is beyond the scope of this chapter to comprehensively delineate treatment strategies, a brief outline of available treatments and references for detailed descriptions of these approaches is provided.

Behavioral Treatments

Many different behavioral treatments have been found to improve subjective ratings of sleep quality and quantity. Unfortunately, studies of behavioral treatment of insomnia using objective measures of sleep as outcome measures are rare. This is problematic since those studies with both objective and subjective measures consistently find discrepancies between these measures [57–64]. In each case, the subjective ratings of sleep quality and quantity are likely to show significant improvement across the group while the objective measures do not. In no instance has total sleep time been shown objectively to increase with behavioral treatment over the entire treatment group, despite subjective reports to the contrary. This is confusing since most of these studies employ active placebo conditions or counterdemand instructions to ensure against a placebo effect. One possible explanation for these results is that patients are not selected and matched to a specific behavioral approach. Any one behavioral treatment is not going to work for all patients with insomnia, even when only one diagnostic category is studied. This view is supported by a study that found that by matching the type of biofeedback to patient characteristics (tense versus relaxed), both groups exhibited objectively improved sleep [65]. This is in contrast to an earlier study of the same biofeedback techniques that had not preassigned subjects to treatment groups and did not demonstrate group differences on objective measures of sleep [61].

Behavioral treatment is the primary treatment for diagnoses of inadequate sleep hygiene, psychophysiologic insomnia, circadian rhythm disorders, and possibly insomnia secondary to an anxiety disorder. Behavioral treatment also should be at least an adjunct treatment for patients in all other diagnostic categories. It is a rare patient who has not accumulated some sleep habits that are contributing to the insomnia. Therefore, even a patient being treated for depression with tricyclic antidepressants should be instructed on the importance of maintaining a regular sleep-wake schedule, avoiding daytime naps, and so forth.

The following is a list of those behavioral treatment approaches that have been studied most. A reference is provided that provides detailed instructions on how to administer the procedure.

Stimulus control therapy teaches the patient not to increase arousal in the bedroom. This approach is especially helpful with patients who have very long awakenings during the night [66].

Sleep restriction therapy manipulates the amount of time in bed to try to consolidate sleep time. One caution is that this treatment has been shown to lead to significant increases in daytime sleepiness [67].

Electromyographic biofeedback seeks to teach the patient to lower his or her tension level in order to promote sleep [61].

Progressive relaxation training teaches muscle relaxation through a series of exercises that the patient must practice. This is typically better suited to patients who primarily have difficulty initiating sleep [68].

Chronotherapy adjusts the circadian phase of patients with delayed sleep-phase syndrome. This is achieved through rigid scheduling of the sleep-wake schedule [69].

Pharmacologic Treatment

While pharmacologic treatment is generally reserved for transient and short-term insomnia, there is a role for hypnotics in patients with chronic insomnia. Use of hypnotics may be helpful for patients with insomnia secondary to restless legs syndrome and/or PLMD, anxiety disorders, severe psychophysiologic insomnia, or certain medical conditions. For many patients, hypnotics should only be considered when their insomnia has been shown to be refractory to other treatments.

Studies of various benzodiazepine hypnotic medications have shown improved sleep in patients with chronic insomnia [70–72]. Effects on sleep include decreased sleep-onset latency, decreased wake after sleep onset, and increased total sleep time. Studies of tolerance to the hypnotic effect of benzodiazepines in insomniac patients have reported evidence to support both the development of tolerance and continued efficacy [73, 74].

Daytime side effects occur with benzodiazepines having a long half-life and also with short-acting drugs taken in high dosages. Performance decrements and anterograde amnesia have been reported, and severity of these side effects is dose related [75–77]. These side effects must be monitored, and if present, they must be weighed against the therapeutic gains in deciding if treatment will be continued.

Once a decision is made to use hypnotic medication, selection of an appropriate drug should take into account the duration of sedation, the rate of absorption, and the type of drug metabolism. The varous benzodiazepines vary markedly, and the drug must be matched to the patient's need. Patient characteristics of importance in selecting a hypnotic include age, diagnosis, timing of wakefulness at night (i.e., when do they most require sedation), and level of daytime anxiety. Detailed information regarding this topic is available elsewhere [78–81].

Patients should be given specific instructions of how to use the medication. The efficacy of the treatment depends in large part on the rules the patient follows in use of the medication. A list of the rules for medication use in the treatment of insomnia and their rationale has been presented by Stepanski et al [82]. If a patient escalates the dosage without consulting the clinician, then that patient is not a candidate for pharmacologic treatment. Other contraindications for use of hypnotic medication are (1) a history of alcohol or drug abuse, (2) a history of psychosis, (3) pulmonary illness that may lead to more severe hypoxemia with sedation, and (4) liver disease that may alter drug metabolism.

One brief recommendation is made regarding treatment of depression in a patient with severe insomnia. Sedating tricyclic antidepressants (e.g., doxepin, amitriptyline), taken at bedtime, are suggested over use of other antidepressants [83].

Summary

Insomnia is one of the most common clinical complaints seen by physicians. The primary care doctor is in a unique position to initiate evaluation and treatment in many of these patients. In some cases improved sleep habits or medication alterations are sufficient to alleviate insomnia. In other cases a referral to a sleep disorders center is necessary. When patients with chronic insomnia are referred to a sleep disorders center for evaluation they often have a complex combination of factors influencing their sleep problem. A careful assessment of medical, psychiatric, and behavioral factors is needed before a diagnosis can be made. Preferably this assessment is made by a multidisciplinary team of practitioners, who also have expertise in sleep disorders medicine. Behavioral and/or medication changes may be needed as part of the evaluation process, and this process may take several weeks to complete. PSG may be required before a definite diagnosis can be made. Once the primary cause of the patient's insomnia is determined, then a treatment plan can be formulated. The treatment should be aimed at remediating the direct cause(s) of the insomnia, although at times only symptomatic treatment may be possible.

References

1. Mellinger G, Balter M, Uhlenhuth: Insomnia and its treatment. *Arch Gen Psych* 42:225–232, 1985
2. Ford D, Kamerow D: Epidemiologic study of sleep disturbances and psychiatric disorders. An opportunity for prevention? *JAMA* 262:1479–1484, 1989
3. Association of Sleep Disorder Centers: Diagnostic classification of sleep and arousal disorders, ed 1. Prepared by the Sleep Disorders Classification Committee. *Sleep* 2:1–137, 1979
4. National Institute of Mental Health, Consensus Development Conference: Drugs and insomnia: The use of medications to promote sleep. *JAMA* 251:2410–2414, 1984
5. Ancoli-Israel S, Kripke D, Mason W, et al: Sleep apnea and nocturnal myoclonus in a senior population. *Sleep* 4:349–358, 1981
6. Stepanski E, Glinn M, Zorick F, et al: Predisposition to and reliability of the first night effect. *Sleep Res* 18:307, 1989
7. Stepanski E, Glinn M, Fortier J, et al: Physiological reactivity in chronic insomnia. *Sleep Res* 18:306, 1989
8. Monroe LJ: Psychological and physiological differences between good and poor sleepers. *J Abnorm Psychol* 72:255–264, 1967
9. Freedman R, Sattler H: Physiological and psychological factors in sleep-onset insomnia. *J Abnorm Psychol* 91:380–389, 1982
10. Stepanski E, Zorick F, Roehrs T, et al: Daytime alertness in patients with chronic insomnia compared with asymptomatic control subjects. *Sleep* 11:54–60, 1988
11. Zarcone VP: Sleep and alcoholism. *In* Weitzman E (ed): Sleep Disorders: Intersections of Basic and Clinical Research, vol 8. Advances in Sleep Research. New York, Spectrum Press, 1982
12. Adamson J, Burdick J: Sleep of dry alcholics. *Arch Gen Psychiatry* 28:146–149, 1973
13. Coleman R, Roffwarg H, Kennedy S, et al: Sleep-wake disorders based upon a polysomnographic diagnosis: A national cooperative study. *JAMA* 247:997–1003, 1982
14. American Sleep Disorder Association: The International Classification of Sleep Disorders. Rochester, MN, ASDA, 1990
15. Fleetham J, West P, Mezon B, et al: Sleep, arousals, and oxygen desaturation in chronic obstructive pulmonary disease. The effect of oxygen therapy. *Am Rev Respir Dis* 126:429–433, 1982
16. Phillipson E, Goldstein R: Breathing during sleep in chronic obstructive pulmonary disease. State of the art. *Chest* 85S:24S–30S, 1984
17. Power J, Stewart I, Connaughton J, et al: Nocturnal cough in patients with chronic bronchitis and emphysema. *Am Rev Respir Dis* 130: 999–1001, 1984
18. George CF, Kryger MH: Sleep in restrictive lung disease. *Sleep* 10:409–418, 1987
19. Moldofsky H, Scarisbrick P, England R, et al: Musculoskeletal symptoms and non-REM sleep disturbance in patients with "fibrositis syndrome" and healthy subjects. *Psychosom Med* 37:341–351, 1975
20. Wittig R, Zorick F, Blumer D, et al: Disturbed sleep in patients complaining of chronic pain. *J Nervous Mental Dis* 170(7):429–431, 1982
21. Moldofsky H, Lue F, Smythe H: Alpha EEG sleep and morning symptoms in rheumatoid arthritis. *J Rheumat* 10:373–379, 1983
22. Mahowald MW, Mahowald ML, Bundlie SR, et al: Sleep fragmentation in rheumatoid arthritis. *Arthritis Rheum* 32:974–983, 1989
23. Vitiello M, Prinz P: Alzheimer's disease. Sleep and sleep-wake patterns. *Clinics Geriatr Med* 5(2):289–299, 1989
24. Prinz P, Peskind E, Vitaliano P, et al: Changes in the sleep and waking EEG in nondemented and demented elderly. *J Am Geriatr Soc* 30:86–93, 1982
25. Kales A, Ansel R, Markham C, et al: Sleep in patients with Parkinson's disease and normal subjects prior to and following levodopa administration. *Clin Pharmacol Ther* 12:397–406, 1971
26. Rabey S, Vardi J, Glaubman H, et al: EEG sleep study in parkinsonism patients under bromocryptine treatment. *Eur Neurol* 27: 345–350, 1978
27. Nicholson A, Stone B: Heterocyclic amphetamine derivatives and caffeine on sleep in man. *Br J Clin Pharmacol* 9:195–203, 1980
28. Nicholson A, Stone B, Jones M: Wakefulness and reduced REM sleep: Studies with prolintane and pemoline. *Br J Clin Pharmacol* 10:465–472, 1980
29. Rechtshaffen A, Marion L: The effect of amphetamine on the sleep cycle. *Electroencephalogr Clin Neurophysiol* 16:438–445, 1964
30. Curatolo P, Robertson D: The health consequences of caffeine. *Ann Intern Med* 98(5): 641–653, 1983

31. Rhind G, Connaughton J, McFie J, et al: Sustained release choline theophyllinate in nocturnal asthma. *Br Med J* 291:1605–1607, 1985
32. Fleetham J, Fera T, Edgell G, Jamal K: The effect of theophylline therapy on sleep disorders in COPD patients. *Am Rev Respir Dis* 127(supp):A85(Abstract), 1983
33. Berry R, Desa M, Branum J, Light R: Effect of theophylline on sleep and sleep-disordered breathing in patients with chronic obstructive pulmonary disease. *Am Rev Respir Dis* 143: 245–250, 1991
34. Rosen R, Kostis J, Taska L, et al: Beta-blocker effects on objective and subjective measures of sleep in normotensive male subjects. *Sleep Res* 15:42, 1986
35. Betts T, Alford C: Beta-blockers and sleep: A controlled trial. *Eur J Clin Pharmacol* 28 (suppl):65–68, 1985
36. Dietrich B, Herrmann W: Influence of cilazapril on memory functions and sleep behaviour in comparison with metoprolol and placebo in healthy subjects. *Br J Clin Pharmacol* 27: 249S–261S, 1989.
36a. Kostis J, Rosen R, Holzer B, et al: CNS side effects of centrally-active antihypertensive agents: A prospective, placebo-controlled study of sleep, mood state, and cognitive and sexual function in hypertensive males. *Psychopharmacology* 93:163–170, 1990
37. Cove-Smith R, Kirk C: New drugs: beta blockers and sympathomimetics. *Br Med J* 286: 1650–1651, 1983
38. Cooper GL: The safety of fluoxetine—An update. *Br J Psychiatry* 153:77–86, 1988
38a. Medical economics data. *Physicians' Desk Reference for Nonprescription Drugs.* Oradell, NJ: Medical Economics Company, 1991
39. Reynolds C, Kupfer D: Sleep research in affective illness: State of the art circa 1987. *Sleep* 10:199–215, 1987
40. Gillin J, Duncan W, Pettigrew K, et al: Successful separation of depressed, normal, and insomniac subjects by EEG sleep data. *Arch Gen Psychiatry* 36:85–90, 1979
41. Reynolds C, Shaw D, Newton T, et al: EEG sleep in outpatients with generalized anxiety: A preliminary comparison with depressed outpatients. *Psychiatry Res* 8:81–89, 1983
42. Williams D, MacLean A, Cairns J: Dose-response effects of ethanol on the sleep of young women. *Journal of Studies on Alcohol* 44:515–523, 1983
43. Greenberg R, Pearlman C: Delirium tremens and dreaming. *Am J Psychiatry* 124:133–142, 1967
44. Mello N, Mendelson J: Behavioral studies of sleep patterns in alcoholics during intoxication and withdrawal. *J Pharmacol Exp Ther* 175:94–112, 1970
45. Roehrs T, Conway W, Wittig R, et al: Sleep-wake complaints in patients with sleep-related respiratory complaints. *Am Rev Respir Dis* 132:520–523, 1985
46. Carskadon M, Dement W: Respiration during sleep in the aged human. *J Gerontol* 36:420–423, 1981
47. Zorick FJ, Roth T, Hartze KM, et al: Evaluation and diagnosis of persistent insomnia. *Am J Psychiatry* 138:769–773, 1981
48. Coleman R, Pollak C, Weitzman E: Periodic movements in sleep (nocturnal myoclonus): Relation to sleep-wake disorders. *Ann Neurol* 8:416–421, 1980
49. Callaghan N: Restless legs syndrome in uremic neuropathy. *Neurology* 16:359–361, 1966
50. Frankel B, Patten B, Gillin C: Restless legs syndrome. *JAMA* 230:1302–1303, 1974
51. Read D, Feest T, Nassim M: Clonazepam: Effective treatment for restless legs syndrome in uraemia. *Br Med J* 283:885, 1981
52. Lutz E: Restless legs, anxiety and caffeinism. *J Clin Psychiatry* 39:693–698, 1978
53. Ware JC, Brown FW, Moorad PJ, et al: Nocturnal myoclonus and tricyclic antidepressants. *Sleep Res* 13:72, 1984
54. Guilleminault C, Raynal D, Takahashi S, et al: Evaluation of short-term and long-term treatment of the narcolepsy syndrome with chlorimipramine hydrochloride. *Acta Neurol Scand* 54:71–78, 1976
55. Hauri P, Fisher J: Persistent psychophysiologic (learned) insomnia. *Sleep* 9:38–53, 1986
56. Weitzman E, Czeisler C, Coleman R, et al: Delayed sleep phase syndrome: A chronobiologic disorder with sleep onset insomnia. *Arch Gen Psychiatry* 38:737–746, 1981
57. Borkovec T, Grayson J, O'Brien G, et al: Relaxation treatment of pseudoinsomnia and idiopathic insomnia: An electroencephalographic evaluation. *J Appl Behav Anal* 12: 37–54, 1979
58. Borkovec T, Weerts T: Effects of progressive relaxation on sleep disturbance: An electroencephalographic evaluation. *Psychosom Med* 38: 173–180, 1976
59. Freedman R, Papsdorf J: Biofeedback and progressive relaxation. Treatment of sleep-onset insomnia: A controlled, all-night investigation. *Biofeedback Self Regul* 1:253–271, 1976
60. Coursey R, Frankel B, Gaarder K, et al: A comparison of relaxation techniques with electrosleep therapy for chronic, sleep-onset insomnia. A sleep EEG study. *Biofeedback Self Regul* 5:57–73, 1980
61. Hauri P: Treating psychophysiologic insomnia with biofeedback. *Arch Gen Psychiatry* 38:752–758, 1981
62. Anderson M, Zendell S, Rosa D, et al: Comparison of sleep restriction therapy and stimu-

lus control in older insomniacs: An update. *Sleep Research* 17:141, 1988
63. Morin C, Kowatch R, Berry T, et al: Cognitive-behavioral treatment of late-life insomnia. *Sleep Research* 19:263, 1990
64. Rubenstein M, Rothenberg S, Maheswaren S, et al: Modified sleep restriction therapy in middle-aged and elderly chronic insomniacs. *Sleep Res* 19:276, 1990
65. Hauri P, Percy L, Hellekson C, et al: The treatment of psychophysiologic insomnia with biofeedback: A replication study. *Biofeedback Self Regul* 7:223–234, 1982
66. Bootzin RR, Nicassio PM: Behavioral treatments for insomnia. *In* Hersen M, Eissler R, Miller P (eds): Progress in Behavior Modification, vol 6. New York, Academic Press, 1978, pp 1–45
67. Spielman AJ, Saskin P, Thorpy MJ: Treatment of chronic insomnia by restriction of time in bed. *Sleep* 10:45–56, 1987
68. Bernstein D, Borkovec T: Progressive Relaxation Training. Champaign, IL, Research Press, 1973
69. Czeisler C, Richardson G, Coleman R, et al: Chronotherapy: Resetting the circadian clocks of patients with delayed sleep phase insomnia. *Sleep* 4:1–21, 1981
70. Vogel G, Barker K, Gibbons P, et al: A comparison of the effects of flurazepam 30 mgs and triazolam 0.5 mgs on the sleep of insomniacs. *Psychopharmacologia* 47:81–86, 1976
71. Roth T, Hartse KM, Saab PG, et al: The effects of flurazepam, lorazepam, and triazolam on sleep and memory. *Psychopharmacology* 70: 231–237, 1980
72. Mitler M, Browman C, Menn S, et al: Nocturnal myoclonus: Treatment efficacy of clonazepam and temazepam. *Sleep* 9:385–392, 1986
73. Greenblatt D, Shader R: Dependence, tolerance, and addiction to benzodiazepines: Clinical and pharmacokinetic considerations. *Drug Metab Rev* 8:13–28, 1978
74. Oswald I, French C, Adam K, et al: Benzodiazepine hypnotics remain effective for 24 weeks. *Br Med J* 284:860–863, 1982
75. Roehrs T, Kribbs N, Zorick F, et al: Hypnotic residual effects of benzodiazepines with repeated administration. *Sleep* 9:309–316, 1986
76. Roehrs T, Zorick F, Sicklesteel J, et al: Effects of hypnotics on memory. *J Clin Pharmacol* 3:310–313, 1983
77. Johnson LC, Chernik DA: Sedative-hypnotics and human performance. *Psychopharmacology* 76:101–114, 1982
78. Nicholson AN: Hypnotics: Clinical pharmacology and therapeutics. *In* Kryger MH, Roth T, Dement WC (eds): Principles and Practice of Sleep Medicine. Philadelphia, W.B. Saunders, 1989, pp 219–228
79. Nicholson AN: The use of short- and long-acting hypnotics in clinical medicine. *Br J Clin Pharmacol* 11:61S–69S, 1981
80. Greenblatt D, Shader R, Divoll M, et al: Benzodiazepines: A summary of pharmacokinetic properties. *Br J Clin Pharmacol* 11:11S–16S, 1981
81. Woods JH, Katz JL, Winger G: Use and abuse of benzodiazepines: Issues relevant to prescribing. *JAMA* 260:3476–3480, 1988
82. Stepanski E, Zorick F, Roth T: Pharmacotherapy of insomnia. *In* Hauri P (ed): Case Studies in Insomnia. Plenum Publishing Corporation, 1991, pp 115–129
83. Ware JC: Tricyclic antidepressants in the treatment of insomnia. *J Clin Psychiatry* 44: 25–28, 1983
84. Bixler E, Kales A, Soldatos C, et al: Prevalence of sleep disorders in the Los Angeles metropolitan area. *Am J Psychiatry* 136:1257–1262, 1979
85. Karacan I, Thornby JI, Anch M, et al: Prevalence of sleep disturbance in a primarily urban Florida county. *Social Science and Medicine* 10:239–244, 1976
86. Karacan I, Thornby J, Williams R: Sleep disturbance: A community survey. *In* Guilleminault C, Lugaresi E (eds): Sleep/Wake Disorders: Natural History, Epidemiology and Long-Term Evolution. New York, Raven Press, 1983, pp 37–60
87. Lugaresi E, Cirignotta F, Zucconi M, et al: Good and poor sleepers: An epidemiological survey of the San Marino population. *In* Guilleminault C, Lugaresi E (eds): Sleep/Wake Disorders: Natural History, Epidemiology and Long-Term Evolution. New York, Raven Press, 1983, pp 1–12
88. Partinen M, Kaprio J, Koskenvuo M, et al: Sleeping habits, sleep quality and use of sleeping pills: A population study of 31,140 adults in Finland. *In* Guilleminault C, Lugaresi E (eds): Sleep/Wake Disorders: Natural History, Epidemiology and Long-Term Evolution. New York, Raven Press, 1983, pp 29–35
89. Welstein L, Dement W, Redington D, et al: Insomnia in the San Francisco Bay Area: A telephone survey. *In* Guilleminault C, Lugaresi E (eds): Sleep/Wake Disorders: Natural History, Epidemiology and Long-Term Evolution. New York, Raven Press, 1983, pp 73–85

Pulmonary Diseases in Pregnancy

Scott B. Ransom, Randall Kelly, and Federico Mariona

This chapter reviews the maternal anatomic and physiologic changes of the respiratory system during pregnancy. The review discusses the pathophysiology, diagnosis, and treatment of various pulmonary disorders in pregnancy.

Maternal Pulmonary Anatomy and Physiology

Pulmonary changes in pregnancy begin early in the first trimester. The subcostal angle increases from the normal 68 degrees to 103 degrees by term, causing an increased transthoracic diameter of approximately 2 cm [1]. This is a physiologic adaptation since the angle begins to increase before any direct anatomic changes occur from uterine growth.

Hyperventilation is characteristic in the first trimester due to a minimally increased respiratory rate and a 40% to 50% increase in tidal volume [2]. This causes an increased minute ventilation of 40% to 50% (minute ventilation = respiratory rate × tidal volume). The hyperventilation enables arterial oxygen tension range from 90 up to 106 mm Hg [3], while causing a decrease in PCO_2 to 30 mm Hg. This results in a respiratory alkalosis and increase in arterial pH from 7.40 to 7.44. The kidneys compensate by decreasing plasma bicarbonate by 4 mEq/L to 18 or 19 mEq/L, resulting in a compensated respiratory alkalosis [5, 69].

Ueland et al, showed that oxygen consumption during pregnancy increases by 32 to 58 mL/min [4].

While the tidal volume is increased during pregnancy, the total lung capacity and vital capacity remain unchanged. The functional residual capacity, residual volume, and expiratory reserve volume in gravid patients are gradually decreased throughout pregnancy by 500, 300, and 200 mL, respectively [6, 7]. These physiologic changes may be attributed to an elevation of the diaphragm and relatively smaller alveoli, which results in increased work required to expand the pregnant woman's lungs.

The diffusing capacity of the lung in pregnancy is increased possibly due to increases in capillary blood volume or red cell mass [3]. These physiologic changes may be affected by alterations in levels of estrogen, progesterone, cortisol, prostaglandins, and histamine associated with pregnancy [8]. Specifically, progesterone elicits a 50% decrease in pulmonary resistance due to its action in the bronchiole muscle fiber. The effects of progesterone may cause an increase in ventilation and an associated decrease in PCO_2 during pregnancy [9].

Pulmonary Function Testing in Pregnancy

Spirometry is an excellent means to assess respiratory function during pregnancy. Spirometry has no limitations or contraindications during pregnancy and should be used as in any other patient. Although spirometry can be completed safely in pregnancy, the clinician should fully correlate the pulmonary testing findings with the normal anatomic and physiologic changes during pregnancy.

Pulmonary function assessment before surgical procedures in pregnancy is an uncommon requirement; however, significant obstructive airway disease is associated with a decreased cough efficiency and an increased risk for atelectasis and postoperative pneumonia. Similarily, invasive pulmonary tests such as bronchoscopy and biopsy can be completed in pregnancy. Nevertheless, the possible risks of the complications of any procedure must be outweighed by the benefit any given procedure will promote in the decision to treat the patient.

Asthma in Pregnancy

Asthma is a disease characterized by dyspnea and wheezing due to obstruction of airflow. The obstruction affects expiration more than inspiration, which results in air trapping and hyperinflation of the lungs. The obstruction of airflow is secondary to contraction of bronchial smooth muscle, mucous hypersecretion, and mucosal edema induced by some factor such as molds, pollens, animal danders, cold air, stress, tobacco smoke, drugs, exercise, and respiratory infections [3]. See Chapter 8 for a detailed discussion of asthma. It is a common occurrence for the first episode of significant bronchospasm to be associated with an upper respiratory tract infection.

Asthma complicates 0.4% to 1.3% of pregnancies [10, 11], which makes it important for the primary care physician to be familiar with the diagnosis and treatment. The goal of therapy in the pregnant patient includes adequate control of asthma symptoms and reduction of risks to the fetus from the treatment of the disease.

The outcome of pregnant patients with asthma is highly variable. Gluck and Gluck [12] reviewed reports of 1087 pregnancies and found no change in asthma in 48% of patients, 23% became worse, and 29% improved during pregnancy. The study revealed that patients improved in pregnancy if their level of IgE decreased and patients tended to become worse if their asthma was severe before pregnancy or their IgE levels increased. An elevation in serum cortisol during pregnancy may account for some improvement of asthma symptoms; however, this cannot account for the entire improvement [13]. Progesterone seems to aid smooth muscle relaxation, reducing bronchomotor tone, and improve asthma in pregnancy [13].

The effects of asthma on pregnancy showed an increase in the incidence of hyperemesis, toxemia, complications of labor, prematurity, low birth weight, hemorrhage, and neonatal death in one study [14]. Gordon et al [15] observed an increased rate of fetal mortality associated with uncontrolled asthma; however, Greenberger and Patterson [11] showed that successful control of asthma was associated with no increase in maternal or fetal morbidity or mortality. Congenital malformations are not increased with maternal asthma [8].

Diagnosis

A complete history, including the duration of the asthmatic attack, current medications, events preceding the attack, and general medical history, are important in the initial evaluation of the asthmatic patient. The physical examination should assess signs of respiratory distress, including flaring nostrils and the use of accessory muscles of respiration. Cyanosis and pulsus paradoxus are evident in a severe attack. Wheezing and a prolonged expiratory phase of respiration are characteristic of asthma. A laboratory evaluation of complete blood count, serum electrolytes, and arterial blood gas determination must be performed. In addition, a Gram stain of sputum must be completed if infection is suspected. Spirometry and chest roentgenography should be used to assess baseline status and exclude bronchopneumonia [5]. There are no established risks to the fetus for a single chest roentgenogram.

The severity of asthma can be judged by the clinical evaluation; however, the need for hospitalization can be assessed by using the index of seven items, each with a score of one point if present. When the total score is four or more, the patient requires hospitalization. The seven items include the following:

1. heart rate greater than 120 beats per minute,
2. respiratory rate of 30 per minute,
3. pulsus paradoxus of 18 mm Hg or more,
4. peak expiratory flow rate of 120 L/min or less,
5. moderate or severe dyspnea,
6. moderate or severe wheezing, and

7. moderate or severe use of accessory respiratory muscles.

While three of the seven criteria are very subjective, the index has been widely used to assess the severity of an asthmatic attack [5].

Arterial blood gas evaluation can aid in the assessment of the severity of an asthmatic attack. Specifically, the combination of low PO_2, low pH, and a PCO_2 above normal is the worst combination, indicating a severe attack; a low PO_2, normal pH, and normal PCO_2 indicates a moderate asthma attack; and an elevated pH, low PCO_2, and normal PO_2 indicates a mild asthma attack. Fetal hypoxia exists when the maternal PO_2 is below 60 mm Hg [5].

Therapy

The management of asthma in pregnancy is the same as for the nonpregnant patient. The physician must identify all potential precipitating factors of the asthmatic condition, appropriately use bronchodilating agents and antibiotics, avoid potentially dangerous drugs to the mother and fetus, maintain adequate oxygenation, and avoid respiratory and metabolic alkalosis. Agents that are considered safe during pregnancy include methylxanthines, β-agonists, anticholinergics, cromolyn sodium, and corticosteroids [8, 70]. While these drugs are considered relatively safe, no drug is absolutely safe and must be used only if absolutely necessary. The use of drugs during the first trimester of pregnancy is of particular importance due to the increased probability of fetal malformations. Nevertheless, the pregnant patient must be treated effectively in order to prevent uncontrolled asthma and acute respiratory failure, which may injure both mother and fetus.

Methylxanthine bronchodilators appear to be safe in pregnancy. While Heinonen et al [16] have revealed no increase of teratogenic effects in humans, Mintz [10] presented evidence of digital malformations in laboratory animals. The xanthines increase levels of cAMP (cyclic adenosine monophosphate) via inhibition of phosphodiesterase. While the xanthines are transferred across the placenta, the theophylline concentrations in neonatal and cord blood are similar to those in maternal blood [17]. Labovitz and Spector [18] showed no changes in Apgar scores by administration of theophylline. Theophylline metabolism may be altered during pregnancy due to an increased absorption of the drug or reduced hepatic metabolism. Theophylline clearance has been reported to be reduced between 20% and 35% during the third trimester of pregnancy [19]. Because of the increased risk of theophylline toxicity, serial theophylline levels should be obtained in patients on methylxanthine therapy during pregnancy.

Sympathomimetic bronchodilators are relatively safe in pregnancy; however, studies have shown vasocontrictive effects of epinephrine on the uterine vessels, which may reduce the uteroplacental circulation. In addition, the Collaborative Perinatal Project showed an increased incidence of malformations with the use of epinephrine during pregnancy [3]. Conversely, terbutaline has been shown to preserve or increase blood flow of the uterine vessels, and terbutaline has not been associated with any congenital malformations [17].

Administration of corticosteroids during pregnancy has remained highly controversial. A number of studies, including Fitzsimons et al [20], Schatz et al [21], and Greenberger and Patterson [11], have shown no increase in congenital malformations with steroid use; however, an animal study by Fainstat [22] has shown an increased risk of cleft palate with steroid use. In human pregnancy, any association of cleft palate due to steroids would occur before the 12th week of gestation since closure of the palate is then complete [22]. While neonates should be evaluated for adrenal suppression, the complication is extremely rare. If the benefits of corticosteroid use for the asthmatic patient are greater than the possible risks, steroid therapy should be implemented [20].

Cromolyn sodium has been considered reasonably safe for use during pregnancy by Greenberger and Patterson [11], despite the manufacturer discouraging use of the drug in pregnancy. The drug has been very effective in patients with asthma and should be considered as a reasonable treatment modality.

The asthmatic mother should be able to breast feed her infant. A regimen of an inhaled β_2-agonist, theophylline in the therapeutic range, and oral or inhaled corticosteroids should be safe and effective for the mother and her baby.

Sarcoidosis in Pregnancy

Sarcoidosis is a multisystem granulomatous disease of unknown etiology. (See Chapter 11) It most commonly affects the lungs; however, sarcoidosis can involve lymph nodes, skin, eyes, heart, and liver. A noncaseating granuloma, with no specific etiologic agent initiating the granuloma, is the characteristic feature of sarcoidosis. It is a rare complication of pregnancy, affecting at most 0.05% of pregnancies [23, 24]. In the U.S. there is a prevalence of sarcoidosis in blacks higher than the caucasian population.

Diagnosis

Many patients are asymptomatic with an abnormal chest radiograph. Other patients may have significant respiratory symptoms including dyspnea and nonproductive cough. Common roentgenographic features of the disorder include bilateral hilar adenopathy and/or interstitial infiltrates. Some asymptomatic patients with typical features of the disorder (symmetrical bilateral hilar adenopathy) may be diagnosed clinically. Other methods of diagnosis when the chest is involved include bronchoscopic transbronchial biopsy, mediastinoscopy, or open-lung biopsy [25].

The course of sarcoidosis during pregnancy is thought to be similar to that in the nonpregnant state. Agha et al [26] reviewed 35 pregnancies in 18 patients with sarcoidosis. In nine patients, there was no effect; in six there was clinical and roentgenographic improvement, and in three there was a deleterious effect on the disease process. No relapse of disease was noted in 15 of the patients; however, three patients experienced a continuation of the disease after pregnancy [26]. Similarly, Haynes de Regt [25] presented a review of 15 patients with sarcoidosis that showed 11 patients who remained stable, two with progression of disease, and two who died from complications of sarcoidosis. Most studies have suggested that pregnancy does not adversely affect the course of disease, with most patients improving or remaining stable. In fact, Scadding [27] suggested that the usual course of the disease in pregnancy remained unchanged from the prepregnant disease progression. Specifically, if the disease was resolving before pregnancy, it seemed to resolve in pregnancy; if the chest radiograph showed inactive disease before pregnancy, this finding generally continued during pregnancy. Many patients with active disease seem to improve during pregnancy, perhaps due to an increase in free plasma cortisol as well as the total cortisol level [28]. The disease progression seems to be adversely affected by pulmonary parenchymal lesions, advanced roentgenologic staging, advanced maternal age, low inflammatory activity, requirement for drug therapy other than steroids, and presence of extrapulmonary sarcoidosis [29].

Treatment

The standard therapy for symptomatic sarcoidosis is corticosteroids. While the actual effectiveness of steroids remains unclear, patients with disease affecting the myocardium, eyes, or the central nervous system should be placed on these agents. Therapy for pulmonary sarcoidosis should be related to functional impairment and symptoms instead of radiographic findings. The initial dose of corticosteroid ranges from 40 to 60 mg of prednisone per day for at least 6 months, followed by a gradual tapering of the drug. During pregnancy, the dose of prednisone should remain constant or decreased if improvement of disease is evident [25, 28].

Cystic Fibrosis in Pregnancy

Cystic fibrosis is the most common serious genetic disorder in caucasians. The gene frequency in caucasians has been found to be 1 in 20. Homozygous patients suffer from the condition at an overall incidence of 1 in 1600 births, with heterozygous patients remaining asymptomatic [22]. It is characterized by an abnormality in exocrine gland secretions, leading to pancreatic and lung disease. Specifically, the pancreas is associated with ductal obstruction and pancreatic enzyme deficiency secondary to abnormally thick mucus [30, 31]. Lung disease is associated with airway plugging, inflammation, bronchiectasis, and recurrent pulmonary infections. Pulmonary disease is the most serious problem, with respiratory failure being the usual cause of death. Cirrhosis from progressive hepatic disease has accounted for a small number of deaths [32].

Diagnosis

Patients with cystic fibrosis usually present with recurrent or persistent respiratory symptoms, including a chronic cough and sputum production, chest radiographic abnormalities, obstructive pulmonary function studies, and abnormal arterial blood gas levels. Other signs may include hemoptysis, pneumothorax, bronchiectasis, and cor pulmonale. Gastrointestinal tract dysfunction and a positive family history for respiratory disease suggest the diagnosis. Nevertheless, the quantitative pilocarpine iontophoresis (sweat chlorides) must be performed to establish the diagnosis [31]. The pulmonary pathology usually is a mixed picture of obstructive and restrictive disease.

Cohen et al [33] produced a national survey in 1980 and found 129 pregnancies in women with cystic fibrosis. The complications included congestive heart failure in 13%, low weight gain in 41%, prematurity in 27%, and perinatal death in 11%. It was found that an 18% mortality existed within 2 years after delivery, but this was found to be similar to the rate of nongestational women with cystic fibrosis at similar ages. The study showed 97 completed pregnancies and 86 viable infants. Fifteen of 84 women died within the first 6 months postpartum, and none died during pregnancy [33]. With couples at risk, preconception counseling may be of great benefit. Additionally, in utero diagnosis of cystic fibrosis may be determined by DNA testing.

Therapy

Johnson et al [34] presented guidelines for treatment of cystic fibrosis during pregnancy including a general history, with emphasis on pulmonary and gastrointestinal symptoms. Studies should include chest radiography, pulmonary function studies, arterial blood gas measurements, and sputum culture. Liver function studies and a glucose tolerance test should be completed as well as serum electrolytes, hemoglobin and hematocrit, urinalysis, electrocardiography, and echocardiography to assess right ventricular function. Follow-up visits should continue every 2 weeks until 26 weeks gestation, then weekly thereafter. Pulmonary function studies, arterial blood gas measurements, sputum culture, weight, and blood count should be assessed monthly. Ultrasound should be completed early for assessment and dating of the fetus. In addition, fetal surveillance by nonstress tests (NSTs) should begin in the third trimester at biweekly visits.

Adequate hydration and chest physiotherapy three to four times daily will aid in mobilizing secretions. A vigorous aerobic exercise program has been shown to aid the bronchial toilet. Prolonged bed rest should be avoided. If pulmonary infection is suspected or if pulmonary function study results deteriorate, proper sputum cultures must be obtained. The most common organisms associated with cystic fibrosis are *Pseudomonas aeruginosa, Hemophilus influenzae,* and *Staphylococcus aureus.* An organism-specific treatment regimen must be developed. Specifically, *Staphylococcus* should be treated with a penicillinase-resistant penicillin or cephalosporin. Ampicillin, amoxicillin, or carbenicillin is appropriate for *H. influenzae.* A parenteral therapy usually must be used for *Pseudomonas.* Both gentamicin or tobramycin are effective [34]. However, combinations of an aminoglycoside with a third-generation cephalosporin such as ceftazadime or a newer semisynthetic penicillin such as piperacillin may be more effective. Drug sensitivity studies are usually necessary to use antibiotics most effectively. Oral agents are sometimes used when pseudomonas is chronically present in the sputum and include cefaclor and ciprofloxacin.

If there is evidence of pancreatic insufficiency, pancreatic extracts should be considered, which may reduce the chance of cholelithiasis, improve nutritional status, and reduce the chance of meconium ileus. A low-fat diet is helpful [30].

An increased incidence of premature labor seems to be present in women with cystic fibrosis. Tocolysis is not ordinarily contraindicated unless marked cor pulmonale is present. Labor and delivery management should include all ordinary precautions for women with known cardiac and pulmonary problems. The patient must be adequately hydrated in labor. Epidural anesthesia is preferable to general anesthesia. The duration of second stage labor can be reduced by performing a forceps delivery. Cesarean section should be considered only for obstetric reasons [34].

Pulmonary Embolus During Pregnancy

Deep venous thrombosis (DVT) of the lower extremities occurs in 0.018% to 0.29% of deliveries. The incidence varies widely depending on the time relative to delivery [35]. Specifically, DVT is three to five times more common postpartum than antepartum and 3 to 16 times more common in cesarean versus vaginal deliveries. Pulmonary embolus occurs in 15% to 24% of patients with untreated DVT, resulting in a 12% to 15% mortality. With appropriate therapy, pulmonary embolus occurs in 4.5% of DVTs, with an overall mortality of 0.7% [36, 37].

The increase in the incidence of embolus in pregnancy is associated with the acquired hypercoagulable state due to the increased potential for coagulation and thrombosis. Clotting factors V, VIII, IX, X, XII, and fibrinogen levels increase during pregnancy, while factor XI and XIII levels decrease. In addition, the placenta produces inhibitors of fibrinolysis [37]. Therefore, the increased potential for thrombosis is due to increased coagulation factors and decreased fibrinolysis. These changes occur most markedly at term and the immediate puerperium in order to physiologically control blood loss after placental separation [37].

The diagnosis and treatment of DVT and pulmonary embolus is the same as in the nonpregnant state (see Chapter 10). Most commonly, the signs and symptoms of DVT include pain, tenderness, swelling, edema, Homans' sign, change in limb color, and a palpable cord. In clinically suspicious cases, venography is the most accurate test for evaluation and can be used even in pregnancy because the benefit of the diagnosis far outweighs any possible side effects or complications [37]. Doppler ultrasound is a noninvasive method of detection of DVT and can detect thrombosis in about 90% of cases according to Markisz [38]. This is the most common method to make the diagnosis during pregnancy. The ^{125}I-labeled fibrinogen is used commonly for identification of DVT, but is contraindicated during pregnancy because unbound ^{125}I crosses the placental barrier to enter the fetal circulation and collects in the fetal thyroid [38].

Pulmonary embolism may present with many symptoms and signs including dyspnea, pleuritic chest pain, apprehension, cough, tachypnea, tachycardia, rales, hemoptysis, fever, diaphoresis, pleural friction rub, and cyanosis. The initial evaluation should include arterial blood gas measurement, chest radiography, and electrocardiography. In addition, any patient suspected of having pulmonary embolism should undergo a lung scan. In pregnancy, no adverse fetal effects have been reported with nuclide ventilation-perfusion scanning [39].

Heparin is the anticoagulant most commonly used in pregnancy because it does not pass the placental barrier [39]. Conversely, warfarin crosses the placenta easily and has been found to be associated with embryopathy including nasal hypoplasia, depression of the bridge of the nose, and epiphyseal stippling in the first trimester, and central nervous system and ophthalmologic abnormalities in the second two trimesters [37, 40]. Therefore, in cases requiring anticoagulant therapy, heparin should be used exclusively in the pregnant patient. Heparin anticoagulation is discussed in Chapter 11.

Amniotic Fluid Embolism

Amniotic fluid embolus is unique to pregnancy. It is associated with a small amount of amniotic fluid which is forced into the maternal circulation with labor and/or delivery. Specifically, amniotic fluid, fetal squamae, lanugo hairs, meconium, fat, mucin, and bile enters the circulation, which results in an embolization into the pulmonary vasculature [41]. Although this is a rare problem affecting only 1 in 8000 to 1 in 80,000 pregnancies, up to 10% to 15% of all maternal deaths are associated with amniotic fluid embolus and over 80% of cases of amniotic fluid embolus are fatal [42]. The risk factors of amniotic fluid embolus include advanced maternal age, multiparity, intrauterine death, use of uterine stimulants, tumultuous labor with tetanic contractions, and meconium in the amniotic fluid. The amniotic fluid is thought to enter the maternal circulation by way of open uterine veins during cervical dilatation, caesarean section or hypertonic contractions and at the placental site when there is placenta previa, premature separation of the placenta, or uterine rupture [43, 44].

Diagnosis

Dyspnea and chest pain followed by cyanosis, loss of consciousness, pulmonary edema, and shock may appear suddenly around the time of delivery. The progression of disease includes respiratory distress, cardiovascular collapse, and disseminated intravascular coagulation. Resnik et al [45] made a definitive diagnosis by detecting squamous cells and cellular debris in blood drawn from a central venous pressure line. Similarly, Shapiro and Wessely [41] used rhodamine B fluorescence for detection of squamae in maternal amniotic fluid embolus. Lung scanning has not proved to be helpful in the diagnosis due to the diffuse peripheral distribution of the disease and the difficulty in differentiation from thromboembolic disease versus amniotic fluid embolus.

Therapy

Therapy is based on circulatory and respiratory support. It is frequently necessary to provide intubation for ventilatory support with positive end-expiratory pressure. In the acute phase, the patient requires fluid resuscitation with monitoring of pulmonary artery and capillary wedge pressures. Chung et al [46] suggested heparinization for control of disseminated intravascular coagulation. Finally, Rodgers and Heymach [42] presented a case in which cryoprecipitate was administered to a patient with amniotic fluid embolus, who showed marked improvement in cardiopulmonary and hematologic status.

Tuberculosis in Pregnancy

Pulmonary tuberculosis is now a rare complication during pregnancy in developed countries. The acid fast bacillus, *Mycobacterium tuberculosis,* has been noted to have undergone a tremendous decline in developed countries due to effective chemotherapeutic agents. In the United States, the majority of the tuberculosis has been associated with a reactivation of the original disease. The disease can present with low-grade fever, night sweats, malaise, cough, sputum production, hemoptysis, and anorexia. Chest radiography can show upper lobe infiltrates, with or without cavitation. A primary infection can present with signs of pneumonia, including parenchymal infiltrates, adenopathy, and pleural effusion.

Diagnosis

The diagnostic algorithm for tuberculosis as in pregnancy is the same for the non-gravid person and may be reviewed in chapter 18. Tuberculin skin testing is valuable in determining if the patient has been infected, although a positive test does not necessarily denote active disease. Skin testing may be positive in up to 80% of patients with reactivation disease and therefore remains a very useful diagnostic tool in the pregnant patient. [47] The definitive diagnosis of tuberculosis is made by positive sputum smear or culture.

Most studies of the effects of tuberculosis on pregnancy conclude that gestation is not altered by tuberculosis. Selikoff et al [48] showed that 600 out of 616 pregnancies resulted in 602 normal live infants, seven cases of early spontaneous abortion, and nine cases of antepartum or intrapartum fetal death. However, Bjerkedal et al [49] presented a large study that showed a higher frequency of pre-eclampsia (7.4% versus 4.7%), vaginal hemorrhage (4.1% versus 2.2%), need for labor induction (14.6% versus 9.1%), spontaneous abortion (20.1 versus 2.3 per 1000), and interventions during labor (12.6% versus 7.7%) in patients with tuberculosis than in control subjects. The study also presented no differences between gestational ages at delivery, prematurity, hyperemesis, or low birth weights in tuberculosis patients versus control patients [49].

Therapy

The problem of managing a patient with tuberculosis in pregnancy is not the potential maternal respiratory impairment but the possible fetal effects of the chemotherapeutic agents. In general, the pregnant patient is treated the same as the nonpregnant patient, with a good understanding of the possible fetal effects of the chemotherapeutic agents. Therapy with two drugs is instituted at standard doses, and the treatment is not altered by the patient's pregnancy [50, 51]. Isoniazid (INH) has been widely used in pregnancy. While it crosses the placenta, it has not shown any teratogenic side effects. Snider [52] presented a study of 16 abnormal fetuses in 1480 pregnancies in which INH was given, which was found to be lower than the normal pregnant population. INH is known to cause peripheral neuritis, which can present as a potential problem during pregnancy. The American Thoracic Society/Centers for Disease Control statement for preventive therapy during pregnancy follows:

> Although no harmful effects of isoniazid to the fetus have been observed, its use during pregnancy generally is for those with tuberculous disease. INH preventive therapy generally should be delayed until after delivery. There does not appear to be any substantial increment in tuberculosis risk for women during pregnancy. An exception is with the pregnant women likely to have been recently infected. Then INH preventive therapy should begin when the infection is documented, but after the first trimester [53].

When INH is used in the pregnant patient, supplemental pyridoxine is recommended in view of the increased need for this vitamin in pregnancy [47].

The use of ethambutol (EMB) during pregnancy has been reported in several series and does not appear to be contraindicated during pregnancy. Snider [52] showed no relationship between the use of EMB during pregnancy and subsequent fetal abnormalities or any other adverse maternal or fetal effects. Lewitt et al [54] presented 655 pregnancies treated with EMB, with only 14 infants or fetuses with any abnormalities. This drug can be considered safe in pregnancy.

Rifampin (RIF) has the ability to inhibit DNA-dependent RNA polymerase and can cross the placental barrier. While no adverse fetal effects have been cited, it should be used with caution until further data become available [54].

Streptomycin was at one time thought to be safe in pregnancy; however, a study by Snider [52] showed a 15% risk of eighth cranial nerve damage. While most effects in the offspring of treated mothers are minor vestibular and auditory impairment, cases of severe and bilateral hearing loss and marked vestibular abnormalities have been reported by Robinson et al [51a].

Therefore, there is no evidence that pregnancy has an adverse effect on tuberculosis. The prognosis of pregnancy is good with early diagnosis and prompt, effective chemotherapy. Preventive therapy should be given in the second and third trimesters in patients at high risk of developing progressive disease. The preferred treatments are INH-EMB, INH-RIF, or INH-EMB-RIF. The use of antituberculosis chemotherapy in the mother after delivery is compatible with nursing [52].

Pneumonia in Pregnancy

The diagnosis and treatment of pneumonia in pregnancy is similiar to that of the nonpregnant patient. The infectious diseases that affect the lung during pregnancy include viruses, mycoplasma, funguses, and bacterial pathogens. Oxorn [55] showed a high incidence of premature delivery (70%) in pneumonia even with antibiotic support. Benedetti et al [56] revealed a perinatal mortality of 40 per 1000 and no maternal deaths in their study of antipartum pneumonia in pregnancy. In addition, Benedetti et al showed no significant change of preterm delivery in patients with pneumonia. This may be because of improved antibiotic therapy since the earlier study [56]. The most common bacterial pneumonia is *Streptococcus pneumoniae,* which accounted for 13 of 21 cases of culture proven bacterial pneumonia in pregnancy [56]. The clinical presentation of bacterial pneumonia in pregnancy is similar to that of the nonpregnant patient. The pneumococcal vaccine is now recommended in high-risk non gravid patients; however, the vaccine is contraindicated in normal pregnancies until futher studies can be completed on its safety [57, 69].

Mycoplasma pneumoniae is very common in the pregnant population and seems to present very gradually. The patient presents with sore throat, nonproductive cough, headache, and fever. Chest radiography reveals patchy infiltrates with occasional consolidation. The patients generally do not have leukocytosis and sputum Gram stain is usually not revealing [58].

Fungal infections are very rare in pregnancy; however, coccidioidomycosis was reviewed by Harris [59]. Of the 50 cases of coccidioidomycosis, 22 became disseminated. The risks of dissemination in pregnancy seem to be 20% for those patients who acquire the disease before pregnancy, while that of the nonpregnant patient seems to be 0.2%. The risk of dissemination was higher in patients who contracted coccidioidomycosis during pregnancy, particularly in the second and third trimesters [59]. Powell et al [60] presented a possible explanation for the increased dissemination and found an increased rate of the growth of fungus and release of endospores in the presence of estradiol and progesterone. Binding proteins for progesterone and estradiol have been identified in the cytosol of the fungus. Nevertheless, coccidioidomycosis seems to present no hazard to the mother or fetus in the undisseminated form; however, in untreated pregnant patients dissemination has a 100% mortality compared with a 50% mortality in nonpregnant patients. The use of amphotericin B has not been shown to have any detrimental effects on the fetal or neonatal course, but relatively few cases have been reported [61].

The use of antibiotics in pregnancy presents a challenge to the clinician. The physician must weigh the benefits of the drug against the possible toxicity or teratogenicity. Table 24-1 summarizes commonly used antibiotics in pregnancy and reports the possible problems.

Pulmonary Edema Associated with Sympathomimetic Therapy

Numerous reports of pulmonary edema have been reported associated with sympathomimetic therapy. Tocolytic agents, which are used to suppress premature uterine contractions, include terbutaline, isoxsuprine, ritodrine, and salbutamol. The β-adrenergic agonists are commonly used tocolytic agents that act by increasing intracellular cAMP. C-AMP decreases the activity of myosin light-chain kinase, the rate-limiting enzyme in the signal, leading to uterine contractions [62, 63]. The physiologic responses of β-agonists include tachycardia, hyperglycemia, hypokalemia, and antidiuresis.

When pregnant women assume the supine position, the excretion of sodium and water may decrease by as much as 60%. Aldosterone secretion increases during pregnancy, leading to increased sodium retention. Tocolytic agents increase secretion of antidiuretic

Table 24-1. Antibiotics in Pregnancy

Penicillin	Safe
Cephalosporins	Safe
Erythromycin	Safe
Erythromycin estolate	Reversible maternal hepatitis in late pregnancy
Nitrofurantoin	Hemolysis in G6PD deficiency in fetus and neonate
Isoniazid	Hepatotoxicity
Sulfonamides	Hyperbilirubinemia if given late in pregnancy
Nalidixic acid	Increased intracranial pressure in newborn
Metronidazole	Carcinogenesis in animals, safe in human pregnancy after first trimester
Clindamycin	Maternal pseudomembranous colitis
Tetracyclines	Dysplasia of teeth and inhibition of bone growth
Chloramphenicol	Blood dyscrasias
Aminoglycosides	Ototoxicity in fetus
Trimethoprim/ Sulfamethoxazole	Teratogenesis, hyperbilirubinemia, megaloblastic anemia

hormone causes further sodium retention and hypotonicity [63, 64]. The resultant hypervolemic and hypo-oncotic state predisposes to pulmonary edema. In addition, several other hypotheses have been used to explain pulmonary edema, seen with use of tocolytic agents, including myocardial failure, postcapillary venoconstriction and the capillary leak syndrome.

Women with pulmonary edema associated with tocolytic therapy may present with dyspnea, chest roentgenography revealing unilateral or bilateral alveolar infiltrates, evidence of hemodilution (decreased hematocrit or hypokalemia), and a rapid clinical response to treatment with diuretics and oxygen. An important feature of this disease is the exclusion of other serious pathology including pulmonary embolus, amniotic fluid embolus, pneumonia, and cardiomyopathy [62].

Treatment of pulmonary edema includes the discontinuation of tocolytic therapy, diuresis (usually with furosemide), and administration of oxygen for hypoxemia. Intubation and mechanical ventilation may be required under severe conditions. A rapid clinical response to treatment is characteristic of pulmonary edema associated with tocolytic therapy [65, 66].

Kyphoscoliosis

Kyphoscoliosis in pregnancy rarely interrupts the normal sequence of labor and delivery; however, in the case of hypoxemia and pulmonary hypertension, the disease process must be controlled. A cesarean delivery may be indicated in these patients due to abnormalities in the bony pelvis. Epidural anesthesia is usually indicated unless severe spinal deformities exist.

Sleep Apnea in Pregnancy

The relationship of sleep apnea to pregnancy is unknown; however, pregnancy could expose a woman to severe hypoxemia during sleep due to a reduced residual volume and cardiac output in the supine position. A recent study of sleep in women of 36 weeks gestation through postpartum periods indicated no difference in severe hypoxemia between the two periods. In fact, hypopneas and apneas were less frequent during pregnancy, probably due to the respiratory stimulatory effects of progesterone [67, 68]. However, snoring and obesity are risk factors for the development of sleep apnea and this diagnosis should be entertained in the at risk mother who develops excessive daytime sleepiness.

References

1. Thompson KJ, Cohen ME: Studies on the circulation in normal pregnancy. *Surg Gynecol Obstet* 66:591, 1938
2. Anderson GJ, James GB, et al: The maternal oxygen tension and acid base status during pregnancy. *J Obstet Gynaecol Br Commonw* 76: 16, 1969
3. Greenberger PA: Asthma in pregnancy. *Clin Perinatol* 12:571, 1985
4. Ueland K, Novy MJ, Metcalfe J: Cardiorespi-

ratory responses to pregnancy and exercise in normal women and patients with heart disease. *Am J Obstet Gynecol* 115:4, 1973
5. Huff RW: Asthma in pregnancy. *Med Clin North Am* 73:653, 1989
6. Lind T: Maternal Physiology. Washington, DC, CREOG, 1985
7. Cugell DW, Frank NR, et al: Pulmonary function in pregnancy. *Am Rev Tuberc* 67:568, 1953
8. Weinstein AM, Dubin, BD, Padleski WK, et al: Asthma and pregnancy. *JAMA* 241:1161, 1979
9. Skatrud JB, Dempsey JA, Kaiser DG: Ventilatory response to medroxyprogesterone acetate in normal subjects: Time course and mechanism. *J Appl Physiol* 44:939, 1978
10. Mintz S: Pregnancy and asthma. *In* Weiss EB, Segal MS (eds): Bronchial Asthma: Mechanisms and Therapeutics. Boston, Little, Brown, 1976, pp 971–982
11. Greenberger PA, Patterson R: Management of asthma during pregnancy. *N Engl J Med* 312:897, 1985
12. Gluck JC, Gluck PA: The effects of pregnancy on asthma: A prospective study. *Ann Allergy* 37:164, 1976
13. DiMarco AF: Asthma in the pregnant patient: A review. *Ann Allergy* 62, 1989
14. Bahna, SL, Bjerkedal T: The course and outcome of pregnancy in women with bronchial asthma. *Acta Allergol* 27:397, 1972
15. Gordon M, Nisrander KR, Berendes H, et al: Fetal morbidity following potentially anoxigenic obstetric conditions: Bronchial asthma. *Am J Obstet Gynecol* 106:645, 1984
16. Heinonen OP, Slone D, Shapiro S, et al: Birth defects and drugs in pregnancy. Littleton, MA, Publishing Science Group, 1977, pp 388–389
17. Mawhinney H, Spector SL: Optimum management of asthma in pregnancy. *Drugs* 32: 178, 1986
18. Labovitz E, Spector S: Placental theophylline transfer in pregnant asthmatics. *JAMA* 247: 786, 1982
19. Carter BL, Driscoll CE, Smith GD: Theophylline clearance during pregnancy. *Obstet Gynecol* 68:555, 1986
20. Fitzsimons R, Greenberger PA, Patterson R: Outcome of pregnancy in women requiring corticosteroids for severe asthma. *J Clin Immunol* 78:349, 1986
21. Schatz, M, Harden K, Forsythe A, et al: The course of asthma during pregnancy, post partum, and with successive pregnancies: A prospective analysis. *J Clin Immunol* 81:509, 1988
22. Fainstat: Cortisone-induced congenital cleft palate in rabbits. *Endocrinology* 55:502, 1954
23. O'Leary: Ten-year study of sarcoidosis and pregnancy. *Am J Obstet Gynecol* 84:462, 1962
24. Gallagher JP, Douglas LH: Sarcoidosis and pregnancy. *Obstet Gynecol* 2:590, 1953
25. Haynes de Regt, R: Sarcoidosis and pregnancy: Improvement in pulmonary function. *JAMA* 200:726, 1967
26. Agha FP, Vade A, Amendola MA, et al: Effects of pregnancy on sarcoidosis. *Surg Gynecol Obstet* 155:817, 1982
27. Scadding. Sarcoidosis. London, Eyre and Spottiswoode, 1967
28. Grossman JH 3rd, Littner MR: Severe sarcoidosis in pregnancy. *Obstet Gynecol* 50 (suppl):81, 1977
29. Dines DE, Banner EA, et al: Sarcoidosis in pregnancy: Improvement in pulmonary function. *JAMA* 200:726, 1967
30. Corkey CW, Newth CJ, Larey M, et al: Pregnancy in cystic fibrosis: A better prognosis in patients with pancreatic function. *Am J Obstet Gynecol* 140:737, 1981
31. Grand RJ, Talamo RC, di Sant'Agnese PA, et al: Diagnosis of maternal cystic fibrosis during pregnancy. *Obstet Gynecol* 61(suppl):2S, 1983
32. Palmer JD, Dillon-Baker C, Tecklin JS, et al: Pregnancy in patients with cystic fibrosis. *Ann Intern Med* 99:596, 1983
33. Cohen LF, Agnese PA, Friedlander J, et al: Cystic fibrosis and pregnancy: A National Survey. *Lancet* 2:842, 1980
34. Johnson SR, Varner MW, Yates SJ, et al: Diagnosis of maternal cystic fibrosis during pregnancy. *Obstet Gynecol* 61(3 suppl):2S–7S, 1983
35. Bonnar J: Venous thromboembolism and pregnancy. *Clin Obstet Gynecol* 8:455, 1981
36. Bergquist A, Bergquist D, Hallbrook T: Acute deep vein thrombosis (DVT) after cesarean section. *Acta Obstet Gynecol Scand* 58:473, 1979
37. Rutherford SE, Phelon JP: Thromboembolic disease in pregnancy. *Clin Perinatol* 13:719, 1986
38. Markisz: Radiologic and nuclear medicine diagnosis. *In* Goldhaber (ed): Pulmonary Embolism and DVT. Philadelphia, WB Saunders, 1985
39. Bratt G, Tiornebalm E, Lackner D, et al: A human pharmacological study comparing conventional heparin and a low molecular weight heparin fragment. *Thromb Haemost* 53:208, 1985
40. Holm HA, Abildgaard U, Kalvenes S: Heparin assays and bleeding complications in treatment of DVT with reference to retroperitoneal bleeding. *Thromb Haemost* 53:278, 1985
41. Shapiro SH, Wessely Z: Rhodamine B fluorescence as a stain for amniotic fluid squames in maternal pulmonary embolism. *Ann Clin Lab Sci* 18:151, 1988
42. Rodgers GP, Heymach GJ: Cryoprecipitate therapy in amniotic fluid embolization. *Am J Med* 76:916, 1984

43. Courtney LD, Amniotic fluid embolism. *Obstet Gynecol Surv* 29:169, 1974
44. Peterson, Taylor: Amniotic fluid embolism: An analysis of 40 cases. *Obstet Gynecol* 35:787, 1970
45. Resnick R, Swartz WH, Plumer MH, et al: Amniotic fluid embolism with survival. *Obstet Gynecol* 47:295, 1976
46. Chung AF, Merkatz IR: Survival following amniotic fluid embolism with early heparinization. *Obstet Gynecol* 42:809, 1973
47. Weinstein AM, Murphy: Antituberculous therapy in pregnancy: Risks to the fetus. *West J Med* 127:195, 1977
48. Selikoff IJ, Dorfman HC, et al: Medical, Surgical and Gynecologic Complications of Pregnancy. Baltimore, MD, Williams & Wilkins, 1965
49. Bjerkedal T, Bahna SL, Lehmann EH: Course and outcome of pregnancy in women with pulmonary tuberculosis. *Scand J Respir Dis* 56:245, 1975
50. Good JT, Iseman MD, Davidson PT, et al: Tuberculosis in association with pregnancy. *Am J Obstet Gynecol* 140:492, 1981
51. Snider DE: Pregnancy and tuberculosis. *Chest* 86:10S-13S, 1984
51a. Robinson GC, Cambon KG. Hearing loss in infants of tuberculous mothers treated with streptomycin during pregnancy 271:949, 1964
52. Snider DE, Powell, KE: Should women taking antituberculosis drugs breastfeed? *Arch Intern Med* 144:589, 1984
53. American Thoracic Society/CDC: Treatment of tuberculosis. *Am Rev Respir Dis* 127:790, 1983
54. Lewitt T, Nebal L, Terrocina S, Karman S: Ethambutol in pregnancy. *Chest* 66:25, 1974
55. Oxorn H: The changing aspects of pneumonia complicating pregnancy. *Am J Obstet Gynecol* 70:1057, 1955
56. Benedetti TJ, Valle R, Ledger WJ: Antepartum pneumonia in pregnancy. *Am J Obstet Gynecol* 144:413, 1982
57. Austrian R: Pneumococcal vaccine, development and prospects. *Am J Med* 67:547, 1979
58. Murray HW, Masur H, Senterfit LB, et al: The protean manifestations of mycoplasma pneumonia infection in adults. *Am J Med* 58:229, 1975
59. Harris RE: Coccidioidomycosis complicating pregnancy. *Obstet Gynecol* 28:401, 1966
60. Powell BL, Drutz DJ, Huppert M, et al: Relationship of progesterone and estradiol binding proteins in *Coccidioides immitis* to coccidioidal dissemination in pregnancy. *Infect Immun* 40:478, 1983
61. Ellinoy BR: Amophotericin B usage in pregnancy complicated by cryptococcosis. *Am J Obstet Gynecol* 115:285, 1973
62. Pissani RJ, Rosenow EL: Pulmonary edema associated with tocolytic therapy. *Ann Intern Med* 110:714, 1989
63. Benedetti TJ, Harglove JC, Rosene KA: Maternal pulmonary edema during premature labor inhibition. *Obstet Gynecol* 59(suppl):33S, 1982
64. Gleicher N, Bazile F, Elrad H: Pulmonary edema after ritodrine therapy in a patient with preeclampsia. *N Engl J Med* 306:174, 1982
65. Benedetti TJ, Kater R, Williams V: Hemodynamic observations in severe preeclampsia complicated by pulmonary edema. *Am J Obstet Gynecol* 152:330, 1985
66. Berkowitz RL, Rafferty TD: Invasive hemodynamic monitoring in critically ill pregnant patients: Role of Swan-Ganz catheterization. *Am J Obstet Gynecol* 137:127, 1980
67. Brownell LG, West P, Dryger MH: Breathing during sleep in normal pregnant women. *Ann Rev Respir Dis* 133:38–41, 1986
68. Conti M, Izzo V, Muggiasca ML, et al: Sleep apnoea syndrome in pregnancy: A case report. *Eur J Anaesthesiol* 5:151–154, 1988
69. Maccato M: Respiratory insufficiency due to pneumonia in pregnancy. *Obstet Gynecol Clinic North Am* 18(2):289–299, 1991
70. Schatz M: Asthma during pregnancy: Interrelationships and management. *Ann of Allergy* 68:123–133, 1992

Preoperative Pulmonary Evaluation

Ernest L. Yoder, John Haapaniemi, and Barry Lesser

Surgically related pulmonary complications persist as a significant cause of perioperative morbidity and mortality [1]. Many factors such as acute or chronic lung disease, congestive heart failure, smoking, obesity, and abnormal pulmonary function studies are associated with a high complication rate. Newer methods for assessing risk have become available, but frequently are either very expensive or carry significant risk due to invasiveness. As a result it is necessary for the managing physician to have a logical approach to identification and assessment of those patients at risk for respiratory-related perioperative morbidity or mortality. Coverage of preoperative cardiac clearance and cardiac surgery itself are beyond the scope of this chapter. What is offered here is a practical, logical approach to preoperative identification and assessment of patients at risk for perioperative pulmonary complications. The goals of evaluation are to identify patients at risk, treat reversible risk factors preoperatively, identify and anticipate problems for treatment early in the intraoperative periods, and identify patients for whom risks outweigh the potential benefits.

Pathophysiology of Intraoperative and Postoperative Pulmonary Alterations

Functional, physiologic, and anesthetic drug-related changes have all been implicated in the pathogenesis of perioperative complications. Intraoperative and postoperative changes in chest wall and diaphragmatic motion, as well as development of regions of microatelectasis and macroatelectasis as causes of altered ventilation-perfusion ratio, have been described [2]. Additionally, inhalational anesthetics have been shown to impair normal, hypoxic pulmonary vasoconstriction [2, 3]. These effects may persist for many hours and appear to be accentuated in elderly, obese, and very ill patients [4]. Tisi [3] lists perioperative declines in forced vital capacity, functional residual capacity, expiratory reserve volume, tidal volume, and sigh frequency, along with an increase in respiratory rate in relationship to the previously noted functional ventilatory changes. Falk et al [5] have demonstrated significant intraoperative declines in oxygen consumption, cardiac index, oxygen delivery, and increased lactate production in the face of stable mixed venous saturation, arteriovenous oxygen content difference, and pulmonary capillary wedge pressure, implying impaired cellular oxygen utilization. Contributors to the previously noted physiologic alterations are inhaled anesthetic agents, drugs that impair cough, the anatomic site of the operation, postoperative pain, tightness of bandages, altered level of consciousness, altered sensation, and immobilization of patients in the supine position [3].

Complications of Surgery and Anesthesia

Among the most common reported complications of surgery and anesthesia are atelectasis, infection, acute respiratory failure, and cardiac decompensation [6–10]. In most studies, advanced age and chronic lung disease are listed as important contributing factors. Impaired cough, retained secretions, decreased tidal volume, and diminished sigh result in decreased expiratory reserve volume, airway closure, and atelectasis [3]. As a result of atelectasis and impaired mucociliary clearance (chronic lung disease and anesthesia), bacterial colonization descends well below the carina, contributing to exacerbation of chronic obstructive pulmonary disease and development of pneumonia. Acute respiratory failure is commonly heralded by increasing dyspnea, cough, purulent sputum production, bronchospasm, and arterial blood gas abnormalities [3].

Patients at Risk for Complications of Surgery and Anesthesia

Patient characteristics and factors related to the type of surgery contribute to the risk of perioperative complications. Table 25-1 lists, along with references, patient characteristics that have been identified as indicative of increased surgical risk. Types of surgery that increase the risk of postoperative pulmonary complications include chest surgery, upper abdominal surgery, aortic surgery, and procedures requiring prolonged anesthesia. In each case there are factors contributing to a quantitatively greater degree of atelectasis as well as a greater drug load [5, 11]. From a pulmonary point of view, local anesthesia is preferred over general. However, spinal anesthesia is not necessarily advantageous relative to general anesthesia. If the abdominal muscles are required to assist breathing, as is often the case in chronic obstructive pulmonary disease (COPD), a high spinal block may carry more risk [11a].

Identifying Patients at Risk

Preoperative evaluation should assess the risk of morbidity and mortality and predict the need for prolonged postoperative ventilatory support and the ability of the patient to withstand pulmonary resection. Screening begins with a thorough history and physical examination. Jewell and Persson [10], in their discussion of the Dripps classification of anesthetic risk and the New York Heart Association classification of heart disease, provides excellent examples of the importance of this data base. Mortality increases as one ascends to the higher classes within either of these schemes. The Dripps classification includes five levels: 1, normal healthy individuals; 2, mild-to-moderate systemic disease; 3, severe systemic disease with limited activity, but not incapacitating; 4, incapacitating, life-threatening disease; and 5, moribund, not expected

Table 25-1. Patient Characteristics Increasing Risk of Perioperative Complications

Risk Factor	*Indicator(s)*	*Reference(s)*
Smoking history	More than 10 pack-years	1–4, 6, 7, 11, 32
Obesity	20% overweight	1–4, 6, 11, 32
Elderly	Age >60 years	1–4, 6, 11, 32
Lung disease		
Acute	Recent signs or symptoms	1–4, 6, 11, 32
Chronic	Obstructive or restrictive Abnormal spirometry	
Decreased strength	Dynamometry	4
Chest wall abnormality	Kyphosis, scoliosis, other	32
Liver disease	Childs' classification, ascites, jaundice, elevated PT or PTT, recent hepatitis	33–35
Cardiac disease	History of congestive heart failure, angina, myocardial infarction, ECG shows myocardial infarction, blocks, premature ventricular contractions Chest radiographic cardiomegaly Aortic stenosis	9, 10, 26
Vascular disease	Carotid bruits, transient ischemic attack	32

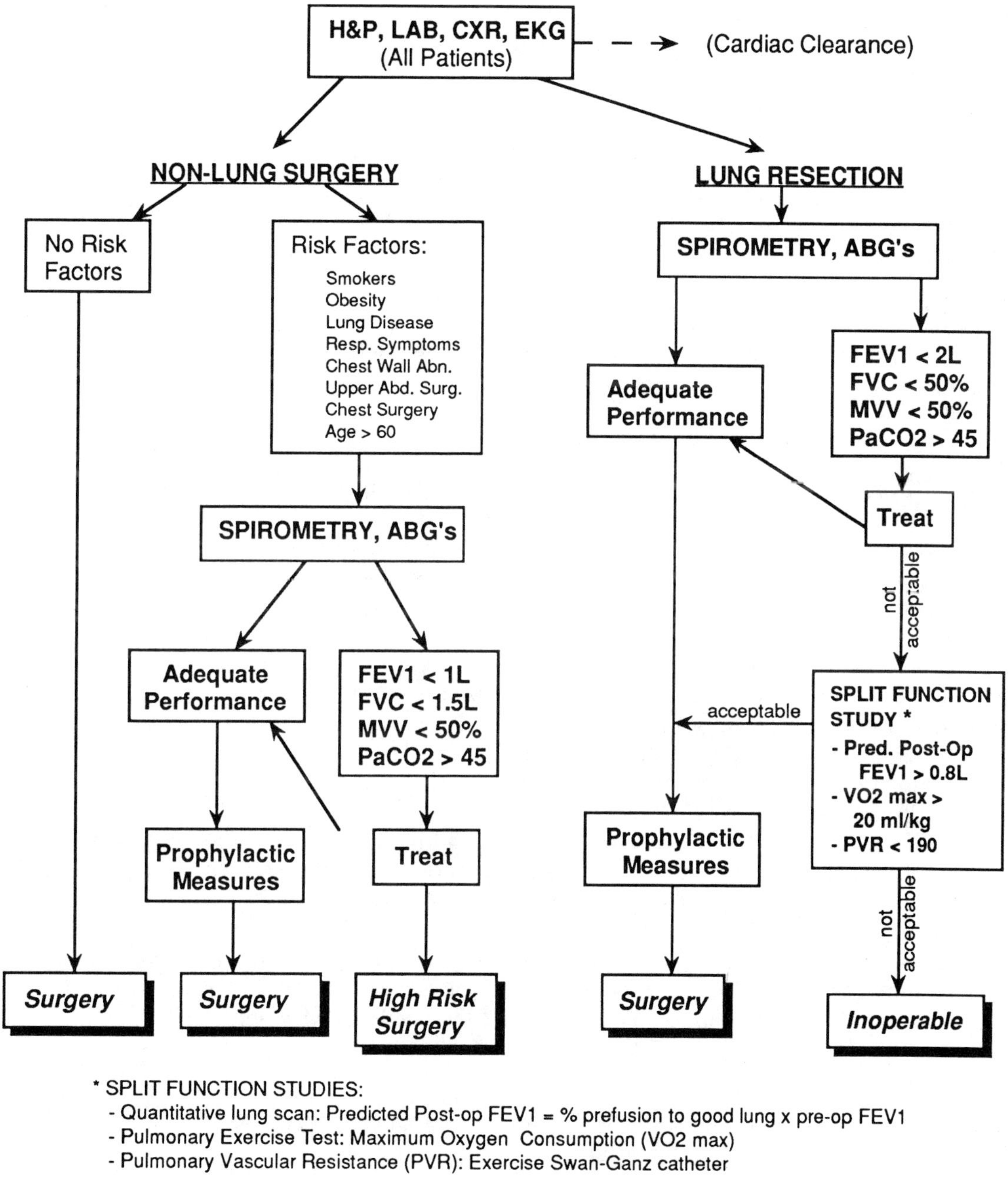
H&P, LAB, CXR, EKG
(All Patients)
(Cardiac Clearance)
NON-LUNG SURGERY
LUNG RESECTION
No Risk Factors
Risk Factors:
Smokers
Obesity
Lung Disease
Resp. Symptoms
Chest Wall Abn.
Upper Abd. Surg.
Chest Surgery
Age > 60
SPIROMETRY, ABG's
Adequate Performance
FEV1 < 1L
FVC < 1.5L
MVV < 50%
PaCO2 > 45
Prophylactic Measures
Treat
Surgery
Surgery
High Risk Surgery
SPIROMETRY, ABG's
FEV1 < 2L
FVC < 50%
MVV < 50%
PaCO2 > 45
Adequate Performance
Treat
not acceptable
acceptable
SPLIT FUNCTION STUDY *
- Pred. Post-Op FEV1 > 0.8L
- VO2 max > 20 ml/kg
- PVR < 190
Prophylactic Measures
not acceptable
Surgery
Inoperable
* SPLIT FUNCTION STUDIES:
- Quantitative lung scan: Predicted Post-op FEV1 = % prefusion to good lung x pre-op FEV1
- Pulmonary Exercise Test: Maximum Oxygen Consumption (VO2 max)
- Pulmonary Vascular Resistance (PVR): Exercise Swan-Ganz catheter

Fig. 25-1. Preoperative evaluation of the pulmonary patient.

to live 24 hours. The New York Heart Association classification can be applied to patients with either angina or congestive heart failure and includes four functional levels: 1, symptoms on supranormal activity; 2, symptoms on normal activity; 3, symptoms on climbing one flight or walking two blocks; and 4, symptoms at rest or on minimal activity [10].

Following the history and physical examination, screening proceeds depending on the type of surgery planned for the patient (Fig. 25-1). Spirometry, chest radiography, electrocardiography, and arterial blood gas measurements may be initially indicated. In the most extreme cases, such as resection of functional lung in a patient with underlying lung

Table 25-2. Screening Pulmonary Function Tests

Study	*Operable Range*	*Possibly Inoperable*	*Reference*
Forced vital capacity	>1.5 L (nonlung surgery) >50% (lung resection)	<1.5 L (nonlung surgery) <50% (lung resection)	2, 3, 6, 11
Forced expiratory volume in 1 second	>1 L (nonlung surgery) >2 L (lung resection)	<1 L (nonlung surgery) <2 L (lung resection)	2, 4, 6, 11
Maximum voluntary ventilation	>50% predicted	<50% predicted	6, 11
Arterial blood gases ($PaCO_2$)	<45 mm Hg	>45 mm Hg	4

If patient falls into inoperable category they are either high risk for nonlung surgery, or need further evaluation for lung surgery.

disease, more extensive investigation is performed as indicated. This may include split function testing such as quantitative nuclear lung scans, measurement of pulmonary vascular resistance, or cardiopulmonary exercise testing. Table 25-2 summarizes the screening pulmonary function values, which predict operability and inoperability for both lung resection and nonthoracic surgery.

Table 25-3 shows the split function studies or more extensive work-up, which may be useful in further defining risk in marginal patients. Lung scans may be viewed *qualitatively* such as in predicting oxygenation improvement after removal of a shunt (perfused, but unventilated lung) [2]. Figure 25-2 shows a *quantitative* perfusion lung scan used to predict postoperative forced expiratory volume in 1 second [12]. Cardiopulmonary exercise testing is performed by analyzing exhaled gases during graded exercise. Of the multiple parameters measured during this test, the maximum oxygen consumption (VO_2 max) has been shown to predict survival in patients undergoing lung resection [13]. Pulmonary vascular resistance measured with a Swan-Ganz catheter during exercise has also been used to predict risk in this group of patients [14].

Prophylactic Measures

In addition to preoperative evaluation, many authors recommend prophylactic measures to improve each high-risk patient's chances of a successful operative outcome [1–4, 6, 9–11, 14–21]. Patients may occasionally be "converted" from inoperative to operative by functional improvement of their pulmonary or cardiac status through carefully planned

Table 25-3. Split Function Studies for Marginal Patients Undergoing Lung Resection

Study	*Operable Range*	*Inoperable Range*	*Reference*
Quantified perfusion lung scan (FEV_1-PPO)*	>800 cc (>40% predicted)	<800 cc (<40% predicted)	6, 11, 20
Cardiopulmonary exercise test (VO_2 max)	>20 mL/kg/min	<15 mL/kg/min	11–13, 20, 25, 30, 31, 36
Pulmonary vascular resistance (after exercise)	<190 dynes-sec-cm^{-5}	>190 dynes-sec-cm^{-5}	14

*PPO, predicted postoperative FEV_1, calculated for pneumonectomy; FEV_1-PPO = [Preoperative FEV_1 × (% perfusion to remaining lung)]/100.

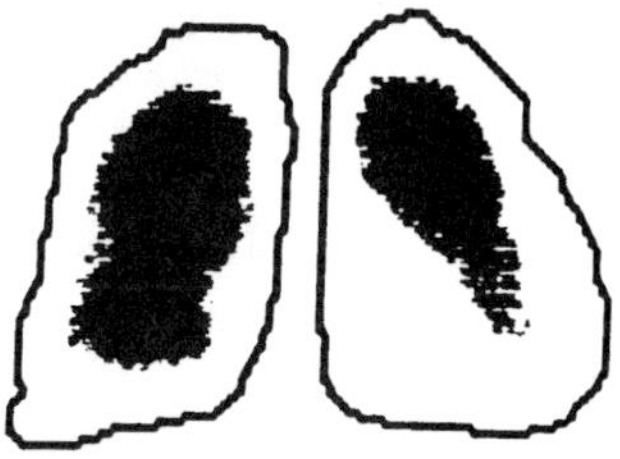
RIGHT LUNG
LEFT LUNG
Pixel count
253,960
Percent flow
57%
Pixel count
192,898
Percent flow
43%

Fig. 25-2. Quantified perfusion lung scan (anterior view) showing percentage of blood flow to each lung. This can then be used in conjunction with the pulmonary function test to calculate a predicted postoperative FEV1 to determine resectability.

preparatory programs. Methods of prophylaxis and preparation are detailed in Table 25-4 and include preoperative, intraoperative, and postoperative components. Some methods are as simple as patient education, while others involve more elaborate measures.

Incentive spirometry (forced inspiratory maneuver) has been shown to increase lung volume postoperatively and has better results when the patient is instructed preoperatively. Other methods such as intermittent positive pressure breathing, forced expiratory maneuvers, and ventilatory stimulants are less effective than incentive spirometry [22]. Patient education is a very important adjunct to successful preoperative preparation and intraoperative and postoperative management. Patients should be carefully instructed as to the reasons for all therapeutic modalities and lifestyle changes [23]. Physician motivation can be a most effective incentive for patient compliance. Patients with abnormal spirometry results and/or a history of acute or chronic lung disease should have a preoperative course of appropriate therapy. This may include methylxanthines, inhaled β-agonists, antibiotics, and even corticosteroids [18]. After a period of therapy or subjective improvement, the patient should be reassessed. Intraoperatively, patients require adequate ventilation, monitoring as indicated [24], and the shortest possible period of anesthesia. Postoperative techniques include early ambulation, pain control, incentive spirometry, and deep breathing and cough exercise [15, 18]. Some authors have demonstrated the benefits of continuous positive airway pressure and positive end-expiratory pressure, but as with intermittent positive pressure breathing, deleterious cardiovascular and pulmonary side effects make them of questionable utility [15–17, 19, 25].

Preparation for Surgery Not Involving Lung Resection

Patients slated for nonthoracic surgery who fall into a potentially high-risk group (smoking, obesity, lung disease, pulmonary symptoms, chest wall abnormality, upper abdominal surgery, chest surgery, age >60, cardiac disease) should, in addition to the routine studies mentioned in the previous section, undergo screening spirometry and arterial blood gas measurement. If the results are good on these preliminary, simple, inexpensive tests, the patient may be an acceptable risk for undergoing surgery. In the case of cardiac symptoms, exercise testing or cardiac catheterization may be indicated [15, 24]. If these studies demonstrate adequate performance, proceed with the planned operation. If the results of either the pulmonary or cardiac evaluation are inadequate, therapeutic and prophylactic measures are indicated (Fig. 25-1, Table 25-4). These recommendations are an attempt to quantify our evaluation of risk versus benefit in predicting the pulmonary complications of surgery. Even though this is the case, the decision to operate will be a clinical judgment.

Preparation for Surgery Involving Lung Resection

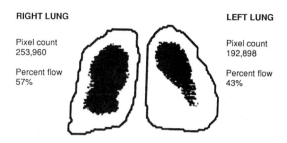

Resection of functioning lung in a patient with preexisting lung disease places the patient at the most extreme risk for developing pulmonary complications. Unfortunately, this is not an uncommon scenario since patients are frequently seen with the combination of chronic obstructive pulmonary disease and lung cancer due to cigarette smoking. In

Table 25-4. Prophylactic and Therapeutic Measures and Indications

Measure	*Indication/Goal*	*References*
Preoperative		
Patient education	All patients for compliance	18
Smoking cessation	Improve lung volumes	7, 23
Incentive spirometry	Improve lung volumes Reduce atelectasis	15, 17, 36
Bronchodilator therapy	Improve lung volumes Treat bronchospasm Reduce secretions	6, 18
Weight reduction	Reduce operative risk	2–4, 6, 18
Secretions control	Reduce pneumonia risk Prevent atelectasis Improve lung volumes	18
Exercise	Improve functional status	15, 18
Intraoperative		
Monitoring	Cardiac disease, lung resection	24
Postoperative		
Early ambulation	Prevent decreased lung volumes	18
Pain control	Improve ventilation	18
Encourage cough	Improve lung volumes	15, 25
Continuous positive airway pressure	Improve lung volumes	16, 19, 25
Positive end-expiratory pressure	Improve lung volumes	16, 25
Intermittent positive-pressure breathing	Improve lung volumes Prevent collapse	15

the evaluation of a patient for lung resection, the worst case scenario (pneumonectomy) is generally anticipated. First, the extent of resection (lobectomy versus pneumonectomy) cannot be known for certain until the chest is explored. Second, pulmonary function in the immediate postoperative period is generally similar to a pneumonectomy. If less extensive surgery can be performed, of course that is preferable. No perfect single predictive test exists for prognosticating patient success in surgery of any site. What is proposed here is a logical, systematic approach, somewhat eclectic, but broad-based enough to distinguish, in most cases, the operable from the inoperable.

In all cases, the patient must have a thorough history and physical examination, baseline screening laboratory data (complete blood count, transaminase levels, blood urea nitrogen, creatinine, bilirubin, serum albumin, urinalysis), chest radiography, electrocardiography [9, 26], spirometry, and arterial blood gases [11, 27]. If results are acceptable (Table 25-2), then proceed with routine care and prophylactic measures. If predictive values (forced vital capacity, forced expiratory volume in 1 second, maximal voluntary ventilation, and $PaCO_2$) demonstrate an inadequate performance (Table 25-2) [10, 11], proceed with aggressive treatment of the underlying pulmonary or cardiac disease and reassess the patient. If the reevaluation indicates operability, then proceed with the planned operation.

If the patient again is assessed as being inoperable, more information is required [11, 28]. The term *split function studies* came about from older tests. In the past bronchospirometry and unilateral balloon occlusion of a pulmonary artery were performed to try to predict how the patient might function with one lung [3]. Lung scans are much less invasive and provide information about split function. Other more "global" studies are also considered in this category. These include quantitative nuclear scanning [11, 20, 29–31], pulmonary artery catheterization [14], and cardiopulmonary exercise testing [14, 31]. One of the critical considerations is the amount of pulmonary vascular bed to be resected. When an animal is sacrificed by progressive lung resection it will die because of loss of pulmonary vascular bed and limited cardiac output. Evaluation of ventilatory parameters as a predictor of postoperative morbidity and mortality is an oversimplification of the complex stresses placed on an individual with surgery. The cardiopulmonary system functions as a unit, and it is somewhat artificial to give "cardiac" or "pulmonary clearance" for surgery. The result of this last tier of studies helps indicate operability and guide the final recommendations on risk presented to the patient.

Summary

This chapter has been an attempt to describe pulmonary-related perioperative risks and complications, the types of patients who are at risk for these complications, how to go about identifying the patient at risk, and how to evaluate these patients. Essentially two groups of patients are at risk: those who are candidates for thoracic surgical procedures and those with pulmonary disease being considered for major surgical procedures of any type. Practical approaches have been detailed for patient identification, evaluation, preoperative preparation, and postoperative management.

References

1. Zibrak JD, O'Donnell CR, Marton K: Indications for pulmonary function testing. *Ann Intern Med* 112:763, 1990
2. Weiner-Kronish JP, Matthay MA: Preoperative evaluation. *In* Murray JF, Nadel JA (eds): Textbook of Respiratory Medicine. Philadelphia, WB Saunders, 1988, pp 683–698
3. Tisi GM: Preoperative identification and evaluation of the patient with lung disease. *Med Clin North Am* 71:399, 1987
4. Stein M: Preoperative evaluation. *In* Wilson AF (ed): Pulmonary Function Testing: Indications and Interpretations. New York, Grune & Stratton, 1985, pp 311–329
5. Falk JL, Rackow EC, Weil MH: Impaired oxygen utilization during anesthesia and surgery. *J Crit Care* 1:150, 1986
6. Jackson CV: Preoperative pulmonary evaluation. *Arch Intern Med* 148:2120, 1988
7. Morton HJV, Camb DA: Tobacco smoking and pulmonary complications after operation. *Lancet* 1:368, 1944
8. Latimer G, Dickman M, Clinton D, et al: Ventilatory patterns and pulmonary complications after upper abdominal surgery determined by preoperative and postoperative computerized spirometry and blood gas analysis. *Am J Surg* 122:622, 1971
9. Goldman L, Caldera DL, Southwick F, et al: Cardiac risk factors and complications in non-cardiac surgery. *Medicine* 57:357, 1978
10. Jewell ER, Persson AV: Preoperative evaluation of the high risk patient. *Surg Clin North Am* 65:3, 1985
11. Gass GD, Olsen GN: Preoperative pulmonary function testing to predict postoperative morbidity and mortality. *Chest* 89:127, 1986
11a. Green NM: Physiology of Spinal Anesthesia, 3rd ed. Baltimore: Williams & Wilkins, 1981, pp 163–165
12. Lawrence VA, Page CP, Harris GD: Preoperative spirometry before abdominal operation. *Arch Intern Med* 149:280, 1989
13. Smith TP, Kinasewitz GT, Tucker WY, et al: Exercise capacity as a predictor of post-thoracotomy morbidity. *Am Rev Respir Dis* 129:730, 1984
14. Fee HJ, Holmes EC, Gewirtz HS, et al: Role of pulmonary vascular resistance measurements in preoperative evaluation of candidates for pulmonary resection. *J Thorac Cardiovasc Surg* 60:519, 1978
15. Celli BR, Rodriguez KS, Snider GL, et al: A controlled trial of intermittent positive pressure breathing, incentive spirometry, and deep breathing exercises in preventing pulmonary complications after abdominal surgery. *Am Rev Respir Dis* 130:12, 1984
16. Ricksten SE, Bengtsson A, Soderberg C, et al: Effects of periodic positive airway pressure by mask on postoperative pulmonary function. *Chest* 92:774, 1986
17. Gale GD, Sanders DE: Incentive spirometry, its value after cardiovascular surgery. *Can Anaesth Soc J* 27:475, 1980

18. Luce JM: Preoperative evaluation and perioperative management of patients with pulmonary disease. *Postgrad Med* 67:201, 1980
19. Lindner KH, Lotz P, Ahnefeld FW: Continuous positive airway pressure effect on residual capacity, vital capacity, and its subdivisions. *Chest* 92:66, 1987
20. Markos J, Mullan BP, Hillman DR, et al: Preoperative assessment as a predictor of mortality and morbidity after lung resection. *Am Rev Respir Dis* 139:902, 1989
21. Gersen MC, Hurst JM, Hertzberg VS, et al: Prediction of pulmonary complications related to elective abdominal and non-cardiac thoracic surgery in geriatric patients. *Am J Med* 88:101, 1990
22. Van De Water JM: Preoperative and postoperative technique in the prevention of pulmonary complications. *Surg Clin North Am* 60: 1339, 1980
23. Warner MA, Offord KP, Warner ME, et al: Role of preoperative cessation of smoking and other factors in postoperative pulmonary complications. *Mayo Clin Proc* 64:609, 1989
24. Archie JP, Feldtman RW: Intraoperative pulmonary and arterial monitoring devices in high risk surgical patients. *Surg Gynecol Obstet* 153:831, 1981
25. Torrington KG, Henderson CJ: Perioperative respiratory therapy. *Chest* 93:946, 1988
26. Hertzler N: Complications: Pulmonary, cardiovascular. *Audio Digest* 32:9, 1985
27. Miller JI, Grossman GD, Hatcher CR: Pulmonary function test criteria for operability and pulmonary resection. *Surg Gynecol Obstet* 153: 893, 1981
28. Olsen GN, Block AJ, Swenson EW, et al: Pulmonary function evaluation of the lung resection candidate: A prospective study. *Am Rev Respir Dis* 111:379, 1975
29. Ali MK, Mountain C, Miller JM, et al: Regional pulmonary function before and after pneumonectomy using 133 xenon. *Chest* 68: 288, 1975
30. Boysen PG, Harris JO, Block AJ, et al: Prospective evaluation for pneumonectomy using perfusion scanning. *Chest* 80:2, 1981
31. Olsen GN, Weiman DS, Bolton JWR, et al: Submaximal invasive exercise testing and quantitative lung scanning in the evaluation for tolerance of lung resection. *Chest* 95:267, 1989
32. Vodinh J, Bonnet F, Touboul C, et al: Risk factors of postoperative pulmonary complications after vascular surgery. *Surgery* 105:360, 1989
33. Sirinek KR, Burk RR, Brown M, et al: Improving survival in patients with cirrhosis undergoing major abdominal operations. *Arch Surg* 122:271, 1987
34. Zimmerman JE, Knaus WA: Outcome prediction in adult intensive care. *In* Shoemaker WC, Ayres A, et al (eds): Textbook of Critical Care. Philadelphia, WB Saunders, 1989, p 1447
35. Friedman LS, Maddrey WC: Surgery in the patient with liver disease. *Med Clin North Am* 71:453, 1987
36. Eisenbacher WL, Manniva A: An algorithm for the interpretation of cardiopulmonary exercise test. *Chest* 97:263, 1990

Basic Chest Radiograph Interpretation

David S. Yates and Mark Lukens

The recent introduction of sophisticated imaging techniques, including diagnostic ultrasound, computed tomography (CT) and magnetic resonance imaging, have caught the imagination of physician and public alike. Although these modalities are of great use in selected instances, the plain chest radiograph is the least expensive and most informative initial diagnostic imaging technique for the primary care practitioner. In a busy office practice, knowledge of basic chest roentgenographic interpretation saves time and improves patient care. The following is basic information and in no way substitutes for the trained eye of the radiologist to ultimately review chest radiographs done in the office.

Fundamentals

The ideal evaluation of chest radiographs begins with proper technique. The basic chest study should consist of posteroanterior (PA) and lateral projections. The lateral view can be extremely helpful in patients with thoracic disease. Routine office roentgenography performed by the primary care practitioner should include both the PA and lateral views. The films should be performed with high voltage technique (high kilovolts) to allow adequate penetration and visualization of mediastinal and retrocardiac structures. A well-penetrated film results in clear delineation of the dorsal spine through the cardiac silhouette (Figs. 26-1A and B). Overpenetrated films may occasionally be necessary to better assess some pathology. An underpenetrated chest film results in poor visualization of structures and a nondiagnostic film (Figs. 26-1C).

There are many additional views that may be helpful in certain cases. Apical lordotic views are commonly obtained when there is suspicion of a lesion or mass in the lung apex. Oblique views can be used to better evaluate small questionable pulmonary densities. Evaluation of pleural effusions frequently consists of lateral decubitus views. Inspiration and expiration films can be helpful to detect small pneumothoraces. These techniques can easily be performed with the basic chest radiographic equipment.

Interpretation of the chest film requires a systematic approach that should be followed with each case. The interpreter must establish his or her own method to evaluate the heart and vascular structures, mediastinum, lung fields, bony thorax, and soft tissues. It is important to follow the same systematic approach on every film and inspect all parts of the film. Often, if obvious pathology is visible, there is a tendency to deviate from the interpreter's normal method of evaluation. Therefore, it is helpful to ignore the obvious pathology initially and return to it following evaluation of the remainder of the chest.

Normal Anatomy

Adequate roentgenographic interpretation requires understanding of the normal anatomic structures of the lungs and mediastinum. Lobar anatomy is important to localize lesions (Fig. 26-2). The right lung consists of three lobes: (1) upper, with apical, anterior, and posterior segments, (2) middle, with medial and lateral segments, and (3) lower, with superior, anterior basal, posterior basal, medial basal, and lateral basal segments. The left lung consists of two lobes: (1) upper, with apical/posterior, anterior, superior lingular, and

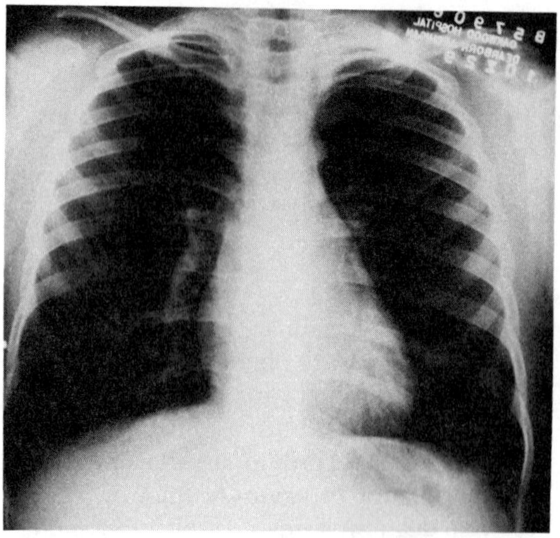

A

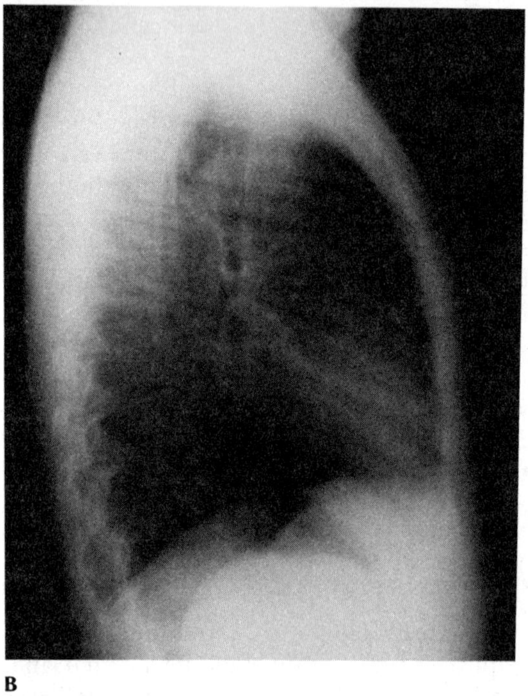

B

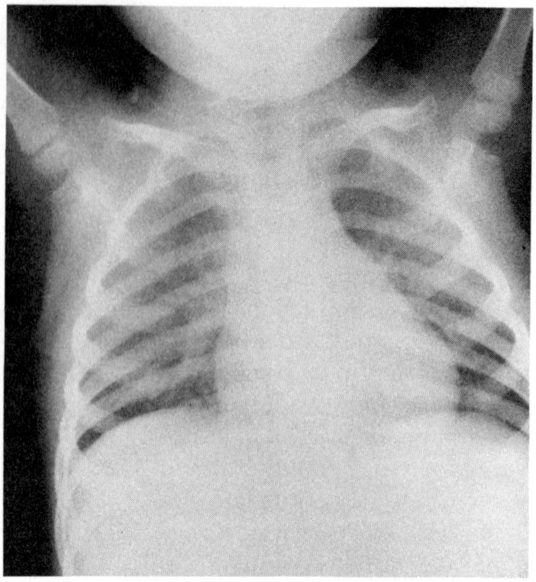

C

Fig. 26-1. (A) Normal PA chest radiograph (optimal high kilovolt technique). (B) Normal lateral chest (optimal high kilovolt technique). (C) Underpenetrated PA chest. Lung markings are accentuated and mediastinal and retrocardiac structures are obscured.

inferior lingular segments, and (2) lower, with superior, anteromedial basal, posterior basal, and lateral basal segments.

Radiographically, the pulmonary hilar shadows are formed by the pulmonary arteries and the left is normally slightly higher than the right. Upper lobe pulmonary veins also contribute to the hilar density.

The mediastinum can be divided in several ways. From a radiologic point of view, the simplest method is to designate anterior, middle, and posterior compartments based on the lateral film (Fig. 26-3). The anterior mediastinum extends from the anterior chest wall to an imaginary line extending along the anterior margin of the trachea and continuing along the posterior cardiac border. The middle mediastinum extends from here to an imaginary line drawn 1 cm posterior to the anterior margins of the dorsal vertebrae. The posterior mediastinum then continues posteriorly [1].

Cardiac size should be evaluated on an upright PA film in full inspiration. Supine anteroposterior and expiratory films magnify the cardiac size. The most widely accepted standard is that the transverse diameter of the heart should not exceed 50% of the greatest internal diameter of the chest. There is, however, wide variation and considerable

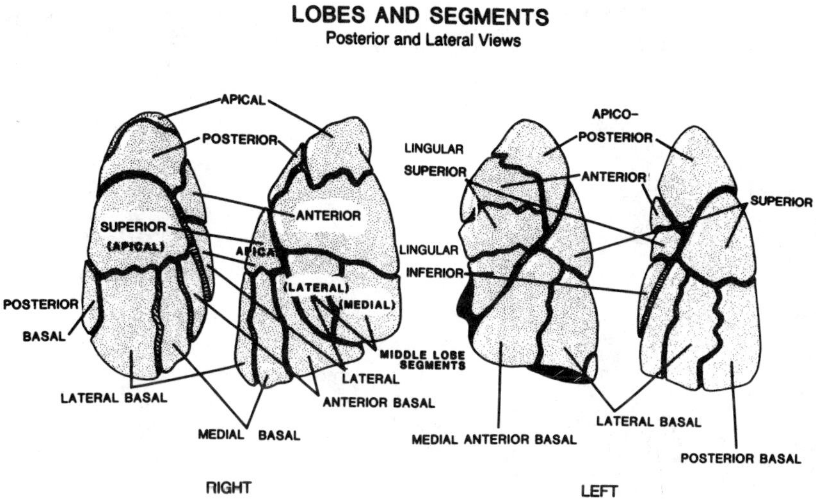
LOBES AND SEGMENTS
Posterior and Lateral Views
APICAL
POSTERIOR
SUPERIOR
(APICAL)
ANTERIOR
LINGULAR
SUPERIOR
APICO-
POSTERIOR
ANTERIOR
SUPERIOR
LINGULAR
INFERIOR
(LATERAL)
(MEDIAL)
POSTERIOR
BASAL
MIDDLE LOBE
SEGMENTS
LATERAL
LATERAL BASAL
ANTERIOR BASAL
MEDIAL BASAL
MEDIAL ANTERIOR BASAL
LATERAL BASAL
POSTERIOR BASAL
RIGHT
LEFT

Lobes and segments: posterior view. Adapted from drawings, courtesy of Henry Ford Hospital.

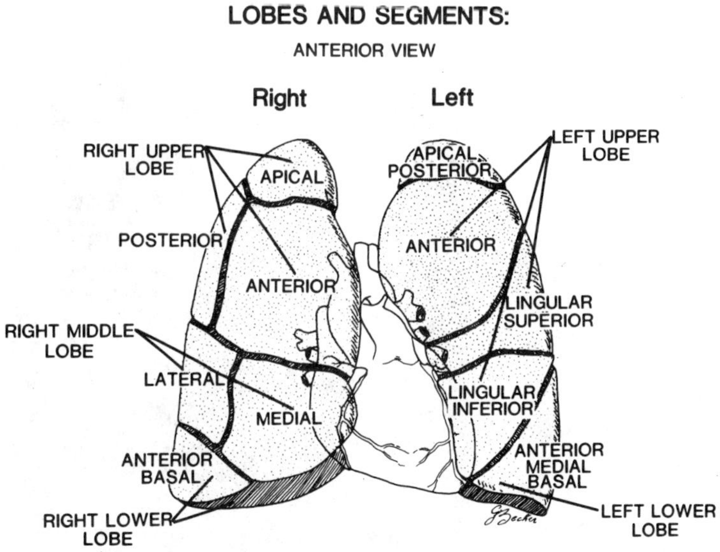
LOBES AND SEGMENTS:
ANTERIOR VIEW
Right
Left
RIGHT UPPER
LOBE
APICAL
POSTERIOR
ANTERIOR
RIGHT MIDDLE
LOBE
LATERAL
MEDIAL
ANTERIOR
BASAL
RIGHT LOWER
LOBE
APICAL
POSTERIOR
LEFT UPPER
LOBE
ANTERIOR
LINGULAR
SUPERIOR
LINGULAR
INFERIOR
ANTERIOR
MEDIAL
BASAL
LEFT LOWER
LOBE

Lobes and segments: anterior view. Adapted from drawings, courtesy of Henry Ford Hospital.

Fig. 26-2. Pulmonary segmental anatomy. (Reprinted from Atlas of Critical Care Chest Roentgenography by L.D. Victor, pp. 3–4, with permission of Aspen Publishers, Inc., © 1985.)

subjectivity. A significant percentage of normal patients have hearts greater than 50%, and many patients with hearts less than 50% may have cardiomegaly when compared with that patient's normal state [2]. Heart failure may be present without cardiomegaly in patients with significant obstructive airways disease associated with hyperinflated lungs, which tend to make the heart appear more vertical (Fig. 26-31A on page 515).

Infection

One of the most common indications for chest radiography is to rule out pneumonia. Acute pneumonia has a variety of patterns

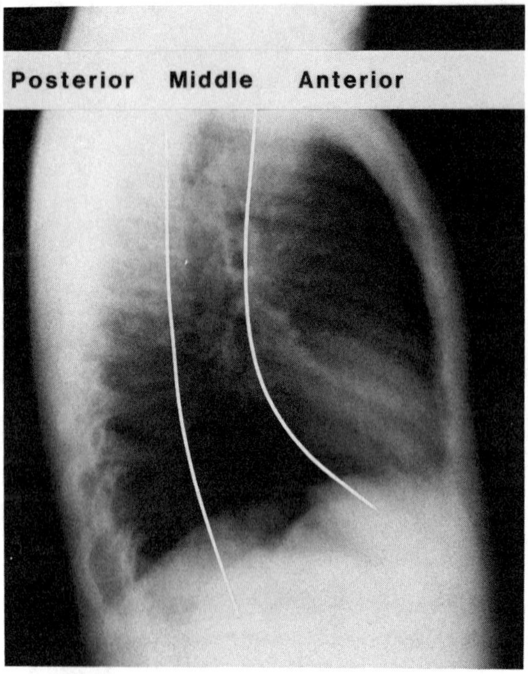
Posterior
Middle
Anterior

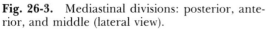

Fig. 26-3. Mediastinal divisions: posterior, anterior, and middle (lateral view).

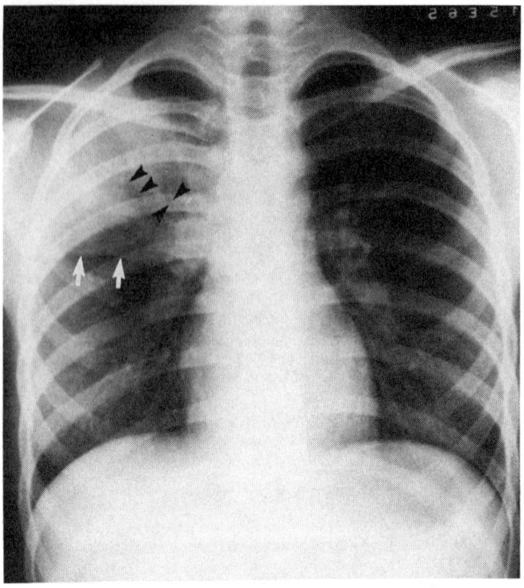

A

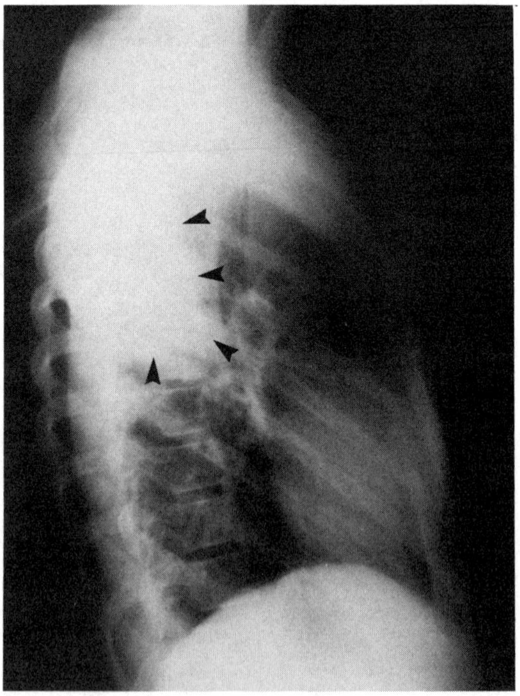

B

Fig. 26-4. Right upper lobe pneumococcal pneumonia. (A) PA view. Notice air bronchograms (black arrows). (See text.) The infiltrate is delineated inferiorly by the right minor fissue (white arrows). (B) Lateral view. Infiltrate is seen to involve the posterior segment of the right upper lobe (black arrows).

on the chest film, depending on the type of organism, mechanism of infection, and patient age, condition, and immune status. Most pulmonary infiltrates appear as an alveolar, bronchial, interstitial, or mixed pattern.

Alveolar pneumonia is an airspace consolidative process, resulting in "fluffy" homogeneous infiltrates in a peripheral nonsegmental distribution. The infiltrates tend to spread centrally. Pneumococcal pneumonia is the classic offending organism (Fig. 26-4).

Bronchopneumonia is the result of an inflammatory process beginning in the bronchi and extending into the peribronchial tissues. These infiltrates may be impossible to distinguish radiographically from an alveolar process. The typical organism is *Staphylococcus* (Fig. 26-5). An alveolar process caused by *Staphylococcus* is shown in Fig. 26-6.

Interstitial pneumonias are typically caused by viral infections, resulting in a fairly nonspecific pattern. Generally, the infiltrates are more diffuse and less confluent than the other types (Fig. 26-7).

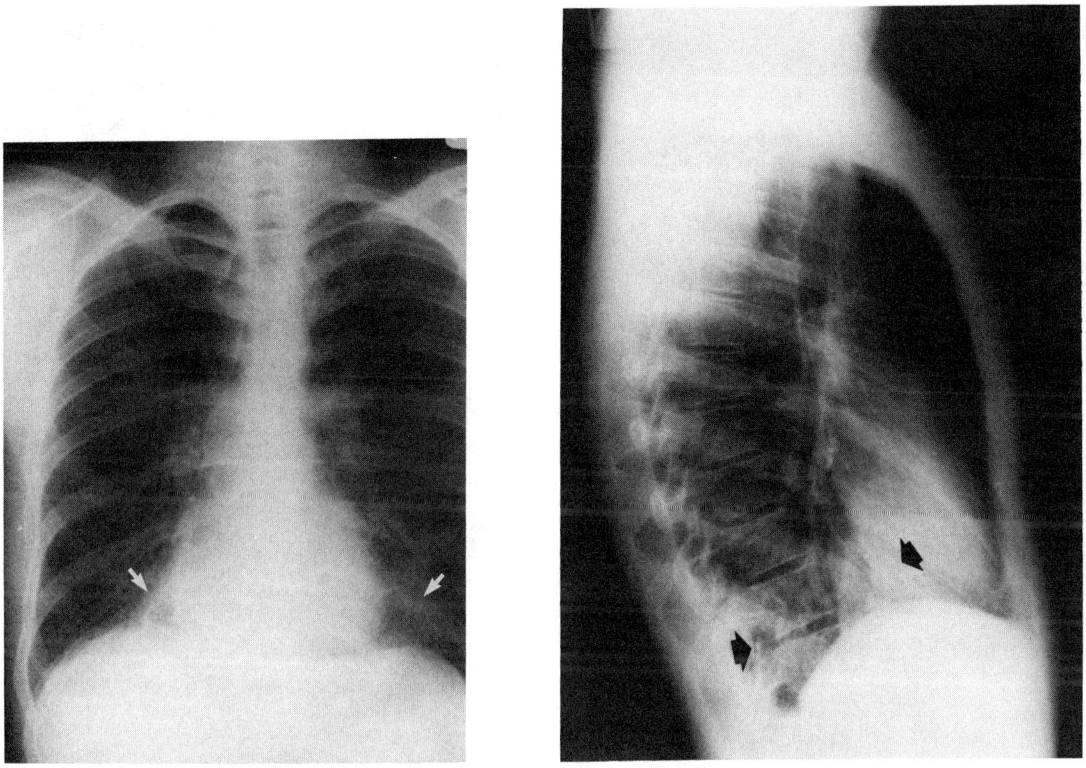
A
B

Fig. 26-5. Bronchopneumonia. (A) PA view. Bilateral basilar infiltrates (white arrows). (B) Lateral view. Poorly defined basilar infiltrates (black arrows) that superimpose on the dorsal spine, causing the vertebral bodies to appear whiter. Normally the spine becomes darker inferiorly on the lateral film.

Air bronchograms result from pulmonary infiltrates that involve the alveoli and peribronchial tissues, leading to clear visualization of the air-filled bronchi (Fig. 26-4) [1]. Another important sign when localizing pulmonary infiltrates or masses is the silhouette sign. This refers to a phenomenon where if two tissues of similar density and makeup are contiguous, the interface between them will be obliterated [3]. This sign is invaluable in locating pulmonary pathology, e.g., a right middle lobe process will obliterate or silhouette the right heart border, while a right lower lobe process will silhouette the diaphragm. Pathology can frequently be localized on a single view based on this diagnostic sign (Figs. 26-6, 26-8, and 26-9).

The presentation of lung infections also varies with the patient's condition. For example, the immunocompromised patient may present with unusual mixed patterns, without any specific appearance. Aspiration pneumonia typically involves the lower lobes, especially right, in the upright patient (Fig. 26-10). In the supine patient, aspiration may result in upper lobe with infiltrates in the apical posterior segment.

Lung abscess may result from a hematogenous infection; however, more commonly it is bronchogenic in origin or a result of aspiration. The abscess will appear as a spherical soft tissue mass with or without central lucency. An air–fluid level may be seen if there is a bronchial communication or if it is caused by a gas-forming organism (Fig. 26-11). The most important differential diagnostic con-

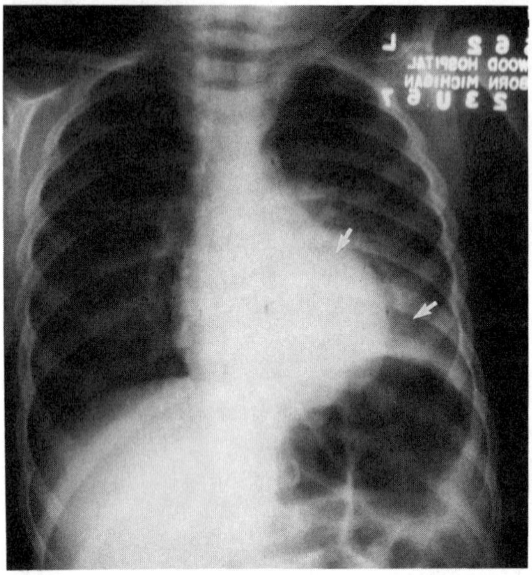

A

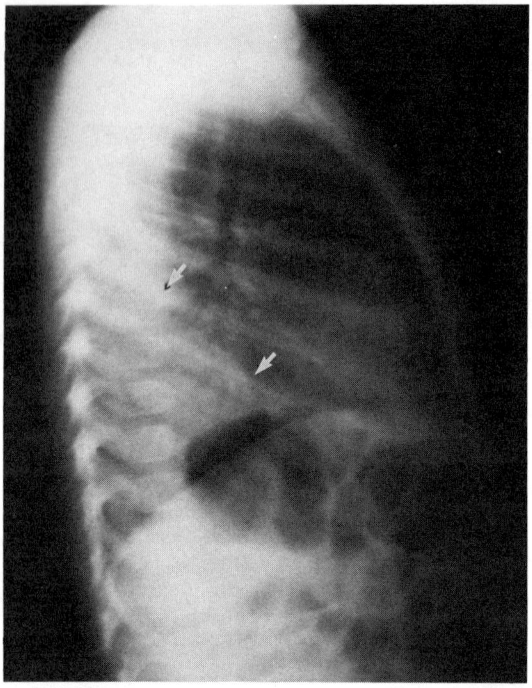

B

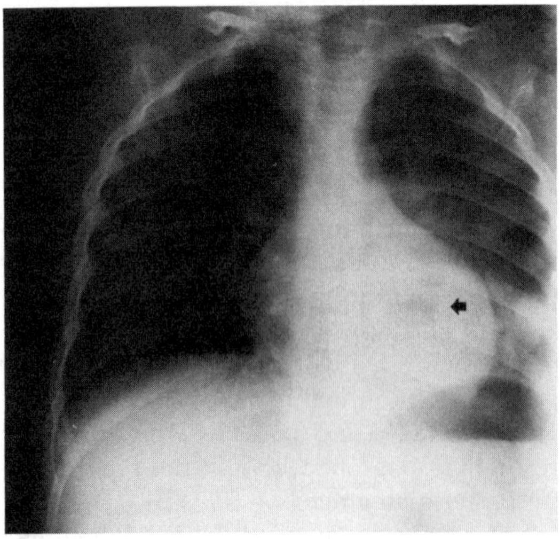

C

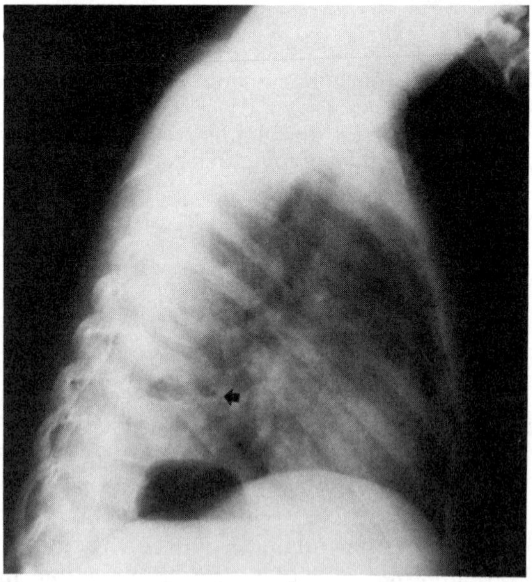

D

Fig. 26-6. Staphylococcal pneumonia. (A) PA views. Left lower lobe infiltrate (white arrows) that largely obscures the left hemidiaphragm (silhouette sign) but preserves the left heart border. (B) Lateral view. Left lower lobe infiltrate seen posteriorly (white arrows). Note multiple air bronchograms anterior, inferior and posterior to arrows. (C and D) Follow-up films 2 weeks later show development of pneumatoceles, small air collections within the consolidation (arrows). This is a fairly common complication in children with staphylococcal pneumonia.

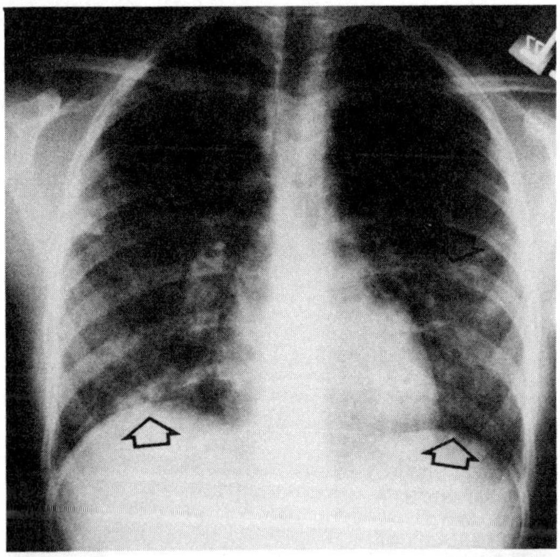

A

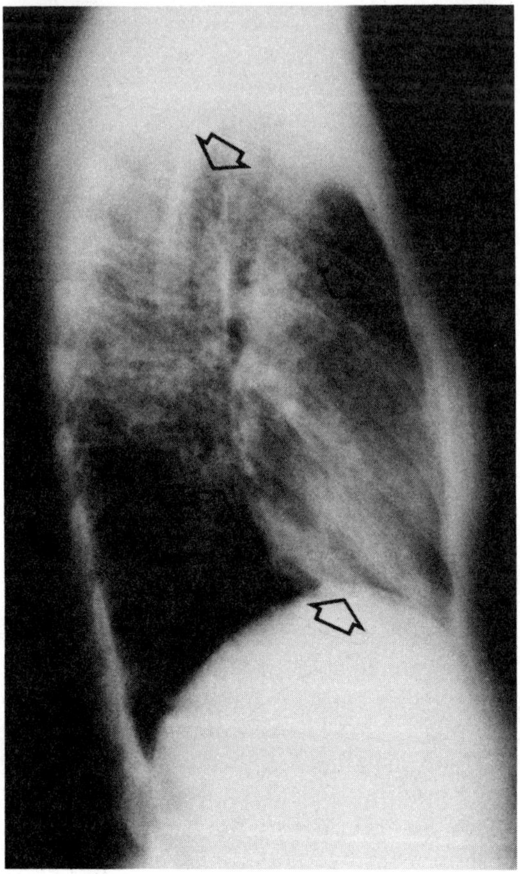

B

Fig. 26-7. Viral pneumonia. (A and B) Diffuse pattern of infiltrates with some reticular or linear densities as well as some areas of ill-defined nodularity. Open arrows outline infiltrates.

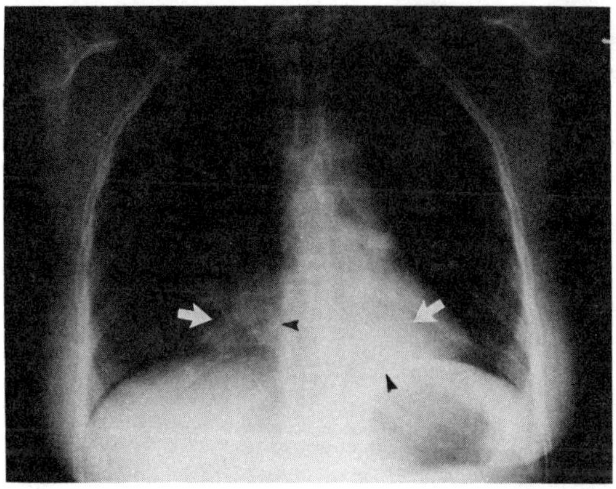

A

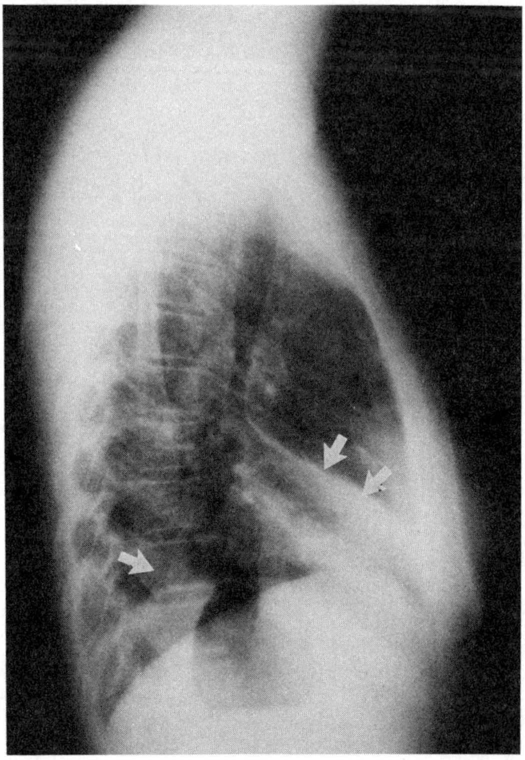

B

Fig. 26-8. Bilateral pneumonia. (A and B) Right middle and left lower lobe infiltrates (white arrows). The right heart border and medial portion of left hemidiaphragm are obscured by the adjacent infiltrates-silhouette sign on the PA view (small black arrows).

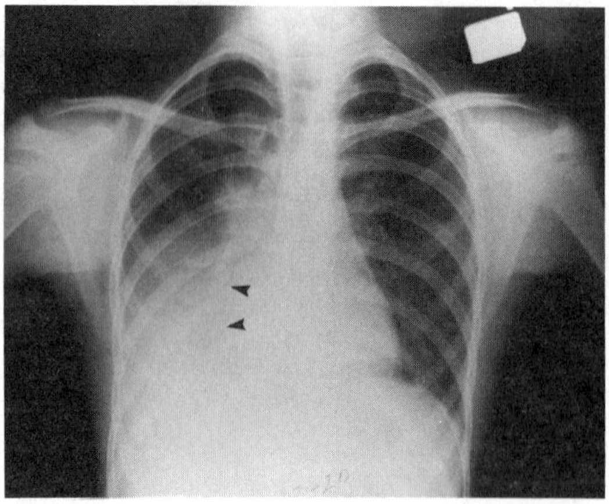

A

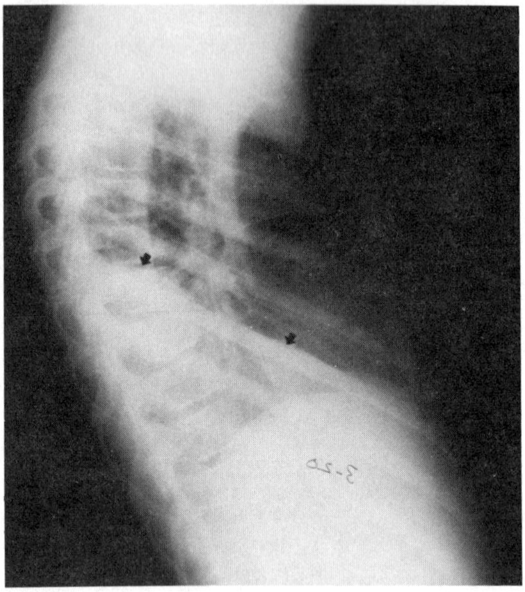

B

Fig. 26-9. Right lower lobe pneumonia. (A) PA view. Right diaphragm is obscured (silhouette sign) but the right heart border can be seen (small arrows), suggesting that the right middle lobe has been spared. (B) Lateral view. Right lower lobe infiltrate delineated anteriorly by the major fissure (arrows).

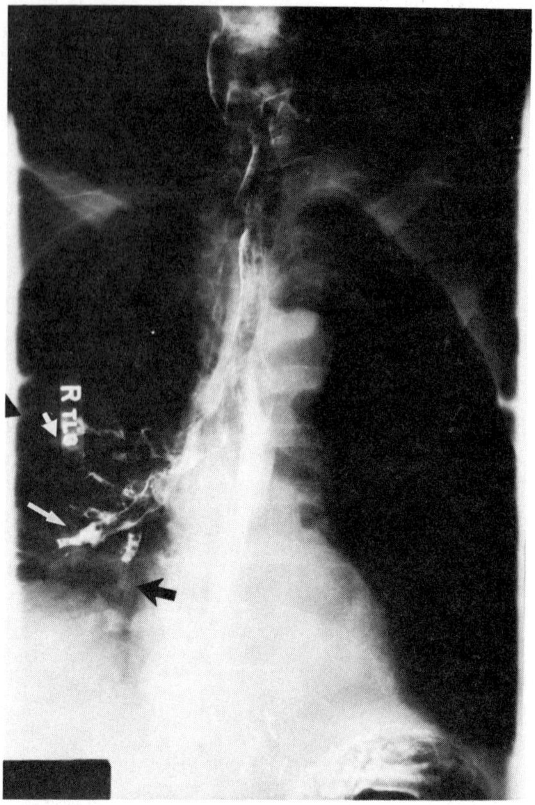

Fig. 26-10. Aspiration pneumonia. This patient aspirated barium during an esophagram, resulting in coating of bronchi in the right middle and lower lobes (white arrows). This corresponds to areas of pulmonary infiltrate (black arrows).

sideration is neoplasm with central necrosis (Fig. 26-12).

Pleural Effusions

Pleural effusions are another common source of abnormality detectable on chest radiography. Large amounts of pleural fluid are not difficult to identify, although it may be difficult to differentiate from other pathology. Small amount of fluid can be a greater diagnostic problem. Less than 100 mL of fluid may be detectable on good quality radiographs. The earliest change seen with small amounts of fluid is blunting of a posterior costophrenic angle on the lateral film. Much larger amounts of pleural fluid are required, at least 300 mL, before the lateral costophrenic angles become obscured (Fig. 26-13). Lateral decubitus views are helpful to confirm small pleural effusions, as well as to evaluate for free versus loculated fluid. Free fluid will layer along the dependent portion of the chest wall [4]. When evaluating right pleural effusions, a right side down or right lateral

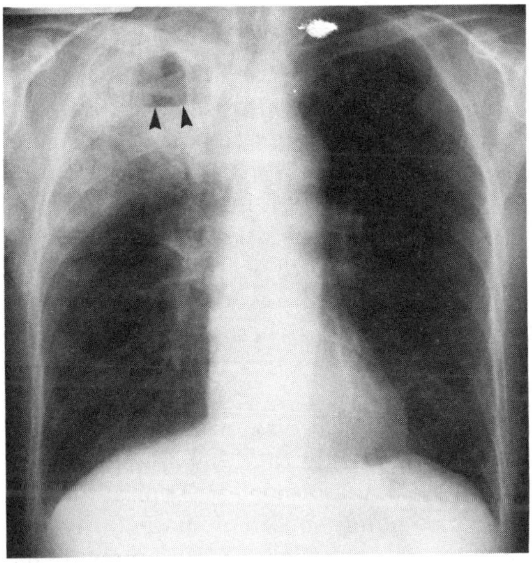

Fig. 26-11. Abscess right upper lobe infiltrate containing an air collection with air–fluid levels (arrows), indicating abscess formation.

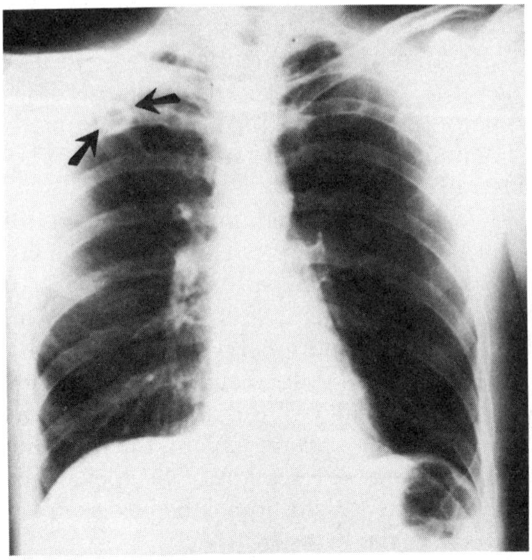

Fig. 26-12. Right upper lobe abscess. Thick-walled cavitary lesion that would be very difficult to differentiate from cavitary neoplasm.

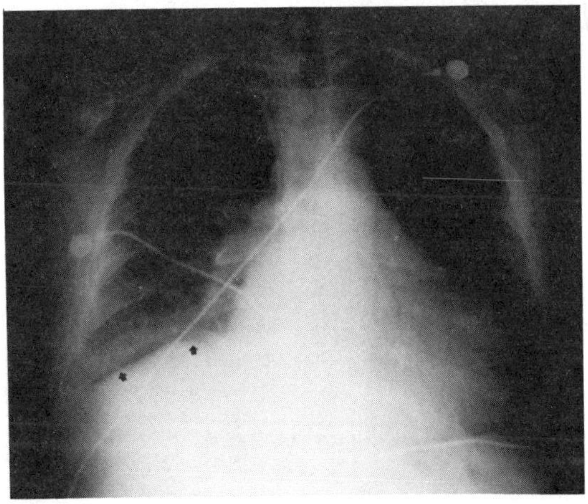

A

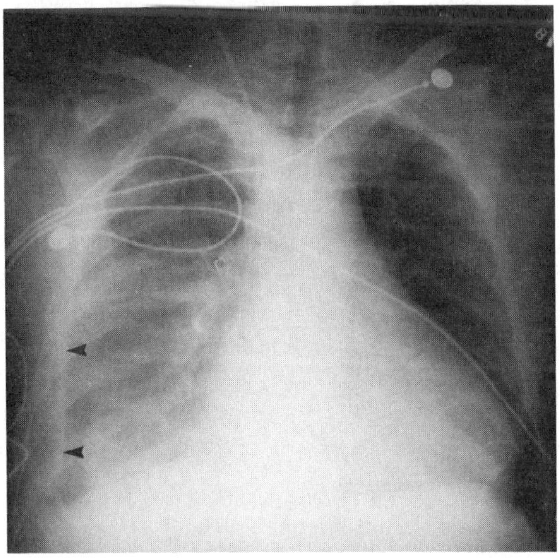

B

Fig. 26-13. Right pleural effusion. (A) In the upright patient the fluid collects at the base or in a subpulmonic location (arrows). Note loss of right costophrenic angle. (B) In the supine patient the fluid layers posteriorly, resulting in diffuse haziness and fluid tracking along the lateral aspect of the lung (arrowheads).

decubitus film is obtained (Fig. 26-14), and vice versa for left side effusions.

Detection of pleural effusions in the supine patient can be more difficult. The fluid in this case layers posteriorly, and it may take at least 500 mL before the fluid is detected. The typical appearance is a hazy density overlying the lung field, which may or may not obscure the costophrenic angles or diaphragm (Fig. 26-13). The fluid may be seen on a cross-table lateral film.

Large amounts of pleural fluid result in mass effect, with shift of the mediastinal structures to the opposite side. This helps to distinguish opacified lung fields due to pleu-

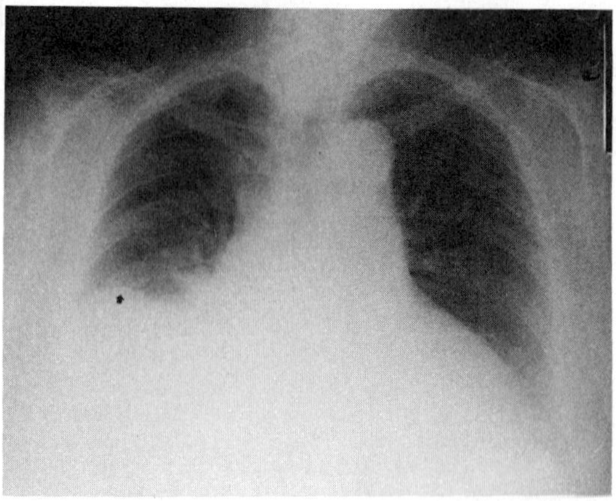

A

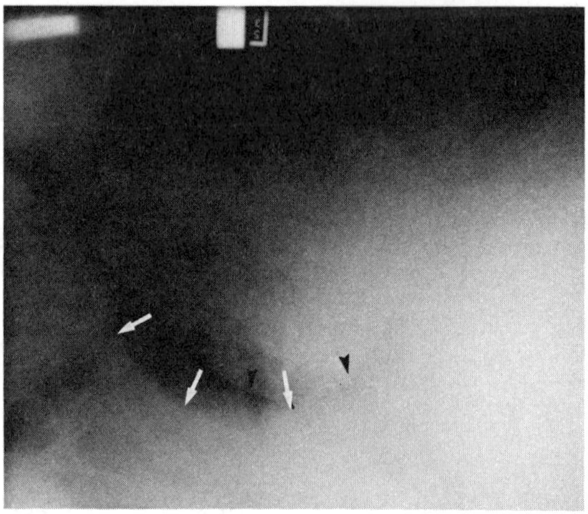

B

Fig. 26-14. Subpulmonic pleural effusion. (A) PA view. Fluid is in a subpulmonic location, resulting in apparent elevation of the right hemidiaphragm and lateral displacement of the apparent diaphragmatic dome (arrow). (B) A right lateral decubitus film (patient right side down) shows the fluid layering between the lung and rib cage (white arrows). Breast shadow outlined by black arrows. Loculated fluid may not layer with changes in positioning. (See text.)

ral fluid from opacification due to pneumonia or atelectasis.

Subpulmonic effusions are another problem encountered occasionally. In this case, the fluid remains inferior to the lung, without causing blunting of the costophrenic angles. This may be suspected when there is apparent elevation of a hemidiaphragm, shift of the dome of the diaphragm laterally, or increased distance between the apparent diaphragm and adjacent abdominal structures. Confirmation frequently requires performing decubitus views to demonstrate the fluid gravitating (Fig. 26-14) [5, 6]. Loculated fluid may not gravitate laterally on decubitus films because of obstruction to flow from inflammatory adhesions, tumor, etc. If intrathoracic fluid is suspected, but not demonstrated to be mobile by decubitus chest radiography, then ultrasonography or CT scanning may be necessary.

Pleural fluid may also present as loculated fluid within a fissure resulting in a "mass like" density or pseudotumor [7]. Typically, pseudotumors change in size or shape fairly rapidly and may change with variations in patient position (Fig. 26-15).

Pneumothorax

Chest radiographs are often obtained on patients presenting with chest pain or shortness of breath to rule out pneumothorax. Air may enter the pleural space spontaneously, as a result of trauma, or in the presence of underlying pulmonary disease such as cancer or eosinophilic granuloma.

Detection of a pneumothorax consists of identifying the thin line representing the visceral pleura with hyperlucency and lack of lung markings peripherally (Figs. 26-16 and 26-17). A small, marginal pneumothorax may be very subtle, and the diagnosis can be aided with an expiratory film that accentuates the findings. In the upright patient, the pneumothorax space is best seen over the apex, while in the supine patient, it may be best seen laterally or at the base.

A common diagnostic problem is the presence of a skin fold that can simulate a pneumothorax. Skin folds often do not parallel the rib cage as might be expected with the visceral pleural line of a pneumothorax. Other features of a skin fold not associated with a pneumothorax include extension beyond the rib cage and the visibility of lung markings peripheral to the line (Fig. 26-18).

The small pneumothorax may require no

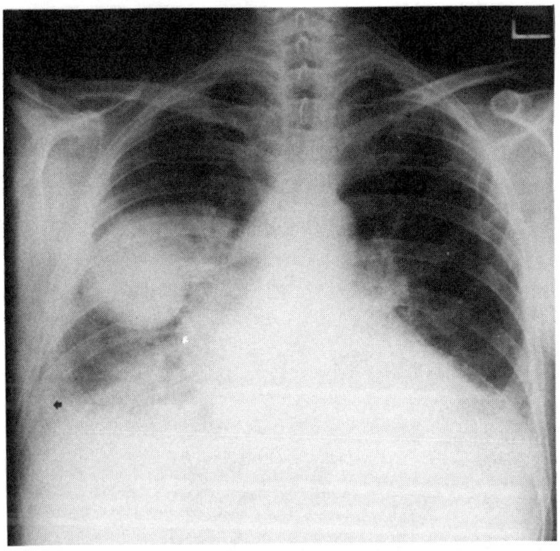

A

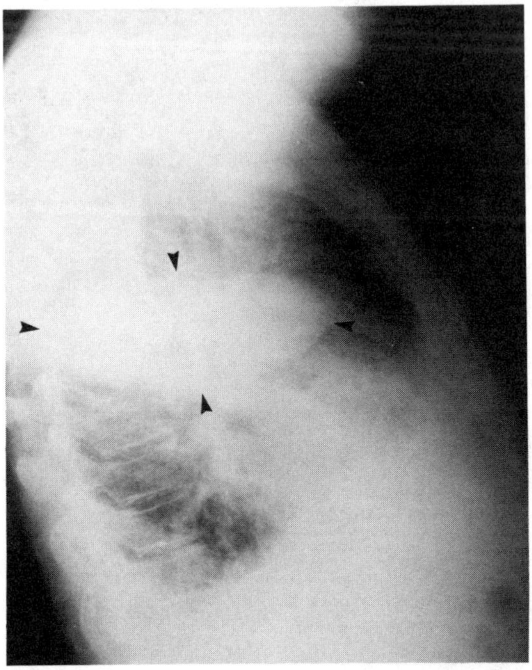

B

Fig. 26-15. Pseudotumor. (A) PA view. Mass-like opacity in the right midlung. Note blunting of right lateral costophrenic angle (arrow). (B) Lateral view. Large opacity (arrows) that represents pleural fluid loculated within the right minor fissure.

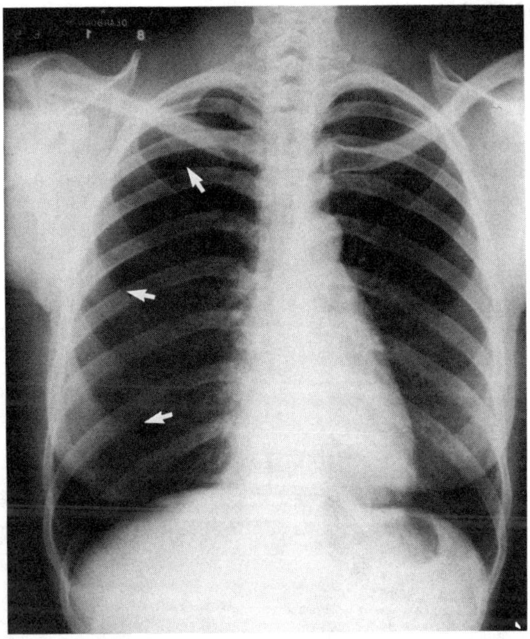

Fig. 26-16. Right pneumothorax. A faint line representing the visceral pleual surface can be visualized (arrows). Notice the lack of lung markings peripheral to this line.

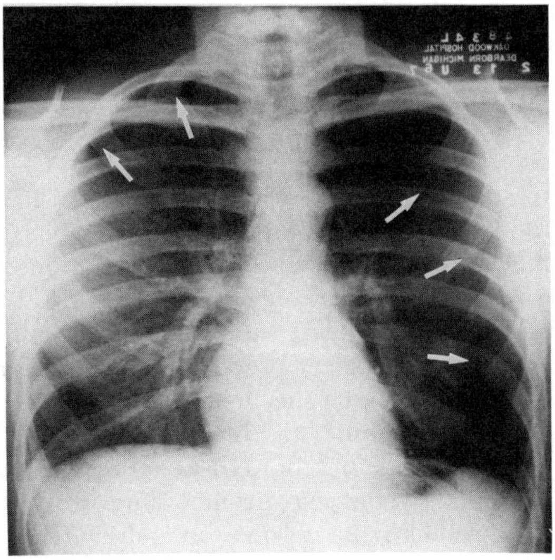

Fig. 26-17. Bilateral pneumothoraces, large on left and small on right (arrows).

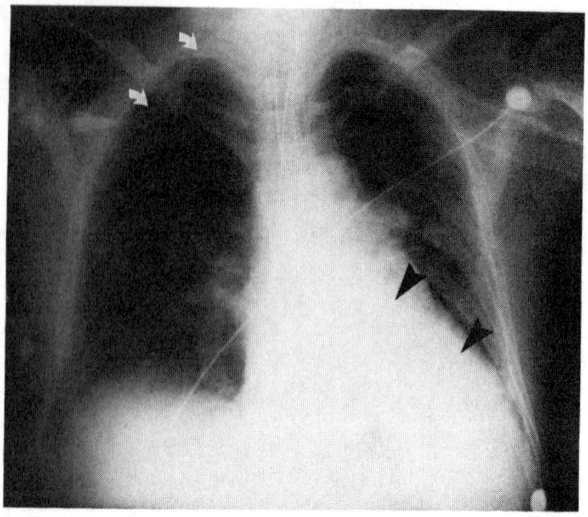
A

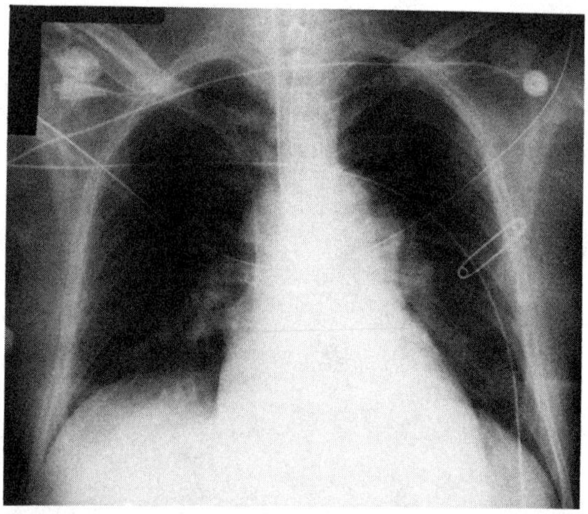
B

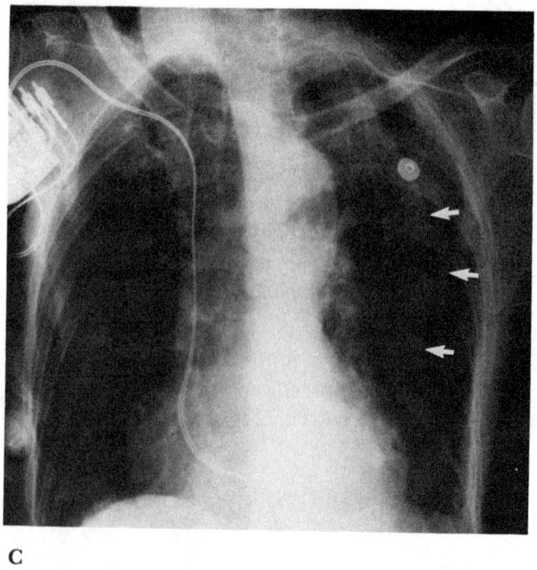
C

Fig. 26-18. Skin fold simulating pneumothorax. (A) Faint line overlies right upper lung; however, this is seen to extend superiorly past the rib cage (white arrows). Notice also atelectasis or consolidation of the left lower lobe (black arrows). (B) Short-term follow-up film fails to reproduce the line. (C) Another example of skin folds on the left (white arrows).

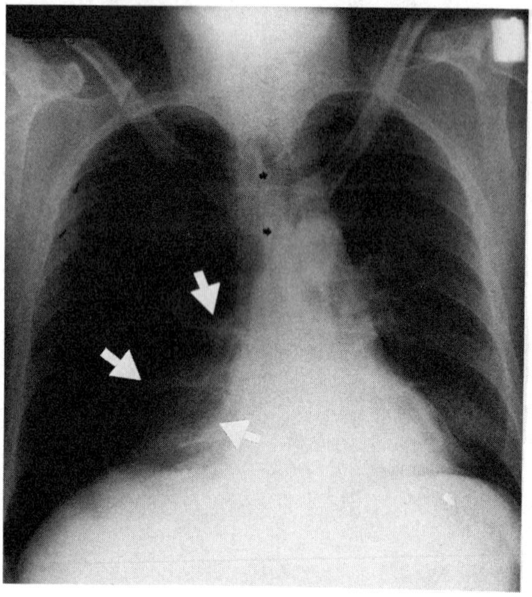

Fig. 26-19. Tension pneumothorax. Right pneumothorax with complete collapse of the lung (white arrows). Mediastinal shift is best seen here by displacement of the trachea to the left (broad black arrows). This pneumothorax was posttraumatic, caused by multiple rib fractures (thin black arrows).

treatment other than follow-up films, while the larger pneumothorax necessitates placement of a chest tube. Some people attempt to estimate the size of a pneumothorax by assigning percentages; however, this tends to vary widely between observers. Others prefer to simply describe the pneumothorax space as small, moderate, and large [8, 9].

Tension pneumothorax is a more serious condition, requiring prompt intervention. This results from a "one-way valve" effect, allowing air to enter but not escape from the pleural space. Air continues to accumulate under greater than atmospheric pressure.

When this occurs, there is mass effect and resulting mediastinal shift to the contralateral side, depression of the diaphragm, and widening of the rib interspaces (Fig. 26-19).

Atelectasis

Atelectasis results from diminished aeration of all or a portion of a lung. If a large portion is involved, i.e., an entire segment or lobe, roentgen signs of volume loss may be seen. The classic signs are elevation of the diaphragm, bowing or displacement of a fissure, mediastinal shift, or narrowed rib interspaces (Fig. 26-20). Lesser degrees of atelectasis (subsegmental) lead to small linear or plate-like densities, typically at the bases (Fig. 26-21).

Fig. 26-20. Total atelectasis of right lung. This overpenetrated film is not adequate for evaluating the left lung; however, it does demonstrate opacification of the right hemithorax and mediastinal shift to the right side. Notice occlusion of right mainstem bronchus (large arrow) and narrowing of left bronchus (small arrow) due to neoplasm.

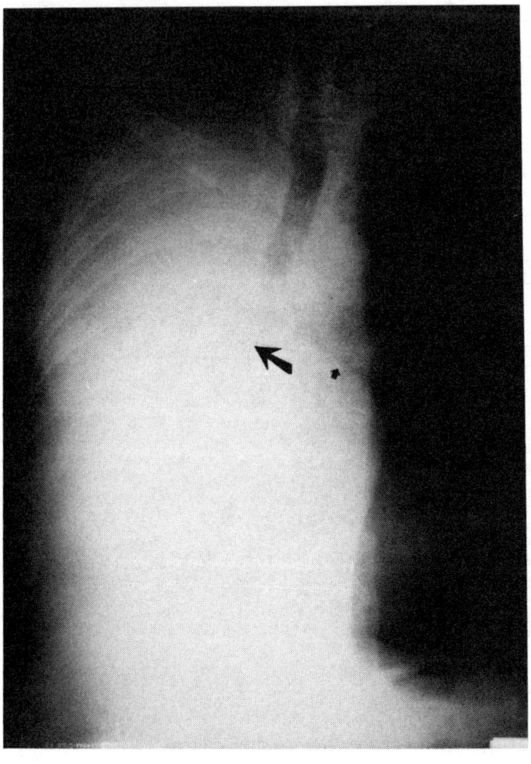

A common diagnostic problem in the presence of a basilar lung density is to differentiate atelectasis from pleural fluid or consolidated lung. Atelectasis leads to mediastinal shift to the ipsilateral side, while pleural effusion results in contralateral shift. Consolidated lung usually causes no shift.

There is an additional type of atelectasis that may simulate a mass lesion, so-called rounded atelectasis [10]. This usually presents as a poorly defined opacity adjacent to a pleural surface, generally lower lobe. Curvilinear density adjacent to the atelectatic lung has been likened to the appearance of a comet tail.

Neoplasia

Lung neoplasms may present as parenchymal mass lesions, nodules, or mediastinal or pleural masses. Parenchymal densities may initially appear to represent pneumonia; however, if the density fails to clear on follow-up films, neoplasm should be considered. Distinguishing benign and malignant densities can be very difficult and the most important diagnostic aid is prior chest roentgenograms. If there are old films, which show a nodule to be unchanged in a year or more, this is likely

Fig. 26-21. Plate-like atelectasis right lung base (small arrows). This patient also demonstrates free intraperitoneal air beneath the diaphragms (large arrows) due to recent abdominal surgery.

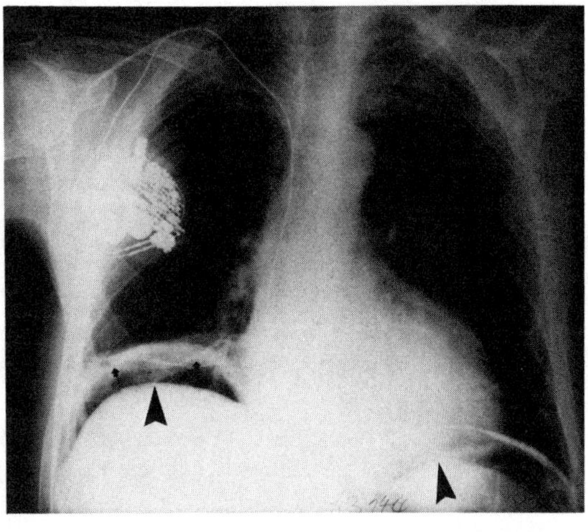

to be a benign lesion. Conversely, if there is appreciable change in size or shape of a lesion when compared with prior films, malignancy is suspected. Most benign lesions show no growth or very slow growth (slow doubling rate) on follow-up films. Rarely, a benign lesion grows very fast (fast doubling rate) [11].

The presence or absence of calcification is also helpful for diagnosis. A uniformly calcified lesion (Fig. 26-24) or one with a central nidus of calcification is likely benign, while a noncalcified lesion or calcification eccentrically located may be malignant or benign (Figs. 26-22, 26-23 and 26-25). CT scanning is extremely helpful to detect small amounts of calcification. Studies have shown that nodules with CT density measurements of greater than 160 to 200 Hounsfield units have a high likelihood of being benign [12].

Margins of the mass may be useful. Malignant lesions are more likely to have spiculated, ill-defined, or lobulated margins (Fig. 26-25). Benign lesions tend to have smooth, sharp margins (Fig. 26-22). Unfortunately, however, these signs are not always reliable. Cavitary nodules may be the result of abscesses or cavitation within malignant neoplasm (Fig. 26-26).

Frequently, the actual neoplasm itself is not

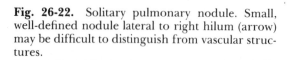

Fig. 26-22. Solitary pulmonary nodule. Small, well-defined nodule lateral to right hilum (arrow) may be difficult to distinguish from vascular structures.

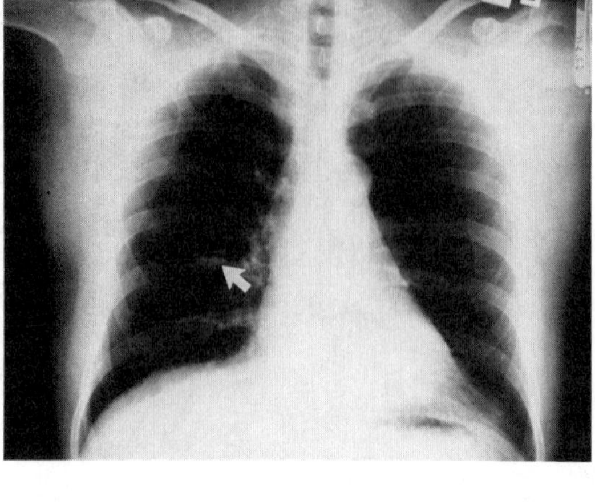

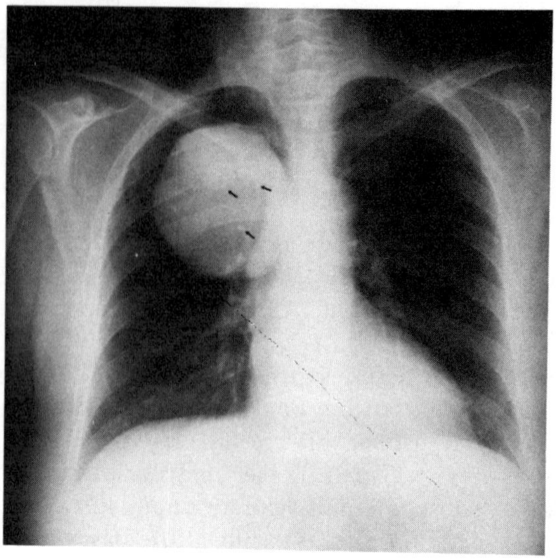

Fig. 26-23. Hamartoma. Large mass with smooth, sharply defined margins, giving a benign appearance except for its large size. Notice small flecks of calcification (arrows).

Fig. 26-24. Granuloma. Small well-defined nodule containing dense, central calcification (arrow).

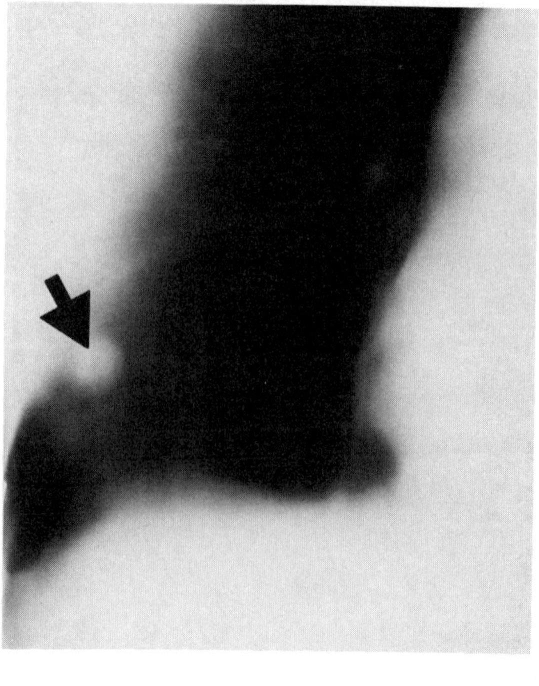

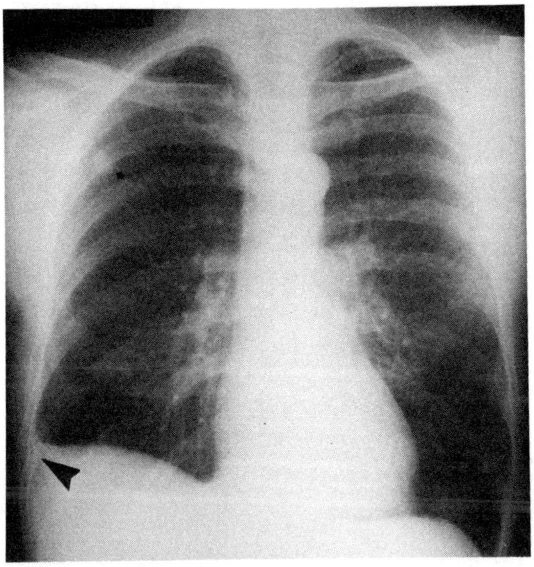

A

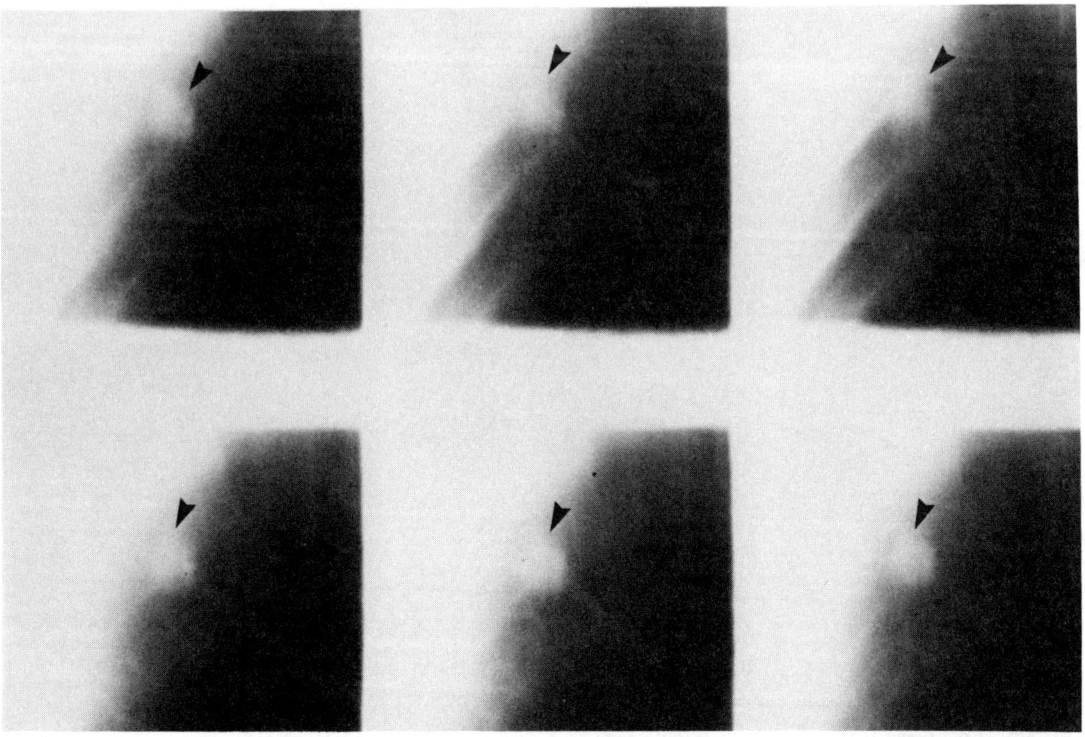

B

Fig. 26-25. Malignant nodule. (A) Small irregular nodule (small arrow) with no calcification. Notice small right pleural effusion (large arrow). (B) Plain film tomograms confirm irregular, spiculated margins and absence of calcification (arrows).

Fig. 26-26. Malignant cavitary neoplasm. (A) Thin-walled cavity with irregular, spiculated margins (white arrows). (B) Tomograms showing irregular margins to better advantage.

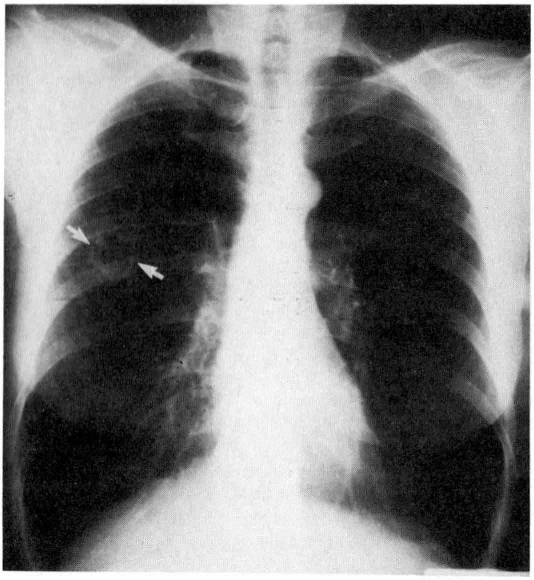

A

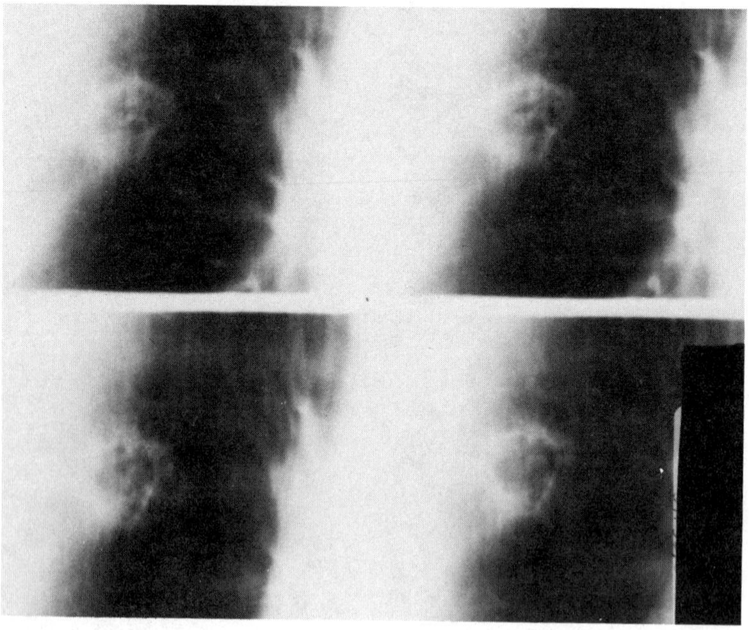

B

seen on the chest film, but rather the result of the lesion (Fig. 26-27). Small central or endobronchial lesions may lead to atelectasis or persistent infiltrates that fail to clear on follow-up examinations. This should lead to further evaluation by means of bronchoscopy or CT scanning.

Enlargement of a hilum or mediastinal widening should lead the interpreter to suspect neoplasm or lymphadenopathy until proven otherwise (Figs. 26-27, 26-28, 26-29, and 26-30). These findings may also be related to normal structures such as vascular shadows, thyroid or thymic tissue, and CT scanning is frequently necessary to distinguish these shadows.

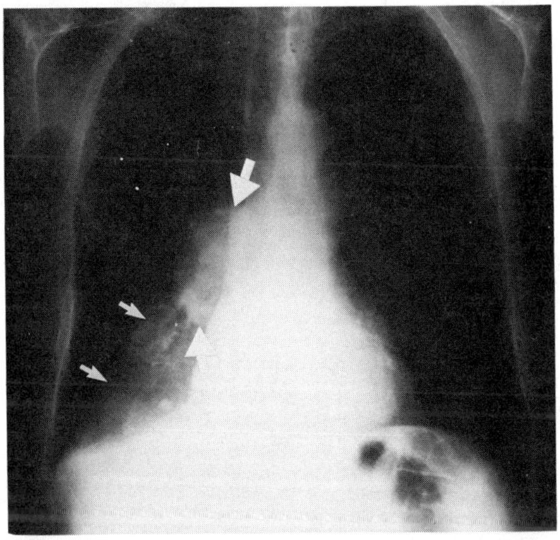

A

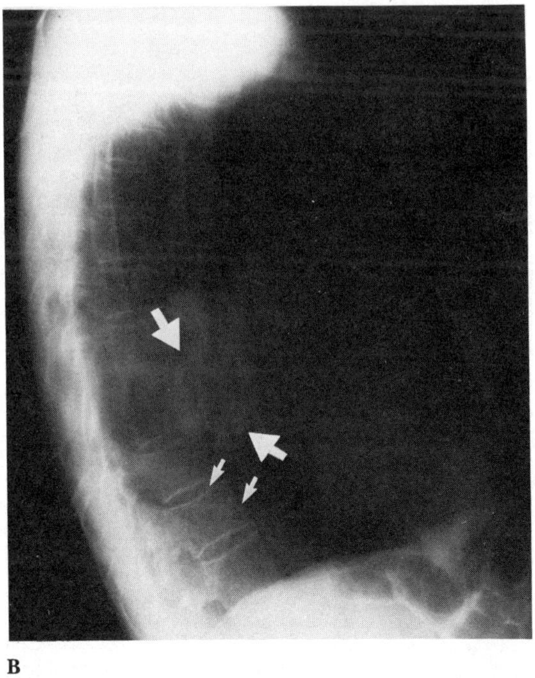

B

Fig. 26-27. Hilar neoplasm. (A and B) Large mass involving the right hilum seen on PA and lateral views (large arrows). There is also an associated right lower lobe atelectasis (small arrows) due to obstruction of the lower lobe bronchus.

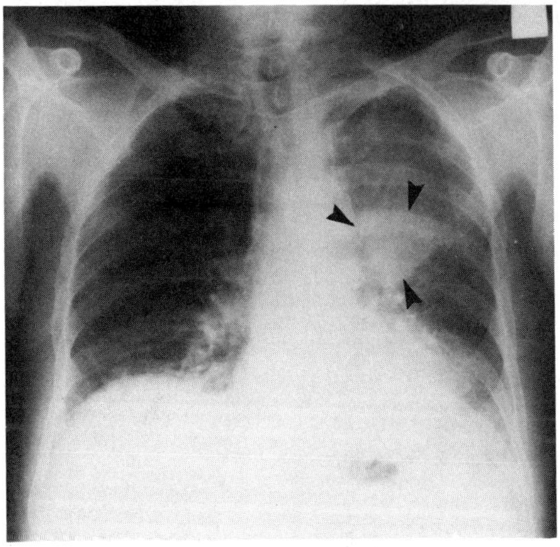

A

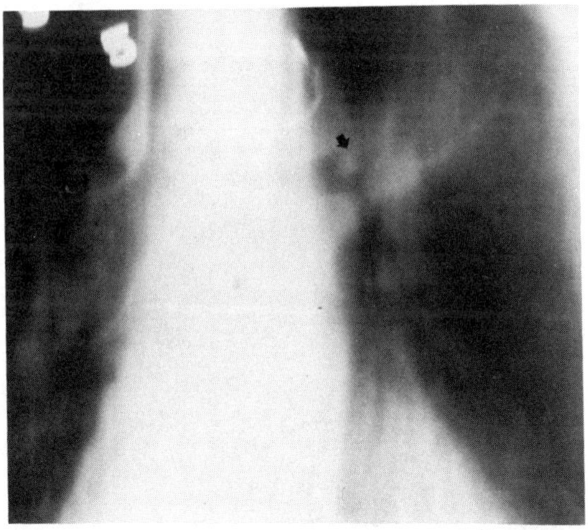

B

Fig. 26-28. Hilar neoplasm. (A) Large mass left hilum (arrows) with hazy infiltrate peripherally due to postobstructive pneumonitis. (B) Tomogram showing obstruction of the left upper lobe bronchus by mass (arrow).

Chronic Obstructive Pulmonary Disease

Pulmonary emphysema presents in many forms and results from many diseases. Roentgenographically, the findings are due to air-space enlargement. The classic signs are (1) flattening of the diaphragm, (2) increased retrosternal clear space, (3) hyperlucency of

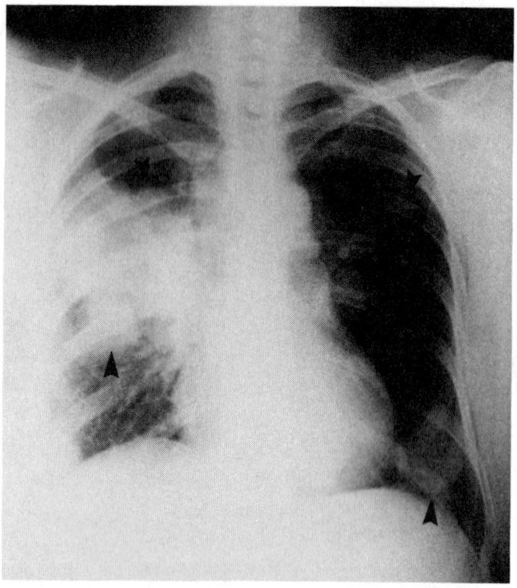

A

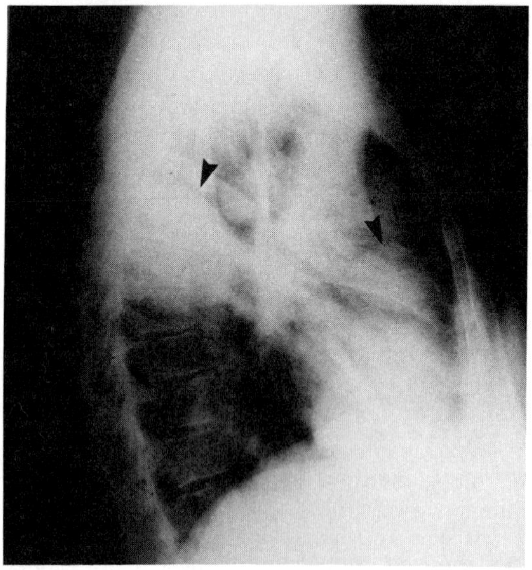

B

Fig. 26-29. CA breast with lung metastasis. (A and B) Multiple pulmonary nodules secondary to metastatic neoplasm (arrows). Notice hyperlucency of left lung due to absence of overlying breast shadow (postmastectomy).

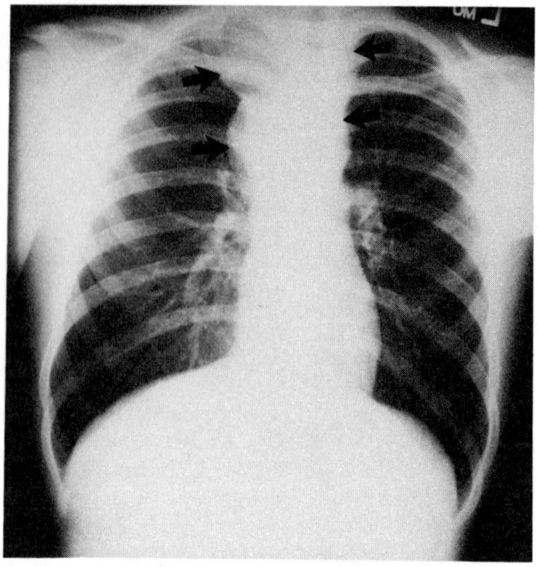

A

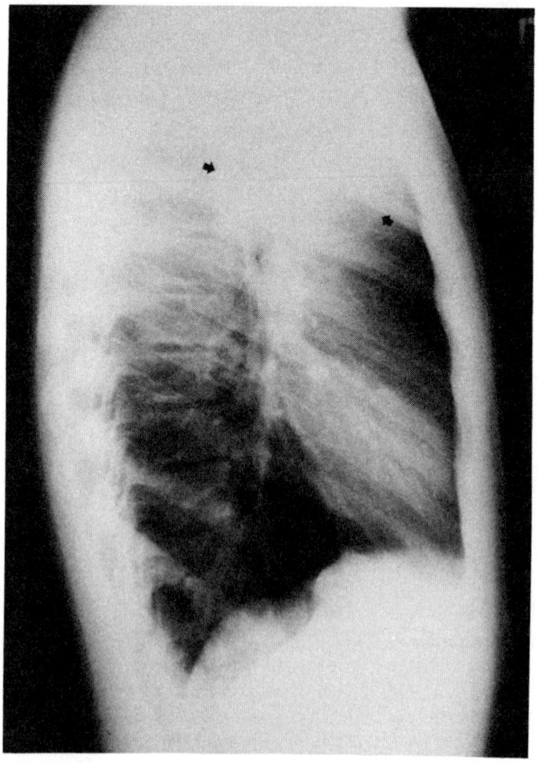

B

Fig. 26-30. Hodgkin's disease. (A) Soft tissue fullness in upper mediastinum with lobulated margins (arrows) due to mass. (B) Mass involves the anterior and middle mediastinum of lateral film (arrows).

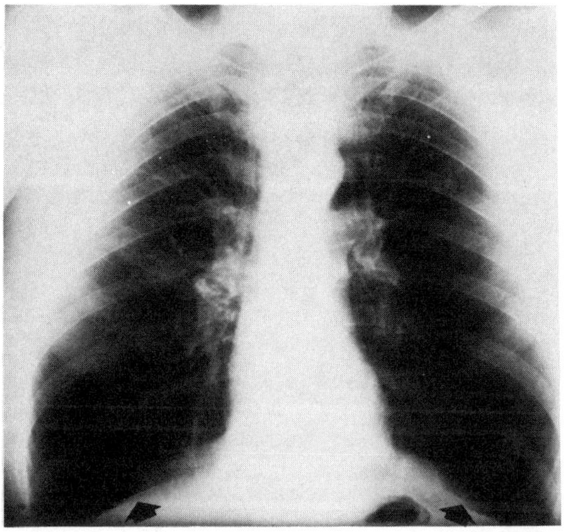

A

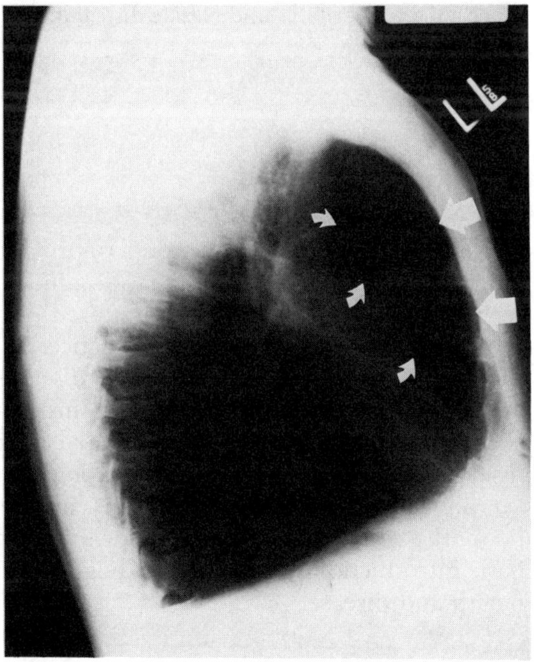

B

Fig. 26-31. Chronic obstructive lung disease. (A) Hyperlucent lungs with depression of the diaphragms (arrows). Large central pulmonary arteries and attenuation or "pruning" of peripheral vessels suggests the presence of pulmonary hypertension. (B) Large, lucent retrosternal clear space (arrows) seen on lateral films.

the lungs and blebs or bullae, and (4) a small, vertically oriented heart. More severe disease leads to enlargement of the central pulmonary arteries and decreased size of peripheral vessels ("pruning"). This is a sign of pulmonary hypertension or cor pulmonale (Fig. 26-31). Obstructive airway disease may also be seen acutely in asthmatic patients or in children following foreign body aspiration.

Congestive Heart Failure and Pulmonary Edema

One of the most common reasons to perform chest radiography in the symptomatic adult patient is to rule out congestive heart failure. Early congestive heart failure can be difficult to detect on chest radiographs and prior films may be helpful for comparison. Enlargement of the cardiac silhouette is accompanied by redistribution of pulmonary arterial blood flow to the upper lung fields, or "cephalization" (Fig. 26-32). Also, early findings are blurring of the normally sharp edges of the vessels due to perivascular edema. More severe failure results in pulmonary edema.

Fig. 26-32. Congestive heart failure. Early roentgen sign of heart failure is redistribution of pulmonary blood flow to the upper lobes or cephalization (arrows). Perivascular edema also leads to fuzzy vessel margins.

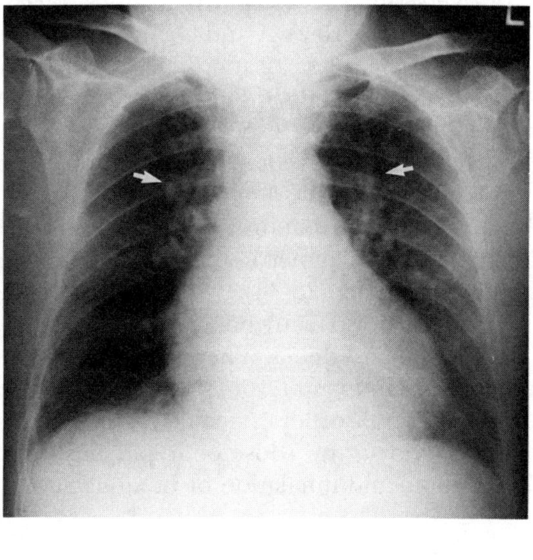

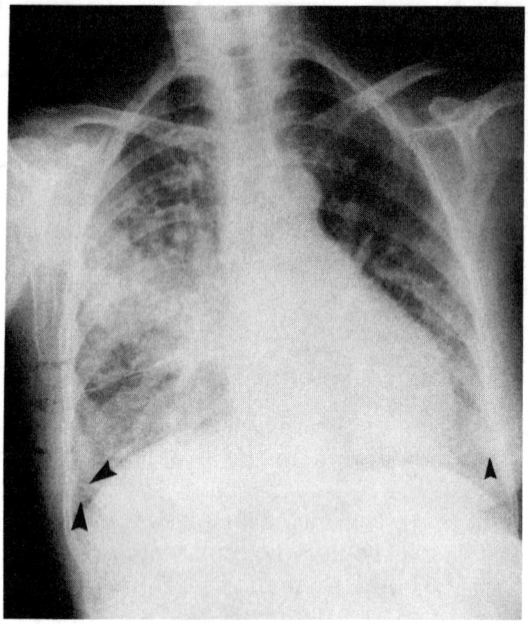

Fig. 26-33. Congestive heart failure. Increasing severity of heart failure leads to interstitial edema. This appears as thickening of the interlobular septae or Kerley's B lines (arrows).

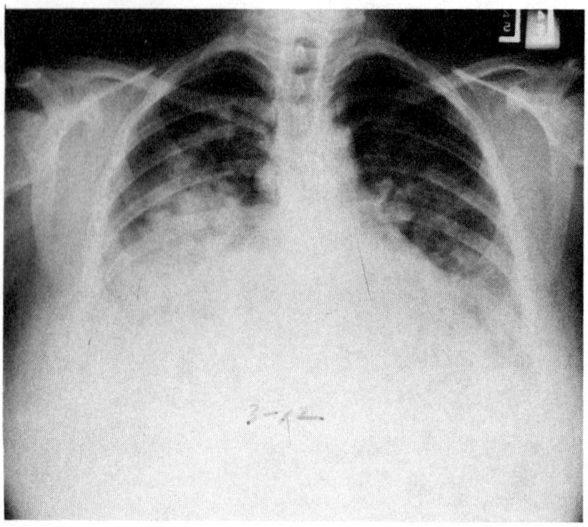

Fig. 26-34. Severe congestive heart failure with pulmonary edema. Note fluffy, alveolar infiltrates, especially in a perihilar and basilar distribution.

Pleural effusions may be present bilaterally; however, if unilateral, it is usually right sided.

Pulmonary edema can present as an interstitial or alveolar process. Interstitial edema leads to thickening of the interlobular septa, forming Kerley's B lines. These are fine, transverse lines at the peripheral lung bases (Fig. 26-33). Kerley's A and C lines are a similar process in other locations [13]. Interstitial edema may be indistinguishable from other interstitial diseases, especially fibrosis, without old films. Alveolar edema appears as more patchy, fluffy densities, particularly in a perihilar distribution. These changes are usually fairly symmetric but are occasionally asymmetric (Fig. 26-34).

There are also many noncardiogenic causes of pulmonary edema. The most common of these are adult respiratory distress syndrome, neurologic disorders, renal disease, fluid overload, drug overdose or hypersensitivity, aspiration, and inhalation of noxious gases.

Conclusion

In this chapter, we have attempted to provide basic introductory chest roentgenographic interpretation for commonly encountered pulmonary illnesses in primary care practice. Radiographs of other commonly seen diseases are to be found in other chapters in this text such as on tuberculosis and interstitial lung disease. After reading this chapter, and observing the other roentgenograms in this book, the primary care physician will have a basic introduction to the chest radiograph in health and disease.

References

1. Felson B: Chest Roentgenology. Philadelphia, W.B. Saunders, 1973
2. Simon G: Principles of Chest X-ray Diagnosis, ed 3. London, Butterworth, 1971
3. Felson B, Felson H: Localization of intrathoracic lesions by means of the PA roentgenograms: The silhouette sign. *Radiology* 55:363, 1950
4. Rigler LG: Roentgen diagnosis of small pleural effusions: A new roentgenographic position. *JAMA* 96:104, 1931

5. Fleischner FG: Atypical arrangement of free pleural effusion. *Radiol Clin North Am* 1: 347, 1963
6. Peterson JA: Recognition of intrapulmonary pleural effusion. *Radiology* 74:34, 1960
7. Higgins JA, Juergens JL, Bruwer AJ, et al: Loculated interlobar pleural effusion due to congestive heart failure. *Arch Intern Med* 96:180, 1955
8. Axel L: A simple way to estimate the size of a pneumothorax. *Invest Radiol* 16:165, 1981
9. Rhea JT, DeLuca SA, Greene RE: Determining the size of a pneumothorax in the upright patient. *Radiology* 144:733, 1982
10. Schneider HJ, Felson B, Gonzalez LL: Rounded atelectasis. *Am J Roentgenol* 134: 225, 1980
11. Nathan MH, Collins VP, Adams RA: Differentiation of benign and malignant pulmonary nodules by growth rate. *Radiology* 79:221, 1962
12. Siegelman SS, Zerhouni EA, Leo FP, et al: CT of the solitary pulmonary nodule. *AJR* 135:1, 1980
13. Heitzman ER, Ziter FM, Markarian B, et al: Kerley's interlobular septal lines, roentgen pathologic correlation. *Am J Roentgenol* 100: 578, 1967

Pulmonary Physiology at Altitude and Depth

Michael S. Eichenhorn

It is not at all unusual for individuals with or without intrinsic lung disease to encounter variation in ambient atmospheric pressure when involved in air travel, mountain vacationing, or scuba diving. Predictable alterations in pulmonary function can be expected in each of these situations, varying on the basis of our understanding of simple physics, gas laws, and/or adaptive changes to hypoxia. Given the mobility of today's society and its broad avocational interests, some knowledge of the effects of these changes is essential for the primary care provider. The intent of this chapter is to provide such a physiologic background and to address the common questions raised therein.

Alterations at Altitude

Unlike the circumstances associated with underwater descent, wherein pressure change itself contributes to altered physiology, ascent results in hypobaric hypoxia. However, the lessening of pressure at altitude generally is of no significant role. Very rapid ascent theoretically may actually lead to intravascular bubble formation and is preventable by oxygen inhalation but is not of significance in any usual mode of ascent, though it may have more bearing in space flight conditions [1]. Although the concentration of oxygen in air does not decrease with altitude, the associated decrease in barometric pressure does lead to a decrease in ambient and hence inspired oxygen concentration. This decrease in alveolar oxygen leads to a subsequent decrement in arterial and eventually mixed venous oxygen [2] (Fig. 27-1). The magnitude of the decrement in inspired PO_2 can be deduced from Table 27-1 [3] or calculated from the simple relationship of $PIO_2 = 0.21$ (barometric pressure, 47) mm Hg.

The resulting decrease in arterial PO_2 leads to stimulation of the peripheral chemoreceptors, thus increasing minute ventilation. This is achieved primarily by increments in tidal volume, with lesser increases in respiratory rate. As carbon dioxide levels decrease with hyperventilation, arterial oxygen levels increase. Acutely, this effect is noted once elevations of 3000 m are reached (with a resultant PaO_2 of 60 mm Hg) although lesser elevations of 500 m also produce increased minute ventilation when sustained for 3 to 4 days. Much of this initial hyperventilatory response is mediated through the carotid bodies, with their resection minimizing or eliminating any acute response to hypoxia.

However, the resultant hypocapnic alkalosis limits the acute response to hypoxia. When altitude is simulated, but isocapnia is preserved, a greater ventilatory response is seen than when hypocapnia also develops (Fig. 27-2) [2]. As hours to days of hypoxic altitude exposure continues, the inhibitory effects of hyperventilation lessen, a process referred to as ventilatory acclimatization.

Simplistic thinking suggested that hypocapnic alkalosis led to decreases in cerebrospinal fluid (CSF) hydrogen concentrations, which limited ventilation. As hours to days passed, an active transport of hydrogen ion into the CSF, together with a renal wasting of bicarbonate, led to decreases in CSF pH, stimulating the central chemoreceptors and allowing minute ventilation to increase further [4].

Unfortunately, it is now recognized that

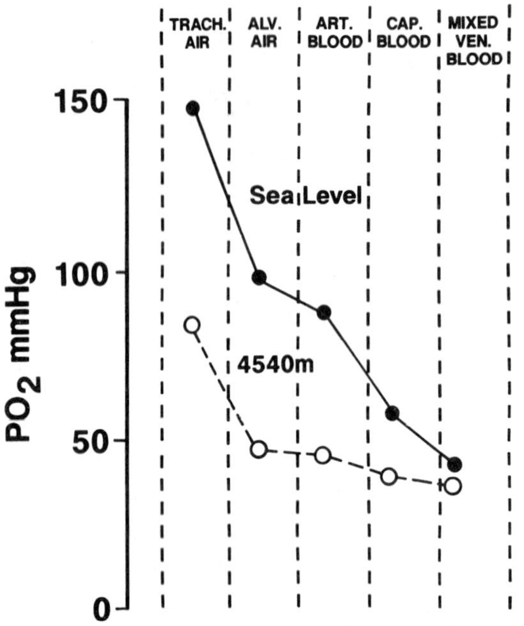
TRACH. AIR
ALV. AIR
ART. BLOOD
CAP. BLOOD
MIXED VEN. BLOOD
150
100
50
0
PO2 mmHg
Sea Level
4540m

Fig. 27-1. Oxygen-tension (PO_2) cascade at low and high altitude. At high altitude, decrease in PO_2 for each step from tracheal or inspired air to venous circulation is decreased. One of the greatest decreases is that from inspired to alveolar air, which largely reflects increased ventilation at high altitude. (*From* Weil JV: Ventilatory control at high altitude. Handbook of Physiology, Section 3, The Respiratory System. Bethesda, MD, American Physio Soc, 1986; with permission.)

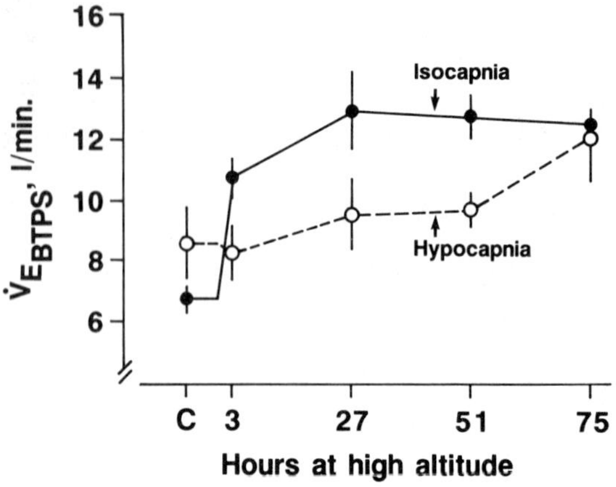
16
14
12
10
8
6
V̇EBTPS, l/min.
Isocapnia
Hypocapnia
C
3
27
51
75
Hours at high altitude

Fig. 27-2. Alteration in time course of ventilatory acclimatization to high altitude when hypocapnia is prevented. Four subjects were exposed to simulated high altitude. In one study, hypocapnia was allowed to develop (broken line). In another it was prevented by addition of CO_2 to ambient air (solid line). Under isocapnic conditions, ventilatory response to altitude was more rapid in onset and was virtually complete by 27 hours in contrast to a gradual increase in ventilation typical of altitude acclimatization, which was seen in hypocapnic group. V_E, expired ventilation. (*From* Nunn JF (ed): Applied Respiratory Physiology, ed 3. Boston, Butterworth, 1987; with permission.)

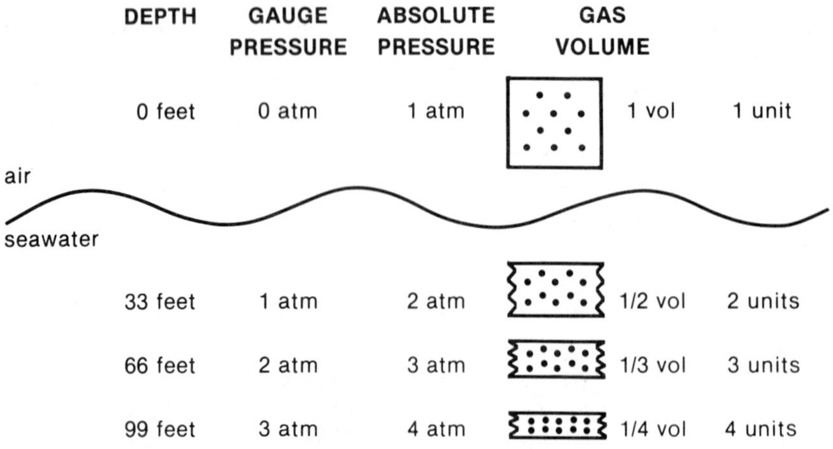
DEPTH
GAUGE PRESSURE
ABSOLUTE PRESSURE
GAS VOLUME
0 feet
0 atm
1 atm
1 vol
1 unit
air
seawater
33 feet
1 atm
2 atm
1/2 vol
2 units
66 feet
2 atm
3 atm
1/3 vol
3 units
99 feet
3 atm
4 atm
1/4 vol
4 units

Fig. 27-3. Gas volume decreases as absolute pressure increases. Gauge pressure is zero at the surface. Thus, gauge pressure equals absolute pressure less 1 atmosphere. (*From* Strauss RH (ed): Diving Medicine. New York, Grune & Stratton, 1976; with permission.)

these persumed alterations in pH develop too slowly to entirely explain acclimatization. While still unclear, it may be that the observed heightened ventilatory response is secondary to increased sensitivity of the central chemoreceptors stimulated by hypoxia and/or augmented activity of the reticular activating system somehow results.

With a lengthy residence at hypoxic altitudes, hypoxic desensitization may occur, wherein further hypoxic exposures fail to produce the expected augmentation of ventilation that would have been anticipated with acute altitude change [5]. Chronic, unchanging altitude exposure may also lead to a similar lessening in the minute ventilation noted as compared with that developing subacutely. Natives at high altitudes demonstrate this desensitization to hypoxic stimuli. Both the duration of the hypoxic exposure and the time in life at which it occurs influence the magnitude of desensitization. Children born at high altitudes who remain there for their early childhood may never attain a normal responsiveness to hypoxia. The more protracted the exposure, the greater the degree of hypoxic desensitization. Thus, recent sojourners show more hyperventilation than do long-term sojourners than do natives; all of whom still have higher minute ventilation than natives at sea level when exposed to a hypoxic environment. With descent, hypoxic desensitization may persist, although some degree of reversibility has at times been demonstrated. The mechanism by which hypoxic desensitization occurs is unclear, with some hereditary predisposition considered likely but not fully accounting for the phenomenon.

The development of polycythemia at altitude can be attributed to the arterial hypoxemia and the increases in erythopoietin that result. Increased levels of 2,3-diphosphoglycerate also occur and shift the hemoglobin oxygen dissociation curve rightward, favoring unloading of oxygen at the tissue level. While polycythemia increases arterial oxygen content, it does not increase PaO_2. Thus, the presence of polycythemia does not explain the development of hypoxic desensitization. In fact, polycythemia may not occur regularly in altitude-exposed individuals in whom hypoxic desensitization is known to exist, as commonly seen in the Sherpas of Tibet [6]. Alternatively, polycythemia may resolve with descent, although hypoxic desensitization still persists.

At best, there is no fully acceptable explanation of late hypoxic desensitization at altitude, though similar effects are also noted in chronically hypoxic individuals at sea level, such as those with end-stage chronic obstructive pulmonary disease or congestive heart failure. These chronically hypoxic individuals also fail to increase ventilation to further induced hypoxia and likewise may show paradoxic suppression of ventilation with oxygen administration.

Additional compensatory factors develop in response to altitude-induced hypoxia. These include increased mitochondrial number and density and increased capillary density in a variety of tissues, combining to enhance the ability of peripheral tissues to extract oxygen despite limited supply. The diffusing capacity for carbon monoxide increases, due to both the increase in red blood cell volume (polycythemia) together with the increase in pulmonary capillary surface area seen in natives attributable to increased alveolar number [5]. Expiratory flow rates and lung volumes are increased in high altitude natives. Similar changes can be induced in rats exposed to hypoxic environments from birth.

Abnormal Adaptation to Altitude

While in the past, gradual exposure to altitude lessened the likelihood of altitude-related illness, more rapid aircraft access has placed significantly greater numbers of individuals at risk. Moore [7] reported estimates of acute mountain sickness from 10% of men traveling to Vail, Colorado (2500 m) to a 42% to 67% incidence in men at 4268 m in Nepal, with adult males more likely to be affected than other age groups.

Acute Mountain Sickness

Acute mountain sickness (AMS) and high altitude pulmonary edema (HAPE) represent two forms of acute failure to acclimatize to high altitude. Some authors view them as distinct entities; others believe that HAPE is an exaggeration of the features of AMS. It should be noted that hyperventilation and tachycardia represent expected responses to acute hypoxia and as such are not abnormal. These two symptoms abate with oxygen administration unlike the symptoms of AMS.

Two thousand Indian soldiers reported by Singh et al [8] during a conflict in the Himalayas in 1965 comprise the largest group studied with AMS. There was a lag between the acute arrival at altitude and the onset of symptoms, extending anywhere from 6 to 96 hours. The severity of the illness was likely to be mild and the duration variable, with abatement generally seen within 2 to 5 days, although up to 4 or more weeks may be required before the individual is entirely asymptomatic [9]. Neuropsychiatric symptoms of disinterest, weakness, headache, and insomnia are characteristic and probably related to mild increases in CSF pressure, as is the typical anorexia, nausea, and vomiting. Dyspnea, cough, chest discomfort, and tachycardia make up the cardiorespiratory symptom complex and are less common.

Singh et al [8] believed that hypoxia led to a redistribution of flow from the periphery and splanchnic systems to the high capacitance pulmonary tree, producing varying degrees of pulmonary congestion that may lead on occasion to high altitude pulmonary edema. Hypoxia leads to hyperventilation characterized by an increased tidal volume with a near-normal respiratory rate. When the respiratory rate also increased, significant pulmonary congestion was present and was likely to be associated with more severe forms of AMS. The reduced splanchnic flow also was thought to lead to renal vasoconstriction, which in turn produced oliguria and a tendency toward sodium retention.

The stress of severe hypoxia also leads to an outpouring of steroids and antidiuretic hormone, which worsens the oliguria. This oliguria and the resultant antidiuresis may amount to a retention of up to 5 L over 24 to 72 hours that is then eventually excreted. This is the opposite of what is experienced by individuals who tolerate exposure to altitudes well and who note the passing of copious amounts of dilute urine or "Hohendiurese." Here the volume receptors of the dilated left atrium inhibit antidiuretic hormone output, rather than lead to a massive outpouring from hypoxic insult. Individuals with AMS also develop tachycardia and mild decreases in systolic blood pressure that may contribute to their symptomatology.

Retinal hemorrhage at times accompanied by papilledema also occurs with AMS. This is thought to arise from the increased intracranial pressure that compromises venous and lymphatic return. Most often, visual acuity is restored on descent.

Though it would seem to follow, in light of the marked fluid retention characteristic of AMS, that diuretic therapy would be advantageous, the literature does not completely support such a conclusion. Singh et al [8] employed furosemide in dosages of 80 mg every 12 hours for 2 days both to treat cases of AMS and to prevent its occurrence. Other authors have thought that many of Singh's cases are more appropriately classified as HAPE and hence tolerated such vigorous therapy. In addition, it has been pointed out that Singh et al supplemented the use of furosemide with beclomethasone to control cerebral symptoms and with morphine, which likely aided the redistribution of pulmonary vascular congestion. Gray et al [10] found in a 1971 study that the use of prophylactic furosemide in 40 mg twice daily doses worsened the symptoms of AMS despite improving urine output. They believed that despite the fluid retention experienced by individuals with AMS, this most often occurred in the face of intravascular depletion, which diuretics worsened. This intravascular depletion at times reached 20% of plasma volume and resulted from a lack of access to palatable drinking water. Potent diuretics also could theoretically aggravate the already established respiratory alkalosis by superimposing a component of contraction alkalosis.

Spironolactone is thought to be advantageous in doses of 25 mg three times a day, beginning 2 days before ascent because it combats the hyperaldosteronism induced by intravascular depletion and thus lessens overall fluid accumulation that leads to the symptoms of AMS [11]. Spironolactone has also been shown to be effective as a prophylaxis against AMS, but is limited to a lesser degree as is furosemide by its diuretic potential.

Dexamethasone has also been used in the prophylaxis and treatment of AMS [12–14]. Theoretically it reduces the vasogenic cerebral edema presumed to be present. In fact, both unpaired and paired studies showed it to be more effective prophylaxis than acetazolamide, with the latter limited in part by nausea and tiredness not experienced by the dexamethasone group. More recently, however, it has been suggested that the enhanced benefit seen with high-dose steroid use was tied more to the euphoric effects of the drug, and acetazolamide more directly reversed the pathophysiologic abnormalities that were seen [14, 15].

Acetazolamide has been the most widely studied prophylactic and when used at doses of 250 to 500 mg twice a day for 2 days before ascent and 2 days after seems to ameliorate many of the symptoms of AMS [15–17]. Though some believe its efficacy is due to its mild diuretic action, most believe that this is an insufficient explanation. Rather, the metabolic acidosis produced by acetazolamide is thought to offset the respiratory alkalosis that results from hypoxic hyperventilation. By increasing the CSF hydrogen concentration, an increased ventilatory response occurs that further elevates PaO_2. The most effective regimen for the avoidance of AMS thus far appears to be a combination of a staged ascent and acetazolamide usage. Staging for 3 to 4 days at 1600 m before ascent to higher altitudes has led to 20% to 25% improvement in symptoms. Staging coupled with acetazolamide use reduced the severity of AMS by about 85% in 35 volunteers studied by the Army in 1976 and has become the recommended course when time permits [16]. For established AMS, oxygen administration, descent, and acetazolamide are recommended. Whether combined treatment with acetazolamide and dexamethasone for established AMS will be more effective than use of a single agent remains to be studied.

Some individuals progress from AMS to dyspnea, tachypnea, and chest discomfort accompanied by bibasilar crepitance that becomes more widespread, a syndrome known as HAPE [18]. In other individuals, respiratory symptomatology may occur first and predominate in the clinical picture. Individuals who develop HAPE are either poorly acclimatized newcomers to altitude or natives or long-term sojourners who return to high altitude after a period of time at sea level. The onset may occur in as little as 3 hours or as late as 10 days after ascent and usually follows moderate exertion. Once present, the syndrome is likely to recur. Retrospective studies on Indian soldiers have suggested that individuals susceptible to HAPE were distinguishable from their normal counterparts by having higher heart rates, smaller lung volumes, and higher pulmonary arterial pressures. Moreover, they desaturated more significantly to hypoxic stimuli and tended to raise their pulmonary artery pressures to a greater extent in response. Low-grade fever and mild leukocytosis are common in established HAPE [18, 19].

The pathogenesis of HAPE is not entirely settled. However, it is apparent that whatever the mechanism, it must explain the marked hyperreactivity of the pulmonary arterial tree to hypoxia, the normal wedge pressure, and the marked desaturation, which is not entirely corrected with oxygen. Currently, it is thought that the hypoxic stress leads to a nonuniform arteriolar constriction that in turn leads to an intensification of ventilation-perfusion abnormalities. The nonuniformity contributes to the resultant patchy radiographic appearance.

HAPE appears to be an increased permeability type of pulmonary edema, but the inciting mechanism is not clear. HAPE also appears to differ from established adult respiratory distress syndrome, at least insofar as bronchoalveolar lavage fluid studies suggest [20]. HAPE fluid reveals evidence of the presence of leukotriene B_4, complement activation, and macrophage chemotaxis, but leukotriene C_4 and D_4 (slow-reacting substance of anaphylaxis) and neutrophil chemotaxis are absent. Elastase and increased oxidant activity characteristic of adult respiratory distress syndrome were also absent. These findings are consistent with the clinical observation of rapid resolution that most often occurs. This is consistent with the concept of Shapiro et al [21] of noncardiogenic edema as a manifestation of pulmonary capillary endothelial dysfunction, with adult respiratory distress syndrome being associated with alveolar epithelial cell dysfunction as well.

It may well be that the combination of hypoxic pulmonary arterial vasoconstriction together with augmented flow through the pulmonary vasculature leads to a mechanical disruption of endothelial cell pores and extrusion of protein-rich plasma. The absence of polymorphonuclear neutrophils suggests that an inflammatory reaction is not likely a primary pathophysiologic event.

The treatment of HAPE includes the administration of oxygen at high concentrations together with evacuation to a lower altitude. HAPE can be prevented by a gradual ascent and the avoidance of marked physical activity. Individuals with a prior history of HAPE, natives returning from sea level after 2 or more weeks, and young people constitute the groups most apt to benefit. It is not clear that other agents are effective in ameliorating the symptoms of HAPE once they have developed or that prophylaxis with acetazolamide has any real effect here as it would appear to have in AMS.

Chronic Mountain Sickness

Monge's disease or chronic mountain sickness (CMS) [2, 22, 23] is an exaggeration of the changes that typically accompany life at higher altitudes and can be divided into three distinct clinicopathologic types. First, there is the sea level resident who moves to high altitude and never acclimatizes. Second, there is a group perhaps more appropriately referred to as Monge's syndrome or secondary CMS who have been acclimatized and then develop another disease such as obesity, kyphoscoliosis, chronic obstructive pulmonary disease (COPD), or neuromuscular disorders that lead to further hypoventilation. Last, there are those with true Monge's disease, who for no apparent reason develop difficulties. It is of interest that Monge's disease appears to be limited almost exclusively to the Andes, with an occasional case from the United States, but no cases from the Himalayas. There are no clear explanations for this variation although some authors have suggested that increased dust exposure in the Andes as a result of the intensive mining accounts for the difference. If this were the case, it would raise the question as to whether Monge's disease as such really exists. A hereditary basis is not likely in that sojourners and natives are both susceptible.

In any case, for reasons that are not clear, those individuals who develop CMS hypoventilate relative to their well counterparts, and Monge's disease has been referred to as an example of the primary hypoventilation syndrome occurring at high altitude. Individuals with CMS, in addition to exaggerating their established loss of hypoxic ventilatory drive, also develop markedly decreased sensitivity to carbon dioxide. Voluntary apnea is also prolonged and results in a higher than normal PCO_2 and lower than normal PO_2 before breaking. Arterial blood gases reveal marked oxygen desaturation averaging 70% as compared with healthy highlander saturations of 81%. Carbon dioxide levels are also increased to 39 mm Hg compared with 32 mm Hg for healthy natives. With exercise, further deterioration in oxygen saturation develops.

Individuals with CMS have more marked pulmonary hypertension than healthy highlanders. Pulmonary artery capillary wedge pressures remain normal. It would appear that in addition to a more intense muscularization of the pulmonary arterial tree, there is also an accentuated vasoconstrictive response to hypoxia so that oxygen administration decreases pulmonary artery pressures significantly more than the 15% to 20% seen in acclimatized individuals.

The worsened hypoxia experienced by those with CMS leads to an exaggerated erythropoietic response, with hematocrits and hemoglobin averaging 79% and 25 g/dL, respectively, compared with healthy natives' values of 59% and 20 g/dL. This polycythemia and the attendant hyperviscosity also contribute to the pulmonary hypertension. Likewise there is an increased diastolic blood pressure in CMS that is thought to be related to the same factors and is the only significant difference in the systemic circuit in CMS, though with marked hypoxia, some left ventricular dysfunction has been noted.

The net effect of these physiologic alterations is to produce an individual with decreased exercise tolerance and fatigability, often with headaches, dizziness, parethesia, and somnolence, which in extreme cases may progress to coma. On examination, marked cyanosis is evident, with the mucous membranes being almost black. Clubbing and splinter hemorrhages are often found. Findings compatible with pulmonary hypertension, with or without right-sided failure, are noted. The treatment of CMS consists of moving to a lower altitude. In all cases, the previously mentioned changes receded within 2 months of sea level residence to practically normal. The administration of O_2 or phlebotomy may provide transient relief. With return to high altitude, symptoms usually recur.

In addition to these well-established clinical syndromes of altitude exposure, Moore [7] has highlighted the concept of altitude-aggravated illness. While focusing largely on pregnancy, wherein increased oxygen demand at sea level is aggravated by a decreased oxygen availability at altitude, she acknowledges an even greater number of individuals with diminished supply due to preexisting cardiac and pulmonary disease worsening at altitude. With regard to pregnancy, infant mortality has been shown to be increased at altitude. There is a lower average birth weight and higher incidence of hyperbilirubinemia. The latter may be tied to higher hematocrits that were seen and increased hemoglobin turnover. Additionally, preeclampsia was increased at altitude when all other factors were controlled. This points out the apparent tenuousness of our adaptive mechanisms to altitude-induced hypoxia.

Sleep at altitude is also apparently disturbed at least in sojourners. There are no systematic studies of sleep in high altitude natives to suggest widespread abnormalities, although some accentuation of the expected desaturation with hypopneas and apneas that are normally seen would be expected given the ambient decreases in oxygen concentration. Poor sleep quality is common with acute ascent [2], and dysrhythmic breathing may be predictive of the development of AMS, though causality cannot be determined [24]. Increased light sleep, decreased deep sleep, frequent arousals, and little change in rapid eye movement sleep characterize the sleep pattern seen with acute ascent [25]. Hypocapnic alkalosis may account for these abnormalities, and treatment with acetazolamide reduces arousals and irregular breathing patterns [26, 27].

Renzetti et al [28] established a worsened prognosis for patients with established COPD living at altitude compared with sea level residents. Kryger et al [29] found that symptomatic COPD predisposed to CMS, and that exaggerated polycythemia was seen in the COPD population compared with those with normal lung function.

The effects of short-term hypoxic exposure in COPD in association with air travel have been the subject of considerable investigation. Graham and Houston [30] exposed individuals with moderate COPD to 1920 m elevation for 4 days and found that PaO_2 decreased from 66 to 51.5 mm Hg acutely, increasing to 54.5 mm Hg with acclimatization. With exercise, more significant hypoxemia developed (46.5 mm Hg). Despite this, there were no apparent cardiovascular complications and only minimal symptoms of fatigue. While this seemingly established the safety of air travel for individuals with mild disease, concern rightfully exists for those with more severe disease and concomitant cardiovascular disease, especially angina pectoris.

With more severe disease and higher achieved altitudes, more significant decreases in arterial oxygenation could well be expected [31]. While some have suggested preflight hypoxic gas inhalation to ascertain the likelihood of altitude desaturation, often the exact altitude for the planned flight and detailed cabin pressurization characteristics cannot be established with certainty before departure. More practically, Cottrell [32] suggests that an appropriate 20 mm Hg decrease in PaO_2 can be expected from flights of 6214 feet or 1894 m, a typical midelevation for domestic flights. Thus, prearranged supplemental oxygen should probably be available for those with sea level PaO_2s of 65 to 70 mm Hg, if altitude simulation is not performed. Certainly all individuals requiring supplemental oxygen at sea level should not have it interrupted. Though at times troublesome to arrange, air carriers are obliged to provide oxygen when prescribed.

Diving Medicine

In the same fashion as is the case with the hypobaric exposure of altitude, alterations in inspired oxygen concentration can be easily predicted from the sample relationship, $PIO_2 = 0.21$ (barometric pressure $-$ 47 mm Hg), or from Table 27-1. While marked increases in altitude are necessary before physiologic disturbances occur due to altitude-induced hypoxemia, alterations below sea level occur much more quickly. Thus, descent to only 33 feet doubles atmospheric pressure, essentially doubling the inspired concentration of oxygen in ambient air. At greater than 3 atmospheres depth (99 feet), the inspired oxygen concentration is such that potential oxygen toxicity with protracted exposure may occur.

The toxicity of oxygen in high concentrations has been well studied [33–35]. It increases both as durations of exposure and inspired concentration increase. In fact, early work with diving medicine during World War II effectively established that using compressed oxygen as an inspired gas at depths of 99 or more feet was hazardous in that oxygen-induced seizures were universally seen [36]. Premonitory symptoms suggestive of central nervous system (CNS) oxygen toxicity including muscle twitching, especially facial, paresthesia, confusion, and euphoria, may not occur. Hyperthermia, activity, and hyperventilation (hypocapnia) increase the likelihood of CNS toxicity. Once present, lessening the inspired oxygen concentrations leads to cessation of seizure activity. Given the potential universality of oxygen-induced CNS toxicity, detailed evaluation of the CNS is not necessary after seizures unless other clinical features also are present and suggestive of organic disease. Similarly, anticonvulsive therapy is not required. The safety of compressed air as a short-term recreational diving mixture has been established, though greater depths and dive durations have led to the use of alternate gas mixtures. For example, nitrox (nitrogen-oxygen) mixtures suitable for use at 300 foot depths (10 atmospheres) would require only 2% oxygen in order to supply the requisite 20% oxygen available in room air at depth. The complexities of such diving theory is beyond the scope of this chapter, and the interested reader is referred to the many comprehensive reviews of this subject [36, 37].

Though oxygen-induced seizures are clearly the most common risk of oxygen inhalation at depth, pulmonary toxicity with tracheobronchitis proceeding to direct alveolar injury with pulmonary edema may also occur. This is manifest in the loss of vital capacity that occurs progressively over time, not at all dissimilar from the intensive care unit experience with protracted oxygen exposures. Again, this is seldom a problem with recreational diving, given the limited time generally spent at depth. Alterations in inspired gas density generally do not contribute to respiratory symptomatology at depth, even though elevations in PCO_2 may be seen. The importance of this effect is generally insignificant in recreational divers, but of more importance in saturation or protracted dives at very substantial depths. Again, the interested reader is referred to diving physiology texts for a more comprehensive review of these issues. Immersion per se may also directly reduce vital capacity and pulmonary compliance as well as increase trapped gas, but these effects are also generally negligible.

Table 27-1. Barometric Pressure Relative to Altitude

Altitude		*Barometric Pressure*		*Inspired Gas PO_2*		*Equivalent Oxygen % at Sea Level*	*Percentage Oxygen Required to Give Sea Level Value of Inspired Gas PO_2*
feet	*meters*	*kPa*	*mm Hg*	*kPa*	*mm Hg*		
0	0	101	760	19.9	149	20.9	20.9
2000	600	94.3	707	18.4	138	19.4	22.6
4000	1220	87.8	659	16.9	127	17.8	24.5
6000	1830	81.2	609	15.7	118	16.6	26.5
8000	2440	75.2	564	14.4	108	15.1	28.8
10,000	3050	69.7	523	13.3	100	14.0	31.3
12,000	3660	64.4	483	12.1	91	12.8	34.2
14,000	4270	59.5	446	11.1	83	11.6	37.3
16,000	4880	54.9	412	10.1	76	10.7	40.8
18,000	5490	50.5	379	9.2	69	9.7	44.8
20,000	6100	46.5	349	8.4	63	8.8	49.3
22,000	6710	42.8	321	7.6	57	8.0	54.3
24,000	7320	39.2	294	6.9	52	7.3	60.3
26,000	7930	36.0	270	6.3	47	6.6	66.8
28,000	8540	32.9	247	5.6	42	5.9	74.5
30,000	9150	30.1	226	4.9	37	5.2	83.2
35,000	10,700	23.7	178	3.7	27	3.8	—
40,000	12,200	18.8	141	2.7	20	2.8	—
45,000	13,700	14.8	111	1.8	13	1.9	—
50,000	15,300	11.6	87	1.1	8	1.1	—
63,000	19,200	6.3	47	0	0	0	—

100% oxygen restores sea level inspired PO_2 at 10,000 m (33,000 feet).
From Nunn JF (ed): Applied Respiratory Physiology, ed 3. Boston, Butterworths, 1987; with permission.

Likewise, cardiovascular changes induced by a lessening of gravitational effects on blood flow are also minimal.

Compounding the effects of high concentration of oxygen at depth are the pressure changes that occur with descent and ascent. These are readily predictable from Boyle's law, which states that the product of pressure and volume must remain constant for a given amount or concentration of gas. Henry's law establishes that increases in pressure across a liquid are distributed evenly by that liquid. Hence, fluid-like organs do not experience change with altered pressure. However, those areas with liquid–gas interface are affected. A doubling of pressure leads to a halving of the volume of a gas contained in or by a liquid medium [38] (Fig. 27-3). Thus, the volume of gas in the lungs, sinuses, intestines, and middle ear are likely to be affected.

With descent, the volume of gas decreases and generally causes little difficulty except potentially with the equalization of pressure across the middle ear or ear squeeze. With compression, if the eustachian tube fails to open to equalize pressure between the middle ear and nasopharynx, middle ear pressure becomes less than ambient. A 60 mm Hg pressure gradient is seen with descent to only 2.6 feet. This is perceived as fullness or pain in the ear. With descent to 39 feet, a 90 mm Hg pressure gradient exists, which may cause the tympanic membrane to rupture. The predisposition to rupture generally occurs between 4.3 and 17.4 feet of descent (Fig. 27-4) [39]. Even without rupture, conductive hearing loss, tinnitus, and possibly vertigo may be seen. Avoidance of this problem can be accomplished by avoiding diving during upper respiratory tract infections or with prior dem-

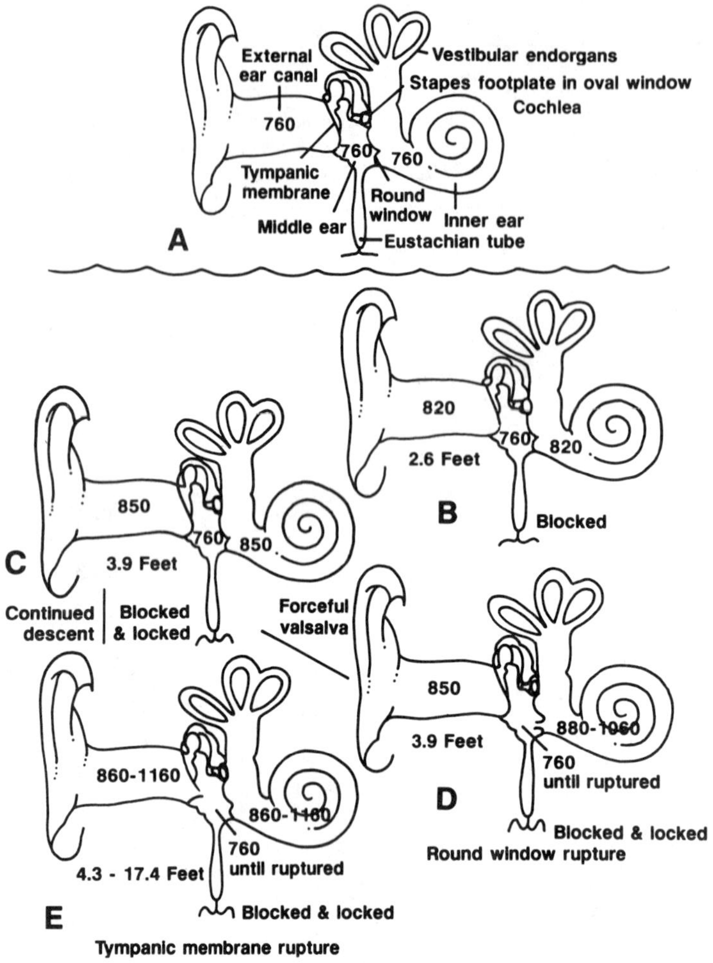
External
ear canal
760
Vestibular endorgans
Stapes footplate in oval window
Cochlea
760
760
Tympanic
membrane
Round
window
Inner ear
Middle ear
Eustachian tube
A
820
760
820
2.6 Feet
B
Blocked
850
760
850
3.9 Feet
C
Continued
descent
Blocked
& locked
Forceful
valsalva
850
3.9 Feet
880-1060
760
until ruptured
D
Blocked & locked
Round window rupture
860-1160
860-1160
760
until ruptured
4.3 - 17.4 Feet
E
Blocked & locked
Tympanic membrane rupture

Fig. 27-4. Otologic barotrauma of descent. Theoretical sequence of changes in the right ear of a diver who does not equilibrate middle ear pressure during descent. Pressures are shown in mm Hg. (A) Surface condition with equal pressures (760 mm Hg) throughout and a patent eustachian tube with a normally closed nasopharyngeal ostium. (B) Depth of approximately 2.6 feet after diver failed to open the eustachian tube on entering the water. Pressure differential of 60 mm Hg exists. Tympanic membrane and round window are bulging into the middle ear. Diver notices pain and pressure in the ear, with a conductive hearing loss and possible vertigo. (C) Depth of approximately 3.9 feet with 90 mm Hg pressure differential and blocked and locked eustachian tube. (D) Forceful Valsalva maneuver can lead to rupture of the round window, with resulting leak of perilymph into the middle ear. The exact pressure differentials at which rupture occurs in humans are unknown. Studies in cats have indicated that round window ruptures occur when a pressure of 120 to 300 mm Hg is added to the CSF space at 1 ata. (E) Continued descent can lead to tympanic membrane rupture at pressure differentials of 4.3 to 17.4 feet. The actual rupture point is quite variable. (*From* Ear and sinus problems in diving. *In* Farmer JC, Bovie AE, Davis JC (eds): Diving Medicine, 2nd ed. Philadelphia, PA, W.B. Saunders, 1990; with permission.)

onstrated difficulties. Pretreatment with nasal or systemic decongestants may be useful. Otologic findings should be normal before diving is resumed. The middle ear and sinuses may also be affected though less commonly with ascent when increased air volume leads to symptom development.

It is the lung with ascent that poses the most potentially serious clinical problem, however. As pulmonary gas volume increases with ascent, exhaled volume in turn increases. Divers returning to the surface in essence must maintain an open glottis to permit this constant exhalation. If this is not done, dramatic increases in intrapulmonary pressures result, predisposing to pneumothorax and potential air embolism if the dissecting gas enters the circulation. The likelihood of these events is increased in the presence of abnormal air cavities within the parenchyma such as blebs or bulla. While these structures may shrink somewhat with descent, they often do not communicate well, if at all, with the tracheobronchial tree to decompress as their volumes increase with ascent.

Similarly, individuals with asthma or chronic obstructive lung disease may not equalize pressure readily due to the increased resistance posed by inflamed or hyperreactive airways, predisposing them to barotrauma despite normal parenchyma. It is important to note that the greatest volume changes occur closest to the surface, and pneumothorax and gas embolism have been described at depths as little as 10 feet below the surface. Hence, individuals interested in recreational diving should be screened for structural abnormalities by chest roentgenography, and advised against diving if abnormalities are recognized. A past medical history of spontaneous pneumothorax should also contraindicate avocational diving.

Likewise, active asthmatic patients should not dive even if seemingly well controlled. The abruptness of an asthmatic attack and its unpredictable nature place these individuals at greater risk for barotrauma and its potentially disastrous consequences. Patients with a remote history of asthma in the past should have spirometry performed and possibly methacholine challenge testing to determine whether any residua remain, placing them at increased risk. While these recommendations may seem extreme, it is the opinion of most authorities that the degree of caution is justified, given the alternative risks. There is debate as to whether or not asthmatic patients are overrepresented in statistics on diving accidents [40, 41]. While active asthma may be denied in many of these cases, subclinical asthma may well be present. Most cases of diving-related gas embolism report normal exhalation during ascent, suggesting that pulmonary overpressurization due either to parenchymal or airways problems must be present in a greater number of individuals than suspected clinically.

As noted, pulmonary overpressurization can lead to barotrauma, with pneumothorax, mediastinal or subcutaneous emphysema, or pneumoperitoneum developing. If the released gas is dispersed into the pulmonary venous circulation, gas embolism into the cerebral circulation may result in coma, contralateral hemicranial signs, brain stem findings, or combinations thereof noted clinically, depending on the portion of the cranial circulation that is affected. Myocardial infarction from coronary artery embolization may also be seen, though the "head up" position of most divers predisposes to cerebral effects given the buoyancy of the intravascular bubbles. Intravascular gas bubbles not only contribute to a physical obstruction to blood flow, but also induce complement activation, inciting a widespread inflammatory reaction.

Similarly, bubble generation and growth are basic to our understanding of decompression illness [42]. While beyond the scope of this chapter, it should be noted that asymptomatic bubbles are formed with most decompressions when studied by ultrasound, but are generally clinically silent. Inert gases pose the greatest clinical hazard, while oxygen and carbon dioxide are metabolized even when found in bubbles, while nitrogen is not. When present, the signs of decompression sickness vary, depending on the site of bubble formation. Joint symptomatology is common, and "pain only" bends occur more frequently than that involving the nervous system wherein either the CNS or spinal cord may be involved. Inattention to prescribed diving tables and/or excessive activity at depth are probably the most common causes of decompression sickness. Recompression shrinks bubbles to preclinical size, and supplemental oxygen augments the concentration gradient, favoring resorption back into circulation. All patients with decompression sickness should be treated with hyperbaric oxygen, fluid resuscitation, and possibly corticosteroids if CNS symptoms are present.

Hyperbaric Oxygen Therapy

While a full discussion of hyperbaric oxygen therapy is also beyond the scope of this chapter, the extension of the discussed physiology of diving medicine to this area is obvious. Oxygen delivered either intermittently or continuously under increased pressure increases the inspired and eventually arterial oxygen content. In fact, at 3 atmospheres pressure, sufficient oxygen can be dissolved within the blood to fully satisfy the body's metabolic demands, even in the absence of hemoglobin. In fact life can be sustained under these conditions, as shown experimentally by Boerema et al [43–48].

This dramatic increase in tissue oxygen levels may be an adjunct to wound healing, particularly in those cases where blood supply is compromised as in chronic refractory osteomyelitis and osteoradionecrosis. Enhanced wound healing might also be expected in certain necrotizing infections, with relatively impaired blood flow. Additionally, high oxygen concentrations may actually inactivate clostridial toxin A, a cause of major tissue damage in gas gangrene and clostridial myonecrosis.

Acutely, high concentrations of oxygen may reverse the tissue hypoxia associated with cyanide or carbon monoxide intoxication, additionally, competitively unbinding the latter from hemoglobin. Most authorities would accept the value of hyperbaric oxygen therapy in severe carbon monoxide intoxication not responding to 100% surface oxygen.

Lastly, hyperbaric oxygen is of value in the treatment of gas embolization. Here, the increases in ambient pressure actually physically shrink the intravascular gas, lessening the physical obstruction that results and minimizing the cascade of mediators created. Additionally, the high concentrations of oxygen create a diffusion gradient, favoring the dissolution of bubble back into the circulation. While some debate persists as to the optimal depth for such treatment, there seems little debate as to the overall efficacy of therapy if a hyperbaric chamber is available. This particular aspect of therapy differs little from that for decompression sickness wherein hyperbaric oxygen therapy is the clearly established treatment of choice.

References

1. Grover RF, Tucker A, Reeves JT: Hypobaria: An etiologic factor in acute mountain sickness. *In* Loeppky JA, Riedesel ML (eds): Oxygen Transport To Human Tissues. North Holland, Elsevier, 1982
2. Weil JV: Ventilatory control at high altitude. Handbook of Physiology, Section 3, The Respiratory System. Bethesda, MD, American Physio Soc, 1986, pp. 703–727
3. Nunn JF: Applied Respiratory Physiology. London, Butterworths, 1987, p 311
4. Severinghaus JW, Mitchell RA, Richardson BW, et al: Respiratory control at high altitude suggesting active transport of CSF pH. *J Appl Physiol* 18:1155–1166, 1963
5. Lenfant C, Sullivan K: Adaptation to high altitude. *N Engl J Med* 284:1298–1309, 1971
6. Lahiri S: Respiratory control in Andean and Himalayan high altitude natives. *In* West JB, Lahiri S (eds): High Altitude and Man. Bethesda, MD, American Physio Soc, 1984
7. Moore LG: Altitude aggravated illness: Examples from pregnancy and prenatal life. *Ann Emerg Med* 16:965–973, 1987
8. Singh I, Khanna PK, Srivastava MC, et al: Acute mountain sickness. *N Engl J Med* 280: 175–184, 1969
9. Johnson TS, Rock PB: Acute mountain sickness. *N Engl J Med* 319:841–845, 1988
10. Gray GW, Bryan AC, Frayser R, et al: Control of acute mountain sickness. *Aerospace Medicine* 42:81–84, 1971
11. Currie TT, Carter PH, Champion WL, et al: Spironolactone and acute mountain sickness. *Med J Aust* 2:168–170, 1976
12. Johnson TS, Rock PB, Fulco CS, et al: Preven-

tion of acute mountain sickness by dexamethasone. *N Engl J Med* 310:683–686, 1984
13. Rock PB, Johnson TS, Larsen RF, et al: Dexamethasone as prophylaxis for acute mountain sickness. *Chest* 95:568–573, 1989
14. Levine BD, Yoshimura K, Kobayashi T, et al: Dexamethasone in the treatment of acute mountain sickness. *N Engl J Med* 321:1707–1713, 1989
15. Ellsworth AJ, Larson EB, Strickland D: A randomized trial of dexamethasone and acetazolamide for acute mountain sickness prophylaxis. *Am J Med* 83:1024–1030, 1987
16. Evans WO, Robinson SM, Horstman DH, et al: Amelioration of the symptoms of acute mountain sickness by staging and acetazolamide. *Aviat Space Environ Med* 47:512–516, 1976
17. Zell SC, Goodman PH: Acetazolamide and dexamethasone in the prevention of acute mountain sickness. *West J Med* 148:541–545, 1988
18. Menon ND: High altitude pulmonary edema. *N Engl J Med* 273:66–73, 1965
19. Kleiner JP, Nelson WP: High altitude pulmonary edema—a rare disease? *JAMA* 234:491–495, 1975
20. Schoene RB: Pulmonary edema at high altitude. *Clin Chest Med* 6:491–507, 1985
21. Shapiro BA, Cane RD, Harrison RA: Positive end expiratory pressure in acute lung injury. *Chest* 83:558–563, 1983
22. Hecht HH: A sea level view of altitude problems. *Am J Med* 50:703–708, 1971
23. Penaloza D, Sime F: Chronic cor pulmonale due to loss of altitude acclimitization (chronic mountain sickness). *Am J Med* 50:728–743, 1971
24. Fujimoto K, Matsuzawa Y, Hirai K, et al: Irregular nocturnal breathing patterns at high altitude in subjects susceptible to HAPE: A preliminary study. *Aviat Space Environ Med* 60:786–791, 1989
25. Miller JC, Horvath SM: Sleep at altitude. *Aviat Space Environ Med* 48:615–620, 1977
26. Sutton JR, Houston CS, Mansell AL, et al: Effect of acetazolamide on hypoxemia during sleep at high altitude. *N Engl J Med* 301: 1329–1331, 1979
27. Weil JV, Kryger MH, Scoggin GH: Sleep and breathing at high altitude. *In* Guilleminault C, Dement WC (eds): Sleep Apnea Syndromes. New York, Liss, 1978, pp 119–136
28. Renzetti AD, McClement JH, Lih BD: The Veteran's Administration cooperative study of pulmonary function: III: Mortality in relation to respiratory function in chronic obstructive lung disease. *Am J Med* 41:115–144, 1966
29. Kryger MR, McCullough R, Doekel R, et al: Excessive polycythemia of high altitude: Role of ventilatory drive and lung disease. *Am Rev Respir Dis* 118:659–665, 1978
30. Graham WG, Houston CS: Short-term adaptation to moderate altitude: Patients with chronic obstructive pulmonary disease. *JAMA* 240:1491–1494, 1978
31. Dillard TA, Berg BW, Rajagopal KR, et al: Hypoxemia during air travel in patients with chronic obstructive pulmonary disease. *Ann Intern Med* 111:362–367, 1989
32. Cottrell JJ: Altitude exposures during aircraft flight: Flying higher. *Chest* 92:81–84, 1988
33. Clark JM, Lambertson CJ: Pulmonary oxygen toxicity: A review. *Pharmacol Rev* 23:37–72, 1971
34. Frank L, Massaro D: Oxygen toxicity. *Am J Med* 69:117–126, 1980
35. Davis WB, Rennard SI, Bitterman PB, et al: Pulmonary oxygen toxicity: Early reversible changes in human alveolar structures induced by hypoxia. *N Engl J Med* 309:878–883, 1983
36. Thom SR, Clark JM: The toxicity of oxygen, carbon monoxide, and carbon dioxide. *In* Bove AA, Davis JC (eds): Diving Medicine. Philadelphia, WB Saunders, 1990
37. Shilling CW, Carlston CB, Mathias RA (eds): The Physician's Guide to Diving Medicine. New York, Plenum Press, 1984
38. Strauss RH: Diving medicine. *Am Rev Respir Dis* 119:1001–1023, 1979
39. Keller AP: A study of the relationship of air pressure to myringo puncture. *Laryngoscope* 68:2015–2029, 1958
40. Neuman TS: Pulmonary disorders in diving. *In* Bove AA, Davis JC (eds): Diving Medicine. Philadelphia, WB Saunders, 1990
41. Vorosmarti J (ed): Fitness to Dive. Bethesda, MD, Undersea and Hyperbaric Medical Society, 1987
42. Vann RD: The physiological basis of decompression. Bethesda, MD, Undersea and Hyperbaric Medical Society, 1989
43. Boerema I, Meijne NG, Brummelkemp WK, et al: Life without blood. *J Cardiovasc Surg* 1:133–146, 1960
44. Davis JC, Hunt TK: Problem Wounds: The Role of Oxygen. New York, Elsevier, 1988
45. Davis JC, Hunt TK: Hyperbaric Oxygen Therapy. Bethesda, MD, Undersea Medical Society, 1986
46. Gabb G, Robin ED: Hyperbaric oxygen: A therapy in search of diseases. *Chest* 92:1074–1982, 1987
47. Davis JC: Hyperbaric oxygen therapy. *J Inten Care Med* 4:55–57, 1989
48. Grim PS, Gottlieb LJ, Boddie A, et al: Hyperbaric oxygen therapy. *JAMA* 263:2216–2220, 1990

Appendix: Health History Questionnaire

IMPORTANT INFORMATION FOR YOUR LUNG SPECIALIST

Dear Patient:

Your doctor has asked me to see you because of a possible lung problem. In order to help you with your difficulty, I must obtain a complete history.

Attached you will find questions about your breathing problem along with a general history.

Please fill these out as completely as possible. If you have difficulty, please ask a family member or nurse to assist you.

Thank you.

Pulmonary Disease Section
Oakwood Hospital

HEALTH HISTORY REVIEW HHR-1
Please Answer All Questions! 1/92

PATIENT
NAME ______________ AGE: ________ DATE: ________
IF SOMEONE OTHER THAN THE PATIENT HELPED FILL OUT THIS FORM:
WHAT IS YOUR NAME: ______________
RELATIONSHIP TO THE PATIENT ______________
What medical problem brought you to our hospital/clinic and why are you seeing a lung or sleep specialist?
____
____
____

Have you ever been evaluated by Doctor ______________ ? .... Yes__ No__ ?__
If so, When? ______________
__Do you have shortness of breath? .... Yes__ No__ ?__
If yes, how long? ______________
__If you have been more short of breath recently, when did it start? ______________
__When you were feeling your usual self a *few months* ago did any of the following make you short of breath?:
__Walking to the bathroom .... Yes__ No__ ?__
__Climbing a flight of stairs .... Yes__ No__ ?__
__Walking a block .... Yes__ No__ ?__
__Walking how far without being short of breath? ______________
__Do you wake up at night:
__Wheezing? .... Yes__ No__ ?__
__Short of breath? .... Yes__ No__ ?__
__How many pillows do you sleep on?
Check: ( ) One ( ) Two ( ) Three ( ) Four
__Do you wheeze or make musical sounds when you:
__Blow your air out at rest? .... Yes__ No__ ?__
__Exercise? .... Yes__ No__ ?__
__Get emotionally upset? .... Yes__ No__ ?__
__Enter cold air on a winter day? .... Yes__ No__ ?__
__How often do you wheeze? Check: ( ) Daily?; ( ) Once a week;
( ) Once a month; ( ) Rarely
__When you enter cold air, do you:
__Cough? .... Yes__ No__ ?__
__Become short of breath? .... Yes__ No__ ?__
__Have you had a fever lately? .... Yes__ No__ ?__
If you have a fever, when did it start? ______________ If yes, how many degrees? ______________
__Have you had chills lately? (The shakes or shivers) .... Yes__ No__ ?__
If so, when did they start? ______________
__Do you sweat at night? .... Yes__ No__ ?__
__Does it involve your whole body? .... Yes__ No__ ?__
__Does it just involve your upper body or neck? .... Yes__ No__ ?__
__How long have you had night sweats? ______________
__Have you ever coughed up blood? .... Yes__ No__ ?__
__If so, when was the last time you coughed up blood? ______________
__Was the blood streaked in your phlegm? .... Yes__ No__ ?__
__Were there blood clots in your phlegm? .... Yes__ No__ ?__
__How much blood did you cough up?
Check:
( ) Teaspoon or less?; ( ) Tablespoon or more?; ( ) Half a cup?;
( ) A cupful or more?

__Have you had a nosebleed lately? .... Yes__ No__ ?__
__Have you had a "cold" recently? .... Yes__ No__ ?__
If so, when did it start? ______________
__Have you had a sore throat recently? .... Yes__ No__ ?__
If so, when did it start? ______________
__Have you had a runny nose recently? .... Yes__ No__ ?__
If so, when did it start? ______________
__Have you had a stuffy nose recently? .... Yes__ No__ ?__
If so, when did it start? ______________
__Have you had a stuffy/runny nose more than three months out of the year? ... Yes__ No__ ?__
__Have you had an earache lately? .... Yes__ No__ ?__
If so, when did it start? ______________
__Do you have a chronic cough? .... Yes__ No__ ?__
__Have you developed a cough recently? .... Yes__ No__ ?__
__Has your cough increased lately? .... Yes__ No__ ?__
__Do you cough up phlegm? .... Yes__ No__ ?__
If so, what color is it? Check one or more:
( ) Clear ( ) White ( ) Yellow ( ) Green ( ) Brown ( ) Black
__Has your phlegm gotten thicker lately? .... Yes__ No__ ?__
__Are you coughing up <u>more</u> phlegm lately? .... Yes__ No__ ?__
__How much phlegm do you cough up in a day?
Check: ( ) A teaspoon or less?; ( )tablespoon or more?;
( ) A half cup?; ( ) A cupful or more?
__Do you cough when you drink fluids or eat solid foods? .... Yes__ No__ ?__
__Do you choke when you drink fluids or eat solid foods? .... Yes__ No__ ?__
__Do you have a hoarse voice? .... Yes__ No__ ?__
If so, when did it start? ______________
__Has your voice changed lately? .... Yes__ No__ ?__
If so, when did it start? ______________
__Do you have swollen ankles? .... Yes__ No__ ?__
__Do you have palpitations or unusual beats of your heart? .... Yes__ No__ ?__
__Do you ever get chest pain or discomfort? .... Yes__ No__ ?__
If yes, is the discomfort: Check all that apply:
( ) Aching?; ( ) Sharp?; ( ) Dull?; ( ) Burning?;
( ) Pressing or Contricting?
If yes, PLEASE ANSWER <u>ALL</u> OF THE FOLLOWING QUESTIONS:
__Do you get the chest discomfort when you exercise? .... Yes__ No__ ?__
What kind of exercise brings on the pain? (Check all that apply)
( ) Walking? ( ) Running? ( ) Climbing stairs? ( ) Having sex?
( ) Stooping over? ( ) Reaching over your head?
__Does the chest discomfort increase with breathing? .... Yes__ No__ ?__
__Does the chest discomfort increase with coughing? .... Yes__ No__ ?__
__Does the chest discomfort increase with twisting or turning of your body? ...... Yes__ No__ ?__
__When you get the discomfort, do you: (Check all that apply)
( ) Sweat? ( ) Get short of breath? ( ) Get scared?
__Does the chest discomfort go into your:
Check: ( ) Jaw ( ) Arm ( ) Back ( ) Stomach ( ) Shoulder
__When you get the discomfort is it always in the same place? .... Yes__ No__ ?__
__Does the pain awaken you from sleep? ______________
__Do any of the following relieve your discomfort? (Check one or more)
( ) Resting? ( ) Nitroglycerine? ( ) Antacids? ( ) Sitting Up?
__Was your chest pain ever evaluated by a doctor? .... Yes__ No__ ?__
What was the doctor's name? ______________
If so, what was the diagnosis? ______________
__Do you get heartburn regularly? .... Yes__ No__ ?__

PLEASE MARK THE SPOT
WHERE YOU HAVE THE MOST PAIN

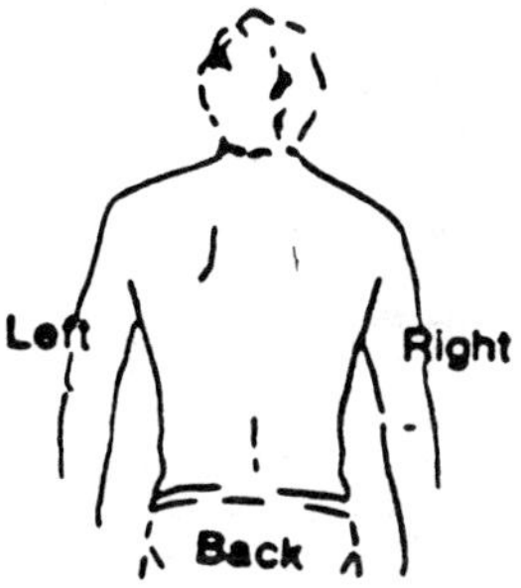
Left
Right
Back

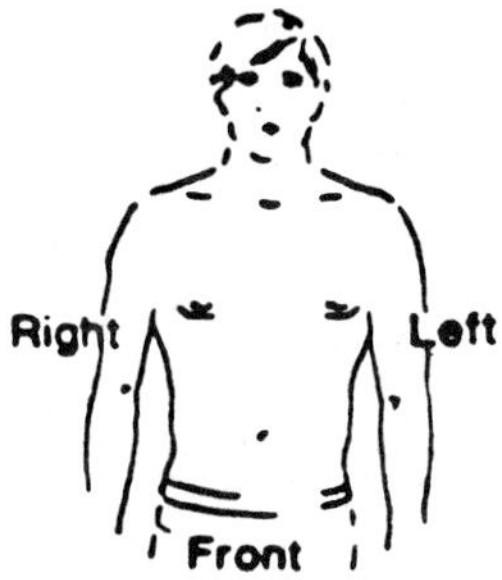
Right
Left
Front

Do you have any abnormal lumps or tumors? .... Yes No_ ?_
Do you have a decreased appetite? .... Yes No_ ?_
Have you lost weight in the last six (6) months? .... Yes No_ ?_
_What did you weigh one year ago? __________ pounds
_What do you weigh now? __________ pounds
Are you excessively sleepy? .... Yes No_ ?_
Have you ever fallen asleep while driving? .... Yes No_ ?_
Do people complain about your snoring? .... Yes No_ ?_
Are you depressed? .... Yes No_ ?_
Do you often feel like crying? .... Yes No_ ?_
Do you have recurrent thoughts of harming yourself? .... Yes No_ ?_
Have you ever seen a psychiatrist or counselor? .... Yes No_ ?_
Are you seeing a psychiatrist or counselor at the present time? .... Yes No_ ?_
Would you like to see a psychiatrist or counselor? .... Yes No_ ?_
Have you ever been told by your doctor or psychiatrist that you have any of the following illnesses: .... Yes No_ ?_
Check where appropriate:
( ) Depression?; ( ) Manic/depression?; ( ) Schizophrenia?;
( ) Nervous exhaustion?
_When was your last skin test for tuberculosis (TB)?
Date: __________ REACTION: Check: ( ) Positive? ( ) Negative?
_If you have ever had tuberculosis, what was the year of your diagnosis?
____

List below any medicines you have taken for tuberculosis and for how long:
Include pills or shots

MEDICINE	HOW OFTEN TAKEN DAILY	HOW LONG TAKEN (MO/YRS)
______	______	______
______	______	______
______	______	______

Have you ever been on a mechanical ventilation (life support) system? .... Yes No_ ?_
If so, how many times? __________ When? __________
If you have great trouble breathing do you wish to be placed on a life support system? .... Yes No_ ?_

LIST ANY OF YOUR PREVIOUS HOSPITALIZATIONS OR SURGERIES EXCEPT FOR NORMAL PREGNANCIES

Date(s)	Reason for Hospitalization	Name/Location	Name of Doctor

LIST HERE ANY DOCTORS YOU HAVE SEEN IN THE PAST FIVE YEARS

Date(s)	Reason	City	Name of Doctor

PAST MEDICAL AND FAMILY HISTORY

Please place an X in box beside any of your illnesses or your family's illnesses	Your Illness	Mother	Father	Your Grand-parents List by name				Your Children List by name					Your Brothers/ Sisters List by name				Your Aunts/ Uncles List by name		
				1.	2.	3.	4.	1.	2.	3.	4.	5.	1.	2.	3.	4.	1.	2.	3.
Present Age																			
Age at Death (if deceased)																			
Cancer																			
Diabetes																			
High Blood Pressure																			
Heart Failure (CHF)																			
Heart Attack (Myocardial Infarction)																			
Angina																			
Rheumatic Fever																			
Ulcers																			
Thyroid Problems																			
Arthritis																			
Gout																			
Liver Disease/Cirrhosis Yellow Jaundice/Hepatitis																			
Allergies																			
Emphysema																			
Asthma																			
Tuberculosis																			
Convulsions (Epilepsy/Fits)																			
Nerve Disease (Polio, MS)																			
Alzheimer's																			
Stroke																			
Mental Illness																			
Suicide Attempt																			
Drug Abuse																			
Alcoholism																			
Bleeding Disorder																			
AIDS/Exposed to AIDS																			
Gonorrhea																			
Syphilis																			

PLACE AN X IN BOX BESIDE ANY OF YOUR MEDICAL PROBLEMS

PROBLEM	YES	NO	DATES
PNEUMONIA How many times have you had pneumonia? ________ Date of last episode			
BRONCHITIS How many times have you had bronchitis? ________ Date of last episode			
THROMBOPHLEBITIS in legs (Blood clot in the veins)			
PULMONARY EMBOLUS (Blood clots in lung)			
HIATAL HERNIA			
REFLUX ESOPHAGITIS (Heartburn)			
BLACK LUNG DISEASE			
Measles Whooping Cough			
THYROID PROBLEMS Low thyroid Yes___ No___ Hyperactive thyroid Yes___ No___			
ANEMIA (Low Blood)			
HEART MURMUR			
BLEEDING ULCERS			
BLOOD TRANSFUSIONS			
DIVERTICULITIS			
COLITIS			
MIGRAINE			
GLAUCOMA			
CATARACTS			
ECZEMA			
KIDNEY STONES			
KIDNEY INFECTIONS			

PLEASE LIST ANY ALLERGIES OR REACTIONS TO MEDICINE

NAME OF MEDICINE	REACTION (rash, wheezing, etc)	DATE

If you need more space to list your allergies or reactions to medicine, please use the back of this sheet.

LIST BELOW ANY MEDICINE YOU ARE NOW TAKING:
(Please include all vitamins, aspirin, pain remedies, laxatives and tranquilizers)

Name of Medicine	Dose (mg)	How Often Taken?	Date Started

Do you use home oxygen?	Yes___ No___	If so, how many liters per minute?________
Do you use a breathing machine (IPPB or nebulizer) at home?	Yes___ No___	If so, how often? ________________
Have you ever had chemotherapy for cancer?	Yes___ No___	If yes, when? ________________
Have you ever had radiation for cancer?	Yes___ No___	If yes, when? ________________

If you need more space to list your medicines, use the back of this sheet.

DO YOU USE ANY OF THE FOLLOWING INHALERS:

INHALER	COLOR		HOW MANY PUFFS?	HOW MANY TIMES A DAY?
ATROVENT	GREEN AND WHITE	Yes___ No___	______	______
BRETHAIRE	YELLOW AND WHITE	Yes___ No___	______	______
ALUPENT	BLUE AND WHITE	Yes___ No___	______	______
PROVENTIL	SOLID YELLOW	Yes___ No___	______	______
VENTOLIN	SOLID BLUE	Yes___ No___	______	______
VANCERIL	SOLID PINK	Yes___ No___	______	______
AZMACORT	SOLID WHITE	Yes___ No___	______	______

HAVE YOU HAD ANY OF THE FOLLOWING LAB TESTS IN THE PAST FIVE (5) YEARS?

TEST	WHAT HOSPITAL OR CLINIC	ORDERING DOCTOR	DATE OF EXAM
GASTROINTESTINAL SERIES			
CAT SCAN OF CHEST			
CAT SCAN OF ABDOMEN			
MRI EXAM			
BLOOD COUNT			
BLOOD CHEMISTRY			
BARIUM ENEMA			
SIGMOIDOSCOPY			
HOLTER MONITOR (device to check your heart beat for 24 hours)			
BRONCHOSCOPY (lighted tube to look at chest and lungs)			
CHEST TUBE (to obtain fluid or air from your chest)			
PULMONARY FUNCTION TESTS			
GASTROSCOPY (lighted tube to look at the stomach)			
MAMMOGRAM			
2D ECHOCARDIOGRAM (probe placed on the heart)			
NUCLEAR SCAN OF HEART (MUGA)			

SOCIAL AND WORK HISTORY
(Please answer all questions)

Marital Status: S M D W (Please circle one)
How many times have you been married? ______
Religious Preference (Optional) ______
RESIDENCES (State or Country): Location(s) as a child– ______
Location(s) as an adult– ______
PRESENT LIVING SITUATION: check: ( ) With Family ( ) Relatives
( ) Friends ( ) Nursing Home ( ) Alone

	Yes No Unsure
__Do you drive a car?	Yes__ No__ ?__
If not, please explain ______	
__Have you ever smoked cigarettes?	Yes__ No__ ?__
If yes:	
How old were you when you had your first cigarette? ______	
How old were you when you had your last cigarette? ______	
When did you have your last cigarette? ______	
How many packs of cigarettes per day did you smoke when you smoked the most, such as at a party? ______	
__Have you ever smoked a pipe?	Yes__ No__ ?__
If yes:	
What was the greatest number of pipes full of tobacco you smoked when you smoked the most? ______	
__Have you ever smoked cigars?	Yes__ No__ ?__
If yes: What was the greatest number of cigars you ever smoked in a day? ______	
__Have you ever had a problem with drinking alcohol?	Yes__ No__ ?__
__When was your last alcoholic drink? (date) ______	
__How many drinks containing alcohol do you drink in a 24 hour period?	

	Weekday	Weekend
Cans of beer	______	______
Glasses of	______	______
Shots of liquor	______	______

__Do you drink much less alcohol now than in the past?	Yes__ No__ ?__
__Do you think you drink too much or feel guilty about drinking?	Yes__ No__ ?__
__Do you drink by yourself?	Yes__ No__ ?__
__Have you been drinking more alcoholic beverages lately?	Yes__ No__ ?__
__Have you had a drunk driving charge?	Yes__ No__ ?__
__How many cups of coffee do you drink per day? ( ) Regular ____ ( ) Decaf ____	
__How many cups of tea do you drink per day? ( ) Regular ____ ( ) Decaf ____	
__Have you ever had a problem with the following drugs? Check: ( ) Sleeping pills? ( ) Heroin? ( ) Cocaine? ( ) Diet pills? ( ) Marijuana?	
__Do you drink more than two soft drinks a day?	Yes__ No__ ?__

__What is, or was your main line of work? ______
__What is, or was your spouse's main line of work? ______
__If you are not presently working: Check one or more:
( ) Are you retired?; ( ) Are you laid off?; ( ) Have you been recently fired?; ( ) Do you receive workman's compensation?;
( ) Are you on disability?
Date any of the above started ______
__If you are on workman's compensation or disability,
please list the reason(s): ______
______
______

IF YOU HAVE HAD ANY OF THESE JOBS/CLASSIFICATIONS, PLEASE CHECK ( ):

( ) ABRASIVE WORKER
( ) ALLOY MAKER
( ) AMMUNITION WORKER
( ) ASBESTOS WORKER
( ) AUTO MECHANIC
( ) BRAKE WORKER
( ) BRICK MAKER/LAYER
( ) CARPENTER
( ) CERAMICS WORKER
( ) COAL MINER
( ) CONSTRUCTION WORKER
( ) COSMETIC WORKER
( ) CUTTING TOOL WORKER
( ) DYNAMITE WORKER
( ) ENAMELLER
( ) FLAME CUTTER
( ) FLUORESCENT LAMP WORKER
( ) FOUNDRYMAN
( ) GLASS MAKER
( ) GRINDER
( ) INSULATION WORKER
( ) METALIZER
( ) MILL WORKER
( ) MINER
( ) NEON SIGN MAKER
( ) NUCLEAR ENERGY WORKER
( ) PAPER MAKER
( ) POLISHER
( ) POTTER
( ) QUARRY MAN
( ) ROOFER
( ) RUBBER WORKER
( ) SANDBLASTER
( ) SHIP BUILDER
( ) SHOT BLASTER
( ) STEAM FITTER
( ) STONE WORKER
( ) SUGAR CANE WORKER
( ) WALL BOARD WORKER
( ) WELDER
( ) WELL DRILLER
( ) X-RAY TUBE MAKER

—Have you ever had problems with the police or law? ( ) Yes ( ) No
If yes, what was the reason?
____

—Are you having financial difficulties? ( ) Yes ( ) No
If yes, please explain ________________________________

—Do you have any of the following pets? (Check all that apply)
( ) Dog ( ) Cat ( ) Bird ( ) Other–What kind of Pet? ______________

Index

The abbreviations f and t stand for figure and table, respectively.

A-a gradient. *See* Alveolar-arterial gradient
Abbreviations, 20t
Abdominal pain, in pneumonia, 352
Abdominal surgery, pleural fluid collections seen after, 294
Abscess(es), 367. *See also* Lung abscess(es)
  epiglottic, 340
  subdiaphragmatic, 299–300
  subphrenic, 299–300
Acceleration/deceleration injury, 401–402
Acebutolol
  cough caused by, 68
  effects on sleep, 448t, 448–449
Acetaminophen, for common cold, 334–335
Acetazolamide, in treatment of acute mountain sickness, 523
Acetylcysteine, 71, 126, 151
Achalasia, 97–98
  tests and findings with, 98t
  treatment of, 98–99
Acid-fast bacilli. *See also Mycobacterium*
  staining for, 391–392
Acquired immunodeficiency syndrome. *See also* Human immunodeficiency virus, infection
  adenovirus infection in, radiographic pattern of, 363t
  mycobacteria causing disease in, 383
  pulmonary disease in, 361–362, 363t
  pulmonary manifestations of, 361–362
Actinobifida dichotomica, hypersensitivity pneumonitis caused by, 309t
Actinomycetes, thermophilic, hypersensitivity pneumonitis caused by, 309t
Activated partial thromboplastin time, 166
Acute mountain sickness, 521–524
Adenocarcinoma, 194f, 410
Adenosine, in asthma, 108t, 109
Adenovirus III, atypical pneumonia syndrome caused by, 360
Adenovirus IV, atypical pneumonia syndrome caused by, 360
Adenovirus VII, atypical pneumonia syndrome caused by, 360
Adenovirus infection, 332, 340
  in acquired immunodeficiency syndrome, radiographic pattern of, 363t
  detection of, 366
Adenylcyclase, 119
Adolescents, with asthma, 131
Adrenergic agents
  for asthma, 119–121
  for chronic obstructive pulmonary disease, 151
α-Adrenergic agonists, effects on sleep, 448t, 448–449
β_2-Adrenergic agonists, 119
  for asthma, 127–128
  side effects of, 120
β-Adrenergic blockers
  cough caused by, 68
  effects on sleep, 448t, 448–449
Adrenergic receptors, 119
Adult respiratory distress syndrome, with alveolar hemorrhage, 82
Advanced sleep-phase syndrome, 471
Adventitial sounds, 46
AeroBid. *See* Flunisolide metered dose inhaler
Aerosol-perfusion scans, 180
Aerosols, radiolabeled, lung scans with, 180
Affective illness
  bipolar, abnormal sleepiness with, 442
  insomnia in, 468–469
Age, and incidence of pulmonary embolus, 159
Aged. *See* Elderly
Agitation, of acute epiglottitis, 337
AIDS. *See* Acquired immunodeficiency syndrome
Air bronchograms, 500f, 501, 502f
Air embolus, 157. *See also* Gas embolism
Airflow, plateau effect of, 12
Airflow limitation
  equal pressure point model for, 12f, 12–13
  waterfall model of, 13, 13f
  wavespeed model of, 13, 13f
Air pollution, 116
  in etiology of lung cancer, 408
  and respiratory morbidity and mortality, 140–141
Air travel, for patients with chronic lung disease, 323, 525–526

Airway management, in epiglottitis, 339–340
Airway obstruction, in asthma, 105–106, 109
Airway opening, pressure at, 7f
Airway resistance, and time constants, 11
Airway smooth muscle, 106
Albuterol
  for asthma, 120
  effects on sleep, 468
  inhaled, 120
  powdered, patient-controlled inhalation of, 319
  in pulmonary function testing, 37
Alcohol, effects on sleep, 447, 464
Alcoholism, insomnia in, 469–470
Aldomet. *See* Methyldopa
Alkylating agents
  lung disease due to, 212–213
  for sarcoidosis, 235
Allergic bronchopulmonary aspergillosis, 130, 236–237
Allergy evaluation, of asthmatic patients, 113–114, 127–128
Allodynia, 100
Alpha motoneurons, 55–56
Alpha-1 protease inhibitor
  deficiency, 143–144, 148
  replacement therapy with, 144–145
Alprazolam, elimination half-life, 450t
ALS. *See* Amyotrophic lateral sclerosis
Alternaria, hypersensitivity pneumonitis caused by, 309t
Altitude
  adaptation to, 519–521, 520f
    abnormal, 521
  barometric pressure relative to, 526, 527t
  ventilatory response to, 519, 520f
Altitude-aggravated illness, 525
Aluminosis, 309
Alupent. *See* Metaproterenol
Alveolar air equation, 15
Alveolar-arterial gradient, 15–16
  in sarcoidosis, 225
Alveolar dead space, with pulmonary embolus, 175
Alveolar hemorrhage syndromes, 81–82
Alveolar hypoxia, vasoconstriction with, 14
Alveolar macrophages
  in asthma, 107
  in idiopathic pulmonary fibrosis, 200–201
  in sarcoidosis, 232
Alveolar oxygen tension, 15
  in acute bronchial asthma, 113
  calculation of, 15
Alveolar pressure, and blood flow, 14
Alveolitis
  with collagen vascular disease, 205
  in idiopathic pulmonary fibrosis, 196–197, 200
  with progressive systemic sclerosis, 208
  in sarcoidosis, 232
  with Sjögren's syndrome, 205
Alveolus(i)
  pressure inside, 7f
  unequal sized, stabilization, 5f, 5–6, 6f
Alzheimer's disease, sleep changes in, 468
Amantadine, 320, 335
Amebiasis, diaphragmatic, 300
American Thoracic Society, standards for spirometry, 23
Aminoglycosides
  indications for, 371
  neuromuscular paralysis caused by, 298
  use in pregnancy, 481, 486t
Aminophylline
  intravenous, 122
    for acute bronchial asthma, 128
  rectal solutions of, 123
Amiodarone, pulmonary toxicity, 68, 214–215
Amitriptyline, sedation with, 449
Amniotic fluid embolism, 157, 165
  deaths from, 483
  diagnosis of, 483
  incidence of, 483
  risk factors for, 483
  therapy for, 483
Amoxicillin
  indications for, 370
  use in pregnancy, 481
Amoxicillin/clavulanic acid, indications for, 370
Amphetamines, effects on sleep, 468
Ampicillin
  indications for, 370
  resistance, 369
  use in pregnancy, 481
AMS. *See* Acute mountain sickness
Amyotrophic lateral sclerosis, 274–275
  respiratory failure in, 297
Anaerobic metabolism, 55, 57
Anaerobic pleuropulmonary infection, 360–361
  antibiotic therapy for, 370–371
Analgesics, effects on sleep, 447–448, 450
Anaphylactic reactions, versus asthma, 115
Anemia
  with alveolar hemorrhage, 81
  dyspnea with, 59
  with hemoptysis, 76
Anesthesia, complications of, 489–490
Angina pectoris, 91–92
  differential diagnosis of, 101–102

Angiography. *See also* Pulmonary angiography
  coronary, in diagnosis of chest pain, 95
Angiotensin converting enzyme, in sarcoidosis, 229, 231–232
Angiotensin-converting enzyme inhibitors, cough with, 68
Ankylosing spondylitis, 49, 269–270
  pulmonary manifestations of, 269–270
  treatment of, 270
Annular plaques, 47
Annulospiral body, 55
Anthrax, 354t
Antibiotics
  for common cold, 335
  for epiglottitis, 340
  for lung abscess, 370–371
  for tracheitis, 343
  use of
    in chronic lung disease, 320
    in pregnancy, 485, 486t
Anticholinergics
  for chronic obstructive pulmonary disease, 151
  for common cold, 334
Anticholinesterase agents, for myasthenia gravis, 277
Anticoagulants
  and alveolar hemorrhage, 82
  hemoptysis with, 76
Anticoagulation. *See also* Heparin, therapy with
  for prophylaxis of deep venous thrombosis, 165–169
  with warfarin, 168, 171–172
Anticonvulsants, effects on sleep, 447–449
Antidepressants, effects on sleep, 447–448, 468
Antihistamines
  in asthma treatment, 126
  for common cold, 333, 334t
  effects on sleep, 447–448
Antihypertensives, effects on sleep, 447–449, 448t, 468
Anti-inflammatory agents, for sarcoidosis, 234–235
Antiplatelet agents
  in deep venous thrombosis prophylaxis, 168–169
  hemoptysis with, 76
Antipsychotic medications, effects on sleep, 450
α1-Antitrypsin, 143–144
Antituberculosis drugs, 392, 392t. *See also specific drug*
  second-line, 393t
Antitussives, 70–71, 71t, 335
Antiviral therapy, for common cold, 335t, 335–336
Anxiety disorders, insomnia with, 469
Anxiolytics, effects on sleep, 447–449
Aortic aneurysm
  chest pain with, 95
  pericardial, 418
Aortic stenosis
  chest pain with, 93
  congenital, 93
  etiology of, 93
Apresoline. *See* Hydralazine
APTT. *See* Activated partial thromboplastin time
Arachidonic acid, in asthma, 108, 108t
Arrhythmias
  in carbon monoxide poisoning, 305
  dyspnea with, 58
  with pericardial disease, 95
Arterial blood gases
  in acute asthma, 113
  with community-acquired pneumonia, 353
  obtaining, in children, 342
Arterial carbon dioxide tension, 15
  in acute bronchial asthma, 113
  elevated, 16
Arteriovenous malformations, pulmonary, 77, 82
AS. *See* Ankylosing spondylitis
Asbestos
  actinolite, 310
  amosite, 310
  amphibole, 310
  anthrophyllite, 310, 312
  chrysotile, 310, 312
  crocidolite, 310, 312
  neoplasms related to, 312
  physical properties of, 310
  serpentine, 310
  tremolite, 310
Asbestos bodies, 310, 310f
Asbestosis, 309–313
  diagnosis of, 311–312
  pleural effusions with, 311
Ascites, in cirrhotic patients, 289–290
Aspergillosis, allergic bronchopulmonary, 130, 236–237
Aspergillus, hypersensitivity pneumonitis caused by, 309t
Aspiration, of oropharyngeal contents, 348, 360
Aspiration pneumonia, 360–361
  anaerobic, antibiotic therapy for, 370–371
  chest x-ray with, 501, 504f
Aspiration syndrome, 69
Aspirin
  and asthma, 117
  for common cold, 334–335

Aspirin—Continued
  for deep venous thrombosis prophylaxis, 168–169
Aspirin hypersensitivity, 139
Aspirin triad, 117–118
Asthma, 105–131, 140f. *See also* Obstructive airway disease
  acute, 128
    emergency treatment of, 125
  adolescents with, 131
  adrenergic drugs for, 119–121
  adult-onset, 110
  after exercise, 128–129
  β_2-agonists for, 127
  airway obstruction of, 105–106, 109
  allergic factors in, 116
  allergy evaluation and therapy for, 113–114, 127–128
  anatomic elements in, 106
  and atopy, 113–114
    in childhood, 110
  atropine and related drugs for, 124
  and breast feeding, 480
  bronchoprovocation for, 37
  cardinal symptoms of, 68
  cellular changes in, 109
  cellular elements in, 107t, 107–108
  challenge testing in, 113
  chest pain with, 111
  chest radiography in, 113
  chief complaint with, 110–111
  childhood, 131
    outcome of, 110
  and chronic eosinophilic pneumonia, 236
  corticosteroids for, 124–127
  cough variant, 68–69
  cough with, 69
  cromolyn sodium for, 123–124, 127
  definition of, 139
  differential diagnosis of, 36
    in adults, 115
    in children, 114–115
  versus diffuse pulmonary disease, 115
  and diving, 529
  dyspnea with, 58, 110–111
  early-onset, 110
  early response in, 106
  end-expiratory grunt of, 111–112
  ephedrine for, 120
  esophageal dysfunction and, 118
  exercise and, 117, 128–129
  extrinsic, 110
  factitious, 115
  factors associated with, 115–118
  forced expiratory volume in 1 second in, 106
  gastroesophageal reflux and, 118
  gross pathology of, 109–110
  history-taking with, 110–111
  hormonal effects modulating, 118
  immunotherapy for, 127–128
  and infection, 116
  versus interstitial fibrosis, 115
  intrinsic, 110
  ipratropium bromide for, 124, 127
  laboratory findings in, 112–114
  versus laryngotracheobronchitis, 111–112, 114
  late or delayed phase of, 106
  long-term considerations with, 131
  management of, in pregnancy, 479–480
  manifestation of, 110–114
  mediators involved in, 108t, 108–109
  medical approach to, 127–128
  medications and, 117
  medications for, 118–127, 119t
  and menses, 118
  methylxanthines for, 121–123
  morbidity of, 105
  mortality due to, 105
  mucus in, 109, 113, 114f, 126
  natural history of, 110
  nocturnal, 129–130
  occult, 37
  occupational, 130–131
    bronchoprovocation studies for, 112
  passive smoking and, 118
  pathophysiology of, 105–109
  patient education about, 131
  pets and, 118
  physical factors in, 116
  physical findings in, 111–112
  prednisone for, 127
  in pregnancy, 478–480
  prevalence of, 105
  pulmonary function testing in, 112
  recurrent, nocturnal pattern of, 106
  respiratory failure in, 111–112
  response to bronchodilators in, 36
  smoking and, 116
  spirometry in, 112
  sputum of patient with, 113
  stress and, 116–117
  theophylline for, 121–123, 127
  treatment of, 118
  triggers of, 115, 115t
    avoidance of, 118
  ventilation-perfusion abnormalities in, 110, 113
  wheezing with, 110–111

Atelectasis, 49, 175
chest radiography/roentgenography with, 509, 509f
plate-like, 509f
postoperative, 294
radiographic findings with, 509, 509f
rounded, 509
total, of right lung, 509f
Atenolol
cough caused by, 68
effects on sleep, 448t, 448–449, 468
Ativan. *See* Lorazepam
Atopy, 139
and asthma, 110, 113–114
and chronic eosinophilic pneumonia, 236
Atropine and related drugs, for asthma, 124
Atrovent. *See* Ipratropium bromide
ATS. *See* American Thoracic Society
Atypical pneumonia syndrome, 353, 355–356
caused by adenovirus, 360
clinical features of, 355t
Aureobasidium pullulans, hypersensitivity pneumonitis caused by, 309t
Auscultation, of chest, 45–46
Azathioprine
for idiopathic pulmonary fibrosis, 202–203
for myasthenia gravis, 277
plus corticosteroids, for idiopathic pulmonary fibrosis, 202–203
for sarcoidosis, 235
Azithromycin, indications for, 370–371
Azmacort. *See* Triamcinolone metered dose inhaler

Bacille Calmette-Guérin, 396
Bactec system, 391
Bacteremia, epiglottitis with, 340
Bacterial tracheitis
clinical features of, 338t, 342–343
complications of, 343
diagnosis of, 343
epidemiology of, 342
etiology of, 342
management of, 343
morbidity of, 343
BAL. *See* Bronchoalveolar lavage
Balloon tamponade, for massive life-threatening hemoptysis, 86
Bamboo spine, 269, 269f
Barometric pressure, relative to altitude, 526, 527t
Barotrauma
otologic, 527–529, 528f
pulmonary, 529
Barrett's esophagitis, 98
Bayes' theorem, 181
BCG. *See* Bacille Calmette-Guérin
Becker's dystrophy, 277–278
Beclomethasone metered dose inhaler, 126
Beclovent. *See* Beclomethasone metered dose inhaler
Bed partner interview, 464–465
Bed rest, and deep venous thrombosis, 158
Belladonna, 124
Bellows, as lung analogy, 2, 2f
Benzodiazepines
for chronic insomnia, 473
daytime side effects of, 473
effects on sleep, 449
elimination half-life, 450t
Benzonatate
commercial preparations of, 71t
dosage, 71t
side effects of, 71t
Bernoulli phenomenon, 13
Bernstein's test, 98
Beryllosis, 310
Beta human chorionic gonadotropin, 412
Bibasilar end-inspiratory (Velcro) rales, 195
Bilateral hilar lymphadenopathy, 223–224
in granulomatous infections, 228
in mycoses, 228
in sarcoidosis, 222–223
significance of, 228–229
in tuberculosis, 228
Biologic clock, 430–434
Biomarker profiles, in lung cancer, 412, 413t
Biopsy. *See also* Lung biopsy; Percutaneous fine needle aspiration biopsy; Transbronchial lung biopsy
bone marrow, in small-cell carcinoma staging, 412
endobronchial, bleeding with, 83
of sarcoidosis, 226–228
Bipolar affective disorder, abnormal sleepiness with, 442
Bitolterol, for asthma, 120
Bleeding. *See also* Alveolar hemorrhage syndrome; Hemoptysis
with endobronchial biopsy, 83
with heparin therapy, 167–168, 170–171, 182–183
with streptokinase, 173, 183–184
with transbronchial lung biopsy, 83
Bleomycin
chronic interstitial pneumonitis/fibrosis caused by, 212
hypersensitivity pneumonitis with, 212

Bleomycin—Continued
  pleural effusions with, 212
  pulmonary toxicity, 68, 212
Blocadren. *See* Timolol
Blood dyscrasias, with alveolar hemorrhage, 82
Blunt chest trauma, 401–405
  with alveolar hemorrhage, 82
  deaths from, 401
  historic perspective on, 401
  mechanisms of, 401–402
  morbidity or disability from, 401
BO. *See* Bronchiolitis obliterans
Bochdalek hernia, 297
Body box. *See* Body plethysmography
Body plethysmography, 38
Bone marrow biopsy, in small-cell carcinoma staging, 412
Bone tumor, chest pain with, 100
BOOP. *See* Bronchiolitis obliterans and organizing pneumonia
Boyle's law, 38, 527
Brachytherapy, 86
  of lung cancer, 413
Bradykinin, in asthma, 108, 108t
Branhamella catarrhalis
  culture, 365
  pneumonia, 354
    antibiotic therapy for, 370
Breast cancer
  lung metastasis, radiographic findings with, 514f
  metastatic, superior vena cava syndrome caused by, 418
Breast feeding, asthma and, 480
Breathing retraining, 320–321
Breath sounds, 44, 46
  vesicular, 45–46
  and vocal resonance, 46
Brethine. *See* Terbutaline
Bricanyl. *See* Terbutaline
Bronchial artery embolus, 78, 86
Bronchial asthma. *See* Asthma
Bronchiectasis, 140f
  computed tomography of, 79
  cough in, 66
  definition of, 139
  hemoptysis with, 73–74, 79
  parapneumonic pleural effusions with, 292
  therapy for, 79
Bronchiolitis obliterans
  bronchoalveolar lavage with, 219–221
  chest radiography with, 217–219, 218f
  clinical findings with, 217
  corticosteroids for, 221–222
  definition of, 217
  fiberoptic bronchoscopy with, 219–221
  histopathology of, 219, 220f
  incidence of, 217
  nomenclature, 217
  physical examination with, 217
  prednisone for, 221–222
  pulmonary function testing with, 219
  reticulonodular and nodular infiltrates in, 218, 218f
  therapy for, 221–222
Bronchiolitis obliterans and organizing pneumonia, 205
  chest radiography in, 218, 218f
  differential diagnosis of, 232
  etiology of, 221
  histopathology of, 219, 220f
  incidence of, 217
  versus interstitial pulmonary fibrosis, 219
  pathogenesis of, 221
  pulmonary function testing with, 219
  therapy for, 221–222
Bronchioloalveolar cell carcinoma, in progressive systemic sclerosis, 207
Bronchitis. *See* Chronic bronchitis
Bronchoalveolar lavage
  with bronchiolitis obliterans, 219–221
  in chronic eosinophilic pneumonia, 239
  with collagen vascular disease, 205–206
  in idiopathic and CVD-associated pulmonary fibrosis, 205
  in idiopathic pulmonary fibrosis, 200–202
  with interstitial lung disease, 193
  in progressive systemic sclerosis, 207–208
  in pulmonary alveolar proteinosis, 252
  with rheumatoid interstitial lung disease, 206–207
  in sarcoidosis, 229–231
Bronchoconstriction, in asthma, 109
  pathways to, 109, 109t
Bronchodilators
  effects on sleep, 468
  methylxanthine, safety in pregnancy, 479
  response to, 36
  sympathomimetic, safety in pregnancy, 479
  in treatment of chronic obstructive pulmonary disease, 151
Bronchogenic carcinoma, 414
  chest radiography with, 67
  cough with, 66–67
  hemoptysis with, 67, 80–81
  histologic types of, 410
  and pleural effusions, 290–291
  superior vena cava syndrome caused by, 418

Broncholithiasis, on chest roentgenography, 75
Bronchophony, 46
Bronchopneumonia, chest x-ray in, 500, 501f
Bronchopneumonic infiltrates, 367
Bronchoprovocation, 21t, 26, 37–38, 112–113
Bronchoscopy. *See also* Fiberoptic bronchoscopy
  in assessing chronic cough, 70
  in diagnosis of neoplastic disorders, 81
  with hemoptysis, 76–77
  hemoptysis with, 83
  indications for, 85–86
  rigid, 77
  with tuberculosis, 79
Bronchospasm, in asthma, 106
Bronkometer. *See* Isoetharine
Bronkosol. *See* Isoetharine
Brucellosis, 354t
Building-related illness, 116
Bullae, 143, 148
Busulfan
  lung disease due to, 212–213
  pleural effusions with, 212

Caffeine, 121
  in beverages, 468, 469t
  effects on sleep, 447, 468
  in nonprescription drugs, 468, 469t
Calcifications
  on chest radiography/roentgenography, 75, 510f
  computed tomography of, 510
Cancer. *See also* Breast cancer; Bronchogenic carcinoma; Carcinoma; Esophageal cancer; Lung cancer
  asbestos-related, 312
Candida albicans, in acquired immunodeficiency syndrome, radiographic pattern of, 363t
Capreomycin, 393t
  side effects of, 396
Captopril, cough associated with, 68
Carbenicillin, use in pregnancy, 481
Carbon monoxide
  environmental exposure to, 305
  half-life of, 306
  occupational exposure to, 305–306
  poisoning, 305
    hyperbaric oxygen therapy for, 530
    treatment of, 306
Carboxyhemoglobin levels, and their corresponding symptoms, 305, 306t
Carcinoembryonic antigen, 412
Carcinoids, bronchial, hemoptysis with, 81
Carcinoma. *See also* Adenocarcinoma; Bronchogenic carcinoma; Cancer; Non–small-cell carcinoma; Small-cell carcinoma
  bronchioloalveolar cell, in progressive systemic sclerosis, 207
  large-cell, 410
  laryngeal, cough with, 67
  in situ, evaluation for, 85
  squamous cell, 410
Cardiac disease
  dyspnea in, 57–58
  orthopnea of, 60
Cardiac output, 57
Cardiac silhouette, cephalization, radiographic appearance of, 515f, 515
Cardiac size, 498–499
Cardiopulmonary exercise test, 21t, 39
Carmustine, interstitial pneumonitis/fibrosis associated with, 213
Cataplexy
  misdiagnosed as epileptic disorder, 449
  of narcolepsy, 445
Catapres. *See* Clonidine
Catheter-related pulmonary embolus, 164–165
Catheter thrombosis, prevention of, 169–170
Cavitary lesions, on chest radiography/roentgenography, 75, 512f
Cavitation, of necrotizing pneumonia, 353
Cefazolin, indications for, 370
Central nervous system dysfunction, insomnia with, 468
Central venous catheter
  complications of, 164
  venous thrombosis with, 169–170
Cephalosporin
  indications for, 370–371
  use in pregnancy, 481, 486t
Cervical spinal cord injuries, 273–274
Cervical spine disease, chest wall pain with, 100
C fiber receptors, 54, 54f
Challenge testing, in asthma, 113
Chalone, 336
Charcot-Leyden crystals, 113
Chemoreceptors, 65
  central, 53
  peripheral, 53, 54f, 56f
Chemotactic factors, in asthma, 108, 108t
Chemotherapy, for lung cancer, 413
Chest. *See also* Blunt chest trauma
  computed tomography of, 78–79
  crush injury to, 402
  diagrammatic view of, seen from back, 44f
  palpation of, 45
Chest clapping. *See* Chest physiotherapy
Chest discomfort. *See* Chest pain

Chest pain, 60, 91–102
  anginal, 91–92
    versus nonanginal, 101–102
  with anxiety disorders, 100
  with aortic stenosis, 93
  with arm movement, 102
  with asbestosis, 311
  with asthma, 110–111
  atypical, 92, 95, 100–101
  with bone tumor, 100
  cardiovascular causes of, 91–95, 102
  causes of, 91, 92t
  with eosinophilic granuloma, 242
  of esophageal origin, 97t, 97–99, 102
  evaluation of, 97
    computer-assisted programs for, 102
  in gastroesophageal reflux disease, 97–98
  gastrointestinal causes of, 97–99
    nonesophageal, 99
  history-taking with, 95
  with idiopathic hypertrophic subaortic stenosis, 93
  with inspiration, 102
  location of, 91
  with mitral stenosis, 93–94
  with mitral valve prolapse, 93–94
  of musculoskeletal origin, 99
  neuromuscular causes of, 99–100
  pathophysiology of, 91
  with pericardial disease, 94–95
  pleuritic, 94–95, 293
    in AIDS patients, 362
    with mixed connective tissue disease, 210
    with pleural effusion, 286
    in progressive systemic sclerosis, 207
    in pulmonary alveolar proteinosis, 249
  in pneumonia, 352
  psychosomatic causes of, 102
  pulmonary causes of, 95–97, 102
  with pulmonary embolus, 96, 174
  with valvular heart disease, 93
Chest physiotherapy, 318, 322–323
Chest radiography/roentgenography, 60
  in asthma, 113
  with atelectasis, 509, 509f, 509, 509f
  with bronchiolitis obliterans, 217–219, 218f
  in bronchiolitis obliterans and organizing pneumonia, 218, 218f
  with bronchogenic carcinoma, 67
  in broncholithiasis, 75
  in bronchopneumonia, 500, 501f
  calcifications on, 510f
  with cavitary lesions, 75, 512f
  in chronic eosinophilic pneumonia, 237, 238f
  with chronic obstructive pulmonary disease, 147–148, 513–515, 515f
  with coagulopathy, 75
  in community-acquired pneumonia, 353
  versus computed tomography, 78–79
  in congestive heart failure, 288, 515–516, 515f–516f
  in drug-induced chronic interstitial pneumonitis/fibrosis, 211
  in emphysema, 513–515, 515f
  with eosinophilic granuloma, 242–244, 243f
  with Goodpasture's syndrome, 75
  with granuloma, 510f
  with hamartoma, 510f
  with hemoptysis, 74t, 75–76
  with hilar neoplasm, 513f
  with Hodgkin's disease, 514f
  with idiopathic hemosiderosis, 75
  in idiopathic pulmonary fibrosis, 195–196, 196f
  interpretation of, 497–516
  lateral view, 497, 498f
  with lung abscess, 501–504, 505f
  with lymphangioleiomyomatosis, 254–255
  with malignant cavitary neoplasm, 512f
  with malignant nodule, 511f
  with mixed connective tissue disease, 210
  with neoplasia, 509–512
  oblique views, 497
  with obstructive airway disease, 515, 515f
  and perfusion scan, clinical utility of, 179
  with pleural effusions, 504–506
  with *Pneumocystis carinii* pneumonia, 362
  in pneumonia, 499–501, 501f–504f
  with pneumothorax, 506–509, 507f–508f
  posteroanterior view, 497, 498f
  in pulmonary alveolar proteinosis, 250, 251f
  with pulmonary edema, 515–516, 516f
  with pulmonary embolus, 75, 175
  with pulmonary hypertension, 186
  in sarcoidosis, 222, 223f, 223–225
  in small-cell carcinoma, 412
  of solitary pulmonary nodule, 415, 510, 510f
  technique for, 497
  in TNM evaluation, 411
  with tuberculosis, 389–390, 390t, 390f
  with Wegener's granulomatosis, 75
Chest wall
  compliance, 275
  configuration of, 48
  diseases of, 265–270
  motion, with diaphragmatic paralysis, 298
  muscular pain, 99
  pain

after thoracotomy, 101
with cervical spine disease, 100
Chest wall syndromes, 48–49. *See also* Restrictive lung disease
Chest wall twinge syndrome, 100
Chest x-ray. *See* Chest radiography/roentgenography
Cheyne-Stokes respirations, 45, 59
CHF. *See* Congestive heart failure
Childhood history, 44
Children
with asthma, 131
pathologic, in children, 451
sleepiness in, 451–452
Chlamydia pneumoniae, 356
microimmunofluorescence for, 366
pneumonia, 358–359
antibiotic therapy for, 371
Chlamydia psittaci, 358
detection of, 366
Chlamydia trachomatis
detection of, 366
pneumonia, antibiotic therapy for, 371
Chlorambucil, 212
for sarcoidosis, 235
Chloramphenicol
indications for, 371
use in pregnancy, 486t
Chlordiazepoxide, elimination half-life, 450t
Chloroquine, for sarcoidosis, 234–235
Chlorpheniramine, 333
Chlorpromazine, pleuritis induced by, 293
Cholecystitis, pain from, 99
Chronic bronchitis, 140f. *See also* Obstructive airway disease
cough with, 66, 69
definition of, 139
hemoptysis with, 79
time constant of lung units in, 11
Chronic eosinophilic pneumonia, 235–241
acute respiratory failure and, 241
chest radiography/roentgenography with, 237, 238f
clinical features of, 236
corticosteroids for, 240
cough in, 236
course of, 236, 240
diagnosis of, 238–239
differential diagnosis of, 232
dyspnea in, 236
epidemiology of, 236
etiology of, 236
fever in, 236
histologic features of, 237–239
histopathology of, 246
laboratory studies in, 236
lung biopsy in, 237–239, 238f–239f
outcome of, 240
pathogenesis of, 239
prednisone for, 240
pulmonary function testing in, 237
radiographic features of, 237, 238f
response to corticosteroid therapy, 237, 239
spontaneous remission of, 240
treatment of, 240
Chronic infections, cough with, 66, 67t
Chronic interstitial pneumonitis
with amiodarone, 214–215
complicating polymyositis/dermatomyositis, 210, 211f
complicating rheumatoid arthritis, 206
drug-induced, 211–217
mechanisms of, 211
with systemic lupus erythematosus, 210
Chronic mountain sickness, 524–526
Chronic obstructive pulmonary disease, 58, 115, 139–152, 186. *See also* Obstructive airway disease
chest radiography/roentgenography with, 147–148, 513–515, 515f
clinical presentation of, 145–146
computed tomography of, 148
cough with, 66, 69, 145
definition of, 139–140
detection of, 19
development of, earliest detectable abnormality in, 22
and diving, 529
dyspnea with, 145
environmental factors in, 149
epidemiology of, 140
forced expiratory volume in 1 second with, 147
hemoptysis with, 145
infections with, 149–150
insomnia with, 466
intermediate probability ventilation-perfusion scan with, 181
laboratory diagnosis of, 146–147
lung transplantation for, 151–152
lung volume with, 147
morbidity and mortality, 19
natural history of, 145–146
pathogenesis of, 140–142
pathology of, 142–143
pharmacotherapy for, 150t, 150–151
physical examination in, 146
prognosis for, at altitude, 525
pulmonary function testing with, 146–147

Chronic obstructive pulmonary disease—Continued
  resistance to airflow in, 142, 146
  risk factors for, 142
  sputum production in, 145
  subspecialty consultation for, 151
  symptomatic therapy for, 150
  theophylline for, 123
  therapeutics, 148–152, 149t
  types of, 139, 140f
Chronotherapy, 473
Churg-Strauss syndrome, 238
Chyliform effusion, 295
Chylothorax, 294–295
Chylous effusions, 286
Circadian rhythm, 430–432
  disorders, 471–472
Cirrhosis, pleural effusions with, 289–290
Clarithromycin, indications for, 370–371
Clavulanic acid. *See* Amoxicillin/clavulanic acid
Clindamycin
  for anaerobic pneumonia, 370
  indications for, 369–371
  use in pregnancy, 486t
Clinical diagnosis, 43–51
Clonidine
  effects on sleep, 448t, 448–449
  transdermal, in tobacco withdrawal, 319
Clorazepate, elimination half-life, 450t
Clubbing, 47–48, 48f, 60
  with asbestosis, 311
  conditions associated with, 47t
  with eosinophilic granuloma, 242
  in idiopathic pulmonary fibrosis, 195
CMS. *See* Chronic mountain sickness
CO. *See* Carbon monoxide
Coagulation profiles, with lytic agents, 183–184
Coagulopathy(ies)
  on chest roentgenography, 75
  hemoptysis with, 76
  management of, 85
  with uremia, 81
Coal worker's pneumoconiosis, 314
Cocaine
  abuse, and hemoptysis, 83
  chest pain and dyspnea with, 101
  effects on sleep, 447, 458
Coccidioides immitis, in acquired immunodeficiency syndrome, radiographic pattern of, 363t
Coccidioidomycosis, 354t
  in pregnancy, 485
Codeine phosphate
  commercial preparations of, 71t
  dosage, 71t
  side effects of, 71t
Codeine sulfate
  commercial preparations of, 71t
  dosage, 71t
  side effects of, 71t
Cold air, and asthma, 116
Collagen vascular disease, 75
  gallium scans with, 205–206
  interstitial pulmonary fibrosis complicating, 205–210
Common cold, 331–337
  antibiotics for, 335
  anticholinergics for, 334
  antihistamines for, 333, 334t
  antiviral therapy for, 335t, 335–336
  complications of, 336
  cost of treatment, 331
  cough with, 66
  epidemiology of, 331–332
  etiologic agents of, 331
  incidence of, 332
  incubation period of, 332
  interferon for, 336
  medications for, 334t
  nonsteroidal antiinflammatory agents for, 334–335
  pathophysiology of, 332
  prevalence of, 331
  susceptibility to, 332–333
  sympathomimetics for, 333–334
  symptomatic treatment of, 333, 336–337
  symptoms of, 332
  therapeutic treatment of, 333–336
  transmission of, 332–333, 337
  vaccine, 336
  vitamin C for, 335
Community-acquired pneumonia, 347–375
  antibiotic prophylaxis for, 375
  antibiotic therapy for, 368–372
  antimicrobial therapy for, empiric, 369t
  arterial blood gases with, 353
  chest radiography in, 353
  clinical presentation of, 351–362, 355t
  epidemiology of, 351
  etiologic agents, 350t, 350–351
  in HIV-positive patients, 362
  hospital admission criteria for, 367–368, 368t
  laboratory diagnosis of, 352–353, 362–367
  management of, 367–372
  mortality from, 351, 367
  pathogenesis of, 347–350
  pathogen prediction by risk category, 351, 352t
  prevention of, 372–375
  risk categories for, 351, 352t
  typical acute, 351–355

Compliance, 2
chest wall, 275
dimensions of, 2
of lung/chest wall system, 3f, 3–4
with medications, 319–320
symbol for, 10
Computed tomography
of bronchiectasis, 79
of calcification, 510
of chest, 78–79
versus chest radiography, 78–79
in chronic obstructive pulmonary disease, 148
with idiopathic pulmonary fibrosis, 196
in small-cell carcinoma, 412
with solitary pulmonary nodule, 415
thin-section, with interstitial lung disease, 193
in TNM evaluation, 411
Computer
logic, for interpretation of spirometry, 30, 31f
in pulmonary function laboratory, 29–30
Conditioning exercises, 321
Conductance
in parallel system, 10–11
symbol for, 10
Confusion
with *Legionella* pneumonia, 357
in pneumonia, 352
Congenital heart disease, 186
Congestive heart failure, 75, 115
chest radiography with, 515–516, 515f–516f
clinical manifestations of, 288
diagnosis of, 288
dyspnea in, 57
fluid collection in, pathophysiology of, 287–288
hypoxemia in, 57
pleural effusions with, 287–289
treatment of, 289
Connective tissue disease, pleural effusions with, 293–294
Consolidation, 45f, 74–75
in pneumonia, 352
Constrictive pericarditis, pleural effusions with, 289
Continuous Oxygen Therapy Trial, 324, 325f
Continuous positive airway pressure, with tracheitis, 343
Control center, of respiration and cyclic inspiratory impulses, 54–55
COPD. *See* Chronic obstructive pulmonary disease
Corgard. *See* Nadolol
Coronary angiography, in diagnosis of chest pain, 95
Coronavirus, 332
Cor pulmonale, 96, 195, 515
with chronic obstructive pulmonary disease, 146
Corticosteroids
for asthma, 124–127
for bronchiolitis obliterans, 221–222
for chronic eosinophilic pneumonia, 240
for eosinophilic granuloma, 248
for idiopathic pulmonary fibrosis, 202–203
inhaled, 125–126
long-acting systemic, 125–126
mechanism of action of, 124
for methotrexate pneumonitis, 214
for myasthenia gravis, 277
for *Pneumocystis carinii* pneumonia, 372
preparations of, 125
progressive systemic sclerosis treated with, 209
for pulmonary complications of mixed connective tissue disease, 210
for pulmonary function testing, 204
for rheumatoid interstitial lung disease, 207
for sarcoidosis, 232–234
short-acting, 125
side effects of, 126
in treatment of chronic obstructive pulmonary disease, 151
use in pregnancy, 479
Costochondritis, 99–100
Cough, 65–72
with acute infections, 66, 67f
with angiotensin-converting enzyme inhibitors, 68
with asbestosis, 311
with asthma, 68–69
in bronchiectasis, 66
with bronchogenic carcinoma, 66–67
cardiovascular etiologies for, 68
character of, 70
chronic, 69
and smoking, 66
with chronic bronchitis, 66, 69
in chronic eosinophilic pneumonia, 236
with chronic infections, 66, 67t
in chronic obstructive pulmonary disease, 66, 69, 145
with common cold, 66
complications of, 69–70
definitive treatment of, 70
diagnostic evaluations with, 70
drug-induced, 68

Cough—Continued
  in drug-induced chronic interstitial pneumonitis/fibrosis, 211
  etiologies of, 66–68
  with foreign body, 68
  function of, 65
  with fungal infections, 66
  with gastroesophageal reflux, 69
  habit, 323
  history and physical examination with, 70
  with idiopathic pulmonary fibrosis, 67, 194–195
  ineffective, 323
  with interstitial lung disease, 67
  in left ventricular failure, 68
  with lung abscesses, 66
  mechanism of, 65–66
  with parenchymal disease, 67
  with pleural effusion, 286
  with pneumonia, 66, 352
  with postnasal drip, 66, 69
  psychogenic, 69
  in pulmonary alveolar proteinosis, 249
  with sarcoidosis, 67
  with sinusitis, 66
  stimuli, 65
  symptomatic treatment of, 71t
  therapy for, 70–71
  timing of, 70
  with tracheobronchitis, 66
  with tuberculosis, 66
  variants, 68–69
Cough preparations, 71, 335
Cough reflex, 348
  mediators of, 65, 66f
  musculoskeletal effectors of, 65, 66f
Cough suppressant, 335
Cough syncope, 69–70
Coxiella burnetii
  pneumonia, 359–360
  serology, 366
Crack cocaine, chest pain and dyspnea with, 101
Crackles, 46
  in drug-induced chronic interstitial pneumonitis/fibrosis, 211
  in pneumonia, 352
Crepitations, with asbestosis, 311
Critical illness, and deep venous thrombosis, 160
Cromolyn sodium
  for asthma, 123–124, 127
  use in pregnancy, 479–480
Croup. *See* Laryngotracheobronchitis
CRP score, with idiopathic pulmonary fibrosis, 197
Cryptococcosis, 354t
Cryptococcus neoformans, in acquired immunodeficiency syndrome, radiographic pattern of, 363t
Cryptostroma corticale, hypersensitivity pneumonitis caused by, 309t
CT. *See* Computed tomography
Cuirass type ventilators, 326
Curschmann's spirals, 113, 114f
CWP. *See* Coal worker's pneumoconiosis
Cyanide antidote kit, 307
Cyanide poisoning, 306–307
Cyanosis, 47
  with asbestosis, 311
  in idiopathic pulmonary fibrosis, 195
Cyclophosphamide
  for idiopathic pulmonary fibrosis, 203–204
  lung disease due to, 212–213
  for pulmonary complications of mixed connective tissue disease, 210
  for rheumatoid interstitial lung disease, 207
  for sarcoidosis, 235
Cycloserine, 393t
  side effects of, 396
Cyclosporine, nephrotoxicity of, 235
Cyclosporine A, for sarcoidosis, 235
Cyst(s)
  bronchogenic, 418
  pericardial, 418
Cystic fibrosis, 115, 186
  in pregnancy, 480–482
Cytomegalovirus
  in acquired immunodeficiency syndrome, radiographic pattern of, 363t
  detection of, 366
  pneumonia, 366
Cytotoxic agents. *See also* Immunosuppressive/cytotoxic agents
  for eosinophilic granuloma, 248
  interstitial pneumonitis caused by, 211–213
Cytoxan. *See* Cyclophosphamide

Dalmane. *See* Flurazepam
Dapsone, for *Pneumocystis carinii* pneumonia, 372
  prophylactic, 375
Daytime sleepiness, 276
Decompression illness, 529–530
  hyperbaric oxygen therapy for, 530
Deep venous thrombosis
  antepartum, 482
  diagnosis of, 161–164
  established, treatment of, 170–174
  incidence of, in general surgical patients, 160–161

lytic therapy for, 173, 173t
pathogenesis of, 157–158
postpartum, 482
postphlebitic syndrome with, 184
prophylaxis, 165–169
mechanical means of, 169
recommendations for, 169
risk factors for, 159t
signs of, 161–162, 162f
sites of, 157, 161
treatment of, in pregnant patient, 172–173
Delayed sleep-phase syndrome, 471
Delta (slow wave) sleep, 426f
in aged, 429
Dementia, sleep changes in, 468
Depression, insomnia in, 468–469
Dermatophagoides, 116, 118
Desquamative interstitial pneumonitis, 194, 197–199, 198f–199f, 205
Dexamethasone
for laryngotracheobronchitis, 342
in treatment of acute mountain sickness, 523
Dextran, in deep venous thrombosis prophylaxis, 168
Dextromethorphan, 71, 71t
commercial preparations of, 71t
dosage, 71t
side effects of, 71t
DHEA. *See* Dihydroergotamine
Diabetes mellitus
neutrophilic alveolitis with, 205
and pulmonary embolus, 159
Diaphragm
anatomy of, 295
congenital cysts, 300
cystic lesions, 300
diseases of, 270–271
endometriosis of, 300
eventration of, 296
functional disturbances of, 296
infections of, 299
metastatic tumors of, 300
parasitic infections of, 300
physiology of, 295–296
traumatic rupture of, 404
tumors of, 300
Diaphragmatic breathing, 321
Diaphragmatic diseases, 295–300
Diaphragmatic dysfunction, 45
Diaphragmatic electrophrenic stimulation, 273–274
Diaphragmatic fatigue, 298–299
Diaphragmatic flutter, 296
Diaphragmatic hernia, 296–297, 418
diagnosis of, 99
pain with, 99
with reflux, 99
traumatic, 404
Diaphragmatic paralysis, 272
bilateral, 270–271, 297
causes of, 297–298
chest wall motion with, 298
dyspnea with, 59
unilateral, 49, 270–271, 298
Diaphragmatic weakness, 271–272
Diarrhea
with oral antimicrobials, 371
in pneumonia, 352
Diazepam, elimination half-life, 450t
Dichloroflavan, 336
Diffuse alveolar infiltrates, with alveolar hemorrhage, 81
Diffuse interstitial fibrosis
with asbestosis, 310–313
functional residual capacity in, 7
pneumoconioses that produce, 309–311
time constant of lung units in, 11
total lung capacity in, 1
Diffuse pulmonary disease, versus asthma, 115
Diffusing capacity for carbon monoxide, 21t
conditions that reduce, 39
in eosinophilic granuloma, 244
with idiopathic pulmonary fibrosis, 196
measurement of, 38–39
with mixed connective tissue disease, 210
in progressive systemic sclerosis, 207–209
in sarcoidosis, 225
Diffusion, 14–15
defect, 17
Dihydroergotamine
contraindications to, 169
and heparin, 169
Diisocyanate, hypersensitivity pneumonitis caused by, 309t
Dilantin. *See* Phenytoin
DIP. *See* Desquamative interstitial pneumonitis
Dipyridamole, for deep venous thrombosis prophylaxis, 168–169
Disability, 20
Disodium cromoglycate. *See* Cromolyn sodium
Disseminated intravascular coagulation, with alveolar hemorrhage, 82
Diuretics, in treatment of acute mountain sickness, 522–523
Diving medicine, 526–530
D_LCO. *See* Diffusing capacity for carbon monoxide

Doppler studies, in diagnosis of deep venous thrombosis, 163
Doxepin, sedation with, 449
Doxycycline, indications for, 370–371
Dreams, 425–426
Dressler's syndrome, pleural effusions with, 294
Dripps classification, of anesthetic risk, 490–491
Drooling, of acute epiglottitis, 337
Drug-induced pneumonitis, 211–217
Drug resistance, and tuberculosis treatment, 393–394
Duchenne type muscular dystrophy, 277
Duplex ultrasound, in diagnosis of deep venous thrombosis, 163–164
Dust, 308
  house
    allergen in, 116
    control of, 118
DVT. *See* Deep venous thrombosis
Dyspnea, 53–61
  with alveolar hemorrhage, 81
  with anemia, 59
  with angina, 92
  with arrhythmias, 58
  with asbestosis, 311
  with asthma, 58, 110–111
  cardiac causes of, 57–58
    versus pulmonary, 60
  in children, 114
  in chronic eosinophilic pneumonia, 236
  with chronic obstructive pulmonary disease, 145
  classification of, 56–57
  with cocaine, 101
  in congestive heart failure, 57
  descriptions of, 53
  diagnosis of, 53
  with diaphragmatic paralysis, 59
  differential diagnosis of, 59–61
  in drug-induced chronic interstitial pneumonitis/fibrosis, 211
  on exertion, 59
  with heart failure, 57–59, 288
  with idiopathic pulmonary fibrosis, 194–195
  with infiltrative disease, 58
  initial evaluation of, 60
  with interstitial fibrosis, 58
  localized, 92
  in lymphangioleiomyomatosis, 254
  with mechanical ventilation, 59
  in mixed connective tissue disease, 209–210
  in muscular dystrophy, 277
  with myocardial infarction, 58
  neurologic causes of, 59
  with obstructive airway disease, 58
  pathophysiology of, 56–59
  with pericardial disease, 58
  physiology of, 53
  with pleural effusion, 59, 286
  with pneumonia, 58
  with pneumothorax, 59
  with postpolio syndrome, 275
  psychological aspects of, 59–61
  in pulmonary alveolar proteinosis, 249
  pulmonary causes of, 58–59
  with pulmonary embolus, 58, 96, 174
  with pulmonary hypertension, 186
  with restrictive disorders, 58
  sources of, 56
  theoretical origins of, 55–56
  unexplained, 51
  with valvular heart disease, 58
Dystrophin, 277–278

Early ambulation, in preventing deep venous thrombosis, 169
Eaton-Lambert syndrome, 277
ECG. *See* Electrocardiography
Echocardiography, in diagnosis of chest pain, 95
Edrophonium chloride, 271
EG. *See* Eosinophilic granuloma
Elastance, 2–3
Elastic recoil
  in emphysema, 3
  pressure of, 2–3, 7
Elavil. *See* Amitriptyline
Elderly, pneumonia in, 348–350
Electrocardiography, 61
  in diagnosis of chest pain, 95
  in pericarditis, 94–95
  with pulmonary embolus, 175
Electroencephalogram, for staging sleep, 425, 426f, 428
Electromyographic biofeedback, 472
Electromyography, 271–272
Electrophrenic pacing, 273–274
ELISA. *See* Enzyme-linked immunosorbent assay
Embolotherapy, for massive hemoptysis, 78, 86
Emery-Dreifuss dystrophy, 277–278
EMG. *See* Electromyography
Emphysema, 58, 140f. *See also* Obstructive airway disease
  anatomic patterns of, 143t
  associated with chronic obstructive pulmonary disease, 143
  definition of, 139
  elastic recoil or elastance of lung in, 3
  functional residual capacity in, 7

hereditary, 143–144
protease-antiprotease theory of, 143–145
pulmonary hyperinflation with, 147–148
radiographic findings with, 513–515, 515f
subcutaneous cervical, 49
time constant of lung units in, 11
total lung capacity in, 1
Empyema(s), 286, 292–293
antibiotic therapy for, 370–371
with esophageal rupture, 293
in tuberculosis, 388
Enalapril, cough associated with, 68
End-expiratory grunt, of asthma, 111–112
Endometriosis, diaphragmatic defects caused by, 300
Endothelial injury, 157–158
Endotracheal tubes, hemoptysis with, 83
Enterovirus, 360
Enviroxime, 336
Enzyme-linked immunosorbent assay, 366
Eosinophilia, 139
Eosinophilic granuloma, 241–248
chest pain with, 242
chest radiographic findings with, 242–244, 243f
in children, 241
course of, 247–248
differential diagnosis of, 232
disseminated, 241
epidemiology of, 241–242
extrapulmonary manifestations of, 241
hemoptysis with, 242
histopathology of, 244–246
immunohistochemical techniques with, 246–247
pathogenesis of, 247
prognosis for, 241, 247–248
pulmonary, 241
clinical manifestations of, 242
incidence of, 241
therapy for, 248
pulmonary function testing with, 244
Eosinophils
in asthma, 107, 109
in idiopathic pulmonary fibrosis, 201
Ephedrine, for asthma, 120
Epidural nerve blocks, indications for, 267
Epiglottic abscesses, 340
Epiglottitis, 114, 337–340
acute, fever of, 337
airway management in, 339–340
antibiotics for, 340
with associated bacteremia, 340
clinical features of, 337–338, 338t
complications of, 340
versus croup, 337, 341
diagnosis of, 339
epidemiology of, 337
etiology of, 339
laryngoscopy in, 338
pneumococcal, 339
prophylactic airway in, 339–340
radiography of, 338–339
treatment of, 339–340
Epinephrine
for asthma, 119–120
for laryngotracheobronchitis, 341
use in pregnancy, 479
Epithelial cells, in asthma, 107t, 109
Epithelial damage, in asthma, 109
Epithelial-derived relaxing factor, in asthma, 108t, 109
Equal pressure point, 12f, 12–13
Ergometer, upper extremity, 321–322, 322f
Erosive esophagitis, 98
ERV. *See* Expiratory reserve volume
Erythema multiforme, 356
Erythema nodosum, 47
in sarcoidosis, 222–223
Erythromycin
indications for, 369–371
use in pregnancy, 486t
Erythromycin estolate, use in pregnancy, 486t
Escherichia coli pneumonia, 354
antibiotic therapy for, 371
Esophageal cancer, 99
Esophageal disease
and asthma, 118
diagnostic tests for, 98–99
management of, 99
Esophageal motility disorders, 97–98
Esophageal pH monitoring, 98
Esophageal rupture
empyema with, 293
pleural effusions with, 293
Esophageal spasm, 98
tests and findings with, 98t
Esophageal syndromes, chest pain in, 97t, 97–99
Esophagitis, 98–99
Estrogens, in lymphangioleiomyomatosis, 254
Ethambutol, 392t, 392
dosage regimens, 394
side effects of, 396
for tuberculosis, 379
use in pregnancy, 484
Ethionamide, 393t
side effects of, 396

Excessive daytime sleepiness, 439–459
  ancillary symptoms of, 443–446
  chief complaint of, 439–441
  disorders of, 440t
  etiology of, 439, 440t
  family history with, 452–453
  onset of symptoms, 441–442
  physical examination for, 453–454
Exercise
  and asthma, 117, 128–129
  conditioning, 321
  program, 321–322
    for postpolio syndrome, 275
Exercise test, 61
  cardiopulmonary, 21t, 39
  in diagnosis of chest pain, 95
Expectorants, 71, 71t, 335
  in asthma treatment, 126
Expiratory muscles, 7–8
Expiratory reserve volume, 1–2, 2f
  measurement of, 22, 23f
Extrapulmonary physical findings, in diagnosis, 47–49
Exudates
  causes of, 285, 287t
  versus transudates, 285–286
    laboratory criteria for, 285, 286t

Family education, 317–318
Family history, 44
Fansidar. *See* Sulfadoxine/pyrimethamine
Fat embolus, 51, 157, 165
Fatigue, with pulmonary hypertension, 186
FEF_{25-75}. *See* Mid-maximal expiratory flow rate
FEF_{max}. *See* Maximum expiratory flow rate
FEV_1. *See* Forced expiratory volume in 1 second
FEV_3. *See* Forced expiratory volume in first 3 seconds
Fever. *See also* Q fever
  of acute epiglottitis, 337
  in chronic eosinophilic pneumonia, 236
  in pneumonia, 352
  Pontiac, 357
  in pulmonary alveolar proteinosis, 249
  rheumatic, 93
  in sarcoidosis, 222–223
FEV_1/FVC. *See* Forced expiratory volume in 1 second to forced vital capacity ratio
FEV_1 percent. *See* Forced expiratory volume in 1 second to forced vital capacity ratio
Fiberoptic bronchoscopy, 76–77, 410
  with bronchiolitis obliterans, 219–221
  in pulmonary alveolar proteinosis, 252
  with pulmonary masses, 417
  with solitary pulmonary nodule, 415
Fibrosarcomas, diaphragmatic, 300
Fibrosis. *See also* Idiopathic pulmonary fibrosis; Interstitial pulmonary fibrosis; Progressive massive fibrosis; Pulmonary fibrosis
  with asbestos exposure, 312
Fibrositis syndrome, sleep abnormalities in, 466–468
Fish proteins, hypersensitivity pneumonitis caused by, 309t
Flail chest, 267
Flexible fiberoptic bronchoscopy, 76–77, 410
Flow
  factors determining, 8, 8f
  laminar, 8, 9f
  resistance to, 8–9
  turbulent, 9, 9f
Flow cytometric analysis, of lung cancer, 412
Flow limitation, 12–14
Flow pressure curves, isovolume, 12f
Flow rates, measurement of, 34
Flow/volume curve, 23
Flow/volume loop(s), 23, 24f, 24–25, 29
  with amyotrophic lateral sclerosis, 274f
  normal, 34, 35f
  obstructed, 33, 33f, 34, 35f
  for pattern recognition, 33, 33f
  restricted, 34, 35f
Flunisolide metered dose inhaler, 126
Fluorescent microscopy, 391–392
Fluoxetine, effects on sleep, 449, 468
Flurazepam, elimination half-life, 450t
FOB. *See* Fiberoptic bronchoscopy
Food allergy, 116
Forced expiratory volume in first 3 seconds, measurement of, 34
Forced expiratory volume in first 3 seconds/forced vital capacity ratio, measurement of, 34
Forced expiratory volume in 1 second
  in asthma, 106
  with chronic obstructive pulmonary disease, 147
  measurement of, 34
  in sarcoidosis, 225
Forced expiratory volume in 1 second to forced vital capacity ratio
  with chronic obstructive pulmonary disease, 147
  to distinguish obstruction from restriction, 34, 36f
Forced vital capacity
  in amyotrophic lateral sclerosis, 274

to distinguish obstruction from restriction, 34, 36f
measurement of, 23, 24f, 34
Foreign body aspiration
in children, 115
cough with, 68
hemoptysis with, 83
FRC. *See* Functional residual capacity
Free running, 430–432
Functional impairment, evaluation of, 20
Functional residual capacity, 1, 2f
in emphysema, 7
measurement of, 22, 23f, 38
in obstructive airway disease, 34
volume of lung at, 7, 8f
Fungal infections, 348
clinical and radiographic features of, 200
cough with, 66
in pregnancy, 485

Gallium scanning
with collagen vascular disease, 205–206
in idiopathic pulmonary fibrosis, 201
with interstitial lung disease, 193
with *Pneumocystis carinii* pneumonia, 362
in sarcoidosis, 229–230
in TNM staging, 411
Gamma loop, function of, 56
Gamma neurons, 55–56
Gas embolism
diving-related, 529
hyperbaric oxygen therapy for, 530
Gastroesophageal reflux
and asthma, 118, 141
chest pain with, 97–98
cough with, 69
diagnosis of, 98
with sleep apnea syndrome, 444
tests and findings with, 98t
treatment of, 98, 142
Gas volume decrease, with absolute pressure increase, 520f, 527
Generalized anxiety disorder, insomnia with, 469
Gentamicin, use in pregnancy, 481
GERD. *See* Gastroesophageal reflux disease
Geriatric patients. *See* Elderly
Ghon's lesion, 384
Glomerulonephritis, with alveolar hemorrhage, 81
Glossopharyngeal breathing, 273
Glucocorticoids, for idiopathic pulmonary fibrosis, 202
Glyceryl guaiacolate, 71, 71t
Goiter, 418
Gold salts, pneumonitis caused by, 211, 213
Golgi tendon organ, 54
Goodpasture's syndrome, 76, 81
on chest roentgenography, 75
Gower's sign, 277
Graham Steell's murmur, 186
Gram-negative bacilli, pneumonia, 353, 355
antibiotic therapy for, 371
Gram-negative pharyngeal colonization, 348
Granuloma. *See also* Eosinophilic granuloma
with chemotherapy-induced lung disease, 214
chest radiography with, 510f
in sarcoidosis, 226, 227f, 232
Granulomatous infection, 232
clinical features of, 228
Granulomatous vasculitis, 232
Greenfield filter, in mechanical prophylaxis for thromboembolic disease, 184
Ground-glass pattern
with bronchiolitis obliterans, 218f, 218–219
with idiopathic pulmonary fibrosis, 196
Guaifenesin, 151, 335
in asthma treatment, 126
commercial preparations of, 71t
dosage, 71t
side effects of, 71t
Guillain-Barré syndrome
etiology of, 276
plasmapheresis in, 276
prognosis for, 276
respiratory failure in, 297
respiratory involvement with, 276

Halcion. *See* Triazolam
Hamartoma, chest x-ray with, 510f
Hamman-Rich syndrome, 195
Hampton's hump, 293
HAPE. *See* High altitude pulmonary edema
Headache, with *Legionella* pneumonia, 357
Heartburn, with sleep apnea syndrome, 444
Heart failure. *See also* Congestive heart failure
high output, dyspnea with, 57–58
and pulmonary embolus, 159
and sleep apnea, 454
Heart murmur
of aortic stenosis, 93
of mitral stenosis, 94
Heart rate, with pulmonary embolus, 175
Heart sounds
in idiopathic pulmonary fibrosis, 195
with pulmonary embolus, 175
Helium dilution, 38
Hemodynamic compromise, with pulmonary embolus, 177–178

Hemophilus influenzae, 348
in acquired immunodeficiency syndrome, radiographic pattern of, 363t
bronchitis caused by, therapy for, 370
culture, 365
epiglottitis caused by, antibiotic regimen for, 340
pneumonia, 353, 355
in acquired immunodeficiency syndrome, 362
antibiotic therapy for, 369–370
tracheitis caused by, 342–343
Hemophilus influenzae type B
detection of, 365
epiglottitis caused by, 339
laryngitis caused by, 337
vaccination against, 150
Hemophilus parainfluenzae, epiglottitis caused by, 339
Hemoptysis, 73–87
with abnormal chest x-ray
etiology of, 74t
management of, 85
and age of patient, 73
with alveolar hemorrhage, 81
anemia with, 76
with anticoagulants, 74
with antiplatelet agents, 76
associated with menses, 83
with bronchial carcinoids, 81
with bronchiectasis, 73–74, 79
with bronchogenic carcinoma, 67, 80–81
bronchoscopy with, 76–77
catamenial, 83
chest roentgenogram with, 74t, 75–76
with chronic bronchitis, 79
with chronic obstructive pulmonary disease, 145
with coagulopathies, 76
cocaine abuse and, 83
diagnosis of, 73
diseases associated with, 79–83
with endotracheal tubes, 83
with eosinophilic granuloma, 242
etiology of, 73, 74t
examination of sputum with, 76
factitious, 83
with foreign body aspiration, 83
versus hematemesis, 75t
history-taking with, 73–74
iatrogenic, 83
initial diagnostic approach and evaluation, 73–76
laboratory assessment with, 76
with *Legionella* pneumonia, 357
in legionnaire's disease, 356
in lymphangioleiomyomatosis, 254
management of, 83–87
massive
balloon tamponade for, 86
embolotherapy for, 78, 86
management of, 84
from metastatic lung cancer, 75
mild-to-moderate, management of, 84
with mitral stenosis, 94
with mycetoma, 80
with neoplastic disorders, 80–81
with normal chest radiograph, 74t, 76
etiology of, 74t
management of, 85
with percutaneous fine needle aspiration biopsy, 83
physical examination with, 74–75
with pneumonia, 79–80, 357
in psittacosis, 356
in pulmonary alveolar proteinosis, 249
pulmonary angiography with, 77–78
with pulmonary embolus, 174
with pulmonary hypertension, 186
with pulmonary infarction, 80
with pulmonary sequestrations, 80
recurrent or life-threatening, management of, 85–86
specific diagnostic studies for, 76–79
time course of, 73
with tracheobronchitis, 79
with tuberculosis, 79
unusual causes of, 83
urinalysis with, 76
Hemosiderosis. *See* Idiopathic hemosiderosis
Hemothorax, 286
Henoch-Schönlein purpura, 81, 186
Henry's law, 527
Heparin
and dihydroergotamine, 169
low molecular weight, 183
therapy with
bleeding complications of, 167–168, 170–171, 182–183
complications of, 166–168, 170–171
full dose, for deep venous thrombosis, 170–171
partial thromboplastin time with, 170
in pregnancy, 172–173
for prophylaxis of deep venous thrombosis, 165–166
for pulmonary embolus, 182–183
thrombotic complications with, 168

Hepatitis, isoniazid-induced, 395
Hepatomegaly, 75
Herpes simplex virus
detection of, 366
pneumonia, 366
Herpes zoster, 100
Hiatal hernia. *See* Diaphragmatic hernia
Hiccup, 296
High altitude pulmonary edema, 521–524
High output heart failure, dyspnea with, 57–58
Hilar neoplasm, chest x-ray with, 513f
Histamine, in asthma, 108, 108t
Histiocytosis X, pulmonary, 241
Histoplasma capsulatum, 228–229
in acquired immunodeficiency syndrome, radiographic pattern of, 363t
Histoplasmosis, 354t
superior vena cava syndrome caused by, 418
History, reliability of, 43
HIV. *See* Human immunodeficiency virus
HNE. *See* Human neutrophil elastase
Hodgkin's disease
chest radiography with, 514f
mediastinal mass in, 417f
superior vena cava syndrome with, 419, 419f
Home oxygen therapy, 323–324
for idiopathic pulmonary fibrosis, 204
Home peak flow monitor, in asthma, 112
Home ventilation, 324–326
psychological aspects of, 279–280
Honeycomb lung, 196–197
Hoover's sign, 49
Horder's spots, 356
Horner's syndrome, 417
Host defenses, respiratory, 347, 348t
Host immune or mechanical defects, in development of community-acquired pneumonia, 347, 348t, 374–375
House dust
allergen in, 116
control of, 118
HP. *See* Hypersensitivity pneumonitis
Human immunodeficiency virus, infection. *See also* Acquired immunodeficiency syndrome
pulmonary manifestations of, 361–362
and tuberculosis, 381, 388, 397–398
Human neutrophil elastase, 143
Humidified air, for laryngotracheobronchitis, 341
HX cells, 245–247
Hyaline membrane disease, 6
Hydralazine
interstitial pneumonitis caused by, 211
pleural effusions with, 212
pleuritis induced by, 294
Hydration, 317–318
Hydrocodone bitartrate
commercial preparations of, 71t
dosage, 71t
side effects of, 71t
Hydrocortisone, for asthma, 125
Hydrogen cyanide, poisoning, 306–307
Hydrogen sulfide, poisoning, 307–308
Hydrothorax, 49
hepatic, 289–290
pelvic tumors associated with, 291
with peritoneal dialysis, 290
Hydroxychloroquine sulfate, for deep venous thrombosis prophylaxis, 168–169
Hyperarousal, and insomnia, 461–462
Hyperbaric oxygen therapy
for carbon monoxide poisoning, 530
for decompression illness, 530
for gas embolism, 530
indications for, 530
and wound healing, 530
Hypercalcemia, in sarcoidosis, 234
Hypercoagulability, and deep venous thrombosis, 158
Hypersensitivity pneumonitis
acute form of, 308
versus asthma, 115
with bleomycin therapy, 212
chronic form of, 308
clinical findings in, 308
drug-induced, 213–217
etiologic agents, 308, 309t
Hypersensitivity vasculitis, 186
Hypersomnolence
idiopathic, 443
diagnosis of, 446
illnesses associated with, 442
Hypertrophic osteoarthropathy, 47–48
Hyperventilation
at altitude, 519
in pregnancy, 477
Hyperventilation provocation test, 101
Hypnogogic hallucinations, with narcolepsy, 445–446
Hypnotics, elimination half-life, 450t
Hypoalbuminemia, pleural effusions with, 289
Hyponatremia, in *Legionella* infection, 356
Hypophosphatemia
with *Legionella* pneumonia, 357
respiratory failure with, 298
Hypoventilation, 186
definition of, 16
Hypoxemia
with alveolar hemorrhage, 81

Hypoxemia—Continued
causes of, 15–17
with community-acquired pneumonia, 353
in congestive heart failure, 57
with diffusion abnormality, 16
due to hypoventilation, 16
with idiopathic pulmonary fibrosis, 196
with kyphoscoliosis, 268
in obesity, 278
in sarcoidosis, 225
shunt, 16
in ventilation/perfusion mismatch, 16
Hypoxia
altitude-induced, compensatory response to, 519–521
in asthma, 111
desensitization to, at altitude, 521
Hysteresis, 6

IC. *See* Inspiratory capacity
Idiopathic hemosiderosis
with alveolar hemorrhage, 82
on chest roentgenography, 75
Idiopathic hypersomnolence, 443
diagnosis of, 446
Idiopathic hypertrophic subaortic stenosis
chest pain with, 93
presenting symptoms of, 93
Idiopathic pulmonary fibrosis, 193–204
alveolar macrophages in, 200–201
alveolitis in, 200
ancillary therapy for, 204
bronchoalveolar lavage in, 200–202
chest radiography in, 195–196, 196f
classification schema, 197–199
clinical signs and symptoms of, 194–195
clubbing in, 195
computed tomography with, 196
cough with, 67, 194–195
cyanosis in, 195
dyspnea with, 194–195
epidemiology of, 193
fibrosis in, 196–197
gallium scanning in, 201
heart sounds in, 195
histopathology of, 197–199, 198f–199f
hypoxemia with, 196
lung biopsy with, 193, 197, 199–200
lung transplantation for, 204
mortality with, 195
natural history of, 195
pathogenesis of, 200–201
prevalence of, 193
pulmonary function testing with, 196–197
radiographic patterns with
acinar, 196
alveolar, 196
ground glass, 196
honeycombing, 196
interstitial, 196
reticular, 196
reticulonodular, 196
synonymous terms for, 193
therapy for, 202–204
I^{125} fibrinogen scans, in diagnosis of deep venous thrombosis, 163
IgE. *See* Immunoglobulin E
ILD. *See* Interstitial lung disease
Immotile cilia syndrome, 115
Immune complex diseases, with alveolar hemorrhage and glomerulonephritis, 81
Immunization, in prevention of respiratory infection, 373
Immunoglobulin E, serum, 113–114, 139
in chronic eosinophilic pneumonia, 236
Immunologic methods, to identify pathogens, 365–366
Immunosuppressive acidic protein, 412
Immunosuppressive agents
for eosinophilic granuloma, 248
for idiopathic pulmonary fibrosis, 202
for myasthenia gravis, 277
Immunosuppressive/cytotoxic agents
for idiopathic pulmonary fibrosis, 204
progressive systemic sclerosis treated with, 209
for sarcoidosis, 234–235
Immunotherapy, for asthma, 127–128
Impedance plethysmography, in diagnosis of deep venous thrombosis, 163
Impotence, 427
Incentive spirometry
postoperative, 493
preoperative preparation for, 493
in restrictive lung disease, 279
Inderal. *See* Propranolol
Indomethacin, for sarcoidosis, 234
Infection(s), 115
acute, cough with, 66, 67f
anaerobic pleuropulmonary, 360–361
chronic, cough with, 66, 67t
with chronic obstructive pulmonary disease, 149–150
cough with, 66, 67f
of diaphragm, 299
fungal, 348
in pregnancy, 485
granulomatous, 232
clinical features of, 228

pleural effusions with, 291–293
pulmonary
diagnosis of, 50
with rheumatoid arthritis, 206
with pulmonary alveolar proteinosis, 249
respiratory tract, epidemiology of, 351
as triggers of acute asthma, 116
upper respiratory tract, 331–344
Infection control, 320
Infiltrative disease, dyspnea with, 58
Influenza, 332
pneumonia with, 360
vaccine, 150, 320, 349, 373, 373t
recommendations for use of, 373t
Influenza A, 340
Influenza virus, detection of, 366
INH. *See* Isoniazid
Inhalants
indoor, 116
outdoor, 116
Insomnia, 461–474
behavior treatments of, 472–473
chronic
model of, 461–462
treatment of, 461, 472
definition of, 461
diagnosis of, 466–472
epidemiology of, 461
evaluation of, 462–466
with inadequate sleep hygiene, 471
with medical illness, 464, 466–468
medication history with, 464
with narcolepsy, 446
ongoing monitoring with, 465
pharmacologic treatment of, 473
predisposition to, 461–462
prevalence of, 461, 462t
with psychiatric illness, 464, 468–471
psychophysiologic, 469, 471
sleep history with, 463
sleep parameters in patients with complaints of, 466, 467t
subjective, 471
symptomatic treatment of, 461
Inspiration, chest pain with, 102
Inspiratory capacity, measurement of, 22, 23f
Inspiratory force meter, 272f
Inspiratory muscles, 7
Inspiratory pressures, measurement of, at bedside, 272
Inspired oxygen tension, 15
calculation of, 15
low, 16
Intal. *See* Cromolyn sodium
Intercostal nerve block, indications for, 267
Intercostal neuralgia, 100
Interferon, for common cold, 336
Interferon intranasal spray, 336
Intermittent positive-pressure ventilation
with kyphoscoliosis, 269
in restrictive lung disease, 279
Internal mammary artery bypass surgery, pain syndrome, 101
Interstitial lung disease. *See also* Restrictive lung disease
causes of, 193
clinical manifestations of, 193
cough with, 67
distinguishing features of, 193
histopathologic features of, 193
insomnia with, 466
lung biopsy with, 193
in progressive systemic sclerosis, 207
rales in, 195
rheumatoid, 206–207
spectrum of, 193
Interstitial pneumonitis. *See also* Chronic interstitial pneumonitis; Usual interstitial pneumonitis
cytotoxic drug-induced, 211–213
desquamative, 194, 197–199, 198f–199f, 205
drug-induced, 211–217
Interstitial pulmonary fibrosis. *See also* Diffuse interstitial fibrosis
associated with collagen vascular disease, 205
versus asthma, 115
complicating collagen vascular disease, 205–210
CVD-associated, histopathologic changes of, 205
differential diagnosis of, 232
dyspnea with, 58
Intrabronchial selective coagulation, 86
Iodinated glycerol, in treatment of chronic obstructive pulmonary disease, 151
IPF. *See* Idiopathic pulmonary fibrosis; Interstitial pulmonary fibrosis
IPG. *See* Impedance plethysmography
Ipratropium bromide
for asthma, 124, 127
for common cold, 334
Irregular sleep-wake pattern, 472
Irritant receptors, 54, 54f
Isoetharine, 120
in pulmonary function testing, 37
Isoniazid, 392t, 392
dosage regimens, 394
pleuritis induced by, 294

Isoniazid—Continued
  preventive therapy with, indications for, 396–397, 397t
  resistance, 393
  side effects of, 395
  for tuberculosis, 379, 381
  use in pregnancy, 484, 486t
Isoproterenol, 120
  in pulmonary function testing, 36–37
Isoxsuprine, pulmonary edema with, 485–486
Isuprel. *See* Isoproterenol

Jet lag, 433
J receptors, 54, 54f

Kanamycin, 393t
  side effects of, 396
Kaposi's sarcoma
  in acquired immunodeficiency syndrome, radiographic pattern of, 363t
  pulmonary, 362
K complexes, 425
Kerley's lines, 516, 516f
Ketotifen, 126
Kininogenase, in asthma, 108, 108t
Kinyoun (Cold Basic Fuchsin Acid-Fast Stain), 391, 391t
Klebsiella pneumoniae, pneumonia, 353
  antibiotic therapy for, 371
  sputum with, 50
Kleine-Levin syndrome, abnormal sleepiness with, 442
K-RAS oncogene, in adenocarcinoma of lung, 412
Kyphoscoliosis, 267–269, 268f
  disorders causing, 267, 267t
  in pregnancy, 486
  surgical treatment of, 269
  treatment of, 268–269
Kyphosis, 267

β-Lactamase, 369–370
Lactate dehydrogenase
  in pleural effusions, 285, 286t
  serum, with pulmonary alveolar proteinosis, 249, 254
LAM. *See* Lymphangioleiomyomatosis
Laminar flow, 8, 9f
Laplace's law, 5, 5f
Large-cell carcinoma, 410
Larks, 434
Laryngeal carcinoma, cough with, 67
Laryngoscopy
  in epiglottitis, 338
  with tracheitis, 343
Laryngotracheal shift, 49
Laryngotracheobronchitis, 340–342
  versus asthma, 111–112, 114
  clinical presentation of, 338t, 340–341
  complications of, 342
  differential diagnosis of, 342
  epidemiology of, 340
  versus epiglottitis, 337, 341
  intubation in, indications for, 342
  treatment of, 341–342
Laser therapy, for lung cancer, 413
Latency. *See* Sleep, onset
Left-sided heart failure, signs of, 288
Left ventricular failure, cough in, 68
Legionella
  in acquired immunodeficiency syndrome, radiographic pattern of, 363t
  culture of, 365
  direct fluorescent antibody staining for, 365–366
  infection, 348
Legionella micdadei, serology, 365
Legionella pneumophila
  pneumonia, 353, 357–368
    antibiotic therapy for, 370
  serology, 365
Legionellosis, 354t
Legionnaire's disease, 356–358
  antibiotic therapy for, 370
  radiographic resolution of, 367
Length-tension disparity, of dyspnea, 55–56, 58
Leptospirosis, 354t
Leukemia, with alveolar hemorrhage, 82
Leukotrienes, in asthma, 108, 108t
Levine's sign, 92
Librium. *See* Chlordiazepoxide
Light stimuli, phase-shifting effects of, 432
Lipid-associated sialic acid plasma, 412
Liquid oxygen systems, 323
Lobar infiltrates, 353
Loefgren's syndrome, in sarcoidosis, 222–223
Lomustine, interstitial pneumonitis/fibrosis associated with, 213
Lopressor. *See* Metoprolol
Lorazepam, elimination half-life, 450t
Lovibond's angle, 47
Lung(s). *See also under* Pulmonary
  anatomy of, 497–499, 499f
  blood flow to, 14, 14f
  dynamic characteristics of, 8–17
  particle deposition in, 308
  perfusion zones of, 14, 14f
  pressure-volume relationship, 2, 3f
  static characteristics of, 1–8
Lung abscess(es), 79, 361

antibiotic therapy for, 370–371
chest x-ray with, 501–504, 505f
cough with, 66
and lung cancer, 361
parapneumonic pleural effusions with, 292
Lung biopsy. *See also* Transbronchial lung biopsy
in chronic eosinophilic pneumonia, 237–239, 238f–239f
with idiopathic pulmonary fibrosis, 193, 197, 199–200
with interstitial lung disease, 193
Lung cancer
and air pollution, 408
anatomic staging of, 411–412
biomarker profiles in, 412, 413t
brachytherapy of, 413
chemotherapy for, 413
clinical manifestations of, 410–411
diagnosis of, 50, 410–411
epidemiology of, 407
etiology of, 407–409
flow cytometric analysis of, 412
follow-up of, 413
histologic types of, 410. *See also* Adenocarcinoma; Non-small-cell carcinoma; Small-cell carcinoma
laser therapy for, 413
metastatic, hemoptysis from, 75
pathogenesis of, 409–410
prognosis for, 407
smoking and, 407–408
and solitary pulmonary nodule, 414
surgery for, 413
therapy for, 413
Lung fluke, 79–80
Lung lavage, with pulmonary alveolar proteinosis, 253–254
Lung resection
preparation for, 493–495
split function studies for marginal patients undergoing, 492, 492t
Lung scan
perfusion, quantitative, 492, 493f
preoperative, 495
in pulmonary embolus, 77
radioisotope perfusion, 178–181, 179f
Lung scintigraphy, with suspected pulmonary embolic disease, 77
Lung transplantation
with end-stage lung disease, 151–152
for idiopathic pulmonary fibrosis, 204
Lung units
parallel, 3f, 3–4
in series, 3f, 3–4
Lung volume(s), 21t
with chronic obstructive pulmonary disease, 147
determination of, 38
diminished, 33–34
measurement of, 22, 23f
in obstructive airway disease, 34
physiologic, 1–2, 2f
in progressive systemic sclerosis, 207–208
in restrictive lung disease, 265
Lupus pernio, 47
Lupus pleuritis, 293–294
Lymphadenopathy, 512. *See also* Bilateral hilar lymphadenopathy
Lymphangioleiomyomatosis, 254–256
chest radiography with, 254–255
dyspnea in, 254
estrogens in, 254
etiology of, 254
hemoptysis in, 254
histologic features of, 255
pleural effusions with, 254
pneumothoraces in, 254
prognosis for, 255–256
pulmonary function testing in, 255
therapy for, 255–256
Lymphangitic carcinomatosis, 194f
Lymphocytes, in collagen vascular disease, 205
Lymphoma
pleural effusions associated with, 291
superior vena cava syndrome caused by, 418
tissue diagnosis of, 417–418
Lytic therapy
contraindications to, 174t, 183
for deep venous thrombosis, 173, 173t
for pulmonary embolus, 182–184
pulmonary hemodynamics with, 183

Macrodantin. *See* Nitrofurantoin
Macrolide antibiotics, indications for, 370
Macrophages, in asthma, 107, 109
Magnetic resonance imaging
in small-cell carcinoma staging, 412
in TNM staging, 411
Main stem bronchi, selective intubation of, 86
Malaise, in pneumonia, 352
Malignancy. *See also* Cancer; Carcinoma
metastatic, pleural effusion with, 291
Malignant cavitary neoplasm, chest x-ray with, 512f
Mantoux test, 385, 386t
Mast cells
activation of, 107
in acute hypersensitivity response, 107
Maxair. *See* Pirbuterol

Maximum breathing capacity, 26, 26f
Maximum expiratory flow rate, 25–26
Maximum voluntary ventilation, 26, 26f
in amyotrophic lateral sclerosis, 274
MBC. *See* Maximum breathing capacity
MCTD. *See* Mixed connective tissue disease
Measles, 340
Mechanical ventilation. *See also* Home ventilation
with cervical spinal cord injuries, 273–274
dyspnea with, 59
in muscular dystrophy, 278
for patients with terminal disease, ethical questions regarding, 326
with postpolio syndrome, 275
in restrictive lung disease, 279
Mechanoreceptors, 53–54, 65
Mediastinal crunch, 49
Mediastinal fibrosis, superior vena cava syndrome caused by, 418
Mediastinal mass
tissue diagnosis of, 417–418
work-up for, 417
Mediastinal neoplasms, 417–418
Mediastinal sounds, 49
Mediastinoscopy, in TNM evaluation, 411
Mediastinum
anatomy of, 417, 497–499, 499f
divisions of, 417, 498, 500f
Medications
and asthma, 117
effects on sleep, 447–448, 464, 468
patient education on, 319–320
Medroxyprogesterone, in lymphangioleiomyomatosis, 255–256
Medullary cough center, 65, 66f
MEF. *See* Maximum expiratory flow rate
Melanoptysis, 314
Melioidosis, 354t
Melphalan, 212
Meningitis, tuberculous, 389
Menses
asthma and, 118
hemoptysis associated with, 81
Mesothelioma
diagnosis of, 312
histologic patterns associated with, 312–313
malignant, 312
Metabolic demands, in obesity, 278
Metaprel. *See* Metaproterenol
Metaproterenol
for asthma, 120
in pulmonary function testing, 37
Metered dose inhalers
of corticosteroids, 126
proper use of, 319
Methacholine, screening challenge, 37–38
Methotrexate
for corticosteroid-dependent asthma, 127
interstitial pneumonitis caused by, 211
pneumonitis caused by, 213–214
pulmonary toxicity, 213
for sarcoidosis, 235
toxicity of, 235
Methyldopa, effects on sleep, 448t, 448–449
Methylphenidate, effects on sleep, 468
Methylprednisolone, 125
pulse, for idiopathic pulmonary fibrosis, 204
Methylxanthine(s)
for asthma, 121–123
safety in pregnancy, 479
Metoprolol, cough caused by, 68
Metoprolol tartrate
cough caused by, 68
effects on sleep, 448t, 448–449, 468
Metronidazole, use in pregnancy, 486t
Mezlocillin, indications for, 371
Micropolyspora faene, hypersensitivity pneumonitis caused by, 309t
Mid-maximal expiratory flow rate, 22, 37
Minute ventilation, in obesity, 278
Mist tent, for laryngotracheobronchitis, 341
Mite allergy, in asthma, 118
Mitomycin, pleural effusions with, 212
Mitral regurgitation, of solitary pulmonary nodule, 415
Mitral stenosis
with alveolar hemorrhage, 82
chest pain with, 93–94
hemoptysis with, 94
Mitral valve prolapse
associated musculoskeletal abnormalities, 93
chest pain with, 93–94
diagnostic criteria for, 94
familial, 93
Mixed connective tissue disease
chest radiography/roentgenography with, 210
clinical features of, 209
neutrophilic alveolitis with, 205
prognosis for, 210
pulmonary fibrosis in, 205
pulmonary involvement in, 209–210
therapy for, 210
Mixed dust pneumoconiosis, 309
MMFR. *See* Mid-maximal expiratory flow rate
Mondor's disease, 100
Monge's disease, 524–526
Monoclonal antibodies, for common cold, 336
Monosodium glutamate, and asthma, 117

Moraxella catarrhalis
pneumonia, 354
tracheitis caused by, 342–343
Morgagni hernia, 297
Motor vehicle accidents
injuries in, 401, 402t
sternal fractures in, injuries associated with, 403t
Mountain sickness. *See* Acute mountain sickness; Chronic mountain sickness
Movement disorders, insomnia secondary to, 470–471
MSLT. *See* Multiple Sleep Latency Test
Mucociliary transport, 348
Mucolytics, 71, 335
in asthma treatment, 126
in treatment of chronic obstructive pulmonary disease, 151
Mucomyst. *See* Acetylcysteine
Mucus
in asthma, 109
casts, in asthmatic sputum, 113, 114f
clearance of, in asthmatic patients, 126
Multiple sclerosis, 49
Multiple Sleep Latency Test, 429, 442, 456, 462, 466
Muscle disorders, 49
Muscle fibers
extrafusal, 55–56
intrafusal, 55–56
Muscle spindle, 54–56, 56f
Muscular dystrophy, 277–278
MVP. *See* Mitral valve prolapse
MVV. *See* Maximum voluntary ventilation
Myasthenia gravis, 49, 276–277
defect in, 276
pulmonary function in, 277
symptoms of, 276
treatment of, 277
Mycetoma, 78, 80f
etiology of, 80
hemoptysis with, 80
therapy for, 80
Mycobacteria
clinical and radiographic features of, 200
infection, 348
in acquired immunodeficiency syndrome, 383
transbronchial lung biopsy in, 228, 229f
nontuberculous, 382–383
classification of, by growth and pigmentation characteristics, 383, 383t–384t
pathogenicity in humans, 383t
Mycobacterium africanum, 382
pathogenicity in humans, 383t
Mycobacterium avium, 382–383
in acquired immunodeficiency syndrome, radiographic pattern of, 363t
pathogenicity in humans, 383t
Mycobacterium bovis, 382
pathogenicity in humans, 383t
Mycobacterium flavescens, 383t
Mycobacterium fortuitum chelonei, pathogenicity in humans, 383t
Mycobacterium gastri, 383t
Mycobacterium gordonae, 383t
Mycobacterium kansasii, 382
pathogenicity in humans, 383t
Mycobacterium leprae, 382
pathogenicity in humans, 383t
Mycobacterium marinum, pathogenicity in humans, 383t
Mycobacterium phlei, 383t
Mycobacterium scrofulaceum, pathogenicity in humans, 383t
Mycobacterium simiae, pathogenicity in humans, 383t
Mycobacterium smegmatis, 383t
Mycobacterium szulgai, pathogenicity in humans, 383t
Mycobacterium terrae, 383t
Mycobacterium triviale, 383t
Mycobacterium tuberculosis, 382–383
in acquired immunodeficiency syndrome, radiographic pattern of, 363t
culture, 391
pathogenicity in humans, 383t
populations of, 394
serology, 391
transmission of, 383–384
Mycobacterium ulcerans, pathogenicity in humans, 383t
Mycobacterium vaccae, 383t
Mycobacterium xenopi, pathogenicity in humans, 383t
Mycoplasma pneumoniae, 356
antibody detection techniques, 366
pneumonia, 356–357
antibiotic therapy for, 371
in pregnancy, 485
radiographic clearing in, 367
serology, 366
Mycoses, bilateral hilar lymphadenopathy in, 228
Myocardial contusion, 405
Myocardial infarction
chest pain associated with, 92
dyspnea with, 58
Myocardial ischemia, in carbon monoxide poisoning, 305
Myoneural disorders, 49

Nadolol, effects on sleep, 448t, 448–449
Nafcillin, indications for, 370
Nalidixic acid, use in pregnancy, 486t
Naps, 443, 446
Narcolepsy, 442–443
  accessory symptoms of, 444t
  age of onset, 441
  familial pattern of, 452
  laboratory diagnosis of, 457
  pediatric, 451, 452t
Nasal cannula, for oxygen, 323–324
Nasotracheal tube, with tracheitis, 343
Nebulizers, proper use of, 319
Neomycin sulfate, respiratory fatigue and failure secondary to, 298
Neoplasia
  chest x-ray with, 509–512
  hemoptysis with, 80–81
Neostigmine, for myasthenia gravis, 277
Nephrotic syndrome, pleural effusions caused by, 289
Nerve cells, in asthma, 107t
Nerve conduction studies, 271
Neurogenic tumors, 418
Neuroleptic medications, effects on sleep, 450
Neurologic diseases, 49
Neuromuscular apparatus, evaluation of, 271
Neuromuscular disease, 271–272. *See also* Amyotrophic lateral sclerosis; Restrictive lung disease
Neurons
  dorsal respiratory group, 54–55
  excitatory, 54
  inhibitory, 54
  ventral respiratory group, 54
Neuron-specific enolase, 412
Neutrophils
  in asthma, 107
  in collagen vascular disease, 205
  in idiopathic pulmonary fibrosis, 201
New York Heart Association, classification of heart disease, 490–491
Nicorette Gum, 318
Nicotine patches, 318–319
Nicotine replacement therapy, 149
Nifedipine, in treatment of achalasia, 98–99
Nitrofurantoin
  interstitial pneumonitis caused by, 211
  pneumonitis caused by, 213, 215–217, 216f
  use in pregnancy, 486t
Nitrogen washout, 38
Nitrosoureas, interstitial pneumonitis/fibrosis associated with, 213
Nocturnal asthma, 129–130
Nocturnal Oxygen Therapy Trial, 324, 325f
Nocturnal ventilation, 326
Non-Hodgkin's lymphoma, in acquired immunodeficiency syndrome, radiographic pattern of, 363t
Nonprescription drugs. *See* Over-the-counter medications
Nonrapid eye movement sleep. *See* NREM sleep
Non–small-cell carcinoma, 410
  extrathoracic evaluation of, 411
  staging of, 411
Nonspecific pneumonitis, in acquired immunodeficiency syndrome, radiographic pattern of, 363t
Nonsteroidal antiinflammatory agents
  aspirin-related, and asthma, 117
  for common cold, 334–335
NREM sleep, 425
NSCC. *See* Non–small-cell carcinoma
NTM. *See* Mycobacteria, nontuberculous
Nutcracker esophagus, 98
  tests and findings with, 98t
Nutrition, 317

OAD. *See* Obstructive airway disease
Obesity
  chest mechanics in, 278
  and pulmonary embolus, 159
  respiratory complications of, 278
Obsessive-compulsive disorder, insomnia with, 469
Obstruction
  extrathoracic, 33, 33f
  intrathoracic, 33, 33f
  versus restriction, 34–36, 36f
Obstructive airway disease, 32–33, 265. *See also* Asthma; Chronic bronchitis; Chronic obstructive pulmonary disease; Emphysema
  chest radiography with, 515, 515f
  diagnosis of, 49–50
  dyspnea with, 58
  reduced flow rates in, 34
Obstructive sleep apnea syndrome, 276, 443–444
  laboratory diagnosis of, 456–457
  pediatric, 451, 452t
  physical findings with, 453, 454f
Occupational asthma, 130–131
  bronchoprovocation studies for, 112
Occupational history, 44
Occupational lung disease, 305–315
Ofloxacin, indications for, 371
Ohm's law, 8

OKT6 common thymocyte antigen, in eosinophilic granuloma, 246
Old tuberculin, 385
Oncogenes, 412
Oophorectomy, in lymphangioleiomyomatosis, 255–256
Open lung biopsy. *See* Lung biopsy
Opportunistic pulmonary infection, with HIV infection, 361
Organidin. *See* Iodinated glycerol
Oropharyngeal colonization, 363, 364f
Oropharyngeal contents, aspiration of, 348, 360
Orthopnea, of cardiac disease, 60
Osler-Weber-Rendu disease, 77, 82, 82f–83f
Osteoarthropathy, 47–48
Osteoporosis, 49
  with heparin therapy, 167
Over-the-counter medications, effects on sleep, 468
Owls, 434
Oxacillin, indications for, 370
Oxazepam, elimination half-life, 450t
Ox protein, hypersensitivity pneumonitis caused by, 309t
Oxygen. *See also* Home oxygen therapy; Hyperbaric oxygen therapy
  supplemental, with pulmonary embolus, 178
  transtracheal, 324, 324f
Oxygenation, with pulmonary embolus, 177–178
Oxygen concentrators, 323
Oxygen consumption, in pregnancy, 477
Oxygen-debt theory, of dyspnea, 55
Oxygen delivery, to tissues, 57
  with pulmonary embolus, 177
Oxygen tension, at altitude, 519, 520f
Oxygen therapy, with tracheitis, 343
Oxygen toxicity
  in high concentrations, 526
  premonitory symptoms of, 526
Oxygen units, portable, 323, 324f

$PaCO_2$. *See* Arterial carbon dioxide tension
Pallor, 47
Palv, 7, 7f
Pancreatic pseudo-cyst, pleuropulmonary abnormalities with, 294
Pancreatitis, pleuropulmonary abnormalities with, 294
P_AO_2. *See* Alveolar oxygen tension
PAP. *See* Pulmonary alveolar proteinosis
Para-aminosalicylic acid, 393t
  side effects of, 396
  for tuberculosis, 379
Paragonimiasis, diaphragmatic, 300
Paragonimus westermani. See Lung fluke
Parainfluenza I, 340
Parainfluenza II, 340
Parainfluenza III, 340
Parainfluenza virus, 332, 360
  detection of, 366
Parallel, definition of, 3
Parallel resistors, 10f, 10–11
Paramalignant effusions, 290–291
Paraneoplastic syndromes, 50
Parapneumonic effusions, 292
Parenchymal diseases, 265
  cough with, 67
Parietal pleura, 283
  hydrostatic forces in, 283
Parkinson's disease, insomnia with, 468
Paroxysmal nocturnal dyspnea, 60
Partial thromboplastin time, with heparinization, 170
Pathogens
  hematogenously seeded, 348
  inhalation of, 348
Patient education, 317–318
P_B. *See* Barometric pressure
PCWP. *See* Pulmonary capillary wedge pressure
Peak expiratory flow, 25–26
Peak flow meter, 25f, 25–26
Pectus carinatum, 49, 265
Pectus excavatum, 48, 265, 266f
PEF. *See* Peak expiratory flow
Pel, 7, 7f
Pellularia, hypersensitivity pneumonitis caused by, 309t
Pelvic tumors, benign, associated with pleural effusions, 291
Pemoline, effects on sleep, 468
D-Penicillamine, progressive systemic sclerosis treated with, 209
Penicillin
  indications for, 369
  resistance, 369–370
  use in pregnancy, 481, 486t
Penicillium, hypersensitivity pneumonitis caused by, 309t
Penile erection (tumescence), with REM sleep, 427
Pentamidine
  adverse reaction to, 371
  aerosolized, 371–372
  for *Pneumocystis carinii* pneumonia, 371
    prophylactic, 375
Peptic ulcer disease, 99
Percent FEV_1. *See* Forced expiratory volume in 1 second to forced vital capacity ratio

Percussion
of chest, 45, 45f
dullness to, 60
hyperresonance to, 60, 74
Percussors, 322–323, 323f
Percutaneous fine needle aspiration biopsy
in diagnosis of solitary pulmonary nodule, 416
hemoptysis with, 83
Perfusion lung scan, quantitative, 492, 493f
Pericardial disease
chest pain with, 94–95
dyspnea with, 58
Pericardial friction rub, 94
Pericarditis, 94–95
constrictive, pleural effusions with, 289
management of, 95
Periodic leg movements, 470
Periodic limb movement disorder, 470–471, 473
Peripheral edema, with heart failure, 288
Peritoneal dialysis, hydrothorax with, 290
Pets, and asthma, 118
PFT. *See* Pulmonary function test(s)/testing
Pharynx, colonization of, 348
Phenylbutazone, for sarcoidosis, 234
Phenylpropanolamine, 333–334
effects on sleep, 468
Phenytoin, pleuritis induced by, 294
Phobias, insomnia with, 469
Phrenic nerve, 295
function, assessment of, 272
palsy, 297–298
paralysis, artificial, 379, 380f
Physical examination, 44–46
in insomnia evaluation, 465
Physiologic dead space, 58
α_1-PI. *See* Alpha-1 protease inhibitor
PIE syndrome, 235
Pig protein, hypersensitivity pneumonitis caused by, 309t
Pindolol, effects on sleep, 448t, 448–449, 468
P_{IO_2}. *See* Inspired oxygen tension
Piperacillin
indications for, 371
use in pregnancy, 481
Pirbuterol, for asthma, 120
Plague, 354t
Plaquenil. *See* Hydroxychloroquine sulfate
Plasma oncotic pressure, 283
Plasmapheresis
in Guillain-Barré syndrome, 276
for myasthenia gravis, 277
Platelet-activating factor, in asthma, 108t, 109
Pleural effusions, 175, 367. *See also* Chylothorax
with ankylosing spondylitis, 269
with asbestos exposure, 311
asymptomatic, 286
bilateral, 287–288
bloody, 286
with bronchogenic carcinoma, 290–291
causes of, 287t
on chest radiography, 504–506
chylous, 286
with cirrhosis, 289–290
with congestive heart failure, 287–289
with connective tissue disease, 293–294
with constrictive pericarditis, 289
cough with, 286
detection of, in supine patient, 505, 505f
with diaphragmatic malignancies, 300
with Dressler's syndrome, 294
in drug-induced chronic interstitial pneumonitis/fibrosis, 211–212
dyspnea with, 59, 286
empyemic, 286
with esophageal rupture, 293
exudative, causes of, 290–295
fungal, 293
with hypoalbuminemia, 289
with infections, 291–293
intra-abdominal causes of, 294–295
lactic dehydrogenase in, 285, 286t
with *Legionella* pneumonia, 357
with lymphangioleiomyomatosis, 254
malignant, 290–291
with mesothelioma, 312
mycoplasmal, 293
from pancreatitis, 294
parapneumonic, 292
parasitic, 293
pathophysiology of, 283–285
pleuritic pain with, 286
with post-myocardial infarction syndrome, 294
postoperative, 294
with post-pericardiotomy syndrome, 294
protein in, 285, 286t
in pulmonary embolus, 293
with radiation therapy, 291
with rheumatoid arthritis, 293–294
right, 504–505, 505f
serosanguinous, 286, 289–290
signs and symptoms of, 286–287
subpulmonic, 506, 506f
with superior vena cava obstruction, 289
with systemic lupus erythematosus, 293–294
tension hydrothorax with, 286
in tuberculosis, 291–292, 388
viral, 293
Pleural fluid, 45f

absorption, 283
and consolidation, 45f
dynamics of, 283–284, 284f
exudative, 284–285
filtration gradient, 283
formation of, causes for, 284–285
loculated within fissure, 506, 507f
movement of, 283–284
oncotic pressure of, 283–284
pH measurement of, 290
transudative, 284–285
Pleural friction rub, 174, 293
with pulmonary infarction, 80
Pleural lymphatica, 283
Pleural plaques, with asbestos exposure, 312
Pleural pressure, 7, 7f
and expiratory effort, 12f
Pleuritic pain. *See* Chest pain, pleuritic
Plombage, 379, 380f
PM/DM. *See* Polymyositis/dermatomyositis
Pneumatic compression devices, 169
in preventing deep venous thrombosis, 169
Pneumatoceles, 502f
Pneumococcal antigen, detection of, 365
Pneumococcal vaccine, 349, 373t, 374, 485
recommendations for use of, 373t
Pneumoconioses, 308–314
definition of, 308
types of, 309
Pneumoconstriction, with pulmonary embolus, 175
Pneumocystis carinii
in acquired immunodeficiency syndrome, radiographic pattern of, 363t
clinical and radiographic features of, 200
identification of, 364–365
pneumonia, 348
antibiotic therapy for, 371–372
in cancer patients, 361
chest radiography/roentgenography with, 362
prophylaxis, 375
Pneumomediastinum, 49, 69
in asthma, 111
with cocaine use, 101
Pneumonia. *See also* Atypical pneumonia syndrome; Bronchiolitis obliterans and organizing pneumonia; Chronic eosinophilic pneumonia; Community-acquired pneumonia
alveolar, chest x-ray in, 500, 500f
anaerobic, 360–361
antibiotic therapy for, 370–371
bacterial, secondary, 360
bilateral, radiographic appearance of, 503f
Branhamella catarrhalis, 354
antibiotic therapy for, 370
chest radiography in, 499–501, 501f–504f
Chlamydia pneumoniae, 358–359
antibiotic therapy for, 371
cough with, 66
Coxiella burnetii, 359–360
cytomegalovirus, 366
diagnosis of, 50
dyspnea with, 58
in elderly, 348–350
Escherichia coli, 354
antibiotic therapy for, 371
factors predisposing to, 348–349, 349t
fever in, 352
gram-negative bacilli, 353, 355
antibiotic therapy for, 371
Hemophilus influenzae, 353, 355
in acquired immunodeficiency syndrome, 362
antibiotic therapy for, 369–370
hemoptysis with, 79–80
incidence of, 347
interstitial, chest x-ray with, 500, 502f
Klebsiella pneumoniae, 353
antibiotic therapy for, 371
sputum with, 50
Legionella, 353, 357–368
antibiotic therapy for, 370
microbiologic diagnosis of, 353
Moraxella catarrhalis, 354
Mycoplasma pneumoniae, 356–357
antibiotic therapy for, 371
nosocomial, 353
prevention of, 374
parapneumonic pleural effusions with, 292
pneumococcal
in acquired immunodeficiency syndrome, 362
chest x-ray in, 500, 500f
radiographic clearing in, 367
Pneumocystis carinii, 348
antibiotic therapy for, 371–372
in cancer patients, 361
chest radiography/roentgenography with, 362
in pregnancy, 485
in progressive systemic sclerosis, 207
radiographic resolution of, 367
radiography with, 366–367
recurrent, 74
right lower lob, 504f
staphylococcal, 353, 355

Pneumonia—Continued
antibiotic therapy for, 370
radiographic appearance of, 500, 502f
sputum with, 50
Streptococcus pneumoniae, 353, 355
antibiotic therapy for, 369
treatment of, patient compliance with, 372
unusual types of, 354t, 355
viral, 360
chest x-ray with, 503f
Pneumonitis. *See also* Chronic interstitial pneumonitis; Hypersensitivity pneumonitis; Interstitial pneumonitis
amiodarone, 214–215, 215f
BCNU-induced, 213
with bleomycin, 212
caused by nitrofurantoin, 215–217, 216f
drug-induced, 211–217
methotrexate-induced, 213–214
nonspecific, in acquired immunodeficiency syndrome, radiographic pattern of, 363t
secondary to cytotoxic agents, 212–213
usual interstitial, 193–194, 197–199, 205
Pneumotachograph, 29
Pneumotaxic center, 55
Pneumothorax, 49, 69, 148. *See also* Tension pneumothorax
with ankylosing spondylitis, 269
in asthma, 111
bilateral, 507f
chest radiography with, 506–509, 507f–508f
with cocaine use, 101
diving-related, 529
dyspnea with, 59
with endometrial deposits, 300
induced, 379, 380f
in lymphangioleiomyomatosis, 254
right, 507f
skin fold simulating, 506, 508f
Pneumovax, 320
Polyarteritis nodosa, 186
Polyarthritis, in sarcoidosis, 222–223
Polymyositis, 49
Polymyositis/dermatomyositis
pulmonary complications of, 210
pulmonary fibrosis in, 205
Polymyxin B, respiratory fatigue and failure secondary to, 298
Polymyxin E, respiratory fatigue and failure secondary to, 298
Polysomnography, 21t, 425, 442, 455–456
drugs affecting, 449–450, 464
with insomnia, 465–466
Pontiac fever, 357
Positive-pressure ventilation, home care using, 326
Postherpetic neuralgia, 100
Posthyperventilation apnea, 59
Post-myocardial infarction syndrome, pleural effusion with, 294
Postnasal drip, cough with, 66, 69–70
Post-pericardiotomy syndrome, pleural effusion with, 294
Postphlebitic syndrome, 184
Postpolio syndrome, 275–276
Postthoracotomy pain syndrome, 101
Posttraumatic stress disorder, insomnia with, 469
Postural drainage, 322
positions for, 322, 322f
Pott's disease, 389
tuberculosis of, 389, 389f
PPD. *See* Purified protein derivative
PPI, 7, 7f
Prednisolone, 125
Prednisone
for asthma, 125, 127
for bronchiolitis obliterans, 221–222
for chronic eosinophilic pneumonia, 240
for chronic obstructive pulmonary disease, 151
for idiopathic pulmonary fibrosis, 202
for pulmonary function testing, 204
for rheumatoid interstitial lung disease, 207
for sarcoidosis, 233
Pregnancy
asthma in, 478–480
management of, 479–480
cystic fibrosis in, 480–482
effects of altitude on, 525
kyphoscoliosis in, 486
maternal pulmonary anatomy and physiology in, 477
pneumonia in, 485
pulmonary diseases in, 477–486
pulmonary embolus in, 482–483
pulmonary function testing in, 477–478
sarcoidosis in, 480
sleep apnea in, 486
spirometry in, 477–478
and thromboembolic disorders, 159–160
treatment of deep venous thrombosis in, 172–173
tuberculosis in, 483–485
use of antibiotics during, 486t
Preoperative pulmonary evaluation, 489–495
Prescription medications, effects on sleep, 447–448
Pretibial rash, 356

Prinzmetal's angina, 92
Procainamide
  interstitial pneumonitis caused by, 211
  pleural effusions with, 212
  pleuritis induced by, 294
Procan. *See* Procainamide
Progesterone, in lymphangioleiomyomatosis, 255–256
Progressive massive fibrosis, 314
Progressive relaxation training, for insomnia, 472–473
Progressive systemic sclerosis
  bronchoalveolar lavage in, 207–208
  interstitial lung disease complicating, radiographic features of, 207
  neutrophilic alveolitis with, 205
  pulmonary fibrosis in, 205
  pulmonary involvement in, 207–208
    prognosis for, 208
    therapy for, 208–209
Prolastin, 144
Pronestyl. *See* Procainamide
Prophylactic measures, perioperative, 492–493, 494t
Propranolol hydrochloride
  cough caused by, 68
  effects on sleep, 448t, 448–449, 468
Prostaglandins, in asthma, 108, 108t
Protamine sulfate, 171
Protein, in pleural effusions, 285, 286t
Prothrombin time
  outpatient monitoring of, 172
  with warfarin, 171
Proventil. *See* Albuterol
Pruning, of peripheral vessels, 186, 515, 515f
Pseudochylus effusion, 295
Pseudoephedrine, 334
  effects on sleep, 468
Pseudotumor, 506, 507f
Psittacosis, 354t, 356, 358
  antibiotic therapy for, 371
  hemoptysis in, 356
  radiographic resolution of, 367
PSS. *See* Progressive systemic sclerosis
Psychiatric history, with insomnia, 464
Psychogenic dyspnea, 59, 61
Psychogenic habit cough, 69
PTT. *See* Partial thromboplastin time
Pulmonary abnormality, degree of, adjectives used to describe, 32, 32t
Pulmonary alterations
  intraoperative, pathophysiology of, 489
  postoperative, pathophysiology of, 489
Pulmonary alveolar proteinosis, 248–254
  chest radiography/roentgenography with, 250, 251f
  clinical features of, 249
  diagnosis of, 252
  differential diagnosis of, 232
  epidemiology of, 249
  etiology of, 248–249
  fever in, 249
  histopathology of, 250–252, 251f
  incidence of, 249
  infections with, 249
  natural history of, 253
  pathogenesis of, 252–253
  pathologic features of, 248
  pulmonary function testing with, 250
  recurrences of, 254
  treatment of, 253–254
Pulmonary angiography, 179, 179f
  for definitive diagnosis of pulmonary embolic disease, 77
  with hemoptysis, 77–78
  indications for, 181
  of pulmonary embolus, 181–182
Pulmonary arterial embolic disease, diagnosis of, 50–51
Pulmonary arteriovenous malformations
  diagnosis of, 82, 82f–83f
  therapy for, 82
Pulmonary artery
  pressure, with pulmonary embolus, 177, 177f
  thrombosis, 157
Pulmonary capillary wedge pressure, with pulmonary embolus, 177, 177f
Pulmonary carcinogens
  environmental, 408
  occupational exposures, 408
Pulmonary complications, perioperative
  pathogenesis of, 489
  patients at risk for, 489, 490t, 490–492
Pulmonary contusion, 267, 404–405
Pulmonary defense mechanisms, 347, 348t
Pulmonary diagnosis, 43–51
  reliability of, 43–44
Pulmonary disease
  chest pain secondary to, 95–97
  development of, earliest detectable abnormality in, 22
  dyspnea of, 58–59
Pulmonary edema. *See also* High altitude pulmonary edema
  associated with sympathomimetic therapy, 485–486
  chest radiography with, 515–516, 516f
  noncardiogenic causes of, 516

Pulmonary edema—Continued
photographic negative of, 237
with tocolytic therapy, 485–486
Pulmonary embolectomy, 184
Pulmonary embolic disease. *See* Pulmonary embolus
Pulmonary embolus, 76
with accidental trauma, 161
associated pleural effusion, 293
atelectasis in, 6
calculated probability of, 181
catheter-related, 164–165
chest pain with, 96, 174
on chest roentgenography, 75
clinical diagnosis of, 174–178
coagulation studies with, 175
diagnostic techniques for, 178–182
dyspnea with, 58, 96, 174
electrocardiography with, 175
heart sounds with, 175
hemodynamic alterations with, 176–178, 178t
hemodynamic support with, 177–178
hemoptysis with, 174
heparin therapy for, 182–183
incidence of, 157, 161
with emergency surgery, 161
laboratory findings with, 175
lung scans in, 77
with malignancy, 159
mortality with, 157, 185
normal radiography with, 85
pathogenesis of, 157–158
perfusion lung scanning with, 179f, 179–181
physiologic changes with, 175–176
in pregnancy, 482–483
pulmonary angiography with, 77–78, 179, 179f, 181–182
recurrent, 96, 184–185
respiratory changes with, 175–176
risk factors for, 159t
in medical patients, 158–160
in surgical patients, 160
sources of, 164–165
treatment of, 182–185
ventilation-perfusion lung scans with, 179–181
wheezing with, 174
Pulmonary fat embolus. *See* Fat embolus
Pulmonary fibrosis. *See also* Idiopathic pulmonary fibrosis; Interstitial pulmonary fibrosis
complicating collagen vascular disease, 205–206
in mixed connective tissue disease, 205
in polymyositis/dermatomyositis, 205
in progressive systemic sclerosis, 205
in rheumatoid arthritis, 205
super-normal flow rates in, 36
Pulmonary function
with kyphoscoliosis, 268
in obesity, 278
Pulmonary function laboratory
setting up, 27–30
tests available in, 19, 21f
Pulmonary function studies. *See* Pulmonary function test(s)/testing
Pulmonary function test(s)/testing, 61, 275
in amyotrophic lateral sclerosis, 274
with ankylosing spondylitis, 270
in assessing chronic cough, 70
in asthma, 112
with bronchiolitis obliterans, 219
with bronchiolitis obliterans and organizing pneumonia, 219
in chronic eosinophilic pneumonia, 237
with chronic obstructive pulmonary disease, 146–147
with chronic pulmonary embolus, 185
computerization of, 29–30
contraindications to, 30
in eosinophilic granuloma, 244
with idiopathic pulmonary fibrosis, 196–197
indications for, 19–22
interpretation of, 22, 32–36, 36f
in lymphangioleiomyomatosis, 255
methods of, 21t
office, 19–39
personnel, 29
predicted normal values, 30–32
in pregnancy, 477–478
with pulmonary alveolar proteinosis, 250
in quadriplegic patients, 273
in sarcoidosis, 225–226
screening, 491–492, 492t
special tests, 36–38
split function studies, 492, 492t
Pulmonary hyperinflation, with emphysema, 147–148
Pulmonary hypertension, 96, 195, 515
causes of, 185–186
chest radiography/roentgenography with, 186
with chronic obstructive pulmonary disease, 146
of mixed connective tissue disease, 209–210
primary, 96, 185
in progressive systemic sclerosis, 207
radiologic findings with, 148
from recurrent pulmonary embolus, 185
secondary, 186

Pulmonary infarction
cough with, 68
hemoptysis with, 80
therapy for, 80
Pulmonary infection, with rheumatoid arthritis, 206
Pulmonary infiltrates, with pneumonia, 367
Pulmonary malignancy, osteoarthropathy with, 47–48
Pulmonary masses, 417
Pulmonary neoplasms, 407–417
Pulmonary physiology, 1–17
dynamic characteristics of, 8–17
static, 1–8
Pulmonary rehabilitation, 149, 317–327
benefits of, 327
goals of, 317
outpatient program, design of, 326–327
Pulmonary review, 43–44
Pulmonary sequestrations, hemoptysis with, 80
Pulmonary thromboembolism
diagnosis of, 50–51
predisposing conditions for, 50
Pulmonary toilet
with fractured ribs, 404
in restrictive lung disease, 279
Pulmowrap, 326
Pulsus paradoxus, 49
in asthma, 111
Pulsus parvus et tardus, 93
Purified protein derivative, 385
Pursed lip breathing, 321
Pyrazinamide, 392t, 392
dosage regimens, 394
side effects of, 396
for tuberculosis, 379, 381
Pyrethrum, hypersensitivity pneumonitis caused by, 309t
Pyridostigmine
for myasthenia gravis, 277
for postpolio syndrome, 275
Pyrimethamine. *See* Sulfadoxine/pyrimethamine
PZA. *See* Pyrazinamide

Q fever, 354t, 356, 359–360
antibiotic therapy for, 371
Quadriplegia, pulmonary function in, 273
Quinidine, pleuritis induced by, 294
Quinolone antibiotics, indications for, 370

R. See Respiratory exchange ratio
R 61837, 336
RA. *See* Rheumatoid arthritis
Radiation therapy
for lung cancer, 413
pleural effusion with, 291
Radiography. *See also* Chest radiography/roentgenography
of epiglottitis, 338–339
with pneumonia, 366–367
Radionuclide bone scan, in small-cell carcinoma staging, 412
Radionuclide superior vena cavagram, 419, 419f
Radon, 409
RADS. *See* Reactive airways dysfunction syndrome
Rales
with asbestosis, 311
basilar, 195
bibasilar, 195
with mixed connective tissue disease, 210
in interstitial lung disease, 195
Rapid eye movement sleep. *See* REM sleep
Rasmussen's aneurysm, 79
Raynaud's phenomenon, with *Mycoplasma pneumoniae,* 356
Reactive airways dysfunction syndrome, 37, 314–315
Referral laboratory, testing in, 38
Reid index, 142
Reliability, of pulmonary diagnosis, 43–44
REM sleep, 425, 426f
hallucinations and paralysis in, 445–446
latency, 428
neurophysiology of, 426f, 426–427
penile erection (tumescence) with, 427
periods, measurement of, 428
tonic and phasic features of, 427, 427t
Renal disease, and alveolar hemorrhage, 81–82
Residual volume, 1–2, 2f
determination of, 38
measurement of, 22, 23f
in obstructive airway disease, 34
Resistance
to flow, 8–9
in Ohm's law, 8
of resistors in series, 9–10
Respiration
control of, 54t
cyclic rhythm of, 55
Respirations, counting, 44–45
Respiratory apraxia, 59
Respiratory exchange ratio, 15
Respiratory failure, 297
acute, and chronic eosinophilic pneumonia, 241
in asthma, 111–112
with hypophosphatemia, 298

Respiratory flow rates, in asthma, 111
Respiratory gases, diffusion of, 14–15, 15f
Respiratory muscle(s), 53
in distribution of ventilation, 12
paralysis of, 59
weakness, 271–272
measurements to determine, 274
in muscular dystrophy, 277
Respiratory rate, 45
in acute bronchial asthma, 113
with pulmonary embolus, 175
Respiratory rhythm, modulation of, 55
Respiratory syncytial virus, 332, 340, 360
enzyme-linked immunosorbent assay for, 366
Respiratory therapy, modalities, 322–323
Respiratory tract infections, epidemiology of, 351
Respiratory viruses, 331–332. *See also specific virus*
Restless legs syndrome, 470–471, 473
Restoril. *See* Temazepam
Restrictive lung disease, 32–33. *See also* Chest wall syndromes; Interstitial lung disease; Neuromuscular disease
definition of, 265
dyspnea with, 58
extrapulmonary causes of, 265–281, 266t
management of, 278–280
mechanical ventilation in, 279
with neuromuscular disease, 271–272
pulmonary function seen in, 265
reduced volume in, 34
with spinal deformity, 49
Rheumatic fever, 93
Rheumatoid arthritis
neutrophilic alveolitis with, 205
pleural effusions with, 293–294
pulmonary complications of, 206–207
pulmonary fibrosis in, 205
sleep fragmentation in, 468
Rheumatologic disease, sleep abnormalities in, 466–468
Rhinovirus, 331–332, 340, 360
Rhonchi. *See* Wheezing
Rib(s)
abnormalities of, 266–267
fractures, 100, 266–267
simple, 403–404
Rifampin, 392t, 392
dosage regimens, 394
side effects of, 395–396
for tuberculosis, 379, 381
use in pregnancy, 484
Right-sided heart failure
dyspnea with, 59
in idiopathic pulmonary fibrosis, 204
signs of, 288
Rigid bronchoscopy, 77
Ritodrine, pulmonary edema with, 485–486
RV. *See* Residual volume

SACE. *See* Angiotensin converting enzyme
Sacroiliitis, of ankylosing spondylitis, 269, 269f
Salbutamol, pulmonary edema with, 485–486
Sarcoidosis, 47, 418
bilateral hilar lymphadenopathy in, 222–223
biopsy of, 226–228
bronchoalveolar lavage in, 229–231
chest radiography with, 222, 223f, 223–225
clinical expression of, 222
corticosteroids for, 232–234
cough with, 67
differential diagnosis of, 232
elastic recoil or elastance of lung in, 3
epidemiology of, 222
erythema nodosum in, 222–223
extrapulmonary involvement with, 222
fever in, 222–223
gallium scanning in, 229–230
histology of, 226
hypercalcemia in, 234
laboratory features in, 223
Loefgren's syndrome in, 222–223
natural history of, 222
newer staging techniques for, 229–232
pathogenesis of, 232
polyarthritis in, 222–223
in pregnancy, 480
prevalence of, 222
prognosis for, 222
pulmonary function testing in, 225–226
pulmonary lesion in, 223
treatment of, 232–235
Sarcoma, diaphragmatic, 300
Scarring, pulmonary, after pneumonia, 367
SCC. *See* Small-cell carcinoma
Schamroth's sign, 47, 48f
Scleroderma. *See* Progressive systemic sclerosis
Scoliosis, 267
in muscular dystrophy, 277
Seat belt injury, 403
Secondary hypercoagulable states, 158
Sectral. *See* Acebutolol
Sedatives
effects on sleep, 447–448
elimination half-life, 450t
Sedentary activities, 439
Seizures, oxygen-induced, 526
Seldane. *See* Terfenadine

Selective bronchial arteriography, with hemoptysis, 77–78, 78f
Selenium, dietary, and risk of lung cancer, 408–409
Semustine, interstitial pneumonitis/fibrosis associated with, 213
Sensors
in control of ventilation, 53–54
peripheral, 54f, 56f
Serax. *See* Oxazepam
Series, definition of, 3
Series resistors, 9f, 9–10, 10f
Shaggy heart appearance, 311–312
Shift work, 433–434, 434f
Shortness of breath. *See* Dyspnea
Shunt(s), 16–17, 17f
intracardiac, with pulmonary embolus, 176
intrapulmonary, with pulmonary embolus, 176
physiologic, 15
Silhouette sign, 501, 502f, 504f
Silica exposure, as lung carcinogen, 408
Silicosis, 309, 313–314, 408
acute, 313–314
chronic, 313–314
clinical and radiographic findings of, 313t, 313–314
Sinequan. *See* Doxepin
Singultus. *See* Hiccup
Sinusitis
and asthma, 117
cough with, 66
Sjögren's syndrome, 205
Sleep. *See also* NREM sleep; REM sleep
in aged, 428–429
at altitude, 525
architecture, 425–428
as biologic rhythm, 429–430
chronically insufficient, 446
continuity, 428
cycle, normal, 425–428
delta (slow wave), 426f
in aged, 429
deprivation, 429
disorders, 439. *See also* Insomnia
primary, 470–471
disorders of initiating and maintaining, 463t
disturbed nocturnal, with narcolepsy, 446
habits, bad, 471
history, 442–443, 463
insufficient, accessory symptoms of, 444t, 446
in normal infant, 428
onset, 428
circadian variation of, 439, 441f
ontogeny of, 428–429
paralysis, 445
purpose of, 434–435
restorative functions of, 429
stages of, 425, 426f, 427–428
Sleep apnea, 10
with postpolio syndrome, 275–276
in pregnancy, 486
Sleep apnea syndrome, 441–443
accessory symptoms of, 444, 444t
familial pattern of, 452
incidence of, 443
physical examination in, 453–454
signs and symptoms of, 443–444
Sleep-inducing areas, 430, 431f
Sleepiness. *See also* Excessive daytime sleepiness
abnormal, of narcolepsy, 444–445
as chief complaint, 439–441
clinical severity of, 439–441
daytime, in pediatric age group, 451–452, 452t
drug and medication effects on, 446–451
due to irregular and/or inadequate sleep, 441–442
laboratory investigation of, 455–458
midday, 429, 447
pathologic, 439–441
Sleep-onset paralysis, with narcolepsy, 445–446
Sleep-related breathing disorders, 470
Sleep restriction therapy, 472
Sleep state misperception, 471
Sleep-wake cycle, physiology of, 425–428
Slow vital capacity, 24–25
Small airways disease, tests for, 22
Small-cell carcinoma, 50, 410
chest radiography/roentgenography with, 412
computed tomography in, 412
extrathoracic evaluation of disease in, 412
staging of, 411–412
therapy for, 413
Smoke, carcinogens, mutagens, and tumor promoters in, 407–408
Smoker's cough, 66
Smoking
and asbestos-related mortality, 312
and asthma, 116
carbon monoxide exposure with, 305
as cause of chronic obstructive pulmonary disease, 140–142
cessation, 149, 318–319, 413
and eosinophilic granuloma, 242
history, 44
and lung cancer, 407–408
passive
and asthma, 118

Smoking—Continued
hazards of, 141
and risk of lung cancer, 408
Snoring, 276, 442
incidence of, 443
Solitary pulmonary nodule, 414f, 414–416
benign
criteria for, 416, 416t
radiographic appearance of, 510, 510f
brachytherapy for, 416
chest radiography/roentgenography with, 415, 510, 510f
computed tomography scan of, 415
diagnosis of, 414
diagnostic menu for, 415–416
differential diagnosis of, 414t, 414–415
etiology of, 414, 414t
fiberoptic bronchoscopy with, 415
local excision of, using yttrium aluminum garnet (YAG) laser, 416
malignant, radiographic appearance of, 510, 511f
radiographic appearance of, 510, 510f
roentgenographic features of, 415
Solu-Medrol. *See* Methylprednisolone
Spacer devices, 319, 319f
Spinal cord disorders, 272–274
Spinal cord injury(ies)
incidence of, 272
pulmonary complications of, 272–273
respiratory failure in, 297
Spinal deformity, restricted lung disease with, 49
Spine, tuberculosis of, 389, 389f
Spirogram(s), 24f
normal, 34, 35f
obstructed, 34, 35f
restricted, 34, 35f
Spirometer(s), 25f, 27–29
accuracy of, 30
American Thoracic Society standards for, 23
computerized, 29–30
graphic display, 27
maintenance of, 30
Spirometry, 21t, 147. *See also* Incentive spirometry
abnormalities on, 34, 35f
in asthma, 112
criteria for, American Thoracic Society, 23
definitions for, 23–26
equipment for, 27–29
flow-sensing devices, 29
good and bad tests, 27, 28f
office, 21–39
prebronchodilator and postbronchodilator, 21t, 26, 36–37
predicted normal values, 30–32
in pregnancy, 477–478
principles of, 22–23
procedures for, 26–27
protocols for, 26
quality control, 30
as screening test, 19
time/volume tracing, 23–24, 24f
volume displacement devices, 29
Spironolactone, in treatment of acute mountain sickness, 522–523
Splenomegaly, 75
Split function studies, 492, 492t, 494–495
Splitting, of rest-activity cycle length, 432
SPN. *See* Solitary pulmonary nodule
Sporotrichosis, 354t
S-100 positive histiocytes, in eosinophilic granuloma, 246–247
Sputum
appearance of, 50
of asthmatic patient, 113
with blood streaking, 79
chronic purulent, 74
with community-acquired pneumonia, 353
culture, 363, 365
in tuberculosis, 391
cytology, 70
examination of
with hemoptysis, 76
with suspected *P. carinii* pneumonia and tuberculosis, 364–365
gram stains, 363–364
in heart failure, 60
in infectious pulmonary process, 60
with oropharyngeal contamination, 363, 364f
purulent, 145
smears, 363–364
Squamous cell carcinoma, 410
markers, 412
Stanford Sleepiness Scale, 429
Staphylococcus aureus
epiglottitis caused by, 339
pneumonia, 353, 355
antibiotic therapy for, 370
sputum with, 50
tracheitis caused by, 342–343
Starling's law, 283
Static lung volumes, measurement of, 38
Status asthmaticus, 128
Sternum
disorders of, 265

fractures of, 402–403
locations of, 402t
Steroids. *See also* Corticosteroids
for edema associated with epiglottitis, 340
for laryngotracheobronchitis, 342
Stimulus control therapy, for insomnia, 472
Stockings, elastic, 169
Stramonium, 124
Streptococcus pneumoniae, 348
in acquired immunodeficiency syndrome, radiographic pattern of, 363t
culture, 365
epiglottitis caused by, 339
with plasma cell dyscrasias and other malignancies, 339
pneumonia, 353, 355
antibiotic therapy for, 369
in pregnancy, 485
sputum with, 50
tracheitis caused by, 342–343
Streptococcus pyogenes, epiglottitis caused by, 339
Streptokinase
allergic reactions to, 173
bleeding complications with, 173, 183–184
clot lysis with, 173
for pulmonary embolus, 183
Streptomycin, 392t, 392
dosage regimens, 394
fetal effects of, 484
resistance, 393
respiratory fatigue and failure secondary to, 298
side effects of, 396
for tuberculosis, 379
Stress, and asthma, 116–117
Stretch receptors, 54, 54f
Striated muscle, architecture of, 55
Stridor, 46, 49
Subclavian vein thrombosis, 164
Subcutaneous emphysema, cervical, 49
Subdiaphragmatic abscess, 299–300
Subphrenic abscess, 299–300
Sulfadoxine/pyrimethamine, prophylactic, for *Pneumocystis carinii* pneumonia, 375
Sulfamethoxazole. *See* Trimethoprim/sulfamethoxazole
Sulfites, and asthma, 117
Sulfonamides, use in pregnancy, 486t
Sulfur dioxide, and asthma, 116–117
Superior vena cava obstruction, pleural effusions with, 289
Superior vena cava syndrome, 417–420
in benign conditions, 419–420
diagnosis of, 418–420
outcome of, 420
signs and symptoms of, 418, 418f
tissue diagnosis in, 419
treatment of, 420
Suprachiasmatic nucleus, 430–433
Supraglottitis, 338
Surface tension, 4–8
Surfactant, 6
loss of, with pulmonary embolus, 176
Surgery
abdominal, pleural fluid collections seen after, 294
complications of, 489–490
involving lung resection, preparation for, 493–495
for lung cancer, 413
for massive life-threatening hemoptysis, 86
not involving lung resection, preparation for, 493
pulmonary complications of, 489
Sus-Phrine. *See* Epinephrine
SVC. *See* Slow vital capacity
SVCS. *See* Superior vena cava syndrome
Sweat chloride determination, 115
Sympathomimetic(s), for common cold, 333–334
Sympathomimetic bronchodilators, safety in pregnancy, 479
Syncope. *See also* Cough syncope
with pulmonary hypertension, 186
Systemic lupus erythematosus, 81, 205
pleural effusions with, 293–294
pleuropulmonary manifestations of, 210
Systemic sclerosis, CREST variant of, 207

Tachycardia
in anemia, 59
in pneumonia, 352
Tachypnea
in anemia, 59
with dyspnea, 51
in pneumonia, 352
Takayasu's arteritis, 186
Tamoxifen, in lymphangioleiomyomatosis, 255–256
Tartrazine, and asthma, 117
TBB. *See* Transbronchial lung biopsy
Telangiectasia, 74–75, 82
Temazepam, elimination half-life, 450t
Temporal arteritis, 186
Tenormin. *See* Atenolol
Tensilon. *See* Edrophonium chloride
Tension hydrothorax, with pleural effusion, 286
Tension pneumothorax, 508f, 508–509
Teratoma, 418

Terbutaline
  for asthma, 120
  effects on sleep, 468
  pulmonary edema with, 485–486
  in pulmonary function testing, 37
  use in pregnancy, 479
Terfenadine, 126
Tetracycline(s)
  indications for, 371
  use in pregnancy, 486t
Theophylline
  and β_2-agonists, potential additive effects of, 120
  for asthma, 121–123, 127
  bioavailability variations, 122
  bronchodilating effects of, 121
  for chronic obstructive pulmonary disease, 123
  dosing regimens, 123
  drug interactions, 122, 122t
  effects of
    on lungs, 121
    outside lungs, 121
    on sleep, 468
  metabolism of, 122
  rapid-release, 122
  rectal suppositories of, 123
  side effects of, 121
  starting patient on, 122–123
  sustained (controlled)-release, 122
  therapeutic blood level, 121
  in treatment of chronic obstructive pulmonary disease, 151
  use in pregnancy, 479
Thermoactinomyces candidus, hypersensitivity pneumonitis caused by, 309t
Thermoactinomyces vulgaris, hypersensitivity pneumonitis caused by, 309t
Thoracic injury
  inventory of, 402
  mechanisms of, 401–402
Thoracic outlet syndrome, 49
Thoracic pain. *See* Chest pain
Thoracic pressures, 6–8, 7f
Thoracoplasty, 270, 379, 381f
Thoracoscopy, indications for, 416
Thoracotomy, chest wall pain after, 101
Thorax, bony, injury to, 402–403
Thorazine. *See* Chlorpromazine
Thrombocytopenia
  with alveolar hemorrhage, 82
  with heparin, 166–167
Thromboembolic disease, sequelae of, 184–185
Thromboxanes, in asthma, 108, 108t
Thymectomy, for myasthenia gravis, 277
Thymoma, 418
Tidal volume, 1, 2f
  measurement of, 22, 23f
  in pregnancy, 477
Tietze's syndrome, 99–100
Time constant, 11, 11f
Time/volume tracing, 23–24, 24f
Timolol, effects on sleep, 448t, 448–449
Tissue plasminogen activator(s)
  lytic therapy with, 173
  for pulmonary embolus, 183
TLC. *See* Total lung capacity
T-lymphocytes, in sarcoidosis, 232
TNM system, tumor staging by, 411
Tobacco, carcinogens, mutagens, and tumor promoters in, 407–408
Tobramycin, use in pregnancy, 481
Tocolytic agents, pulmonary edema with, 485–486
Tornalate. *See* Bitolterol
Total lung capacity, 1, 2f, 7
  determination of, 38
  in emphysema, 1
  with idiopathic pulmonary fibrosis, 196
  measurement of, 22, 23f
  in restrictive lung disease, 265
Toxic shock syndrome, with tracheitis, 343
Tracé alternans, 428
Tracheal shift, 75
Tracheitis. *See* Bacterial tracheitis
Tracheobronchitis
  cough with, 66
  hemoptysis with, 79
Transbronchial lung biopsy
  bleeding with, 83
  in chronic eosinophilic pneumonia, 239
  in evaluation of interstitial lung disease, 200
  indications for, 200
  in mycobacteriosis, 228, 229f
  in sarcoidosis, 226
Transfer factor. *See* Diffusing capacity for carbon monoxide
Transtracheal oxygen, 324, 324f
Transudates
  causes of, 287t, 287–290
    cardiovascular, 287–289
  development of, 285
  versus exudate, 285–286
    laboratory criteria for, 285, 286t
Tranxene. *See* Clorazepate
Trauma. *See* Blunt chest trauma
Triamcinolone metered dose inhaler, 126
Triazolam, elimination half-life, 450t
Trichinosis, diaphragmatic, 300

Tricyclic antidepressants
effects on sleep, 468
sedation with, 449
Trimethadione, respiratory fatigue and failure secondary to, 298
Trimethoprim/sulfamethoxazole
adverse reaction to, in AIDS patients, 371
indications for, 369–371
for *Pneumocystis carinii* pneumonia, 371
prophylactic, 375
use in pregnancy, 486t
Troleandomycin, 127
Tuberculin(s), types of, 385
Tuberculin skin test, 385–388
indications for, 387t
interpretation of, 387–388, 388t
Tuberculomas, 389
Tuberculosis, 379–400
bilateral hilar lymphadenopathy in, 228
cavitary, 390f
chemotherapy for, 379–381
chest radiographic manifestations of, 389–390, 390t, 390f
classification of, 385t
cough with, 66
diagnosis of, 388–392
disseminated (miliary), 388, 390f
drug-resistant, 393–394
epidemiology of, 381–382
extrapulmonary, 388
treatment of, 394
hemoptysis with, 79
historical background of, 379–381
in HIV-infected patients, 362, 381, 388, 397–398
home therapy for, 381
incidence of, 381–382
infection, versus disease, 384–385
of kidney, 389, 389f
microbiology of, 382–384
pathogenesis of, 383–384
pleural effusions in, 291–292
in pregnancy, 483–485
presumptive diagnosis of, 390–391
prevention of, 396–397
signs and symptoms of, 388
and silicosis, 314
transmission of, 383–384
methods to control, 384t
treatment of, 392–397
history of, 379
patient compliance with, 394
Tuberculous pleurisy with effusion, 291–292
Tularemia, 354t
Tumor(s)
bone, chest pain with, 100
cough with, 67
of diaphragm, 300
Tumor markers, 412, 413t
Turbulent flow, 9, 9f
TWAR. *See Chlamydia pneumoniae*

UIP. *See* Usual interstitial pneumonitis
Upper respiratory tract infections, 331–344
Uremia, coagulopathy with, 81
Urinalysis, with hemoptysis, 76
Urokinase, thrombolytic therapy with, 173–174
Usual interstitial pneumonitis, 193–194, 197–199, 205

Vaccination, in HIV-positive patients, 374
Valium. *See* Diazepam
Valvular heart disease, 75
chest pain with, 93
dyspnea with, 58
Vanceril. *See* Beclomethasone metered dose inhaler
Vancomycin, indications for, 370
Vasculitis, 81
hypersensitivity, 186
pulmonary hypertension with, 185–186
Vasodilator agents, with cor pulmonale or pulmonary hypertension complicating idiopathic pulmonary fibrosis, 204
VC. *See* Vital capacity
Vena cava interruption, 184
Venography, for diagnosis of deep venous thrombosis, 162f, 162–163
Ventilation
control of, 53
distribution of, 11–12
mechanical. *See* Home ventilation; Mechanical ventilation
nonuniformity of, 11–12
Ventilation-perfusion abnormalities, 16, 16f
in asthma, 110, 113
with community-acquired pneumonia, 353
with kyphoscoliosis, 268
in obesity, 278
with pulmonary embolus, 176
Ventilation-perfusion ratio, with pulmonary embolus, 175
Ventilation-perfusion scan, 178–181, 179f
of pulmonary embolism, 179–181
with suspected pulmonary embolic disease, 77
Ventilator(s)
Cuirass type, 326
negative pressure, 279
positive pressure, 279

Ventolin. *See* Albuterol
Vinca alkaloids, for eosinophilic granuloma, 248
Viralizer, 337
Viral therapy, 335
Virology, of respiratory tract, 366
Visceral pleura, 283
  fluid movement from, 284
  hydrostatic pressure of, 284
  oncotic pressure gradient of, 284
Visken. *See* Pindolol
Vital capacity, 1–2, 2f, 275
  with idiopathic pulmonary fibrosis, 196
  measurement of, 22, 23f, 272
  reduced, 265
  in restrictive lung disease, 265
Vitamin A, dietary, 413
  and risk of lung cancer, 408–409
Vitamin C, for common cold, 335
Vitamin E, dietary, and risk of lung cancer, 408–409
V_{max}, 12
Vocal cord dysfunction, 115
Vocal fremitus, 45
Vocal resonance, 46
Volume, in pulmonary physiology, 2
Volume-pressure curve(s)
  for air-filled and water-filled lungs, 4f, 4–5
  of normal lung, 6, 7f
  of two different compliant systems, 3f
V/Q. *See* Ventilation-perfusion

Walking, 321
Walking pneumonia, 355
Warfarin
  anticoagulation with, 171
  contraindications to, with pregnancy, 172
  in deep venous thrombosis prophylaxis, 168
  drug interactions, 171–172, 172t
Water-air interface, 5
Wegener's granulomatosis, 74, 76, 81f, 81, 186
  on chest roentgenography, 75
  pleural effusion in, 294
Westermark's sign, 76
Wheezing, 46
  with asthma, 60, 68, 110–111
  with cardiac failure, 60
  causes of, 115
  diffuse expiratory, 74
  with eosinophilic granuloma, 242
  localized, 74
  with obstruction, 49
  in pneumonia, 352
  with pulmonary embolus, 174
Whole lung lavage, with pulmonary alveolar proteinosis, 253–254
Work of breathing, increased, and dyspnea, 55
Wound healing, and hyperbaric oxygen therapy, 530
Wright spirometer, 272

Xanax. *See* Alprazolam
Xanthine, naturally occurring, 121
Xenon washout, 180

Zenker's diverticulum, 99
Ziehl-Nelson and Kinyoun staining, 391
Zinc, for common cold, 336